MW00845444

TEXTBOOK FOR THE ADULT-GERONTOLOGY ACUTE CARE NURSE PRACTITIONER

Valerie J. Fuller, PhD, DNP, AGACNP-BC, FNP-BC, FNAP, FAANP, is an adult-gerontology acute care nurse practitioner and family nurse practitioner who works in the Department of Surgery at Maine Medical Center in Portland, Maine. She is the Region 1 Director to the American Association of Nurse Practitioners, Board Chair and APRN member of the Maine State Board of Nursing, and Past President of the Maine Nurse Practitioner Association. She is actively involved in APRN education, practice, and policy issues at local, state, and national levels. Her clinical and research interests include vascular surgery, wound care, and delirium.

Paula S. McCauley, DNP, ACNP-BC, CMC, CSC, FAANP, is an adult acute care nurse practitioner. She has also served for many years as acute care nurse practitioner in cardiology and critical care at the University of Connecticut Health Center, John Dempsey Hospital. She has served as Associate Dean for Academic Affairs/Associate Clinical Professor/Acute Care Track Coordinator at University of Connecticut School of Nursing. She is actively involved in APRN practice, serving as cochair of the Acute Care Specialty community of the American Association of Nurse Practitioners and chair of the 2022 task force on the American Association of Critical Care Nurses revisions of the Scope and Standards for Acute Care Nurse Practitioners. Her clinical and research interests include advanced practice education, cardiology, cardiovascular surgery, and pain management.

TEXTBOOK FOR THE ADULT-GERONTOLOGY ACUTE CARE NURSE PRACTITIONER

Evidence-Based Standards of Practice

Valerie J. Fuller, PhD, DNP, AGACNP-BC,
FNP-BC, FNAP, FAANP

Paula S. McCauley, DNP, ACNP-BC,
CMC, CSC, FAANP

Editors

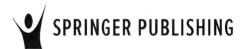

SPRINGER PUBLISHING

Copyright © 2023 Springer Publishing Company, LLC
All rights reserved.

First Springer Publishing edition 2023

No part of this publication may be reproduced, stored in a retrieval system, or transmitted in any form or by any means, electronic, mechanical, photocopying, recording, or otherwise, without the prior permission of Springer Publishing Company, LLC, or authorization through payment of the appropriate fees to the Copyright Clearance Center, Inc., 222 Rosewood Drive, Danvers, MA 01923, 978-750-8400, fax 978-646-8600, info@copyright.com or at www.copyright.com.

Springer Publishing Company, LLC
11 West 42nd Street, New York, NY 10036
www.springerpub.com
connect.springerpub.com/

Vice President and Publisher: Elizabeth Nieginski
Director, Content Development: Taylor Ball
Production Editor: Joseph Stubenrauch
Compositor: Amnet

ISBN: 978-0-8261-5232-9
ebook ISBN: 978-0-8261-5233-6
DOI: 10.1891/9780826152336

SUPPLEMENTS:

A robust set of instructor resources designed to supplement this text is located at **http://connect.springerpub.com/content/reference-book/978-0-8261-6079-9.** Qualifying instructors may request access by emailing **textbook@springerpub.com.**

Instructor PowerPoints ISBN: 978-0-8261-5231-2

23 24 25 26/ 5 4 3 2 1

Medicine is an ever-changing science. Research and clinical experience are continually expanding our knowledge, in particular our understanding of proper treatment and drug therapy. The authors, editors, and publisher have made every effort to ensure that all information in this book is in accordance with the state of knowledge at the time of production of the book. Nevertheless, the authors, editors, and publisher are not responsible for any errors or omissions or for any consequence from application of the information in this book and make no warranty, expressed or implied, with respect to the content of this publication. Every reader should examine carefully the package inserts accompanying each drug and should carefully check whether the dosage schedules therein or the contraindications stated by the manufacturer differ from the statements made in this book. Such examination is particularly important with drugs that are either rarely used or have been newly released on the market.

Library of Congress Cataloging-in-Publication Data

Names: Fuller, Valerie J., editor. | McCauley, Paula S., editor.
Title: Textbook for the adult-gerontology acute care nurse practitioner :
  evidence-based standards of practice / [edited by] Valerie J. Fuller,
  Paula S. McCauley.
Description: First Springer Publishing edition. | New York, NY : Springer
  Publishing Company, 2022. | Includes bibliographical references and
  index.
Identifiers: LCCN 2022020433 (print) | LCCN 2022020434 (ebook) | ISBN
  9780826152329 (paperback) | ISBN 9780826152336 (ebook)
Subjects: MESH: Geriatric Nursing—methods | Acute Disease—nursing | Nurse
  Practitioners | Evidence-Based Nursing
Classification: LCC RC954 (print) | LCC RC954 (ebook) | NLM WY 152 | DDC
  618.97/0231—dc23/eng/20220801
LC record available at https://lccn.loc.gov/2022020433
LC ebook record available at https://lccn.loc.gov/2022020434

Contact sales@springerpub.com to receive discount rates on bulk purchases.

Publisher's Note: **New and used products purchased from third-party sellers are not guaranteed for quality, authenticity, or access to any included digital components.**

Eternal ISBN for reference work: 978-0-8261-6079-9
Printed in the United States of America.

This textbook is dedicated to all Acute Care Nurse Practitioner students and practitioners—may you find within these pages the information you need to improve the health and well-being of your patients and their families.

Valerie J. Fuller
Paula S. McCauley

CONTENTS

* Lead author.

* Lead author.

* Lead author.

---

* Lead author.

---

* Lead author.

CONTRIBUTORS

Al-Zada "Al" Aguilar, DNP, ACNP-BC, CCRN
RWJUH-NB MICU APP Service
Robert Wood Johnson University Hospital
New Brunswick, New Jersey;
Adjunct Clinical Faculty—BSN to AGACNP/DNP
    Program
Rutgers University, School of Nursing
Newark, New Jersey

**Bimbola Akintade, PhD, MBA, MHA, ACNP-BC,
    NEA-BC, FAANP**
Associate Professor and Associate Dean, Master's
    Program
University of Maryland School of Nursing
Baltimore, Maryland

Terri L. Allison, DNP, ACNP- BC, FAANP
Assistant Dean for Academics, Doctoral Nursing Practice
Professor of Nursing
Vanderbilt University School of Nursing
Nashville, Tennessee

Mary Alt, CCRN, MSN, APRN-BC
Grand Canyon University Adjunct Faculty
College of Nursing and Healthcare Professions
Phoenix, Arizona

**Daniel L. Arellano, PhD, RN, APRN, ACNP-BC,
    CCRN, CEN, CFRN, EMT-P, FCCM, FAANP**
Assistant Professor of Nursing–Clinical
Jane and Robert Cizik School of Nursing
University of Texas Health Science Center at Houston
Houston, Texas

Deborah Astemborski, ACNP-C, RNFA, CNRN
Adjunct Faculty AG-ACNP
College of Nursing
Grand Canyon University
Phoenix, Arizona

**Stephanie G. Barnes, MSN, AGPCNP-C, PCCN,
    CHFN**
Clinical Director for Advanced Heart Failure Services
Duke Heart Center
Duke University Hospital
Durham, North Carolina

Amanda Bergeron, MSN, APRN, AGACNP-BC
Advanced Cardiopulmonary Therapies and Transplant
Memorial Hermann Hospital
Houston, Texas

Jennifer Branch, DNP, APRN, NP-C, CCTC, FNKF
The University of Kansas Health System
Kansas City, Kansas

**Steven Branham, PhD, APRN, ACNP-BC, FNP-BC,
    ENP-C, FAANP, CCRN**
Retired Professor
Adult Gerontology Acute Care Nurse Practitioner
    Program
Texas Tech Health Sciences Center—School of Nursing
Lubbock, Texas

Lori Dugan Brien, DNP, ACNP-BC
Assistant Professor
Department of Advanced Nursing Practice
Assistant Director, Adult-Gerontology Acute Care
    Nurse Practitioner Program
Georgetown University School of Nursing and Health
    Studies
Washington, DC

**Camille Brockett-Walker, DNP, AGACNP-BC,
    FNP-BC**
Nell Hodgson Woodruff School of Nursing
Emory University
Atlanta, Georgia

Matthew Buesking, DNP, MSN, AGACNP-BC
Creighton University
Omaha, Nebraska

Roxanne Buterakos, DNP, RN, AG-ACNP-BC, PNP-BC
Assistant Professor
School of Nursing
University of Michigan
Flint, Michigan

Molly Lillis Cahill, MSN, APRN,BC, ANP-C, CNN, FNKF
KC Kidney Consultants
Kansas City, Missouri

Margaret J. Carman, DNP, RN, ACNP-BC, ENP-BC FAEN
Associate Professor
University of North Carolina School of Nursing
Chapel Hill, North Carolina

Brooke Carpenter, MS, AGACNP-BC
Critical Care Nurse Practitioner
California Pacific Medical Center
San Francisco, California

Dawn Carpenter, DNP, ACNP-BC, CCRN
Nurse Practitioner
Department of Trauma and Surgical Critical Care
Guthrie Healthcare System
Sayre, Pennsylvania;
Associate Professor
Graduate School of Nursing
University of Massachusetts Medical School
Worcester, Massachusetts

Monee' Carter-Griffin, DNP, MAOL, APRN, ACNP-BC
Director of Education, Advanced Practice Providers
Dallas Pulmonary and Critical Care (DPACC), PA
Dallas-Forth Worth, Texas;
Assistant Professor, Clinical
Department of Graduate Nursing
University of Texas at Arlington
Arlington, Texas

Ameera Chakravarthy, MS, RN, ACNP-BC, FNP-BC, CNE
Interim Specialty Director
AGACNP-AGCNS DNP Program
University of Maryland School of Nursing
Baltimore, Maryland

Kindra Clark-Snustad, DNP
Teaching Associate
Division of Gastroenterology
University of Washington
Seattle, Washington

Andrea Colburn, DNP, MSN, AGACNP-BC, CCRN
University of Texas Medical Branch–School of Nursing
Galveston, Texas

Rita A. DelloStritto, PhD, APRN, CNS, ENP, ACNP-BC, FAANP
Professor
Texas Woman's University
Nelda C. Stark College of Nursing
Houston, Texas

Latanja L. Divens, PhD, DNP, APRN, FNP-BC
Assistant Professor of Clinical Nursing
Program Coordinator for Adult Gerontology Primary Care Nurse Practitioner
Doctor of Nursing Practice
School of Nursing
Louisiana State University Health Sciences Center
New Orleans, Louisiana

Amy Elliott, BSN, MSN, AGPC, NP-C
University of Michigan
Ann Arbor, Michigan

Ann Eschelbach, RN, MSN, ACNP-BC
University of Michigan
Ann Arbor, Michigan

Stacey Evans, MSN, RN, FNP-BC, AGACNP-BC- CSC
Long Beach Memorial Medical Center
Long Beach, California

Thomas Farley, MS, ACNP
Assistant Clinical Professor of Nursing
University of California San Francisco School of Nursing
San Francisco, California

Jacqueline Ferdowsali, DNP, AGACNP-BC
Associate Professor
Orvis School of Nursing
University of Nevada-Reno
Reno, Nevada

Lisa Fetters, DNP, RN, AG-ACNP, CCNS, CEN
Assistant Professor
School of Nursing
The University of Michigan-Flint
Flint, Michigan

Leanne H. Fowler, DNP, MBA, APRN, AGACNP-BC, CNE
Associate Professor of Clinical Nursing
Director of Nurse Practitioner Programs
Doctor of Nursing Practice
School of Nursing
Louisiana State University Health Sciences Center
New Orleans, Louisiana

R. Brandon Frady, DNP, ACNP-BC, CCRN-CMC
Clinical Assistant Professor
Georgia Baptist College of Nursing
Mercer University
Atlanta, Georgia

Valerie J. Fuller, PhD, DNP, AGACNP-BC, FNP-BC, FNAP, FAANP
Maine Medical Center, Department of Surgery
Assistant Professor of Surgery—Tufts Medical School
Portland, Maine

Alnee Gadberry, MSN, AGACNP-BC, FNP-C
Eskenazi Health
Indianapolis, Indiana

David S. Goede, DNP, ACNP-BC, AACC
Nursing Faculty
Keiser University
Tampa, Florida

Bradley Goettl, DNP, AGACNP-BC, FNP-C, ENP-C, CFRN, LP
Assistant Director, Office of Advanced Practice Providers
UT Southwestern Medical Center
Dallas, Texas

Steven J. Gort, MSN, MS-Microbiology, APNP, CNP, AGACNP-BC, CCRN
Critical Care Nurse Practitioner
Critical Care Unit
Mayo Clinic Health System
Eau Claire, Wisconsin

Donna Gullette, PhD, APRN, AGACNP-BC, FAANP
Associate Dean for Practice
University of Arkansas for Medical Sciences
College of Nursing
Little Rock, Arkansas

Whitney Haley, MSN, AGACNP-BC
Pulmonary Critical Care
Ascension St. Thomas West
Nashville, Tennessee

Mary S. Haras, PhD, MBA, APRN, NP-C, CNN
Associate Professor and Chair
Department of Advanced Nursing Practice
School of Nursing and Health Studies
Georgetown University
Washington, DC

Clare Harris, MSN, RN, ANP-BC
Nurse Practitioner
Multidisciplinary Venous Health Program
Michigan Medicine
Ann Arbor, Michigan

Tara C. Hilliard, PhD, APRN, ACNP-BC
Texas Tech Health Sciences Center—School of Nursing Program
Director Adult Gerontology Acute Care Nurse Practitioner Program
Associate Professor
Lubbock, Texas

Deborah Ann Hoch, DNP, CCRN, ACNP-BC
Clinical Instructor
Tufts University School of Medicine
Maine Medical Center
Division of Nephrology and Transplantation
Portland, Maine

Melinda Hodne, DNP, APRN-BC
Assistant Professor
Rhode Island College
Providence, Rhode Island

Lori Hull-Grommesh, DNP, APRN, ACNP-BC, NEA-BC, FAANP
Cizik School of Nursing
University of Texas
Houston, Texas

Kimberly Ichrist, DNP, AGACNP-BC, CCRN
The Ohio State University Wexner Medical Center
Columbus, Ohio

Kristopher J. Jackson, PhD, MSN, AGACNP-BC
Nurse Practitioner
University of California San Francisco Medical Center
San Francisco, California

Jeffrey D. Jacobs, MD
Clinical Assistant Professor
Division of Gastroenterology
University of Washington
Seattle, Washington

Suzanne James, MSN, RN, FNP-BC
Nephrology Nurse Practitioner
KC Kidney Consultants
Kansas City, Missouri

Vanessa M. Kalis, DNP, APRN, CNS, ACNP-BC, CPNP-AC, CHSE
Associate Professor
University of Massachusetts Global
Irvine, California;
Nurse Practitioner, Adult Congenital Heart Disease
University of California–Los Angeles
Los Angeles, California

Brayden Kameg, DNP, PMHNP-BC
University of Pittsburgh School of Nursing
Pittsburgh, Pennsylvania

Kendra J. Kamp, PhD, MS, RN
Assistant Professor
Department of Biobehavioral Nursing and Health
  Informatics
School of Nursing
University of Washington
Seattle, Washington

Nancy Knechel, PhD, RN, ACNP-BC
Oregon Health and Science University and Asante
  Health System
Ashland, Oregon

Kristina Kordesch, ACNP-AG
Critical Care Nurse Practitioner
Department of Critical Care Medicine
UCSF Medical Center
San Francisco, California

Patrick A. Laird, DNP, APRN, ACNP-BC, NEA-BC
Chief Nursing Officer
Cornerstone Hospital of Conroe
Conroe, Texas

Gail Lis, DNP, ACNP, BC
Assistant Dean Division of Nursing
Professor
Mercy College of Ohio
Toledo, Ohio

Ann Luciano, RN, MSN, ACNP-BC
NP Lead for the Multidisciplinary PAD Program
University of Michigan Health
Ann Arbor, Michigan

Donna Lynch-Smith, DNP, ACNP-BC, APRN, NE-BC, CNL
Associate Professor/AG-ACNP Concentration
  Coordinator, DNP Program
University of Tennessee Health Science Center
Memphis, Tennessee

Genevieve MacDonald, MSN, ACNP-BC
Nurse Practitioner
Surgical First Assistant, Cardiovascular Surgery
Maine Medical Center
Portland, Maine

Adrienne Markiewicz, MSN, RN, AGACNP-BC
Division of Pulmonary and Critical Care
Department of Medicine
Medical College of Wisconsin
Milwaukee, Wisconsin

Jeanne Martin, DNP, ANP-BC
Nurse Practitioner
Department of Urology
Stony Brook University Hospital;
Adjunct Clinical Instructor
Department of Graduate Nursing Studies
Stony Brook University School of Nursing
Stony Brook, New York

Cathy McAtee, DNP, ACNP-BC, CCRN, CNE
Instructor of Clinical Nursing
Faculty, Doctor of Nursing Practice
School of Nursing
Louisiana State University Health Sciences Center
New Orleans, Louisiana

Paula S. McCauley, DNP, ACNP-BC, CMC, CSC, FAANP
Acute Care Nurse Practitioner
Research Professor
University of Connecticut School of Nursing
Manchester, Connecticut

Jaime A. McDermott, DNP, ACNP-BC, CCRN, CHFN
Acute Care Nurse Practitioner
Division of Cardiology
Duke University Hospital
Durham, North Carolina

Diane McLaughlin, DNP, AGACNP-BC, CCRN
Frances Payne Bolton School of Nursing
Case Western Reserve University
Cleveland, Ohio

Beth McLear, DNP, FNP-C, ACNP-BC
Associate Professor
Augusta University College of Nursing
Augusta, Georgia

Alexander Menard, DNP, AGACNP-BC
Nurse Practitioner
Surgical Critical Care
UMASS Memorial Medical Center;
Assistant Professor
Graduate School of Nursing
University of Massachusetts Medical School
Worcester, Massachusetts

Helen Miley, RN, PhD, CCRN, AG-ACNP
Nurse Practitioner, Critical Care
Howell, New Jersey

Barbara Miller, MS, CRNP
APP Clinical Program Manager
Thoracic Surgery, Surgical Oncology, OMFS, ENT
University of Maryland Medical Center
Baltimore, Maryland

Sarah M. Muller, MSN, APRN, AGACNP-BC
Houston Methodist Hospital–Neurosurgical Intensive
    Care Unit
Houston, Texas

Kelly K. Nye, MSN, AGPCNP-BC
Cardiovascular Nurse Practitioner AdventHealth
    Tampa
Tampa, Florida

**Daniel O'Neill, DNP, FNP-C, FACNP,
    FAANP CCRN, CEN**
Staff Hicuity Health Care
Houston, Texas

Jamie L. Oliva, PhD, ANP-BC, BMTCN
Assistant Professor of Clinical Nursing
University of Rochester School of Nursing
Nurse Scientist
Wilmot Cancer Institute
University of Rochester Medical Center
Rochester, New York

Elizabeth Palermo, DNP, RN, ANP-BC, ACNP-BC
Assistant Professor of Clinical Nursing
University of Rochester School of Nursing
Nurse Practitioner
Strong Memorial Hospital Medicine Division
University of Rochester Medical Center
Rochester, New York

Dorota Pawlak, PhD, APRN, ADM-BC
UConn Health Center
Farmington, Connecticut

Richard Pembridge, ACNP, EDD
Grand Canyon University Program Director
College of Nursing and Healthcare Professions
Phoenix, Arizona

LaTricia D. Perry, PhD, MSN, RN, CNE
Associate Dean, School of Nursing
Nevada State College
Henderson, Nevada

Jessica S. Peters, DNP, MS, RN, ACNP-BC
Assistant Professor, Acute and Chronic Care
School of Nursing
Johns Hopkins University
Baltimore, Maryland

Alyssa Profita, DNP, RN, AGACNP-BC
Division of Pulmonary and Critical Care
Department of Medicine
Medical College of Wisconsin
Milwaukee, Wisconsin

Liza Rieke, MSN, APRN, ACNP-BC
U.S. Department of Veterans Affairs
Louis Stokes Cleveland VA Medical Center
Surgical Critical Care
Cleveland, Ohio

Sherry Rivera, DNP, APRN, ANP-C, FNKF
Assistant Professor of Clinical Nursing
Faculty, Doctor of Nursing Practice
School of Nursing
Louisiana State University Health Sciences Center
New Orleans, Louisiana

Karen Salazar, MSN, APRN, AGACNP-BC
Houston Methodist Hospital–Neurosurgical Intensive
  Care Unit
Texas Women's University–Adjunct Faculty
Houston, Texas

**Aaron M. Sebach, PhD, DNP, MBA, AGACNP-BC,
  FNP-BC, NP-C, CP-C, CEN, CPEN, CGNC, CLNC,
  CNE, CNEcl, SFHM**
Associate Professor and Director, Graduate Nursing
  Programs
Wilmington University
New Castle, Delaware;
Hospital Medicine Nurse Practitioner
TidalHealth Peninsula Regional
Salisbury, Maryland

**Susanna (Sue) Sirianni, RN, DNP, ACNP-BC,
  ANP-BC, CCRN**
Lead NP, SICU
Sinai Grace Hospital
Detroit, Michigan;
Associate Adjunct Professor
Madonna University
Livonia, Michigan

Kathryn E. Smith, PharmD, BCPS, BCCCP
Clinical Pharmacy Specialist–Surgery/Trauma Critical
  Care
Department of Pharmacy
Maine Medical Center
Portland, Maine

**L. Douglas Smith, Jr., MSN, APRN, ACNP-BC, CCRN,
  CNRN, SCRN**
Lead Advanced Practice Provider and Critical-Care
  Nurse Practitioner
Intensive Care Consortium at HCA TriStar Centennial
  Medical Center
Instructor of Nursing/Vanderbilt University School of
  Nursing
Nashville, Tennessee

Abbye Solis, DNP, ACNP-BC
Acute Care Nurse Practitioner
Weinberg Surgical Intensive Care Unit
The Johns Hopkins Hospital
Baltimore, Maryland;
Adjunct Faculty
Department of Advanced Practice Nursing
Georgetown University
Washington, DC

Cathy Stepter, DNP, AGACNP-BC, ACNS-BC, CNE
Baptist Health Sciences University
Division of Nursing
Memphis, Tennessee

Amy Stoddard, DNP, ACNPC-AG, CCRN
Contributing Faculty AGACNP Program
Walden School of Nursing
Minneapolis, Minnesota

**Lynda Stoodley, DNP, NP-C, AGACNP-BC,
  AGPCNP-BC, CCRN-CSC**
Cor Healthcare Medical Associates
Torrance, California

**Diane Fuller Switzer, DNP, RN, ARNP, FNP/ENP-BC,
  ENP-C, CCRN, CEN, FAEN, FAANP**
Assistant Clinical Professor
College of Nursing
Seattle University
Seattle, Washington

Carolina D. Tennyson, DNP, ACNP-BC, AACC
Assistant Professor
Duke University School of Nursing
Acute Care Nurse Practitioner
Duke University Hospital
Durham, North Carolina

Maggie Thompson, DNP, RN, AGACNP-BC
Assistant Professor of Clinical Teaching
College of Nursing
University of Colorado Anschutz Medical Campus
Aurora, Colorado

**Kelly A. Thompson-Brazill, DNP, ACNP-BC,
  CCRN-CSC, FCCM**
Associate Professor
Department of Advanced Nursing Practice
Director, Adult-Gerontology Acute Care Nurse
  Practitioner Program
Georgetown University School of Nursing and Health
  Studies
Washington, DC

Catherine C. Tierney, DNP, ACNP-BC
Assistant Professor
Department of Advanced Practice Nursing
Clinical Faculty Director, Adult-Gerontology Acute
    Care Nurse Practitioner Program
Georgetown University School of Nursing and Health
    Studies
Washington, DC

Helena Turner, MS, PMHNP, RN
Assistant Professor of Clinical Nursing
Oregon Health and Science University
Ashland Campus
Ashland, Oregon

Sally M. Villaseñor, DNP, RN, ACNP-BC
Assistant Professor
College of Nursing
Wayne State University
Detroit, Michigan

**Michelle Wade, MSN/Ed, APRN, NP-C, ACNPC-AG,
    FAANP**
Adult-Gerontology Primary Care Nurse Practitioner
Adult-Gerontology Acute Care Nurse Practitioner
Lead Hospitalist—Gifford Medical Center
Randolph, Vermont;
Adjunct Faculty
Vermont Technical College
Randolph, Vermont

Alice X. Wang, PharmD
PGY-1 Pharmacy Resident
Department of Pharmacy
Maine Medical Center
Portland, Maine

Michelle Wang, PharmD
Critical Care Clinical Pharmacist
Department of Acute Care Pharmacy
Beth Israel Deaconess Medical Center
Boston, Massachusetts

**Melissa Diehl Weidner, MSN, CRNP, AGACNP-BC,
    ANP-BC**
Chair, Graduate Nursing Department
Assistant Professor
Misericordia University
Dallas, Pennsylvania

**Chris Winkelman, PhD, ACNP-BC, CCRN-K, CNE,
    FCCM, FAANP**
Frances Payne Bolton School of Nursing
Case Western Reserve University
Cleveland, Ohio

FOREWORD

Increasingly, nurse practitioners (NPs) are becoming the providers of choice for patients across the globe. The number of NPs continues to increase annually and although most NPs practice in primary care, more and more are educated, trained, and board certified to practice in acute care. These NPs provide care for patients who are in acute or critical condition in hospitals, specialty care settings, home-based settings, or via telehealth. In many hospitals, NPs staff the intensive care units (ICUs) around the clock, providing immediate provider response for patient care needs. Acute care NPs partner with other members of a multidisciplinary care team, often serving as first responders and principal coordinators for a patient's care. Working in adult, pediatric, and neonatal ICUs, as well as specialty care areas of practice, acute care NPs are caring for highly complex, critically ill patients with a variety of disease states.

Beyond the ICU, acute care NPs lead rapid response teams, transplant teams, cardiology teams, hospitalist teams, and many other medical and surgical specialty teams. The evolution of acute care NP practice has helped hospital systems achieve critical quality and safety goals. Acute care NPs drive quality indicators such as ideal hospital lengths of stay, reduction in adverse events, reduction in nosocomial infections, reduction in unexpected hospital readmissions, and reduction in unnecessary resource utilization and thereby costs of care. Studies continue to demonstrate the acute care NP's ability to optimize communication and coordination of care, improve handovers between services, and adhere to established standards of care. Their quality of education, experience, evidence-based practice, and multidisciplinary collaboration are paramount, and as thus, acute care NPs have become the mainstay of state-of-the-art acute care hospitals and critical care organizations.

Dr. Valerie J. Fuller and Dr. Paula S. McCauley have carefully compiled the first edition of the *Textbook for the Adult-Gerontology Acute Care Nurse Practitioner* as a comprehensive resource for both instruction and clinical practice. Written by NPs for NPs, the chapters provide an overview of assessment, diagnoses, treatments, and management of care. Succinct information is provided on presenting signs and symptoms, history and physical exam findings, diagnostic considerations, treatment, and clinical pearls for the management of a variety of disorders, general clinical topics, and special considerations for AGACNP nursing practice. The editors have assembled nearly 100 expert authors who discuss the evidence-based gold standards for diagnostics and tests for optimal detection of multisystem disorders, patient management, and transitions of care. In these chapters, learners will gain greater understanding of the etiology and pathophysiology of acute and critical illnesses, and the latest in advanced pharmacologic and nonpharmacologic therapies.

Working in acute care for many years, we are thrilled for this first edition of *Textbook for the Adult-Gerontology Acute Care Nurse Practitioner*. We anticipate this book will be used often in classrooms, in workshops, as a reference for presentations and publications, and as a daily resource guide for acute care NPs practicing across acute and critical care settings. The authors of each chapter are indeed experts in their field and have thoroughly outlined important considerations for AGACNPs. We congratulate the editors and chapter authors for their efforts in developing a clearly outlined and accurate text for AGACNP use that will no doubt impact AGACNP care, to impact patient care outcomes, quality of life, and care delivery—truly the first of its kind.

April N. Kapu, DNP, APRN, ACNP-BC, FAANP, FCCM, FAAN
Associate Dean for Clinical and Community Partnerships, Vanderbilt University School of Nursing
Professor of Nursing, Vanderbilt University School of Nursing
2021–2023 President, American Association of Nurse Practitioners

Ruth Kleinpell, PhD, APRN, ACNP-BC, FAANP, FAAN, MCCM
Associate Dean for Clinical Scholarship, Vanderbilt University School of Nursing
Professor of Nursing, Vanderbilt University School of Nursing
2017 President, Society of Critical Care Medicine

PREFACE

Since the inception of the nurse practitioner (NP) role by Dr. Loretta Ford and Dr. Henry Silver in 1965, NPs have provided high-quality, patient-centered healthcare to individuals of all ages. Originally developed as a primary care role, the NP role expanded to address complex acute and critical patient conditions as well as healthcare workforce needs. The first acute care nurse practitioner (ACNP) education programs began in 1992 and ACNPs are now the fastest growing subset of NPs in the country (Kleinpell et al., 2018). ACNPs can be found in a wide variety of settings including critical care units, outpatient specialty practices, urgent care centers, and inpatient hospital services such as surgery, cardiology, pulmonology, and many others.

We have long recognized the need for a single comprehensive resource for ACNP practice that could be utilized by educational programs, students, and providers alike. Having both served as program directors in ACNP programs, we often had to pull together resources from our medical colleagues which often resulted in numerous textbooks and other information focused on a medical model. To that end, we are very pleased to bring you the first edition of the *Textbook for the Adult-Gerontology Acute Care Nurse Practitioner: Evidence-Based Standards of Practice*.

In an effort to create a resource both concise and comprehensive, we offer coverage of the conditions and challenges common in AGACNP practice and integrate evidence-based standards throughout. Clinical conditions are presented by body system, each organized by consistent headings to guide the practitioner or student to pertinent information related to the evaluation, diagnosis, treatment, and transition of care. Brief and easy-to-find Clinical Pearls and Key Takeaways boxes are included throughout the text, making critical information easy to locate. Additionally, special topics on palliative and end-of-life care, pain, and pain management are discussed in the context of the AGACNP's professional role. Instructors who choose to rely upon *Textbook for the Adult-Gerontology Acute Care Nurse Practitioner* for teaching will have access to valuable supplements in the form of PowerPoint slides to aid lectures or serve as study notes.

To sufficiently address the needs of those whom we hope will come to rely upon this text, we have included the expert perspectives of over 100 authors. These contributors have helped to ensure that this first-of-its-kind text adequately reflects the skills and competencies of the AGACNP specialty, and we are grateful for their work.

Valerie J. Fuller, PhD, DNP, AGACNP-BC, FNP-BC,
FNAP, FAANP
Paula S. McCauley, DNP, ACNP-BC, CMC, CSC, FAANP

REFERENCE

Kleinpell, R., Cook, M., & Padden, D. (2018). American Association of Nurse Practitioners National Nurse Practitioner sample surgery: Update on acute care nurse practitioner practice. *Journal of the American Association of Nurse Practitioners, 30*(3), 140–149.

ACKNOWLEDGMENTS

Writing a textbook of this depth and breadth during one of the worst pandemics in history did not come without its challenges. We are deeply indebted to our esteemed authors who not only worked on the frontlines of this global healthcare crisis but also took the time to share their clinical wisdom and expertise for this text. You rose to the challenge both professionally and personally and we cannot thank you enough.

We also wish to thank our team at Springer Publishing, especially Elizabeth Nieginski, Taylor Ball, and Joseph Stubenrauch. The patience and kindness you exhibited during a time when it was immensely difficult for us to step away from our clinical roles will not soon be forgotten.

INSTRUCTOR RESOURCES

 A robust set of instructor resources designed to supplement this text is located at
http://connect.springerpub.com/content/reference-book/978-0-8261-6079-9.
Qualifying instructors may request access by emailing **textbook@springerpub.com.**

Instructor resources include:

- Chapter-Based PowerPoint Presentations
- AACN Competency Grid

PART I

ROLE, SCOPE, AND STANDARDS OF THE ACUTE CARE NURSE PRACTITIONER

CHAPTER 1

ROLE OF THE ACUTE CARE NURSE PRACTITIONER

Valerie J. Fuller and Paula S. McCauley

ROLE AND DEFINITION OF THE NURSE PRACTITIONER IN ACUTE CARE

ROLE

The acute care nurse practitioner (ACNP) role began in the early 1970s but saw notable expansion during the 1990s in response to the increasing acuity and complexity of hospitalized patients, hospital restructuring, and changes in the resident physician workforce (Kleinpell, 1997; Richmond & Keane, 1992; Shaw et al., 1997). These changes spurred the development of the first ACNP programs in 1992 at Case Western Reserve University, the University of Connecticut, the University of Pittsburgh, and the University of Pennsylvania to prepare nurse practitioners in the care of patients with acute, critical, and complex medical conditions. The first ACNP certification exam was jointly administered in December of 1995 by the American Nurses Credentialing Center (ANCC) and the American Association of Critical-Care Nurses (AACN). In 2020 there were more than 12,700 certified ACNPs in the United States (American Association of Nurse Practitioners [AANP], 2021).

DEFINITION

The AACN Scope and Standards for ACNP practice define the ACNP as,

> "… a registered nurse who has completed an accredited graduate-level educational program that prepares him or her as a nurse practitioner with supervised clinical practice to acquire advanced knowledge, skills, and abilities. This education and training qualifies him or her to independently: (1) perform comprehensive health assessments; (2) order and interpret the full spectrum of diagnostic tests and procedures; (3) use a differential diagnosis to reach a medical diagnosis; and (4) order, provide, and evaluate the outcomes of interventions. The purpose of the ACNP is to provide advanced nursing care across the continuum of health care services to meet the specialized physiologic and psychological needs of patients with acute, critical, and/or complex chronic health conditions. This care is continuous and comprehensive and may be provided in any setting where the patient may be found" (AACN, 2012, p. 6).

ADVANCED PRACTICE REGISTERED NURSE CONSENSUS MODEL

In response to a proliferation of nurse practitioner (NP) specialties along with a lack of standardization around advanced practice registered nurse (APRN) licensure, accreditation, certification, education, and regulation, the APRN Consensus Work Group and the National Council of State Boards of Nursing APRN Advisory Committee published the Consensus Model for APRN Regulation in 2008. The model was endorsed by over 48 professional nursing organizations to promote uniformity and standardization of the four APRN roles while ensuring patient safety and expanding access to care (APRN Consensus Work Group, 2008; Fuller, 2021). There are six population foci outlined in the model (Figure 1.1), with adult-gerontology and pediatrics being delineated as either acute care or primary care and based on competencies obtained through formal education (Doherty et al., 2018). The model also requires a graduate or postgraduate degree from an accredited institution, national certification, use of the APRN title, independent prescribing, independent practice, and both RN and APRN licensure. To date, 18 jurisdictions (16 states plus Guam and the Northern Mariana Islands) have fully adopted the seven key elements of the Consensus Model with the remaining states in varying stages of implementation (Figure 1.2; Buck, 2021).

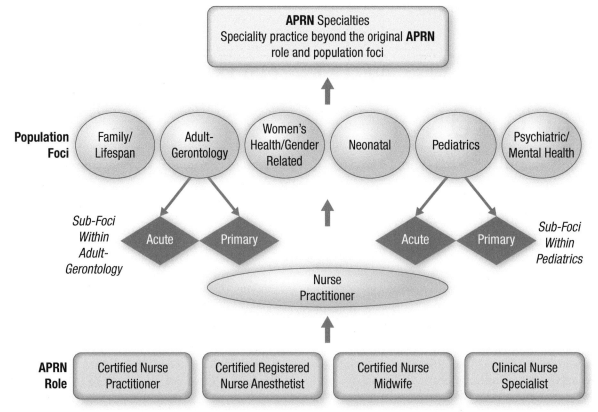

FIGURE 1.1: The advanced practice registered nurse (APRN) regulatory model.
Source: Reproduced with permission from the APRN Consensus Work Group, National Council of State Boards of Nursing APRN Advisory Committee. (2008). *Consensus model for APRN regulation: Licensure, accreditation, certification and education.* NCSBN. https://ncsbn.org/Consensus_Model_for_APRN_Regulation_July_2008.pdf

LICENSURE ACCREDITATION, CERTIFICATION, AND EDUCATION OF THE ADULT-GERONTOLOGY ACUTE CARE NURSE PRACTITIONER

APRN regulation includes the elements of licensure, accreditation, certification, and education (also referred to as the LACE [Licensure, Accreditation, Certification, and Education] model). The four recognized APRN roles include the certified nurse practitioner (CNP), certified nurse midwife (CNM), certified registered nurse anesthetist (CRNA) and clinical nurse specialist (CNS).

Each of the topics that follow is outlined in the Consensus Model for APRN Regulation. For a more in-depth review, the reader is referred to the *Consensus Model for APRN Regulation: Licensure, Accreditation, Certification and Education* which can be found at https://www.ncsbn.org/Consensus_Model_for_APRN_Regulation_July_2008.pdf.

LICENSURE

Licensure is the granting of the authority to practice (APRN Consensus Work Group, 2008, p. 7). The Consensus

Model stipulates that the APRN should carry both an RN license and an APRN license issued by the state Board of Nursing in the state(s) where the adult-gerontology acute care nurse practitioner (AGACNP) intends to practice. Nurse practitioners are licensed and regulated by the Board of Nursing in all states and, in some states with restricted practice environments, nurse practitioners may be jointly regulated by the state Board of Nursing and the state Board of Medicine. The scope and standards for APRNs is outlined in each state's Nurse Practice Act. The "nurse practitioner scope of practice should match patient care needs and is based on the individual NP's role and population education and certification, both of which are derived from nationally vetted competencies" (National Organization of Nurse Practitioner Faculties [NONPF] Task Force, 2021).

The AGACNP should be aware that many states have APRN and RN title protection in their rules and regulations that specify that one cannot present oneself as an APRN or RN unless one holds a valid license in that state.

Licensure rules and regulations vary significantly by state and the AGACNP should refer to their respective state Board of Nursing for further information.

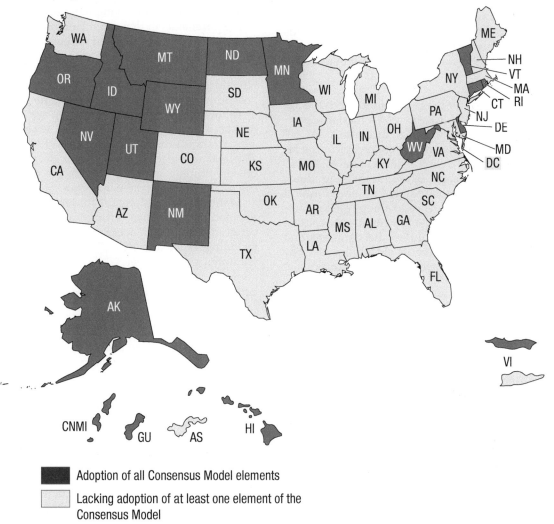

Jurisdictions Aligned With All Seven Elements of the Consensus Model, as of May 2021

■ Adoption of all Consensus Model elements

☐ Lacking adoption of at least one element of the Consensus Model

FIGURE 1.2: Jurisdictions aligned with all seven elements of the APRN Consensus Model, as of May 2021.
Source: Reproduced with permission from Buck, M. (2021). An update on the consensus model for APRN regulation: More than a decade of progress. *Journal of Nursing Regulation, 12*(2), 22–33. https://doi.org/10.1016/S2155-8256(21)00053-3.

ACCREDITATION

Accreditation is the formal review and approval by a recognized agency of educational degree or certification programs in nursing or nursing-related programs (APRN Consensus Work Group, 2008, p. 7). APRN programs must be accredited or undergo a pre-approval process prior to admitting students, and APRN students must graduate from an accredited program to sit for national certification and be eligible for state licensure. The two accrediting organizations for nurse practitioner programs in the United States are the Commission on Collegiate Nursing Education (CCNE) and the Accreditation Commission for Education in Nursing (ACEN). AGACNP students should confirm that their education program is accredited and by whom.

CERTIFICATION

Certification is the formal recognition of the knowledge, skills, and experience demonstrated by the achievement of standards identified by the profession (APRN Consensus Work Group, 2008, p. 7).

The Consensus Model stipulates that the APRN be nationally certified in their role and population, prior to licensure (Buck, 2021). Two states (California and New

York) do not currently require certification for APRNs, but nearly all employers, insurers, and credentialing bodies require national certification as part of their eligibility criteria.

The two organizations that offer national certification for the AGACNP are the ANCC, which awards the AGACNP-BC credential, and the AACN, which awards the ACNPC-AG credential. The purpose of national certification is to ensure that the NP meets minimum competency levels for safe entry into practice (Carpenter et al., 2019).

To be eligible to sit for the certification exam the applicant must hold an RN license; hold a master's, postgraduate certificate, or doctoral degree from an AGACNP program that is nationally accredited; complete the required faculty-supervised clinical hours in the AGACNP role and population; complete three separate graduate courses in Advanced Pharmacology, Advanced Physical Health Assessment and Advanced Pathophysiology (often called the 3Ps); and be able to demonstrate content that covers health promotion, differential diagnoses and disease management (Carpenter et al., 2019, p. 15). The NP's certification must match their formal educational preparation.

EDUCATION

Education is the formal preparation of APRNs in graduate degree–granting or postgraduate certificate programs (APRN Consensus Work Group, 2008, p. 7). Nurse practitioners are educated in the NP role and in one of the six population foci outlined in Figure 1.1 (e.g., the role of a nurse practitioner with a population of adult-gerontology acute care as in the case of the AGACNP). If the APRN changes a role or population, the APRN must complete an accredited graduate program that aligns with the new role or population (APRN LACE Network, 2021). RN or APRN experience or clinical training programs outside of a graduate institution (i.e., residency or fellowship programs) are not a substitute for completion of a formal program in the new role or population (APRN LACE Network, 2021; NONPF Task Force, 2021).

Doctor of Nursing Practice

The concept of the doctor of nursing practice (DNP) discussion began in the nursing community in the 1990s. Clinical doctorates are required for other licensed independent practitioners (LIPs) in healthcare including pharmacists, medical doctors, dentists, podiatrists, and psychologists. Preparing NPs at the doctoral level is recommended to promote parity with other disciplines and further enhance recognition in the healthcare arena. Current discussion among nursing organizations recommends that all NP programs move from a master's to a DNP as entry level by 2025 (NONPF, 2019).

Postlicensure Clinical Training Programs

NPs must graduate from nationally accredited graduate programs that have met rigorous requirements. NPs come out of these programs prepared to be competent, safe practitioners and having met the didactic and clinical requirements in their population foci. Postlicensure clinical hours are not required for entry into practice after graduation. Residency is required to obtain a license to practice for physicians; it is not accurately applied to NP education as the supervision of a preceptor is embedded into the NP education requirements.

Fellowship training has sprung up across the healthcare landscape over the past several years in efforts to support transition into practice for APRNs. Both fellowship and residencies for NPs provide optional postlicensure training, often from healthcare systems, and are essentially extended onboarding programs. They are not a substitute for postlicensure training to move to a new population focus when certification is required, such as between primary and acute care. Nursing organizations including AANP and NONPF do not endorse mandated fellowships or residencies (NONPF, 2019).

SCOPE AND STANDARDS OF PRACTICE

The practice of the AGACNP is not defined by the setting but is determined by the acuity of patient needs and driven by the condition and acuity of the patient. Scope of practice defines the boundaries for the various roles in which the nurse practitioner may practice, describing the who, what, where, when, and why the practitioner functions within a defined role. Scope of practice varies geographically, within institutions, as well as departments, thus designation as a LIP may vary among states or between facilities. Scope of practice is influenced by national certification and regulated by state requirements and laws, institutional rules, specific regulations at the service/departmental level and finally by the individual practitioner (Kleinpell et al., 2014).

The Scope and Standards for the AGACNP are developed by a collective of nursing organizations and experts, are updated every 3 to 5 years, and published by AACN (2022). The formal educational preparation qualifies them to independently (AACN, 2022):

- perform comprehensive health assessments;
- order and interpret the full spectrum of diagnostic tests and procedures;
- formulate a differential diagnosis to reach a diagnosis; and
- order, provide, and evaluate the outcomes of interventions.

It is essential that the AGACNP understands both state practice acts and institutional bylaws. Collaborative practice is the basis of the scope and standards of acute care but has seen major changes over the past several years with attainment of full practice authority in many states. Self-regulation and accountability

BOX 1.1 CURRENT STANDARDS OF CLINICAL PRACTICE FOR THE AGACNP

- Professional practice
- Education
- Collaboration
- Ethics
- Advocacy
- Systems thinking
- Resource utilization
- Leadership
- Collegiality
- Quality of practice
- Clinical inquiry

Source: Data from American Association of Critical-Care Nurses. (2022). *Scope and standards of practice for the acute care nurse practitioner*. American Association of Critical-Care Nurses.

are also imperative in understanding and adhering to scope of practice. The AGACNP autonomously provides patient-centered care and consults and/or collaborates with other members of the interprofessional team. AGACNPs do not require physician supervision or oversight (as may be defined in collaborative practice arrangements) to fulfill their role (AACN, 2022).

Standards of Clinical Practice are statements that describe the level of care or performance common to the practice. The Standards of Clinical Practice for the AGACNP are based on educational preparation and define how the quality of care may be evaluated and apply to the care that the AGACNP provides to all patients within the population. The current standards are included in Box 1.1; full descriptions are available in the 2022 publication from the AACN.

ISSUES AND TRENDS

LEGISLATION

Federal legislation has a direct impact on the role of the AGACNP. Federal legislation allowing APRNs to bill Medicare directly for services was initially passed in 1997. Since then, additional changes have occurred, with full practice authority attained in 26 U.S. states, the District of Columbia, and the U.S. territories of Guam and the Northern Mariana Islands. Medicare laws and rules influence the policy of nongovernmental payers (Loversidge, 2016).

Medicare refers to NPs and PAs as nonphysician providers or NPPs and each provider has an individual Medicare/Medicaid number used to bill for services. NP services are billed at 85% of the physician rate. Currently, NPs are the fastest-growing Medicare designated provider specialty, providing a significant impact on healthcare costs. Advocacy and research are necessary for continued support for NPs' full practice authority for all practitioners and to measure impact and outcomes of NP care (Centers for Medicare & Medicaid Services [CMS], 2019).

REIMBURSEMENT, BILLING, AND CODING

The AGACNP may bill for services rendered if they fall within the nurse practitioner's scope of practice (Hoffman & Guttendorf, 2017). The AGACNP must have an understanding of billing mechanisms as well as policy related restrictions and guidelines that dictate billing practices at their place of employment. Whether an AGACNP bills for services delivered in the hospital inpatient setting depends on how the salary is listed on the hospital's Medicare cost report. AGACNPs who provide inpatient care may bill direct or shared. Direct services are billed under the NPs own National Provider Identifier (NPI) number regardless of setting. If care is provided in the clinic or office setting the AGACNP will bill for the type of visit, level of encounter, new or follow-up visit, and complexity of the visit. Shared or split billing, often used in the inpatient setting, may be done under either the AGACNP's or the physician's NPI number. There needs to be documentation from both providers to support shared billing and the billing is usually done under the physician's number. The disparity here is that NP billing is at 85% of the physician's rate, thus the incentive for billing under the physician's number resulting in the higher rate, increasing healthcare costs.

Documentation is key to reimbursement and must be sufficient to support the billed service. Evaluation and Management (E&M) codes, Current Procedural Terminology (CPT) codes and diagnostic codes from the *International Classification of Diseases,* 10th revision (ICD-10) are utilized and assigned to support the level of care (Lindeke, 2010).

There are four categories of history taking that will designate the level of care:
- problem focused;
- expanded problem focused;
- detailed; and
- comprehensive.

Documentation at any level must include statements of the chief complaint along with seven variables: 1) location, 2) quality, 3) severity, 4) duration, 5) timing, 6) context, 7) modifying factors, and signs/symptoms. The physical examination expands to address the level of care. Problem focused is limited to the system impacted, expanded problem focused adds other symptomatic or related systems, these both require a limited history of present illness (HPI) and review of systems (ROS). Detailed and comprehensive exams may be single-problem focused or include multiple system problems—both require an expanded HPI and ROS, and past, family, and social history.

There are four levels of decision-making:
- straightforward;
- low complexity;

- moderate complexity; and
- high complexity.

Additional components can be used to alter coding and include counseling, coordination of care, complexity, and time.

CRITICAL CARE SERVICES

Detailed information is required for critical care billing, which is billed in time increments. Critical care services are time-based codes, and the initial critical care time (CPT code 99291) is met by a single physician or advanced practice provider (APP). Following the guidelines outlined by the CMS, additional critical care time (CPT code 99292) in the same calendar day can be billed by another provider in the same practice. If there are additional claims made, separate progress notes are required to support the claim and the critical care time documented must match what was submitted on each claim (Dorman et al., 2014; Munro, 2013).

The Coding for Chest Medicine (Chest, 2016) and Coding and Billing for Critical Care—A Practice Tool (Dorman et al., 2014) are helpful references. The CPT provides codes for inpatient and adult critical care services.

PROLONGED SERVICES

When a serious diagnosis requires considerable discussion related to complex treatment options such as terminal illness, palliative care, or prolonged mechanical life support, prolonged service codes may be utilized. Prolonged service codes capture the extended face-to-face time spent with the patient in the inpatient hospital (99356, 99357) setting and are considered companion codes to the E&M codes. Code 99356 is used when there is a medically necessary, direct, face-to-face patient encounter that requires additional time beyond the usual service threshold time. This code may only be used once on a calendar day, and the documented time must be performed by the same provider. Code 99357 is used to report each additional 30 minutes beyond the first hour of prolonged services. The medical record must include documentation of time spent face-to-face with the patient, the content of the medically necessary prolonged service, and the required primary or daily visit documentation (Magdic, 2013).

NURSE PRACTITIONER COST-EFFECTIVENESS

Institutional regulations may dictate how the billing process occurs, but the ACNP should recognize the benefits of billing under their own provider number, providing evidence of the AGACNP's value and worth to the healthcare system. NP cost-effectiveness and high-quality care has been well documented with substantial evidence over the past 50 years. Cost-effectiveness and healthcare savings are appreciated due to lower compensation or salaries for NPs versus physicians, which is especially evident if the NP is practicing independently. Other areas where cost-effectiveness has been demonstrated specific to the AGANCP are through reduced lengths of stay and emergency visits, quality and program enhancements, and reduced overall drug costs for inpatients (Chen et al., 2009; Newhouse et al., 2011).

BARRIERS TO PRACTICE

NPs have practiced on the front lines of the COVID-19 pandemic, providing care across the continuum to all populations. Meeting healthcare needs of patients during COVID-19 demanded flexibility throughout healthcare systems and settings. To provide wider access to care several waivers were issued by the CMS to reduce barriers to care during the pandemic that allowed NPs to practice at the top of their license to the full extent of the education and certification. Several examples include authorizing NPs to perform all mandatory visits in skilled nursing facilities, telehealth services, and home healthcare visits. Implementation of regulatory language that recognizes NPs as authorized practitioners in the Coronavirus Aid, Relief, and Economic Security (CARES) Act removed barriers to care for home healthcare, infusion, and rehabilitative therapies (Snyder & Kerns, 2021). Expanded telehealth services qualified the NP as the primary care provider. Waivers authorized NPs in critical access hospitals to practice to the full extent of their license by removing the physical physician presence requirement and authorizing Medicare hospital patients to be under the care of an NP. The CMS is proposing a permanent authorization for NPs to order and directly supervise cardiac and pulmonary rehabilitation. Nursing organizations are working together to request that these become permanent changes to practice.

AGACNPs also led innovative programs that addressed a multitude of complex issues and the needs of patients during the pandemic—innovations in technology, protocols, and practice as well as education.

TELEHEALTH

Over the past several years, strategies to address the national healthcare provider shortage and limited access to care have driven the broader use of telehealth as an effective strategy. Telehealth includes live and asynchronous types of technology such as remote monitoring and various types of stored information. Telehealth was rapidly moved into the forefront as a necessary option for access to healthcare in 2020 as the rapid spread of the COVID-19 placed the United States in lock down (Snyder & Kerns, 2021). Today it is widely recognized and reimbursed. AGACNPs may utilize telehealth for postacute follow up visits, in specialty clinics for routine visits and follow-ups, for monitoring of special populations such as patients with heart failure or diabetes, wound management, as well as patient and family education programs.

Telehealth has been integrated into NP education, providing knowledge and skills that will empower the AGACNP to meet direct clinical needs and innovative opportunities to address healthcare needs. NP students may find that immersion into telehealth programs may be done in both simulated programs and actual precepted visits (NONPF Statement of Telehealth, 2018).

DIVERSITY, EQUITY, AND INCLUSION

Numerous events over the past several years have brought diversity equity and inclusion (DEI) to the forefront. Social determinants of health, healthcare inequity, and disparity have been identified and recognized across the nursing community. NPs provide access to healthcare services within and among diverse groups and recognition of the need to develop an infrastructure that will achieve and sustain DEI through education, practice and advocacy has been adopted across the profession. Standards for NP education have been broadened to incorporate practices that promote DEI within all educational programs, and nursing organizations have developed advocacy and leadership resources that recruit and promote DEI among their members.

CONCLUSION

Initially developed to provide coverage for the gap in practice in hospital residencies, the AGACNP role has evolved greatly over the past three decades. We have experienced significant recognition and expansion of the role, although not without barriers or turbulence, to the contemporary state of the role recognized as an integral member of the healthcare team for services throughout the acute care population. Expansion of the original AGACNP education requirements to include more comprehensive geriatric competencies provides the current basis of certification for AGACNPs.

Appreciation of the scope and standards, education, and licensure is paramount for safe and effective practice.

We have introduced the basis of these herein along with resources that provide more in-depth description and discussion and encourage readers to access them to better understand the role and responsibilities as well as potential innovative possibilities for the future.

KEY TAKEAWAYS

- APRN regulation includes the elements of licensure, accreditation, certification, and education.
- Scope of practice is impacted by:
  - state requirements and laws;
  - institutional rules and regulations;
  - national certification by professional organizations;
  - service line specific regulations; and
  - individual autonomy.
- AGACNPs must understand common coding and billing practices.
- Billing under individual NPI number demonstrates the AGACNPs value.

A robust set of instructor resources designed to supplement this text is located at **http://connect.springerpub.com/ content/reference-book/978-0-8261-6079-9.** Qualifying instructors may request access by emailing **textbook@springerpub.com.**

REFERENCES

Full list of references can be accessed at http://connect. springerpub.com/content/reference-book/978-0-8261-6079-9

CLINICAL PRACTICE OF THE ACUTE CARE NURSE PRACTITIONER: DISORDERS OF BODY SYSTEMS

CHAPTER 2

HEAD, EYES, EARS, NOSE, AND THROAT DISORDERS

LEARNING OBJECTIVES

- Diagnose and differentiate disorders of the head, eyes, ears, nose, and throat (HEENT).
- Understand and implement clinical practice guidelines and patterns related to quality care in patients diagnosed with HEENT disorders.
- Compare and contrast the etiology and treatment for the pathologies of HEENT.
- Recognize assessment findings consistent with the common HEENT emergencies.
- Demonstrate understanding of appropriate interventions and referrals when indicated for the emergencies.
- Demonstrate understanding of airway management challenges.
- Demonstrate awareness of when to refer to a specialist.

INTRODUCTION

Ear and eye emergencies are commonly seen as primary conditions in urgent care but uncommon in most acute care settings. They can be seen as a primary differential (e.g., acute angle-closure glaucoma) or as a secondary differential as an inpatient acute care setting. Being able to accurately diagnose, treat, and order appropriate consultation is of prime importance regardless of the setting. This chapter discusses the most common head, eyes, ears, nose, and throat (HEENT) disease processes.

CONDITIONS OF THE HEAD

2.1: BELL'S PALSY

L. Douglas Smith, Jr.

Bell's palsy (BP) is an acute onset idiopathic unilateral facial nerve dysfunction with resultant paresis or paralysis of facial muscles (Luu et al., 2021). BP occurs annually in approximately 40 to 53 per 100,000 persons and indiscriminately affects people of all ages or sex (Zhang et al., 2020). The incidence of BP is higher following a recent viral upper respiratory infection (URI), in pregnant women and immunocompromised patients, and in patients who are obese or suffer from chronic diabetes or hypertension (Eviston et al., 2015; Gagyor et al., 2019). The exact pathogenesis of BP is unknown, though many hypotheses discuss facial nerve infection, edema, compression, and autoimmunity as likely causes of the dysfunction (Eviston et al., 2015). Most patients affected by BP fully recover within 4 months, many spontaneously and without treatment, while a minority persist with varying degrees of facial nerve dysfunction (Luu et al., 2021; Shokri et al., 2020). Patients with persistent facial asymmetry and long-term clinical side effects are likely to suffer psychological distress and impaired quality of life (Luu et al., 2021; Zhang et al., 2020).

PRESENTING SIGNS AND SYMPTOMS

Patients present with an evolving acute unilateral facial nerve paresis or paralysis where maximum dysfunction occurs approximately 72 hours after symptom onset (Shokri et al., 2020). Weakness is seen on half of the face through the forehead and eyebrows to the mouth, resulting in significant facial asymmetry (Twoon et al., 2016). Associated complaints include hyperacusis, ipsilateral postauricular pain, dysgeusia, oral droop, loss of facial expression, nasal obstruction, alteration in taste, and dysarthria (Eviston et al., 2015; Twoon et al., 2016).

HISTORY AND PHYSICAL EXAM FINDINGS

For the patient presenting with acute facial palsy, the importance of a thorough history and comprehensive physical exam in establishing the appropriate diagnosis cannot be overstated (Shokri et al., 2020; Twoon et al., 2016). It is imperative to establish a time course for the onset and progression of symptoms (Shokri et al., 2020; Zhang et al., 2020). The patient may also report significant nasal congestion, drooling and biting of the lower lip and mucosa, and an inability to close the eyelid (Shokri et al., 2020).

Physical examination of the face reveals the absence of forehead wrinkles, brow ptosis, incomplete eye closure with lagophthalmos, effaced nasolabial fold, oral incompetence, dental show only on the contralateral side, and significant facial asymmetry at rest and with movement (Shokri et al., 2020). The critical physical exam finding of BP is paresis/paralysis of the forehead (Eviston et al., 2015; Twoon et al., 2016). Guidelines recommend describing the degree of palsy using a validated grading system (i.e., House-Brackmann grading system; Kim & Lee, 2020).

DIFFERENTIAL DIAGNOSIS AND DIAGNOSTIC CONSIDERATIONS

BP is a clinical diagnosis of exclusion requiring the careful consideration of other causes known to produce facial palsy (Zhang et al., 2020). If the presentation, history, and physical examination are consistent with BP, diagnostic testing with laboratory evaluations and diagnostic imaging are unnecessary (Kim & Lee, 2020; Shokri et al., 2020). There is a broad range of differential diagnoses for facial palsy and misdiagnosis is not uncommon (Eviston et al., 2015). Potential causes of acute facial paresis/paralysis include infective (bacterial, viral, and tick-borne), traumatic, neoplastic (intra- and extracranial neoplasm), neurological (encephalomyelitis, Guillain-Barré syndrome), and autoimmune inflammatory or granulomatous conditions (vasculitis, sarcoidosis), which may explain the presentation (Kim & Lee, 2020; Shokri et al., 2020; Zhang et al., 2020). The elimination of acute stroke as the etiology is imperative; paresis/paralysis of the forehead is the crucial discriminator guiding the clinician toward BP (Eviston et al., 2015; Shokri et al., 2020).

TREATMENT

Prompt diagnosis and treatment initiation are critical as delays in diagnosis and treatment result in permanent dysfunction (Gagyor et al., 2019; Luu et al., 2021). A 10-day course of high-dose corticosteroid therapy is the mainstay of treatment (Baugh et al., 2013; Gronseth et al., 2012; Luu et al., 2021; Shokri et al., 2020). Prednisone 60 mg for 5 days followed by a 5-day taper is likely an effective strategy (Baugh et al., 2013; Eviston et al., 2015; Shokri et al., 2020). Antiviral agents combined with corticosteroids may benefit those with severe facial paralysis; however, an antiviral agent as monotherapy is inappropriate (Gagyor et al., 2019; Kim & Lee, 2020; Luu et al., 2021; Shokri et al., 2020). A typical antiviral regimen for BP may include valacyclovir 1.0 to 3.2 g/day for 5 to 7 days (Gagyor et al., 2019; Shokri et al., 2020).

Clinicians should initiate ocular protective measures for patients presenting with eyelid dysfunction to avoid foreign particle invasion and corneal damage (Luu et al., 2021). Effective strategies include the use of physical barriers (protective glasses), artificial tears/ointments, and taping the eyes closed at night (Eviston et al., 2015). The use of an eyelid weight along with a referral to

ophthalmology should be considered early in the treatment course (Eviston et al., 2015; Twoon et al., 2016).

TRANSITION OF CARE

The generalist clinician manages BP. Referral to facial nerve specialists, including neurology and potentially ENT surgery, occurs in the setting of concomitant new or worsening neurological deficit, development of ocular symptoms, or incomplete recovery within 3 months (Baugh et al., 2013; Kim & Lee, 2020; Luu et al., 2021; Shokri et al., 2020).

KEY TAKEAWAYS

- The patient presenting with acute unilateral facial paresis/paralysis is assessed by a thorough history and comprehensive physical examination to exclude identifiable causes.
- High-dose oral corticosteroids, alone or combined with antiviral therapy, should be administered as soon as possible.
- Initiate eye-protective interventions for patients with impaired eye closure.
- Refer patients with ocular symptoms, new or worsening neurological deficit, or incomplete recovery after 3 months to a facial nerve specialist.

EVIDENCE-BASED RESOURCES

Further information regarding BP is available in these evidence-based resources:

Baugh, R. F., Basura, G. J., Ishii, L. E., Schwartz, S. R., Drumheller, C. M., Burkholder, R., Deckard, N. A., Dawson, C., Driscoll, C., Gillespie, M. B., Gurgel, R. K., Halperin, J., Khalid, A. N., Kumar, K. A., Micco, A., Munsell, D., Rosenbaum, S., & Vaughan, W. (2013). Clinical practice guideline: Bell's palsy. *Otolaryngology—Head and Neck Surgery, 149*(Suppl. 3), S1–S27. https://doi.org/10.1177/0194599813505967

Luu, N. N., Chorath, K. T., May, B. R., Bhuiyan, N., Moreira, A. G., & Rajasekaran, K. (2021, January 3). Clinical practice guidelines in idiopathic facial paralysis: Systematic review using the appraisal of guidelines for research and evaluation (agree ii) instrument. *Journal of Neurology.* https://doi.org/10.1007/s00415-020-10345-0

CONDITIONS OF THE EYES

2.2: ACUTE ANGLE-CLOSURE GLAUCOMA

Helen Miley

Acute angle-closure glaucoma (AACG) is an ophthalmic emergency in which there is a severe elevation of the intraocular pressure (IOP) exceeding 40 mmHg.

PRESENTING SIGNS AND SYMPTOMS

The onset of AACG symptoms includes a sudden onset of acute pain, redness of the eye, and blurred vision. Associated symptoms include nausea, vomiting, and profuse sweating. AACG is more common in the older adult and in Inuit and Asian persons (Lin & Biggerstaff, 2019; Tanna, 2020). It is less common in Caucasians and least common in African Americans. Gonioscopy reveals a closed angle without any visible angle structures.

DIFFERENTIAL DIAGNOSIS AND DIAGNOSTIC CONSIDERATIONS

If not properly diagnosed and treated, progressive and permanent ocular damage occurs in a matter of hours to days. Ocular examination shows a very shallow anterior chamber, corneal edema, and a mid-dilated pupil. If the IOP is not reduced blindness will occur. Differential diagnoses include iritis, conjunctivitis, corneal abrasion, uveitis, and keratitis.

TREATMENT

The treatment consists of lowering the pressure within the eye by a combination of optic drops alpha-adrenergic agonists (e.g., brimonidine), beta blockers (e.g., levobunolol and timolol), miotic agents (pilocarpine), and oral medications. An emergency consult with the ophthamologist for a laser iridotomy is necessary.

CLINICAL PEARLS

- Symptoms of ACCG occur rapidly.
- Early aggressive treatment to preserve sight is imperative.

KEY TAKEAWAY

- Emergency consult with ophthalmology.

2.3: BLEPHARITIS

Al-Zada "Al" Aguilar

Among the most common causes of chronic ocular irritation, blepharitis is a chronic eyelid inflammation that is frequently associated with symptoms of ocular surface irritation and dry eye (Amescua et al., 2019; Sung et al., 2018; Tarff & Behrens, 2017). Blepharitis can be classified based on anatomy: Anterior blepharitis affects the eyelid skin, base of the eyelashes, and the eyelash follicles, whereas posterior blepharitis affects the meibomian glands (Amescua et al., 2019).

Anterior Blepharitis

Affecting mainly the anterior eyelid, staphylococcal and seborrheic blepharitis are subtypes of anterior blepharitis (Amescua et al., 2019). Staphylococcal blepharitis is characterized by scaling, crusting (i.e., scurf), erythema and microscopic soap bubbles seen on the eyelid margin along with eyelash loss or misdirection (Amescua et al., 2019; Auran & Casper, 2019). Those with seborrheic blepharitis have greasy scaling of the anterior eyelid and often have associated seborrheic dermatitis elsewhere on the body (e.g., head, scalp; Amescua et al., 2019; Auran & Casper, 2019).

Posterior Blepharitis

One of the most common causes of non-sight-threatening evaporative eye disease, posterior blepharitis affects the meibomian glands (Amescua et al., 2019; Auran & Casper, 2019). Meibomian gland dysfunction (MGD) has been defined as a chronic diffuse abnormality of the meibomian glands, characterized by terminal duct obstruction and/or changes in glandular secretion resulting in tear film alteration, increased bacterial growth on the lid margin, evaporative dry eye, and ocular surface damage and inflammation (Amescua et al., 2019; Bagheri & Wajda, 2017).

PRESENTING SIGNS AND SYMPTOMS

Patients with blepharitis often present with ocular erythema, pruritus, lid swelling, eyelids glued together with crusting along the eyelid margin, foreign body sensation, burning, tearing, madarosis, trichiasis, blurred vision, photophobia, conjunctival injection, and recurrent hordeolum (Amescua et al., 2019; Auran & Casper, 2019; Bagheri & Wajda, 2017; Kaur et al., 2019; Tarff et al., 2017). Individuals may describe worsening symptoms upon awakening or even with reading (Auran & Casper, 2019). Those with posterior blepharitis or MGD may also present with inspissated meibomian glands or expression of turbid, foamy, and even thick cheese-like meibomian discharge at eyelid margins (Amescua et al., 2019; Auran & Casper, 2019; Bagheri & Wajda, 2017).

HISTORY AND PHYSICAL EXAM FINDINGS

Initial evaluation includes comprehensive history taking and eye examination, characteristic bio-microscopic findings, as well as ancillary testing (Amescua et al., 2019; Auran & Casper, 2019; Tarff et al., 2017). History-taking should include age; duration of symptoms; laterality; precipitating factors; co-existent systemic diseases such as rosacea, seborrheic dermatitis, psoriasis, and graft-versus-host disease (GVHD); current or prior topical or systemic medications; and sick contacts (Amescua et al., 2019; Kaur et al., 2019). For instance, risk for seborrheic blepharitis and MGD often increases with age (Amescua et al., 2019). Eye examination includes measurement of visual acuity, external examination, slit lamp bio-microscopy, and measurement of intraocular pressure (IOP) (Amescua et al., 2019). External examination includes visualization of the skin and eyelids (Amescua et al., 2019; Kaur et al., 2019). Slit lamp bio-microscopy includes evaluation of tear film, anterior and posterior eyelid margin, eyelashes, tarsal and bulbar conjunctiva, and the cornea (Amescua et al., 2019; Bagheri & Wajda, 2017).

DIFFERENTIAL DIAGNOSIS AND DIAGNOSTIC CONSIDERATIONS

In patients with chronic blepharitis, especially if unresponsive to conventional treatment, the following differential diagnoses should be considered: aqueous deficient dry eye; demidocosis; viral, (multi-drug resistant) bacterial, and parasitic ocular infection; autoimmune or neoplastic diseases; dermatoses; thyroid eye disease; toxins; and trauma (Amescua et al., 2019; Auran & Casper, 2019). In these circumstances, cultures and eyelid biopsy may help with diagnosis (Amescua et al., 2019; Auran & Casper, 2019). Blepharitis can be differentiated from aqueous tear deficiency as symptoms are typically worse in the morning whereas the latter is worse later in the day (Amescua et al., 2019; Auran & Casper, 2019; Bagheri & Wajda, 2017). Demidocosis or *Demodex folluculorum* infestation should be considered in those with chronic blepharitis and rosacea, especially with severe ocular surface pain and collarettes (cylindrical dandruff-like sleeves along the eyelashes and eyelash base) visualized under microscopic evaluation (Amescua et al., 2019; Auran & Casper, 2019; Bagheri & Wajda, 2017). Benign and malignant eyelid tumors (e.g., basal cell or squamous cell carcinoma, melanoma, or sebaceous carcinoma) or ocular mucous membrane pemphigoid (OMMP) should be considered in those with unilateral chronic blepharitis unresponsive to therapy, especially in the setting of marked asymmetry; conjunctival cicatricial changes; madarosis; atypical eyelid-margin inflammation; or new, non-inflamed, and persistent eyelid masses (Amescua et al., 2019; Auran & Casper, 2019). In consultation with an ophthalmologist and pathologist, an eyelid biopsy should be performed as prompt diagnosis can lead to immediate treatment that can prevent disfigurement and other ocular complications (Amescua et al., 2019; Auran & Casper, 2019).

TREATMENT

Management involves scheduled, long-term, daily eyelid hygiene through the use of warm compresses, eyelid cleansers (e.g., hypochlorous acid 0.01%), and eyelid massage (horizontal and vertical; Amescua et al., 2019; Sung et al., 2018). These are particularly helpful in those with MGD as they facilitate expression of meibomian gland secretions, remove eyelash crusting, and mitigate ocular surface inflammation (Amescua et al., 2019; Auran & Casper, 2019; Bagheri & Wajda, 2017; Kaur et al., 2019). Topical and/or systemic antibiotics along with topical anti-inflammatory agents such as corticosteroids or even cyclosporine may be used (Amescua et al., 2019; Auran & Casper, 2019; Bagheri & Wajda, 2017; Tarff et al., 2017). Topical (i.e., ointment or suspension) antimicrobials include bacitracin, erythromycin, azithromycin, and tobramycin/

dexamethasone (Amescua et al., 2019; Bagheri & Wajda, 2017; Kaur et al., 2019). If those with MGD have inadequate symptom relief despite sustained eyelid hygiene, daily oral tetracyclines (e.g., doxycycline, tetracycline) or even macrolides (e.g., azithromycin, erythromycin) may be used (Amescua et al., 2019; Bagheri & Wajda, 2017; Kaur et al., 2019). In combination with 0.1% topical tacrolimus, oral azithromycin can be an alternative to tetracyclines (Amescua et al., 2019; Bagheri & Wajda, 2017).

Adjunct treatment includes use of topical cyclosporine, site-specific corticosteroids, artificial tears, and even omega-3 fatty acids. Because of their ability to decrease eyelid or ocular surface inflammation, a brief course of topical cyclosporine or site-specific corticosteroid eye drops or ointments (e.g., loteprednol etabonate, fluorometholone) may be helpful in providing symptom relief in those with blepharitis (Amescua et al., 2019; Auran & Casper, 2019; Bagheri & Wajda, 2017). To prevent complications such as increased IOP and cataracts, the minimal effective dose of corticosteroids should be used, and long-term therapy should be avoided if possible (Amescua et al., 2019). Nonetheless, patients on corticosteroid therapy should be re-evaluated within a few weeks to determine response, compliance, and measure IOP (Amescua et al., 2019). In those with tear dysfunction or dry eyes, preservative-free artificial tears can be used as an adjunct to eyelid cleansing and medications (Amescua et al., 2019; Bagheri & Wajda, 2017). By altering lipid meibum composition, omega-3 fatty acids have been able to stabilize the tear film and suppress inflammation to prevent blockage of meibomian gland ducts and improve tear stability, and therefore have been implicated in the management of mild-to-moderate MGD (Auran & Casper, 2019; Bagheri & Wajda, 2017). Other treatments include procedures that unclog the inspissated meibomian gland orifices using intense pulsed light (IPL) or mechanical interventions such as meibomian gland probing, vectored thermal pulsation (VTP), and microblepharoexfolation (Amescua et al., 2019; Auran & Casper, 2019; Bagheri & Wajda, 2017).

Consultation and patient follow-up with an ophthalmologist is indicated in those with co-existent ocular disorders; recurrence and/or lack of response to therapy; worsening clinical manifestations such as moderate to severe pain, severe or chronic erythema, orbital involvement, and visual loss; or require corticosteroid taper for symptom relief (Amescua et al., 2019)

KEY TAKEAWAYS

- Blepharitis is a chronic ocular inflammation that can be categorized based on anatomy—anterior (e.g., staphylococcal or seborrheic) and posterior (e.g., MGD).
- Topical or systemic antimicrobials and scheduled long-term daily eyelid hygiene remain the cornerstones in the management of blepharitis.

EVIDENCE-BASED RESOURCE

Amescua, G., Akpek, E. K., Farid, M., Garcia-Ferrer, F. J., Lin, A., Rhee, M. K., Varu, D. M., Musch, D. C., Dunn, S. P., Mah, F. S., & American Academy of Ophthalmology Preferred Practice Pattern Cornea and External Disease Panel. (2019). Blepharitis preferred practice Pattern®. *Ophthalmology, 126*(1), P56–P93. https://doi.org/10.1016/j.ophtha.2018.10.019

2.4: CHALAZION

Al-Zada "Al" Aguilar

Chalazia are one of the most common, chronic lipogranulomatous sterile lesions affecting the eyelids, usually below the lid margin (Auran & Casper, 2019; Aycinena et al., 2016; Fukuoka et al., 2017; Jin et al., 2017; Kaur et al., 2019; Wu et al., 2018). Chalazia often occur as a result of meibomian gland (MGD) or gland of Zeis dysfunction from prior hordeola (stye) or micro-abscesses (Auran & Casper, 2019; Aycinena et al., 2016; Fukuoka et al., 2017; Jin et al., 2017; Kaur et al., 2019; Wu et al., 2018). Risk factors include chronic blepharitis, MGD, seborrheic dermatitis, gastritis, and smoking (Jin et al., 2017). Sequelae of chalazion include conjunctivitis, cellulitis, cosmetic disfigurement, corneal abrasion, and, if large enough, visual disturbances such as hyperopia or corneal pressure-induced astigmatism (Aycinena et al., 2016; Jin et al., 2017; Wu et al., 2018).

PRESENTING SIGNS AND SYMPTOMS

Patients are usually asymptomatic but may present with acute or chronic eyelid lump and eyelid erythema, swelling, or tenderness (Bagheri & Wajda, 2017; Kaur et al., 2019). Associated signs and symptoms related to acne rosacea, blepharitis, and MGD may also be present (Bagheri & Wajda, 2017).

HISTORY AND PHYSICAL EXAM FINDINGS

Initial evaluation should include taking a comprehensive health history and performing an eye examination. History taking involves asking about prior ocular surgery, trauma, co-existent ocular disorders, and the presence of eyelid lesions (Bagheri & Wajda, 2017). Eye examination includes external examination and slit lamp examination. A visible or palpable, well-defined subcutaneous eyelid nodule may be present, but may not be identifiable in some cases (Bagheri & Wajda, 2017). Eyelid eversion may reveal madarosis, white lashes due to loss of melanin (poliosis), and ulceration (Bagheri & Wajda, 2017). Slit lamp examination of the meibomian glands may reveal inspissation (Bagheri & Wajda, 2017).

DIFFERENTIAL DIAGNOSIS AND DIAGNOSTIC CONSIDERATIONS

The following differential diagnoses should be considered when evaluating a patient for possible chalazion: pre-septal cellulitis, pyogenic granuloma, and sebaceous carcinoma (Bagheri & Wajda, 2017). Those with pre-septal cellulitis will present with both eyelid and periorbital erythema and edema, whereas chalazion typically affects the eyelid, below the lid margin (Auran & Casper, 2019; Aycinena et al., 2016; Bagheri & Wajda, 2017; Fukuoka et al., 2017; Jin et al., 2017; Kaur et al., 2019; Wu et al., 2018). In older patients with recurrent chalazia, especially with concomitant chronic unilateral blepharitis, madarosis, or eyelid thickening, an eyelid biopsy should be performed to rule out sebaceous carcinoma (Bagheri & Wajda, 2017). A benign, deep-red, pedunculated lesion, pyogenic granuloma is often associated with trauma, surgery, or chalazion (Bagheri & Wajda, 2017).

TREATMENT

Chalazia may disappear spontaneously in up to 43% of lesions (Aycinena et al., 2016). Therefore, initial management involves daily scheduled eyelid hygiene such as hot compresses, saltwater soaks, and digital massages (Aycinena et al., 2016; Bagheri & Wajda, 2017; Kaur et al., 2019). In those with chalazia lasting less than 2 months, eyelid hygiene has been associated with resolution rates ranging from 25% up to 87% (Aycinena et al., 2016, 10). This approach has such a varied and wide range of success because it is highly dependent on patient education and compliance (Aycinena et al., 2016). Invasive methods such as chalazion excision or incision and curettage (I&C), transcutaneous or transconjunctival intralesional corticosteroid injections, or both, may be considered (Aycinena et al., 2016; Fukuoka et al., 2017; Jin et al., 2017; Wu et al., 2018). Such methods are preferred in older individuals with chronic (>2 months), large chalazia that do not heal despite conservative methods as these likely have developed into suppurative granulomas (Aycinena et al., 2016; Bagheri & Wajda, 2017; Fukuoka et al., 2017; Jin et al., 2017; Kaur et al., 2019; Wu et al., 2018). Patients are not routinely seen after medical intervention unless the lesion persists over 4 weeks (Bagheri & Wajda, 2017). Those who have had an invasive procedure such as an incision and drainage (I&D) are usually re-evaluated in 1 week or as needed (Bagheri & Wajda, 2017).

KEY TAKEAWAYS

- Chalazia are often caused by MGD or gland of Zeis dysfunction and are one of the most common, chronic lipogranulomatous sterile lesions affecting the eyelids.
- If there is no resolution after 4 weeks of scheduled daily eyelid hygiene, intralesional corticosteroid injections or I&D may be implemented to treat chalazion.

EVIDENCE-BASED RESOURCE

Aycinena, A. R., Achiron, A., Paul, M., & Burgansky-Eliash, Z. (2016). Incision and curettage versus steroid injection for the treatment of chalazia: A meta-analysis. *Ophthalmic Plastic and Reconstructive Surgery, 32*(3), 220–224. https://doi.org/10.1097/IOP.0000000000000483

2.5: CONJUNCTIVITIS

Al-Zada "Al" Aguilar

Conjunctivitis is an inflammation of the bulbar (muous membrane covering the globe) and palpebral (mucous membrane covering the inside of the eyelid) conjunctiva (Auran & Casper, 2019; Azari & Arabi, 2020; Frings et al., 2017; Tarff & Behrens, 2017; Tarff et al., 2017; Varu et al., 2019; Yeu & Hauswirth, 2020). Conjunctivitis is classified based on etiology, chronicity, surrounding tissue involvement, and severity (Azari & Arabi, 2020).

Types include infectious and noninfectious (Azari & Arabi, 2020; Varu et al., 2019). The most common infectious cause is viral, accounting for 80% of cases, followed by bacterial (Azari & Arabi, 2020; Varu et al., 2019; Yeu & Hauswirth, 2020). Noninfectious forms include allergic forms, affecting 40% of the U.S. population, as well as less common forms such as mechanical/irritative/toxic, immune-mediated, and neoplastic (Azari & Arabi, 2020; Varu et al., 2019; Yeu & Hauswirth, 2020). In terms of chronicity, conjunctivitis is divided into acute (<4 weeks) and chronic (>4 weeks; Azari & Arabi, 2020; Tarff & Behrens, 2017). If acute, conjunctivitis is most likely to be infectious, allergic, or related to a systemic reaction such as Stevens-Johnson syndrome (SJS) or toxic epidermal necrolysis (TEN; Azari & Arabi, 2020). If chronic and/or recurrent, it is typically noninfectious and is usually associated with allergies, toxins, or systemic diseases (Azari & Arabi, 2020; Kaur et al., 2019; Tarff & Behrens, 2017; Yeu & Hauswirth, 2020). If the cornea or eyelid margins are affected, then it is kerato-conjunctivitis and blepharo-conjunctivitis, respectively (Azari & Arabi, 2020). Severity is determined by signs and symptoms such as pain, visual deficits, and presence of drainage (Azari & Arabi, 2020).

Viral Conjunctivitis

Types of viral conjunctivitis include adenovirus, herpes simplex virus (HSV), and varicella (herpes) zoster virus (VZV; Azari & Arabi, 2020; Kaur et al., 2019; Tarff & Behrens, 2017; Yeu & Hauswirth, 2020). Human adenoviruses (HAdV) account for up to 90% while the remainder are caused by HSV (5%), VZV, and *Molluscum contagiosum* (Azari & Arabi, 2020; Kaur et al., 2019; Tarff & Behrens, 2017; Yeu & Hauswirth, 2020). HAdV, specifically the HAdV-D species, is highly contagious, especially in the presence of concurrent upper respiratory infection with transmission risk up to 50% via direct or indirect contact through shared items (Auran & Casper, 2019; Azari & Arabi, 2020; Kaur et al., 2019; Varu et al., 2019; Yeu & Hauswirth, 2020). It is particularly contagious for 10 to 12 days from onset as long as there is conjunctival erythema and/or active discharge (Bagheri & Wajda, 2017; Tarff & Behrens, 2017). It is self-limiting, improving within 14 days, although longer with corneal involvement (Auran & Casper, 2019; Azari & Arabi, 2020; Bagheri & Wajda, 2017; Kaur et al., 2019; Varu et al., 2019; Yeu & Hauswirth, 2020). Severe cases can progress to pharyngo-conjunctivitis and epidemic kerato-conjunctivitis (EKC; Azari & Arabi, 2020; Bagheri & Wajda, 2017; Tarff & Behrens, 2017; Yeu & Hauswirth, 2020). Predisposing factors for HSV conjunctivitis include exposure to an infected person or prior HSV infection (Varu et al., 2019; Yeu & Hauswirth, 2020). Reactivation may be triggered by stress such as trauma, ultraviolet (UV) exposure, and other viral illnesses (Auran & Casper, 2019; Varu et al., 2019; Yeu & Hauswirth, 2020). Unless complications occur (e.g., EKC), HSV conjunctivitis is typically self-limiting and resolves within 7 days (Varu et al., 2019; Yeu & Hauswirth, 2020). Predisposing factors for VZV conjunctivitis include active chicken pox or exposure to an individual with active chicken pox or recurrent VZV (Varu et al., 2019; Yeu & Hauswirth, 2020). Potential complications include increased intraocular pressure (IOP) associated with uveitis, corneal scarring or vascularization, keratitis, and ectropion (Varu et al., 2019; Yeu & Hauswirth, 2020).

Bacterial Conjunctivitis

If mild, bacterial conjunctivitis is typically nongonococcal and often self-limiting, lasting up to 10 days without treatment (Varu et al., 2019; Yeu & Hauswirth, 2020). However, severe infections may persist for greater than 4 weeks if left untreated (Varu et al., 2019; Yeu & Hauswirth, 2020). If *Haemophilus influenza* is the causative organism (especially in children), this may also be associated with meningitis, pharyngitis, or otitis media (Azari & Arabi, 2020; Bagheri & Wajda, 2017; Varu et al., 2019). *Chlamydia trachomatis* may cause a variety of ocular surface infections such as trachoma and inclusion conjunctivitis (Azari & Arabi, 2020). Usually caused by *C. trachomatis* serotypes D-K, inclusion conjunctivitis typically presents with unilateral eye involvement and concurrent genital infection (e.g., cervicitis, vaginitis, urethritis) in at least 50% of those infected (Azari & Arabi, 2020; Bagheri & Wajda, 2017). Usually occurring due to *C. trachomatis* serotypes A-C in developing countries in crowded areas with poor sanitation, trachoma may cause mucopurulent drainage, but at later stages, may cause conjunctival, corneal, and eyelid scarring, potentially leading to vision loss (Azari & Arabi, 2020; Bagheri & Wajda, 2017). Also known as hyperacute bacterial conjunctivitis for its rapid onset and progression (within 24 hours), gonococcal conjunctivitis is often caused by *Neisseria gonorrhoaea* (Azari & Arabi, 2020; Bagheri & Wajda, 2017; Kaur et al., 2019; Tarff & Behrens, 2017; Varu et al., 2019; Yeu & Hauswirth, 2020).

Allergic Conjunctivitis

Allergic conjunctivitis is usually triggered by environmental allergens, seasonal recurrences (e.g., spring/summer), outdoor air pollution, or animal dander and existing hypersensitivity conditions (e.g., asthma, atopy, dermatitis) without seasonal correlation (Auran & Casper, 2019; Azari & Arabi, 2020; Bagheri & Wajda, 2017; Frings et al., 2017; Kaur et al., 2019; Tarff & Behrens, 2017; Varu et al., 2019; Yeu & Hauswirth, 2020).

Mechanical/Irritative Conjunctivitis

Examples of mechanical or irritative conjunctivitis include contact-lens–related kerato-conjunctivitis, giant papillary conjunctivitis (GPC), contact dermato-conjunctivitis, and toxic conjunctivitis (Azari & Arabi, 2020; Varu et al., 2019). Contact-lens–related and GPC are characterized by worsening intolerance of contact lenses, conjunctival injection, and corneal neovascularization (Auran & Casper, 2019; Varu et al., 2019). Those who wear contact lenses, especially reusable soft contact lens, are at risk for developing kerato-conjunctivitis, microbial keratitis, or even GPC (Auran & Casper, 2019; Varu et al., 2019). They can be differentiated from one another based on symptom onset—contact-lens–related kerato-conjunctivitis typically has subacute to acute onset of symptoms whereas GPC has chronic gradual increase in symptoms and signs with contact lens wear (Varu et al., 2019). Contact dermato-conjunctivitis is a type IV delayed hypersensitivity reaction that occurs via antigen and T-cell interaction leading to cytokine release. It is typically triggered by poison ivy, poison oak, and latex. It may cause itching, follicular inflammation, lid swelling, keratitis, and even cicatrization at later stages (Azari & Arabi, 2020). Long-term use of topical eye medications, specifically those with preservative benzalkonium chloride, may cause toxic conjunctivitis resulting in symptoms such as conjunctival inflammation, congestion, GPC, and dry eyes to subconjunctival fibrosis and scarring, and even pseudo-pemphigoid in those with underlying glaucoma (Azari & Arabi, 2020).

Immune-Mediated Secondary Conjunctivitis

Immune-mediated triggers of secondary conjunctivitis include graft-versus-host disease (GVHD), thyroid eye disease, Stevens-Johnson syndrome (SJS)/toxic epidermal necrolysis (TEN), and vasculitis (Azari & Arabi, 2020; Varu et al., 2019). Given it is systemic, GVHD can be present in other organ systems such as the skin, GI tract, and lungs (Varu et al., 2019). Although rare, patients who have undergone allogeneic stem cell transplantation are at risk (Azari & Arabi, 2020; Varu et al., 2019). GVHD conjunctivitis may occur acutely 3 months' post-stem cell transplantation; however, it tends to occur much later in the chronic phase (Varu et al., 2019). Nevertheless, its presence portends severe systemic disease and an overall poor prognosis (Azari & Arabi, 2020). Another form of secondary conjunctivitis occurs in those with thyroid eye disease from Graves' disease or Hashimoto's thyroiditis (Varu et al., 2019). Another form of immune-mediated conjunctivitis occurs as a result of vasculitides such as sarcoidosis, varying forms of granulomatosis with polyangiitis, Kawasaki disease, as well as drug-induced or infection-induced vasculitis. Given

that it is systemic, vasculitides can be present in other organ systems such as the skin, lymph nodes, kidneys, and lungs (Varu et al., 2019).

PRESENTING SIGNS AND SYMPTOMS

Clinical signs and symptoms that are helpful in the diagnosis of infectious conjunctivitis include ocular discharge, conjunctival injection, presence of red eye(s), eyelashes stuck together in the morning, eyelid or conjunctival edema, and history of sick contacts with conjunctivitis (Azari & Arabi, 2020; Bagheri & Wajda, 2017; Kaur et al., 2019; Tarff & Behrens, 2017). Signs and symptoms may be exacerbated by other ocular disorders such as dry eye or blepharitis (Varu et al., 2019).

Viral Conjunctivitis

Viral conjunctivitis initially presents unilaterally and progresses bilaterally with the following symptoms: tearing, itching, burning, foreign body sensation, and ocular discharge (Auran & Casper, 2019; Bagheri & Wajda, 2017; Frings et al., 2017).

Bacterial Conjunctivitis

Accounting for approximately 30% of acute infectious conjunctivitis, patients with acute bacterial conjunctivitis present with rapid onset of unilateral or bilateral conjunctival hyperemia along with either mucopurulent discharge or sticky eyelids upon awakening and chemosis (Auran & Casper, 2019; Azari & Arabi, 2020; Bagheri & Wajda, 2017; Frings et al., 2017; Kaur et al., 2019; Varu et al., 2019; Yeu & Hauswirth, 2020). There is typically no adenopathy or follicle formation, but there may be papillae or tiny, clear, bleb-like nodules (Auran & Casper, 2019).

Allergic Conjunctivitis

Most cases of allergic conjunctivitis present with bilateral ocular symptoms such as the hallmark symptom of ocular pruritus as well as hyperemia, dryness, watery or mucoid discharge, conjunctival edema (chemosis), injection, periocular hyperpigmentation, rhinorrhea, and, less commonly, foreign body sensation (Auran & Casper, 2019; Azari & Arabi, 2020; Bagheri & Wajda, 2017; Frings et al., 2017; Kaur et al., 2019; Tarff & Behrens, 2017; Varu et al., 2019; Yeu & Hauswirth, 2020). The degree of chemosis is often disproportionate to conjunctival redness (Azari & Arabi, 2020; Tarff & Behrens, 2017). Moreover, some patients may have well-delineated, sterile gray-white infiltrate with overlying epithelial defect or a "shield ulcer" (Bagheri & Wajda, 2017).

Mechanical/Irritative Conjunctivitis

Those with rosacea may also present with ocular manifestation in the form of conjunctivitis (Azari & Arabi, 2020). Clinical findings include papillary and follicular conjunctival reaction, interpalpebral conjunctival redness, conjunctival granuloma, phlyctenule, pinguecula, and in some cases cicatrization, entropion, and trichiasis leading to conjunctival scarring (Azari & Arabi, 2020).

Immune-Mediated Secondary Conjunctivitis

In the acute phase of GVHD, conjunctivitis is often ulcerative, presenting with purulent drainage, conjunctival hemorrhage, pseudo-membrane formation, and scarring (Azari & Arabi, 2020). In the chronic form of GVHD, up to three quarters of patients suffer from dry eyes, with its severity correlating with the severity of GVHD (Azari & Arabi, 2020). Thyroid-eye-disease–related conjunctivitis typically occurs spontaneously or within 18 months of diagnosis along with bilateral, and, less commonly, asymmetric ocular signs (Varu et al., 2019). These include periorbital and conjunctival edema and erythema, exposure keratopathy, upper eyelid retraction, and eyeball protrusion (proptosis; Varu et al., 2019). Ocular clinical findings are typically unilateral or bilateral in vasculitides-associated conjunctivitis and include conjunctival nodules or granuloma, proptosis, scleritis, keratitis, corneal ulcers, iris or trabecular meshwork nodules, uveitis, and even optic disc swelling (Varu et al., 2019). Associated self-limiting clinical signs include conjunctival redness with purulent drainage, which usually lasts between 1 and 4 weeks (Azari & Arabi, 2020). Occurring in up to 88% of cases, ocular clinical findings of SJS and TEN range from conjunctival redness to near-complete sloughing of palpebral conjunctiva and lid margins (Azari & Arabi, 2020). Long-term sequelae include severe dry eyes, symblepharon formation, and corneal scarring (Azari & Arabi, 2020).

HISTORY AND PHYSICAL EXAM FINDINGS

Initial evaluation should include a comprehensive health history and physical examination. History taking includes asking about sign and symptom description, onset, and duration; precipitating, alleviating, and exacerbating factors; laterality; presence of constitutional signs and symptoms; sick contacts; prior ocular surgery or trauma; co-existent ocular and systemic disorders (e.g., upper respiratory infection, autoimmune or hypersensitivity disorders); immunocompromised states and conditions (e.g., diabetes, HIV, cancer); contact lens use; social and medication history (Azari & Arabi, 2020; Bagheri & Wajda, 2017; Kaur et al., 2019; Tarff & Behrens, 2017; Varu et al., 2019). Physical examination should include the following: measurement of visual acuity, external examination, and slit-lamp bio-microscopy (Azari & Arabi, 2020; Bagheri & Wajda, 2017; Kaur et al., 2019; Varu et al., 2019). External examination includes evaluation of the eyelid, orbits, pupils, conjunctiva, cornea, and skin for abnormalities as well as the presence of ocular discharge or regional lymphadenopathy (e.g., preauricular or submandibular). Slit-lamp bio-microscopy includes evaluation of the cornea, eyelid margins, eyelashes, lacrimal puncta, and canaliculi; tarsal, forniceal, and bulbar conjunctiva; and the anterior chamber or iris (Azari & Arabi, 2020; Varu

et al., 2019) and provides a more detailed visualization of the conjunctival epithelium, allowing for differentiation between infectious and noninfectious forms of conjunctivitis. Moreover, the addition of fluorescein staining can be useful to highlight the corneal and anterior chambers to evaluate for inflammation or injury (Yeu & Hauswirth, 2020). See Table 2.1 for a summary of signs, symptoms, and physical findings in conjunctivitis.

DIFFERENTIAL DIAGNOSIS AND DIAGNOSTIC CONSIDERATIONS

For patients presenting with severe pain, anisocoria, painful pupillary reaction, and/or orbital signs, diagnoses such as uveitis, keratitis, glaucoma, scleritis, and ocular trauma from foreign bodies should be considered as potential alternatives (Auran & Casper, 2019; Azari & Arabi, 2020; Yeu & Hauswirth, 2020). Blurred vision and photophobia suggest corneal involvement (Auran & Casper, 2019; Bagheri & Wajda, 2017; Frings et al., 2017). Dry eye disease may mimic acute infectious conjunctivitis through signs and symptoms such as grittiness, hyperemia, and stinging (Yeu & Hauswirth, 2020).

Bacterial Conjunctivitis

For acute bacterial forms of conjunctivitis, the most common pathogens include *Staphylococcus* species, *Streptococcus* species, *Haemophilus influenzae*, *Moraxella catarrhalis*, and gram-negative (intestinal) bacteria (Azari & Arabi, 2020; Kaur et al., 2019; Yeu & Hauswirth, 2020). As they are rarely helpful in determining treatment course and are not cost-effective, routine bacteriological exams are typically not performed (Varu et al., 2019). However, cultures may be helpful in those who have a high probability of having gonococcal, chlamydial, or resistant staphylococcal infections (e.g., methicillin-resistant *Staphylococcus aureus* [MRSA])i, methicillin-resistant *Staphylococcus epidermidis* [MRSE]),such as the immunocompromised and/or those with moderate/severe, hyperacute and/or bacterial conjunctivitis with copious mucopurulent discharge refractory to conventional treatment (Azari & Arabi, 2020; Bagheri & Wajda, 2017; Kaur et al., 2019; Tarff & Behrens, 2017; Varu et al., 2019; Yeu & Hauswirth, 2020). The most hyperacute form of bacterial conjunctivitis is caused by either *Neisseria gonorrhoeae* or *Chlamydia trachomatis* (Yeu & Hauswirth, 2020). In suspected cases, immunofluorescent antibody test and enzyme-linked immunosorbent assay (ELISA) can be used to confirm suspected cases of chlamydial conjunctivitis, whereas Gram stains and cytology can be used for suspected cases of gonococcal conjunctivitis (Kaur et al., 2019; Varu et al., 2019; Yeu & Hauswirth, 2020).

Viral Conjunctivitis

Viral conjunctivitis should be considered if a patient has an associated upper respiratory infection or known sick contacts (Auran & Casper, 2019; Bagheri & Wajda, 2017; Varu et al., 2019; Yeu & Hauswirth, 2020). Viral diagnostic

TABLE 2.1: Signs, Symptoms, and Physical Findings in Conjunctivitis

| | BACTERIAL | | | VIRAL | | | ALLERGIC |
	NON-GONOCOCCAL	**GONOCOCCAL**	**CHLAMYDIAL**	**ADENOVIRUS**	**HSV**	**VZV**	
Laterality	Unilateral or bilateral	Unilateral or bilateral	Unilateral or bilateral	Unilateral (early) → bilateral (late)	Unilateral	Unilateral (early) → bilateral (late)	Bilateral
Conjunctival findings	Papillary	Papillary; conjunctival injection (marked)	Follicular (lymphoid); conjunctival injection; subepithelial infiltrates	Follicular (lymphoid); pseudomembrane; conjunctival injection; subepithelial infiltrates	Follicular; conjunctival injection; branching lesions with end bulbs; *presence of dendrites*	Follicular (mild); conjunctival injection; branching lesions without end bulbs	*Papillary (cobblestone) with chemosis (edema); conjunctival injection; eosinophilic changes*
Ocular discharge	Scant, mucopurulent	*Copious, hyperpurulent*	Scant, stringy/ mucopurulent *(glued eyelids upon wakening)*	Serous with epiphora (tear overflow)	Serous	Serous	Serous or mucoid
Ocular signs and symptoms	-------	*Blurred vision, pain, photophobia*	-------	-------	-------	-------	*Severe pruritus (hallmark)*
Extra-ocular signs and symptoms (e.g., LN, fever, sore throat, skin lesions)	Fever/sore throat; occasional LN uncommon; no skin lesions	LN uncommon; skin lesions— periorbital, oropharyngeal, genitoperineal	LN uncommon; *skin lesions— periorbital, oropharyngeal, genito-perineal*	*Fever/sore throat common;* LN present; no skin lesions	LN present; *skin lesions— vesicular, periorbital*	No extraocular signs or symptoms	

HSV, herpes simplex virus; LN, lymphadenopathy; VZV, varicella zoster virus.

Source: Data from Auran, J., & Casper, D. S. (2019). Blepharitis and conjunctivitis. In *The Columbia Guide to basic elements of eye care* (pp. 97–104). Springer International Publishing. https://doi.org/10.1007/978-3-030-10886-1_9; Azari, A. A., & Arabi, A. (2020). Conjunctivitis: A systematic review. *Journal of Ophthalmic and Vision Research, 15*(3), 372–395. https://doi.org/10.18502/jovr.v15i3.7456; Bagheri, N., & Wajda, B. N. (2017). *The wills eye manual: Office and emergency room diagnosis and treatment of eye disease* (7th ed). Wolters Kluwer; Frings, A., Geerling, G., & Schargus, M. (2017). Red eye: A guide for non-specialists. *Deutsches Ärzteblatt International, 114*(17), 302–312. https://doi.org/10.3238/arztebl.2017.0302; Kaur, S., Larsen, H., & Nattis, A. (2019). Primary care approach to eye conditions. *Osteopathic Family Physician, 1*(2). https://ofpjournal.com/index.php/ofp/article/view/581; Varu, D. M., Rhee, M. K., Akpek, E. K., Amescua, G., Farid, M., Garcia-Ferrer, F. J., Lin, A., Musch, D. C., Mah, F. S., Dunn, S. P., & American Academy of Ophthalmology Preferred Practice Pattern Cornea and External Disease Panel. (2019). Conjunctivitis preferred practice Pattern®. *Ophthalmology, 126*(1), P94–P169. https://doi.org/10.1016/j.ophtha.2018.10.020; Yeu, E., & Hauswirth, S. (2020). A review of the differential diagnosis of acute infectious conjunctivitis: Implications for treatment and management. *Clinical Ophthalmology, 14*, 805–813. https://doi.org/10.2147/OPTH.S236571

testing is rarely used in practice due to the cost of equipment and training; however, it may be useful in preventing misdiagnosis, disease spread, and unnecessary antibiotic use, while decreasing healthcare costs and loss of productivity (Azari & Arabi, 2020; Varu et al., 2019; Yeu & Hauswirth, 2020).

Allergic Conjunctivitis

Allergy skin testing such as skin prick testing, pollen immunoglobulin E (IgE) detection, and high serum IgE levels have been implicated in confirming the diagnosis and assessing the severity of allergic conjunctivitis (Azari & Arabi, 2020; Varu et al., 2019).

Immune-Mediated Secondary Conjunctivitis

Early, mild manifestations of immune-mediated conjunctivitis are similar in acute infectious conjunctivitis such as redness, tearing, clear discharge, and conjunctival injection. They differ based on time course as immune-mediated tends to be prolonged (Yeu & Hauswirth, 2020). As the gold standard, biopsy of the conjunctiva or extraocular tissue can be used for diagnostic confirmation (Varu et al., 2019). Other helpful tests in the diagnosis of secondary conjunctivitis include CT scan, thyroid function and antibody, liver enzyme and anti-neutrophil cytoplasmic antibodies (ANCA) (Varu et al., 2019).

TREATMENT

Bacterial Conjunctivitis

Acute mild bacterial conjunctivitis is typically self-limiting and resolves within 5 to 10 days in up to 60% of immune-competent adults; therefore, use of antibiotics should be delayed when possible (Azari & Arabi, 2020; Tarff & Behrens, 2017; Varu et al., 2019; Yeu & Hauswirth, 2020). However, it may be reasonable to initiate a 5- to 7-day course of antibiotic drops or ointments to facilitate recovery and therefore reduce transmissibility (Auran & Casper, 2019; Tarff & Behrens, 2017; Varu et al., 2019). Antimicrobial selection should be determined based on patient allergies, culture and sensitivities, resistance patterns, cost, and patient compliance (Azari & Arabi, 2020; Kaur et al., 2019; Tarff & Behrens, 2017; Varu et al., 2019). In those patients with moderate to severe bacterial conjunctivitis, ophthalmic and, in some cases, systemic antimicrobial therapy should be initiated (Azari & Arabi, 2020; Bagheri & Wajda, 2017; Varu et al., 2019). Moreover, concern for resistant strains (e.g., MRSA, MRSE), refractory, and/or chronic forms of bacterial conjunctivitis all require consultation with an ophthalmologist and infectious disease specialist (Azari & Arabi, 2020; Bagheri & Wajda, 2017; Kaur et al., 2019). Given the rapid onset and progression of hyperacute bacterial conjunctivitis, which is often caused by *N. gonorrhoeae*, immediate treatment is warranted to prevent corneal involvement and potential perforation (Azari & Arabi, 2020; Bagheri &

Wajda, 2017; Yeu & Hauswirth, 2020). Expert consultation (i.e., ophthalmologist, infectious disease specialist) should be obtained in all cases of gonococcal conjunctivitis (Bagheri & Wajda, 2017). Daily then every 2 to 3 day follow-up is recommended until the condition resolves (Azari & Arabi, 2020; Bagheri & Wajda, 2017; Kaur et al., 2019). Severe gonococcal conjunctivitis, lack of improvement in 3 to 4 days, and/or corneal involvement warrants hospitalization for closer monitoring, initiation of IV ceftriaxone (1–2 g/day), and expert consultation (Azari & Arabi, 2020; Bagheri & Wajda, 2017; Kaur et al., 2019; Varu et al., 2019). The mainstay of treatment for chlamydial conjunctivitis is systemic antibiotics; however, the addition of topical antibiotics facilitates resolution (Azari & Arabi, 2020; Bagheri & Wajda, 2017; Kaur et al., 2019; Varu et al., 2019; Yeu & Hauswirth, 2020). If severe, a 2 to 3-day follow-up is recommended; otherwise, a 2 to 3-week follow-up is sufficient in patients with inclusion chlamydial or trachoma conjunctivitis (Bagheri & Wajda, 2017). Sexual contacts of those with confirmed gonococcal and/or chlamydial infections should also be informed, evaluated, appropriately referred, and, if warranted, treated (Azari & Arabi, 2020; Bagheri & Wajda, 2017; Kaur et al., 2019; Varu et al., 2019). See Table 2.2 for details on the management of bacterial conjunctivitis.

Viral Conjunctivitis

Adenoviral Conjunctivitis

Given that viral conjunctivitis is highly contagious, preventive infection control measures such as hand hygiene and avoiding close contact with those with active infection are emphasized to prevent further spread of disease (Auran & Casper, 2019; Azari & Arabi, 2020; Bagheri & Wajda, 2017; Frings et al., 2017; Kaur et al., 2019; Varu et al., 2019; Yeu & Hauswirth, 2020). Antibiotics are not indicated and topical and/or oral antiviral medications do not appear to be useful (Azari & Arabi, 2020; Tarff & Behrens, 2017; Varu et al., 2019; Yeu & Hauswirth, 2020). Cold compresses, chilled artificial tears, oral analgesics, and topical antihistamines (e.g., epinasatine 0.05% 2 times per day) are useful in mitigating symptoms (Auran & Casper, 2019; Azari & Arabi, 2020; Bagheri & Wajda, 2017; Kaur et al., 2019; Tarff & Behrens, 2017; Varu et al., 2019; Yeu & Hauswirth, 2020). If mild, patients can be observed while implementing supportive measures; if severe with visual changes, photophobia, and/or presence of pseudo- and/or true membranes, topical steroids or steroid-sparing preservative-free agents (e.g., cyclosporine or tacrolimus eye drops) may help reduce symptoms and scarring (Auran & Casper, 2019; Azari & Arabi, 2020; Bagheri & Wajda, 2017; Varu et al., 2019; Yeu & Hauswirth, 2020). Topical corticosteroids should be used judiciously; short-term use can prolong viral shedding while long-term use may increase IOP and risk for cataract and glaucoma (Auran & Casper, 2019;

TABLE 2.2: Management of Bacterial Conjunctivitis

	MILD	MODERATE/SEVERE	GONOCOCCAL	CHLAMYDIAL
Antimicrobial management	**Standard:** Trimethoprim/polymyxin B or fluoroquinolone QID **If Haemophilus:** Amoxicillin/clavulanate (20–40 mg/kg/day TID)	**Potential microbes:** Staphylococcus (MRSA/MRSE), Streptococcus, Haemophilus **Standard:** Vancomycin-fortified or besofloxacin	**Standard:** Ceftriaxone IM (250–1000 mg × 1 dose) *plus* zithromax PO (1 g × 1 dose) *or* doxycycline (100 mg BID × 7 days) **If cephalosporin allergy:** Zithromax PO (2 g × 1 dose) *plus* gemifloxacin PO (320 mg × 1 dose) *or* zithromax PO (2 g × 1 dose) *plus* gentamicin IM (240 mg × 1 dose) **If corneal involvement and/or contact lens:** Fluoroquinolone ointment QID or drop q1–2h (e.g., besofloxacin, ciprofloxacin, gatifloxacin, levofloxacin, moxifloxacin) **If severe:** Ceftriaxone IV (1–2 g)	**For inclusion conjunctivitis (standard):** Zithromax PO (1 g × 1 dose), doxycycline (100 mg BID × 7–14 days), *or* erythromycin (500 mg QID × 6 days) **If severe:** 6 wees doxycycline **Consider adding:** 2–3 week topical erythromycin *or* tetracycline TID **For trachoma (standard):** Zithromax PO (20 mg/kg) *plus* 2–3 week doxycycline (100 mg PO BID) *or* Erythromycin *plus* 3–6-week tetracycline *or* erythromycin ointment (BID-QID)
Adjunct	Warm compress	Warm compress	Saline lavage	-------
Referral	Optional	Ophthalmologist (recommended)	Ophthalmologist, infectious disease (recommended) **If severe:** *Hospitalize* Evaluate +/− treat sexual contacts	Ophthalmologist, infectious disease (recommended) Evaluate +/− treat sexual contacts

BID, 2 times per day; TID, 3 times perday; QID, 4 times day; MRSA, methicillin resistant *Staphylococcus aureus*; MRSE, methicillin resistant *Staphylococcus epidermidis*.

TABLE 2.3: Management of Viral Conjunctivitis

	VIRAL		
	ADENOVIRAL	**HSV**	**VZV**
Treatment / symptom management	**If mild/moderate:** • Cold compress • Chilled artificial tears (4–8 times day) • PO analgesics • Topical antihistamines (e.g., epinasatine 0.05% BID) **If severe (visual changes and/or photophobia +/− pseudo- and/or true membranes):** Add topical steroids (loteprednol 0.2%–0.5% BID or prednisolone acetate 0.5% QID) or steroid-sparing, preservative-free drops (cyclosporine [CsA] 1–2% or tacrolimus) or povidone-iodine 0.4% +/− dexamethasone 0.1% ****Infection control measures****	**Topical antivirals:** Ganciclovir 0.05%–0.15% (3–5 times per day), trifluridine 1% solution (5–8 times per day) and/or **PO antivirals:** Acyclovir (200–400 mg 5 times per /day), valacyclovir (500 mg BID-TID), or famciclovir (250 mg BID) • Can use warm compress ****Corticosteroids are contraindicated****	**PO antivirals:** Acyclovir (800 mg 5 times per day for 7 days), valacyclovir (1000 mg q8h for 7 days), or famciclovir (500 mg TID for 7 days) Add lubricating eye drops ****Consider long-term prophylaxis and VZV vaccine if immunocompromised and/or with chronic disease****
Referral	Ophthalmologist (recommended) ****Especially if severe, corneal ulcer or infiltrates or membranous conjunctivitis, on corticosteroids, worsening vision**	Ophthalmologist (recommended)	Ophthalmologist (recommended)

Azari & Arabi, 2020; Varu et al., 2019; Yeu & Hauswirth, 2020). Ophthalmology referral and follow-up should occur in 1 week in individuals with severe disease, with corneal subepithelial ulceration/infiltrates or membranous conjunctivitis, on corticosteroids, or have symptoms such as worsening pain and/or vision (Azari & Arabi, 2020; Bagheri & Wajda, 2017).

Herpes Simplex Virus Conjunctivitis

Unless complications occur, HSV conjunctivitis is typically self-limiting and subsides within 7 days (Varu et al., 2019; Yeu & Hauswirth, 2020). To reduce duration of illness, viral shedding, and the development of keratitis (especially in those with suspected corneal involvement), topical antivirals can be administered (Auran & Casper, 2019; Azari & Arabi, 2020; Bagheri & Wajda, 2017; Tarff & Behrens, 2017; Varu et al., 2019; Yeu & Hauswirth, 2020). Topical corticosteroids are contraindicated because they will worsen not only HSV, but also corneal or conjunctival diseases (Bagheri & Wajda, 2017; Varu et al., 2019; Yeu & Hauswirth, 2020). Warm compresses can also be applied for relief (Bagheri & Wajda, 2017).

Varicella Zoster Virus Conjunctivitis

Just like HSV, VZV conjunctivitis typically lasts for only a few days (Yeu & Hauswirth, 2020). Because topical antivirals alone are not typically effective in treating VZV conjunctivitis, oral antivirals and lubricating drops can

be added (Auran & Casper, 2019; Varu et al., 2019; Yeu & Hauswirth, 2020). Used with caution, the addition of topical corticosteroids can be considered if the preceding regimen is ineffective (Auran & Casper, 2019; Tarff & Behrens, 2017; Yeu & Hauswirth, 2020). Those who are immunocompromised, have chronic disease, or other sequelae may require prolonged and more aggressive treatment or possibly long-term prophylaxis (Varu et al., 2019). The Centers for Disease Control and Prevention recommends administration of VZV vaccine (i.e., zoster vaccine live [ZVL] or recombinant zoster vaccine [RZV]) in patients 50 years or older to reduce incidence of VZV and associated sequelae such as conjunctivitis (Varu et al., 2019). See Table 2.3 for details on the management of viral conjunctivitis.

Allergic Conjunctivitis

Management of allergic conjunctivitis includes protection or avoidance of allergens,; limiting eye rubbing, artificial tears and cold compresses, topical or oral antihistamines, mast cell inhibitors, and even topical cyclosporine (0.05%) if recurrent or persistent (Auran & Casper, 2019; Azari & Arabi, 2020; Bagheri & Wajda, 2017; Frings et al., 2017; Kaur et al., 2019; Tarff & Behrens, 2017; Varu et al., 2019; Yeu & Hauswirth, 2020). For mild cases, artificial tears (4–8 times per day) are helpful as they dilute and even flush the ocular surface clean of allergens and inflammatory mediators while providing a barrier (Azari & Arabi, 2020; Bagheri & Wajda, 2017; Tarff & Behrens, 2017). For moderate cases, antihistamines and/or mast cell stabilizer drops are helpful as they can stabilize mast cell membranes, provide histamine receptor antagonist effects, and modify the action of eosinophils (Azari & Arabi, 2020; Bagheri & Wajda, 2017; Frings et al., 2017; Kaur et al., 2019; Tarff & Behrens, 2017). For cases in which symptoms are severe and refractory and in which corneal involvement and HSV infection have been ruled out, adding a 1- to 2-week course of mild topical corticosteroids or even cyclosporine may be helpful (Auran & Casper, 2019; Azari & Arabi, 2020; Bagheri & Wajda, 2017; Frings et al., 2017; Varu et al., 2019; Yeu & Hauswirth, 2020). Regardless, corticosteroids should be used with caution given the tendency to increase IOP, and risk for cataracts and glaucoma (Tarff & Behrens, 2017). NSAIDs such as diclofenac and ketorolac (0.5% 4 times per day) may help reduce inflammation but should be used cautiously given increased risk of corneal toxicity with chronic use (Azari & Arabi, 2020; Bagheri & Wajda, 2017).

The presence of a shield ulcer would warrant monitoring every 1 to 3 days along with immediate referral to ophthalmologist for scraping to prevent re-epithelization (Bagheri & Wajda, 2017). In general, those difficult-to-control despite topical medications and oral antihistamines should be referred to an ophthalmologist and/or allergist (Varu et al., 2019). Otherwise, follow-up should occur in 2 weeks, especially in those on topical steroids for tapering and side-effect monitoring (e.g., increased IOP; Bagheri & Wajda, 2017).

Mechanical/Irritative Conjunctivitis

Limiting toxin and/or chemical exposure with use of protective eye gear, and if possible, discontinuing the offending agents will facilitate resolution (Azari & Arabi, 2020; Tarff & Behrens, 2017; Varu et al., 2019). However, if there is persistent conjunctivitis despite the preceding measures, a brief course of preservative-free topical steroids may be indicated (Varu et al., 2019). In those with contact lens-induced or chronic GPC, switching to 1-day single use contact lenses or contact lens abstinence is recommended. If severe enough, treatment can also include topical antihistamines, mast cell stabilizers, and in certain cases, a 1- to 2-week course of topical steroids with topical cyclosporine 0.05% (Auran & Casper, 2019; Varu et al., 2019). Associated abnormalities such as aqueous tear deficiency and MGD should also be addressed. At follow-up evaluation, contact lens care regimen, fit, and type should be reviewed while considering alternatives to contact lenses such as eyeglasses or refractive surgery to allow for recovery (Varu et al., 2019).

Immune-Mediated Secondary Conjunctivitis

Treatment of any form of immune-mediated secondary conjunctivitis often involves addressing the underlying systemic disorder (Table 2.4). Therefore, treatment of GVHD in allogeneic stem cell transplant patients, superior limbic kerato-conjunctivitis (SLK) in those with thyroid disorders, or those with vasculitis will usually address the conjunctival inflammation. Referral to an appropriate medical specialist should be considered in those with conjunctivitis appearing as a manifestation of systemic disease (Varu et al., 2019).

KEY TAKEAWAYS

- Conjunctivitis can be classified based on etiology, chronicity, severity, and extraocular manifestations.
- Clinical findings such as severe pain, anisocoria, painful pupillary reaction, and/or orbital signs should prompt the AGACNP to look for non conjunctival ocular diseases (e.g., keratitis).
- Cultures should be obtained in the immunocompromised and/or those with moderate/severe, hyperacute and/or bacterial conjunctivitis with copious purulent discharge refractory to conventional management.
- Symptom control, minimizing ocular damage, restoring or maintaining normal visual function, and, if applicable, detection and treatment of the underlying systemic disease are cornerstones for the management of any form of conjunctivitis (Azari & Arabi, 2020; Varu et al., 2019).
- Antimicrobial selection should be determined based on patient allergies, culture and sensitivities, resistance patterns, cost, and patient compliance (Azari & Arabi, 2020; Bagheri & Wajda, 2017; Tarff & Behrens, 2017; Varu et al., 2019).
- Given the high risk for severe keratitis and corneal perforation, patients with gonococcal (e.g., hyperacute bacterial) conjunctivitis should be monitored closely, treated aggressively, and referred to an ophthalmologist.
- Adenoviral conjunctivitis is highly contagious; therefore, strict isolation and hand hygiene measures should be implemented to limit disease transmission.
- Allergic conjunctivitis is usually caused by seasonal allergies and can be easily treated with antihistamines and mast cell stabilizers (Azari & Arabi, 2020).
- Topical corticosteroids should not be used in HSV conjunctivitis. If HSV is ruled out, it should be used cautiously as it can prolong the infectious period, increase IOP acutely, and increase risk for

TABLE 2.4: Management of Noninfectious Conjunctivitis

	ALLERGIC	MECHANICAL/ IRRITATIVE	IMMUNE-MEDIATED/ SECONDARY (E.G., GVHD, THYROID DISORDER, VASCULITIDES)
Treatment / symptom management	**If mild**: Limit allergens and eye rubbing, add artificial tears (4–8 time per day) and cold compress **If moderate**: Add topical antihistamines Daily dosing: Olopatadine (0.2% or 0.7%) and alcaftadine (0.25%) BID dosing: Bepotastine (1.5%), nedocromil sodium (2%), epinastine (0.05%), ketotifen OTC (0.025%), olopatadine (0.1%) QID dosing: Iodoxamide (0.1%), pemirolast (0.1%) *and/or* PO antihistamines: Loratadine (10 mg daily) *or* fexofenadine > diphenhydramine (25 mg TID-QID) *plus* Mast cell inhibitors (initiate weeks prior to antigen exposure) **If recurrent/persistent**: Can add topical cyclosporine (0.05–2% BID-QID) **If severe and/or refractory**: Add topical corticosteroids (loteprednol (0.2%) or fluorometholone (0.1%) QID) ****contraindicated in HSV conjunctivitis and/or if corneal involvement**** • **For analgesia**: Can add topical NSAIDs (diclofenac, ketorolac 0.5% QID)	**Nonpharmacological:** • Limit toxic/chemical exposure • Discontinue offending agents (e.g., contact lens, eye drops) • Use protective eye gear **If mild/moderate**: Can use topical antihistamines, mast cell stabilizers **If severe/refractory**: Add topical corticosteroids (1–2 weeks) +/− topical CsA	****Treat underlying systemic disorder**** **GVHD**: Ocular lubrication; topical cyclosporine and steroids **Vasculitides**: topical and/or peri-ocular corticosteroids; (consider systemic therapy if bilateral ocular involvement and/or advanced vision loss)
Referral	Ophthalmologist and/or allergist (recommended) ***Especially if difficult-to-control or in the presence of a "shield ulcer"*	• Ophthalmologist (recommended)	• Ophthalmologist and medical specialist (recommended)

GVHD, graft=versus-host disease; NSAIDs, non-steroidal anti-inflammatory drugs.

cataracts or glaucoma if used chronically (Auran & Casper, 2019; Azari & Arabi, 2020; Bagheri & Wajda, 2017; Tarff & Behrens, 2017; Varu et al., 2019).

■ In those with chronic conjunctivitis, the possibility of systemic disease involvement should be investigated (Azari & Arabi, 2020).

EVIDENCE-BASED RESOURCES

Azari, A. A., & Arabi, A. (2020). Conjunctivitis: A systematic review. *Journal of Ophthalmic and Vision Research, 15*(3), 372–395. https://doi.org/10.18502/jovr.v15i3.7456

Varu, D. M., Rhee, M. K., Akpek, E. K., Amescua, G., Farid, M., Garcia-Ferrer, F. J., Lin, A., Musch, D. C., Mah, F. S., Dunn, S. P., & American Academy of Ophthalmology Preferred Practice Pattern Cornea and External Disease Panel. (2019). Conjunctivitis preferred practice Pattern®. *Ophthalmology, 126*(1), P94–P169. https://doi.org/10.1016/j.ophtha.2018.10.020

2.6: CORNEAL ABRASION

Al-Zada "Al" Aguilar

A corneal abrasion results from shearing forces causing micro-trauma and superficial scratches of the corneal epithelium (Fay & Suh, 2019; Kaye et al., 2019; Tarff & Behrens, 2017; Wakai et al., 2017). They most commonly occur due to direct minor mechanical trauma from foreign bodies (e.g., fingernail, vegetable matter), corneal drying, contact lens use, and occupational and/or environmental hazards (Fay & Suh, 2019; Fusco et al., 2019; Kaye et al., 2019; Tarff & Behrens, 2017). Corneal abrasions can occur as long as normal protective eye mechanisms such as complete lid closure, autonomic reflexes (e.g., Bell's phenomenon), corneal blink reflex, reflex tearing, and tear production are compromised or have been removed (Fay & Suh, 2019; Kaye et al., 2019; Malafa et al., 2016; Small et al., 2019). Therefore, they can occur in the hospital in the perioperative and critical care settings.

PRESENTING SIGNS AND SYMPTOMS

Signs and symptoms include acute pain, worsening with extraocular muscle movement; photophobia; foreign body sensation; excessive lacrimation; blepharospasm; blurred vision; and headache (Bagheri & Wajda, 2017; Fay & Suh, 2019; Fusco et al., 2019; Kaur et al., 2019; Kaye et al., 2019; Malafa et al., 2016; Thiel et al., 2017; Wakai et al., 2017). Size of the corneal abrasion affects the patient's clinical presentation; smaller abrasions may present with the preceding findings, whereas larger abrasions may result in corneal erosion or scarring that will lead to bacterial keratitis or even blindness if not addressed (Kaye et al., 2019; Small et al., 2019; Thiel et al., 2017; Wakai et al., 2017).

HISTORY AND PHYSICAL FINDINGS

Obtaining a detailed but focused history and physical that is suggestive of a recent, unilateral, and mechanical ocular trauma will help direct the AGACNP to a diagnosis of corneal abrasion (Fay & Suh, 2019; Fusco et al., 2019; Tarff & Behrens, 2017; Wakai et al., 2017). In general, advanced age, co-existent ocular disorders (e.g., dry eye, proptosis, exophthalmos), and prior or recent history of ocular surface injury (e.g., prior corneal trauma) contribute to an increased risk for corneal abrasions (Kaye et al., 2019; Malafa et al., 2016; Papp et al., 2019; Small et al., 2019). However, corneal abrasions that occur in the perioperative and critical care settings are usually the sequelae of other factors that compromise existing eye protective mechanisms. Perioperative risk factors include prolonged surgery (>60–90 mins) and positioning (Kaye et al., 2019; Malafa et al., 2016; Papp et al., 2019; Small et al., 2019). Prolonged surgery results in prolonged general anesthesia, which predisposes patients to incomplete eyelid closure (lagophthalmos) while suppressing protective eye mechanisms (Kaye et al., 2019; Malafa et al., 2016; Papp et al., 2019). Moreover, patient positioning such as proning, recumbency, and Trendelenburg result in choroidal blood vessel compression, diminished venous outflow, and increased intraocular pressure (IOP) which then decreases ocular perfusion pressure and oxygenation. Moreover, the dependent eye is exposed, which then leads to an increased risk for ischemia, edema, and surface fragility, therefore, predisposing these patients to corneal abrasions (Kaye et al., 2019; Malafa et al., 2016; Papp et al., 2019; Small et al., 2019). In critical care, lagophthalmos occurs and protective eye mechanisms are diminished due to neurological injury such as a stroke, periorbital edema due to facial trauma, or iatrogenic disease due to sedatives and/or paralytics (Small et al., 2019). Diminished protective eye mechanisms then lead to exposure keratopathy and corneal abrasion, which may then be worsened with drying effects of oxygen masks or mechanical ventilation (Kaye et al., 2019; Malafa et al., 2016; Small et al., 2019).

Physical examination should include measurement of visual acuity; pupil and extraocular muscle examination; and slit-lamp with fluorescein dye examination (Fay & Suh, 2019; Fusco et al., 2019; Malafa et al., 2016). Eye examination begins by administration of a topical anesthetic (e.g., tetracaine 1%, proparacaine 0.5%; Fay & Suh, 2019; Kaye et al., 2019). Next, eyelids are everted to remove any foreign bodies with irrigation or a cotton swab and topical anesthetic (Bagheri & Wajda, 2017; Kaur et al., 2019; Fay & Suh, 2019; Malafa et al., 2016). Visual acuity should then be tested; diminished visual acuity suggests a central corneal abrasion (Fay & Suh, 2019).

Slit lamp evaluation would be helpful as it can help better visualize the extent of a corneal abrasion along with any deeper laceration or perforation compromising the stroma (Bagheri & Wajda, 2017; Fay & Suh, 2019; Kaur et al., 2019; Kaye et al., 2019; Tarff & Behrens, 2017). Additionally, an opacified cornea may suggest an infection (e.g., infectious keratitis; Bagheri & Wajda, 2017; Fay & Suh, 2019). Fluorescein dye examination of the ocular surface under cobalt blue light is helpful in confirming the presence of a corneal epithelial defect, which shows as a fluorescent green or yellow linear or epithelial defect pattern (Bagheri & Wajda, 2017; Fay & Suh, 2019; Kaye et al., 2019; Malafa et al., 2016; Small et al., 2019). If the fluorescein dye is visualized leaking from the anterior chamber, this is known as a positive Seidel test (Bagheri & Wajda, 2017; Fusco et al., 2019; Tarff & Behrens, 2017). A positive Seidel test indicates the presence of a full thickness corneal laceration potentially compromising the stroma and is considered an ophthalmologic emergency (Bagheri & Wajda, 2017; Fusco et al., 2019; Tarff & Behrens, 2017). If negative, it may indicate a self-sealed full-thickness or partial-thickness laceration (Bagheri & Wajda, 2017). In general, IOP measurement should be avoided in full thickness laceration and even in a negative Seidel test (i.e., previously self-sealed full-thickness laceration) to prevent exacerbating an existing laceration (Bagheri & Wajda, 2017). Therefore, an opacified cornea and/or a positive Seidel test would warrant an emergent referral to an ophthalmologist (Bagheri & Wajda, 2017; Fay & Suh, 2019; Kaur et al., 2019; Kaye et al., 2019; Tarff & Behrens, 2017). Persistent visual deficit postinjury is atypical and, therefore, the anterior chamber (i.e., chamber depth, normal iris, and round pupil) should then be evaluated as disruption may indicate a perforating injury due to an intraocular foreign body (Fay & Suh, 2019; Malafa et al., 2016).

DIFFERENTIAL DIAGNOSIS AND DIAGNOSTIC CONSIDERATIONS

Differential diagnoses include infectious keratitis or corneal ulcer, especially in those who wear contact lenses; herpes simplex keratitis; recurrent erosion syndrome; UV keratopathy or Welder's eye photokeratosis (corneal flash burn); or severe dry eye syndrome (Bagheri & Wajda, 2017; Fay & Suh, 2019).

TREATMENT

Most traumatic or perioperative abrasions heal within 1 to 3 days; however, they may be associated with symptoms such as significant pain, photophobia, and foreign body sensation warranting aggressive interventions (Wakai et al., 2017; Malafa et al., 2016). Widely accepted corneal abrasion management includes topical antibiotics such as chloramphenicol or trimethoprim/polymyxin; oral analgesics such as acetaminophen, NSAIDs, and even opioids in severe cases; and ocular lubricants such as artificial tears (Bagheri & Wajda, 2017; Thiel et al., 2017; Wakai et al., 2017).

Prophylactic topical antibiotics (solution or ointment) are recommended for all corneal abrasions to prevent secondary infection and progression to ulceration (Fusco et al., 2019; Malafa et al., 2016). A 2- to 3-day course of topical antibiotics has been recommended (Malafa et al., 2016). Although it may cause temporary blurred vision, an ointment 4 times per day is preferred over the solution as it can provide sustained lubrication in the eye while acting as a film to prevent tear evaporation and therefore providing more pain relief. First-line therapy includes the following ophthalmic preparations: bacitracin ointment, erythromycin 0.5% ointment, polymyxin B/trimethoprim, and sulfacetamide 10% (Bleph-10; Allergan; Bagheri & Wajda, 2017; Fusco et al., 2019; Kaye et al., 2019). In those with contact lenses or those who sustain injury from a foreign body (e.g., fingernail or vegetable matter), a 5- to 7-day course of topical antibiotics with gram negative, specifically, anti-pseudomonal coverage would be preferred such as ofloxacin 0.3%, moxifloxacin hydrochloride 0.5%, or gentamicin 0.3% (Bagheri & Wajda, 2017; Fay & Suh, 2019; Frings et al., 2017; Fusco et al., 2019; Kaye et al., 2019; Malafa et al., 2016; Tarff & Behrens, 2017). Moreover, those who wear contact lenses should avoid contact lens wear for at least 1 week beyond full recovery and completion of a full antibiotic course (Bagheri & Wajda, 2017; Fay & Suh, 2019). If the abrasion is caused by organic matter (e.g., tree branches), it is also important to monitor the patient for delayed-onset fungal keratitis (Fay & Suh, 2019). Preservative-free methylcellulose lubricant drops such as Refresh (Allergan) or Systane PF (Alcon) can be used to provide comfort and consistent ocular surface moisture (Kaye et al., 2019; Malafa et al., 2016).

In general, traumatic corneal abrasions with confirmed foreign body should not be removed by the AGACNP (Kaur et al., 2019). A plastic or metal eye shield should be placed, and the patient should be referred to an ophthalmologist for foreign body removal and ocular surgical repair while a CT scan of the orbits is expedited (Frings et al., 2017; Kaur et al., 2019; Malafa et al., 2016; Tarff & Behrens, 2017). As the corneal abrasion is a portal of infection, tetanus prophylaxis and antibiotics with antipseudomonal coverage should be administered (Fusco et al., 2019; Kaur et al., 2019).

Due to its lack of ability to improve patient discomfort as well as delayed healing from diminished corneal oxygenation, eye patching is no longer recommended for corneal abrasions (Bagheri & Wajda, 2017; Fay & Suh, 2019; Kaye et al., 2019; Malafa et al., 2016; Tarff & Behrens, 2017; Thiel et al., 2017; Wakai et al., 2017). There are mixed recommendations regarding use of topical anesthetics, NSAIDs, and cycloplegics for ocular pain related to corneal abrasions. Topical anesthetics (e.g., tetracaine hydrochloride 1%, proparacaine 0.5%, bupivacaine 0.75%) provide ocular analgesia without adversely affecting corneal healing and epithelialization in the short term; however, prolonged use has been associated with delayed healing leading to corneal infections, scarring, and ulceration (Kaye et al., 2019; Malafa et al., 2016; Thiel et al., 2017; Wakai et al., 2017). Topical NSAIDs (e.g., diclofenac 0.1%, ketorolac 0.4%–0.5% 4 times per day) are not recommended as first-line analgesia for corneal abrasion as they are weaker, more expensive than anesthetics, and have been associated with adverse corneal effects with prolonged use such as conjunctival hyperemia and corneal ulcerations, especially in those with co-existent ocular disease (Bagheri & Wajda, 2017; Kaye et al., 2019; Malafa et al., 2016; Thiel et al., 2017). If necessary, as an adjunct for breakthrough pain, a short 1- to 2-day course has been recommended (Malafa et al., 2016). Short-term use of topical cycloplegics (e.g., cyclopentolate [0.5%–2% 1 drop 2–3 times per day]; homatropine m [2.5%–5% 1 drop daily]) have been associated with reduction in pain and photophobia in traumatic iritis and large corneal abrasions, but prolonged use can precipitate acute glaucoma and other anticholinergic symptoms (Bagheri & Wajda, 2017; Fay & Suh, 2019; Kaye et al., 2019; Malafa et al., 2016; Thiel et al., 2017). General consensus advises against use of any steroid-containing preparations due to impaired epithelial healing and increased susceptibility to infection (Bagheri & Wajda, 2017; Fay & Suh, 2019; Kaur et al., 2019; Kaye et al., 2019; Malafa et al., 2016).

Implementation of eye protection strategies can be instituted to prevent perioperative corneal abrasion. Strategies include implementation of an assessment tool evaluating the severity of lagophthalmos along with use of preservative-free methylcellulose-based ointment and eyelid closure devices such as tape (e.g., 3M Durapore) or bio-occlusive dressings (e.g., 3M Tegaderm Film or Opsite) if needed (Kaye et al., 2019; Malafa et al., 2016; Papp et al., 2019; Small et al., 2019).

Uncomplicated, peripheral, and/or small (4 mm or less) abrasions with associated pain are expected to resolve by 1 to 3 days whereas central and/or large abrasions with associated pain may take up to 5 days, although improvement in pain and epithelial defect should begin in 1 day (Bagheri & Wajda, 2017; Kaye et al., 2019; Malafa et al., 2016; Tarff & Behrens, 2017). Follow-up should occur every 1–3 days to ensure appropriate healing (Bagheri & Wajda, 2017; Fay & Suh, 2019; Malafa et al., 2016; Tarff & Behrens, 2017). Deviation from this or an atypical clinical course usually suggests problematic wound healing and/or missed diagnosis and would warrant immediate ophthalmologic consultation (Malafa et al., 2016). Other indications for ophthalmologic consultation are as follows: worsening pain or vision; pupillary and/or corneal abnormalities (e.g., laceration, opacification, perforation); embedded foreign body in the ocular surface; presence of a corneal abrasion without any identifiable or discrete injury; IOP elevation; and contact lens-related abrasions (Fay & Suh, 2019; Frings et al., 2017; Fusco et al., 2019; Kaur et al., 2019; Malafa et al., 2016; Tarff & Behrens, 2017).

KEY TAKEAWAYS

- Corneal abrasions occur once protective eye mechanisms have been compromised, allowing shearing forces to cause microtrauma and superficial scratches on the cornea.
- Slit-lamp test with fluorescein dye examination can determine the degree of corneal abrasion and rule out stromal involvement (e.g., positive Seidel sign), which is an ocular emergency warranting emergent ophthalmologic consultation.
- Treatment guidelines for management of corneal abrasion include prophylactic topical antibiotics, oral analgesics, and preservative free methylcellulose lubricant drops.
- Use of eye patching, topical steroids and topical NSAIDs is not recommended due to limited pain relief and, in certain instances, long-term corneal complications such as delayed corneal healing and infectious sequelae.

EVIDENCE-BASED RESOURCE

Malafa, M. M., Coleman, J. E., Bowman, R. W., & Rohrich, R. J. (2016). Perioperative corneal abrasion: Updated guidelines for prevention and management. *Plastic and Reconstructive Surgery, 137*(5), 790e–798e. https://doi .org/10.1097/PRS.0000000000002108

2.7: CORNEAL ULCER

Al-Zada "Al" Aguilar

Corneal ulcer, also referred to as ulcerative keratitis, is a potentially sight-threatening corneal epithelial defect with underlying inflammation that causes corneal thinning, tissue loss, and even stromal damage and necrosis (Farahani et al., 2017; Fay & Suh, 2019; Joag et al., 2017; Tarff & Behrens, 2017). Corneal ulcers are caused by both infectious and noninfectious causes, with bacterial causes being the most common (Bagheri & Wajda, 2017; Fay & Suh, 2019; Farahani et al., 2017; Joag et al., 2017). Other types include viral, fungal, and parasitic (Fay & Suh, 2019; Tarff & Behrens, 2017). Viral keratitis is typically caused by herpes simplex virus (HSV) and less commonly varicella zoster virus (VZV) and cytomegalovirus

(CMV; Austin et al., 2017). Fungal keratitis is typically caused by yeasts such as *Candida*, *Aspergillus*, and *Fusarium* (Farahani et al., 2017; Fay & Suh, 2019). Corneal trauma and contact lens use have been dominant risk factors in the development of infectious keratitis, including fungal keratitis (Austin et al., 2017; Bagheri & Wajda, 2017; Farahani et al., 2017; Fay & Suh, 2019; Joag et al., 2017; Mahmoudi et al., 2018; Ung et al., 2019). Noninfectious causes include allergic, autoimmune, iatrogenic, neurotrophic, and toxic causes (Fay & Suh, 2019; Frings et al., 2017). In general, keratitis occurs due to altered immunity, innervation, corneal structure, and protective eye mechanisms (e.g., complete lid closure, corneal blink reflex, tear production; Fay & Suh, 2019; Joag et al., 2017). Timely diagnosis and management are critical as any delay may result in irreversible vision loss, corneal perforation, and even loss of the eye (Fay & Suh, 2019; Farahani et al., 2017; Frings et al., 2017; Ung et al., 2019).

PRESENTING SIGNS AND SYMPTOMS

Clinical findings are typically unilateral and include pain, eyelid and conjunctival erythema and edema, photophobia, foreign body sensation, and decreased or blurry vision (Bagheri & Wajda, 2017; Fay & Suh, 2019; Farahani et al., 2017; Frings et al., 2017; Mahmoudi et al., 2018; Tarff & Behrens, 2017). Bacterial ulcers typically cause rapid onset of pain, photophobia, and conjunctival injection (Farahani et al., 2017). Viral, specifically, herpetic ulcers cause complaints similar to bacterial ulcers (Farahani et al., 2017). In those with fungal ulcers, pain is severe and disproportionate to slit lamp findings (Farahani et al., 2017). In those with ulcers related to *Acanthamoeba*, clinical findings include a several week history of severe ocular pain out of proportion to exam findings and severe photophobia (Bagheri & Wajda, 2017; Farahani et al., 2017; Fay & Suh, 2019). A decrease in vision is influenced by location of corneal infiltrate (especially if central); degree of anterior chamber reaction; and presence of secretions (Farahani et al., 2017; Fay & Suh, 2019; Mahmoudi et al., 2018). Except for contact lens-associated keratitis, noninfectious keratitis may be asymptomatic or minimally symptomatic (Fay & Suh, 2019).

HISTORY AND PHYSICAL FINDINGS

Obtaining a comprehensive yet focused history of present illness will direct the AGACNP to diagnosing and differentiating types of keratitis. Population demographics, geographical location, climate, occupation, symptom onset, precipitating factors, co-existent ocular (e.g., lagophthalmos, tear insufficiency) or systemic disorders (e.g., diabetes, immunocompromised states, autoimmune disorders), ocular history (e.g., contact lens wear, eye surgery) as well as certain medications (e.g., ophthalmic steroids, NSAIDs, or anesthetics) may help determine the cause of the keratitis (Bagheri & Wajda, 2017; Farahani et al., 2017; Fay & Suh, 2019; Joag et al., 2017; Mahmoudi et al., 2018; Tarff & Behrens, 2017; Ung et al., 2019).

TABLE 2.5: Approach to Comprehensive Ocular Examination

EXAM	DETAILS
External examination Evaluate eyelid, lash, and periorbital skin	**Skin**: Seborrhea, rosacea **Eyelid**: Lagophthalmos (e.g., ectropion, entropion, floppy lid syndrome); evert to rule out foreign body
Visual acuity (use Snellen chart)	Affected by location of lesion and extended anterior chamber inflammation → miosis
Intraocular pressure (IOP) (use Tono-pen)	Do *not* measure if corneal perforation with stromal involvement Elevated from inflammation of trabecular meshwork (e.g., HSV)
Lacrimal system evaluation	Rule out underlying canaliculitis or dacryocystitis
Slit lamp evaluation Evaluate cornea, epithelium, endothelium, stroma	Rule out conjunctival or scleral injection Evaluate cornea (size and location of corneal infiltrate; opacification; sensation using cotton-tipped applicator) Evaluate anterior chamber (high magnification: cell, flare, or hypopyon [layered collection of inflammatory cells])
Fluorescein Stain Evaluation **(under cobalt blue light illumination)** (use topical anesthetic) Evaluate ulcers, foreign bodies, corneal epithelial defects	**Positive Seidel test**: Green fluorescein stain present in corneal stroma and anterior chamber (i.e., full thickness defect or corneal perforation) ***Ophthalmic emergency!!***

HVS, herpes simplex virus.

Source: Data from Bagheri, N., & Wajda, B. N. (2017). *The Wills eye manual: Office and emergency room diagnosis and treatment of eye disease* (7th ed). Wolters Kluwer; Farahani, M., Patel, R., & Dwarakanathan, S. (2017). Infectious corneal ulcers. *Disease-a-Month, 63*(2), 33–37. https://doi.org/10.1016/j.disamonth.2016.09.003; Fay, J., & Suh, L. H. (2019). Corneal trauma, infection, and opacities. In *The Columbia guide to basic elements of eye care* (pp. 137–147). Springer International Publishing. https://doi.org/10.1007/978-3-030-10886-1_12; Joag, M. G., Sayed-Ahmed, I. O., & Karp, C. L. (2017). The corneal ulcer. In *Cornea* (4th ed., pp. 241–245). https://doi.org/10.1016/B978-0-323-35757-9.00020-0; Tarff, A., & Behrens, A. (2017). Ocular emergencies: Red eye. *Medical Clinics of North America, 101*(3), 615–639. https://doi.org/10.1016/j.mcna.2016.12.013; Ung, L., Bispo, P. J. M., Shanbhag, S. S., Gilmore, M. S., & Chodosh, J. (2019). The persistent dilemma of microbial keratitis: Global burden, diagnosis, and antimicrobial resistance. *Survey of Ophthalmology, 64*(3), 255–271. https://doi.org/10.1016/j.survophthal.2018.12.003

A comprehensive ocular examination should include the following: external examination (e.g., eyelids, lashes, periorbital skin); measurement of visual acuity and IOP; pupillary exam; tear function exam; slit lamp with fluorescein stain evaluation (e.g., conjunctival or scleral injection; size and location of corneal infiltrate; corneal opacification and sensation; anterior chamber); and, if needed, Gram stain and culture (Austin et al., 2017; Bagheri & Wajda, 2017; Farahani et al., 2017; Fay & Suh, 2019; Joag et al., 2017; Tarff & Behrens, 2017; Ung et al., 2019). See Table 2.5 for the approach to comprehensive ocular examinations. Slit lamp evaluation can be helpful in differentiating infectious from noninfectious forms of keratitis (Table 2.6).

Next, topical anesthetic and fluorescein dye should be applied to the ocular surface and then visualized under cobalt blue illumination to highlight any ulcers, foreign bodies, or corneal epithelial defects. Fluorescein dye examination of the ocular surface under cobalt blue light is helpful in confirming the presence of a corneal epithelial defect, which shows as a fluorescent green or yellow linear or epithelial defect pattern (Bagheri & Wajda, 2017; Fay & Suh, 2019; Farahani et al., 2017). If the fluorescein dye is visualized leaking from the anterior chamber or corneal stroma, this is known as a positive Seidel test, which indicates the presence of a full thickness corneal laceration potentially compromising the stroma and is considered an ophthalmologic emergency (Bagheri & Wajda, 2017; Farahani et al., 2017).

DIFFERENTIAL DIAGNOSIS AND DIAGNOSTIC CONSIDERATIONS

Differential diagnoses for ulcerative keratitis include ocular conditions that present with redness, pain, and photophobia such as conjunctivitis (allergic, bacterial, or viral), contact lens-associated keratopathy corneal abrasion, iritis, ocular chemical injury, corneal foreign body, pterygium, blepharitis, medication-induced ocular toxicity, and dry eye syndrome (Bagheri ,& Wajda, 2017; Fay & Suh, 2019; Austin et al., 2017).

To date, the mainstay in the diagnosis of infectious keratitis is still microscopic examination along with staining, culture, and susceptibility of corneal samples via scraping (Austin et al., 2017; Bagheri & Wajda, 2017; Joag et al., 2017; Mahmoudi et al., 2018; Ung et al., 2019). Culturing infiltrates are typically indicated if they are in the visual axis; larger than 1 to 2 mm; unresponsive to initial treatment; or if there is a suspicion for an unusual causative organism based on history and examination (Bagheri & Wajda, 2017). If the suspected infection is from contact lens wear, contact lens culture would be helpful (Bagheri & Wajda, 2017; Frings et al., 2017; Joag et al., 2017). For those with progression of disease despite negative corneal culture and/or adequate coverage, a corneal biopsy would be warranted for further diagnostic information and to rule out infectious crystalline keratopathy (ICK), parasitic keratitis, and noninfectious

TABLE 2.6: Differentiating Forms of Keratitis Based on Slit-Lamp Evaluation

BACTERIAL	VIRAL	FUNGAL	MISCELLANEOUS INFECTIONS	NEUROTROPHIC	TOXIC	POST-TREATED INFECTION	NON INFECTIOUS IMMUNE-RELATED
Staphylococcus: Well-circumscribed lesion *Streptococcus:* Well-circumscribed lesion; acute highly suppurative; deep central stromal ulcer with advancing edge of infection; sterile hypopyon; infectious crystalline keratopathy (ICK) (paucity of inflammatory cells) [hallmark] *Gram-negative bacteria (e.g., Pseudomonas):* Less discreet infiltrates; copious mucopurulent conjunctival discharge; hypopyon	*HSV:* Increased IOP; dendritic lesions with subdendritic stromal edema and terminal bulbs at the end of each dendritic branch; corneal stromal opacification without epithelial defect; endothelilitis → corneal edema *VZV:* punctate keratitis and pseudodendrites (5%–51%) without terminal bulbs; epithelial keratitis → stromal keratitis (increased risk for vision loss)	*Filamentous (e.g. Fusarium or Aspergillus):* Corneal ulcer with dry, raised necrotic/ slough surface; deep stromal infiltrate with feathery borders with satellite lesions; anterior chamber inflammation (e.g., hypopyon) *Nonfilamentous (e.g., Candida):* Gray-white stromal infiltrate; diffuse punctate epithelial +/− dendritic lesions	*Acanthamoeba:* Ring-shaped stromal infiltrate; radial peri-neuritis *Mycobacterium, Nocardia:* central "cracked wind-shield"; peripheral "brush fire"	Persistent central oval epithelial defect with rolled epithelial edge lesion	Diffuse epitheliopathy	Resolved epithelial defect or defect healing over area of prior dense infiltration	Varied degrees of stromal infiltration; localized scleritis, episcleritis, or iritis; peripheral marginal melts with or without epithelial defects *Rheumatologic disorders:* Peripheral corneal thinning, ulceration

HSV, herpes simplex virus; ICK, infectious crystalline keratopathy; IOP, intraocular pressure; VZV, varicella zoster virus.

Source: Data from Bagheri, N., & Wajda, B. N. (2017). *The Wills eye manual: Office and emergency room diagnosis and treatment of eye disease* (7th ed). Wolters Kluwer; Farahani, M., Patel, R., & Dwarakanathan, S. (2017). Infectious corneal ulcers. *Disease-a-Month, 63*(2), 33–37. https://doi.org/10.1016/j.disamonth.2016.09.003; Fay, J., & Suh, L. H. (2019). Corneal trauma, infection, and opacities. In *The Columbia guide to basic elements of eye care* (pp. 137–147). Springer International Publishing. https://doi.org/10.1007/978-3-030-10886-1_12; Frings, A., Geerling, G., & Schargus, M. (2017). Red eye: A guide for non-specialists. *Deutsches Ärzteblatt International, 114*(17), 302–312. https://doi.org/10.3238/arztebl.2017.0302; Joag, M. G., Sayed-Ahmed, I. O., & Karp, C. L. (2017). The corneal ulcer. In *Cornea* (4th ed., pp. 241–245). https://doi.org/10.1016/B978-0-323-35757-9.00020-0; Li, L, Lu, C., Wang, L., Chen, M., White, J., Hao, X., McLean, K. M., Chen, H., & Hughes, T. C. (2018). Gelatin-based photocurable hydrogels for corneal wound repair. *ACS Applied Materials & Interfaces, 10*(16), 13283 -13292. https://doi .org/10.1021acsami.7b17054; Mahmoudi, S., Masoomi, A., Ahmadikia, K., Tabatabaei, S.A., Soleimani, M., Rezaie, S., Ghahvechian, H., & Banafsheafshan, A. (2018). Fungal keratitis: An overview of clinical and laboratory aspects. *Mycoses, 61*(12), 916–930. https://doi.org/10.1111/myc.12822

causes of keratitis (Bagheri & Wajda, 2017; Joag et al., 2017; Mahmoudi et al., 2018).

The overall yield from culture and stain is unsatisfactory due to suboptimal sensitivity (27.4%–61.6%) from technical difficulties, prior antibiotic use, and timely susceptibility and resistance data (Ung et al., 2019). As a result, there has been a rise in alternative molecular diagnostic tests. Given its high sensitivity (up to 86.8%) and specificity (up to 85.9%), in vivo confocal microscopy is helpful not only for diagnosing microbes, but also monitoring treatment efficacy (Austin et al., 2017; Farahani et al., 2017; Joag et al., 2017; Mahmoudi et al., 2018; Ung et al., 2019). Given its high sensitivity (70%–98%) and specificity (94.7%–98%) when supplemented with clinical diagnosis and culture data as reference standards, polymerase chain reaction (PCR) testing has also been useful in the diagnosis of viral (e.g., HSV, VZV, CMV), bacterial, fungal, and parasitic (e.g., *Acanthamoeba*) keratitis (Austin et al., 2017; Bagheri & Wajda, 2017; Farahani et al., 2017; Ung et al., 2019). In noninfectious (e.g., peripheral ulcerative keratitis), disease-specific testing is performed to rule out potential causes such as collagen-vascular and granulomatous disorders (Fay & Suh, 2019).

TREATMENT

Topical antibiotics remain the first-line treatment for bacterial keratitis (Austin et al., 2017; Robaei et al., 2016; Tarff & Behrens, 2017). For treatment of viral and fungal keratitis, treatment principles include use of topical and in some cases, systemic agents (Austin et al., 2017; Bagheri & Wajda, 2017; Farahani et al., 2017; Fay & Suh, 2019; Mahmoudi et al., 2018). *Acanthamoeba* is the most difficult to treat and there are currently no FDA-approved drugs as the available drugs are often associated with significant ocular surface toxicity (Farahani et al., 2017; Fay & Suh, 2019; Tarff & Behrens, 2017). Recommendations have been made based on proven in vitro and clinical efficacy (Farahani et al., 2017). See Table 2.7 for antimicrobial treatment recommendations for infectious keratitis.

Treatment Efficacy, Failure, and Adjunctive Therapy

Lack of worsening or stabilization suggests effective therapy as corneal healing takes time (Joag et al., 2017). Indicators of clinical improvement include decreasing size and density of the corneal infiltrate, inflammation, and associated pain as well as resolution of the epithelial defect and anterior chamber reaction (Bagheri & Wajda, 2017; Joag et al., 2017). Reduced pain is often the first sign of treatment response (Bagheri & Wajda, 2017). If improving, antibiotics should be adjusted based on culture and sensitivities and gradually tapered over 4 to 6 weeks (Bagheri & Wajda, 2017).

Unfortunately, some cases of infectious keratitis are difficult to treat and others, despite appropriate antimicrobial coverage, develop inflammatory sequelae that result in the following poor clinical outcomes: scleral extension, endophthalmitis, corneal melting and/or scarring leading to permanent visual loss, and even corneal perforation (Austin et al., 2017; Bagheri & Wajda, 2017; Fay & Suh, 2019; Robaei et al., 2016). In the case of treatment failure, management may require high risk procedures such as excision and therapeutic penetrating keratoplasty (Austin et al., 2017; Bagheri & Wajda, 2017; Fay & Suh, 2019; Frings et al., 2017; Joag et al., 2017). Other adjunctive therapy such as anticollagenases, corticosteroids, and analgesics have been described in the literature in the management of infectious keratitis. See Table 2.8 for adjunctive treatment recommendations for infective keratitis.

Consultation with an ophthalmologist is indicated in the following: obtaining tissue diagnosis for Gram stain, culture, and/or biopsy; difficult-to-treat corneal ulcer; worsening symptoms (i.e., increased pain or ulcer size when looking in the mirror, decreased vision); corneal ulcer associated with contact lens use; or ocular complaints post-LASIK (Bagheri & Wajda, 2017; Farahani et al., 2017; Fay & Suh, 2019; Frings et al., 2017; Joag et al., 2017). Consultation with a medical specialist is warranted if the underlying cause is attributed to a systemic disorder such as collagen-vascular and/or granulomatous diseases (Fay & Suh, 2019). Hospital admission is indicated in the following: vision-threatening or impending corneal perforation; high likelihood of noncompliance; suspected medication abuse; need for parenteral antibiotics; and gonococcal, fungal, and/or atypical mycobacterial keratitis given rapid onset and increased risk for sequelae (Bagheri & Wajda, 2017).

> ### KEY TAKEAWAYS
>
> - Corneal trauma and contact lens use have been dominant risk factors in the development of infectious keratitis, including fungal keratitis.
> - Slit-lamp evaluation along with fluorescein staining are helpful in differentiating infectious from noninfectious keratitis, but also in ruling out ophthalmologic emergencies such as corneal perforation (i.e., positive Seidel test).
> - Timely diagnosis, management, and expert referral are critical as any delay may result in irreversible vision loss, corneal perforation, and even loss of the eye.
> - Antimicrobial treatment is determined based on coverage, pharmacodynamics and pharmacokinetics, area-specific epidemiology of pathogens and resistance patterns, as well as cost and availability.

EVIDENCE-BASED RESOURCE

Joag, M. G., Sayed-Ahmed, I. O., & Karp, C. L. (2017). The corneal ulcer. In *Cornea* (4th ed., pp. 241–245). https://doi.org/10.1016/B978-0-323-35757-9.00020-0

TABLE 2.7: Antimicrobial Treatment Recommendations for Infectious Keratitis

BACTERIAL	VIRAL	MISCELLANEOUS
Low risk of visual loss and/or small peripheral ulcer (<2 mm) • <u>No contact lens</u>: Topical fourth-generation fluoroquinolone (i.e., gatifloxacin and moxifloxacin hourly drop) *or* Polymyxin B/trimethoprim (q1-2h while awake) • <u>Contact lens</u>: Fluoroquinolones +/− Polymyxin B/trimethoprim drops q1-2h while awake +/− tobramycin or ciprofloxacin (1-4×/day); proper ocular (i.e., contact lens) hygiene **Borderline risk of visual loss and/or medium size peripheral ulcer (1-1.5 mm) and/or <1 mm with epithelial defect, mild anterior chamber reaction, and/or moderate discharge** Fluoroquinolones Gram-positive coverage: Moxifloxacin, esofloxacin *Pseudomonas, Serratia* coverage: Gatifloxacin, ciprofloxacin *plus* Polymyxin B/trimethoprim q1h **Vision-threatening, central, and/or larger ulcer (>1.5-2 mm)** ***Obtain corneal culture (by ophthalmologist)** • <u>Standard</u>: Fortified aminoglycosides (tobramycin or gentamicin 15 mg/mL q1h) *plus* Cefazolin 50 mg/mL (If MRSA, hospital/antibiotic exposure, poor treatment response, and/or allergy to PCN/cephalosporin: substitute with vancomycin 25 mg/mL q1h) • <u>If severe with Pseudomonas</u>: Fortified tobramycin q30mins plus cefazolin q1h +/− fortified ceftazidime q1h ***Loading doses recommended if severe and/or vision-threatening: 1 drop q5min then q30-60min ATC until midnight then q1h after* <u>**Additional considerations:**</u> • <u>If scleral involvement and/or impending corneal perforation</u>: Add oral fluoroquinolones (ciprofloxacin 500 mg BID, moxifloxacin 400 mg daily) • <u>If Neisseria with corneal or conjunctival involvement</u>: Add ceftriaxone 1 g q12-24h • *If Haemophilus* (increased risk for otitis media, pneumonia, meningitis): Add amoxicillin/clavalunate 20-40 mg/kg/day TID	**HSV:** • 10-14 days topical trifluridine or ganciclovir gel • Add antibiotics if epithelial defect • If stroma involved: PO acyclovir +/− topical corticosteroids (HEDS I) • Consider PO acyclovir prophylaxis if recurrence, immunocompromised (HEDS II) **CMV:** Valacyclovir PO (1 g TID) **VZV:** • Topical ganciclovir 0.15% • To limit ocular toxicity, can substitute PO form (i.e., valacyclovir 1 g TID, famciclovir 500 mg TID, or acyclovir 800 mg 5×/day) • Administer VZV vaccine	**Fungal:** • <u>Filamentous fungi</u> (e.g., Aspergillus): Topical natamycin 5% • <u>If deep ulcer and/or suspected endophthalmitis</u>: Fluconazole or itraconazole 200-400 mg PO load dose then 100-200 mg PO daily *or* voriconazole 200 mg PO BID ***Consider mechanical debridement (increased infection load, better topical penetration) and/or intrastromal administration* **Acanthamoeba:** • <u>Standard</u>: 3-12 months biguanides (e.g., polyhexamethylene biguanide) • <u>Alternatives</u>: Aminoglycosides (e.g., neomycin), azoles (e.g. voriconazole) ** *Obtain ophthalmology and/or infectious specialist consultation!* **Atypical mycobacterium:** • Increased risk with prior LASIK • <u>Standard</u>: Prolonged treatment with clarithromycin 500 mg PO BID with fluoroquinolone, amikacin (15 mg/ml), clarithromycin (1-4%), or tobramycin (15 mg/mL) ointments

ATC, around the clock; CMV, cytomegalovirus; HEDS, Herpetic Eye Disease Study; HSV, herpes simplex virus; MRSA, methicillin-resistant *Staphylococcus aureus*; PCN, penicillin; VZV, varicella zoster virus.

Source: Data from Bagheri, N., & Wajda, B. N. (2017). *The Wills eye manual: Office and emergency room diagnosis and treatment of eye disease* (7th ed). Wolters Kluwer; Farahani, M., Patel, R., & Dwarakanathan, S. (2017). Infectious corneal ulcers. *Disease-a-Month, 63*(2), 33–37. https://doi.org/10.1016/j.disamonth.2016.09.003; Fay, J., & Suh, L. H. (2019). Corneal trauma, infection, and opacities. In *The Columbia guide to basic elements of eye care* (pp. 137–147). Springer International Publishing. https://doi.org/10.1007/978-3-030-10886-1_12; Frings, A., Geerling, G., & Schargus, M. (2017). Red eye: A guide for non-specialists. *Deutsches Ärzteblatt International, 114*(17), 302–312. https://doi.org/10.3238/arztebl.2017.0302; Joag, M. G., Sayed-Ahmed, I. O., & Karp, C. L. (2017). The corneal ulcer. In *Cornea* (4th ed., pp. 241–245). https://doi.org/10.1016/B978-0-323-35757-9.00020-0; Li, L., Lu, C., Wang, L., Chen, M., White, J., Hao, X., McLean, K. M., Chen, H., & Hughes, T. C. (2018). Gelatin-based photocurable hydrogels for corneal wound repair. *ACS Applied Materials & Interfaces, 10*(16), 13283–13292. https://doi.org/10.1021/acsami.7b17054; Mahmoudi, S., Masoomi, A., Ahmadikia, K., Tabatabaei, S. A., Soleimani, M., Rezaie, S., Ghahvechian, H., & Banafsheafshan, A. (2018). Fungal keratitis: An overview of clinical and laboratory aspects. *Mycoses, 61*(12), 916–930. https://doi.org/10.1111/myc.12822

TABLE 2.8: Adjunctive Treatment Recommendations for Infectious Keratitis

EXAMPLE	DETAILS
Anti-collagenases (e.g., high-dose systemic tetracycline [i.e., doxycycline])	Stabilize corneal healing, decreased complications (e.g., corneal perforation)
Corticosteroids (systemic or topical)	Controversial • <u>Advantages</u>: Decreased discomfort and inflammation • <u>Disadvantages</u>: Delayed epithelial healing, immunosuppression Can add if the following criteria are met: • After at least 2 days of appropriate antimicrobial coverage • Culture and sensitivities known • Adequate source control: Infiltrate improving, epithelial defect becoming smaller • Culture-positive non-*Nocardia*, nonfungal, nonparasitic keratitis Taper to lowest amount needed for symptom control, decreased inflammation (Note: Long-term use increases risk for cataract and/or glaucoma) **If considering starting, can defer to ophthalmologist**

Miscellaneous	• Eye shield protection without eye patch: prevent corneal perforation
	• Avoid contact lens wear
	• Administer doxycycline 100 mg PO BID and ascorbic acid 1–2 g daily: decreased connective tissue breakdown, decreased risk of corneal perforation
	• Analgesics PO as needed
	• Treat increased IOP
	• Administer cycloplegic drops
	  o Atropine 1% BID–TID: If hypopyon present
	  o Cyclopentolate 1% TID: Decreased discomfort, prevent synechiae formation

IOP, intraocular pressure.

Source: Data from Austin, A., Lietman, T., & Rose-Nussbaumer, J. (2017). Update on the management of infectious keratitis. *Ophthalmology, 124*(11), 1678–1689. https://doi.org/10.1016/j.ophtha.2017.05.012; Bagheri, N., & Wajda, B. N. (2017). *The Wills eye manual: Office and emergency room diagnosis and treatment of eye disease* (7th ed). Wolters Kluwer; Farahani, M., Patel, R., & Dwarakanathan, S. (2017). Infectious corneal ulcers. *Disease-a-Month, 63*(2), 33–37. https://doi.org/10.1016/j.disamonth.2016.09.003; Fay, J., & Suh, L. H. (2019). Corneal trauma, infection, and opacities. In *The Columbia Guide to basic elements of eye care* (pp. 137–147). Springer International Publishing. https://doi.org/10.1007/978-3-030-10886-1_12; Frings, A., Geerling, G., & Schargus, M. (2017) Red eye: A guide for non-specialists. *Deutsches Ärzteblatt International, 114*(17), 302–312. https://doi.org/10.3238/arztebl.2017.0302; Joag, M. G., Sayed-Ahmed, I. O., & Karp, C. L. (2017). The corneal ulcer. In *Cornea* (4th ed., pp. 241–245). https://doi.org/10.1016/B978-0-323-35757-9.00020-0; Li, 2018; Mahmoudi, S., Masoomi, A., Ahmadikia, K., Tabatabaei, S. A., Soleimani, M., Rezaie, S., Ghahvechian, H., & Banafsheafshan, A. (2018). Fungal keratitis: An overview of clinical and laboratory aspects. *Mycoses, 61*(12), 916–930. https://doi.org/10.1111/myc.12822; Robaei, D., Carnt, N., & Watson, S. (2016). Established and emerging ancillary techniques in management of microbial keratitis: A review. *British Journal of Ophthalmology, 100*(9), 1163–1170. https://doi.org/10.1136/bjophthalmol-2015-307371

2.8: ORBITAL CELLULITIS

Al-Zada "Al" Aguilar

Orbital cellulitis is a serious infection and inflammation of the postseptal orbital tissues (Casper & Cioffi, 2019; Gordon & Phelps, 2020; Maeng & Winn, 2019; Tsirouki et al., 2018; Yen & Johnson, 2018). Types include posttraumatic, especially in the cases of intraorbital foreign bodies (IOrbFBs), postsurgery, infectious, malignancy and/or treatment-related (Casper & Cioffi, 2019; Maeng & Winn, 2019; Yen & Johnson, 2018). The Chandler criteria is an established staging system in which stages of orbital cellulitis have been categorized based on severity, location, and extension (Table 2.9). Ocular complications include retinovascular, scleral, or choroid occlusion or infarction, anterior or posterior optic neuropathy, exposure keratopathy leading to corneal ulcers, exudative retinal detachment, papilledema, and glaucoma (Tsirouki et al., 2018; Yen & Johnson, 2018). In certain cases, intracranial complications such as brain abscess (e.g., epidural and subdural empyema), meningitis, and even strokes can occur via direct vascular extension, retrograde thrombophlebitis, or hematogenous spread via the sinus-intracranial venous system (Bagheri & Wajda, 2017; Casper & Cioffi, 2019; Tsirouki et al., 2018; Yen & Johnson, 2018). Other complications include periorbital necrotizing fasciitis, orbital bone osteomyelitis, and septicemia (Maeng & Winn, 2019; Tsirouki et al., 2018; Yen & Johnson, 2018).

PRESENTING SIGNS AND SYMPTOMS

Ocular and facial findings include severe, deep orbital pain; eyelid edema and erythema; limited extraocular movements; visual changes such as diplopia; ophthalmoplegia; proptosis and (downward) globe displacement; ptosis; conjunctival chemosis; periorbital tissue erythema; discharge; and trigeminal and facial nerve paresthesias (in fungal orbital cellulitis; Bagheri & Wajda, 2017; Casper & Cioffi, 2019; Gordon & Phelps, 2020; Maeng & Winn, 2019; Tsirouki et al., 2018; Yen & Johnson, 2018). Early signs include periocular pain or pain with eye movement as well as globe injection (Yen & Johnson, 2018). Later signs include proptosis, extraocular motility restriction, optic disc

TABLE 2.9: Chandler's Classification of Orbital Cellulitis

Stage 1: Preseptal cellulitis	Infection of periorbital structures anterior to the orbital septum and the eyelid
Stage 2: Orbital cellulitis	Infection of periorbital structures posterior to the orbital septum
Stage 3: Subperiosteal abscess (SPA)	Infected fluid collection between orbital bones (i.e., frontal, ethmoid, or maxillary) and periorbital structures (most common type of orbital collection)
Stage 4: Orbital abscess	Infected fluid collection within the orbit itself due to ocular surgery, penetrating injury and penetrating injury
Stage 5: Cavernous sinus thrombosis (CST)	Thrombus formed after phlebitis developed extending posteriorly to the cavernous sinus; rare; may lead to cranial nerve palsies (III, V, VI)

Source: Data from Chen, R. W. S., & Cioffi, G. A. (2019). Ocular emergencies. In: *The Columbia guide to basic elements of eye care* (pp. 63–69). Springer International Publishing; Gordon, A. A., & Phelps, P. O. (2020). Management of preseptal and orbital cellulitis for the primary care physician. *Disease-a-Month, 66*(10), 101044. https://doi.org/10.1016/j.disamonth.2020.101044; Maeng, M. M., & Winn, B. J. (2019). Orbital infections and inflammations. In *The Columbia guide to basic elements of eye care* (pp. 355–371). Springer International Publishing. https://doi.org/10.1007/978-3-030-10886-1_32; Tsirouki, T., Dastiridou, A. I., Ibánez Flores, N., Cerpa, J. C., Moschos, M. M., Brazitikos, P., & Androudi, S. (2018). Orbital cellulitis. *Survey of Ophthalmology, 63*(4), 534–553. https://doi.org/10.1016/j.survophthal.2017.12.001; Yen, M. T., & Johnson, T. E. (2018). *Orbital cellulitis and periorbital infections.* Springer International Publishing. https://doi.org/10.1007/978-3-319-62606-2

swelling, and decreased vision (Maeng & Winn, 2019; Tsirouki et al., 2018; Yen & Johnson, 2018). Signs of optic neuropathy such as dyschromatopsia and afferent pupillary defect may occur in severe cases (Bagheri & Wajda, 2017). Constitutional findings include fever, fatigue, toxic appearance, nasal or sinus congestion, purulent nasal discharge, and loss of appetite (Yen & Johnson, 2018). Increasing eyelid edema, fixed globe displacement, severe pain, and worsening visual acuity are highly suggestive of an abscess (Gordon & Phelps, 2020; Yen & Johnson, 2018). Bilateral eye findings, prostration, cranial nerve palsy (IV–VI), severe loss of visual acuity, and meningeal signs should raise concern for cavernous sinus thrombosis (CST) and/or meningitis (Tsirouki et al., 2018; Yen & Johnson, 2018).

HISTORY AND PHYSICAL EXAM FINDINGS

Obtaining a comprehensive yet focused history and physical examination will direct the AGACNP to a diagnosis of orbital cellulitis. History taking should highlight risk factors such as: (older) age; (winter or spring) seasonal occurrence; recent ocular and/or otolaryngological infection, surgery, or trauma; presence of extra-ocular infections and/or signs or symptoms; systemic diseases (e.g., diabetes); history of immunosuppression (e.g., HIV, chronic steroid use, malignancy); and (recent) dental history (Bagheri & Wajda, 2017; Casper & Cioffi, 2019; Gordon & Phelps, 2020; Hamed-Azzam et al., 2018; Maeng & Winn, 2019; Tsirouki et al., 2018; Yen & Johnson, 2018). Moreover, due to the shared interface and venous system of the paranasal sinuses with the orbit, cavernous sinus, and face, (chronic bacterial, usually frontal or ethmoid) sinusitis is the leading predisposing risk factor for developing orbital cellulitis (Bagheri & Wajda, 2017; Casper & Cioffi, 2019; Hamed-Azzam et al., 2018; Maeng & Winn, 2019; Tsirouki et al., 2018; Yen & Johnson, 2018). A comprehensive yet focused physical exam should include the following: measurement of globe position; visual acuity;

pupillary reaction; color vision; visual field; evaluation of cornea, retina, optic nerve, and extraocular muscle; presence of pre-auricular or cervical lymphadenopathy; nasal passages; and measurement of intraocular pressure (IOP; Bagheri & Wajda, 2017).

DIFFERENTIAL DIAGNOSIS AND DIAGNOSTIC CONSIDERATIONS

A complete blood count (CBC) along with blood cultures should be drawn prior to initiation of therapy, although blood cultures are typically low-yielding (Bagheri & Wajda, 2017; Gordon & Phelps, 2020; Maeng & Winn, 2019; Tsirouki et al., 2018; Yen & Johnson, 2018). Cultures from orbital abscess postdrainage or direct aspiration of an infected sinus are most reliable; however, they are not routinely performed (Tsirouki et al., 2018). Therefore, cultures from nasal or throat swabs and ocular secretions are acceptable alternatives (Gordon & Phelps, 2020; Tsirouki et al., 2018; Yen & Johnson, 2018). A lumbar puncture may even be considered if meningeal signs are present (Gordon & Phelps, 2020).

CT scan is the imaging modality of choice in the diagnosis of orbital cellulitis and its associated complications (Bagheri & Wajda, 2017; Gordon & Phelps, 2020; Tsirouki et al., 2018; Yen & Johnson, 2018). Orbital CT scan, specifically a thin-section axial scan (between 1 and 3 mm) with contrast enhancement can determine which cases can be managed medically (i.e., antibiotics) or surgically (i.e., abscess drainage and orbit decompression) while facilitating diagnoses of intracranial complications (Casper & Cioffi, 2019; Gordon & Phelps, 2020; Tsirouki et al., 2018; Yen & Johnson, 2018). It is typically warranted in the following: atypical presentation and/or difficult to diagnose; worsening clinical course with new orbital and/or central nervous system signs; and nonresolving pyrexia over 36 hours despite antibiotic therapy (Bagheri & Wajda, 2017; Maeng & Winn, 2019; Tsirouki et al., 2018; Yen & Johnson, 2018).

MRI can also be used to supplement CT, preferably with contrast (i.e., gadolinium) to elucidate pathology, especially when there is a suspicion for subperiosteal or orbital abscesses or intracranial involvement and when CT findings are unclear (Gordon & Phelps, 2020; Tsirouki et al., 2018; Yen & Johnson, 2018). MRI is safer than CT (as it limits radiation exposure), but its use is limited due to decreased availability and increased scanning time (Tsirouki et al., 2018).

After the introduction of *Haemophilus influenzae* and pneumococcal vaccines, the prevalence of *H. influenzae* and *Streptococcus pneumoniae* orbital cellulitis have markedly declined (Gordon & Phelps, 2020; Yen & Johnson, 2018). Nontypeable *H. influenzae, Staphylococcus aureus,* and *Streptococcus* are now emerging as the most common causative organisms (Casper & Cioffi, 2019; Gordon & Phelps, 2020; Hamed-Azzam et al., 2018; Maeng & Winn, 2019; Tsirouki et al., 2018; Yen & Johnson, 2018). *S. aureus* is most common among posttraumatic and postsurgical orbital infection, although mixed bacterial, gram negative, and anaerobic infections can also occur (Bagheri & Wajda, 2017; Yen & Johnson, 2018). Sinusitis-related orbital cellulitis is usually caused by *S. aureus*, *Streptococcus*, and even anaerobes (Yen & Johnson, 2018). There is also a rising incidence (21%–72%) of methicillin resistant *S. aureus* (MRSA; Gordon & Phelps, 2020; Tsirouki et al., 2018; Yen & Johnson, 2018). *Mucor* fungi and *Aspergillus* are also common causes of fungal orbital cellulitis, especially in the immunocompromised (Bagheri & Wajda, 2017; Maeng & Winn, 2019; Tsirouki et al., 2018; Yen & Johnson, 2018).

Differential diagnoses include preseptal cellulitis; non infectious orbital inflammation (e.g., immune-mediated); frontal bone osteomyelitis; contact dermatitis; other cutaneous infections (e.g., periorbital necrotizing fasciitis; erysipelas); malignancy (e.g., T-cell lymphoma, orbital metastasis, malignant melanoma); and autoimmune manifestations (e.g., sickle-cell disease, systemic lupus erythematosus (SLE), rheumatologic disorders; Casper & Cioffi, 2019; Maeng & Winn, 2019; Tsirouki et al., 2018; Yen & Johnson, 2018). Orbital cellulitis can be differentiated from preseptal cellulitis as the former occurs posterior to the orbital septum, whereas the latter occurs anteriorly (Casper & Cioffi, 2019). Periorbital necrotizing fasciitis can be differentiated from orbital cellulitis given its rapid progression; severe and disproportionate pain that initially presents with rose-violet, dermatomal (V1–V3) skin changes with anesthesia and crepitus that progress to gangrene within 4 to 5 days; and suppuration and skin sloughing within 8 to 10 days (Casper & Cioffi, 2019; Maeng & Winn, 2019; Tsirouki et al., 2018; Yen & Johnson, 2018).

TREATMENT

Management of orbital cellulitis, especially in those with neuro-ocular abnormalities warrants hospital admission, early implementation of systemic antibiotics, as well as oculoplastic consultation (Figure 2.1; Casper & Cioffi, 2019; Gordon & Phelps, 2020; Tsirouki et al., 2018; Yen & Johnson, 2018). Antibiotic regimens chosen are based on existing comorbidities, drug–drug interactions, prior antimicrobial exposure, local epidemiology of resistance, microbiology and susceptibilities, rapidity of symptom onset, presence of features suggestive of adjacent fungal sinusitis, neurological sequelae, as well as geographic and economic variables (Tsirouki et al., 2018; Yen & Johnson, 2018). Antibiotics used should have activity against *S. aureus* (including MRSA), *Streptococcus*, gram-negative bacillus, and anaerobic bacteria (Bagheri & Wajda, 2017; Gordon & Phelps, 2020; Maeng & Winn, 2019). Parenteral antibiotics are typically continued for an average of 4 days and transitioned to a 1- to 4-week course of outpatient oral antibiotics postdischarge (Bagheri et al., 2017; Maeng & Winn, 2019; Yen & Johnson, 2018). Medication noncompliance is a common reason for failure to improve or recurrence. Therefore, the oral antibiotic regimen should be individualized for ease of use and affordability, with use of effective generic alternatives to brand name when possible (Bagheri & Wajda, 2017). Surgical drainage is warranted in situations highly suggestive of abscess formation such as lack of treatment response with worsening orbital signs and symptoms or retained foreign body, especially in older patients who are more likely to have polymicrobial abscesses (Bagheri & Wajda, 2017; Casper & Cioffi, 2019; Gordon & Phelps, 2020; Tsirouki et al., 2018; Yen & Johnson, 2018). Although controversial, corticosteroids can be considered after 3 days of antibiotics as it reduces postinfectious inflammation, resulting in decreased proptosis and pain (Bagheri & Wajda, 2017; Tsirouki et al., 2018; Yen & Johnson, 2018); however, corticosteroid use is contraindicated in those with fungal infections or the immunocompromised as they will worsen immunosuppression while delaying or preventing resolution of the orbital cellulitis (Tsirouki et al., 2018). Signs of improvement are often gradual in patients with orbital cellulitis, particularly in those with severe disease and/or who are older (Yen & Johnson, 2018). Moreover, systemic signs may improve prior to orbital signs (Casper & Cioffi, 2019; Yen & Johnson, 2018). See Table 2.10 for recommended management of orbital cellulitis.

An ophthalmologist should be consulted in all patients with orbital, especially fungal, cellulitis (Gordon & Phelps, 2020; Maeng & Winn, 2019). Oculoplastic surgical consultation is recommended in patients with (large, atypical, nonmedial) SPA requiring drainage or those with cavernous sinus thrombosis (CST; Gordon & Phelps, 2020; Maeng & Winn, 2019). Infectious disease consultation is warranted in those with severe, atypical, or unresponsive orbital cellulitis (i.e., suspected multidrug resistance; Bagheri & Wajda, 2017; Yen & Johnson, 2018) Otolaryngology consultation should be requested in the presence of co-existent otolaryngological infections (i.e., paranasal sinusitis); (large, atypical, nonmedial) subperiosteal abscess (SPA); CST;

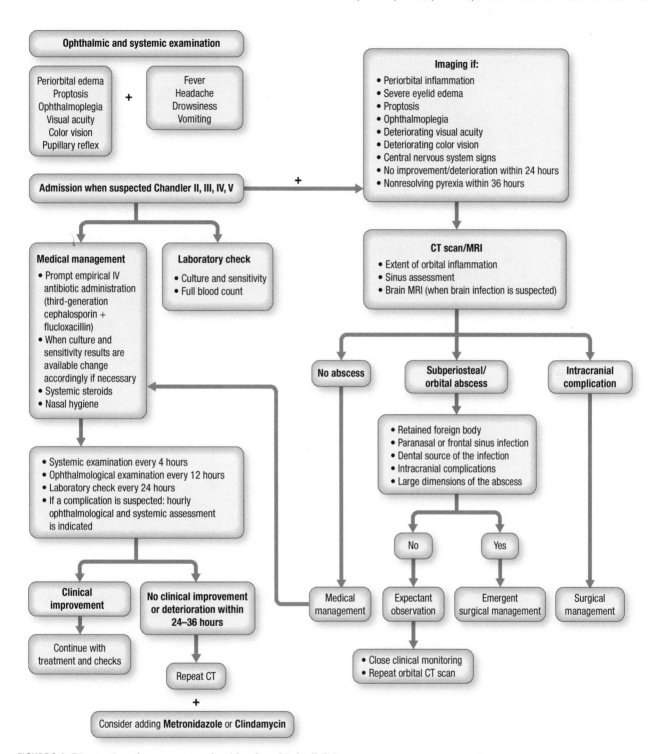

FIGURE 2.1: Diagnostic and management algorithm for orbital cellulitis.
Source: Adapted with permission from Elsevier, Inc. (2018). Orbital cellulitis. *Survey of Ophthalmology, 63*(4), 546.

TABLE 2.10: Recommendations for Management of Orbital Cellulitis

Antimicrobials *Parenteral* *(average 4 days) up to 1–2 weeks → Oral (1–4 week course)*	**Parenteral** (Gram-positive [MRSA] *plus* gram-negative coverage) Gram-positive coverage (MRSA) • Vancomycin IV 15 mg/kg q12h (normal renal function) if: (a) penicillin or cephalosporin allergy; (b) MRSA; (c) severe case; (d) skin source; (e) failed conventional therapy; (f) complicated (i.e., sinusitis, SPA) • Alternatives: Tetracycline derivatives, trimethoprim/sulfamethoxazole, clindamycin (watch given increased resistance) Gram-negative/-positive or community acquired (i.e., no recent hospitalization, nursing home): Ampicillin-sulbactam (3 g IV q6h) *or* piperacillin-tazobactam (4.5 g IV q8h *or* 3.375 g IV q6h) • If penicillin allergy: fluorquinolones (levofloxacin 750 mg IV daily, ciprofloxacin 400 mg IV q12h, *or* moxifloxacin 400 mg IV daily) Standard: Vancomycin (15 mg/kg q12h) *plus* 3rd generation cephalosporin (i.e., ceftriaxone 1–2 g IV daily) Severe: Vancomycin *plus* ceftriaxone 2 g IV daily *plus* metronidazole 500 mg IV q6-8h If intracranial involvement, ongoing pyrexia 24–36h, and/or complicated (i.e., sinusitis, SPA): Add anaerobic coverage (i.e., clindamycin *or* metronidazole) If unresponsive to standard therapy and high risk (e.g., immunocompromised): Add antifungal (i.e., amphotericin B, azoles); consider surgical debridement **Oral** Standard: Amoxicillin/clavulanate 875 mg PO q12h *or* cefpodoxime 200 mg PO q12h If MRSA suspected: (a) doxycycline 100 mg PO q12h (contraindicated in pregnancy); *or* (b) trimethoprim/sulfamethoxazole (160/800 mg) 1–2 tabs PO q12h; *or* (c) clindamycin 450 mg PO q6-8h; *or* (d) linezolid 600 mg PO BID
Corticosteroids	Advantages: Decreased postinfectious inflammation, proptosis, and pain Disadvantages: Fungal etiology, immunocompromised (delay healing, worsen immunosuppression)
Adjunct	If concomitant sinusitis: Consider adding (a) nasal hygiene; (b) nasal decongestants (e.g., oxymetazoline nasal spray BID); (c) intranasal corticosteroids If corneal exposure and chemosis: Consider adding erythromycin or bacitracin ointment QID If increased IOP, tight orbit and/or optic neuropathy: Consider cantholysis or canthotomy
Surgical Drainage	Approach: Conjunctival, percutaneous, or intranasal Indications: Presence of abscess (i.e., SPA) especially with (a) lack of clinical improvement 24–48h; (b) worsening orbital s/sx (e.g., ocular motility and pupillary abnormalities; optic or retinal nerve compromise); (c) intracranial complications; (d) co-existent ocular and otolaryngological infections; and/or (e) retained foreign body

IOP, intraocular pressure; MRSA, methicillin-resistant *Staphylococcus aureus*; SPA, subperiosteal abscess; s/sx, signs and symptoms.

Source: Data from Bagheri, N., & Wajda, B. N. (2017). *The Wills eye manual: Office and emergency room diagnosis and treatment of eye disease* (7th ed). Wolters Kluwer; Chen & Cioffi, 2019; Gordon, A. A., & Phelps, P. O. (2020). Management of preseptal and orbital cellulitis for the primary care physician. *Disease-a-Month, 66*(10), 101044. https://doi .org/10.1016/j.disamonth.2020.101044; Maeng, M. M., & Winn, B. J. (2019). Orbital infections and inflammations. In *The Columbia guide to basic elements of eye care* (pp. 355–371). Springer International Publishing. https://doi.org/10.1007/978-3-030-10886-1_32; Tsirouki, T., Dastiridou, A. I., Ibánez Flores, N., Cerpa, J. C., Moschos, M. M., Brazitikos, P., & Androudi, S. (2018). Orbital cellulitis. *Survey of Ophthalmology, 63*(4), 534–553. https://doi.org/10.1016/j.survophthal.2017.12.001; Yen, M. T., & Johnson, T. E. (2018). *Orbital cellulitis and periorbital infections*. Springer International Publishing. https://doi.org/10.1007/978-3-319-62606-2

and mucormycosis (Bagheri & Wajda, 2017; Gordon & Phelps, 2020; Maeng & Winn, 2019; Yen & Johnson, 2018). Oromaxillofacial surgery should be consulted if a dental source is suspected as it may be aggressive, potentially vision threatening, and may spread into the cavernous sinus (Bagheri & Wajda, 2017). A multidisciplinary approach involving oculoplastic surgeons, otolaryngologists, infectious disease experts, and neurosurgeons is required in those with intracranial complications (Tsirouki et al., 2018).

KEY TAKEAWAYS

■ Ophthalmoplegia, proptosis, and (downward) globe displacement are strongly suggestive of orbital cellulitis. However, the AGACNP should be aware of ocular signs (e.g., worsening visual acuity and pain) that may suggest abscess formation and extraocular signs (e.g., meningisms, cranial nerve palsies) that may suggest neurologic alinvolvement.

■ A CT scan is the gold standard for the diagnosis of orbital cellulitis and its complications.

■ Empiric antimicrobials should provide gram-positive (preferably including MRSA), gram-negative, and anaerobic coverage.

■ Abscess drainage is usually indicated if the patient is unresponsive to therapy, especially in the elderly who are at risk for developing polymicrobial abscess.

■ Corticosteroid use is controversial.

■ A multidisciplinary approach with expert consultation is necessary to facilitate recovery and mitigate complications in orbital cellulitis, especially in the presence of extraocular manifestations.

EVIDENCE-BASED RESOURCE

Tsirouki, T., Dastiridou, A. I., Ibánez Flores, N., Cerpa, J. C., Moschos, M. M., Brazitikos, P., & Androudi, S. (2018). Orbital cellulitis. *Survey of Ophthalmology, 63*(4), 534–553. https://doi.org/10.1016/j.survophthal.2017.12.001

2.9: RETINAL DETACHMENT

Helen Miley

Retinal detachment is an ophthalmologic emergency, caused by separation of the retina from the epithelium. The most common etiology is a retinal break called rhegmatogenous detachment. Risk factors include myopia, cataract surgery, and ocular trauma.

PRESENTING SIGNS AND SYMPTOMS

Retinal detachment causes no associated pain, and the patient often describes it as a "curtain" that causes loss of vision. It occurs suddenly and photopsias may also be present. Indirect ophthalmoscopy is necessary to diagnosis the detachment; direct funduscopy may not be sufficient to see the detachment.

DIFFERENTIAL DIAGNOSIS AND DIAGNOSTIC CONSIDERATIONS

Other possible etiologies for the preceding symptoms include abnormalities involving the vitreous, such as hemorrhage or inflammation. Examining the eye for an intraocular foreign body is also part of the differential. Direct funduscopic examination is a useful screening tool, but peripheral retinal detachments can be missed. Slit lamp testing with the eye in extreme positions of gaze is also helpful and should be done. Indirect ophthalmoscopy with pupillary dilation will assist with the diagnosis. Regardless of the possibilities, urgent consult is necessary with an ophthalmologist.

TREATMENT

There are several options for treatment: sealing agents, scleral buckling, pneumatic retinopexy or vitrectomy, all which require expertise of an ophthalmologist.

CLINICAL PEARLS

- Emergent consult with an ophthalmologist is indicated.

KEY TAKEAWAYS

- Any degree of retinal detachment will cause blurred vision and urgent consultation is necessary.

2.10: UVEITIS

Helen Miley

Uveitis is an inflammation of the intraocular uveal track that can be distinguished by location: anterior, intermediate, posterior, or panuveitis. More than 50% of the cases are idiopathic. Trauma, infection, and autoimmune diseases (e.g., spondyloarthropathies, herpes simplex or zoster virus, multiple sclerosis, sarcoidosis, tuberculous, syphilis, Lyme disease) are other etiologies that are noted (LaMattina, 2020).

PRESENTING SIGNS AND SYMPTOMS

The presenting symptoms include decreased vision, achy feeling in the eye, accompanied by redness and photophobia. Floaters may also be present. The symptoms can occur suddenly, have a variable duration, and may lead to chronicity (Table 2.11).

DIFFERENTIAL DIAGNOSIS AND DIAGNOSTIC CONSIDERATIONS

The diagnosis of uveitis is by clinical examination and symptomatology. Slit lap examination and ophthalmoscopy after pupillary dilation are recommended. The most frequent complication is the development of cataracts, glaucoma, retinal detachment, neovascularization of the retina, optic nerve or iris, macular edema and hypotony. Differential diagnoses include corneal inflammation, episcleritis, scleritis, and acute closed-angle glaucoma.

TREATMENT

Depending on the cause, uveitis is typically treated with topical or locally injected steroids (prednislone acetate) and a topical cycloplegic-mydriatic (e.g., cyclopentolate) drug. In the most severe cases, immunosuppressive drugs may be indicated, such as methotrexate. Complications include cataract, glaucoma, retinal detachment, neovascularization, edema, and hypotony.

TABLE 2.11: Signs and Symptoms of Uveitis

TYPE OF UVEITIS	SYMPTOMS	SIGNS
Anterior uveitis	Ocular ache Redness Photophobia Decreased vision	Hyperemia of the conjunctiva Slit lamp findings include clumping of WBCs
Intermediate uveitis	Floaters Decreased vision	Primary sign is the presence of cells in the vitreous humor "snowballs"
Posterior uveitis	Diverse symptoms	Signs include retinitis and optic disc edema
Panuveitis	Any combination of the preceding	

CLINICAL PEARLS

- Referral, treatment, and follow-up by an ophthalmologist is necessary.

KEY TAKEAWAYS

- Most cases are idiopathic but may be due to preexisting autoimmune diseases or infectious processes.

CONDITIONS OF THE EARS

2.11: HERPES ZOSTER OTICUS (RAMSAY-HUNT SYNDROME)

Helen Miley

Ramsay-Hunt syndrome is a major otologic complication of the reactivation of a varicella zoster viral infection that includes ipsilateral facial paralysis, ear pain, and the presence of vesicles in the auditory canal and auricle.

PRESENTING SIGNS AND SYMPTOMS

Clinically, the patient presents with a triad of ipsilateral facial paralysis, unilateral ear pain and hearing loss, headache, and vesicles in the auditory canal and auricle. Facial paralysis is often more severe than Bell's palsy , is attributed to herpes simplex virus (HSV), and has a decreased probability of complete recovery.

DIFFERENTIAL DIAGNOSIS AND DIAGNOSTIC CONSIDERATIONS

Diagnosis is made by physical exam and the presence of vesicles. Laboratory studies may include elevated WBC and erythrocyte sedimentation rate (ESR), plus viral cultures. If central nervous system (CNS) involvement is suspected, then spinal tap and CT/MRI of the cranium may be indicated to rule out structural lesions. Differential diagnoses include Bell's palsy, postherpetic neuralgia, and trigeminal neuralgia.

TREATMENT

Treatment includes oral corticosteroids and antiviral medications, pain control, and meticulous eye care. If severe, then systemic medications may be indicated.

CLINICAL PEARLS

- Prompt treatment of the HSV is the cornerstone of treatment.

KEY TAKEAWAY

- Hearing loss and facial paralysis are usually reversible with proper treatment.

2.12: MALIGNANT OTITIS EXTERNA

Helen Miley

Malignant otitis externa (MOE) is a life-threatening infection that involves migration to the temporal bone and other structures frequently occurring in immunocompromised patients and diabetics. MOE is a rare but aggressive disease that has been associated with a mortality rate of up to 80% (Danishyar & Ashurst, 2020; Isaacson, 2020; Shirai & Preciado, 2019).

PRESENTING SIGNS AND SYMPTOMS

The symptoms of MOE begin with ear pain and may progress to cranial nerve abnormalities (especially the 7th CN). Once that occurs, the prognosis is poor. The prominent physical examination finding is the presence of granulation tissue in the external auditory canal. The organism most commonly implicated in MOE is *Pseudomonas aeruginosa*. In patients who are immunocompromised, the most commonly implicated organisms includ, *Aspergillus*, *Staphylococcus aureus*, *Proteus mirabilis*, *Klebsiella oxytoca*, and *Candida* species. Imaging studies include CT and MRI. Fluoroquinolones (e.g., ciprofloxacin) must be initiated early, which may increase survival.

DIFFERENTIAL DIAGNOSIS AND DIAGNOSTIC CONSIDERATIONS

The path to diagnosis is clinical examination and CT of the temporal bone with biopsy. The AGACNP must rule out malignant tumors, such as squamous cell carcinoma.

TREATMENT

Treatment includes systemic antibiotics, topical antibiotic/steroid cream, and, in extreme cases, surgical debridement.

CLINICAL PEARLS

- Prompt diagnosis and treatment is necessary to prevent complications and decrease mortality.

KEY TAKEAWAYS

- Suspect this diagnosis in patients with severe relenting ear pain who are immunocompromised or have diabetes mellitus.

2.13: MASTOIDITIS

Donna Gullette

Acute mastoiditis is a complication of both acute (AOM) and chronic otitis media (COM) related to middle-ear infections that more commonly occur in pediatric populations rather than adults (Schwam et al., 2020). COM can lead to purulent infections of the middle ear, causing the bacteria to spread from the posterior section of the middle ear to the adjacent air space of the mastoid cavity (Laulajainen-Hongisto et al., 2016; Olaf & Duguet, 2019). The middle-ear and mastoid air spaces are continuous, thus creating a pathway for bacteria from AOM to cause mastoiditis. The proximity of the mastoid, eustachian tube, and middle ear is the key in the pathogenesis of mastoiditis. Purulent material trapped within the mastoid cavity causes acute mastoiditis with periostitis (inflammation of the periosteum). During this stage of infection, the patient will complain of fever, otolgia, postauricular tenderness, and/or upper respiratory symptoms. During physical examination of the affected ear, there may be erythema, bulging tympanic membranes (TMs), and swelling or protrusion of the auricle. If the acute infection does not clear, then the patient may develop coalescent mastoiditis.

With coalescent mastoiditis, the pneumatic cells can coalesce into larger cavities filled with purulent material, causing an abscess to develop (Tsementzis, 2019). The abscess can drain on its own if the patient has had a previously perforated TM. Coalescent mastoiditis can be diagnosed with a temporal bone CT that reveals erosion of the mastoid walls (Tsementzis, 2019).

In addition to mastoiditis, some of the other intratemporal complications include petrositis (inflammation of the petrous portion of the temporal bone), facial paralysis, and labyrinthitis. Further intracranial complications can develop, causing meningitis, abscesses, or sinus thrombosis (Tsementzis, 2019).

Since the advent of antibiotics, there have been fewer complications of intracranial abscesses associated with otitis media and less chronic otitis media (COM). Acute otitis media (AOM) can be successfully treated with oral amoxicillin and nasal decongestants. Amoxicillin is given orally, 1 g every 8 hours for 5 to 7 days. Other antibiotics—such as amoxicillin clavulanate 875/125 mg or 2 g ER orally every 12 hours for 5 to 10 days, or cefuroxime 500 mg orally every 12 hours for 5 to 7 days—may be used as alternatives to amoxicillin, particularly if resistance is suspected. The most common causative organisms associated with AOM in adults are *H. influenzae, S. pneumoniae, and S. pyrogens* (Lustig & Schindler, 2021, p. 215). However, not all patients with AOM will have a positive culture.

In a study of 160 adult patients hospitalized for treatment of mastoiditis, 38% had AOM, and 33% had acute mastoiditis (Laulajainen-Hongisto et al., 2016). The most common organism found among those with AOM and acute mastoiditis was *S. pyrogens*. Patients who cultured positive for Group A *Streptococcus* had more severe cases and required hospitalization (Laulajainen-Hongisto et al., 2016). All patients received parenteral antimicrobials including cefuroxime, ceftriaxone, and/or metronidazole (Laulajainen-Hongisto et al., 2016). Forty-four percent of patients had a mastiodectomy related to latent mastoiditis, defined as COM longer than 1 year with previous treatment with oral antibiotics (Laulajainen-Hongisto et al., 2016).

PRESENTING SIGNS AND SYMPTOMS

Acute Otitis Media

AOM generally occurs after an upper respiratory infection. Adults present with otalgia, fullness in the affected ear, and decreased hearing, and may have fever. Physical findings are erythema of the tympanic membrane (TM), which may bulge outward if the infection is severe, and decreased mobility. Severe bulging may represent TM rupture. The rupture provides instant relief of pain, accompanied with otorrhea.

Chronic Otitis Media

COM and mastoiditis develop from recurrent otitis media and can result from trauma. Patients with otitis media present with otalgia, otorrhea, fever, and headache (Heah et al., 2016). COM can cause benign intracranial hypertension secondary to the spreading inflammation into the sinuses. The infective organisms are different from AOM. The most common organisms that cause COM are *P. aeruginosa, Proteus* species, and mixed anaerobic bacteria. The hallmark characteristic of COM is purulent otorrhea from the affected ear (Heah et al., 2016). Pain is typically not present with COM but hearing loss may be present.

Most cases of COM will require removal of infected particles, use of ear plugs to prevent water from entering the area, and topical antibiotics such as ofloxacin 0.3% solution or ciprofloxacin with dexamethasone. If the culture is positive for *Pseudomonas*, ciprofloxacin 500 mg orally, twice daily for 1 to 6 weeks, will help dry the drainage from the ear.

Mastoiditis in adults presents with severe otalgia, fever, and headache. Physical examination reveals postauricular erythema, warmth, tenderness, and protrusion. The otoscopic examination shows swelling of the auditory canal, bulging and purulence behind the TM (Sahi et al., 2020). In cases where the TM is normal, this usually eliminates the diagnosis of acute mastoiditis.

HISTORY AND PHYSICAL FINDINGS

Patents who have eustachian tube dysfunction secondary to an upper respiratory tract infection (URI) can develop AOM. Compression of the eustachian tube can lead to accumulation of fluid, which traps bacteria and causes a middle-ear effusion. Adults with AOM present without fever but with otalgia, erythema of the TM, and hearing loss. The TM may be bulging or appear cloudy, yellowish, or opaque (Schwam et al., 2020). The ear canal, if obstructed with cerumen, should be removed with curettage to clearly visualize the TM.

In COM, patients present with purulent drainage from the ear, otalgia, with or without fever. The facial

TABLE 2.12: Medical Management of Otitis Media and Mastoiditis

CONDITION	TREATMENT[a]	COMPLICATIONS	REFERRAL
Acute otitis media	Amoxicillin-clavulanate 875 mg/125 orally twice daily for 7–10 days. High dose amoxicillin may be needed for those with high-risk comorbidities.[a] If allergic, use cefuroxime 500 mg orally twice daily. If allergic to cephalosporins, use doxycycline 100 mg every 12 hours or azithromycin 500 mg orally for 1 day then 250 mg orally for 5 days.	May be recurrent; leads to chronic otitis media or mastoiditis.	Surgical drainage (myringotomy or mastoidectomy) by a qualified surgeon.
Chronic otitis media	Removal of purulent material; ofloxacin 0.30% drops or ciprofloxacin with dexamethasone; or ciprofloxacin 500 mg orally twice daily for 1 to 6 weeks.	Mastoiditis; antibiotics help dry up drainage.	Referral to ENT specialists for treatment and surgery.
Mastoiditis	IV cefazolin 0.5–1 g every 6 to 8 hours.	Results from inadequate antimicrobial therapy.	Surgical drainage mastoidectomy if no improvement in 48 hours.
Petrous apictitis	Prolong antimicrobial therapy directed at the culture results.	Persistent infection and drainage from the middle ear; foul-smelling drainage; retroorbital pain; facial paralysis 6th cranial nerve; meningitis.	Surgical drainage—pertrous apcicectomy.

[a]Treatment recommendations data from Gilbert, D. N., Chambers, H. F., Eliopoulos, G. M., Saag, M. S., & Pavia, A. T. (2020). *The Sanford guide to antimicrobial therapy 2020* (50th ed.). Antimicrobial Therapy, Inc.; Limb, C. J., Lustig, L. R., & Durand, M. L. (2021). *Acute otitis media in adults*. UpToDate. http://www.uptodate.com

nerve can be involved with COM, and therefore an examination of the facial nerves should be performed. Some of the complications associated with COM include TM perforation, conductive hearing loss, labyrinthitis, facial nerve paralysis, acute mastoiditis, and intracranial infections (Laulajainen-Hongisto et al., 2016).

In acute mastoiditis, patients present with otalgia, fever, postauricular erythema, swelling, and tenderness. A CT should be obtained to determine the extent of bone damage. An emergent ENT consultation should be requested, and the patient admitted to the hospital for IV vancomycin and ceftriaxone. Patients being treated for acute mastoiditis should be monitored carefully during the first 48 hours for deterioration; should that occur, then surgical intervention of mastoidectomy is required (Sahi et al., 2020).

DIFFERENTIAL DIAGNOSIS AND DIAGNOSTIC CONSIDERATIONS

The differential diagnoses for AOM include cellulitis, otitis media with effusion (OME), COM, external otitis (otitis externa), herpes zoster infection, lymphadenopathy, trauma, tumor, or head and neck infections (Sahi et al., 2020). OME can be misdiagnosed as AOM. The difference between AOM and OME is that, in OME, fluid is present in the middle ear, but there are no signs of infection. OME is generally associated with eustachian tube dysfunction and a feeling of fullness. Most of the cases of OME resolve without antibiotics in 12 weeks. In adults, seasonal allergies can induce OME. These patients benefit from nasal saline, decongestants, nasal steroids (such

as fluticasone), or a combination of these. Patients should avoid airline travel because of potential trauma to the ear during flight. Patients who fail to achieve resolution of the effusion in 12 weeks should be referred for evaluation by otologists.

Diagnostic Testing

Patients presenting with mastoiditis may need additional laboratory work including CBC, ESR, and C-reactive protein (CRP). It is not uncommon to find leukocytosis with a shift to the left. CT imaging of the mastoid may demonstrate bony separation, extension of infection, fluid, thickening of periosteum, and/or abscess (Sahi et al., 2020).

TREATMENT

Depending on the type of otitis media, different oral and IV antibiotics, steroids, and topical agents are used. Table 2.12 outlines the recommended medical management for these conditions.

TRANSITION OF CARE

Patients with mastoiditis should be instructed to go to an emergency department that has ENT specialists on staff since most patients will require hospitalization. Patients with mastoiditis requiring surgical mastoidectomy must be treated with IV antibiotics for an average of 4 days (Laulajainen-Hongisto et al., 2016). The patient will be discharged home with oral antibiotics based on culture results.

Patients, once discharged from the hospital, should follow up with an ENT provider for evaluation. These patients should also have immunizations, particularly the pneumonia vaccine, updated by their primary care provider.

CLINICAL PEARLS

- Timely and appropriate treatment of inner-ear infections prevents complications of mastoiditis.
- Use of ultrasound in screening for mastoiditis may be of benefit in early diagnosis prior to CT scanning and help to control cost.
- Diabetes mellitus increases the risk for development of mastoiditis and otitis media.

2.14: VERTIGO, BENIGN PAROXYSMAL POSITIONAL

Helen Miley

Benign paroxysmal positional vertigo (BPPV) is a common form of vertigo, accounting for nearly one half of patients with peripheral vestibular dysfunction present. The incidence increases with age (over 60 years) and it is more common in women. It is most commonly attributed to calcium debris within the posterior semicircular canal, known as canalithiasis. While symptoms can be troublesome, the disorder usually responds to treatment with particle-repositioning maneuvers, an office-based procedure and one that patients can be taught to perform at home (Power et al., 2020; Yoon et al., 2018).

PRESENTING SIGNS AND SYMPTOMS

Recurrent episodes of vertigo that last 1 minute or less, provoked by head movements such as looking up, getting up from bed, rolling over in bed is the most common symptom. It can be associated with nausea and vomiting. The vertigo lasts less than 60 seconds.

DIFFERENTIAL DIAGNOSIS AND DIAGNOSTIC CONSIDERATIONS

Observing nystagmus during a provoking maneuver (Dix-Hallpike maneuver) solidifies the diagnosis of BPPV with the typical history. The Dix-Hallpike maneuver is simple to perform. With the patient sitting up, extend the neck to one side. Then rapidly place the patient supine, so that the head hangs off the bed for 30 seconds. Look for nystagmus. If no nystagmus is observed, return the patient to the upright position and repeat on the opposite side. If no nystagmus is noted when the head is turned to either side, then the test is negative for BPPV.

Differential diagnoses will include postural hypotension, chronic unilateral vestibular hypofunction, vestibular paroxysmia, vestibular migraines, central positional vertigo, or rotational vertebral artery syndrome.

TREATMENT

Treatment options for BPPV involves canalith repositioning maneuvers that involve moving the head through a series of specific positions intended to return the errant canalith to the utricle.

CLINICAL PEARLS

- BBPV is a common cause of peripheral vertigo.
- Observing nystagmus is the key diagnostic tool.
- No medication is effective; best to treat with repositioning maneuvers.

KEY TAKEAWAYS

- Occurs secondary to otoconial crystal in the semicircular canal.
- Symptoms are exacerbated by head movements.
- Canalith-repositioning maneuvers will alleviate the symptoms.

CONDITIONS OF THE NOSE

2.15: EPISTAXIS

R. Brandon Frady

Epistaxis is estimated to have a single lifetime occurrence in 60% of people in the United States (Pallin et al., 2005). Approximately 6% of those with a nosebleed will seek medical care resulting in 1.7 ED visits per 1000 U.S. residents (Pallin et al., 2005). Epistaxis is bimodal, occurring young in life and recurring at higher rates after the fifth decade of life. Patients 70 to 79 years have a sixfold increase in epistaxis episodes compared to 20- to 39-year-olds (Pallin et al., 2005). Of patients seen in the ED, approximately 27,000 hospitalizations occur annually (Pallin et al., 2005). The likelihood of hospitalization for epistaxis increases on average 1.4% with each decade of life (Pallin et al., 2005). Epistaxis mortality rates trend low. However, morbidity rates are higher in patients 70 years and older, especially those with cardiovascular comorbidities (Krulewitz & Fix, 2019; Tunkel et al., 2020a). Over 85% of epistaxis cases are atraumatic in nature (Pallin et al., 2005). A recent study from the United Kingdom suggests a 30-day all-cause mortality rate. Those who died were admitted to the hospital and had cardiovascular comorbidities, diabetes, or bleeding diathesis (Integrate [The National ENT Trainee Research Network], 2018). The direct mortality cause was not the epistaxis but the underlying comorbid condition (Integrate [The National ENT Trainee Research Network], 2018).

Epistaxis occurs in the anterior or posterior area of the nasopharynx. The distinction between anterior and posterior is essential to the assessment and interventions of epistaxis. Anterior origins of bleeding are more common, and posterior epistaxis is more challenging to treat and is often associated with arterial bleeding (Krulewitz & Fix, 2019). Anterior bleeding at Kiesselbach's plexus occurs in 80% to 90% of patients. Anterior bleeding occurs more often in the healthcare setting, but posterior bleeding more often results in hospitalization. The posterior bleeds arise from sphenopalatine and the terminal branches of the maxillary arteries. In addition to the location of bleeding, the classification of primary versus secondary is vital to the management of epistaxis (Krulewitz & Fix, 2019).

Primary epistaxis is often iatrogenic, occurring spontaneously. It may be associated with environmental factors such as living in colder climates or drier winter months. The reduced humidity and increased heating in the home contribute to drier air and increased evaporation in the nasal passages leading to epistaxis (Krulewitz & Fix, 2019). Eighty-five percent of anterior epistaxis is associated with the primary classification. Secondary epistaxis is associated with trauma, metabolic disorders, autoimmune disorders, vascular abnormalities, neoplasms, inflammation, congenital nasal malformations, anticoagulation, and antiplatelet medications (Krulewitz & Fix, 2019). One study found that 87% of syndromes associated with platelets, blood vessels, and coagulation factors had related epistaxis (Guha et al., 2019). Some patients have a high risk for the development of epistaxis. Box 2.1 outlines common predisposing factors for epistaxis.

PRESENTING SIGNS AND SYMPTOMS

Patients with epistaxis typically present to the hospital with overt bleeding from their nasal cavity. Patients with anterior bleeding typically have blood from a single nare compared to posterior bleeding from both nares. The development of blood clots may worsen the symptoms of shortness of breath and/or difficulty in breathing. Patients may have hematemesis or hemoptysis if large amounts of blood in the posterior pharynx region

are aspirated or swallowed. Hemodynamic assessment may reveal tachycardia, hypotension, and or delayed capillary refill in patients experiencing hemodynamic compromise. Patients with frequent or recurrent epistaxis may complain of persistent dry nose, frequent nasal infections, difficulty breathing through the nose, and difficulty with smell and taste.

HISTORY AND PHYSICAL EXAM FINDINGS

History and physical exam is focused initially on the rapid treatment of epistaxis. AGACNPs should focus on the location of bleeding, the onset of bleeding, estimation of blood loss (based on patient reporting), and chronicity of epistaxis (Morgan & Kellerman, 2014). A more comprehensive history and physical examination should focus on conditions that make bleeding worse or increase bleeding frequency once the patient is stabilized.

Chief Complaint and History of Present illness

Chief complaints are associated with active nose bleeding but may include coughing up blood and/or vomiting blood. The history of present illness should consist of the onset of bleeding, the length of time of bleeding, and any intervention that was attempted before arrival and was successful in stopping the bleeding for any time. Additionally, the assessment of comorbid conditions is essential to the ongoing treatment of epistaxis. Hypertension, anticoagulation, and antiplatelet therapies increase the bleeding frequency and significance (Khan et al., 2017).

Review of Systems

Pertinent positives include nose bleeding and may contain hematemesis, hemoptysis, nausea, vomiting, and diarrhea. If the epistaxis is significant, the patient may have airway compromise and exhibit shortness of breath and difficulty breathing. While evaluating the patient, it is essential to establish a pattern and frequency of epistaxis. Additional historical findings are bleeding disorders, bleeding after surgery, NSAID use, anticoagulation use, nasal spray use, cocaine use, oxygen use (especially without humidification), and trauma. Patients with significant or prolonged bleeding and a history of cardiovascular or pulmonary problems may develop worsening of shortness of breath, dyspnea, chest pain/pressure, arm or jaw pain, and syncope.

Physical Exam

Physical exam findings should rapidly focus on airway, breathing, and circulation to confirm the patient is able to protect the airway, have effective breathing, and are hemodynamically stable. After initial stabilization, the location of bleeding (anterior vs. posterior) position the patient for nasal rhinoscopy. The AGACNP needs to ensure that personal protective equipment (PPE) is used during the rhinoscopy. PPE should include standard precautions plus eye shielding. It may be necessary to place a pledget soaked with a vasoconstrictor and anesthetic

BOX 2.1 PREDISPOSING RISK FACTORS FOR EPISTAXIS

- Nasal trauma
- Rhinitis
- Nasal mucosal drying (Unhumidified oxygen, winter weather, low humidity)
- Deviated septum
- Atherosclerotic heart disease
- Hereditary hemorrhagic telangiectasia
- Inhaled cocaine use
- Alcohol use
- Trauma
- Anticoagulation medications
- Antiplatelet medications

agent to control bleeding and enhance the nasal passage assessment (Krulewitz & Fix, 2019; Morgan & Kellerman, 2014; Tunkel et al., 2020a). If blood clots obscure the visualization, asking the patient to blow their nose may clear clotting and improve visualization.

DIFFERENTIAL DIAGNOSIS AND DIAGNOSTIC CONSIDERATIONS

The differential diagnoses for epistaxis include associations with trauma, metabolic derangements, autoimmune disorders, vascular abnormalities, iatrogenic causes, and idiopathic, neoplasm, inflammatory, and congenital disorders (Krulewitz & Fix, 2019; Morgan & Kellerman, 2014; Tunkel et al., 2020a). Box 2.2 provides an expanded list of differentials.

Diagnostic Data

Patients with epistaxis do not routinely require laboratory or diagnostic studies. For patients that are on vitamin K antagonist, the international normalized ratio (INR) may be beneficial. If the patient is on a direct oral anticoagulant (DOAC), the INR may not be as helpful as the INR could be falsely elevated. For the patient with excessive bleeding and or instability, a CBC, comprehensive metabolic panel, and type and screen are reasonable (Krulewitz & Fix, 2019; Morgan & Kellerman, 2014).

Patients who continue to experience bleeding after compression, nasal packing, and nasal cautery may need a CT angiogram to determine if a supply artery's embolization is necessary to control bleeding (Krajina & Chrobok, 2014; Tunkel et al., 2020a).

TREATMENT

Initial epistaxis management should focus on rapid assessment and determination of airway maintenance, hemodynamic stability, and bleeding severity or significance (Morgan & Kellerman, 2014; Tunkel et al., 2020a). Treatment for epistaxis focuses on control of the bleeding (Figure 2.2). All patients presenting with a nosebleed should have external compression of the nares for a minimum of 5 minutes. AGACNPs treating patients with hemodynamic compromise and or severe bleeding will initiate IV fluid resuscitation, CBC, and type and cross match for blood product administration along with nasal compression (Morgan & Kellerman, 2014). There is significant variation in external compression timing literature (Iqbal et al., 2017; Khan et al., 2017; Krulewitz & Fix, 2019; Tunkel et al., 2020a). Apply compression to the cartilage region of the nose just below the bone. In addition to external compression, the patient is seated leaning forward to minimize swallowing and or aspirating blood. A key component to treating epistaxis is the visualization of the nares to determine the source of bleeding. Differentiating between anterior and posterior bleeding is key to the overall management of epistaxis. The bleeding location is not always exact

---

BOX 2.2 EXPANDED DIFFERENTIAL DIAGNOSES FOR EPISTAXIS

- Trauma
  - Digital
  - Facial
  - Foreign body
  - Septal perforation
  - Barotrauma
- Metabolic derangements
  - Hepatic dysfunction
  - Renal failure
  - Uremia
  - Alcohol
- Autoimmune disorders
  - Hemophilia
  - Leukemia
  - von Willebrand disease
- Vascular abnormalities
  - Hereditary hemorrhagic telangiectasia
  - Cardiovascular disease
  - Diabetes
  - Hypertension
  - Granulomatosis with polyangiitis

- Iatrogenic
  - Post-surgical
  - Nasal tube passage
- Medications
  - Anticoagulation
  - Antiplatelet
  - NSAIDs
- Idiopathic
  neoplasm
  - Juvenile angiofibroma
  - Nasopharyngeal carcinoma
  - Squamous cell cancer
  - Paranasal tumor
- Inflammatory
  - Rhinosinusitis
  - Nasal polyps
- Congenital
  - Septal deviation
  - Septal spur

Source: Data from Krulewitz, N. A., & Fix, M. L. (2019). Epistaxis. *Emergency Medicine Clinics of North America, 37*(1), 29–39. https://doi.org/10.1016/j.emc.2018.09.005

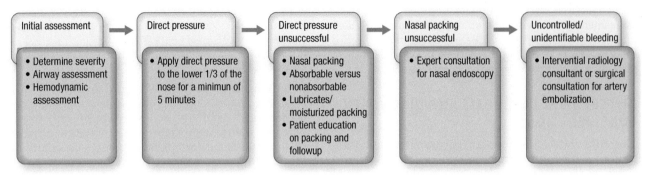

FIGURE 2.2: Epistaxis treatment algorithm.

on presentation and may not be appreciable during the initial management.

Anterior Bleeding

The majority of nose bleeds are anterior. After manual compression for a minimum of 5 minutes, the evaluation of ongoing bleeding, development of blood clots in the nose, and revaluation of continued bleeding are essential to the continued management of anterior bleeding. After hemostasis, the patient may need to blow their nose to clear clotting to allow for visual inspection for the location of bleeding. If there is residual bleeding, or if overt bleeding resumes while attempting to identify the source, the AGACNP should consider the use of intranasal topical vasoconstrictors, topical anesthetics, and moisturizing agents to control bleeding. Topical vasoconstrictors may be directly sprayed into the nose, placed on cotton balls, or placed on pledgets and placed into the nose to assist with control and assessment of the location of bleeding. Box 2.3 outlines recommended topical vasoconstrictors. In addition to topical vasoconstrictors, topical anesthetics are useful if patients have discomfort during the hemostasis process or nasal examination process. If anterior bleeding is not controlled, nasal packing with an absorbable or nonabsorbable packing soaked with a vasoconstrictor, moisture/lubricating agent, and an anesthetic agent may control bleeding (Krulewitz & Fix, 2019; Morgan & Kellerman, 2014; Tunkel et al., 2020a; Williams et al., 2017). If compression and

---

BOX 2.3 COMMON TOPICAL MEDICATIONS FOR EPISTAXIS

Oxymetazoline 0.05%
Phenylephrine 0.5%
Epinephrine 1:1000
Cocaine 4%
Tranexamic acid

Source: Data from Krulewitz, N. A., & Fix, M. L. (2018). Epistaxis. *Emergency Medicine Clinics of North America*, 37(1), 29–39. https://doi.org/10.1016/j.emc.2018.09.005

---

topical vasoconstriction fail to achieve hemostasis, nasal cautery is the next appropriate intervention.

Cautery can be either chemical with silver nitrate or electrical. A silver nitrate stick is touched to the site of bleeding (Krulewitz & Fix, 2019; Morgan & Kellerman, 2014). Any cautery techniques should be limited to the smallest area possible and the shortest time possible. There is a risk of septal perforation with prolonged use of cautery techniques (Krulewitz & Fix, 2019). If cautery fails, anterior packing is the next best approach. Packing with resorbable (preferred in patients with antiplatelet or anticoagulation therapy) or nonresorbable material is currently accepted to treat persistent bleeding. Traditional packing is falling out of favor for more commercially available nasal tampon packing devices. These products are generally easy to insert and are readily available in the ED. Anterior packing should be lubricated with antibiotic ointment or petroleum jelly prior to insertion to aid in the insertion and to help prevent toxic shock syndrome associated with *Staphylococcus aureus*. Packing should remain in the nares for a minimum of 24 hours. Common side effects associated with nasal packing include pain, nasal crusting, and compromised breathing.

Packing soaked with tranexamic acid (TXA) is an option for patients that need nasal packing after failed or incomplete cautery. A 2016 systematic literature review reported limited studies on TXA use in epistaxis; however, there is an increasing body of literature on the use of topical TXA in the treatment of epistaxis (Kamhieh & Fox, 2016). With nasal packing, patient education should include the length of time the packing remains in place if nonresorbable. For resorbable packing, patient education includes how long the packing will take to dissolve. Additionally, patient education should be provided on the signs and symptoms of toxic shock symptoms (Krulewitz & Fix, 2019). If the patient continues to bleed despite the preceding interventions, posterior bleeding should be considered as the epistaxis source and expert consultation should be sought.

Posterior Bleeding

The posterior bleeding diagnosis is made if bleeding is uncontrolled by anterior treatment strategies, bleeding is from both nares, and there is hematemesis, hemoptysis, nausea, and vomiting. Treatment of posterior bleeding includes a balloon tampon (using a Foley catheter or similar), nasal tampons designed for posterior use, or inflatable balloon catheters (Krulewitz & Fix, 2019; Morgan & Kellerman, 2014; Tunkel et al., 2020b). Posterior packing is painful and may require procedural sedation and pain management. Generally, these balloons are inserted, inflated, and retraction is applied to seat the balloon in the posterior oropharynx. Ensuring lubrication to facilitate insertion and prevent toxic shock during posterior bleeding management is a cornerstone of therapy. Patients requiring intervention for posterior bleeding should be hospitalized for observation and ongoing management. The patient should be monitored for airway, breathing, and hemodynamic compromise while the nasal tampon or balloon is in place. Posterior bleeding patients are more challenging to control and may require angiogram and arterial embolization by an interventional radiologist (Krajina & Chrobok, 2014). Embolization of the distal branches of the bilateral internal maxillary artery and ipsilateral distal branches of the facial artery is preferred (Krajina & Chrobok, 2014).

The initial evaluation of patients with epistaxis should include a CBC, coagulation studies (including prothrombin time, partial thromboplastin time, international normalized raio [INR], fibrinogen, type, and cross or screen depending on the hemodynamic stability and the significance of bleeding). Patients that fail compression, nasal packing, nasal cautery, or have posterior bleeding should be referred to an ear, nose, and throat (ENT) specialist.

Once hemostasis is achieved, patients should be educated on avoiding straining, sneezing, vigorous exercise, avoidance of hot, dry environments, and prevention of nasal trauma for 3 to 5 days. Based on the instrumentation needed to control bleeding, patients may need a 5-day antibiotic course focused on treating staphylococcal organisms.

CLINICAL PEARLS

- Epistaxis requires rapid assessment and intervention.
- The initial management for epistaxis is nasal compression.
- Assess for anterior bleeding versus posterior bleeding.
- If compression, cautery, and nasal packing fail, consult ENT.

KEY TAKEAWAYS

- The majority of epistaxis is related to trauma.
- Epistaxis is bimodal, occurring in the young and the elderly.
- Initial treatment of epistaxis should be direct nasal pressure.
- Early consultation with ENT.

EVIDENCE-BASED RESOURCE

Clinical Practice Guideline: Nosebleed (Epistaxis) (Tunkel et al., 2020a).

2.16: RHINITIS, ALLERGIC AND NONALLERGIC

Leanne H. Fowler

Rhinitis is an inflammatory condition of the nasal mucosa that can be categorized into allergic or nonallergic etiological types (Table 2.13). Presentations of rhinitis are allergic, nonallergic, or a combination of both allergic and nonallergic causes of rhinitis. Allergic rhinitis (AR) is the most common type of rhinitis and is one of the most common chronic medical conditions in the United States. The highest prevalence of AR is among children; however, adolescents, adults, and older adults are also affected. AR can be intermittent (formerly known as seasonal) or persistent (formerly known as perennial), affects over 19.2 million adults (18 years old and older), and is responsible for over 12 million provider office visits annually (Centers for Disease Control and Prevention [CDC], 2018a). Nonallergic rhinitis can be an acute or chronic medical condition and can be subcategorized as infectious, eosinophilic, vasomotor, or miscellaneous etiological type (Shah & Emanuel, 2020). AGACNPs may encounter patients ranging from adolescents to older adults suffering complex chronic, acute, or acute on chronic presentations of rhinitis. This section explores the evaluation and evidence-based management of rhinitis, and pertinent implications for AGACNP practice in any healthcare setting.

TABLE 2.13: Allergic and Nonallergic Types of Rhinitis

RHINITIS TYPE	ETIOLOGY
Allergic rhinitis	Intermittent (seasonal) Persistent (perennial) Mixed (seasonal and perennial)

Nonallergic rhinitis	Infectious
	  Viral
	Chemical exposure
	  Cigarette smoke, garden sprays, ammonia, occupational chemicals, cocaine, etc.
	Vasomotor
	  Odors, temperature changes, chemical exposures, alcohol use, etc.
	Eosinophilic (NARES)
	  Polyposis
	Medicamentosa
	  Chronic over-the-counter nasal vasoconstriction sprays
	Miscellaneous
	  Pregnancy-induced

NARES, nonallergic rhinitis with eosinophilia.

The nose serves as an anatomical structure of the upper airway providing the warming, humidifying, and cleaning of the air inspired while using less energy than if a person were mouth breathing. The nose is a structure comprised of cartilage and turbinate bones that are all lined with ciliated mucosa made of columnar epithelium with stromal and inflammatory cells, nerves, blood vessels (fed from the internal and external carotid arteries), and seromucous glands. Nasal mucus consists of two layers overlying the epithelial surface. The deep layer of mucus is thin whereas the superficial layer is more viscous and acts to trap inhaled particles, infectious agents, and foreign substances. The superficial layer of mucus is rich with inflammatory mediators and leukocytes acting to protect the individual from infection or other foreign matter.

PRESENTING SIGNS AND SYMPTOMS

Allergic and nonallergic rhinitis involve acute and/or chronic inflammatory processes that are triggered by allergens or other foreign matter from the environment. In the pathophysiology of the acute and chronic inflammatory processes already described, the only difference is the duration of inflammation. Inflammation associated with rhinitis lasting longer than 2 weeks is considered chronic (Huether & McCance, 2019). Regardless of the duration, the basic functions of the inflammatory processes in persons with rhinitis occur as a part of a human's innate immunity and defense mechanisms in response to cellular or tissue damage. Within seconds of the injury, the process of inflammation causes (a) vasodilation which aids to increase rich immunocompetent blood flow to the area; (b) increased vascular permeability which facilitates edema and increased blood flow of immunocompetent cells and chemicals into the injured tissue; and (c) white blood cell adherence to vessel walls to help protect the site of injury (Huether & McCance, 2019). The inflammatory processes are responsible for many of the signs and symptoms patients who are experiencing allergic or nonallergic rhinitis have.

Allergic Rhinitis

The symptoms characteristically associated with AR include sneezing, nasal itching, nasal congestion, and rhinorrhea. AR is most prevalent in males younger than 20 years of age and all genders younger than 40 years of age (Shah & Emanuel, 2020). Etiological factors associated with AR occur secondary to an overactive immune response to repeated contact with substances such as pollen, mold spores, pet dander, dust mites, stinging insects, and some foods. The allergic response causes an excessive IgE-mediated reaction (atopic response) to allergens and induces an inflammatory response. Although AR is not a life-threatening illness, the effects of the illness can range from being annoying to being disabling to an individual by negatively affecting sleep, energy levels, and enjoyment of social activities.

Furthermore, AR is often associated with other chronic conditions that can be disabling such as asthma, rhinosinusitis, nasal polyposis, or otitis media with effusion (OME). AR can be classified as intermittent or persistent.

Intermittent Allergic Rhinitis

Patients presenting with intermittent AR report symptoms of sneezing, watery and red eyes, watery rhinorrhea, itchy eyes, ears, nose, and throat, and nasal congestion during high pollinated or high mold seasons. Symptoms can be worse in the morning and exacerbated by dry and windy conditions.

Persistent Allergic Rhinitis

The signs and symptoms associated with persistent AR are usually constant, present for more than 4 weeks, and vary in intensity during certain seasons (Seidman et al., 2015). Patients most often present with chronic nasal congestion and/or blockage and postnasal drip. Complaints of itchy, red, and watery eyes, sneezing, or a runny nose are less common but can occur during season exacerbations or an increased exposure to allergens (e.g., pet dander, dust mites). Food allergies can contribute to persistent AR but are most often associated with GI or anaphylaxis symptoms. Persistent AR triggered by food allergies are more common during infancy and childhood (Shah & Emanuel, 2020).

Nonallergic Rhinitis

A variety of etiological factors contribute to the presentation of nonallergic rhinitis. Infectious nonallergic rhinitis is most often caused by viruses associated with the common cold and can present with watery clear or white rhinorrhea, sneezing, and nasal congestion. Viral rhinitis is also often associated with nonnasal symptoms of a headache, malaise, body aches, sore throat, and nonproductive cough.

Chemical exposures causing nonallergic rhinitis can present with clear and runny rhinorrhea, sneezing, reduced airflow, or nasal dryness. Cigarette smoke exposure, especially repeated exposure seen with persons living with chronic tobacco use disorder, causes chronic decreased ciliary function placing the person at a higher risk for chronic nonallergic rhinitis, infection, and other upper airway disorders. Removal or avoidance of smoke exposure contributes to the person regaining ciliary function of the nasal mucosa.

Vasomotor rhinitis is a nonallergic type of rhinitis that has a similar presentation to the type caused by chemical exposures but is thought to be secondary to abnormal autonomic regulation of the nose (Shah & Emanuel, 2020). Persons with vasomotor rhinitis experience symptoms with environmental temperature changes, the eating of spicy foods, strong odors or inhalation of chemicals, and alcohol consumption.

Nonallergic rhinitis with eosinophilia (NARES) presents as a syndrome of symptoms and is associated with obstructive sinusitis secondary to polyposis. Patients can present with acute on chronic symptoms including nasal congestion, nasal obstruction, headache, and sinus pain to name a few. Nasal smears yield marked eosinophilia when the patient does not produce allergies to inhaled allergens during skin or in vitro testing.

Rhinitis medicamentosa is directly related to the patient's use of over-the-counter vasoconstricting nasal sprays to self-medicate for nasal congestion. With repeated use or increased doses of nasal decongestants beyond the recommended timeframe and doses, tachyphylaxis occurs. Consequently, the patient experiences rebound rhinitis and worsening nasal congestion that can lead to severe nasal obstruction when the effect of the medication subsides.

There are multiple miscellaneous types of nonallergic rhinitis. This section focuses on the type associated with pregnancy. Nonallergic rhinitis during pregnancy is most common during the second and third trimesters of pregnancy. Hyaluronic acid levels rise within the nasal mucosa secondary to the rise in estrogen during pregnancy and cause an increase of nasal edema, nasal mucus production, and decreased cilia function. Consequently, the pregnant female experiences nasal congestion and obstruction that can lead to mouth breathing and snoring during sleep.

HISTORY AND PHYSICAL FINDINGS

Patient History

Obtaining a detailed history hinges upon asking the right questions and actively listening to patients tell their story about the complaint. The AGACNP can obtain a meaningful history by listening for clues lending suspicion for genetic, allergic, or nonallergic environmental factors contributing to the patient's symptoms of nasal congestion, rhinorrhea, watery eyes, and scratchy throat (primary symptoms of rhinitis). The patterns of onset, duration, progression, and severity of symptoms can help the AGACNP distinguish between acute or chronic illness, and whether the patient has allergic or nonallergic characteristics of rhinitis. For example, an increase of symptoms at night are often associated with AR. Additionally, constant and recurrent allergic symptoms (persistent) are often associated with allergies to nonseasonal allergens such as dust mites or pet dander. Quality of life can be greatly impacted by the patterns of symptoms associated with rhinitis. A thorough allergy history (e.g., known or suspected triggers, onset and duration of reactions, resolution of symptoms) is necessary to identify the cause and differentiate intermittent from persistent AR.

Review of Systems

A review of systems (ROS) should include investigation of constitutional symptoms of fever, chills, or fatigue and then by system such as the eyes, ears, nose, throat, and neck. Because AR is closely associated with comorbidities such as rhinosinusitis and asthma, it would be prudent to expand the investigation to include inquiry of the frequency, onset, duration, and severity of (a) skin rashes associated with atopic dermatitis; (b) shortness of breath, coughing, and wheezing often associated with asthma; and (c) facial pain, nasal obstruction and headache associated with rhinosinusitis. If patients present with signs and symptoms of systemic illness such as fever, chills, or unintentional weight loss or gain, a more comprehensive ROS should be performed. Pertinent positive and negative symptoms associated with rhinitis are listed in Table 2.14. Symptoms of complications associated with rhinitis include those associated with acute or chronic rhinosinusitis (CRS) and otitis media. Other signs and symptoms of complications associated with rhinitis include fever, dental pain, dental caries, or gingivitis associated with excessive mouth breathing, eustachian tube dysfunction, and insomnia.

Past Medical History

Symptoms of environmental allergies are most prevalent in childhood but can persist into adolescence, adulthood, and even in some older adults. Obtaining a thorough personal history of allergy-related symptoms can inform the AGACNP as to the duration and triggers of AR. AR is very often associated with a history of asthma, rhinosinusitis, and/or atopic dermatitis or eczema. The AGACNP should also inquire about the complications associated with chronic rhinitis such as recurrent infections, epistaxis, and symptoms of eustachian tube dysfunction.

Home Medications

Home medications obtained should include over-the-counter supplements, antihistamines, analgesics, cold medications, and other therapies used to support the patient's symptoms. The AGACNP should be careful to obtain the patient's frequency of use of any medications and the patient's adherence to a prescribed regimen. Patients with a history of chronic rhinitis often have a home treatment regimen including saline nasal irrigation, oral or nasal antihistamines daily (with AR), topical nasal steroids, and/or topical nasal decongestants. Identifying which medications provide the patient with some relief can help the AGACNP distinguish between the type of rhinitis the patient is experiencing. For example, patients with AR often gain relief from the use of antihistamines and/or topical nasal steroid use. Gaining an understanding of the patient's frequency of using nasal decongestants and/or cold medications can lend the AGACNP insight into the frequency and duration of infectious or obstructive complications of chronic rhinitis. The AGACNP should also anticipate a patient with a medical history of asthma may also be prescribed a rescue bronchodilator in the home treatment regimen.

Family History

A family history of asthma, allergies, and atopic dermatitis in first-degree relatives is common among patients diagnosed with AR. A family history of persons who smoke

TABLE 2.14: Pertinent Symptoms Associated With Rhinitis

SYSTEM	PERTINENT POSITIVES	PERTINENT NEGATIVES
Constitutional	Fatigue	Fever, chills, general weakness
Eyes	Watery drainage, itchy, redness	Swelling, pain
Ears, nose, mouth, throat	Nasal congestion, sneezing, watery and clear rhinorrhea, nasal itching, pharyngeal erythema or edema	Ear pain or fullness, epistaxis, dental pain, trismus, sore throat, hoarseness
Cardiovascular	-----	-----
Respiratory	Nonproductive cough	Productive cough, dyspnea, wheezing
Gastrointestinal	-----	Odynophagia, dysphagia, nausea, vomiting, abdominal pain
Genitourinary	-----	-----
Musculoskeletal	-----	Arthralgia, myalgia, joint swelling
Skin, hair, nails (including breasts)	Rash, itching, dry or scaly patches	-----
Neurological	Headache, anosmia	Hearing loss, vision changes or loss
Psychiatric	Insomnia	-----
Endocrine	-----	Unintentional weight loss or gain
Hematologic/lymphatic	Enlarged, painful nodes	Node or glandular swelling

cigarettes or other forms of tobacco living in the same home as the patient when the patient was a child or during the visit are also associated with the patient developing both AR and nonallergic rhinitis (Brozek et al., 2017).

Social and Occupational History

Tobacco use or direct and repeated tobacco smoke exposure can trigger acute exacerbations or perpetuate chronic rhinitis. Additionally, alcohol use, vaping, or snorted illicit drug use are other important factors to investigate as potential triggers for nonallergic rhinitis. Living with, sleeping in the same bed with, or other exposure to pets is a piece of history that can reinforce suspicions the AGACNP may have for AR. Occupational hazards can include the patient being exposed to chemicals or gases in the work environment that could be the cause of nonallergic rhinitis.

Physical Examination

The data collected during a patient's history are strengthened by the data collected during the physical examination during the development of differential diagnoses for patients with rhinitis. Examination of the head and neck focused on the patient's general appearance, eyes, ears, nose, mouth, and pharynx are pertinent for uncomplicated rhinitis that is not associated with extra-nasal conditions. Expanding the examination to the glands of the neck, lymphatics of the neck, lungs, skin, and abdomen are all areas to also evaluate for acute or chronic illness lending suspicion for rhinitis-associated

conditions such as atopic dermatosis, rhinosinusitis, migraine headaches, asthma, or upper respiratory infections. The AGACNP should be vigilant to evaluate patients for the differing findings associated with AR and nonallergic rhinitis. Pertinent examination findings in the patient with rhinitis are noted in Table 2.15.

TABLE 2.15: Physical Examination Findings Associated With Rhinitis

AREAS	EXPECTED PHYSICAL EXAMINATION FINDINGS
Vitals signs	Afebrile, hemodynamic stability, nonhypoxic
Constitutional	Nontoxic, in no acute respiratory distress
Eyes	Bilateral injection, small to moderate clear watery drainage, "allergic shiners"
Ears, nose, mouth, and throat	Chronic otitis media with clear effusions Pale nasal membranes
Respiratory	Unlabored respirations, clear bilateral breath sounds, no cyanosis or clubbing (wheezing is only expected in uncontrolled asthma)
Gastrointestinal	Soft and nontender abdomen, no organomegaly, no pulsatile mass
Musculoskeletal	Full range of motion, no synovitis, no myositis
Skin	Areas of dry patches of skin, eczema plaques can be present

DIFFERENTIAL DIGANOSIS AND DIAGNOSTIC CONSIDERATIONS

A clinical diagnosis can be made for most patients with rhinitis. The AGACNP should make the clinical diagnosis of AR for patients with a history of one or more allergic symptoms such as a runny nose, itchy nose, nasal congestion, or sneezing; or physical examination findings of a pale nasal mucosa, clear rhinorrhea, or watery, bilateral conjunctival injection (Seidman et al., 2015). A clinical diagnosis can also be made for patients with nonallergic rhinitis and differentiated from AR by the absence of the allergic symptoms of itchy nose, rhinorrhea, and bilateral conjunctival injection.

Differential diagnoses should consider the varying etiologies of rhinitis and extranasal conditions. Differential diagnoses can be classified by acute or chronic illness, allergic or nonallergic, and obstructive or nonobstructive (Box 2.4). A rhinitis diagnosis should be differentiated from infectious, vasomotor, medication-induced, pregnancy-related, NARES, and obstructive etiologies. Obstructive etiologies of rhinitis can be caused by tumors, nasal polyposis, or structural defects. Obstructive etiologies are indications for surgical evaluation for treatment.

Diagnostic Tests

Most patients diagnosed with rhinitis do not undergo diagnostic testing. Patients who experience symptoms despite nonsurgical treatment are referred to otolaryngology for surgical management or an allergy/immunology specialist for advanced immunotherapy.

Allergy Testing

Allergy testing helps to identify the causative allergens responsible for the symptoms patients have with AR. In adolescents and adults, a screening battery of testing should include 10 to 12 allergens such as mold, pollens, pet dander, and dust mites from the local environment. Testing can be performed through skin-prick testing, intradermal testing, or through in vitro serum assays (Shah & Emanuel, 2020).

BOX 2.4 DIFFERENTIAL DIAGNOSES FOR RHINITIS

Acute Rhinitis
- Viral rhinitis
- Intermittent allergic rhinitis
- Vasomotor nonallergic rhinitis
- Chemical nonallergic rhinitis

Chronic Rhinitis
- Persistent allergic rhinitis
- Nonallergic rhinitis with eosinophilia

Obstructive Rhinitis
- Chronic rhinitis with septal deviation
- Chronic rhinitis with septal perforation
- Chronic rhinitis with turbinate hypertrophy

Imaging

Other than direct visualization of the internal structures of the nose via rhinoscopy, radiographic imaging is not indicated in the patient with rhinitis. Additionally, AR guidelines recommend against the use of radiographic imaging (Seidman et al., 2015).

TREATMENT

Nonpharmacologic Therapies

Avoiding the known triggers of rhinitis (e.g., perfumes, pet dander, dust mites, cigarette smoke, grasses, or pollens) is the first-line therapy for conservative treatment and is often referred to as environmental control, especially in AR. If patients are not able to avoid known triggers, such as those within the work environments, wearing a particulate mask is helpful in limiting the patient's exposure and thereby reducing the severity of symptoms experienced.

Saline irrigation is another nonpharmacological therapy that helps to reduce nasal crusting and mucous stasis. Saline irrigation is most often used as adjunctive therapy with nasal steroid use and works to enhance its effectiveness and improve ciliary function within the nose (Shah & Emanuel, 2020).

Pharmacotherapies

There are multiple oral and/or topical intranasal pharmacotherapies that can be used as monotherapy or as combination therapy in the treatment of patients with rhinitis. Differentiating allergic from nonallergic rhinitis is important in the use of oral antihistamines such as loratadine, cetirizine, or diphenhydramine. Second-generation antihistamines are considered first line therapies for AR and have fewer sedating effects (Seidman et al., 2015). However, diphenhydramine, a first-generation antihistamine is useful in patients with acute allergy symptoms and in patients with acute or chronic allergy symptoms that are coupled by insomnia. Although older adult patients (over 65 years old) are less affected by allergy-related conditions, those who have AR should not be prescribed oral antihistamines due to the secondary anticholinergic effects upon the brain, eyes, bladder, prostate, and bowel (American Geriatric Society [AGS], 2019). Additionally, any patients with a history of narrow-angle glaucoma, prostatic hypertrophy, or bladder neck obstruction also have contraindications for anticholinergic agents (Shah & Emanuel, 2020).

Intranasal Steroids

Patients experiencing AR and nonallergic rhinitis symptoms (acute or chronic) can be treated with topical intranasal steroids such as fluticasone, triamcinolone, beclomethasone, or budesonide. Guidelines for AR strongly recommend topical intranasal steroid treatment for patients with symptoms that affect the patient's quality of life (Seidman et al., 2015). Topical intranasal steroids work to reduce the inflammatory response within the nasal mucosa, thereby reducing nasal edema and symptoms of nasal congestion, nasal itching, and rhinorrhea.

Intranasal Antihistamines

Topical intranasal antihistamines, such as azelastine or olopatadine, can be offered to patients diagnosed with AR and are indicated for use with intranasal steroid treatment in these patients (Seidman, 2015). Due to the anticholinergic effects of intranasal antihistamines, they should be avoided in patients with narrow-angle glaucoma, prostatic hypertrophy, or bladder neck obstruction (Shah & Emanuel, 2020).

Nasal Decongestants

The nasal congestion associated with nonallergic rhinitis can be treated with adrenergic agents such as oral pseudoephedrine and intranasal phenylephrine. These pharmacotherapies work to constrict the capillaries within the nose to reduce nasal congestion. Adverse effects of these medications are often dose-related and can include tachycardia, hypertension, urinary retention, and irritability. Therefore, patients with a history of hypertension, severe coronary artery disease, or use of monoamine oxidase inhibitors should not use nasal decongestants. The adverse effects directly associated with topical intranasal adrenergic agents are related to the overuse of the medication and can causes rebound congestion after withdrawal of the therapy (rhinitis medicamentosa). To prevent the adverse effect of rhinitis medicamentosa, patients should be cautioned not to use topical intranasal adrenergic agents for longer than 5 days (Shah & Emanuel, 2020).

Immunotherapy

Patients who do not respond well to pharmacotherapy and environmental control can be referred to an allergy/immunology specialist for desensitization therapy to allergens. Immunotherapy involves administering small doses of the allergen(s) over a period of a few years to desensitize the patient and theoretically reduce symptoms of AR.

Surgical Therapies

Surgical treatment for patients with rhinitis focuses on correcting structural abnormalities such as septal deviation, perforated septum, or nasal obstruction related to turbinate hypertrophy or septal defects. Referral to an otolaryngologist is indicated in patients with recurrent symptoms related to these structural abnormalities identified. Septoplasty involves the reconstruction of cartilaginous or bony structures of the septum causing deviation. Septal perforations contributing to increased nasal crusting or epistaxis are corrected by the placement of flap closures, septal buttons, or auto harvest of other free tissue (Shah & Emanuel, 2020).

TRANSITION OF CARE

The AGACNP's encounter with the patient with rhinitis might take place in an emergency department during the episodic acute exacerbation of chronic disease or acute infection. The AGACNP practicing in the allergy or otolaryngology specialty areas would also encounter patients diagnosed with rhinitis. Transitioning the care of patients with rhinitis from a primary care provider to specialists most often occurs when the disease is refractory to medical treatments or is obstructive. Transitioning the care of patients with rhinitis from an emergency setting to a primary care provider is important to establish a long-term management plan. Fortunately, patients living with acute or chronic rhinitis do not require hospitalization. Even those patients undergoing surgical interventions are most often treated on an outpatient basis and have minimal complications warranting hospitalization.

2.17: RHINOSINUSITIS

Leanne H. Fowler

Rhinosinusitis (formerly known as sinusitis) is the symptomatic inflammation of the paranasal sinuses and nasal cavity. The condition's name evolved from being called sinusitis to rhinosinusitis because the inflammation of the sinuses is also commonly associated with the inflammation of the nasal mucosa and can be classified as acute or chronic. Acute rhinosinusitis (ARS) involves a duration of illness lasting no more than 4 weeks. Whereas chronic rhinosinusitis (CRS) involves a duration of illness greater than 12 weeks and can have a significant impact upon a patient's quality of life. ARS can be further classified as acute bacterial rhinosinusitis (ABRS) or viral rhinosinusitis (VRS; Rosenfeld et al., 2015).

Rhinosinusitis is one of the most common conditions diagnosed in the United States (approximately 29 million persons) and accounts for about 4.1 million primary care office visits and over 234,000 emergency department visits (Centers for Disease Control and Prevention, 2018b). Rhinosinusitis is diagnosed more than rhinitis, chronic obstructive pulmonary disease, and bronchitis combined (Rosenfeld et al., 2015). Patients with CRS are estimated to visit the doctor's office two times more often than patients without CRS (Rosenfeld et al., 2015).

The structure and function of the nose are discussed more in the rhinitis section. There are six paranasal sinuses lined with the same mucociliary epithelium with which the nose and lower airways are lined. The mucociliary epithelial layer of inflammatory cells, nerves, and blood vessels work to protect and rid the nose and parasinuses from environmental particles, infectious germs, and foreign substances (Huether & McCance, 2019). Therefore, the role of acute and chronic inflammation is involved in the acute and chronic disease of rhinosinusitis. Inflammation of the mucosa can lead to the accumulation of mucus in the sinuses due to the obstruction caused by edematous mucous membranes. Acute infections of the nose and sinuses are usually caused by *Haemophilus influenzae* or *Streptococcus pneumoniae* (McGinnis, 2020). Chronic infections of the nose and sinuses are most commonly associated with chronic inflammation and intermittent infections with anaerobic germs, gram-negative bacteria, or *Staphylococcus aureus* that exacerbates CRS symptoms (Zenga & Harris, 2020). Patients with CRS and recurrent infections can be associated with drug resistant germs (DeMuri & Wald, 2020). Patients with immunocompromising conditions with CRS can also develop fungal infections with *Aspergillus, Fusarium,* or *Mucorales* germs (McGinnis, 2020; Zenga & Harris, 2020).

PRESENTING SIGNS AND SYMPTOMS

Patients presenting with ARS and CRS can have varying presenting symptoms. ARS is usually caused by an infectious etiology and can mimic the signs and symptoms of the common cold (viral upper respiratory illness [URI]). The duration of ARS is usually no more than 4 weeks but can extend up to 12 weeks and can follow a recent URI (McGinnis, 2020). Acute infectious rhinosinusitis should be differentiated from bacterial and viral. Patients with CRS are commonly affected by chronic allergic symptoms and should be evaluated for recurrent ARS and for obstructive CRS from nasal polyps. Rhinosinusitis symptoms persisting greater than 12 weeks is a defining characteristic for CRS (Zenga & Harris, 2020).

Acute Infectious Rhinosinusitis

Patients with infectious and uncomplicated ARS complain of nasal congestion, rhinorrhea, facial pain or pressure in the areas overlying the sinuses, tooth pain, halitosis, and frontal headache (McGinnis, 2020). Profuse watery and clear drainage with the other symptoms mentioned is most common with viral ARS. Viral ARS is more common than ABRS. The cardinal signs of ABRS include purulent nasal drainage that is coupled with facial pain or fullness or nasal obstruction that does not improve or worsens over the period of 10 days (Rosenfeld et al., 2015). The presenting findings of patients with complicated ARS can include complaints of headache, a growing mass on the nose and/or face, and progressive severity of dental or ear pain.

Chronic Rhinosinusitis

Patients presenting with CRS complain of a combination of persistent symptoms of mucopurulent drainage, nasal obstruction, facial pain or pressure, and hyposmia or anosmia that varies in severity and intensity intermittently and whether acute infection is involved. Because the symptoms of rhinosinusitis (acute or chronic) are closely similar to symptoms associated with upper respiratory illness, identifying the onset of symptom severity and the duration of severe symptoms is important in differentiating CRS from ABRS. Patients living with CRS can also experience viral ARS. Similar to the patient without CRS, ABRS should be highly suspected when symptoms do not improve after 10 days of increased severity of chronic illness. Fever is not a common finding in patients

with ARS, ABRS, or CRS. However, when it is present, patients can appear and feel severely ill (DeMuri & Wald, 2020). It is important for AGACNPs to distinguish ARS from CRS, CRS from ABRS, and CRS with obstructive nasal polyposis or by another sinonasal structural defect (Rosenfeld et al., 2015). In rare circumstances, AGACNPs must also have an increased index of suspicion for fungal infections in the patient with CRS.

Fungal Sinusitis

Patients with CRS can have allergic fungal sinusitis or mycetoma (also known as a fungal ball). Patients that develop mycetoma are most commonly associated with obstructed mucous flow that leads to the accumulation of colonized growth of fungal elements. In chronic allergic fungal sinusitis, the colonizing and accumulation of fungal elements occurs secondary to the thick eosinophilic mucin, nasal polyps, and bony remodeling that occurs in patients with CRS associated with nasal polyposis. Patients can have the same presenting symptoms as patients with obstructive CRS. These forms of fungal sinusitis are considered less severe disease when compared to invasive fungal sinusitis (Zenga & Harris, 2020).

Patients presenting with invasive fungal sinusitis are most commonly immunocompromised by chemotherapy for cancer or when there is a history of uncontrolled diabetes mellitus. The AGACNP should have a high index of suspicion in patients with immunocompromising illnesses because early stages of the disease can be associated with subtle symptoms. As the disease progresses, patients can complain of facial pain, headache, rhinorrhea, loss of smell or other sensations of the nose or face, or mental status changes (Zenga & Harris, 2020).

HISTORY AND PHYSICAL EXAM FINDINGS

A thorough history and physical examination of the patient with rhinosinusitis is crucial to the development of timely, appropriate, and prioritized differential diagnoses and the development of a safe and effective management plan. Depending on the acuity of the patient, a focused or expanded problem-focused approach to the history and physical is appropriate. When patients have presenting symptoms of systemic illness (e.g., fever, chills, generalized weakness) or have a history of an immunocompromising illness, the AGACNP should complete a comprehensive history and physical examination.

Patient History

The ROS for the patient with rhinosinusitis should include inquiry of at least constitutional, head, ears, eyes, nose, and throat (HEENT), neck, and respiratory. If the patient has risk factors or a history of chronic lung or cardiac disease, it is reasonable to expand the ROS interview to these systems. Patients with a personal or family history of other allergic conditions (e.g., rhinitis, eczema, asthma) may also present with skin rashes that need examination.

Patients with a history of immunocompromising illnesses should have a comprehensive interview of their history.

Home Medications

The AGACNP should be sure to inquire about patients prescribed home medications to manage chronic allergic or asthmatic illness. Inquiring about patient adherence to the home medication regimen can also help the AGACNP determine if the patient's treatment plan is effective or needs to be modified.

Social and Occupational History

Patients with a history of CRS and recurrent ABRS can experience exacerbated symptoms if environmental triggers in the workplace or home are not controlled. A personal history of tobacco use or other smoke exposure should prompt the AGACNP to initiate tobacco cessation counseling. Patients within an environment of tobacco smoke or pet dander exposure should also be counseled to eliminate or control these triggers as much as possible in an effort to avoid or reduce repeated exacerbations.

Physical Examination

The patient's overall appearance is important to observe during the physical examination to identify whether the patient is in acute respiratory distress or has a toxic appearance suggesting a systemic and more severe illness. AGACNPs should also be careful to inspect the face and mucous membranes of patients with ARS for swelling, erythema, and drainage. Patients with ARS can have pain and tenderness with palpation or percussion over the sinuses. Inspection of the nasal mucus should also include determining patency of the nares. Inspection of the oral mucosa should include evaluating the patient for associated tonsillitis, pharyngitis, or dental disease. The AGACNP should also palpate the neck to evaluate the patient for anterior cervical or submandibular adenitis, and to evaluate the neck for focal tenderness that could be indicative of deep neck space infection or adenitis.

Invasive Fungal Sinusitis

The AGACNP should make careful inspections of the face, nose, and mouth in patients suspected to have invasive fungal sinusitis. The nasal turbinates may have dark ulcers seen during inspection of the nose. The lateral nasal walls, septum, or palate may have decreased to no sensation upon palpation and the patient may have cranial nerve deficits in late stages of the disease.

DIFFERENTIAL DIAGNOSIS AND DIAGNOSTIC CONSIDERATIONS

Determining the etiology of ARS is crucial in informing the patient's therapy. Distinguishing ABRS from VRS hinges upon the history and physical examination findings to establish a clinical diagnosis. When establishing the diagnosis of a patient with rhinosinusitis it is also important to determine if the condition is complicated

TABLE 2.16: Diagnostic Criteria for Chronic Rhinosinusitis With Nasal Polyposis

Two or more symptoms of inflammation (One symptom should be nasal congestion/blockage or nasal discharge)	Nasal obstruction or congestion
	Nasal discharge
	Facial pain or pressure
	Hyposmia or anosmia
	Endoscopic or CT evidence of nasal polyps

or uncomplicated. Complicated rhinosinusitis involves the extended inflammation or infection from the parasinuses into neurological, ophthalmological, or other surrounding soft tissue (Rosenfeld et al., 2015). Differential diagnoses for patients with complicated ARS include migraine headache, foreign body retention (especially if postprocedural or postsurgical), dental caries, or craniofacial neoplasm (McGinnis, 2020).

Diagnostic Tests

Most patients with ARS or CRS are diagnosed during the clinical encounter without the use of diagnostic laboratory or radiographic tests. Diagnostic criteria (Table 2.16) are used for patients with CRS with nasal polyps using subjective and objective clinical findings (Hopkins, 2019).

Imaging

Radiographic imaging of the patient with uncomplicated ARS is not recommended by clinical guidelines unless the AGACNP suspects the patient has complicated ARS or an alternative differential diagnosis (Rosenfeld et al., 2015). Direct visualization of the nose and sinuses via anterior rhinoscopy or nasal endoscopy is indicated for confirming the diagnosis and is most often performed by an otolaryngology specialist for patients with obstructive CRS or recurrent ABRS. Patients suspected to have complicated ARS can benefit from CT imaging with contrast to localize the obstruction and/or exclude intracranial extension of disease (Rosenfeld et al., 2015). CT imaging is also useful in visualizing mycetoma associated with fungal sinusitis or invasive disease extending beyond the nose and parasinuses (Zenga & Harris, 2020).

Histology

In patients with suspected invasive fungal sinusitis, a biopsy of the darkened ulcerated tissue should be obtained for pathologic examination. The pathologist should be informed of the suspicion of a fungal sinusitis to ensure fungal stains are performed. The lack of bleeding at the biopsy site should lend higher suspicion for tissue infarction and an invasive fungal sinusitis (Zenga & Harris, 2020).

TREATMENT

Treatment for patients with rhinosinusitis should be differentiated as acute or chronic, uncomplicated, or complicated, and obstructive or nonobstructive. Uncomplicated

ARS is effectively treated with supportive therapies such as nasal saline irrigation, nasal decongestants, and/or nasal steroids to reduce symptoms. Antibiotic therapies should be reserved for patients with the cardinal findings of ABRS or recurrent ABRS in the setting of CRS.

Chronic Rhinosinusitis

The primary goals of treating patients with CRS is to reduce and stabilize inflammation and minimize symptoms with supportive therapies. The supportive therapies include saline nasal irrigations, topical nasal steroids, and avoidance of allergy triggers. Patients with recurrent ARS and a history of CRS, are indicated for antibiotic therapy in addition to supportive therapies in the treatment plan.

Obstructive Chronic Rhinosinusitis

AGACNPs should evaluate the patient with recurrent ABRS in the setting of obstructive CRS for nasal polyps. Topical nasal steroids or oral steroids in addition to antibiotics are indicated for treatment in such patients to facilitate the shrinkage of nasal polyps and subsequently allow drainage of the sinuses. In the event these medical therapies do not control the patient's symptoms, surgical interventions may be indicated to remove the obstruction of nasal drainage. Post surgical intervention, patients with CRS should continue maintenance medical therapy aimed at reducing inflammation and CRS symptoms. The functional endoscopic sinus surgery (FESS) is a surgical intervention used to remove obstructed mucoid secretions and decompress or open sinonasal tracts to prevent further obstruction and facilitate drainage. In patients with CRS related to allergies, it is vital to continue long-term topical glucocorticoid therapy postoperatively to maintain patent sinonasal tracts (Zenga & Harris, 2020).

TRANSITION OF CARE

The AGACNP's encounter with the patient with rhinosinusitis could take place in an emergency department for patients presenting with ARS or CRS with recurrent ABRS. The AGACNP practicing in allergy or otolaryngology specialty areas could also encounter patients diagnosed with varying forms of rhinosinusitis. The AGACNP practicing in other specialty clinics (e.g., pulmonology, cardiology, endocrinology) who manage the complex chronic care of other systems may also encounter the patient seeking care or experiencing ARS or CRS symptoms. Transitioning the care of patients with rhinosinusitis from the ED or specialty clinic to a primary care provider or to allergy/immunology or otolaryngology specialists should occur for patients in need of follow-up and chronic disease management. Fortunately, patients living with acute or CRS do not require hospitalization. Even those patients undergoing surgical interventions are most often treated on an outpatient basis and have minimal complications warranting hospitalization.

CLINICAL PEARLS

- Most ARS is caused by viral infection and should not persist beyond 10 days.
- ARS symptoms that persist beyond 10 days is often caused by bacterial infection and should be treated by antibiotics.
- Patients with obstructive rhinosinusitis and recurrent acute bacterial infections should be evaluated by Otolaryngology for surgical intervention when the patient is refractory to medical therapies.

CONDITIONS OF THE THROAT

2.18: ANGIOEDEMA

Thomas Farley

Angioedema is a clinical syndrome characterized by swelling of the lips, tongue, larynx, and face with associated nausea, vomiting, and abdominal pain. Angioedema is differentiated from standard edema because it is non-pitting, transient, and subcutaneous or submucosal (Bernstein & Moellman, 2012). Angioedema is a common emergency department (ED) complaint in the United States (Bernstein & Moellman, 2012).

Two broad types of angioedema exist: histamine-mediated and bradykinin-mediated.

The initial approach to both types of angioedema is first to create a plan for airway management. The diagnostic workup should continue while the airway is being monitored or secured. Angioedema of the tongue or larynx is associated with a high risk of progressive airway loss (LoVerde et al., 2017). Standard direct laryngoscopy may not be sufficient to perform intubation. No commercially available rapid point of care test is available to differentiate between the two types (Bernstein et al., 2017). Angioedema is a clinical diagnosis and select serum studies may help distinguish between bradykinin mediated subtypes (Bernstein, 2018).

Histamine mediated angioedema is treated with standard therapy for anaphylaxis. A thorough history is necessary to determine the possible trigger and prevent further episodes. The bradykinin mediated type has several subtypes including hereditary angioedema (HAE) and angiotensin converting enzyme inhibitor (ACEi) triggered. Several FDA-approved drugs are available for treatment of HAE and are used off label to treat other bradykinin mediated subtypes (Lawlor et al., 2018).

PRESENTING SIGNS AND SYMPTOMS

Features common to both types of angioedema include:
- Swelling of the lips or tongue
- Laryngeal swelling
- Facial swelling

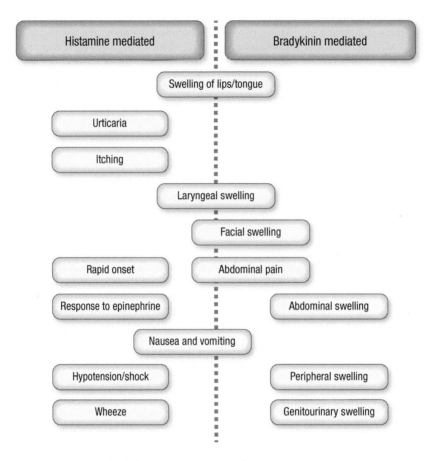

FIGURE 2.3: Distinguishing histamine- versus bradykinin-mediated angioedema.
Source: Reproduced from Bernstein, J. A., Cremonesi, P., Hoffmann, T. K., & Hollingsworth, J. (2017). Angioedema in the emergency department: A practical guide to differential diagnosis and management. *International Journal of Emergency Medicine, 10*(1), 15. https://doi.org/10.1186/s12245-017-0141-z, Fig. 3.

- Abdominal pain
- Nausea and vomiting

Urticaria and itching are not associated with bradykinin-mediated angioedema (Bernstein et al., 2017)

HISTORY AND PHYSICAL FINDINGS

History

- Exposure to NSAIDs.
- Exposure to ACEi or angiotensin receptor blocker drugs (ARB).
- Exposure to recombinant tissue plasminogen activator (rTPA).
- Exposure to antibiotics.
- Exposure to gliptins (Long et al., 2019).
- Exposure to mammalian target of rapamycin (mTOR) inhibitors (Long et al., 2019).
- Family history of HAE.
- Prior episodes of angioedema.
- Exposure to known allergen.
- Recent trauma.

Physical Examination

Refer to Figure 2.3 for physical exam findings that distinguish histamine- versus bradykinin-mediated angioedema.

DIFFERENTIAL DIAGNOSIS AND DIAGNOSTIC CONSIDERATIONS

It is crucial to distinguish between histamine versus bradykinin mediated angioedema.

The histamine type resolves within 24 to 48 hours; bradykinin type angioedema can take up to 7 days to resolve (Long et al., 2019).

Figure 2.4 illustrates a diagnostic algorithm for angioedema in the ED.

Patients presenting with a chief complaint of abdominal pain are challenging. Complaints of abdominal pain with swelling may suggest HAE (Bork et al., 2006).

Diagnostic Tests

Serum for C1-INH concentration, C1-INH function, C4 concentration, and tryptase concentration should be

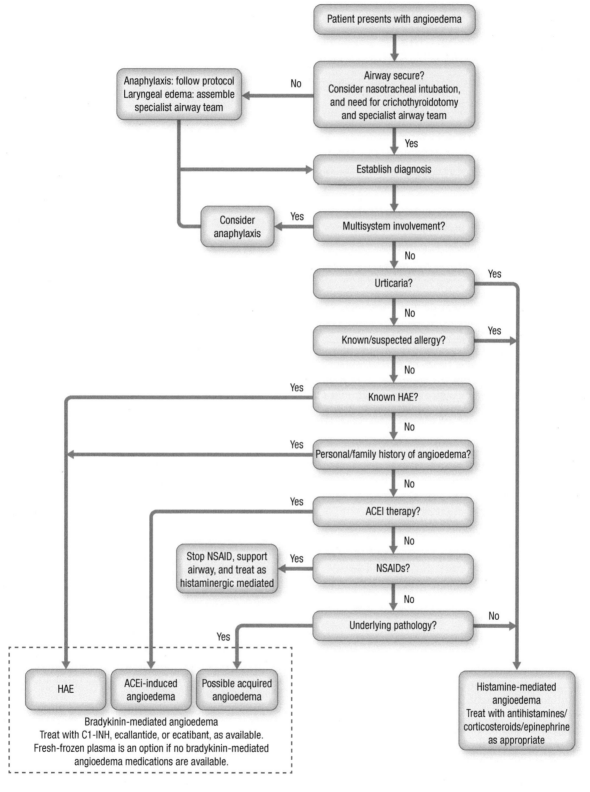

FIGURE 2.4: Flow diagram of diagnosis of angioedema in the emergency department. ACEi angiotensin-converting enzyme inhibitor, HAE hereditary angioedema.

Source: Reproduced from Bernstein, J. A., Cremonesi, P., Hoffmann, T. K., & Hollingsworth, J. (2017). Angioedema in the emergency department: A practical guide to differential diagnosis and management. *International Journal of Emergency Medicine, 10*(1), 15. https://doi.org/10.1186/s12245-017-0141-z, Fig. 2.

TABLE 2.17: Results of Diagnostic Tests to Help Distinguish Among Angioedema Types

	C1-INH CONCENTRATION	C1-INH FUNCTION	C4 CONCENTRATION	TRYPTASE CONCENTRATION*
HAE type I	Low	Low	Low	Normal
HAE type II	Normal or high	Low	Low	Normal
HAE with normal C1-INH	Normal	Normal	Normal	Normal
Acquired AE	Low	Low	Low	Normal
ACEi-induced AE	Normal	Normal	Normal	Normal
Histamine-mediated anaphylaxis	Normal	Normal	Normal	Normal or Elevated

*In blood drawn within 4–6 h of onset of attack.

ACEi, angiotensin converting enzyme inhibitor; AE, angioedema; C1-INH, C1 inhibitor; HAE, hereditary angioedema.

Source: Reproduced from Bernstein, J. A., Cremonesi, P., Hoffmann, T. K., & Hollingsworth, J. (2017). Angioedema in the emergency department: A practical guide to differential diagnosis and management. *International Journal of Emergency Medicine, 10*(1), 15. https://doi.org/10.1186/s12245-017-0141-z, Table 1

obtained once immediate treatment is complete. ACEi caused angioedema cannot be confirmed with serum tests (Bernstein et al., 2017).

Table 2.17 lists various diagnostic tests and their value in differentiating between types of angioedema.

HAE has several subtypes differentiated by quantity of functional C1-INH or presence of dysfunctional C1-INH (Bernstein, 2018). Consultation with an allergy specialist is recommended when attempting to determine the subtype of HAE.

Differential Diagnoses

Differential diagnoses of clinical entities that mimic angioedema include:

- Anaphylaxis
- Acquired C1-INH deficiency from B-cell lymphoma (Bernstein, 2018)
- Anasarca
- Myxedema
- Superior vena cava syndrome

TREATMENT

Immediate Management

From time of initial presentation, the AGACNP's focus should be on establishing an airway management plan. Angioedema is a clinical diagnosis and labs do not guide initial management. Treatment for the histamine-mediated form is:

- H_1 and H_2 blockade with antihistamines
- Epinephrine 0.3–0.5 mg IM
- Glucocorticoids methylprednisolone 125 mg IV

Specific Management

If angioedema is determined to be the bradykinin-mediated type:

- Any possible offending drugs or triggers should be discontinued and avoided.

- HAE can be effectively treated by a selection of targeted therapies that seek to increase serum levels of C1-INH, block bradykinin receptors, or inhibit kallikrein.
- Review of studies shows median time of onset relief to range from 15 min to 2 hr (Bork et al., 2016).
- Systemic review of the literature indicates off-label use of drugs approved for HAE in other bradykinin-mediated subtypes of angioedema specifically ACEi associated (Lawlor et al., 2018).
- Additional meta-analysis demonstrated no benefit of bradykinin receptor blockers over placebo in ACEi-associated angioedema with few adverse side effects (Jeon et al., 2019).

Table 2.18 lists the four targeted medications approved by the FDA to treat HAE.

Consider transfusion of fresh frozen plasma that contains C1-INH. Use is limited due to varying effectiveness and potential transmission of blood=borne pathogens (Loverde et al., 2017).

TRANSITION OF CARE

Disposition will depend on response to therapies and ability to maintain patent airway. Many patients will require critical care for airway management and ventilator management.

Patients diagnosed with histamine type should be discharged with an emergency epinephrine injector.

CLINICAL PEARLS

- Hypotension, urticaria, and bronchospasm are atypical in a bradykinin-mediated attack (Long et al., 2019).
- Angioedema of the tongue or larynx is associated with high risk of progressive airway loss.

TABLE 2.18: Angioedema Medications

MEDICATION (TRADE NAME)	MECHANISM	ROUTE	DOSE	TIME TO ONSET	MINOR SIDE EFFECTS	SERIOUS SIDE EFFECTS
Plasma derived C1-INH (Berinert, Cinryze)	C1-INH protein replacement	IV	Berinert 20 units/kg; Cinryze 1000 units	Median 30–48 min	Dysgeusia	Hypersensitivity, thrombosis, blood-borne infection
Recombinant C1-INH (Ruconest)	C1-INH protein replacement	IV	50 units/kg	Median 90 min	Pruritis, rash, sinusitis	Hypersensitivity, anaphylaxis
Ecallantide (Kalbitor)	Kallikrein inhibitor	SQ	30 mg	Median 67 min	Headache, injection site reactions, nausea, fever	Hypersensitivity, anaphylaxis
Icatibant acetate (Firazyr)	Bradykinin B2 receptor antagonist	SQ	30 mg	Median 2 hr	Elevated LFTs, injection reaction, dizziness, headache, nausea, fever	Theoretical worsening of an ongoing ischemic event
Fresh frozen plasma	C1-INH protein replacement (various amounts)	IV	15 mg/kg	Min to hr		Hypersensitivity, worsening angioedema, transfusion infection

C1-INH, C1 inhibitor; LFTs, liver function tests.

Source: Long, B. J., Koyfman, A., & Gottlieb, M. (2019, July). Evaluation and management of angioedema in the emergency department. *Western Journal of Emergency Medicine,* *20*(4), 587–600. https://doi.org/10.5811/westjem.2019.5.42650

- Bradykinin-mediated attacks can last up to 7 days if not treated.
- Treat suspected histamine-mediated form with standard anaphylaxis therapies.
- Anaphylaxis therapies are not effective in bradykinin-mediated forms.
- Obtaining a thorough history is key to determining possible triggers or if subtype is hereditary.
- Obtain expert consultation to aid in determining if bradykinin-mediated subtype.
- Trial of approved HAE therapies in ACEi-caused angioedema may be warranted.

KEY TAKEAWAYS

- Angioedema can be fatal.
- Devise a plan for securing the airway while determining cause.
- Angioedema is a clinical diagnosis.
- Histamine- or bradykinin-mediated type often determined by history and physical.
- Labs only assist in determining subtype of bradykinin-mediated variety.

2.19: DENTAL ABSCESSES

Nancy Knechel

Dental pain or a severe toothache is almost always the chief complaint for a dental abscess. On exam, the abscess appears as a shiny, smooth, red papule that is sensitive to the touch. AGACNPs may also find increased tooth mobility and regional lymphadenopathy. Diagnosis can usually be made from the history and physical exam. In most acute care settings, imaging is not necessary unless the infection is severe. A dental abscess will not go away spontaneously and the primary treatment is incision and drainage (I&D) with broad-spectrum antibiotics for at least 10 days and pain control. While most dental abscesses can be treated in the outpatient setting, the AGACNP should be aware it can be a source of sepsis. Since most AGACNPs have limited training in managing dental problems, it is often appropriate to refer the patient to a dentist, dental surgeon, or maxillofacial surgeon after initial treatment and depending on the extent of disease.

PRESENTING SIGNS AND SYMPTOMS

An abscess is a collection of purulent exudate and in the case of a dental abscess, it occurs near the base of an infected tooth. A dental abscess is caused from bacteria entering the innermost part of the tooth, the dental pulp, through a cavity, crack, or chip, and can spread down to the root. The dental pulp contains the nerve, and since it provides sensory innervation through a tooth's nerve, an infection here will cause pain. The dental abscess can be periapical (tip of the root) or periodontal (in the gums and the side of root; Gould, 2019; Loureiro et al., 2019). Regardless of type, the cardinal symptom of a dental abscess is pain. A dental abscess should always be considered when a patient reports a severe toothache or dental pain, particularly in the setting of poor dental hygiene or a history of unrepaired dental trauma (Sanders & Houck, 2019). Although patients can often identify the painful tooth, sometimes the pain can be difficult to attribute to a specific tooth, and may be described as mouth, face, or jaw pain. If the infection is more severe, patients may also report neck or ear pain. The pain can be throbbing or sharp, and it is often worse when lying down. Patients may also report gingivitis, a loose or partial tooth, difficult mastication, difficulty sleeping on affected side, and sensitivity to heat/cold or sweets, decreased oral intake, gingival bleeding, and fever (Robertson et al., 2015). If the abscess spontaneously ruptures, patients may report drainage near the painful tooth, a foul or salty taste, and a putrid smell in the mouth that persists despite brushing teeth (Gould, 2019).

HISTORY AND PHYSICAL EXAM FINDINGS

The history should be focused on the duration and development of the pain, and any associated symptoms. Dental abscesses will often present as localized dental pain that progresses over hours to days (Gould, 2019). It is also important to gather information regarding routine dental care, most recent visit to the dentist, and history of any recent dental trauma or injury for which treatment was not sought.

On exam, AGACNPs will find the gingiva to have increased warmth, edema, and erythema. There will be tenderness with palpation of the gum line and a fluctuant mass may be visible and palpable. Sometimes it can be difficult to visualize or locate the abscess by visual inspection, but if visualized it usually looks like a single soft reddish papule. The gums may appear shiny due to inflammation. The abscess is often on the buccal side of the gum line, and the lower posterior teeth are the most frequently involved. AGACNPs may also find increased tooth mobility, regional lymphadenopathy, and tenderness with tapping the tooth, the latter is particularly true in periapical abscesses (Gould, 2019).

In cases of a more severe infection, patients may have dysphagia, trismus, face and neck swelling, difficulty breathing, and signs of dehydration (Gould, 2019). A severe dental infection should be recognized as a potential source of sepsis. AGACNPs should assess for signs and symptoms suggesting a spreading infection. Signs of systemic infection include fever, tachycardia, tachypnea, hypotension, lymphadenopathy, cellulitis, and difficulty with fully opening the mouth.

DIFFERENTIAL DIAGNOSIS AND DIAGNOSTIC CONSIDERATIONS

Diagnosis can usually be made exclusively from the history of present illness and physical exam. Imaging is generally not needed or helpful in the case of an uncomplicated dental abscess (Gould, 2019). Dedicated mandible radiographs, orthopantomograms, are usually available in hospitals and provide panoramic views of the maxilla and teeth. While this allows the AGACNP to evaluate the gross anatomy and general dental health, it may not provide sufficient detail to evaluate for periapical changes unless the periodontal disease is advanced (Robertson et al., 2015). Dental radiographs can provide adequate imaging to confirm diagnosis, but this is often only available to dental providers. CT imaging is sensitive for bony structures, so this modality may be useful in cases where evaluation of osseous involvement is necessary (Chow, 2020). In more severe or complicated dental abscess cases, a CBC, blood culture, and CT with IV contrast can provide valuable additional information on the extent of the infection.

Differential diagnoses to consider include dental caries, dental trauma/root fracture, gingival abscess (abscess of the gum tissue only and does not involve the tooth), sinusitis, temporomandibular joint (TMJ) disorders, parotitis (parotid salivary gland infection), peritonsillar abscess, peridontitis (infection of the supporting structures of the tooth), buccal bifurcation cyst, or eosinophilic granuloma. Pulpitis, an inflammatory condition of the dental pulp, can be a noninfectious inflammation as a result of trauma or dental repair, or the inflammation may be because it is infected, thus increasing a practitioner's suspicion for a dental abscess. Less common diagnoses include Langerhans cells histiocytosis, lateral periodontal cyst, osteomyelitis, periapical granuloma, or cyst. Deciding the diagnosis will require consideration of the history of present illness and physical exam including tapping on the teeth to narrow down the location. It is also important to recognize that some differential diagnoses may be as a result of an untreated dental abscess, and thus co-exist (e.g., osteomyelitis, sinusitis, pulpitis).

TREATMENT

A dental abscess will not self-resolve. The primary treatment is I&D. Needle aspiration may be an appropriate alternative, particularly in anatomically difficult locations. Whenever possible, a wound culture of the fluid should be obtained to guide antibiotic treatment (Stephens et al., 2018).

Odontogenic infections are polymicrobial (Bayetto et al., 2020), and gram-negative and anaerobes are abundant. Antibiotic therapy needs to be sufficiently broad to cover a variety of bacteria and should be at least 10 days. Augmentin (amoxicillin-clavulanate) 875 mg orally every 12 hours is the most commonly-prescribed antimicrobial. Alternatives include clindamycin 300 mg to 450 mg three times a day, or levofloxacin plus metronidazole (Chow, 2020; Gould, 2019; Sanders & Houck, 2019).

Another aspect of the treatment care plan is pain control. NSAIDs should be part of the pain control regimen. However, pain control for a dental abscess will almost always require opioids (Stephens et al., 2018). To avoid painful stimuli while healing, a room-temperature soft diet is usually recommended (Gould, 2019).

Admission to a hospital is often not required, unless the infection is severe with a fever, difficulty breathing, or evidence of sepsis. In such cases patients should be admitted for IV antibiotics, and fluid resuscitation and establishment of a secure airway, if appropriate. The preferred antibiotic treatment choice for most patients is Unasyn (ampicillin-sublactam) 3 g IV every 6 hours.

TRANSITION OF CARE

Since most AGACNPs have limited training and experience in managing dental problems, it is often preferable to consult or refer the patient to a specialist for definitive care after determining the diagnosis, stabilizing the patient, and initiating treatments. If the abscess is uncomplicated, follow up with a dentist in 1 to 2 days is appropriate for tooth extraction or root canal. If the abscess is complicated, a dental surgeon or a maxillofacial surgeon is more appropriate once infection control measures and/or a sepsis protocol is initiated (Robertson et al., 2015).

KEY TAKEAWAYS

- Dental abscesses will not self-resolve.
- A dental abscess is often the result of poor oral hygiene and progression of dental decay.
- Dental abscesses can lead to sepsis.
- The gold standard of treatment is I&D.
- Consultation or referral to a specialist after stabilization, if appropriate.

2.20: EPIGLOTTITIS

Thomas Farley

Epiglottitis is defined as an infection of the epiglottis with resultant inflammation and edema. Epiglottitis may present as an airway emergency requiring airway intubation. Adjacent structures of arytenoids, vocal cords, and aryepiglottic folds are often involved. Epiglottitis is less common in children due to the widespread use of childhood *Haemophilus influenzae* type B (Hib) vaccine. Today it is predominately a disease of unvaccinated adults (Dowdy & Cornelius, 2020). Associated risk factors are male sex, tobacco smoke exposure, hypertension, and diabetes (Hanna et al., 2019; Sideris et al., 2020; Tsai et al., 2018).

Epiglottitis is caused by a variety of bacterial and viral pathogens, including SARS-COV2. This disorder can rapidly progress to complete airway obstruction. Approximately 11% of patients with epiglottitis will need an artificial airway (Sideris et al., 2020). Stridor is a late sign and highly correlated with loss of airway. Clinicians need to ensure that providers capable of performing cricothyrotomy are available when creating the airway plan. Treatment is IV antimicrobials. IV steroids and epiglottic abscess drainage are of unproven benefit (Dowdy & Cornelius, 2020; Sideris et al., 2020).

PRESENTING SIGNS AND SYMPTOMS

Signs and symptoms of epiglottitis include:
- Sore throat
- Fever
- Dyspnea
- Dysphagia
- Odynophagia
- Hoarseness of voice
- Stridor

HISTORY AND PHYSICAL FINDINGS
History

History relevant to epiglottitis may include:
- Exposure to e-cigarette or cannabis vapor.
- Exposure to tobacco smoke.
- Increased incidence with male sex, hypertension, COPD, advanced age, obesity, pre-existing epiglottic cyst, and diabetes (Hanna et al., 2019; Tsai et al., 2018).

Physical Examination

Physical examination findings include:
- Tachycardia
- Tachypnea
- Hypoxia
- Tripod stance
- Posterior oropharynx edema
- Enlarged tonsils
- Cervical lymphadenopathy
- If visualized the epiglottis is bright red and edematous/
- CT findings with epiglottic enlargement and pre-epiglottic edema
- Lateral neck radiograph can show the "thumb" sign (Figure 2.5; Angirekula & Multani, 2015).

DIFFERENTIAL DIAGNOSIS AND DIAGNOSTIC CONSIDERATIONS
Differential Diagnoses

Differential diagnoses include:
- *Epiglottic abscess.* An abscess may require surgical drainage.
- *Croup or laryngotracheobronchitis.* Upper airway infection that results in narrowing of the glottis. Often caused by viral infection. Associated with barking cough and stridor. Generally effects children under the age of 3.
- *Tracheitis.* Often develops as secondary bacterial infection complicating viral laryngotracheobronchitis. Caused by *Staphylococcus aureus, Haemophilus. influenzae,* alpha hemolytic streptococcus, and group A strep. Patients present with a history of upper respiratory tract illness, followed by high fever and malaise. Odynophagia and dysphagia are absent. Tracheitis generally affects children under the age of 8.

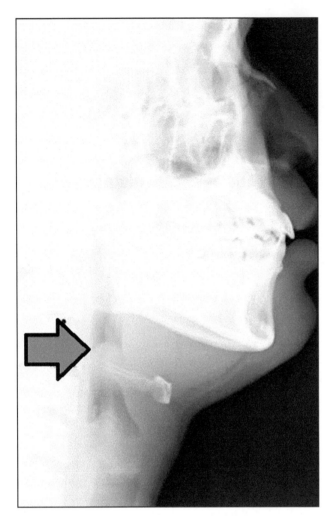

FIGURE 2.5: Lateral x-ray reveals "thumb sign" that indicates a swollen epiglottis, suggestive of epiglottitis. *Source*: Courtesy of Med Chaos.

- *Noninfectious causes:*
  - Thermal injury
  - Ingestion of caustic agents
  - Foreign body

Diagnostic Considerations

The most common cause is bacterial infection from the following:
- *Streptococcus pneumoniae*
- *Streptococcus pyogenes*
- *Staphylococcus aureus* (Harris et al., 2012)
- *Streptococcus viridians*
- *Neisseria meningitides*
- *Haemophilus influenzae B*
- *Serratia marcescens* (Musham et al., 2012)

Case reports of viral infections including (Fondaw et al., 2020)
- Coronavirus

Surface swab cultures are often negative so antibiotic therapy is empiric.

TREATMENT

Humidified, high flow oxygen should be delivered via mask or nasal cannula. Securing the airway may require video-assisted or fiberoptic visualization. Consider percutaneous cricothyroidotomy in lieu of an endotracheal tube. IV steroids such as dexamethasone 4 mg IV every 8 hours lack proven benefit but may decrease edema. Consider inhaled racemic epinephrine to treat mucosal edema. Treat infection with IV antibiotics such as a third-generation cephalosporin and include methicillin-resistant *Staphylococcus aureus* (MRSA) coverage with vancomycin. Patients with penicillin allergy should receive a quinolone antibiotic plus vancomycin (Dowdy & Cornelius, 2020). Consider *Haemophilus influenzae* type b (HiB) vaccination in high-risk unvaccinated adults.

TRANSITION OF CARE

Daily examination of supraglottic structures can help guide removal of the artificial airway and evaluate for abscess formation (Dowdy & Cornelius, 2020).

CLINICAL PEARLS

- Consider admission to critical care unit for continuous airway observation.
- Evaluate for impending airway obstruction.
- Stridor is a late sign.
- Anticipate and plan for difficult airway.
- Start empiric antibiotics immediately.

KEY TAKEAWAYS

- Epiglottitis is an infection of the epiglottis by a spectrum of infective organisms.
- Epiglottitis can evolve into an airway emergency.
- Metanalysis data show that approximately 11% of patients will require intubation.
- Assume that intubation will be difficult. Consult airway experts.

2.21: LARYNGITIS

R. Brandon Frady

Laryngitis is an inflammation of the larynx that is associated with a variety of conditions. Laryngitis has common presentations of acute or chronic, infective, or inflammatory, an isolated disorder, or a systemic disorder. Upper respiratory tract infections are a common cause of laryngitis. It is important to note that laryngitis may be a symptom of systemic disease.

The larynx is an organ that protects the airway, safe swallowing, and the creation of positive pressure. The larynx is essential for cough, straining, and swallowing.

The term laryngitis is defined as inflammation. Laryngitis is broken into an acute process and a chronic process. Acute laryngitis is typically self-limiting and is most commonly due to viral upper respiratory tract infection. In addition to URI, acute voice strain leading to trauma is a cause of acute laryngitis. Chronic laryngitis is associated with irritant exposure, gastroesophageal reflux, and habitual voice misuse.

Acute Laryngitis

Acute laryngitis is commonly caused by viral, bacterial, fungal, or trauma. Inflammation and edema are contributing to impaired vibration of vocal cord folds resulting in presenting symptoms. Inflammation may involve all areas of the larynx. Viral presentations include blisters, especially in cases of herpes, erythema, and pain disproportionate to mucosal appearance. Viruses are the most common cause of acute laryngitis. The most prevalent viruses are rhinovirus, adenovirus, influenza, and parainfluenza. Patients who are immunocompromised may have laryngitis secondary to herpes virus, HIV, or coxsackievirus. Viral laryngitis is rarely severe in nature.

Bacterial Laryngitis

Acute bacterial laryngitis is challenging to distinguish from viral causes, and both may exist simultaneously. Frequently encountered bacteria are *Haemophilus influenzae, Streptococcus pneumoniae, Staphylococcus aureus, Beta hemolytic streptococcus, Moraxella catarrhalis,* and *Klebsiella pneumoniae.* Typically, these bacteria create a pseudomembrane cast, purulence, erythema, and involvement with distant sites like the lungs and tonsils.

Fungal Laryngitis

Patients with fungal laryngitis are often underdiagnosed. Fungal laryngitis can be seen in both immunocompromised and immunocompetent patients. It is reported that fungal laryngitis is present in up to 10% of cases. The use of antibiotics and inhaled corticosteroids are risk factors. Laryngeal candidiasis may mimic other disorders like hyperkeratosis, leukoplakia, or malignancy. Biopsies are confirmatory for fungal infections but are often very difficult to obtain.

Phonotrauma

Phonotrauma is associated with acute or chronic vocal misuse. The vocal folds are forced together, causing trauma and inflammation. Examples of vocal stressors are screaming, forceful singing, and straining the voice. Phonotrauma can be acute or chronic.

Chronic Laryngitis

Chronic laryngitis is defined as symptoms that last longer than 3 weeks. Chronic laryngitis is associated with inflammatory processes, including allergies, laryngopharyngeal reflux, autoimmune disorders, and granulomatous conditions. In patients with chronic laryngitis, the glottis needs to be visualized; therefore, referral to

otolaryngology is essential. In a 2013 study by Stein et al., the rate of chronic laryngitis was approximately 3.47 per 1000 people. Over the last several years, there has been increased awareness of the extraesophageal symptom of laryngitis as a part of gastroesophageal reflux disease (GERD). Extensive population studies have demonstrated that patients with GERD are at risk for laryngeal and pulmonary complications.

PRESENTING SIGNS AND SYMPTOMS

Laryngeal symptoms can have many causes. When assessing the patient with laryngitis, it is essential to perform an airway assessment to determine airway patency and to quickly identify patients with stridor and/or respiratory distress. The rapid assessment and treatment of airway compromise is the primary intervention for patients with laryngitis with airway compromise. Laryngitis signs and symptoms include dysphonia, excessive air loss from incomplete closure of vocal cords, pain, or discomfort in the anterior neck. The primary presenting symptom is hoarseness. Additional symptoms may include cough, throat clearing, feeling of a lump in the throat, fever, myalgia, and dysphagia. It is key to ask the patient about dysphagia, otalgia, reflux, globus pharyngeal, weight loss, pulmonary status, and choking.

Additionally, an evaluation of lifestyle, smoking, diet, and hydration should be performed. Patients who have had recent neck surgery, recent endotracheal intubation, radiation to the neck, unintentional weight loss, or dysphagia, or have a history of smoking should be emergently or urgently referred. Odynophagia, dysphagia, hoarseness, drooling, and stridor are classic findings of a compromised airway and need immediate attention.

Patients with chronic laryngitis are likely to exhibit hoarseness, dysphagia, odynophagia, globus pharyngis, chronic cough, and repetitive throat clearing. Additionally, laryngeal reflux has been associated with premalignant and malignant conditions.

HISTORY AND PHYSICAL FINDINGS

The physical examination of the patient with laryngitis should include a general inspection and palpation of the head and neck, including the oral cavity and oropharynx, and a voice assessment. There are numerous scales available to assess phonation.

DIFFERENTIAL DIAGNOSIS AND DIAGNOSTIC CONSIDERATIONS

The differential diagnoses for laryngitis include sinusitis, pulmonary conditions, allergies, stridor, malignancy, otic etiologies, rhino etiologies, and aspiration. There are limited diagnostic considerations for laryngitis. Typically, the diagnosis is based on clinical presentation and examination of the patient's larynx. The suspicion of laryngitis, clinical assessment, and presumptive treatment aids in the confirmation of laryngitis.

TREATMENT

The management of laryngitis is based on the etiology and presentation of the patient. The most critical first step is to assess the airway patency and breathing of the patient. Patients with airway compromise should be evaluated for airway patency and emergent endotracheal intubation. In addition to intubation, corticosteroids, IV antibiotics for bacterial infections, and nebulized epinephrine are other possible treatments. Acute laryngitis is self-limiting and resolves within 2 weeks. Management of acute laryngitis includes vocal hygiene which consists of vocal rest, hydration, humidification, and caffeine intake limitation.

Antibiotics for acute laryngitis are often overprescribed. Patients with fever for greater than 48 hours, purulent sputum, presence of pseudomembranes or systemic symptoms should receive antimicrobial therapy. Antibiotic selection is based on the suspected causative organism. A 2014 study by Wood et al. suggested that the use of erythromycin improved vocal disturbance within 1 week and improvement in cough within 2 weeks. Fungal treatment with oral antifungals and monitoring for the resolution of signs and symptoms are the bases of treatment for fungal laryngitis. Treatment for chronic laryngeal reflux is focused on high-dose proton pump inhibitors, dietary modifications, and recommendations consistent with GERD management.

CLINICAL PEARLS

- Laryngitis causes are numerous and varied.
- Acute laryngitis is common and self-limited.
- Initial assessment of the patient must include airway assessment.
- Patients with immunocompromised states are at risk for infectious causes of laryngitis.
- Laryngopharyngeal reflux is associated with chronic laryngitis.

2.22: LUDWIG'S ANGINA

Thomas Farley

Ludwig's angina is an infectious disorder characterized by neck and perimandibular cellulitis with severe edema. Edema from the infection can lead to loss of airway from compression on lingual, epiglottic, or hypopharyngeal structures. The syndrome is named after a German surgeon and the sensation of strangulation associated with severe disease. Risk factors for developing Ludwig's angina include HIV infection and diabetes (Botha et al., 2015). Infections are often caused by dental caries, untreated oral infections, or trauma (Joshua et al., 2018).

A major challenge in Ludwig's angina is standard direct laryngoscopy, which is difficult to impossible to perform since the tongue cannot be displaced due to edema of the mandibular structures. AGACNPs must prepare for surgical airway access, which is required in up to 60% of patients (Botha et al., 2015). Retrospective reviews do not support IV antibiotics alone even in early-stage disease (Edetanlen & Saheeb, 2018). Approach to definitive treatment involves a CT scan of the neck with IV contrast and consultation with a head and neck surgeon. Anticipate and plan for goal-directed treatment of severe sepsis including IV fluids and vasopressors.

PRESENTING SIGNS AND SYMPTOMS

Signs and symptoms of Ludwig's angina include the following:
- Dysphagia
- Odynophagia
- Trismus
- Neck pain
- Fever
- Muffled or hoarse voice
- Stridor

HISTORY AND PHYSICAL FINDINGS

History

Ludwig's angina is seen with increased incidence in men. Relevant history includes diabetes, hypertension, HIV infection, alcoholism, and tobacco use.

Physical Examination

Physical examination findings may include the following:
- Firm, "woody" sub-mandible or neck on palpation
- Tachycardia
- Tachypnea
- Hypoxia
- Tripod stance
- Cervical lymphadenopathy

DIFFERENTIAL DIAGNOSIS AND DIAGNOSTIC CONSIDERATIONS

Differential Diagnoses

Differential diagnoses include:
- Salivary gland lithiasis with abscess. May mimic invasive soft tissue infection. Evaluate with CT neck with IV contrast.
- Mediastinitis if the infection invades the mediastinum. Evaluate with CT chest with IV contrast.
- Lemierre's syndrome, which is caused by tonsillitis or endometritis with hematogenous dissemination. Surgery is rarely required (Vallée et al., 2020).

TREATMENT

CT scanning with IV contrast imaging should be used to evaluate for tissue necrosis, fascial gas, drainable abscess, and infection margins (Joshua et al., 2018). Up to 60% of patients will require surgical airway interventions (Botha et al., 2015). Antibiotic therapy should cover oral flora including anaerobes. Ampicillin plus sulbactam is an adequate choice (Joshua et al., 2018). Consider adding methicillin-resistant *Staphylococcus aureus* (MRSA) and resistant gram-negative bacteria coverage in immunocompromised patients. Prognosis improves with combined surgical drainage and appropriate antibiotics (Edetanlen & Saheeb, 2018; Walia et al., 2014). A retrospective analysis by Botha et al. (2015) suggests that the most frequent complications include mediastinitis and necrotizing fasciitis (Botha et al., 2015).

TRANSITION OF CARE

Patients evaluated in the ED for suspected disease should have surgical consultation without delay. Admission may be directly to the operating room.

CLINICAL PEARLS

- Assess for underlying comorbidities and dental disease.
- Standard direct laryngoscopy is often impossible due to edema.
- Plan for fiberoptic nasopharyngeal or surgical airway.
- Give IV antibiotics to cover oral flora
- Therapy should include surgical drainage.
- Resuscitate with fluids as needed for sepsis. Measure lactate.

KEY TAKEAWAYS

- Syndrome has a high fatality rate even when reated appropriately with surgical drainage and IV antibiotics.
- Plan immediately for airway control with fiberoptic nasal approach or cricothyrotomy.
- Start IV antibiotics, consider CT imaging of neck with contrast, and consult a surgeon for drainage.
- Be vigilant for signs and symptoms of progressive sepsis and shock.

2.23: PAROTITIS

Helen Miley

Parotitis is an inflammation of the parotid glands. It can be noted as a local symptom or as a manifestation of a systemic process. Predisposing factors include anything that may interfere with salivation, such as dehydration, immunosuppression, and medications. It is commonly caused by *Staphylococcus aureus*, but *Streptococcus viridans*, *Escherichia coli*, and anaerobic oral flora may also be culprits. Autoimmune diseases such as Sjogen's syndrome or rheumatoid arthritis may also predispose a patient to parotitis (Wilson & Pandey, 2020).

PRESENTING SIGNS AND SYMPTOMS

The signs and symptoms of parotitis are progressive in nature. Enlargement is noted is one or both parotid glands, along with pain, especially with mastication, that subsides within 1 hour after eating. Physical examination will not reveal an enlarged, edematous, and tender gland.

DIFFERENTIAL DIAGNOSIS AND DIAGNOSTIC CONSIDERATIONS

There is little imaging that is diagnostic for parotitis. Ultrasound of the gland may demonstrate an abscess. Inflammatory markers may be elevated but are nonspecific. If there is drainage, a Gram stain may be helpful with speciation of the organism. Differential diagnoses include sialolithiasis, tumors, and sarcoidosis.

TREATMENT

Treatment is nonspecific and includes local heat application, massage of the gland and adequate hydration. If the pain is bothersome, anti-inflammatories agents, such as acetaminophen can be used. In immunocompromised patients, antibiotics are necessary. If the gram stain demonstrates an organism, the antibiotics should be tailored accordingly. If the parotitis is refractory to treatment, consultation with an otolaryngologist for incision and drainage may be considered.

CLINICAL PEARLS

- Parotitis is a clinical diagnosis. If chronic or relenting, then consultation for surgery is necessary.

KEY TAKEAWAYS

- *S. aureus* is the most common etiology.
- Parotitis has a favorable prognosis, but the underlying disease must also be treated.

2.24: PERITONSILLAR ABSCESS

Helen Miley

Peritonsillar cellulitis and abscess (PTA) are uncommon infections, but when noted, are very serious.

PRESENTING SIGNS AND SYMPTOMS

The usual presentation of a patient with PTA is a unilateral sore throat that is severe in nature. There is a muffled voice and the presence of drooling. Trismus (spasm of the jaw) may be noted in more than half of the patients. Secondary signs and symptoms include decreased oral intake, fatigue, and irritability.

DIFFERENTIAL DIAGNOSIS AND DIAGNOSTIC CONSIDERATIONS

Clinical examination and a thorough history are typically the only tools needed to make an accurate diagnosis. If drooling is present, suspect epiglottitis, and avoid being aggressive with the oral cavity examination. Imaging and examination in the operating room should be done if this is suspected. Other differentials include retropharyngeal or parapharyngeal abscesses, and severe tonsillitis.

TREATMENT

Antibiotics are the cornerstone of treatment. Surgical intervention is only necessary if there is airway compromise. Drainage of the abscess can be helpful.

CLINICAL PEARLS

- Not commonly seen in the adult population.
- Suspect if pain is unilateral, severe, with or without drooling.

KEY TAKEAWAYS

- Treatment with antibiotics is the cornerstone of treatment.

2.25: PHARYNGITIS

Nancy Knechel

Sore throat, tonsillar exudate, tender anterior cervical lymph nodes, and fever are highly suggestive of acute pharyngitis, particularly of bacterial etiology. If rhinorrhea, cough, conjunctivitis, hoarseness, and/or malaise are present, acute pharyngitis of viral etiology is more likely. The primary diagnostic test is a rapid antigen detection test and/or throat culture via a throat swab, although this will only identify bacterial pharyngitis, not viral. Other differential diagnoses to consider are mononucleosis, retropharyngeal/peritonsillar abscess, epiglottitis, Lemierre's syndrome, acute retroviral syndrome due to HIV, airway obstruction, allergic rhinitis (AR), head and neck neoplasias, gastroesophageal reflux disease (GERD), diphtheria, and herpes simplex virus (HSV). Viral and bacterial pharyngitis are typically self-limiting and can resolve without treatment. If a throat swab test is positive for group A beta-hemolytic streptococcal pharyngitis, treatment with an effective antibiotic, usually penicillin, for 10 days is accepted as the treatment of choice. Pain relief can be via systemic oral analgesia or topical anesthetics.

PRESENTING SIGNS AND SYMPTOMS

Sore throat and sudden onset of fever are the classic signs and symptoms for acute pharyngitis. The majority of viral pharyngitis cases are caused by respiratory viruses, such as adenovirus, coronavirus, and rhinovirus, and thus the signs and symptoms often include those of an upper respiratory tract infection (Chow & Doron, 2020). Symptoms that are overtly viral include rhinorrhea, cough, conjunctivitis, hoarse voice, malaise, and/or oral ulcers or vesicles (Shapiro et al., 2017). In the absence of these viral features, bacterial etiology is more likely. Patients may also report a headache and chills.

HISTORY AND PHYSICAL FINDINGS

The history and physical examination should focus on differentiating a chief complaint of sore throat due to uncomplicated acute pharyngitis from other etiologies (Wolford et al., 2018). In history taking, it is important to note the onset, duration, progression, and severity of the symptoms. Symptoms are usually described as sudden or acute in onset. It is also important to determine if there is a history of exposure to *Streptococcus* within the last 2 weeks.

On exam, AGACNPs are likely to find pharyngeal erythema, edema, engorged uvula, patchy tonsillar or pharyngeal exudate, enlarged tonsils, petechial eruption on the soft palate, and prominent and tender anterior cervical lymphadenopathy. There may be a scarlatiniform rash and a strawberry tongue (Chow & Doron, 2020).

Warning signs of complicated pharyngitis that is compromising the airway include drooling, muffled voice, stridor, dyspnea, tachypnea, and tripod positioning. Complications may also involve deep neck space infections, as evidenced by asymmetric bulging of the pharyngeal wall or soft palate, stiff or painful neck, trismus, fevers/chills, and neck crepitus (Chow & Doron, 2020).

DIFFERENTIAL DIAGNOSIS AND DIAGNOSTIC CONSIDERATIONS

Most cases of pharyngitis are viral. When it is bacterial, group A beta-hemolytic *Streptococcus* is the most common etiology. However, even differentiating between these two solely based on clinical signs and symptoms can be difficult. Furthermore, the signs and symptoms of pharyngitis overlap significantly with many other infectious sources, making diagnosis difficult when exclusively based on signs and symptoms (Choby, 2009; Shapiro et al., 2017).

Although group A beta-hemolytic *Streptococcus* is the most common cause for bacterial pharyngitis, group B, C, or G *Streptococcus* can also cause acute pharyngitis. More rare causes include *Arcanobacterium haemolyticum, Fusobacterium necrophorum, Mycoplasma pneumoniae, Chlamydia pneumoniae, Corynebacterium diptheriae, Francisella tularensis, Neisseria gonorrhoeae, Treponema pallidum,* and HIV (Wolford et al., 2018).

Obtaining a throat culture is the best way to distinguish viral from bacterial pharyngitis. It will also identify the pathogen, facilitating diagnosis to guide appropriate antibiotic therapy (Mustafa & Ghaffari, 2020). Rapid antigen detection tests are widely available, which provide highly specific results much faster, but test sensitivity varies from 70% to 90% (Wolford et al., 2018). The pharyngotonsillar swabs are collected at the point of care, and a positive throat culture can confirm the diagnosis. Obtaining lab tests only serves as an adjunct, and imaging, such as a chest or lateral neck x-ray, is generally unnecessary unless there is concern for pulmonary involvement or possible airway compromise. Likewise, a CT scan would be unnecessary unless there is concern for a mass or abscess (Wolford et al., 2018).

Mononucleosis is a pharyngeal infection with the Epstein-Barr virus and often presents similarly, with sore throat, fever, pharyngeal exudates, soft palate petechia, and malaise. One common feature of infectious mononucleosis that should make this diagnosis less likely is if posterior cervical lymphadenopathy is absent. Patients with mononucleosis may also have hepatosplenomegaly, which would not be present in pharyngitis.

Other differentials to consider are retropharyngeal abscess or peritonsillar abscess, epiglottitis, Lemierre's syndrome or internal jugular vein thrombophlebitis, acute retroviral syndrome due to HIV, airway obstruction, AR, head and neck neoplasias, GERD, diphtheria, and HSV (Wolford et al., 2018).

TREATMENT

Both viral and bacterial pharyngitis are self-limiting and can resolve without treatment. Untreated group A beta-hemolytic *Streptococcus* generally lasts 7 to 10 days, although when bacterial pharyngitis goes untreated, it extends the length of illness, extends the length of communicability, and increases the chances for complications, such as peritonsillar abscess or rheumatic fever. Evidence-based recommendations for treatment are mixed, with inconclusive research on whether to prescribe antibiotics to patients to reduce the risk of rheumatic fever, or to forego prescriptions to minimize antibiotic resistance (Oliver et al., 2018). Treatment with an effective antibiotic for 10 days is usually accepted for swab-positive group A beta-hemolytic streptococcal pharyngitis. Oral penicillin is the antibiotic of choice. Alternatively, amoxicillin, cephalosporins, and macrolides may also be used. For patients with a penicillin allergy, azithromycin or clindamycin can be used (Wolford et al., 2018).

Patients often seek pain relief from the sore throat. Treatment may be topical or systemic oral analgesics. Over-the-counter systemic therapy is recommended and generally sufficient, such as NSAIDs, aspirin, or acetaminophen. For those with contraindications, at high risk of side effects from systemic analgesics, or those wishing to avoid systemic therapy, topical therapies via lozenges or sprays, are a reasonable option (Stead, 2020).

TRANSITION OF CARE

There is generally no need to transfer care to a specialist for uncomplicated acute pharyngitis. Most AGACNPs have access to the pharyngeal swab tests and can appropriately manage pharyngitis independently.

CLINICAL PEARLS

- Antibiotics are often overprescribed since the majority of acute pharyngitis cases (50%–80%) are viral.
- Clinicians often believe antibiotics are the most important treatment sought by patients; however, research has shown more than 80% of patients are primarily interested in pain relief and reassurance.

KEY TAKEAWAYS

- The chief complaint for acute pharyngitis is most commonly a sudden onset of a sore throat.
- A rapid antigen detection test and throat culture are the primary diagnostic tools.
- Penicillin V 500 mg BID or TID for 10 days is the treatment of choice for group A *Streptococcus* pharyngitis.

2.26: SIALADENITIS

R. Brandon Frady

Sialadenitis is an inflammation of the salivary glands. The major salivary glands include paired parotid, submandibular, and sublingual glands. While there are thousands of minor glands, these major glands account for 95% of saliva production. Men are more likely to develop sialolithiasis than women, with an occurrence between 30 and 60 years of age. The majority (75%) of sialadenitis cases are unilateral, with 25% being bilateral (Cascarini & McGurk, 2009). In a recent study (877 cases) 73% of obstructive sialadenitis was associated with calculi and 26% was associated with stricture (Cascarini & McGurk, 2009). Risk factors associated with the development of sialadenitis or sialolithiasis are hypovolemia, diuretics, anticholinergic medications, gout, trauma, smoking, nephrolithiasis, and chronic periodontal disease (Wilson et al., 2014).

The pathogenesis of sialadenitis or sialolithiasis is not fully known. Theoretically, stagnation of salivary flow and elevated salivary calcium levels are thought to be significant contributors. Inflammation of the salivary gland or duct along with localized injury are often contributing factors. Sialadenitis is classified as acute, chronic, or sialosis (Wilson et al., 2014).

Acute Unifocal Salivary Gland Swelling

Acute sialadenitis is a sudden, painful enlargement of the affected gland. Typically, acute sialadenitis is associated with obstruction, infection, inflammation, or stricture. The classification of acute unifocal salivary gland swelling is determined by the duration lasting less than a few weeks. The onset and duration are based on the etiology. Etiologies include obstruction, infection, ductal stricture, ductal foreign body, pneumoparotitis, or external duct compression with obstruction secondary to sialolithiasis (salivary stone) being the most common.

Sialadenitis Infection

For patients with acute unifocal salivary gland swelling, the evaluation for infection is essential. Bacterial infections are classified as primary and secondary. Primary bacterial sialadenitis develops over a few hours to days and is associated with fever, gland tenderness, and purulent drainage. A complete look at the signs, symptoms, and treatment is discussed later. Secondary bacterial sialadenitis occurs secondary to ductal obstruction. The patient may have obstructive symptoms days before the development of infectious symptoms.

Obstructive Sialadenitis

Sialadenitis is frequently associated with salivary gland obstruction. The cause of obstructive sialadenitis is associated with salivary stones or strictures. Classically, patients have intermittent gland swelling around the time of salivary gland stimulation. Mechanical obstruction causes the gland to swell. Obstruction is associated with sialolithiasis (stones), ductal stricture, ductal foreign body, pneumoparotitis, and external compression. Sialolithiasis is the most common cause of obstruction and sialadenitis. Risk factors for salivary stones include hypovolemia, diuretic use, anticholinergic medications, trauma, gout, smoking, and chronic periodontal disease.

Salivary duct strictures or foreign bodies are also potential causes of sialadenitis. Ductal strictures often present like salivary stones. While ultrasound may aid in the diagnosis of stricture, sialography is more sensitive compared to ultrasound. Causes of stricture are attributed to irradiation, trauma, prior infection, autoimmune disease, or unknown etiologies. Foreign bodies in the salivary gland(s) are infrequent but may be associated with the retrograde entrance of a foreign body into the duct. Ultrasound and CT may not effectively detect foreign bodies, so sialography is used to diagnose ductal foreign bodies.

Pneumoparotitis

Pneumoparotitis happens as a result of air entering into the duct or gland. This typically occurs when air is forced under pressure into the oral cavity. Noninvasive positive pressure or continuous positive airway pressure can lead to pneumoparotitis. In patients with pneumoparotitis, the drainage from the affected gland will appear bubbly. Treatment is associate with limiting or removal of the positive pressure. Pneumoparotitis sustained for an extended period can lead to chronic duct changes and possible chronic infections.

Inflammation

Patients may develop sialadenitis secondary to inflammatory processes. Inflammation is most often associated with postradiation sialadenitis. The swelling and pain will usually subside within weeks to months after the discontinuing of radiation therapy. Damage can be to the duct, or the gland itself, is the root cause of inflammatory sialadenitis.

Acute Multifocal Salivary Gland Swelling

Acute multifactorial salivary gland swelling is associated with a viral illness, inflammation, juvenile recurrent parotitis, drug-induced sialadenitis, and acute sialadenitis of bulimia nervosa. Viral sialadenitis is most often associated with mumps, but it may be secondary to adenovirus, enterovirus, parvovirus, and herpes virus type 6.

In addition to a viral illness, inflammation of the salivary glands is associated with radioiodine treatment (131-I) for thyroid carcinoma or hyperthyroidism and iodinated contrast dye. Patients receiving 131-I will have pain, swelling, and xerostomia that is worse with higher doses of radiation. Symptoms may develop within hours of exposure and last for several days. Finally, contrast-induced sialadenitis is a rapid and painless enlargement of a salivary gland that may occur shortly after infusion of iodinated contrast. Contrast-induced sialadenitis occurs with high iodine loads and in patients with renal dysfunction. Less rare conditions associated with multifocal salivary gland swelling are drug-induced and in bulimia patients that stop vomiting. For both of these cases, patients have a short duration of swelling and are supported with NSAIDs.

PRESENTING SIGNS AND SYMPTOMS

When evaluating patients with sialadenitis, consider whether symptoms are persistent, intermittent, or recurrent. Consider the duration of symptoms to determine acute versus chronic status and consider the location and number of glands involved to determine categorization. Patients may present with discomfort in the area of swelling, foul taste in the mouth, aggravation of symptoms secondary to a stimulus (eating or salivary stimulants), fever, prodromal viral illness, weight loss, joint pain, dry eyes, or dry mouth (Cascarini & McGurk, 2009).

Acute Unifocal Presentation

Patients with acute unifocal sialadenitis are assessed first for infection by evaluating patients for fever, significant gland tenderness, and purulent saliva expression. Timing of symptoms is often helpful in determining if the infection is primary or secondary (Wilson et al., 2014). Primary infections may develop over hours to days, with fever present at the time of swelling. Additionally, patients may complain of a foul taste in the mouth, or ductal massage reveals purulent saliva. If secondary bacterial sialadenitis is present, the obstructive symptoms will be present for days before infectious symptoms. Infection is secondary to obstruction and presents with swollen glands with tenderness or pain, purulent saliva if the duct is partially obstructed, and fever.

In the absence of an infection, patients with acute sialadenitis associated with obstruction present with enlarged, tender glands without erythema or warmth at the gland site (Cascarini & McGurk, 2009). The onset of swelling often occurs within seconds of salivary gland stimulation.

Finally, it is important to note sialadenitis can be chronic. Table 2.19 compares acute versus chronic causes of sialadenitis. Some common causes are tumors, immune-mediated process, infectious nature, and infiltrative process.

TABLE 2.19: Comparison of Acute Versus Chronic Sialadenitis

ACUTE	CHRONIC
Acute Unifocal: <ul><li>Obstruction</li><li>Ductal stricture</li><li>Pneumoparotitis</li><li>External compression of duct</li><li>Infectious</li><li>Inflammation</li></ul>	**Chronic Unifocal:** <ul><li>Tumor</li><li>Polycystic parotid disease</li></ul>
Acute Multifocal: <ul><li>Viral infections<ul><li>Mumps</li><li>Other viral conditions</li></ul></li><li>Inflammation<ul><li>Radiation treatment (131-I)</li><li>Contrast-induced</li></ul></li><li>Juvenile recurrent parotitis</li><li>Drug-induced</li><li>Bulimia nervosa</li></ul>	**Chronic Multifocal:** <ul><li>Metabolic causes</li><li>Immune-mediated<ul><li>Sjogren's syndrome</li><li>IgG4 disease</li><li>Kussmaul disease</li></ul></li><li>Granulomatous<ul><li>Sarcoidosis</li><li>Anti-neutrophilic cytoplasmic autoantibodies (ANCA) vasculiti</li><li>HIV-related</li></ul></li><li>Infiltrative causes</li><li>Amyloidosis</li></ul>

HISTORY AND PHYSICAL FINDINGS

When assessing the salivary gland(s), the essential starting point is evaluating the duration of symptoms and the number of glands involved. Additional information necessary to diagnosing sialadenitis is the number of glands, gland size, texture, tenderness, erythema of the surrounding skin, foul taste in the mouth, symptoms associated with eating or salivary stimulants, fever, viral illness, weight loss, joint pain, and dry eyes or mouth (Ugga et al., 2017). Comorbid conditions of alcohol use, diabetes, bulimia, autoimmune disease, liver disease, local external beam radiation, recent IV contrast injection, and any new medications are included in the initial workup.

The physical exam offers valuable information aiding in the diagnosis of sialadenitis. Essential elements of the physical exam include the number of gland(s) involved, size of the gland(s), the texture of the gland(s), tenderness of the gland, erythema of skin surrounding the gland, massaging the gland to express saliva or purulent output, and otologic evaluation in patients with ear pain (Ugga et al., 2017). The number of the gland(s) determines if there is a unifocal condition or multifocal condition. Gland(s) size of normal, atrophic, or enlarged is essential to the physical exam. Palpation of the gland provides information about the texture, whether smooth, sift, firm, nodular, or a distinct mass. Salivary discharge may be thin and watery (normal), mucoid, purulent, bubbly, and reduced or absent. Additionally, a focused cranial nerve V (trigeminal nerve) and VII (facial nerve) are included with gland(s) swelling (Ugga

et al., 2017). Finally, careful attention should be given to the surrounding structure adjacent to the gland(s) as these structures may be causing the salivary gland(s) symptoms and require evaluation during the physical examination.

DIFFERENTIAL DIAGNOSIS AND DIAGNOSTIC CONSIDERATIONS

Differential diagnoses include viral illness, HIV, Sjogren's syndrome, sarcoidosis, salivary gland tumors, benign and malignant tumor, and vascular conditions (Chen et al., 2013).

Imaging is an essential part of the diagnostic process for salivary disorders. Diagnostic considerations include ultrasound, CT, MRI, and sialendoscopy (Ugga et al., 2017). Ultrasound or CT with contrast are the most commonly used diagnostic testing for patients with salivary gland disorders. If a patient has a contraindication to the contrast, then noncontrast is acceptable for salivary gland(s) assessment (Ugga et al., 2017). For patients suspected of neoplasms or vascular conditions of the salivary gland(s), MRI is the most appropriate diagnostic tool. Other techniques for evaluating salivary gland(s) are sialography and sialendoscopy (Ugga et al., 2017). Otolaryngologists generally perform these procedures.

TREATMENT

The treatment of sialadenitis is based on the etiology. In this section acute management is the focus of treatments as these patients may present to the healthcare system for care. Initial management consists of conservative management with the possibility of consultation to otolaryngology.

Acute

Sialadenitis is considered acute when the duration is less than a few weeks. Acute unifocal salivary gland swelling is the most common cause (Cascarini & McGurk, 2009). Treatment is focused initially on sialagogues (salivary stimulants) such as sour candy, local heat, oral hydration, and massage of the involved salivary gland as the initial treatment for acute unifocal sialadenitis. This initial conservative treatment is most successful in patients with partial obstructions (Wilson et al., 2014). Patients with complete obstruction may experience pain with salivary stimulation. In cases where patients develop pain with sour candy, treatment referral to otolaryngology is appropriate.

The treatment for sialadenitis from stone obstruction is focused on the nonpharmacological treatment of tart sour candy, discontinuing offending medications if able, pain control with NSAIDs, and, if infections are suspected antistaphylococcal antibiotics for 7 to 10 days (Wilson et al., 2014). If there is no improvement with these methods, then referral to an otolaryngologist is needed.

CLINICAL PEARLS

- Salivary gland swelling may be due to many causes.
- Determining the timing, duration, and infectious nature is essential to diagnosing sialadenitis.
- First-line imaging is ultrasound or CT.
- Consultation to otolaryngology is needed for cases unresponsive to conservative methods or recurrent sialadenitis.

2.27: UPPER RESPIRATORY INFECTION/ COUGH

Beth McLear

The common cold is an acute upper respiratory infection usually caused by a viral pathogen. It is one of the most common infections encountered in the United States (Harris et al., 2016). Most cases are minor and self-limiting with symptoms lasting 7 to 10 days (Arroll & Kenealy, 2018). Rhinoviruses and adenoviruses are the most common viral pathogens, although over 200 viruses can cause colds (CDC, n.d.). Because of these common viruses' numerous serotypes, patients are susceptible to the common cold throughout the life span. Treatment is based on the alleviation of symptom duration and severity. Occasionally, the common cold is implicated in developing and exacerbating other diseases such as acute bacterial sinusitis, acute otitis media (AOM), bronchitis, asthma, and cystic fibrosis.

PRESENTING SIGNS AND SYMPTOMS

Common cold symptoms usually appear 2 to 3 days after inoculation. Patients typically present with rhinorrhea, nasal congestion, sore throat, cough, general malaise, and occasionally a low-grade fever. Sore throat, rhinorrhea, sneezing, nasal congestion, or obstruction of nasal breathing are common early in the course. The severity and type of symptoms will vary with individuals and factors related to the infective pathogen. A cough is common and typically develops on the fourth or fifth day and outlasts other cold symptoms. The cough is caused by laryngeal involvement or may be related to upper airway syndrome related to nasal secretions from postnasal drip (Druce et al., 2016).

HISTORY AND PHYSICAL FINDINGS

History

Rhinorrhea is more common and characteristic of a viral infection than a bacterial infection. Secretions often evolve from clear to opaque white to green to yellow within 2 to 3 days of symptom onset in a viral URI. For that reason, it is important not to use color and opacity to distinguish viral from bacterial illness unless they persist for more than 10 to 14 days (Chow, 2012). Other symptoms include sore throat, sneezing, mild body aches, low-grade fever, and cough.

Physical Exam

Fever, if present, is low grade. Typically, the nasal mucous membranes have a glistening, glassy appearance, but mild erythema or edema may also be present. The pharynx appears normal, without any erythema, exudate, or ulceration. If the infection is secondary to adenovirus, mild pharyngeal edema is present. If there is marked erythema, edema, exudates, or small vesicles are observed in the oropharynx, consider other etiologies such as Epstein-Barr virus (EBV) or group A beta hemolytic Streptococcal (GAS) infection. Occasionally mildly enlarged, nontender cervical lymph nodes are present. Chest auscultation may reveal rhonchi.

DIFFERENTIAL DIAGNOSIS AND DIAGNOSTIC CONSIDERATIONS

Differential Diagnoses

Many symptoms of the common cold may overlap with other conditions. It is important to distinguish the common cold from these more serious or treatable disorders. Differential diagnoses for the common cold include COVID-19, influenza, allergic rhinitis, isolated pharyngitis, bacterial sinusitis, pertussis, and acute bronchitis, which generally has a longer duration, with a mean of 18 days in adults (Ebell et al., 2013). Table 2.20 provides a summary of distinguishing features that may be considered when distinguishing the common cold from other diagnoses.

Diagnostic Considerations

If a thorough history and physical exam indicate a viral etiology consistent with the common cold, an aggressive workup is not necessary. If influenza or COVID-19 are suspected, then specific viral testing should be performed. A CBC may be considered but is of little value in the diagnosis of the common cold. If other bacterial or viral infections are suspected, screening and cultures should be performed.

TREATMENT

Explaining the self-limited nature of the common cold to patients can assist with managing expectations, limiting antibiotic use, and avoiding over-the-counter purchases that may not help. Antibiotics are not indicated in the treatment of the common cold and should not be prescribed (Spurling et al., 2017). Therapy aimed at reducing the severity and duration of symptoms is the mainstay of treatment of the common cold in the immunocompetent adult. These therapies include analgesics, decongestants with or without antihistamines, intranasal ipratropium, and zinc.

Analgesics

NSAID drugs reduce headache, ear pain, muscle pain, joint pain, and sneezing but do not improve cough, cold duration, or total symptom score (Kim et al., 2015;

TABLE 2.20: Distinguishing Features of Common Cold, Influenza, COVID-19, Allergic Rhinitis, and Acute Bronchitis

	COMMON COLD	INFLUENZA	COVID-19	ALLERGIC RHINITIS	ACUTE BRONCHITIS
Onset	Gradual	Rapid	Varies	Gradual	Gradual
Cough*	Common, dry	Common, dry	Common	Common, chronic	Prominent, persistent, wet, or dry
Rhinorrhea	Common	Sometimes	Uncommon	Common	Uncommon
Sore throat	Common	Sometimes	Uncommon	Sometimes, on awakening	Common
Fever or chills*	None or low grade	Common, high	Common	Uncommon	uncomon
Aches and pains	Mild	Common	Common	Uncommon	Sometimes
Shortness of breath	Uncommon	Uncommon	Sometimes	Uncommon	Sometimes, mild
Sneezing	Common	Sometimes	Uncommon	Common	Uncommon
Congestion	Common	Sometimes	Uncommon	Common	Uncommon
Loss of taste or smell*	Sometimes	Uncommon	Sometimes, sudden	Uncommon	No
Headache	Common, mild	Common	Sometimes	Uncommon	Uncommon
Nausea or vomiting	Uncommon	Sometimes	Uncommon	No	Uncommon
Diarrhea	Uncommon	Sometimes	Uncommon, except in children	No	Uncommon

*Fever, chills, loss of taste or smell and cough are common in COVID-19.

Source: Data from World Health Organization. (2020). *Q&A: Influenza and COVID-19–similarities and differences*. https://www.who.int/westernpacific/news/q-a-detail/q-a-similarities-and-differences-covid-19-and-influenza; Centers for Disease Control and Prevention. (n.d.). *Cold versus flu*. https://www.cdc.gov/flu/symptoms/coldflu.htm; Seidman, M. D., Gurgel, R. K., Lin, S. Y., Schwartz, S. R., Baroody, F. M., Bonner, J. R., Dawson, D. E., Dykewicz, M. S., Hackell, J. M., Han, J. K., Ishman, S. L., Krouse, H. J., Malekzadeh, S., Mims, J. W., Omole, F. S., Reddy, W. D., Wallace, D. V., Walsh, S. A., Warren, B. E., … Guideline Otolaryngology Development Group. AAO-HNSF. (2015). Clinical practice guideline: Allergic rhinitis. *Otolaryngology–Head and Neck Surgery, 152*(1, Suppl.), S1–S43. https://doi.org/10.1177/0194599814561600; Dykewicz, M. S., Wallace, D. V., Amrol, D. J., Fuad M Baroody, F. M., Bernstein, J. A., Craig, T. J., Dinakar, C., Ellis, A. K., Finegold, I., Golden, D. B. K., Greenhawt, M. J., Hagan, J. B., Horner, C. C., Khan, D. A., Lang, D. M., Larenas-Linnemann, D. S. S., Lieberman, J. A., Meltzer, E. O., Oppenheimer, J. J., … Steven, G. V. (2020). Rhinitis: A practice parameter update. *The Journal of Allergy and Clinical Immunology, 146*(4), 721–767. https://doi.org/10.1016/j.jaci.2020.07.007

Malesker et al., 2017). Acetaminophen has been shown to provide a short-term reduction of rhinorrhea and nasal congestion, but has no effect on a sore throat, malaise, sneezing, or cough (Li et al., 2013; Malesker et al., 2017).

Decongestants and Antihistamines

Oral and topical nasal decongestants relieve nasal congestion, but there is no evidence to support that they relieve cough (Deckx et al., 2016; Malesker et al., 2017). Topical oxymetazoline, which is included in many common over-the-counter intranasal decongestants, reduces the duration and severity of nasal congestion after multiple doses but is associated with the risk of rhinitis medicamentosa when used for more than 3 days (Reinecke & Tschaikin, 2005). Antihistamines combined with oral decongestants and/or analgesics may provide some relief of cold symptoms, with a limited effect on cough. Evidence does not support antihistamine monotherapy for relief of cold symptoms, including cough (DeSutter et al., 2015).

Intranasal Ipratropium

Ipratropium, an anticholinergic, inhibits secretions from the serous and seromucous glands lining the nasal mucosa and provides relief from rhinorrhea (AlBawalii et al., 2013).

Zinc

Several meta-analysis and systematic reviews suggest that taking at least 75 mg of zinc acetate or gluconate lozenges per day relieves cough and nasal discharge more quickly when treatment is started within 24 hours of symptom onset (Hemilä, 2017; Hemilä & Chalker, 2015; Science et al., 2012).

Other Common Treatments

There are many other common treatments that are often utilized that show little to no benefit in treating the common cold. Nasal irrigation with saline is effective for the treatment of chronic rhinosinusitis (CRS). However, only low-quality evidence supports its benefit in upper respiratory infections (URIs; King et al., 2015). Intranasal steroids are not more effective than placebo for reducing symptom duration or severity in the common cold. The use of vitamin C and D supplements has not shown improvement in the severity or duration of symptoms (Hemilä & Chalker,

2013; Murdoch et al., 2012). Commonly recommended antitussives and expectorants have little benefit in the treatment of cough due to the common cold and are not recommended for use by the American College of Chest Physicians (Malesker et al., 2017)

CLINICAL PEARLS

- Analgesics, decongestants with or without antihistamines, and intranasal ipratropium provide symptomatic relief.
- Intranasal steroids and antihistamine monotherapy are not recommended.
- Zinc, when started within 24 hours of symptom onset, may provide relief from cough and nasal congestion duration.

KEY TAKEAWAYS

- Acute URI due to the common cold is usually a self-limiting disease.
- Do not treat with antibiotics.
- Provide suggestions for symptomatic relief.

 SPRINGER PUBLISHING CONNECT™

A robust set of instructor resources designed to supplement this text is located at **http://connect.springerpub.com/content/ reference-book/978-0-8261-6079-9.** Qualifying instructors may request access by emailing **textbook@springerpub.com.**

REFERENCES

Full list of references can be accessed at http://connect .springerpub.com/content/reference-book/978-0-8261-6079-9

CARDIOVASCULAR DISORDERS

INTRODUCTION

Disorders of the cardiovascular (CV) system are some of the most commonly encountered conditions across the acute care population and have evolved into a specialty within healthcare. The AGACNP must have a solid foundation of the structure, function, and physiology of the CV system in order to appreciate and recognize pathophysiology. Disorders of the CV system are complex and include coronary artery disease (CAD), hypertension, cardiomyopathy, structural heart disorders, arrhythmias, and infectious and inflammatory conditions. This chapter provides a brief but comprehensive introduction to the CV system and reviews common disorders, current therapeutic guidelines, and treatments for each diagnosis.

3.1: CORONARY ARTERY DISEASE

Lynda Stoodley

Coronary artery diseae (CAD), otherwise known as atherosclerotic cardiovascular disease (ASCVD) remains the leading cause of mortality and morbidity in the United States (*The ABCs of Primary Cardiovascular Prevention: 2019 Update*, 2019).

The development of CAD begins in childhood and can progress with time. The rate of progression varies and can accelerate due to various factors, such as endothelial dysfunction, dyslipidemia, inflammatory, and immunologic factors, plaque rupture, and smoking (Zhao, 2020). Atherosclerosis causes narrowing of arteries and when it occurs in the coronary vessel, the coronary artery lumen diminishes in size and can lead to ischemia of the myocardium. This occurs as a result of a mismatch of oxygen demand versus supply. If the lumen becomes completely obstructed, a myocardial infarction (MI) may occur (Figure 3.1). The extent of myocardial consequence is impacted by the location, degree, and disease burden (Anderson, 2016).

CAD can lead to acute coronary syndrome (ACS), which may be fatal if untreated. ACS includes ST-elevation myocardial infarctions (STEMI), non-ST-elevation myocardial infarctions (NSTEMI), and unstable angina (Singh et al., 2020).

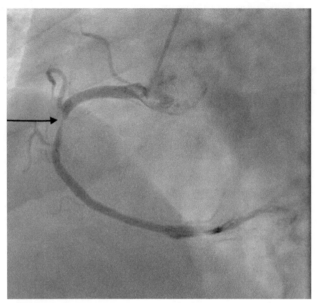

FIGURE 3.1: Right coronary artery occlusion.

PRESENTING SIGNS AND SYMPTOMS

Patients with CAD may be asymptomatic until progression leads to a mismatch between oxygen demand and supply which may cause a patient to develop symptoms. A common sign of CAD is chest pain, which may or may not radiate down either arm, or into the jaw, and may occur with or without exertion. The sensation may be described as pain, pressure, crushing, tightness, or squeezing. The patient may also present with a combination of shortness of breath (SOB), diaphoresis, palpitations, fatigue, and nausea and vomiting. Patients with diabetes, the elderly, and women may present with vague symptoms (Singh et al., 2020). Symptoms that occur with exertion and resolve with activity cessation should be treated as a red flag for CAD.

HISTORY AND PHYSICAL FINDINGS

History

Certain modifiable and nonmodifiable risk factors increase a patient's likelihood for developing CAD. Obtaining a thorough history to identify risk factors for CAD is vital when the AGACNP is evaluating a patient suspected of having CAD.

Nonmodifiable Risk Factors

CAD prevalence increases after 35 years of age (Sanchis-Gomar et al., 2016). Males have a higher risk although the risk narrows significantly in postmenopausal females (Brown et al., 2020). Additionally, Blacks, Hispanics, Latinos, and Southeast Asians are at higher risk

of developing CAD (Carnethon et al., 2017; Rodriguez et al., 2014; Volgman et al., 2018). Lastly, family history of premature CAD, which is defined as occurring prior to age 50, increases a person's chances of CAD.

Modifiable Risk Factors

Modifiable risk factors include hypertension, hyperlipidemia, diabetes mellitus, obesity, smoking, poor diet, and a sedentary lifestyle (Brown et al., 2020). Socioeconomic factors such as financial strain, lack of affordable and nutritious food, exposure to domestic violence, and inadequate housing also place the patient at risk of CAD (Brown et al., 2020).

Physical Findings

Physical findings may be absent or minimal in patients with stable CAD. As the disease progresses and/or becomes unstable, findings may be present on physical exam. If the disease becomes unstable and ACS develops, the patient may appear anxious and be diaphoretic, often rubbing their chest. If the patient has congestive heart failure (CHF), they may present with crackles and have extra heart sounds, such as an S3. Murmurs may be present if chordae or papillary muscles are ruptured. Lower extremity edema may be present if the right and/or left ventricle begin to fail. Blood pressure and heart rate may be high or low. Arrythmias such as atrial fibrillation, ventricular tachycardias (VTs), or complete heart block may occur.

DIFFERENTIAL DIAGNOSIS AND DIAGNOSTIC CONSIDERATIONS

Differential diagnoses of CAD include gastroesophageal reflux disease (GERD), which may have symptoms similar to CAD. If chest discomfort is relieved by antacids, the symptoms are most likely gastrointestinal (GI) in origin. Musculoskeletal disorders, such as costochondritis or arthritis, may also cause chest pain. If the patient is able to pinpoint the discomfort or if it is localized to one area, a cardiac disorder is less likely as cardiac ischemia discomfort is usually diffuse across the chest. Anxiety may also cause chest discomfort or shortness of breath (SOB); anxiety should be considered if the patient has minimal or no risk factors for CAD or is very young. Pericarditis may cause chest pain and the patient may report relief in symptoms when leaning forward and/or the ECG will show global ST segment elevation in all leads. Lastly, pneumonia can cause pleuritic chest pain or SOB, similar to cardiac ischemic symptoms.

Life-threatening disorders that may also cause chest discomfort are pulmonary embolism or aortic dissection, which can be diagnosed by CT angiogram. Diagnosing these disorders quickly is imperative for any clinician.

TREATMENT

Primary Prevention

Measures to decrease the incidence of atherosclerotic heart disease begin with primary prevention. According to Arnett et al. (2019), this can be accomplished by promoting a healthy lifestyle. In 2015, approximately 630,000 Americans died from heart disease, with 366,000 dying from CAD (Arnett et al., 2019), most likely due to suboptimal implementation of prevention strategies and uncontrolled ASCVD risk factors (Arnett et al., 2019; Johnson et al., 2014; Weir et al., 2016). Lifestyle recommendations include consuming a healthy diet, engaging in at least 150 minutes of moderate intensity physical activity a week, and tobacco cessation. Comorbid conditions such as diabetes, hyperlipidemia, and hypertension should be controlled, with pharmacological agents if needed. Aspirin is not recommended in the routine primary prevention of ASCVD (Arnett et al., 2019).

In addition to lifestyle changes, determining ASCVD is recommended for adults 40 to 75 years of age (Arnett et al., 2019). This allows the clinician to work with the patient and develop the most appropriate plan of care (Arnett et al., 2019). The American College of Cardiology (ACC) ASCVD Risk Estimator Plus, estimates the 10-year risk, the impact of different interventions on risk, and can be reassessed over time to aid in clinical decision-making. An ABCDE checklist, developed by the ACC, may be used to help clinicians guide patients (Figure 3.2).

Secondary Prevention

Patients with known CAD need aggressive risk factor modification. This includes smoking cessation, excellent blood pressure control with a target of less than 130/80 mmHg, lipid lowering strategies, weight reduction, if necessary, routine physical activity, and excellent blood glucose control.

Control of ischemic symptoms, if present, can be accomplished with nitrates, beta blockers (BB), and calcium channel blockers. Other medical therapy includes aspirin and high intensity statin therapy. Revascularization with percutaneous interventions (PCI) or coronary artery bypass grafting may be warranted if medical therapy does not control symptoms.

TRANSITION OF CARE

Newly diagnosed CAD requires a multidisciplinary approach with frequent monitoring to ensure risk factor modification occurs.

CLINICAL PEARLS

- Symptoms such as chest pain, SOB, fatigue, palpitations, or dizziness that occur with exertion are red flags for CAD.

KEY TAKEAWAYS

- In patients 40 to 75 years of age, ASCVD risk calculation should be completed routinely.
- Once diagnosed with CAD, aggressive risk factor modification is imperative.
- CAD prevention utilizing the ABCDE checklist will guide clinicians in addressing risk factors.
- Secondary prevention of CAD includes ASA, statin therapy, if needed, utilizing pharmacological therapy to obtain excellent blood glucose and blood pressure control.

EVIDENCE-BASED RESOURCES

2019 ACC/AHA Guideline on the Primary Prevention of Cardiovascular Disease: Executive Summary: A Report of the ACC/American Heart Association Task Force on Clinical Practice Guidelines.

2012 ACCF/AHA/ACP/AATS/PCNA/SCAI/STS Guideline for the Diagnosis and Management of Patients with Stable Ischemic Heart Disease: A Report of the ACC Foundation/American Heart Association Task Force on Practice Guidelines, and the American College of Physicians, American Association for Thoracic Surgery, Preventive Cardiovascular Nurses Association, Society for Cardiovascular Angiography and Interventions, and Society of Thoracic Surgeons.

2014 ACC/AHA/AATS/PCNA/SCAI/STS Focused Update of the Guideline for the Diagnosis and Management of Patients with Stable Ischemic Heart Disease: A Report of the ACC/American Heart Association Task Force on Practice Guidelines, and the American Association for Thoracic Surgery, Preventive Cardiovascular Nurses Association, Society for Cardiovascular Angiography and Interventions, and Society of Thoracic Surgeons.

3.2: DYSLIPIDEMIA

Monee' Carter-Griffin

Heart disease is the leading cause of death in the United States. A major risk factor contributing to heart disease is dyslipidemia. Dyslipidemia is defined as an elevated plasma cholesterol, elevated triglycerides, and/or low high-density lipoprotein cholesterol (HDL-C) levels (Davidson, 2019). Primary (e.g., genetics) and secondary (e.g., sedentary life, diet, and diabetes mellitus) causes contribute to the development of dyslipidemia, with secondary causes being the most important and prevalent in the United States (Davidson, 2019). A heart-healthy lifestyle reduces risk across all stages, while a 50% or greater reduction of low-density lipoprotein cholesterol (LDL-C) levels reduces risk in patients with clinical ASCVD (Grundy et al., 2019).

Top highlights for primary ASCVD prevention		
	• Adopting a team-based care approach improves the quality and maintenance of care. • Engaging patients in shared-decision making helps identify and address potential barriers to treatment.	
A	**ASSESS RISK** • For adults who are 40 to 75 years of age, clinicians should use the Pooled Cohort Equations (PCE) to estimate 10-year ASCVD risk but should also acknowledge that PCE may either significantly overestimate or underestimate ASCVD risk in selected patients. • Risk-enhancing factors and coronary artery calcium scores may help refine risk assessment in adults, when there is uncertainty about the reliability of the 10-year ASCVD risk estimation. **ANTIPLATELET THERAPY** • Aspirin should be used infrequently for primary ASCVD prevention and should be reserved for high risk individuals after other risk factors have been addressed.	
B	**BLOOD PRESSURE** • Lifestyle interventions are recommended for all those with elevated blood pressure and hypertension. • For those requiring antihypertensive medications, the goal blood pressure should be <130/80 mmHg.	
C	**CHOLESTEROL** • Statins are recommended for adults 40 to 75 years of age with 10-year ASCVD risk of >7.5%, diabetics and those with LDL-C > 190 mg/dL. • Risk-enhancing factors and a coronary artery calcium score may guide statin therapy when there is uncertainty about the reliability of ASCVD risk estimation. **CIGARETTE SMOKING** • For those who use tobacco, a combination of behavioral intervention plus pharmacotherapy should be recommended to assist quitting. • Having a dedicated trained staff to tobacco treatment in every instruction can facilitate tobacco cessation.	
D	**DIABETES** • Metformin remains the first line therapy for patients with type 2 diabetes. • In diabetic patients with other ASCVD risk factors who require additional glucose lowering, the addition of a sodium-glucose cotransporter-2 inhibitor or glucagon-like peptide-1 receptor agonist is reasonable. **DIET AND WEIGHT** • A diet rich in vegetables, fruits, legumes, nuts, whole grains, and fish is recommended. • Intake of trans and saturated fats should be avoided. • For overweight or obese adults, reducing daily caloric intake by 500 kCal/day from baseline and increasing physical activity to >150 min of brisk activity per week are reasonable for initial intervention.	
E	**EXERCISE** • Clinicians should encourage adults to engage in at least 150 minutes of moderate-intensity exercise or 75 minutes of vigorous-intensity exercise weekly. • Sedentary behavior should be avoided especially in those who achieve the least amount of recommended moderate-to-vigorous intensity exercise. **ECONOMIC AND SOCIAL FACTORS** • Clinicians should routinely explore socioeconomic barriers to following therapy recommendations and tailor advice to individual patient cirumstances.	

FIGURE 3.2: Top highlights for primary ASCVD prevention.
Source: Reproduced with permission from ABCDE of Primary Prevention: Lifestyle Changes and Team-Based Care, Figure 1. https://www.acc.org/latest-in-cardiology/articles/2019/03/21/14/39/abcs-of-primary-cv-prevention-2019-update-gl-prevention © 2019 American College of Cardiology Foundation

PRESENTING SIGNS AND SYMPTOMS

Dyslipidemia is usually asymptomatic; however, it can contribute and/or lead to symptomatic CV disease such as coronary artery disease (CAD), peripheral arterial disease, and stroke (Davidson, 2019). Dyslipidemia presenting with significantly elevated triglyceride levels greater than 500 mg/dL can cause other disease states and/or symptoms such as (Davidson, 2019):

■ Acute pancreatitis
■ Xanthomas (flat or slightly raised yellow patches on the skin)
■ Paresthesias (>2000 mg/dL)

- Dyspnea (>2000 mg/dL)
- Confusion (>2000 mg/dL)

HISTORY AND PHYSICAL FINDINGS

The history should focus on risk factors for developing dyslipidemia and/or conditions resulting from dyslipidemia (Grundy et al., 2019):

- Recent history of acute coronary syndrome (ACS; within the past 12 months) and/or overall history of myocardial infarction (MI).
- Past medical history of ischemic stroke, diabetes mellitus, hypertension, chronic kidney disease, and/or heart failure (HF).
- Elevated triglycerides and/or LDL-C levels despite appropriate medical management.
- Symptomatic peripheral arterial disease.
- History of familial disease including genetic disorders and premature ASCVD.
- Social history of sedentary lifestyle, excessive dietary intake of calories, saturated fat and trans-fat, alcohol abuse, and smoking.
- In women, a history of premature menopause and pregnancy conditions such as pre-eclampsia.

Physical exam findings resulting solely from dyslipidemia may not be present unless there are significantly elevated triglyceride levels (Davidson, 2019). Patients may present with physical exam findings of other disease states, for which dyslipidemia is a contributing factor such as CAD, pancreatitis, peripheral arterial disease, and/or stroke.

If presenting triglyceride levels are >500 mg/dL, the AGACNP may observe:

- Hepatosplenomegaly
- Xanthomas (flat or slightly raised yellow patches on the skin)
- Creamy white appearance of retinal arteries and veins (>2000 mg/dL)
- Milky appearance to blood plasma (>2000 mg/dL)

DIFFERENTIAL DIAGNOSIS AND DIAGNOSTIC CONSIDERATIONS

Differential Diagnoses

Differential diagnoses include:

- Familial lipid disorders (e.g., familial combined hyperlipidemia)
- Primary biliary liver disease and other cholestatic liver diseases
- Nephrotic syndrome
- Hypothyroidism
- Alcohol abuse/heavy alcohol use
- Diabetes mellitus

Diagnostic Tests

Dyslipidemia is diagnosed by obtaining a fasting lipid profile (Box 3.1). Lipoprotein (a) levels should be drawn in patients with premature ASCVD, CV disease with

---

BOX 3.1 FASTING LIPID PROFILE RANGES

Total cholesterol
- Ideal is <200 mg/dL
- Borderline is 200–239 mg/dL
- High is >240 mg/dL

HDL-C levels
- Ideal is >60 mg/dL
- Borderline is 40–59 mg/dL (females) and 50–59 mg/dL (males)
- Low is <40 mg/dL (females) and 50 mg/dL (males)

LDL-C levels
- Ideal is <100 mg/dL
- Borderline is 130–159 mg/dL
- High is 160–189 mg/dL, with very high >190 mg/dL

Triglycerides
- Ideal is <150 mg/dL
- Borderline is 150–199 mg/dL
- High is 200–499 mg/dL, with very high >500 mg/dL.

---

normal or near normal lipid levels, and/or high LDL-C levels refractory to medication management (Davidson, 2019). C-reactive protein (CRP) may also be measured in these patients.

Other diagnostic considerations include tests to identify the underlying cause for dyslipidemia such as:

- Hemoglobin A1c
- TSH level
- Liver function tests
- Urinalysis

Further workup may be required for patients with confirmed dyslipidemia and signs and symptoms consistent with other disease states.

TREATMENT

Risk Assessment

In lower risk primary prevention patients, an ASCVD risk assessment is recommended for adults aged 40 to 75 years with LDL-C levels equal to or greater than 70 mg/dL. The ASCVD risk assessment should not be completed in those receiving treatment for secondary prevention, LDL-C greater than 190 mg/dL, and/or those aged 40 to 75 years with diabetes.

AGACNPs should assess for other risk factors that influence or increase ASCVD risk such as family history of premature ASCVD, primary hypercholesterolemia, chronic kidney disease, chronic inflammatory conditions (e.g., rheumatoid arthritis), and metabolic syndrome (Grundy et al., 2019).

Lifestyle Modifications

The AGACNP should review lifestyle habits such as diet, physical activity, and tobacco use. A heart-healthy lifestyle should be emphasized to all patients regardless of age and/or risk factors for developing ASCVD (Grundy et al., 2019).

Primary Prevention

Treatment recommendations for adults aged 20 to 39 years are:
- Risk assessment
- Encourage heart-healthy lifestyles
- Consider medication management with statin therapy if family history of premature ASCVD and LDL-C level equal to or greater than 160 mg/dL.

Treatment recommendations for adults aged 40 to 75 years and LDL-C levels equal to or greater than 70 mg/dL to less than 190 mg/dL without diabetes mellitus are:
- Risk assessment
- If low risk, emphasize lifestyle modifications
- If intermediate risk plus risk enhancers (e.g., metabolic syndrome, chronic kidney disease), initiate moderate-intensity statin
- If high risk, initiate statin therapy

Patients with very high LDL-C levels are recommended to start a high-intensity statin. Patients with diabetes mellitus and aged 40 to 75 years should be initiated on a moderate-intensity statin (Grundy et al., 2019).

Secondary Prevention

Patients with clinical ASCVD but not at high risk who are <75 years in age are recommended to start a high-intensity statin with a goal to decrease the LDL-C by equal to or greater than 50%. If patients are unable to tolerate a high-intensity statin, a moderate-intensity statin is recommended. If on maximal statin therapy and LDL-C levels are >70 mg/dL, ezetimide can be added. For patients with clinical ASCVD but not at high risk who are >75 years, a high-intensity statin should be continued or a moderate- to high-intensity statin initiated.

A high-intensity or maximal statin is recommended for patients with clinical ASCVD and identified as high risk (e.g., ACS within 12 months, history of MI, symptomatic peripheral disease, hypertension, smoking).

For patients with primary severe hypercholesterolemia, an LDL-C level equal to or greater than 190 mg/dL, maximal statin therapy is recommended (Grundy et al., 2019).

Statin Therapy

- High-intensity statin therapy (Grundy et al., 2019) with the goal to lower LDL-C levels by 50% or greater
- Atorvastatin 80 mg
  - Rosuvastatin 20 mg
- Moderate-intensity statin therapy with the goal to lower LDL-C levels between 30% and 49%.
- Atorvastatin 10 mg
- Rosuvastatin 10 mg
- Simvastatin 20–40 mg
- Pravastatin 40 mg
- Low-intensity statin therap with the goal to lower LDL-C levels by 30% or less
- Simvastatin 10 mg
- Pravastatin 10–20 mg
- For patients with elevated triglycerides, fibrates, niacin, and omega-3 supplements can be prescribed (or added) to decrease triglyceride levels
- Additional treatment may be required pending the underlying cause for dyslipidemia

TRANSITION OF CARE

Pending the underlying etiology and associated treatment will dictate further care; however, solely treating dyslipidemia can be managed on an outpatient basis.

CLINICAL PEARLS

- Monitor for side effects associated with statin therapy such as elevated liver enzymes, myalgias, and/or rhabdomyolysis.
- Current recommendations are to obtain a baseline liver function test and creatine kinase (CK) level prior to statin initiation.
- If a patient is unable to tolerate statin therapy, attempt dose reduction of the prescribed statin or prescribe a different statin.
- Recheck lipid levels approximately 8 to 12 weeks after starting or changing medication management. Once the lipid levels are stabilized, the provider can check lipid levels one to two times annually.

KEY TAKEAWAYS

- Often, there are no overt signs or symptoms of dyslipidemia unless the patient is presenting with another symptomatic condition and/or disease.
- Providers should emphasize a heart-healthy lifestyle (e.g., diet, exercise, weight control) to all individuals regardless of age, gender, and/or race.
- Some degree of statin therapy is recommended for all patients with clinical ASCVD, regardless of the patient's risk.

EVIDENCE-BASED RESOURCES

Grundy, S. M., Stone, N. J., Bailey, A. L., Beam, C., Birtcher, K. K., Blumenthal, R. S., Braun, L. T., de Ferranti, S., Faiella-Tommasino, J., Forman, D. E., Goldberg, R., Heidenreich, P. A., Hlatky, M. A., Jones, D. W., Lloyd-Jones, D., Lopez-Pajares, N., Ndumele, C. E., Orringer, C. E., Peralta, C. A., … Yeboah, J. (2019). 2018 AHA/ACC/AACVPR/AAPA/ABC/ACPM/ADA/AGS/APHA/ASPC/NLA/PCNA guideline on the management of blood cholesterol: A report of the American College of Cardiology/American Heart Association Task Force on Clinical Practice Guidelines. *Circulation, 139*, e1082–e1143. https://doi.org/10.1161/CIR.0000000000000625

3.3: ACUTE CORONARY SYNDROMES

Carolina D. Tennyson, Stephanie G. Barnes, and Jaime A. McDermott

Acute coronary syndrome (ACS) is an operational term that refers to a spectrum of conditions consistent with acute myocardial ischemia and/or infarction related to a reduction in coronary blood flow. The hallmark of ACS is the imbalance between myocardial oxygen consumption and demand, most commonly due to coronary artery obstruction or coronary embolism. Rapid assessment, diagnosis, and treatment are the cornerstone for improving morbidity and mortality related to ACS (Thygesen et al., 2018). Treatment pathways are based on symptoms, elevation of cardiac biomarkers, ECG findings, and heart dysfunction. ST-segment elevation or a new left bundle-branch block on ECG is an indication for immediate coronary angiography due to concern for ST-elevation myocardial infarction (STEMI). The absence of ST-elevation, while reassuring, does not preclude further workup and a trend of biomarkers.

Acute myocardial infarction (MI) can sometimes lead to myocardial dysfunction, cardiogenic shock, and even cardiac arrest. When this occurs, the priority is immediate advanced cardiac life support (ACLS) and achievement of timely coronary reperfusion. It is important for the AGACNP to think critically about the etiology of the patient's ischemia and recognize the types of MI, as this will guide management (Thygesen et al., 2018).

PRESENTING SIGNS AND SYMPTOMS

Possible ischemic symptoms include various combinations of chest, mandibular, or epigastric pain during exertion or at rest. These symptoms are not specific for MI, so a full evaluation should be done to rule out other critical illness. While chest pain is a common symptom, MI can also occur with atypical symptoms like sudden cardiac death (SCD), or without any symptoms at all (Thygesen et al., 2018). Anginal equivalents include dyspnea, nausea, or fatigue.

Angina can be categorized as stable or unstable. Stable angina is experienced predictably during exertion while unstable angina is acute, unexpected, progressive, and unrelenting. Stable angina is a chronic condition that should be monitored closely and can be managed with medications. Of note, stable coronary heart disease and angina are not commonly associated with acute ECG changes or elevation of cardiac biomarkers (Ferraro et al., 2020).

When the patient endorses acute chest pain, clinicians should begin a prompt workup including a history and physical exam to understand the location, onset, and duration of chest pain. Aggravating or alleviating factors in chest pain should be evaluated. An early 12-lead ECG and cardiac biomarkers are obtained which assist in differentiating cardiac from noncardiac chest pain. In patients with ACS, there are distinct features obtained during the history and physical exam that assist clinicians in making a diagnosis.

HISTORY AND PHYSICAL FINDINGS

A prompt and expeditious history and physical exam is imperative in clinical scenarios in which a patient is complaining of angina or its equivalent. Relevant history includes cardiac risk factors such as coronary disease, hypertension, hyperlipidemia, diabetes, or metabolic syndrome. Cigarette smoking and a family history of CAD are other risk factors for ACS. Physical exam may be benign; however, consideration should be made for patients who are exhibiting signs of cardiogenic shock on presentation. These signs and symptoms include hypotension, tachycardia, decreased mentation or ventricular arrhythmias. The skin evaluation (warm vs. cool, dry vs. wet) can be insightful when investigating for signs of heart failure (HF).

DIFFERENTIAL DIAGNOSIS AND DIAGNOSTIC CONSIDERATIONS

AGACNPs should be familiar with the common differential diagnoses for ACS (Table 3.1). Arriving at a final diagnosis is dependent on a thorough history and physical exam including the nature of the pain, associated symptoms, precipitating and aggravating factors,

TABLE 3.1: Differential Diagnosis for Acute Coronary Syndrome

ORGAN SYSTEM	DIFFERENTIAL DIAGNOSES
Cardiac	Heart failure, hypertension, mitral valve prolapse, myocarditis, endocarditis, pericarditis, aortic dissection or aneurysm
Pulmonary	Pulmonary embolism, pneumonia, pleurisy, pneumothorax, pulmonary hypertension
Gastrointestinal	Gastroesophageal reflux disease (GERD), peptic ulcer disease (PUD), esophagitis, esophageal spasm, hiatal hernia, gallbladder disease
Musculoskeletal	Muscle strain or overuse, trauma, diaphragmatic hernia, fibromyalgia, cervical radiculopathy
Inflammatory	Costocondritis, Teitze syndrome
Other	Psychiatric disorders (anxiety, depression), illicit drug use (cocaine, amphetamines)

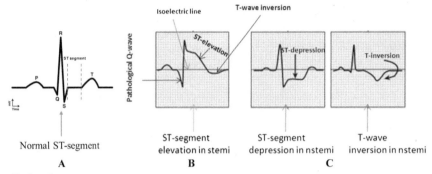

FIGURE 3.3: ECG signs of ischemia.
Source: Reproduced with permission from Chowdhury, M. E. H., Alzoubi, K., Khandakar, A., Khallifa, R., Abouhasera, R., Koubaa, S., Ahmed, R., & Hasan, M. A. (2019). Wearable real-time heart attack detection and warning system to reduce road accidents. *Sensors, 19*(12), 2780. https://doi.org/10.3390/s19122780

ameliorating factors, and diagnostic and physical findings. Diagnostic tests will direct your assessment of the type of myocardial injury the patient is experiencing.

The use of diagnostic tests can assist in determining inclusion or exclusion of ACS. When ACS is suspected, initial evaluation with resting and/or exercise standard 12-lead ECG should be done within 10 minutes of arrival to evaluate for ST segment depression or elevation, new T-wave inversion, left ventricular (LV) hypertrophy, or bundle branch blocks with repolarization (Figure 3.3; Amsterdam et al., 2014; Panchal et al., 2020; Patel et al., 2017). Ancillary evaluation with posterior leads (V7–V9) can also be considered (Amsterdam et al., 2014). Serial ECG evaluation at specified intervals or with current symptoms is sometimes necessary (Amsterdam et al., 2014).

Cardiac troponin (cTn) is a component of myocardial cells and is expressed exclusively by the heart. Elevation of this biomarker reflects injury to myocardial cells but does not indicate the underlying mechanism for the injury. Blood samples for the measurement of cTn should be drawn immediately at the first suspicion of ACS and repeated 3 to 6 hours later to assess a trend. Sampling beyond 6 hours may be necessary if further ischemic episodes occur. Additional laboratory evaluation includes brain natriuretic peptide (BNP) or NT-pro-BNP and a comprehensive metabolic profile for end-organ function (Amsterdam et al., 2014).

Imaging for ACS should begin with noninvasive testing that maximizes diagnosis, based on initial evaluation with ECG and cardiac biomarkers. Thoughtful consideration of patient factors including associated symptoms and end-organ function should be considered when deciding additional noninvasive and invasive testing. Initial imaging should include a chest x-ray to evaluate for cardiac and pulmonary structure abnormalities. Transthoracic or transesophageal echocardiography can provide a relatively rapid evaluation of ventricular wall motion abnormalities. Echocardiography can also be useful in identifying ejection fraction, right ventricular (RV) strain, pericardial effusion, and valvular disease. Additional noninvasive imaging which may aid in diagnosis includes CT coronary angiography for low-

risk patients and myocardial perfusion imaging or stress testing for intermediate-risk patients (Patel et al., 2017). Left heart catheterization with or without coronary angiography is considered the gold standard for diagnosis and treatment of CAD (Panchal et al., 2020; Patel et al., 2017). In patients who are chest-pain free and ruled in for ACS, angiography is considered nonurgent. Urgent evaluation with angiography should be considered in patients with STEMI or refractory chest pain, arrhythmias in the setting of ischemia, and/or hemodynamic instability (Panchal et al., 2020; Patel et al., 2017).

Myocardial injury is defined as a detection of an elevated cTn value above the 99th percentile of upper reference limit (URL). That injury is considered acute if there is a rise and/or fall of cTn values. The Universal Definition of Myocardial Infarction (UDMI) has undergone a fourth iteration and MIs are classified as Type 1 to 5. Type 1 MI is myocardial injury believed to be due to acute coronary thrombus. Non-ischemic causes of myocardial injury are numerous and include myocarditis, catheter ablation cardiac contusion, coronary vasospasm, severe anemia, critical illness, and pulmonary embolism. Abnormalities in cTn and a nonischemic cause of oxygen supply and demand imbalance is defined as a Type 2 MI. Type 2 MI has been documented to occur more often in women (Thygesen et al., 2018). The diagnostic criteria for Type 1 and 2 MI are described in Table 3.2. As mentioned, patients can present atypically with SCD and die before biomarkers and imaging can be obtained. When the suspicion for an acute myocardial ischemic event is high, even when biomarker and imaging evidence of MI is lacking, the diagnosis is deemed a Type 3 MI. Type 4 is associated with PCI and postcoronary artery bypass graft (CABG) surgery, occuring within 48 hours after the procedure.

TREATMENT

Treatment of ACS includes pharmacological therapies, lifestyle changes, and aggressive management of comorbid conditions such as diabetes and hypertension. The risk of major adverse cardiovascular events is relatively low in patients without a history of CAD presenting

TABLE 3.2 DIAGNOSTIC CRITERIA FOR TYPE 1 AND 2 MYOCARDIAL INFARCTION

Type 1 MI *Detection of a rise and/or fall of cTn values with at least one value above the 99th % of upper reference limit and one of the following:*	Type 2 MI *Detection of a rise and/or fall of cTn values with at least one value above the 99th % of upper reference limit and evidence of an imbalance between myocardial oxygen supply and demand unrelated to acute coronary thrombosis and one of the following:*
Symptoms of ischemia	Symptoms of ischemia
New ST-segment changes or a left bundle branch block	New ST-segment changes or a left bundle branch block
Development of pathological Q waves on the ECG	Development of pathological Q waves on the ECG
Imaging study showing new regional wall motion abnormality	Imaging study showing new regional wall motion abnormality
Presence of an intracoronary thrombus at autopsy or angiography	

with stable chest pain. The management goals in patients with stable angina are to improve event-free survival and improve symptoms. Guidelines for ACS support the use of pharmacological therapies including lipid-lowering therapies, antithrombotics, blood pressure and diabetes control (Ferraro et al., 2020). Lifestyle changes such as cessation of cigarette smoking, low fat and low cholesterol diets, and increased activity can have a substantial impact on patient outcome. Anti-inflammatory treatment is a novel therapy to consider for secondary prevention (Ferraro et al., 2020).

Pain Control

Opioids and sublingual nitroglycerin can be used for pain control in the setting of stable or unstable angina. Nitroglycerin is a potent venodilator and reduces preload as well as an arterial dilator, dilating the coronary arteries, improving blood flow and therefore myocardial blood flow and oxygenation. Side effects may include hypotension and flushing and hemodynamic instability; cardiogenic shock is a contraindication to nitroglycerin administration. Nitroglycerin can be given by multiple routes including intravenous and transdermal.

Antiplatelet Therapy

All patients with STEMI and NSTEMI should immediately be given aspirin 160 to 325 mg to chew and started on IV heparin infusion to maintain therapeutic activated clotting times. The AHA/ACC ACS task force identifies chronic dual anti-platelet therapy (DAPT), or aspirin in addition to a P2Y12 inhibitor like clopidogrel or ticagrelor, as a Class 1 Recommendation (Amsterdam et al., 2014) for patients with NSTEMI. Coronary anatomy and PCI stent choice will influence the duration of these therapies and is managed by a cardiology specialist.

Beta Blockade and Renin-Angiotensin-Aldosterone System

Oral beta blockade should be initiated in the first 24 hours in patients with STEMI who do not have signs of HF or evidence of a low output state. Angiotensin-converting enzyme (ACE) inhibitors or angiotensin receptor blockers (ARBs) should also be prescribed for patients with acute MI, particularly if their ejection fraction is less than 40%. Studies have established the benefit of an aldosterone antagonist, eplerenone, in patients after infarction complicated by LV dysfunction and HF (Pitt et al., 2003). For more on medical therapy for patients with depressed ejection fraction and HF after MI, refer to Section 3.7, "Heart Failure" in this chapter.

Thrombolytics/Percutaneous Coronary Intervention

Timely primary percutaneous coronary intervention (PCI) is the preferred strategy for patients with STEMI and a transfer to a PCI-capable hospital is the appropriate triage approach for these patients. In hospitals without PCI capabilities or in cases where a patient does not have access to PCI within 120 minutes, fibrinolytic therapy should be administered within 30 minutes of the patient's presentation (O'Gara et al., 2013). Fibrinolytic agents such as tenecteplase, reteplase, or alteplase can be given only in the absence of contraindications such as intracranial hemorrhage (ICH), recent surgery, or trauma. In hospitals that have capability for rapid reperfusion, guidelines indicate that the patient should be receiving PCI within 90 minutes of presentation (O'Gara et al., 2013). This "door-to-balloon" time is a performance measure that is evaluated regionally and nationally for quality improvement initiatives.

Cardiogenic Shock

When myocardial ischemia causes cardiogenic shock, inotropes and mechanical circulatory support may be required to maintain adequate cardiac output. Intra-aortic balloon pump counterpulsation can be useful for patients in cardiogenic shock after STEMI (O'Gara et al., 2013). Alternative assist devices like extracorporeal membrane oxygenation (ECMO) or ventricular assist devices may be considered in eligible patients with refractory shock.

Cardiac Arrest

In and out of hospital cardiac arrest is associated with a high mortality rate; however, data show that there has been improvement in survival over the past two decades

TABLE 3.3: Reversible Causes of Cardiac Arrest

Hs	Ts
Hypovolemia	Tension pneumothorax
Hypoxia	Tamponade, cardiac
Hydrogen ion (acidosis)	Toxins
Hypo-/hyperkalemia	Thrombosis, pulmonary
Hypothermia	Thrombosis, coronary

with recent large studies reporting around 20% chance of survival (Andersen et al., 2019). There are well-recognized reversible causes of cardiac arrest, known as the Hs and Ts (Table 3.3). Acute coronary thrombosis is one of these differentials. Of note, both defibrillation and chest compressions will increase a patient's Troponin level, so this biomarker is often unhelpful if measured during or after resuscitation.

According to American Heart Association Guidelines, the mainstays of cardiac arrest management are early recognition, high-quality chest compressions, early defibrillation, administration of epinephrine, and treating reversible causes (Panchal et al., 2020). Interventions proven to increase recovery of spontaneous circulation and survival to hospital discharge are early administration of epinephrine and concurrent high-quality CPR (Panchal et al., 2020).

Postcardiac arrest care is a critical component of the Chain of Survival (Berg et al., 2020) and timely initiation of targeted temperature management (TTM), head CT scan and electroencephalogram (EEG) monitoring is indicated for patients who do not follow commands after return of spontaneous circulation (ROSC). TTM between 32° and 36° Celsius and prevention of fever for at least 24 hours are currently recommended. This induced hypothermia is achieved by transcutaneous or intravenous cooling technologies. Physiologically, TTM is thought to decrease cerebral and total body oxygen demand postarrest. Research on this therapy is evolving, but some trials have demonstrated a favorable effect on neurological outcomes (Nielson et al., 2013; Panchal et al., 2020).

Treating Risk Factors

Treatment with statins in patient stabilized after ACS lowers the risk of coronary heart disease death, recurrent MI, stroke, and the need for coronary revascularization. Baseline fasting lipid profile should be tested and a high-intensity statin therapy should be initiated in all patients (even those with LDL-C levels <70 mg/dL). Renin angiotensin aldosterone system (RAAS) inhibitors can reduce major CV events in patients with STEMI and should be prescribed as soon as possible (O'Gara et al., 2013). The magnitude of clinical benefit with RAAS inhibitors is greatest in high-risk patients. Be sure to consider this adjunct medical management when preparing patients for discharge.

TRANSITION OF CARE

Standardized interventions using a discharge protocol should be provided during hospitalization, in addition to posthospitalization interventions to improve the quality of care and prevent adverse events following hospital discharge (Amsterdam et al., 2014; Panchal et al., 2020). Discharge planning should include completion of risk assessment for factors associated with re-hospitalization. Patient and/or caregiver education should be aimed at various aspects of ACS including diet modification, medication adherence, and physical activity. These are further addressed with a referral to a comprehensive CV rehabilitation program. Medication reconciliation should be performed at admission and on discharge. Written discharge instructions should be provided to the patient and/or caregiver on discharge and should include a contact phone number for emergencies. Telephone and clinical follow-up with a cardiology provider should be performed. Communication with the patient's other providers should be done to ensure proper handoff. Consideration of home health follow-up to assist the patient with home needs, smoking cessation, and hypertension, hyperlipidemia, and/or diabetes management should be considered.

CLINICAL PEARLS

- ACS includes the spectrum of myocardial ischemia, Types 1–4 MI.
- BB, RAAS inhibitors, and statins are recommended for all patients after STEMI.
- STEMI can lead to cardiogenic shock and cardiac arrest if left untreated.

KEY TAKEAWAYS

- ST-segment elevation, depression, and T wave inversion can be ECG findings of an acute event.
- Comprehensive evaluation with cardiac enzymes, diagnostics, and imaging is vital to differentiating ACS from alternative diagnoses.
- To reduce the risk of post-ACS complications, a standardized transition of care model should be undertaken.
- Timely PCI or thrombolysis is the most important intervention for patients with STEMI.
- Patients who are not neurologically intact after ROSC should undergo TTM to decrease cerebral and systemic oxygen demand in the postarrest phase.

3.4: ACUTE INFLAMMATORY DISEASE

Andrea Colburn

Cardiac infections can be severe, life-threatening, and may involve the heart valves (endocarditis), heart muscle (myocarditis), and the pericardium (pericarditis). Inflammation and infection of the heart can be caused by viral, bacterial, or fungal infections or as a result of medical conditions such as turbulent blood flow due to congenital heart disease (Levinson et al., 2020). Although uncommon, infective endocarditis (IE) is a potentially lethal disease associated with increased morbidity and mortality and a potential for multiorgan involvement, thus more attention is given to this disease as early recognition and prompt treatment are paramount to survival (Baddour et al., 2015).

INFECTIVE ENDOCARDITIS

The epidemiologic profile of IE has changed substantially due to a decline in rheumatic heart disease, antibiotic resistance, and changes in pathogens (Cahill et al., 2017). IE is classified according to valve characteristics as in native valve endocarditis (NVE), acute and subacute; prosthetic valve endocarditis (PVE), or intravenous drug use (IVDU) endocarditis, and according to site involved as in right-sided endocarditis, common in IVDU, or the more common left-sided endocarditis (Wang & Holland, 2020). Infection of the endothelium lining the cardiac valve leaflets often begins with formation of microscopic, noninfected platelet-fibrin thrombi on damaged leaflet surfaces called nonbacterial thrombotic endocarditis (NBTE; see Figure 3.4; Crawford & Doernberg, 2017). It is theorized that initial valve damage occurs from minor trauma due to turbulent blood flow as in valvular disorders, rheumatic heart disease, direct injury (e.g., foreign body), or repeated IV drug injections which can damage

cardiac valves leaving the endothelium vulnerable to pathogens (Levinson et al., 2020). Infection of thrombi formations can occur as a result of seeding by transient circulating blood-borne organisms such as after tooth brushing, dental procedures, defecating, or mucous membrane manipulation (Brenner et al., 2020).

Acute IE is an aggressive disease marked by severe febrile illness developing over days to 2 weeks, rapidly damaging cardiac structures which leads to an acute onset of congestive heart failure (CHF); death can occur within weeks if acute IE is left untreated (Miller, 2020). Subacute endocarditis is discernable by its slow, indolent course over weeks to months with gradual destruction of cardiac structures (Miller, 2020). It is marked by low-grade fever, anorexia, weight loss, flu-like symptoms, and syndromes similar to polymyalgia and rheumatic fever (Brusch, 2021).

Common pathogens include *Staphylococcus*, *Streptococci* (viridians group), and *Enterococcus* species; *Staphylococcus aureus* is the single most common organism in native and prosthetic valve, and IVDU with the highest rates for death (Brenner et al., 2020). Cases of IE associated with negative blood cultures are commonly due to prior antibiotic therapy; however, incidence of IE without prior antibiotic administration are increasing and often due to fastidious organisms in the HACEK group (*Haemophilus*, *Actinobacillus*, *Cardiobacterium*, *Eikenella*, and *Kingella*), *Bartonella* species, or *Coxiella burnetii* (Brenner et al., 2020).

Risk Factors

Risk factors include native valve disease, prosthetic valve, or cardiac implantable electronic devices (CIEDs), hemodialysis, venous catheters, immunosuppression, IVDU, homelessness, recent hospitalization or long-term care stay, and older/frail patients with multiple comorbidities (Cahill et al., 2017).

PRESENTING SIGNS AND SYMPTOMS

IE often presents as a constellation of symptoms with the most common clinical manifestations listed in Table 3.4 (Brenner et al., 2020; Brusch, 2021).

HISTORY AND PHYSICAL FINDINGS

Physical manifestations of IE can be highly variable as patients can present with acute/fulminant symptoms or vague, nonspecific constitutional complaints (Brusch, 2021). Obtaining a thorough patient history is critical to distinguishing between acute and subacute IE. Targeted questioning should determine the interval of onset of symptoms, recent history of invasive procedures, indwelling catheters, implanted cardiac devices, oral surgeries or dental procedures, respiratory infection, or recreational IVDU (Brenner et al., 2020; Brusch, 2021).

Physical exam findings may include the following (Crawford & Doernberg, 2017; Vilcant & Hai, 2020):

■ Fever is the most common symptom, often lasting several weeks.

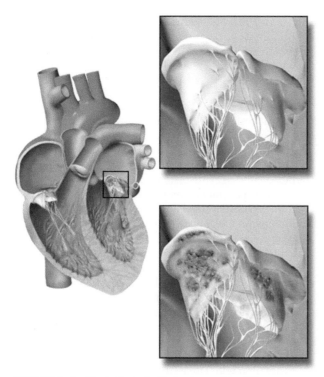

FIGURE 3.4: An illustration of mitral valve endocarditis.
Source: Courtesy of BruceBlaus.

TABLE 3.4: Key Clinical Manifestations of Infective Endocarditis

Fever >38°C [100.4°F]	*Most common symptom*; may not be present in the elderly or immunocompromised
Chest pain	Precordial or localized "pleuritic"; may intensify with coughing, inspiration, or recumbent position, relieved by sitting forward
New cardiac murmur Syncope, heart block	50%–85% Atrioventricular (AV) nodal conduction abnormalities
Shortness of breath	Due to heart failure, significant valve destruction
Skin findings	*Petechiae* on mucous membranes (mouth). Common but nonspecific *Splinter hemorrhages* (dark red linear lesions under the nail bed resembling splinters) *Osler nodes* (antigen-antibody deposition from uncontrolled infection resulting in small, painful nodules on fingers and toes) *Janeway lesions* (small hemorrhagic painless nodules on palms or soles; usually represent IE due to *Staphylococcus aureus* infection) *Roth spots* – Rare (pale-centered retinal hemorrhages arising from immune-mediated vasculitis)

Source: Adapted from Brenner, D., Marco, C., & Rothman, R. (2020). Endocarditis. In *Tintinalli's emergency medicine: A comprehensive study guide* (9th ed.). McGraw-Hill. https://accessmedicine-mhmedical-com.libux.utmb.edu/content.aspx?bookid=2353&sectionid=220292705, Copyright 2020 by McGraw-Hill.

TABLE 3.5: Overview of Antibiotic Therapy for Infective Endocarditis

UNCOMPLICATED HISTORY	COMPLICATED HISTORY*	PROSTHETIC HEART VALVE
ceftriaxone 1–2 g IV, *or* nafcillin 2 g IV, *or* oxacillin 2 g IV, *or* vancomycin 15 mg/kg ***plus*** gentamicin 1–3 mg/kg IV, *or* tobramycin 1 mg/kg IV	nafcillin 2 g IV ***plus*** gentamicin 1–3 mg/kg IV ***plus*** vancomycin 15 mg/kg IV	vancomycin 15 mg/kg IV ***plus*** gentamicin 1–3 mg/kg IV ***plus*** rifampin 300 mg PO

*Complicated history is defined as congenital heart disease, IV drug use, nosocomial infections, or methicillin-resistant *Staphylococcus aureus*.

Source: Reproduced with permission from Brenner, D., Marco, C., & Rothman, R. (2020). Endocarditis. In *Tintinalli's emergency medicine: A comprehensive study guide* (9th ed.). McGraw-Hill. https://accessmedicine-mhmedical-com.libux.utmb.edu/content.aspx?bookid=2353&sectionid=220292705, Copyright 2020 by McGraw-Hill.

- Murmur: Patients may have a new systolic murmur from mitral regurgitation (MR) or a diastolic murmur from aortic regurgitation (AR). Acute regurgitation can lead to signs of heart failure (HF) such as shortness of breath (SOB), orthopnea, hypoxia, tachypnea, jugular venous distention, and crackles. Perivalvular abscess can lead to bradycardia and heart block. Valvular vegetations may embolize leading to stroke or infarct to other organs.
- Vascular phenomena associated with IE include cutaneous skin findings as noted in Table 3.4.
- Dyspnea, cough, and chest pain are common in IV drug users (Brusch, 2021).
- Pericardial friction rub is heard best with patient sitting upright and leaning forward.
- Evidence of myocardial ischemia, embolic stroke; 40% of patients may have neurological changes.

DIFFERENTIAL DIAGNOSIS AND DIAGNOSTIC CONSIDERATIONS

The differential for a patient presenting with fever and vague symptoms of systemic illness is broad. Key differentials to consider include acute rheumatic fever, atrial myxoma, systemic lupus erythematosus, venous thromboembolism, vasculitis, myocarditis, fever of unknown origin, and intra-abdominal infections (Vilcant & Hai, 2020) Patients presenting with symptoms of HF should be evaluated for causes of noninfectious endocarditis and nonvalvular HF as well (Hubers et al., 2020).

Diagnostic Testing

Diagnostic testing includes the following (Baddour et al., 2015):

- Echocardiogram: Useful to detect vegetations and cardiac complications
- Blood cultures: Three sets should be obtained via *three* different peripheral venipuncture sites. The first and third sets drawn should be drawn at least 1 hour apart.
- Rheumatoid factor (RF): High RF is associated with IE and should prompt a TTE to differentiate.
- White blood cell (WBC) count: Leukocytosis (not sensitive nor specific in IE).
- Basic metabolic panel (BMP): Renal function may be abnormal in setting of renal artery occlusion.
- Erythrocyte sedimentation rate (ESR)/CRP: Sensitive, but not specific. Elevated in 90% to 100% of cases.
- Brain natriuretic peptide (BNP): May help differentiate cardiac from pulmonary etiology.
- Evaluation with Duke Criteria: The Duke criteria are widely used for diagnosing IE (Figures 3.5 and 3.6).

DEFINITE IE	Possible IE	Major Criteria

Possible IE

- 1 Major and 1 Minor Criterion
- 3 Minor Criterion

Major Criteria

Positive Blood Cultures for IE
- Typical microorganisms consistent with IE from 2 separate blood cultures (BC)
- Persistently positive BC
- Single positive BC for *Coxiella burnetii* or IgG antibody titer >1:800

Evidence of Endocardial Involvement
- Echocardiogram positive for IE
- New valvular regurgitation

DEFINITE IE

Pathologic Criteria
1. Microorganisms - demonstrated by culture or histology of a vegetation, a vegetation that has embolized, or an intracardiac abscess OR
2. Pathologic lesions - vegetation or intracardiac abscess demonstrating active endocarditis on histology

Clinica Criteria
- 2 major criteria OR
- 1 major and 3 minor criteria OR
- 5 Minor criteria

Rejected IE

1. Firm alternate diagnosis explaining evidence of IE
2. Resolution of infection endocarditis syndrome with antibiotic therapy for≤4 days
3. No pathologic evidence of IE at surgery or autopsy, with antibiotic therapy for ≤ 4 days
4. Does NOT meet criteria for possible IE, as described previously

Minor Criteria

- Predisposing heart condition or IDU
- Fever≥ 38°C
- Vascular phenomena
- Immunologic phenomena
- Micro: +BC not meeting a major criterion OR serologic evidence of active infection with organism consistent with IE

FIGURE 3.5: The modified Duke criteria for Infective Endocarditis (IE).
Source: Reproduced with permission from Proposed modifications to the Duke criteria for the diagnosis of infective endocarditis by Li, J. S., Sexton, D. J., Mick, N., Nettles, R., Fowler, V. G., Ryan, T., Bashore, T., & Corey, G. R. (2000). Proposed modifications to the duke criteria for the diagnosis of infective endocarditis. *Clinical Infectious Diseases, 30*(4), 633–638. https://doi.org/10.1086/313753. Copyright 2000 by Oxford University Press.

Definition of Terms Used in the Modified Duke Criteria

Blood culture positive for IE

- Typical microorganisms consistent with IE from 2 separate blood cultures: Viridans streptococci, Streptococcus bovis, HACEK group, Staphylococcus *aureus*; or community-acquired *enterococci* in the absence of a primary focus, OR

  Microorganisms consistent with IE from persistently positive blood cultures defined as follows: at least 2 positive cultures of blood samples drawn >12 h apart or all 3 or a majority of≥4 separate cultures of blood (with first and last sample drawn at least 1 h apart)

Echocardiogram positive for IE

- Oscillating intracardiac mass on valve or supporting structures, in path of regurgitant jets, or on implanted material in the absence of alternative anatomic explanation; abscess: or new partial dehiscence of prosthetic valve or new valvular regurgitation (worsening, changing, or pre-existing murmur is not sufficient)

*TTE as first test EXCEPT TEE is recommended for patients with prosthetic valves or reated at least Possible IE by clinical criteria, OR complicated IE (perivalvular abscess)

Vascular Phenomena

- Major arterial emboli, septic pulmonary infarcts, mycotic aneurysm, intracranial hemorrhage, conjunctival hemorrhages, and Janeway lesions

Immunologic Phenomena

- Glomerulonephritis, Osler nodes, Roth spots, and rheumatoid factor

ABBREVIATIONS

HACEK- Haemophilus species, Aggregatibacter species, Cardiobacterium hominis, Eikenella corrodens, and Kingella species

IDU – injection drug use

IE – infective endocarditis

IgG – immunoglobulin G

TEE – transesophageal echocardiography

TTE – transthoracic echocardiography

FIGURE 3.6: Definitions of terms used in the modified Duke criteria.
Source: Reproduced with permission from Proposed modifications to the Duke criteria for the diagnosis of infective endocarditis by Li, J. S., Sexton, D. J., Mick, N., Nettles, R., Fowler, V. G., Ryan, T., Bashore, T., & Corey, G. R. (2000). Proposed modifications to the duke criteria for the diagnosis of infective endocarditis. *Clinical Infectious Diseases, 30*(4), 633–638. https://doi.org/10.1086/313753. Copyright 2000 by Oxford University Press

Anticoagulation/Antiplatelet Therapy

Although patients with IE are at high risk for both embolic events and bleeding complications, available data suggest neither anticoagulation nor antithrombotic therapy reduces risk of embolism and is not recommended without expert consultation (Wang & Holland, 2020).

Surgical Intervention

Indications for surgical intervention (NVE and PVE):

- HF unresponsive to medical therapy
- IE due to fungal infection or multiresistant organisms
- Persistent sepsis >72 hours after appropriate antibiotic treatment
- Ruptured aneurysm of the sinus of Valsalva; perivalvular abscess; intracardiac fistula
- Conduction disturbances due to septal abscess
- For IE associated with implantable cardiac devices treatment includes antimicrobial therapy and removal of the device (Miller, 2020)

Indications for surgery in patients actively injecting drugs are the same as in NVE and PVE; however, long-term outcomes remain poor due to on-going infection risk (Straw et al., 2019).

TRANSITION OF CARE

- All suspected cases of IE should be hospitalized for further workup and appropriate treatment.
- A repeat TTE should be obtained after completion of antibiotic therapy to provide a new baseline for valve appearance, function, and evaluation of LV function.
- Patients should be educated on the importance of dental hygiene, regular dental examinations, and the role of antibiotic prophylaxis prior to oral procedures including regular cleaning (Brusch, 2021).

CLINICAL PEARLS

- Signs and symptoms of IE can be vague and non-specific. Vigilance is necessary in remaining aware of risk factors and common presenting signs and symptoms of IE.
- Suspect IE in anyone with new onset of cardiac murmur and fever of unknown origin (with or without bacteremia), or bacteremia without a clear etiology, peripheral embolic phenomena, or IVDU.
- Blood cultures and TTE should be performed as quickly as possible in *all* cases of suspected IE.
- *Staphylococcus aureus* is the predominant causative organism and leads to an aggressive form of IE particularly in the elderly or vulnerable populations.
- Signs of HF and valve dysfunction support valve surgery unless IE is due to IVDU.

KEY TAKEAWAYS

- IE is a febrile disease with high morbidity and mortality, thus early recognition and treatment is paramount as untreated IE is always fatal.
- Patients with IE require prompt treatment by a multidisciplinary team including prompt consultations to cardiology, infectious disease, and cardiac surgery specialists.
- Diagnosis is based on the Modified Duke Criteria and differentiated as definite, possible, or rejected IE.
- Blood cultures are collected three times from different peripheral venipuncture sites; the first and second samples taken at least 1 hour apart.
- Management includes empiric antibiotics covering the most common pathogens and consultation with cardiology, infectious disease, and CV surgery particularly if the patient has valvular insufficiency.

MYOCARDITIS

Myocarditis is defined as an inflammatory disease of the heart muscle often manifesting as chest pain, heart failure (HF), and/or arrhythmias (Levinson et al., 2020). Common viral pathogens include *Coxsackie* viruses (most common), cytomegalovirus, Epstein-Barr, parvovirus B19, COVID-19, and influenza viruses; other pathogens linked to myocarditis are *Trypanosoma cruzi* (Chagas' disease), and *Trichinella spiralis* (Levinson et al., 2020). According to the 2019 Global Burden of Disease report (Cooper, 2021), myocarditis affects men and women between the ages of 35 and 39 years with a higher prevalence observed in men. Inflammation or infection of cardiac muscle enlarges and weakens the heart often resulting in cardiac dysfunction and HF (Levinson et al., 2020). Infectious myocarditis often follows an upper respiratory infection (URI); however, a variety of medications, illicit drugs, toxic substances, and systemic disorders are associated with myocarditis (Bashore et al., 2021). General classifications of myocarditis include acute (nonfulminant) with symptoms developing over 3 months or fewer; fulminant myocarditis (FM), an uncommon syndrome characterized by abrupt onset (over 1–2 days) with unexplained severe diffuse cardiac inflammation often leading to death; or subacute/chronic myocarditis characterized by symptoms developing over more than 3 months (Cooper, 2021).

Risk Factors

Risk factors include viral infections, influenza, rubella, polio, HIV; young, healthy, athletic individuals ages puberty to early 30s are considered as high-risk (Myocarditis Foundation, 2021).

PRESENTING SIGNS AND SYMPTOMS

Symptoms are highly variable with common signs being excessive fatigue, chest pain, unexplained tachycardia, fever, and progressive dyspnea and weakness days to weeks after a viral illness (Lakdawala et al., 2020). Patients may present manifesting cardiogenic shock or experience sudden death. Many patients go undiagnosed due to variable clinical manifestations including subclinical, nonspecific signs often attributed to systemic manifestations of an underlying infection or disease process (Cooper, 2021).

HISTORY AND PHYSICAL EXAM FINDINGS

Patients may present days to weeks after onset of an acute febrile illness or respiratory infection and may exhibit early symptoms such as exertional intolerance (with or without chest pain) or fluid retention; however, many exhibit signs of acute uncompensated HF and cardiogenic shock (Selby, 2017).

Physical exam findings may include hypotension, cool extremities, tachycardia, cardiac gallops, rales, distended neck veins, peripheral edema, new cardiomegaly on chest x-ray, heart block or new-onset bundle branch block on ECG (Cooper, 2021).

DIFFERENTIAL DIAGNOSIS AND DIAGNOSTIC CONSIDERATIONS

Differential Diagnoses

Common differential diagnoses to rule out myocarditis in older children and adults include pericarditis, dilated cardiomyopathy, acute coronary syndrome (ACS), and endocarditis. Stress (Takotsubo) cardiomyopathy, unstable angina, and Chagas' disease are other diagnoses to consider. Suspect myocarditis in young patients with or without pre-existing cardiovascular (CV) conditions presenting with history of recent viral URI or enteroviral infection and CV symptoms (Bashore et al., 2021; Selby, 2017).

Diagnostic Testing

There are no specific laboratory findings for myocarditis; however, there is often elevation in markers of inflammation and infection (Bashore et al., 2021).

- ECG: May reveal low QRS voltage due myocardial edema and arrhythmias. Diffuse ST elevation is common in FM but should not delay coronary angiogram to rule out ACS.
- Cardiac biomarkers: Troponin levels are commonly elevated; aids in diagnosis, but absence does not exclude myocarditis. Brain natriuretic peptide (BNP) or N-terminal pro-BNP (NT-proBNP) aid in evaluation of HF.
- Labs: CBC may reveal high eosinophil counts or increased white blood cells (WBCs); increased erythrocyte sedimentation rate (ESR)/C-reactive protein (CRP).
- Chest x-ray: Limited sensitivity; may reveal enlarged heart, pulmonary edema, pleural effusions, pulmonary infiltrates.

- Echocardiogram: Indicated but no specific findings for myocarditis; useful to measure ventricular wall size, thickness, and evaluation of systolic and diastolic function (Selby, 2017).
- Endomyocardial biopsy (EMB): EMB is considered the gold standard for a definitive diagnosis of myocarditis by the World Health Organization/International Society and Federation of Cardiology (WHO/ ISFC; Kociol et al., 2020). Performed via cardiac catheterization, tissue samples are obtained from the right or left ventricle and diagnosis is based on the following histologic and immunohistochemical criteria:
  - Histologic criteria: Presence of myocardial inflammation and necrosis not typical of cardiac ischemia in coronary artery disease (CAD), myocyte degeneration and
  - Immunohistochemical criteria: 14 leukocytes/mm^2 or higher, 7 CD3-positive T-lymphocytes/mm2 or higher.
  - Indications for EMB include new onset HF <2 weeks with hemodynamic compromise or unexplained onset of HF <3 months and demonstrating a dilated LV, new arrhythmias, and conduction disturbances.
  - Coronary angiography: Coronary angiography with EMB is recommended in all patients with clinically suspected myocarditis and is essential in guiding management of patients with new onset HF <2 weeks with hemodynamic compromise (Kociol et al., 2020).
  - Cardiac MRI: Can support diagnosis and is recommended before EMB in unexplained acute cardiomyopathy not requiring inotropic or mechanical circulatory support and responsive to medical management in less than 2 weeks (Kociol et al., 2020).

TREATMENT

There is no known treatment specific to myocarditis. Treatment is primarily supportive with management of HF, cardiogenic shock, arrhythmias, or autoimmune diseases; however, patients may ultimately require heart transplant (Levinson et al., 2020). Patients with myocarditis are typically young with no history of cardiac disease and are often given IV fluids which worsens symptoms of acute HF or leads to cardiogenic shock (Kociol et al., 2020). Antibiotic treatment is targeted at identified infecting organisms and medical therapy directed toward the clinical scenario included treatment of HF with guideline-directed medical therapy (GDMT) such as ACE-inhibitors and beta-blockers if LV ejection fraction is less than 40% (Bashore et al., 2021).

TRANSITION OF CARE

All patients suspected of myocarditis should be admitted to a tertiary care center with consultation to cardiology until a definitive diagnosis can be made. Hemodynamically unstable patients require ICU admission at facilities with ventricular support devices and transplantation options available (Bashore et al., 2021).

CLINICAL PEARLS

- Features supporting suspicion of myocarditis include fever ≥38.0°C at presentation or within the last 20 days; recent viral illness; prior suspected or definite myocarditis; patients with elevated cardiac biomarkers and new or unexplained onset of ECG changes suggesting ischemia or arrhythmias (with or without cardiac symptoms); exposure to toxic agents, or extra-cardiac immune disease.
- Prognosis varies from spontaneous resolution in mild cases to chronic dilated cardiomyopathy, or cardiogenic shock and multiorgan failure with short survival times (Cooper, 2021).

KEY TAKEAWAYS

- A focused history and physical is necessary to evaluate for signs/symptoms of suspected myocarditis
- Acute HF can develop rapidly leading to cardiogenic shock or death; management may require a multidisciplinary team with expertise in advanced circulatory support and transplantation.
- Suspect myocarditis in young patients presenting with recent viral respiratory or GI infection presenting with CV symptoms, new onset of dyspnea at rest or with exercise, arrhythmias, fatigue (with or without signs of HF), and elevated cardiac biomarkers (e.g., troponin) especially in the absence of cardiac risk factors.
- In patients who have not had EMB or cardiac MRI, a clinically suspected myocarditis diagnosis can be made based on clinical presentation and noninvasive diagnostic findings.

ACUTE PERICARDITIS

Defined as inflammation of the pericardium due to inflammation or infection, acute pericarditis is the most common disorder involving the pericardium and is often self-limited and responsive to oral anti-inflammatory medications (Goins et al., 2019). Viral and idiopathic infections are the most common cause of pericarditis in the United States. Common viral pathogens include Coxsackie or echoviruses; influenza A and B, adenoviruses, mumps, Epstein-Barr, HIV, herpes simplex, varicella-zoster, measles, and hepatitis viruses A, B, and C to name a few (Goins et al., 2019). Bacterial infections are often due to *Staphylococcus aureus* and *Streptococcus pneumoniae*; however, *mycobacterium tuberculosis* is the most common cause of pericarditis worldwide (Goins et al., 2019).

Risk Factors

Post-myocardial infarction especially with late presentation, autoimmune disease, trauma/injury, bacterial, viral, and fungal infections, kidney failure, uremia, and dialysis, and rarely, medications (phenytoin and procainamide). Most patients have no identifiable cause and are presumed to have a viral or autoimmune etiology (Imazio, 2019).

PRESENTING SIGNS AND SYMPTOMS

- Chest pain: A predominant symptom characterized by acute onset of sharp or stabbing, pleuritic anterior chest pain. Distinctive characteristics include chest pain made worse with coughing, inspiration, or a supine position; pain improves by leaning forward. Referred pain to the left trapezial ridge is also a distinguishing feature and is due to inflammation of the diaphragmatic pleura.
- Fever: May or may not have fever.
- Dyspnea: Attributed to pain with inspiration (Goins et al., 2019; Levinson et al., 2020).

HISTORY AND PHYSICAL FINDINGS

Patients typically present with chest pain which radiates to the left scapular region and they may complain of low-grade fever or "flu-like" respiratory or GI symptoms (Goins et al., 2019; Levinson et al., 2020).

Physical exam findings may include the following (Figure 3.7):

- Pericardial friction rub: Very specific for pericarditis identified as a scratchy sound best heard along the left sternal border while patient is leaning forward.
- Pericardial effusion: Often small and more common in uremic or malignant pericarditis; severe infection may result in cardiac tamponade or constrictive physiology with symptoms of heart failure (HF).

DIFFERENTIAL DIAGNOSIS AND DIAGNOSTIC CONSIDERATIONS

Differential Diagnoses

Key differential diagnoses to rule out are MI and pulmonary embolus (PE). Chest pain in pericarditis is sharp or stabbing and positional in nature, whereas chest pain in MI is typically pressure-like and includes prior exertional symptoms and lack of variation with respiration or position (Goins et al., 2019).

Clinicians must distinguish between common features of chest pain and ECG changes associated with pericarditis versus MI (Goins et al., 2019). ECG changes of ST elevation are seen in both pathologies; however, ST elevation in MI is typically localized to a vascular bed with reciprocal ST depression; in pericarditis the ST elevations are often diffuse/global, PR segment depression seen in pericarditis is very rare in MI (Goins et al., 2019).

Other disease states that can mimic acute pericarditis involve inflammation of structures in close proximity to the pericardium such as cholecystitis, pancreatitis, and pneumonia (Goins et al., 2019).

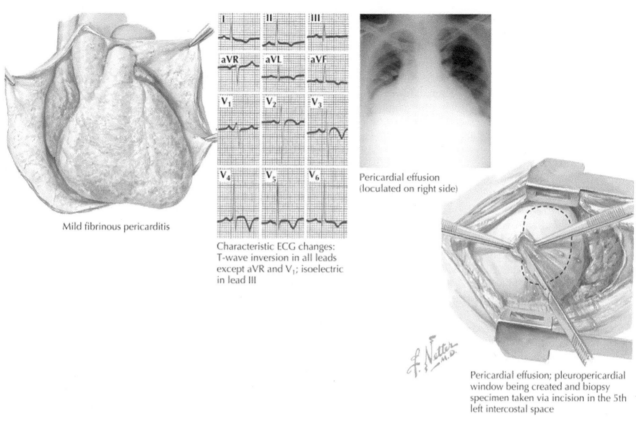

Mild fibrinous pericarditis

Characteristic ECG changes:
T-wave inversion in all leads
except aVR and V₁; isoelectric
in lead III

Pericardial effusion
(loculated on right side)

Pericardial effusion; pleuropericardial
window being created and biopsy
specimen taken via incision in the 5th
left intercostal space

FIGURE 3.7: Diseases of the pericardium: Presentation and treatment of pericarditis.

Source: Reprinted from Goins, A. E., Chiles, C. D., & Stouffer, G. A. (2019). Pericardial disease: Clinical features and treatment. In G. Stouffer, M. S. Runge, C. Patterson, & J. S. Rossi (Eds.), *Netter's cardiology* (3rd ed.). Elsevier. https://www-clinicalkey-com.libux.utmb.edu/#!/content/book/3-s2.0-B978032354726000056X?scrollTo=%23hl0000200, Page 391, Copyright (2019), with permission from Elsevier.

Diagnostic Tests

There are no lab tests sensitive or specific to differentiate pericarditis from MI.

- Pericardiocentesis or pericardial biopsy: Culture of pericardial fluid or tissue may reveal causative bacteria; viruses are rarely isolated.
- ECG: Early ECG changes in acute pericarditis include PR segment depression and diffuse ST elevations without reciprocal changes. In later stages, T-wave inversions appear in all leads except aVR and V1 (see Figure 3.7). Note that a lack of ECG changes does not exclude a diagnosis of pericarditis.
- Chest x-ray: May reveal an enlarged cardiac silhouette.
- WBC: Can be elevated due to stress or MI; used to confirm suspicion of acute pericarditis and monitor responsiveness to treatment.
- Troponin: Can be elevated in both pericarditis and MI.
- CK and troponin: Elevations may indicate concurrent myocarditis (myopericarditis)
- CRP and ESR: Will be elevated; used to confirm suspicion of acute pericarditis and monitor responsiveness to treatment.
- Echocardiogram: May reveal pericardial effusions.

Diagnosis

The European Society of Cardiology (ESC) 2015 guidelines state diagnosis of acute pericarditis must include at least two of the following criteria:

- Chest pain typical of pericarditis (sharp, pleuritic, positional in nature)
- Pericardial friction rub
- Diffuse ST-segment elevation or PR depression on ECG
- New or worsening pericardial effusion per echocardiography

TREATMENT

Most cases are self-limited and respond to combination therapy of nonsteroidal anti-inflammatory drugs (NSAIDs) and colchicine as well as restriction from strenuous exercise (Imazio, 2019):

- Ibuprofen:
  - 600 mg PO Q8h × 10 days, then
  - 400 mg PO Q8h × 10 days, then
  - 200 mg PO Q8h × 10 days
- Aspirin (325 mg) taper dosing:
  - 800 mg PO Q8h × 7–10 days, then

- 650 mg PO Q8h × 10 days, then
- 325 mg PO Q8h × 10 days
- Colchicine:
  - If >70 kg: 0.6 mg PO Q12h × 3 months
  - If <h70 kg: 0.6 mg PO Q24h × 3 months
- Contraindications: Liver disease, renal insufficiency/failure (Cr >2.5 mg/dL), myopathies, blood dyscrasia, inflammatory bowel disease, pregnancy or lactation, women of childbearing age not using contraception.
- Proton pump inhibitor (GI protection): PO Q24h × 3 months (omeprazole or pantoprazole).
- Glucocorticoids: Used only in patients with contraindications to NSAIDs with lowest effective dosages. Steroids should be avoided in all cases due to risk for increased recurrence. Expert consultation is strongly recommended if prescribing.
- Response to treatment is defined as improvement/resolution of symptoms within 1 to 2 weeks of initiation of therapy and normalization of CRP levels, if measured.
- Large pericardial effusions resulting in cardiac tamponade require pericardiocentesis or surgical interventions (e.g., balloon pericardiotomy or pericardial window) to prevent complications such as profound hypotension and death.
- Hospitalization is warranted for patients with fever >38.0°C (100.4°F), evidence of cardiac tamponade, moderate-to-large pericardial effusion, elevated troponin, immunosuppressed patients, or failure to show improvement after 7 days of appropriately dosed NSAIDs and colchicine therapy.

TRANSITION OF CARE

Most patients can be managed as outpatients with close follow-up. Patients appropriate for admission include suspected myocarditis or myopericarditis, large pericardial effusions, tachycardia out of proportion to pain/fever, and significant elevations in troponin.

CLINICAL PEARLS

- Rule out STEMI prior to diagnosing pericarditis.
- Treat pericarditis with combination therapy of NSAID/aspirin/colchicine.
- Presence of large pericardial effusions or tachycardia out of proportion to fever/pain are more likely to have complicated courses.

KEY TAKEAWAYS

- Long-term prognosis is good for patients with acute idiopathic or viral pericarditis.
- Management is based on identifiable causes (e.g., bacterial infection or malignancy) and drainage of pericardial effusion, if necessary.

- Cardiac tamponade is a medical emergency that can lead to death if untreated and may be the first manifestation of malignancy or other disorders in patients with no other history or risk factors for pericardial disease.
- Strenuous activity is avoided until resolution of symptoms due to high risk of recurrent symptoms.

EVIDENCE-BASED RESOURCES

Society Guidelines for Infective Endocarditis (https://www.ahajournals.org/doi/10.1161/CIR.0000000000000923)

Society Guidelines for Myocarditis (https://www.ahajournals.org/doi/10.1161/CIRCRESAHA.118.313578)

Society Guidelines for Acute Pericarditis (https://academic-oup-com.libux.utmb.edu/eurheartj/article/36/42/2921/2293375)

3.5: CARDIAC TAMPONADE

Lynda Stoodley

Cardiac tamponade, also known as pericardial tamponade, is a slow or rapid compression of the heart due to the pericardial accumulation of fluid, pus, blood, clots, or gas. Causes include inflammation, trauma, rupture of the heart or aortic dissection (Adler et al., 2015; Risti et al., 2014; Spodick, 2003). Cardiac tamponade is estimated to occur in two cases per 10,000 and approximately 2% of penetrating injuries are reported to result in cardiac tamponade (Yarlagadda, 2021).

The normal pericardial sac contains approximately 10 to 50 mL of fluid and acts as a lubricant between the pericardial layers (Adler et al., 2015). A pericardial effusion occurs if there is an accumulation of fluid beyond the usual limit in the pericardial sac (Figure 3.8). If there is a gradual increase in fluid accumulation, the

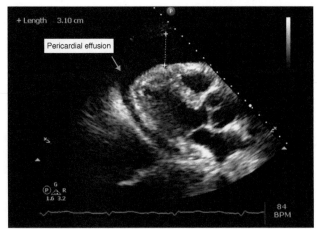

FIGURE 3.8: A pericardial effusion occurs if there is an accumulation of fluid beyond the usual limit in the pericardial sac.

pericardial sac can accommodate up to 1 to 1.5 L of fluid before cardiac output is compromised, but if it accumulates rapidly, tamponade may occur with as little as 150 mL fluid accumulation (Merck Manual, 2020). This excess fluid can cause compression of the cardiac chambers and compromise cardiac function, preventing full force contraction of the heart, thus decreasing cardiac output (Spodick, 2003).

PRESENTING SIGNS AND SYMPTOMS

Patient presentation varies and depends on a variety of factors including the volume of the effusion and its rate of accumulation, etiology of the effusion, the thickness and compliance of the pericardium, and the presence of co-existing heart disease (Hoit, 2017). Many patients are asymptomatic, and effusions are found incidentally on x-ray or echocardiogram performed for other reasons (Adler et al., 2015). All pericardial effusions do not lead to cardiac tamponade.

Patients with cardiac tamponade may present with Beck's triad, which is hypotension, muffled heart sounds, and jugular venous distention (Braunwald, 2018) but these signs may not always be present or easily identifiable. Pulsus paradoxus or paradoxical pulse is a decrease in systolic blood pressure during inspiration of >10 mmHg and is a classic sign of cardiac tamponade (Chen, 2019; Merck Manual, 2020). Another sign is tachycardia as the heart attempts to increase cardiac output. Cardiac tamponade should be considered if the patient is hypotensive and has signs of decreased end organ perfusion such as elevated serum lactate and decreased urine output (McCanny & Colreavy, 2017).

Patients may report shortness of breath (SOB), chest pain, or dizziness. Other less common symptoms may include nausea, dysphagia, hoarseness, and hiccups (related to compression of the stomach, esophagus or phrenic nerve; Adler et al., 2015; Imazio et al., 2010; Risti et al., 2014; Roy et al., 2007).

HISTORY AND PHYSICAL FINDINGS

A comprehensive history can reveal underlying disorders that can lead to pericardial effusions, such as malignancies, connective tissue disorders, renal failure, recent cardiovascular (CV) procedures, such as pacemaker insertion, coronary artery bypass graft (CABG), valvular surgery, and trauma (Chen, 2019; Yarlagadda, 2021).

Physical exam findings may include ECG changes demonstrating reduced QRS and T wave voltage and electrical alternans (Argula et al., 2015), and increased cardiac silhouette on chest x-ray if there is a large effusion (McCanny & Colreavy, 2017). Patients may have signs of hypoperfusion such as cold clammy skin, diaphoresis, altered mentation, and shock if accumulation of the pericardial fluid occurs quickly.

DIFFERENTIAL DIAGNOSIS AND DIAGNOSTIC CONSIDERATIONS

Differential diagnoses for cardiac tamponade include constrictive pericarditis, restrictive cardiomyopathy, tuberculosis, acute right heart failure, severe asthma, tension pneumothorax, superior vena cava obstruction, or extreme obesity (McCanny & Colreavy, 2017). When a pericardial effusion is detected, the first step is to assess its size, presence of cardiac tamponade, and possible associated CV or systemic diseases (Adler et al., 2015). Echocardiography is the single most sensitive diagnostic tool to identify pericardial effusion and provides an estimate of amount, location, and degree of hemodynamic impact.

Echocardiography can determine if there is hemodynamic compromise known as tamponade physiology, which includes (Cosyns et al., 2014; Imazio et al., 2010; Klein et al., 2013, 2020; Risti et al., 2014):

- Collapse of the right atrium (RA) in systole and the right ventricle (RV) in diastole
- Dilatation of the inferior vena cava (>20 mm in an adult size heart) and hepatic veins
- Septal "bounce"
- Respiratory variability seen with Doppler analysis of the LV outflow tract, demonstrating decrease of >10% following deep inspiration

TREATMENT

The treatment of cardiac tamponade is to drain the pericardial fluid, either by needle pericardiocentesis or a pericardial window via a surgical approach (Adler et al., 2015). The intervention is dependent on degree of hemodynamic compromise, as well as relative contraindications and indications for each.(Chen, 2019). Additional interventions include supplemental oxygen, volume expansion, and vasopressors (Chen, 2019).

TRANSITION OF CARE

After the initial treatment and stabilization of the patient, treatment of the underlying cause of the effusion is needed, if identified.

CLINICAL PEARLS

- Cardiac tamponade is a life-threatening compression of the heart due to the pericardial accumulation of fluid, pus, blood, clots, or gas as a result of inflammation, trauma, rupture of the heart, or aortic dissection (Adler et al., 2015; Risti et al., 2014; Spodick, 2003).
- Patients with cardiac tamponade may present with Beck's triad, which is hypotension, muffled heart tones, and jugular venous distention (Braunwald, 2018).
- Echocardiography is the most useful diagnostic tool to identify pericardial effusion providing the best estimate of size and tamponade physiology (Cosyns et al., 2014; Imazio et al., 2010; Klein et al., 2013, 2020; Risti et al., 2014).

■ The treatment of cardiac tamponade requires drainage of the pericardial fluid, by needle pericardiocentesis or a surgical approach (Adler et al., 2015).

KEY TAKEAWAYS

■ Patient presentation varies and depends on a variety of factors including the volume of the effusion and its rate of accumulation, etiology of the effusion, the thickness and compliance of the pericardium, and the presence of co-existing heart disease (Hoit, 2017).

EVIDENCE-BASED RESOURCE

Adler, Y., Charron, P., Imazio, M., Badano, L., Barón-Esquivias, G., Bogaert, J., Brucato, A., Gueret, P., Klingel, K., Lionis, C., Maisch, B., Mayosi, B., Pavie, A., Ristic', A. D., Tenas, M. S., Seferovic, P., Swedberg, K., & Tomkowski, W. (2015). 2015 ESC Guidelines for the diagnosis and management of pericardial diseases. *Kardiologia Polska, 73*(11), 1028–1091. https://doi.org/10.5603/kp.2015.0228

3.6: CARDIOMYOPATHY

Amy Stoddard

Cardiomyopathy is a general term for myocardial (heart muscle) disease. There are four subtypes of cardiomyopathy: dilated, hypertrophic, restrictive, and takotsubo. Each type will be discussed in detail.

Dilated

Dilated cardiomyopathy is left ventricular (LV) or biventricular dilation with systolic dysfunction (Merlo et al., 2018). In dilated cardiomyopathy, there is an absence of apparent volume overload, elevated blood pressure, valvular disease, or coronary disease to explain the ventricular dilation (Merlo et al., 2018). Although primary dilated cardiomyopathy is idiopathic and typically genetic, secondary dilated cardiomyopathy can be due to infection, autoimmune disease, endocrine disease, obstructive sleep apnea, prolonged tachyarrhythmias, toxins or drugs, and irradiation or chemotherapy (Ovidiu et al., 2018).

Hypertrophic

Hypertrophic cardiomyopathy is defined as LV hypertrophy with no LV dilation and a normal to increased ejection fraction without any overload (Marian & Braunwald, 2017). Hypertrophic cardiomyopathy is a genetic condition of the cardiac myocytes, typically occurring from a single gene mutation, and is autosomal dominant (Marian & Braunwald, 2017). Genetic mutations cause a series of events starting with the initial mutation that leads to molecular changes in sarcomere protein structure and function, which causes activation of the hypertrophic signaling pathways of the heart (Marian & Braunwald, 2017).

Restrictive

Restrictive cardiomyopathy is a stiffening of the myocardial tissue that causes impaired ventricular filling; both the right ventricular (RV) and the LV chambers remain standard size with normal systolic function until the later stages of disease (Muchtar et al., 2017). Restrictive cardiomyopathy can be genetic (storage disorders) or acquired through infiltrative diseases (amyloidosis and sarcoidosis), noninfiltrative disease (diabetic, idiopathic, scleroderma), endomyocardial diseases (carcinoid) and secondary to chemotherapy and radiation (Muchtar et al., 2017).

Takotsubo

Takotsubo cardiomyopathy, also known as stress cardiomyopathy or broken heart syndrome, is known for the apical ballooning seen on echocardiography (Medina de Chazal et al., 2018). Takotsubo is a reversible LV systolic and diastolic dysfunction due to physical or emotional stress (Medina de Chazal et al., 2018). In addition, neurological causes such as subarachnoid hemorrhage can also cause takotsubo. The apical ballooning seen on echocardiography resembles the Japanese octopus trap; this is where the name takotsubo originates from (Medina de Chazal et al., 2018).

PRESENTING SIGNS AND SYMPTOMS

Dilated cardiomyopathy patients may present with heart failure (HF) symptomology such as lower extremity edema, orthopnea, paroxysmal nocturnal dyspnea (PND), fatigue, jugular vein distention, pulmonary edema, thromboembolic events, arrhythmias, and, in later stages of the disease, valvular damage (Ovidiu et al., 2018).

Individuals with hypertrophic cardiomyopathy are typically asymptomatic for many years (Marian & Braunwald, 2017). However, when patients present with symptoms, they will include HF symptoms, chest pain, or arrhythmias (Marian & Braunwald, 2017).

Individuals with restrictive cardiomyopathy patients may present with signs of left and right HF (Muchtar et al., 2017). Other common symptoms include dyspnea, fatigue at rest, exercise intolerance, syncope, palpitations, and angina (Rammos et al., 2017).

Symptoms of takotsubo cardiomyopathy include the acute onset of chest pain, shortness of breath (SOB), and dizziness (Medina de Chazal et al., 2018). Individuals may also present after a syncopal episode or describing what appears to be a presyncopal state (Medina de Chazal et al., 2018).

HISTORY AND PHYSICAL FINDINGS

Symptoms of dilated cardiomyopathy include lower extremity edema, orthopnea, jugular venous distention, and crackles (secondary to pulmonary edema). Obtaining a family history is essential to determine if any family members also have dilated cardiomyopathy. Dilated cardiomyopathy is inherited in approximately 20% to 50% of cases and is autosomal dominant primarily (Jain et al., 2021). When taking the family history, one should ask if any first-degree relative has ever been given a diagnosis of dilated cardiomyopathy or if any first-degree relative has passed from sudden cardiac death between the ages of 20 to 60 years old (Jain et al., 2021).

In hypertrophic cardiomyopathy, symptoms are caused by diastolic HF and a LV outflow obstruction (Marian & Braunwald, 2017). On examination, the precordial impulse will be displaced to the left and more forceful than usual; an additional heart sound (S4) can be heard prominently and in those patients with LV outflow tract obstruction (LVOTO), a harsh grade 3 to 4 mid-systolic murmur can be heard (Marian & Braunwald, 2017).

Restrictive cardiomyopathy symptoms include distended jugular veins, lower extremity edema, crackles on auscultation, and possibly S3 and S4 heart sounds (Rammos et al., 2017).

Takotsubo cardiomyopathy patients will typically be in respiratory distress secondary to the pulmonary edema on presentation (Medina de Chazal et al., 2018). On examination, these patients may have jugular vein distention, crackles, S3 gallop, a systolic ejection murmur, tachycardia, and hypotension (Medina de Chazal et al., 2018). If the patient presents with shock-like symptoms, it is life-threatening due to the potential for these patients to decline from rapid progression to cardiogenic shock (Medina de Chazal et al., 2018).

DIFFERENTIAL DIAGNOSIS AND DIAGNOSTIC CONSIDERATIONS

In all cardiomyopathy patients, ischemic heart dysfunction or any valve disorders such as aortic stenosis (AS) will need to be ruled out as the cause of any symptoms (Merlo et al., 2018). Obtaining extended family history is critical as some cardiomyopathies are genetic. Obtaining a past medical history to determine if the patient has any history of diseases that can have cardiac complications such as hypertension or diabetes is essential.

Cardiac MRI is the gold standard for diagnosing dilated cardiomyopathy and used to determine the amount of fibrosis (Ovidiu et al., 2018). Echocardiogram is also used to measure LV size; however, an increase in the LV dimensions may not be seen early with cardiomyopathy (McNally & Mestroni, 2017).

Hypertrophic cardiomyopathy is also diagnosed with cardiac MRI to determine interstitial fibrosis (Marian & Braunwald, 2017). Echocardiography will reveal asymmetric hypertrophy involving the basal interventricular septum (below the aortic valve) and may involve the free wall of the LV (Marian & Braunwald, 2017). Diagnosis is made when the end-diastolic ventricular septal thickness in adults is greater than or equal to 13 mm in diameter (Marian & Braunwald, 2017).

Restrictive cardiomyopathy is diagnosed with transthoracic echocardiogram (TTE), which is essential in determining a diagnosis of restrictive cardiomyopathy versus constrictive pericarditis as the presentation of symptoms is similar (Rammos et al., 2017). In addition, a restrictive filling pattern with normal or almost normal systolic function and decreased diastolic dysfunction are findings typically found on TTE (Muchtar et al., 2017).

Takotsubo cardiomyopathy is diagnosed when LV wall motion abnormalities are seen on TTE that are inconsistent with any coronary artery distribution (Medina de Chazal et al., 2018). The ballooning of the apex seen on TTE is due to apical hypokinesia or akinesia with basal hyperkinesis (Medina de Chazal et al., 2018). These patients typically present with elevated troponins, elevated serum natriuretic peptide (BNP), and ECG changes (Medina de Chazal et al., 2018). Definitive diagnosis is made with a left heart catherization without findings of obstructive CAD.

TREATMENT

Management of dilated cardiomyopathy consists of reducing HF symptoms, arrhythmia surveillance and treatment, and maintaining as much LV function as possible (McNally & Mestroni, 2017; Ommen et al., 2020). Guideline-directed therapy, which consists of angiotensin converting enzymes (ACE) inhibitors or angiotensin II receptor blockers (ARBs), with beta-blockers, and an aldosterone antagonist is used to manage HF symptoms (McNally & Mestroni, 2017). Patients who have refractory HF may require advanced therapies, mechanical circulatory support devices, or possible orthotopic heart transplantation (McNally & Mestroni, 2017).

Hypertrophic cardiomyopathy patients are treated with lifestyle modification since they are mainly asymptomatic; if there is evidence of LVOTO, medication can reduce the LVOTO, or there is a possible need for surgical intervention including septal myectomy/mitral valve interventions (Geske et al., 2018). Lifestyle modifications such as low impact aerobic exercise, low sodium diet, and avoidance of alcohol are all recommendations for patients with hypertrophic cardiomyopathy (Geske et al., 2018). Beta-blockers are the first-line treatment for hypertrophic cardiomyopathy patients (Geske et al., 2018). In addition, dual-chamber pacemakers with an atrioventricular delay are effective for some hypertrophic patients with LVOTO (Geske et al., 2018). SCD is a concern in this population. Extensive LV hypertrophy, excessive late gadolinium enhancement, and the presence of an apical aneurysm place patients at an increased risk of SCD (Geske et al., 2018). The American Cardiology guidelines state that a septal myomectomy is the mainstay of invasive surgical therapy; however, European Cardiology guidelines prefer the alcohol septal ablation procedure (Geske et al., 2018).

Restrictive cardiomyopathy is treated by managing the HF symptoms; however, diuresis remains a challenge

(Muchtar et al., 2017). If there is a treatable underlying condition causing the restrictive cardiomyopathy, such as cancer or sarcoidosis, those conditions must be treated (Muchtar et al., 2017). The restrictive cardiomyopathy patient relies on high filling pressures to maintain cardiac output and adequate tissue perfusion; excessive diuresis can lead to a low cardiac output state (Muchtar et al., 2017). Advanced therapies for refractory HF, such as mechanical circulatory support devices or orthotopic cardiac transplantation, may be necessary (Muchtar et al., 2017).

Takotsubo cardiomyopathy is sometimes treated with watchful waiting and supportive care. Continuous ECG monitoring, treatment of arrhythmias, systemic anticoagulation until LV recovery occurs to present thrombus formation are the mainstays of treatment (Medina de Chazal et al., 2018). The complications from takotsubo such as LVOTO, intramyocardial hemorrhage and rupture, stroke, and acute HF that declines into cardiogenic shock can be fatal (Medina de Chazal et al., 2018). Patients who present with HF symptoms such as pulmonary congestion should be treated with diuretics, venodilators, beta-blockers, and arterial vasodilators (Medina de Chazal et al., 2018). For those patients who develop cardiogenic shock, treatment is based on evidence of LVOTO (Medina de Chazal et al., 2018). In LVOTO, introtropes should be avoided as they may worsen the condition. Treatment should begin with intravenous fluids, beta-blockers, and vasopressors (if needed) (Medina de Chazal et al., 2018). In those patients without LVOTO, inotropes and vasopressors are used for treatment (Medina de Chazal et al., 2018). For those in refractory cardiogenic shock and LVOTO, extracorporeal membrane obstruction (ECMO) support is used; for those in cardiogenic shock without LVOTO, an impella device or intra-aortic balloon pump can be used (Medina de Chazal et al., 2018).

CLINICAL PEARLS

- Patients can present with HF symptomology.
- Cardiac MRI will determine the amount of fibrosis.
- Echocardiogram is used to determine wall thickness.
- Treat HF symptoms with guideline-directed medical therapy.

KEY TAKEAWAYS

- There are four types of cardiomyopathies: dilated, hypertrophic, restrictive, and stress or takotsubo.
- The typical presentation is HF symptoms.
- Echocardiogram and cardiac MRI are vital diagnostic tests.
- Use guideline-directed medical therapy for HF symptoms.
- With refractory HF symptoms, refer to an advanced HF center.

3.7: HEART FAILURE

Carolina D. Tennyson, Jaime A. McDermott, and Stephanie G. Barnes

Heart failure (HF) is a clinical syndrome caused by structural or functional cardiac abnormalities rendering the heart unable to deliver adequate perfusion to the body. The HF syndrome is a major public health crisis affecting more than 25 million patients worldwide (Ambrosy et al., 2014).

Etiologies of HF include acute and chronic syndromes. An ischemic etiology is universally the most common cause of HF. It can also develop secondary to hypertension, heart valve abnormalities, and congenital heart disease (Mentz & O'Connor, 2016). The most common tool used to classify and report HF stages is the New York Heart Association (NYHA) functional classes 1 to 4, which considers symptoms and physical limitations. Guidelines for therapies are largely divided by the HF etiology and whether the ejection fraction is preserved (HFpEF; i.e., >40%) or reduced (HFrEF; <40%).

Neurohormonal activation, venous congestion, myocardial injury, and renal dysfunction are central to the pathophysiology of chronic HF. Fortunately, there is evidence to show that multiple medications in conjunction can significantly improve mortality and symptoms for patients with HF and reduced ejection fraction, known as guideline-directed medicines and therapies (GDMT; Maddox et al., 2021). For those patients who suffer from acute decompensated HF and end organ damage, advanced therapies like IV inotropes, mechanical circulatory support, or cardiac transplantation may be considered.

PRESENTING SIGNS AND SYMPTOMS

HF is a complex syndrome characterized by symptoms such as weight gain, swelling, dyspnea, and activity intolerance. In the setting of a HF exacerbation, some patients demonstrate an intolerance to their HF medications and may have symptomatic hypotension, worsening renal function, or hyperkalemia (Mentz & O'Connor, 2016). Patients may also present with a concomitant process like pneumonia, myocardial ischemia, or heart arrhythmias. Patients with HF often experience sleep-disordered breathing like orthopnea, paroxysmal nocturnal dyspnea (PND) as well as dyspnea with bending over (bendopnea). Clinical history is an important feature in the evaluation of HF.

HISTORY AND PHYSICAL FINDINGS
Review of Systems

Questions related to the baseline symptom burden of patients with HF can give insight into the context of a patient's HF exacerbation. The frequency and duration of congestive symptoms should be evaluated, including progression of dyspnea on exertion (DOE) to dyspnea at rest, progression of activity intolerance, orthopnea, or

PND, all of which are highly sensitive to HF. Pertaining to the history of HF, it is important to inquire about recent changes in diuretic dosing, medication regimen, emergency department visits, or hospitalizations. Consideration should be made for obtaining history of recent medication intolerance or challenges affecting medication adherence. Compliance to a sodium and fluid restricted diet is debated in the literature but a recent intake in high sodium rich foods or excess fluid intake should be reviewed (Yancy et al., 2018). Patients with HF are typically instructed to monitor their weight for fluctuations, so ask about body weight specifically.

If a patient has an internal cardiac defibrillator (ICD), inquire about recent defibrillator shocks because patients with HF with a reduced ejection fraction have a risk of sudden cardiac death. The occurrence of ICD shocks should cue clinicians to investigate for progression of HF and presence of life-threatening arrhythmias like ventricular tachycardia or ventricular fibrillation.

Past Medical History

When obtaining the past medical history for a patient with HF, it is important to understand the onset of the diagnosis and whether it is the initial presentation or a presentation for a known, chronic condition. Consideration should be made to inquire about comorbid conditions such as hypertension, hyperlipidemia, prior myocardial infarction (MI), obesity, sleep apnea, atrial fibrillation, diabetes, thyroid disease, or recent viral illness.

Implantable and wearable device-based technologies can aid in the assessment of HF, but most of the research in this area has been done in the chronic HF population (Mentz & O'Connor, 2016). If available, information from a smart watch or implanted pulmonary artery pressure monitor may be useful to correlate with patient symptoms.

Family History

Obtaining a family history for the presence of SCD, coronary artery disease (CAD), myocardial infarction (MI), hypertension, or presence of known HF should be evaluated.

Social History

When obtaining a social history, consider evaluation for substance or alcohol use or abuse. Evaluation of social support and a focus on social determinants of health should be considered.

Physical Exam

Patients hospitalized with HF are stratified based on the assessment of congestion and degree of perfusion. Those who are hypervolemic or congested may have edema or elevated jugular venous distention and are considered to have a "wet" profile. Patients who are warm to the touch and well perfused are considered "warm" and patients who feel cool to the touch are considered "cold." Other symptoms of poor perfusion might include hypotension, altered mental status, or acute kidney injury. This warm/cold, wet/dry assessment can help assess the degree of compensation which is outlined in Figure 3.9.

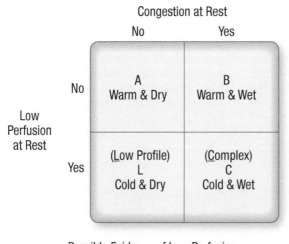

FIGURE 3.9: Stages of decompensated heart failure.

Source: Reproduced with permission from Thenappan, T., Anderson, A. S., & Fedson, S. (2015). Diagnostic testing and the assessment of heart failure. In R. R. Baliga & G. J. Haas (Eds.), *Management of heart failure: Volume 1: Medical* (pp. 31–45). Springer Publishing Company. https://doi.org/10.1007/978-1-4471-6657-3_3.

The priority of the physical exam should be to determine whether the patient is in a low output state or not. A patient who is in cardiogenic shock will display a wet/cold profile and their congestion and perfusion should be addressed immediately. Patients with tachycardia, kidney dysfunction, hypotension, but without shock are considered intermediate risk. Low risk patients have a normal basic metabolic panel (BMP), troponin, blood pressure, and heart rate (Hollenberg et al., 2019). Consider where fluid is accumulating as this reflects whether a patient has left, right, or biventricular HF.

DIFFERENTIAL DIAGNOSIS AND DIAGNOSTIC CONSIDERATIONS

Dyspnea, the most common presenting symptom for HF, can be explained by several etiologies including viral illnesses, pneumonia, chronic obstructive pulmonary disease (COPD) exacerbation, and more. Differential diagnoses to consider are summarized in Table 3.6. Another common complaint, chest pain, has a wide differential list such as pulmonary edema, aortic dissection, or acute coronary syndrome (ACS).

The first steps to differentiate HF from these differentials are diagnostic tests including an ECG to evaluate for cardiac ischemia and a chest x-ray to evaluate for pulmonary opacities, infiltrates, or pneumothorax. Left ventricular (LV) hypertrophy and pulmonary edema are findings consistent with, but not diagnostic of HF. The initial workup may unveil concomitant processes which are not uncommon in patients with HF.

Echocardiography is a noninvasive assessment that should routinely be performed in patients with acute HF to assess for wall motion abnormalities that may indicate ischemia, volume status, and most importantly ejection fraction. If the patient has signs of ischemia on the ECG and has new ventricular wall motion abnormalities on the echocardiogram, continue down the ACS workup and treatment pathway outlined in the ACS section. Additional testing such as a diagnostic right and left heart cardiac catheterization can provide both an evaluation of the coronary arteries as well as measurement

of invasive hemodynamics. Cardiac biopsy may also be indicated if HF due to myocarditis or cardiac amyloidosis is suspected.

Biomarkers such as B-type natriuretic peptide (BNP) concentrations are typically observed as a compensatory response to elevated cardiac wall stress and its trend can be used in risk stratification and assessment of decongestion. Troponins should be evaluated to complete the ischemic workup. A full list of serum evaluation can be found in Table 3.7.

The interdependence of the heart and kidneys has been characterized as cardiorenal syndrome and many patients present with concomitant worsening renal function and HF symptoms. Venous congestion, neurohormonal activation, and inflammation are contributors to renal dysfunction in patients with HF. Be sure to evaluate the renal function and urine output early and often in this patient population.

TABLE 3.6: Differential Diagnoses for Heart Failure

HEART FAILURE TYPE	DIFFERENTIAL DIAGNOSES
Acute	Asthma, carbon monoxide, cardiac tamponade, hiatal hernia, hypotension, pneumonia, aspiration, foreign body obstruction
Chronic	Asthma, chronic obstructive pulmonary disease, interstitial lung disease
Cardiac	Cardiomyopathy, arrhythmias, acute coronary syndrome, pericarditis
Pulmonary	Croup, lung cancer, pulmonary edema, pulmonary fibrosis, sarcoidosis, pneumothorax, bronchitis, tuberculosis, influenza, COVID-19
Other	Anemia, broken ribs, trauma, choking, epiglottis, anxiety, obesity, drugs (e.g., beta-blockers), poor physical conditioning, myasthenia gravis

TABLE 3.7: Diagnostic Testing for Heart Failure

EVALUATION	DIAGNOSTIC TEST
Initial laboratory evaluation	Complete blood count, urinalysis, serum electrolytes (including calcium and magnesium), blood urea nitrogen, serum creatinine, glucose, fasting lipid profile, liver function tests, thyroid-stimulating hormone, BNP or NT-pro-BNP, troponin
Additional laboratory evaluation	HIV, autoimmune disease including antinucleic acid antibodies, C3/C4 complement, and ANA, SPEP/UPEP, serum free light chains, iron studies, routine toxicology
Initial imaging	ECG, chest x-ray, 2-dimensional echocardiogram with Doppler
Additional imaging	Viability assessment, radionuclide ventriculography or MRI, cardiac MRI, right heart catheterization, left heart catheterization with or without coronary angiography, endomyocardial biopsy

ANA, antinuclear antibody; BNP, B-type natriuretic peptide; SPEP + UPEP, serum and urine protein electrophoresis

TREATMENT

Guideline-Directed Medical Therapy (GDMT)

The priorities of treating acute HF are decongestion and optimization of GDMT. GDMT slows the progression of ventricular enlargement or remodeling through minimization of circulatory congestion and vasoconstriction, increasing tissue perfusion, and decreasing neurohormonal activity through inhibition of the RAAS and sympathetic nervous system (Yancy et al., 2018). Decongestion itself does not improve outcomes but improves HF symptoms of volume overload.

Most HF medical therapies are indicated for patients with HF with reduced ejection fraction (HFrEF) and there is little therapy to improve mortality in the preserved ejection fraction population. GDMT for patients with HFrEF is disease modifying and has shown to significantly reduce morbidity and mortality (Bhatt et al., 2021). Modern GDMT includes a beta-blocker, an angiotensin receptor-modifier (ACE/ARB/ARNI), a sodium-glucose cotransporter-2 inhibitor (SGLT2i; Zelniker & Braunwald, 2020), and a mineralocorticoid receptor antagonist (MRA). Initiation and intensification of GDMT can and should be done in the inpatient setting (Bhatt et al., 2021). Initiation and target doses for GDMT are summarized in Table 3.8 (Maddox et al., 2021). Inpatient dose optimization should take place after aggressive decongestion and in a well-perfused hemodynamic state (not in cardiogenic shock).

Decongestion

Decongestion is achieved medically with loop diuretics like furosemide and bumetanide. These diuretics inhibit the reabsorption of sodium or chloride at various sites in the kidney, minimizing fluid retention and increasing urine output to reduce symptom burden associated with HF. An IV diuretic should be continued throughout the hospitalization until effective decongestion warrants transition to oral diuretics prior to discharge (Hollenberg et al., 2019). Major adverse effects associated with diuretics include electrolyte depletion (potassium, magnesium) predisposing patients to cardiac arrhythmias, hypovolemia, hypotension, and azotemia. Initiation and target dosing for IV and oral diuretic therapy are defined in Table 3.9. Targets for decongestion include downtrending B-type natriuretic peptide (by at least 30%), water weight loss, and improvement in clinical symptoms and physical exam. If there is inadequate improvement, IV diuretics can be increased by 50% to 100% until the total diuretic dose exceeds 400 to 500 mg of furosemide in 24 hours. Consider intermittent doses of metolazone, acetazolamide, or other thiazide diuretics as adjunct therapies for decongestion (Hollenberg et al., 2019).

Maintaining Adequate Cardiac Output

Cardiac output is calculated by the patient's heart rate and stroke volume. The stroke volume is affected by variables such as preload, afterload, and contractility. Heart rate is controlled by the autonomic nervous system and is affected by age and hormones. Much of HF treatment can be linked to optimizing these calculations to yield an adequate cardiac output.

Inotropes are an adjunct HF therapy that can be used to increase cardiac output in the acute, chronic, or palliative care setting. Inotropes generally fall into one of three categories: beta-agonists (dobutamine, dopamine, epinephrine); phosphodiesterase III inhibitors (milrinone); and calcium sensitizers (levosimendan). Drug choice is tailored to patient hemodynamics, known drug side effects, and goals of care. All of them are delivered intravenously, preferably into a central vein.

Adjunct Nonpharmacologic Therapies

Patients with an ejection fraction less than 35% are at risk for SCD and are recommended to undergo primary prevention implantation of an ICD (Maddox et al., 2021) after receiving GDMT for at least 6 months. This device has both pacing and defibrillation capability. In addition, chronic resynchronization therapy-defibrillator (CRT-D) may be indicated to improve timing and synchronization of right and LV systole.

TABLE 3.8: Initiation/Target Doses for Guideline-Directed Medical Therapy for Heart Failure

MEDICAL THERAPY	INITIATION/TARGET DOSES
ACE inhibitors	captopril 6.25 mg TID to 50 mg TID enalapril 2.5 mg BID to 10 or 20 mg BID lisinopril 2.5/5 mg daily to 20 or 40 mg daily ramipril 1.25 mg daily to 10 mg daily
ARBs	candesartan 4 or 8 mg daily to 32 mg daily losartan 25 or 50 mg daily to 150 mg daily valsartan 40 mg BID to 160 mg BID
ARNI	sacubitril/valsartan 24/26 mg or 49/51 mg BID to 97/103 mg BID
Beta-blockers	carvedilol 3.125 mg BID to 25 or 50 mg BID (based on weight) metoprolol succinate 12.5 or 25 mg daily to 200 mg daily bisoprolol 1.25 mg daily to 10 mg daily
Aldosterone antagonists	spironolactone 12.5 or 25 mg daily to 25 or 50 mg daily eplerenone 25 mg daily to 50 mg daily
Vasodilators	hydralazine 25 mg TID to 75 mg TID isosorbide dinitrate 20 mg TID to 40 mg TID Combination isosorbide dinitrate/hydralazine 20/37.5 mg TID to 40/75 mg TID
Ivabradine	ivabradine 2.5 or 5 mg BID to 7.5 mg BID
SGLT2i	dapagliflozin 10 mg daily empagliflozin 10 mg daily to 25 mg daily

TABLE 3.9: Adjunct Diuretic Therapy for Heat Failure: Initiation and Target Dosing

	INTRAVENOUS	ORAL
Loop	bumetanide 0.5 to 4 mg once to TID; up to 5 mg/dose bumetanide infusion 0.5 to 2 mg/h; up to 4 mg/h furosemide 40 to 160 mg once TID; up to 200 mg/dose furosemide infusion 5 to 20 mg/h; up to 40 mg/h	bumex 0.5 to 2 mg daily or BID to 10 mg daily furosemide 20 daily or BID to 600 mg daily torsemide 10 daily or BID to 200 mg daily
Thiazide	chlorothiazide 0.5 to 1 g daily or BID to 2 g daily	metolazone 2.5 or 5 mg daily or BID to 20 mg daily hydrochlorothiazide 25 to 50 mg daily to BID to 100 mg daily chlorthalidone 12.5 to 25 mg daily or BID to 100 mg daily

Source: Data from Hollenberg, S. M., Warner Stevenson, L., Ahmad, T., Amin, V. J., Bozkurt, B., Butler, J., Davis, L. L., Drazner, M. H., Kirkpatrick, J. N., Peterson, P. N., Reed, B. N., Roy, C. L., & Storrow, A. B. (2019). 2019 ACC expert consensus decision pathway on risk assessment, management, and clinical trajectory of patients hospitalized with heart failure. *Journal of the American College of Cardiology, 74*(15), 1966–2011. https://doi.org/10.1016/j.jacc.2019.08.001.

Advanced Therapies

A durable left ventricular assist device (LVAD) is a surgically implanted mechanical pump that diverts blood out of the left side of the heart and delivers it directly to the aorta, bypassing the sick ventricle. These pumps are being used more often, but come with a host of complications including stroke, bleeding, infection, and thrombosis. Patients need chronic anticoagulation to prevent pump thrombosis. Patients with LVADs must maintain adequate right ventricular function to deliver blood volume to the pump. LVADs are preload dependent and afterload sensitive. Therefore, hypertension and hypovolemia must be avoided and treated for the pump to support the cardiac output.

Advanced therapies, including heart transplant and mechanical circulatory support (intra-aortic balloon pump, durable LVAD, temporary ventricular assist devices) may be considered when HF is refractory to therapy. Patients undergo a rigorous evaluation by a multidisciplinary team to determine the best therapy for the individual; separate criteria exist for each therapy. Both therapies have been shown to improve quality of life and prolong patient survival.

TRANSITION OF CARE

Key interventions are essential to ensure a seamless transition of care from the inpatient to the outpatient setting to minimize the risk of re-hospitalization. Re-admission risk assessment and medication reconciliation should take place on admission and at discharge (Hollenberg et al., 2019; Yancy et al., 2013). Specialized patient education regarding sodium and fluid restriction, and measurement of daily weights should be performed during the acute care stay and reinforced during follow-up (Yancy et al., 2013). Patients should be counseled on medication adherence, weight loss, exercise training or regular physical activity, and medications which may contribute to HF (NSAIDs, nondihydropyridine calcium channel blockers). Patients and/or caregivers should be provided with written instructions at discharge that outline their treatment plan.

Outpatient providers participating in the patient's care should be updated on the patient's clinical status and any GDMT or medication modifications (Hollenberg et al., 2019). Guidelines recommend a follow-up appointment with a HF provider within 7 to 14 days of hospital discharge (Hollenberg et al., 2019; Yancy et al., 2013). Referral to palliative care or hospice care should be considered for end-stage HF patients who are refractory to medical therapy and not candidates for advanced therapies (Hollenberg et al., 2019).

CLINICAL PEARLS

- Diuresis is symptom management; GDMT improves outcomes.
- The physical assessment for congestion (wet or dry) and perfusion (warm or cold) can help determine if the patient is in a low output state.
- Patients with LVADs are at risk for bleeding, infection, and stroke and require chronic anticoagulation.
- Patients should have postdischarge follow-up within 7 to 14 days after HF hospitalization.

KEY TAKEAWAYS

- It is important to address comorbidities of patients with HF.
- Decongestion and GDMT optimization are the primary goals for patients with HF.
- The cornerstone of HF treatment is inhibition of the renin-angiotensin-aldosteorne system (RAAS) and sympathetic nervous system (SNS).
- GDMT = BB + ARNI + MRA + SGLT2i.
- Patients with LVADs are at risk for bleeding, infection, and stroke and require chronic anticoagulation.
- Reduce the risk of re-hospitalization by communicating with outpatient HF providers and arranging follow-up during transition of care.

EVIDENCE-BASED RESOURCES

Hollenberg, S. M., Warner Stevenson, L., Ahmad, T., Amin, V. J., Bozkurt, B., Butler, J., Davis, L. L., Drazner, M. H., Kirkpatrick, J. N., Peterson, P. N., Reed, B. N., Roy, C.

L., & Storrow, A. B. (2019). 2019 ACC expert consensus decision pathway on risk assessment, management, and clinical trajectory of patients hospitalized with heart failure. *Journal of the American College of Cardiology, 74*(15), 1966–2011. https://doi.org/10.1016/j.jacc.2019.08.001

Maddox, T. M., Januzzi, J. L., Allen, L. A., Breathett, K., Butler, J., Davis, L. L., Fonarow, G. C., Ibrahim, N. E., Lindenfeld, J., Masoudi, F. A., Motiwala, S. R., Oliveros, E., Patterson, J. H., Walsh, M. N., Wasserman, A., Yancy, C. W., & Youmans, Q. R. (2021). 2021 update to the 2017 ACC expert consensus decision pathway for optimization of heart failure treatment: Answers to 10 pivotal issues about heart failure with reduced ejection fraction. *Journal of the American College of Cardiology, 77*(6), 772–810. https://doi.org/10.1016/j.jacc.2020.11.022

Mentz, R. J., & O'Connor, C. M. (2016). Pathophysiology and clinical evaluation of acute heart failure. *Nature Reviews Cardiology, 13*(1), 28–35. https://doi.org/10.1038/nrcardio.2015.134

3.8: HYPERTENSION, HYPERTENSIVE EMERGENCIES AND URGENCIES

Monee' Carter-Griffin

Hypertension is a common disease affecting nearly half of adults in the United States with multiple long-term implications on cardiovascular (CV) health if left untreated (Centers for Disease Control and Prevention [CDC], 2020; Whelton et al., 2018). A potential complication of uncontrolled hypertension is hypertensive urgency or hypertensive emergency. Both hypertensive urgency and hypertensive emergency represent a systolic blood pressure and/or diastolic blood pressure greater than 180/120 mmHg (Whelton et al., 2018). The difference between hypertensive urgency and hypertensive emergency is evidence of acute targeted end-organ damage during a hypertensive emergency, whereas hypertensive urgency has no evidence of such damage (Whelton et al., 2018).

PRESENTING SIGNS AND SYMPTOMS

Often, patients with hypertension are asymptomatic and do not present with signs and symptoms unless their blood pressure is significantly elevated and/or they have prolonged uncontrolled hypertension resulting in targeted end-organ damage (Unger et al., 2020; Whelton et al., 2018).

Patients with hypertensive urgency will present asymptomatic, with severe blood pressure elevation, greater than 180/120 mmHg, but will not have evidence of acute targeted end-organ damage.

Patients with hypertensive emergency will present with signs and symptoms of acute end-organ damage, signs and symptoms of which will vary pending the underlying targeted end-organ damage and may include:

- Neurological end-organ damage: Hypertensive encephalopathy, intracerebral hemorrhage (ICH), and acute ischemic stroke. Neurological end-organ damage may present as confusion, severe headache, visual changes, facial droop, unilateral weakness, and seizures.
- Cardiovascular end-organ damage: Acute myocardial infarction (AMI), acute left ventricular (LV) failure with pulmonary edema, unstable angina pectoris, and dissecting aortic aneurysm. Cardiovascular end-organ damage may present with severe chest and/or upper back pain and shortness of breath (SOB) due to pulmonary edema.
- Renal end-organ damage: Acute renal failure.
- Retinal end-organ damage: Decrease in visual acuity.
- Generalized signs and symptoms such as dizziness, nausea, vomiting, pallor, and so forth may be present. Generalized signs and symptoms may be the result of targeted end-organ damage.

HISTORY AND PHYSICAL FINDINGS

History may include pre-existing hypertension (Box 3.2); however, patients may present with no known prior history of hypertension.

Hypertension

The AGACNP must assess for a history of modifiable (e.g., obesity, sedentary lifestyle, smoking, diabetes mellitus) and nonmodifiable (e.g., advanced age, family history, ethnicity/race) risk factors.

The AGACNP may need to assess for a history of renovascular disease, endocrine disorders (e.g., hyperthyroidism, pheochromocytoma, Cushing's syndrome), obstructive sleep apnea, illicit drug use, and current medications.

Hypertension Urgency and Emergency

The AGACNP must assess for onset and duration of symptoms and potential causes (e.g., nonadherence to antihypertensive medication management, lifestyle changes, illicit drug use or use of medications known to cause elevations in blood pressure).

Assess for a history of known disease states that can manifest as a hypertensive crisis and/or progress in the presence of a hypertensive crisis such as coronary artery disease (CAD), aortic aneurysm, heart failure (HF), prior cerebrovascular accident (CVA), and renal disease.

Other diseases to assess include a history of thyroid disease (e.g., hyperthyroidism), pheochromocytoma, and collagen-vascular diseases (e.g., systemic lupus erythematous).

BOX 3.2 HYPERTENSION STAGES

- Stage I hypertension: Systolic blood pressure of 130–139 mmHg AND/OR diastolic blood pressure of 80–89 mmHg.
- Stage II hypertension: Systolic blood pressure ≥140 mmHg AND/OR diastolic blood pressure ≥90 mmHg.

Physical Findings

Physical exam findings will vary pending the underlying targeted end-organ damage; however, patients presenting with hypertension or hypertensive urgency will not demonstrate *acute* targeted-end organ damage.

- Neurological: Changes in level of consciousness, weakness, cranial nerve deficits, and visual field changes.
- Retinal (eyes): Papilledema, retinal hemorrhages.
- Cardiovascular: Jugular venous distention, peripheral edema, extra heart tones (e.g., S3 heart sound), tachycardia, and asymmetric pulses and/or blood pressure.
- Pulmonary: Crackles and/or rales, tachypnea, and hypoxia.
- Nonspecific symptoms associated with hypertension, without acute targeted-end organ damage, include dizziness, tinnitus, epistaxis, and fatigue.

DIFFERENTIAL DIAGNOSIS AND DIAGNOSTIC CONSIDERATIONS

Differential Diagnoses

Other disease states can manifest and/or present as a hypertension/hypertensive crisis. These disease states include acute ischemic stroke, ICH, dissecting aortic aneurysm, thyrotoxicosis, renal artery stenosis, and pheochromocytoma.

Diagnostic Considerations

Routine diagnostics for patients presenting with hypertension or hypertensive urgency with no evidence of acute targeted end-organ damage include laboratory analysis: lipid panel, electrolytes, fasting blood glucose, urinalysis.

Hypertensive Emergency

Diagnostics may vary pending the patient's presentation and exam findings.

For patients presenting to the hospital with hypertensive emergency, laboratory analysis including complete blood count (CBC) and complete metabolic panel (CMP) should be completed as part of the initial assessment.

For patients presenting with neurological complaints and/or exam findings, a brain CT is warranted to assess for ICH or acute ischemic stroke.

For patients presenting with CV complaints and/or exam findings, an ECG, cardiac enzymes (e.g., troponin), transthoracic echocardiogram (TTE), and chest x-ray may be warranted. A CT-angiography thorax and/or abdomen may be warranted if there is a concern for acute aortic disease. Additional diagnostics such as a urinalysis, B-type natriuretic peptide (BNP) or NT-proBNP, and toxicology screen may be warranted pending the patient's history and presentation (Unger et al., 2020).

TREATMENT

Nonpharmacologic therapy including diet and exercise is recommended for patients with elevated blood pressure and/or diagnosed with Stage I or Stage II hypertension (Whelton et al., 2018).

Pharmacologic Considerations

Pharmacologic therapy is indicated for patients presenting with (Unger et al., 2020):

- Stage I hypertension and underlying CV disease OR Stage II hypertension with no history of CV disease.
- Primary or first-line oral anti-hypertensives include thiazide diuretics, calcium channel blockers, and angiotensin-converting enzyme (ACE) inhibitors or angiotensive receptor blockers (ARBs).
- For patients requiring more than one oral anthypertensive for blood pressure control, two first-line oral antihypertensives are recommended. Medications from the same drug class should not be prescribed. hypertensive for blood pressure control, two first-line oral anti-hypertensives are recommended. Medications from the same drug class should not be prescribed.
- Secondary oral antihypertensives include loop diuretics, aldosterone antagonists, beta-blockers, alpha-1 blockers, central alpha$_2$ agonist, and direct vasodilators.
- For patients with hypertension and comorbid conditions such as HF, guidelines recommend prescribing according to goal directed medical therapy.

Patients with hypertensive urgency and who are otherwise stable with no acute evidence of targeted end-organ damage can be started on or resume oral anti hypertensive therapy. If the patient is currently on oral antihypertensive medications, therapy should be intensified. Rapid-acting antihypertensive medications such as clonidine and captopril can be administered. The patient should receive an antihypertensive in the presence of a healthcare provider and monitored to ensure blood pressure is improving. Outpatient treatment is recommended for patients with hypertensive urgency.

Patients with hypertensive emergency require ICU admission and initiation on IV antihypertensive therapy. Blood pressure should be reduced no more than 25% over the first hour, then to 160/100 mmHg over the next 2 to 6 hours, then to normal over the next 24 to 48 hours. Based on the disease state, there may be a preferred drug for lowering blood pressure(Peixoto, 2019):

- Aortic dissection: esmolol, labetalol
- Acute pulmonary edema: clevidipine, nitroglycerin, and nitroprusside
- Acute coronary syndrome (ACS): esmolol, labetalol, nicardipine, and nitroglycerin
- Acute renal failure: clevidipine, fenoldopam, and nicardipine
- Catecholamine excess states: clevidipine, nicardipine, and phentolamine
- Acute ischemic stroke: labetalol, clevidipine, and nicardipine

- Acute ICH: labetalol, clevidipine, and nicardipine
- Dihydropyridine calcium channel blocker
  - Nicardipine initial dose of 5 mg/h with a maximum dose of 15 mg/h.
  - Clevidipine initial dose of 1 to 2 mg/h with a maximum dose of 32 mg/h.
- Vasodilators
  - Sodium nitroprusside initial dose of 0.3 to 0.5 mcg/kg/min with a maximum dose of 10 mcg/kg/min.
  - Nitroglycerin initial dose of 5 mcg/min with a maximum dose of 20 mcg/min.
  - Hydralazine initial 10 mg IV push with a maximum initial dose of 20 mg. Can repeat every 4 to 6 h.
- Adrenergic blockers
  - Esmolol loading dose of 500 to 1000 mcg/kg/min, followed by 50 mcg/kg/min with a maximum dose of 200 mcg/kg/min.
  - Labetalol initial dose of 0.3 to 1.0 mg/kg IV push (maximum 20 mg) or 0.4 to 1.0 mg/kg/h with a maximum cumulative dose of 300 mg.
  - Phentolamine initial dose of 5 mg IV push with bolus doses every 10 min for target blood pressure control.
- Dopamine receptor selective agonist
  - Fenoldopam initial dose of 0.1 to 0.3 mcg/kg/min with a maximum dose of 1.6 mcg/kg/min.
- ACE Inhibitor
  - Enalaprilat initial dose of 1.25 mg with a maximum dose of 5 mg. Can repeat every 6 hours.

Adjunctive Therapy

Patients with hypertension or hypertensive urgency do not require additional therapy. Patients experiencing hypertensive emergency will require continuous cardiac monitoring and may require intra-arterial blood pressure monitoring while on IV antihypertensive therapy. Patients may also require additional interventions pending the underlying targeted end-organ damage including cardiac catheterization for acute myocardial infarction (MI), or tissue plasminogen activator (tPA) for acute ischemic stroke (Peixoto, 2019).

TRANSITION OF CARE

Patients with hypertension and hypertensive urgency can be managed in the outpatient setting with follow-up after resuming or intensifying antihypertensive therapy.

Patients with hypertensive emergency can be transitioned to oral antihypertensive therapy once the goal blood pressure is achieved.

CLINICAL PEARLS

- Patients with hypertensive urgency managed in the outpatient setting should follow up with their provider within 24 to 72 hours following the initiation, intensification, or resumption of medication therapy.
- Consider the pharmacokinetics and adverse effects of the antihypertensive drug prior to prescribing, especially with underlying comorbid conditions (e.g., HF, aortic stenosis [AS]).

- The choice of oral antihypertensive therapy to start, intensify, and/or transition may vary pending the race of the patient (e.g., African Americans initial antihypertensive treatment should include thiazide diuretic or calcium channel blocker [CCB]).
- Certain disease states such as aortic dissection and acute ischemic stroke require blood pressure reductions outside of the parameters listed within this section.

KEY TAKEAWAYS

- Hypertensive urgency is a systolic and/or diastolic blood pressure greater than 180/120 mmHg *with no* acute evidence of targeted end-organ damage.
- Hypertensive urgency is treated with oral antihypertensive therapy in the outpatient setting.
- Hypertensive emergency is a systolic and/or diastolic blood pressure greater than 180/120 mmHg *with* evidence of targeted end-organ damage.
- Hypertensive emergency requires hospitalization and prompt blood pressure management with IV antihypertensive therapy to prevent and/or reduce further end-organ damage.

EVIDENCE-BASED RESOURCES

2017 ACC/AHA/AAPA/ABC/ACPM/AGS/APhA/ASH/ASPC/NMA/PCNA Guideline for the Prevention, Detection, Evaluation, and Management of High Blood Pressure in Adults.

3.9: STRUCTURAL HEART DEFECTS: ACQUIRED AND CONGENITAL

Vanessa M. Kalis

Structural heart disease can encompass a wide range of diagnoses. Specific topics covered in this section include atrial septal defect (ASD), ventricular septal defect (VSD), patent ductus arteriosus, hypertrophic cardiomyopathy, and arrhythmogenic right ventricular cardiomyopathy (ARVC). Many patients with these defects will need long-term follow-up for continued monitoring at specialized centers.

ATRIAL SEPTAL DEFECT

An ASD is a communication between the right and left atrium. It is estimated that 7% of all congenital heart disease are ASDs (Akagi, 2015). The shunting of blood from the left atrium (LA) to the right atrium (RA) causes right-sided heart enlargement and right ventricular (RV) dysfunction over time (Oster et al., 2018). Long term, this can also lead to paradoxical embolisms or atrial arrhythmias (Stout et al., 2018). In addition, some patients will develop pulmonary arterial hypertension (PAH), evidenced by right to left shunting of blood across the atrium due to high pulmonary pressures (Oster et al., 2018). While ASDs can occur in conjunction with other congenital heart anomalies, they can also occur in isolation (Stout et al., 2018).

PRESENTING SIGNS AND SYMPTOMS/ HISTORY AND PHYSICAL FINDINGS

Patients with ASDs can remain asymptomatic for some time, depending on the size of the defect. When patients present with symptoms, they can have shortness of breath (SOB), fatigue, atrial dysrhythmias, and/or right-sided heart failure (HF). Some patients also present with supraventricular arrhythmias such as atrial fibrillation or atrial flutter (Stout et al., 2018). Patients with ASDs can be diagnosed due to a murmur noted on physical examination. Auscultation can reveal a fixed, split-second heart sound (S2) without respiratory variation and a systolic murmur in the pulmonary area. In an adult, there may be pulmonary hypertension due to longstanding increased left to right blood flow with concomitant dilation of the RA, right ventricle (RV), and pulmonary artery (Stout et al., 2018).

DIFFERENTIAL DIAGNOSIS AND DIAGNOSTIC CONSIDERATIONS

Differentials for patients presenting with a murmur and signs of right-sided HF include cardiomyopathy, other valve abnormalities such as pulmonary stenosis and aortic stenosis (AS), or other congenital heart defects including a ventricular septal defect (VSD), tetralogy of Fallot, or atrioventricular canal. Diagnostic testing can include an ECG, chest radiograph, and echocardiography. An ECG may show atrial arrhythmias and signs of RV overload and a chest radiograph may reveal enlargement of the pulmonary arteries and cardiomegaly. An echocardiogram demonstrates the type of ASD and the direction of blood flow (Stout et al., 2018).

TREATMENT

Treatment for an ASD will depend on the size of the defect and age at diagnosis (Stout et al., 2018). Treatment of ASDs often involves closure of the defect, which can be done surgically for all types of ASDs or percutaneously for secundum ASDs. In adults with secundum ASDs, a device closure is often done through a transcatheter approach unless other surgical procedures are required (such as other concomitant heart defects that need to be repaired or during another open-heart surgery such as a coronary artery bypass grafting [CABG]). Cardiac catheterization with a transesophageal echocardiogram is done at the time of percutaneous device closure to measure hemodynamics, including pulmonary artery pressures and shunt magnitude (Stout et al., 2018). There are times when the decision is made not to close the ASD due to the small size of the shunt or due to the development of pulmonary

hypertension with right to left shunting seen in the atrium. Severe PAH is a contraindication to closure of the ASD. Patients do report improvement in their symptoms after ASD closure (Akagi, 2015). Long-term outcomes are better in those patients who undergo ASD closure (Stout et al., 2018).

VENTRICULAR SEPTAL DEFECTS

VSDs are the most common congenital heart disease at birth, but many small VSDs will close spontaneously over time. Small defects commonly close during infancy. The determinants of symptoms as well as long-term consequences include size of the defect, pulmonary vascular resistance, and function of the ventricles.

PRESENTING SIGNS AND SYMPTOMS/ HISTORY AND PHYSICAL FINDINGS

Adults presenting with undiagnosed VSDs can present without any symptoms, but with a holosystolic murmur heard on auscultation. These are often what are termed restrictive VSDs, which are small. For patients with larger VSDs, they can present with dyspnea, exercise intolerance, and cyanosis. In addition, sometimes the VSD can be found when patients present with infectious endocarditis (IE; Stout et al., 2018). Patients with larger VSDs will have progressive PAH which and can have LV overload with significant aortic valve regurgitation, which is heard as an early diastolic murmur, or tricuspid valve regurgitation, which has a holosystolic murmur. A prominent RV impulse is present, and assessment of the jugular venous pressures shows a prominent "a" wave.

DIFFERENTIAL DIAGNOSIS AND DIAGNOSTIC CONSIDERATIONS

An ECG can show biventricular hypertrophy and a chest radiograph may show increased pulmonary vascular markings in patients with large VSDs. Echocardiography will show the defect and can assess the location of the defect(s), chamber sizes, ventricular function, and severity of LV volume overload. Many asymptomatic patients will have small VSDs with small left to right shunting and no LV volume overload or PAH on echocardiogram (Stout et al., 2018). Patients with moderate-sized VSDs will have mild to moderate LV volume overload and mild or no PAH. Large VSDs cause LV volume overload and PAH (Maagaard et al., 2018).

TREATMENT

Treatment of patients with VSDs varies based on the size of the defect. Small, restrictive VSDs can be monitored over time without intervention (Stout et al., 2018). Patients who have moderate to large VSDs can be treated with VSD closure via surgery or a transcatheter approach when there is only mild to moderate pulmonary hypertension (Stout et al., 2018). Patients with large, nonrestrictive VSDs that have not been treated will be cyanotic due to pulmonary hypertension should be treated with pulmonary vasodilator therapy (Stout et al., 2018).

PATENT DUCTUS ARTERIOSUS

A patent ductus arteriosus is a connection between the aorta and pulmonary artery that is normally present in a fetus and usually closes shortly after birth. However, sometimes this connection does not close and persists (Stout et al., 2018).

PRESENTING SIGNS AND SYMPTOMS/HISTORY AND PHYSICAL FINDINGS

As with other congenital heart defects, the clinical manifestations depend on the PDA size as well as systemic and vascular resistances. Patients with small PDAs will often go undetected as they will not have any symptoms and their exam will be normal. Patients with moderate to large PDAs can present with exercise intolerance as the amount of blood shunting causes LV dilation and dysfunction (Stout et al., 2018). Over time, this can cause increased pulmonary pressures and PAH. Patients with PDAs can have a continuous murmur peaking in late systole upon auscultation. Patients with moderate or large PDAs can present with dyspnea, palpitations from atrial arrhythmias, and cyanosis.

DIFFERENTIAL DIAGNOSIS AND DIAGNOSTIC CONSIDERATIONS

Differential diagnoses of patients with dyspnea and palpitations are numerous. Diagnosis of a PDA can be made through an echocardiogram as the PDA can be identified, the volume of shunting can be documented, and measurements of pulmonary pressures can be taken. In addition, pulse oximetry can be used to assess for the presence of right to left shunting by measuring oxygen saturation in the feet and both hands.

TREATMENT

For adults with a patent ductus arteriosus, treatment options include catheter based or surgical intervention. PDA closure is indicated if there is left-sided enlargement (left atrium or left ventricle) with PA pressures less than half systemic pressure with PVR less than one-third systemic. Closure of the PDA can prevent further progression of pulmonary artery hypertension.

ARRHYTHMOGENIC RIGHT VENTRICULAR CARDIOMYOPATHY

ARVC is an inherited disorder characterized by replacement of the myocardium with fibrous or fibrofatty tissue, resulting initially in regional wall abnormalities and progressing to global RV dilation and thinning of the walls. This results in ventricular arrhythmias that originate from the RV (Elliott et al., 2019).

PRESENTING SIGNS AND SYMPTOMS/HISTORY AND PHYSICAL FINDINGS

Patients with ARVC can remain asymptomatic for years. Symptoms can include palpitations, syncope, atypical chest pain, dyspnea, HF, and even cardiac arrest. Many patients present with palpitations given the abnormal RV myocardium resulting in ventricular dysrhythmias. However, some patients suffer a cardiac arrest as their first presentation of the disease (Corrado et al., 2020). Many patients with ARVC can present with ventricular arrythmias. The ventricular arrhythmias can range from isolated premature ventricular contractions (PVCs) to sustained VT or even ventricular fibrillation and cardiac arrest (Corrado et al., 2020).

DIFFERENTIAL DIAGNOSIS AND DIAGNOSTIC CONSIDERATIONS

Patients who present with palpitations, chest pain, and syncope can have a variety of diagnoses. When an echocardiogram is done showing decreased function of the RV, the differential diagnosis should include cardiac sarcoidosis, Brugada syndrome, congenital heart diseases such as Ebstein's anomaly, and PAH. Initial evaluation should include an echocardiogram showing regional wall abnormalities and a cardiac MRI is recommended for definitive diagnosis and better characterization of the disease. Common findings on 12-lead ECG can include negative T waves in the right precordial leads, low QRS voltages in the limb leads, and/or a right bundle branch block (Corrado et al., 2020). Endometrial biopsy (EMB) is indicated for patients whose final diagnosis depends on histologic exclusion of other potential diagnoses such as sarcoidosis. Genetic testing is indicated to help identify a pathogenic mutation in patients who fit the diagnostic criteria for ARVC to help detect carriers among family members (Corrado et al., 2020).

TREATMENT

The goal of treatment for ARVC is to prevent ventricular dysrhythmias and improve HF symptoms. Patients are typically treated with beta-blockers or amiodarone for the dysrhythmias and considered for an implantable cardioverter-defibrillator. Patients are usually given exercise restrictions, especially with competitive sports. Finally, patients who have refractory arrhythmias or HF can be considered for heart transplantation (Corrado et al., 2020).

KEY TAKEAWAYS

■ Patients with congenital heart disease need long-term follow-up, even after closure of septal defects and should be seen by a specialized center.

■ For patients with regional wall abnormalities seen on echocardiogram, consider structural heart abnormalities such as hypertrophic cardiomyopathy and ARVC.

3.10: SYNCOPE

Monee' Carter-Griffin

Syncope is "a symptom resulting in abrupt, complete loss of consciousness, with the inability to maintain postural tone, with rapid and spontaneous recovery" (Shen et al., 2017, p. e46). Syncope is presumed to result from transient cerebral hypoperfusion and should not be associated with other clinical features of nonsyncope causes (e.g., seizures; Moya & Fumero, 2020; Shen et al., 2017). Syncope is divided into two categories: cardiac and noncardiac. Cardiac syncope is the result of cardiac disease, whereas noncardiac syncope is the result of reflex (neurally mediated) syncope or orthostatic hypotension-induced syncope (Williford & Olshansky, 2020).

PRESENTING SIGNS AND SYMPTOMS

Patients will present with a transient loss of consciousness. Signs and symptoms consistent with a transient loss of consciousness include:

■ Amnesia: Inability to remember events during the syncopal episode
■ Loss of responsiveness
■ Short duration: Defined as 5 minutes or less
■ Self-limited: Spontaneous recovery with no required medical intervention
■ Abnormal motor control resulting in falls and/or loss of muscle tone or an increase in muscle tone

Depending on the etiology, cardiac versus noncardiac, of the syncopal episode, patients may report other symptoms such as abdominal pain, chest pain, diaphoresis, dizziness, double vision, fatigue, headache, nausea with/without vomiting, pallor, or palpitations. Patients may report lightheadedness, "tunnel vision," and altered consciousness with the complete loss of consciousness prior to the syncopal episode (Shen et al., 2017, p. e46). These symptoms are commonly referred to as presyncope (near-syncope).

HISTORY AND PHYSICAL FINDINGS

History

The history should focus on the following (Shen et al., 2017):

■ Preceding circumstances (e.g., physical activity, meals, standing to sitting)
■ Presence of a prodrome (symptoms prior to the syncopal episode) or postdrome (symptoms after the syncopal episode)

■ Events during the syncopal episode (e.g., color, any noted movements)
■ Duration of the syncopal episode
■ Past medical history, especially history of heart disease (ischemic heart disease, heart failure [HF], structural heart disease, and/or prior arrhythmias)
■ Family history, especially history of syncope and/or sudden cardiac death (SCD)
■ Current prescriptions and over-the-counter medications

Bystanders present during the event are important for obtaining a thorough history as the patient is unaware of the syncopal event (Shen et al., 2017).

Physical Exam

The patient should receive a detailed cardiovascular and neurological exam.

Pending the etiology of the syncopal episode, physical exam findings will vary and may include blood pressure and/or heart rate changes from lying to sitting, bradyarrhythmias, tachyarrhythmias, long pauses between heart beats, murmurs, and gallops. The patient may present with no abnormal physical exam findings or findings outside of their baseline.

The AGACNP must assess for traumatic injuries such as bruises, abrasions, and so forth due to falling and loss of muscle tone during the syncopal episode.

DIFFERENTIAL DIAGNOSIS AND DIAGNOSTIC CONSIDERATIONS

Differential Diagnoses

Differential diagnoses potentially manifesting as syncope are:

■ Acute aortic dissection
■ Arrhythmias (e.g., third-degree atrioventricular heart block, atrial fibrillation, prolong QT syndrome, paroxysmal VT, sick sinus syndrome)
■ Dehydration
■ Hypoglycemia
■ Hypoxemia
■ Medication toxicities (e.g., calcium channel blocker, BB)
■ Myocardial infarction
■ Narcolepsy
■ Pulmonary embolism
■ Seizure disorders
■ Valvular heart disease (VHD)

Syncope is a usually a symptom due to an underlying etiology. The AGACNP must complete a thorough workup to identify the etiology.

Diagnostic Considerations

Diagnostic evaluation is highly dependent on the suspected etiology for syncope (Shen et al., 2017).

■ A 12-lead ECG should be a part of the initial evaluation for all patients with syncope.

- A risk assessment evaluating for short- and long-term morbidity and mortality risk is recommended.
  - Risks include male sex, greater than 60 years of age, no prodrome, history of heart disease, family history of SCD, palpitations prior to loss of consciousness, cerebrovascular disease, abnormal ECG, and high CHADS-2 score.
- Common blood tests are:
  - Electrolytes
  - Complete blood count
  - Glucose
  - Biomarkers such as troponin and NT-proBNP
- Transthoracic echocardiography (TTE) may be warranted in patients with suspected structural heart disease.
- An electrophysiological (EP) study may be warranted in patients with suspected arrhythmias.
- Stress testing if an ischemic etiology is possible.
- Cardiac CT and/or MRI.
  - Should be ordered if a cardiac etiology is suspected based on the history, physical exam, and/or ECG.
- Cardiac monitoring (e.g., Holter monitor and external loop recorder) can be used to evaluate patients in the ambulatory setting with suspected arrhythmias.
- Tilt-table testing may be warranted in patients with suspected noncardiac syncope, specifically vasovagal and orthostatic hypotension syncope.
- If a suspected neurological etiology, simultaneous electroencephalogram (EEG) and hemodynamic evaluation during tilt-testing may be warranted and useful to differentiate syncope from seizures.
- Routine neurological evaluation (e.g., MRI and/or CT head, carotid artery imaging, and EEG) is not recommended in the absence of focal neurological findings.

TREATMENT

Treatment is largely dependent on the etiology of syncope.

Cardiac Syncope

- Arrhythmias (Shen et al., 2017)
  - Goal directed medical therapy is recommended for patients with syncope due to bradyarrhythmias, supraventricular tachycardia (SVT), atrial fibrillation, and ventricular arrhythmias.
  - Beta-blocker therapy is indicated as first-line therapy for patients with long QT syndrome and syncope.
  - An implantable cardioverter defibrillator (ICD) may be considered in patients with Brugada syndrome, short QT syndrome, and long QT syndrome plus syncope.
  - For catecholamine-associated arrhythmias, exercise restriction and medication management with a beta-blocker are recommended.
- Structural heart disease (Shen et al., 2017)
  - Goal directed medical therapy is recommended for patients with VHD, with hypertrophic cardiomyopathy, ischemic cardiomyopathy, and nonischemic cardiomyopathy.

- An implantable cardioverter-defibrillator (ICD) is recommended for patients with right ventricular cardiomyopathy with associated arrhythmias and syncope.

Noncardiac Syncope

- Reflex syncope (Shen et al., 2017)
  - Vasovagal syncope
    - Education on diagnosis and prognosis is recommended.
    - Physical countermaneuvers (e.g., leg crossing) may be useful.
    - Fluid and salt intake may be appropriate pending no contraindications.
    - If recurrent vasovagal syncope, medication management with midodrine, fludrocortisone, a beta-blocker, and selected serotonin reuptake inhibitors (SSRIs) may be appropriate pending no contraindications.
    - A dual-chamber pacemaker may be reasonable in patients 40 years and older, with recurrent vasovagal syncope and prolonged spontaneous pauses.
  - Carotid sinus syndrome (Shen et al., 2017)
    - Cardiac pacing may be warranted in patients with associated pauses, atrioventricular (AV) block, or a 50 mmHg or more drop in the systolic blood pressure during carotid massage.
- Orthostatic hypotension (Shen et al., 2017)
  - If neurogenic, acute water ingestion, counter-pressure maneuvers, midodrine, fludrocortisone, salt and fluid intake, and octreotide may be reasonable pending no contraindications.
  - If drug-induced, removal or reducing the dosage may be warranted.
  - If dehydration, acute water ingestion or IV fluid administration pending the degree of dehydration is recommended.

TRANSITION OF CARE

Patients identified as low risk with an initial clear evaluation do not require further evaluation and/or hospitalization. Patients with an unclear evaluation and/or serious medical conditions may require ongoing observation or hospitalization. Patients can be discharged from observation or the hospital pending the etiology and treatment for syncope.

CLINICAL PEARLS

- Presyncope may progress to syncope or could terminate with no syncopal episode (Shen et al., 2017, p. e46).
- Certain characteristics (e.g., older age, male sex, and underlying heart disease) are more commonly associated with a cardiac etiology of syncope (Shen et al., 2017, p. e46).

- It is important for the provider to use the history and physical exam findings to differentiate between syncope and nonsyncope causes.
- Patients should have a normal baseline mental status following a syncopal episode. Altered mental status, abnormal behavior, confusion, lethargy, and/or somnolence should not be attributed to syncope and further investigated for other nonsyncope-related causes (Morag & Brenner, 2017).
- A syncope workup may reveal an undetermined etiology and is a common problem during syncope evaluation.

KEY TAKEAWAYS

- Syncope can be the result of multiple causes, diagnoses, and/or mechanisms.
- The transient loss of consciousness experienced in syncope should not be associated with trauma or other nonsyncopal causes such as a seizure or intoxication (Moya & Fumero, 2020).
- The primary goal for syncope evaluation is identifying a cause, determining the possibility of recurrence, and assessing the risk of adverse outcomes.

EVIDENCE-BASED RESOURCES

Brignole, M., & Benditt, D. G. (Eds.). (2020). *Syncope: An evidenced-based approach*. Springer Publishing Company.

Shen, W. K., Sheldon, R. S., Benditt, D. G., Cohen, M. I., Forman, D. E., Goldberger, Z. D., Grubb, B. P., Hamdan, M. H., Krahn, A. D., Link, M. S., Olshansky, B., Raj, S. R., Sandhu, R. K., Sorajja, D., Sun, B. C., & Yancy, C. W. (2017). 2017 ACC/AHA/HRS guideline for the evaluation and management of patients with syncope. *Journal of the American College of Cardiology, 70*, e39–e110. https://doi.org/10.1016/j.jacc.2017.03.003

3.11: TACHYARRHYTHMIAS AND CARDIAC RHYTHM DISTURBANCES

Vanessa M. Kalis

This section discusses common cardiac dysrhythmias including atrioventricular (AV) nodal reentrant tachycardia (AVNRT), AV reciprocating tachycardia (AVRT), atrial tachycardia, atrial flutter, atrial fibrillation, conduction defects, and ventricular tachycardia (VT). Common presenting clinical manifestations are reviewed as well as findings on ECG and treatment of each dysrhythmia.

SUPRAVENTRICULAR DYSRHYTHMIAS

Supraventricular dysrhythmias (SVTs) include all tachyarrhythmias that originate from or incorporate tissue above the AV node (Page et al., 2016). Types of SVT that

are discussed in this section include AVNRT, AVRT, and atrial tachycardia, atrial flutter, and atrial fibrillation. AVNRT is more common in women and is usually seen in individuals over age 30, while AVRT is seen more commonly in younger individuals (Page et al., 2016). AVNRT is a reentrant rhythm that has two distinct pathways that creates a "circuit" with repeat activation (Page et al., 2016) and the tachycardia is contained in the AV node. In AVRT, the electrical connection includes the atrium, a second accessory pathway, and the ventricle (Page et al., 2016). In both AVNRT and AVRT, the p waves are usually not well seen.

Atrial tachycardia represents about 10% of SVTs and has increased incidence with age and in patients with structural heart disease. In atrial tachycardia, the dysrhythmia originates from an area in the atrium outside the sinus node. This results in a different p wave morphology seen on ECG. Atrial tachycardia can be unifocal (coming from one site) or multifocal (arising from multiple areas within the atrium). The exact cause of atrial tachycardia is not known but is more frequently seen in patients with coronary artery disease (CAD), valvular heart disease (VHD), congenital heart disease, and cardiomyopathies (Page et al., 2016). The p waves are seen in atrial tachycardia and are distinctly different than sinus p waves in morphology.

Atrial flutter is an atrial dysrhythmia with a large reentrant circuit and the ECG is characterized by regular repetitive flutter waves and constant p-wave morphology (Page et al., 2016). The atrial rate is usually between 250 and 350 beats per minute. Typical atrial flutter has negative sawtooth flutter waves in ECG leads II, III, and aVF (Page et al., 2016). However, up to half of the patients who have atrial flutter will later have atrial fibrillation (Page et al., 2016).

Atrial fibrillation is a rhythm disorder characterized by chaotic electrical activity in the atrium without a discernable atrial rate and variable ventricular rate (January et al., 2014). It is the most common dysrhythmia in the world that increases in prevalence as people age (January et al., 2014). It is often associated with structural heart disease and other chronic conditions and has significant morbidity and mortality related to frequent hospitalizations, hemodynamic alterations, and thromboembolic events (January et al., 2014).

PRESENTING SIGNS AND SYMPTOMS/ HISTORY AND PHYSICAL FINDINGS

While some patients with atrial dysrhythmias can be asymptomatic, patients with SVT can present with palpitations, dizziness, shortness of breath (SOB), dizziness, near syncope, syncope, chest pain, and/or fatigue. Some patients can even present with cardiomyopathy and heart failure (HF; Page et al., 2016). Patients with SVT can report intermittent tachycardia, increasing in frequency and/or duration over time. Others present for evaluation with the tachycardia. Exam findings may be normal for patients with a history of tachycardia. Those with higher heart rates may be symptomatic, with abnormal blood pressures (low or high depending on their level of compensation). Exam findings can include a regular or irregular pulse, variations in heart sounds and possible irregular jugular venous pulsations, depending on the type of atrial dysrhythmia (January et al., 2014).

DIFFERENTIAL DIAGNOSIS AND DIAGNOSTIC CONSIDERATIONS

For patients reporting symptoms concerning for a tachycardia, differential diagnoses include rhythm disturbances such as an SVT, ventricular dysrhythmias, as well as sinus tachycardia due to another cause, including infection and sepsis, hyperthyroidism, electrolyte abnormalities, and more. For patients who present with ongoing tachycardia, a 12-lead ECG can confirm the diagnosis. Other diagnostic testing can include ambulatory monitoring for patients who report symptoms concerning for SVT but have normal resting 12-lead ECGs. Diagnostic testing also includes an echocardiogram to assess cardiac structures and document cardiac function. For patients with atrial fibrillation, stress testing should be done to rule out cardiac ischemia.

TREATMENT

Treatment for all SVTs can be divided into acute and long-term treatment. Immediate treatment of AVNRT, AVRT, and atrial tachycardia can include synchronized cardioversion if unstable (Page et al., 2016). For patients who are stable, vagal maneuvers can slow the heart rate and sometimes convert the patient back to sinus rhythm. Adenosine can be given as it can help diagnose the dysrhythmia and sometimes even terminate the tachycardia (Page et al., 2016). Beta-blockers and calcium channel blockers can be given intravenously to help slow the ventricular rate (Page et al., 2016). Immediate treatment for atrial fibrillation will depend on symptoms and estimated episode duration. Patients who present with a duration of symptoms less than 24 to 48 hours can undergo synchronized cardioversion to convert them back to sinus rhythm. For patients with an unknown duration of atrial fibrillation and significant symptoms, a transesophageal echocardiogram is done to rule out any thrombus in the atrial appendage or atrium prior to cardioversion (January et al., 2019). Patients with atrial fibrillation often need anticoagulation (Amerena & Ridley, 2017). A CHA2DS2-VASc risk score should be determined (1 point each for HF, hypertension, age 65 to 74, diabetes, vascular disease, and female, and 2 points for age >75 or history of stroke/TIA/thromboembolism) and a score of 3 or higher indicates oral anticoagulation should be initiated (Heidenreich et al., 2020).

Long-term treatment for SVT includes medications and catheter ablation (Page et al., 2016). Beta-blockers and calcium channel blockers can be prescribed to help slow the heart rate during SVT episodes (Page et al., 2016). However, rate control medications such as beta-blockers and calcium channel blockers are not highly effective at controlling the heart rate in atrial flutter (Page et al., 2016). More aggressive therapy includes antiarrhythmic medications which are designed to restore and maintain sinus rhythm, thereby minimizing patient symptoms. The choice of antiarrhythmic medication is based on patient and provider choice. Options include flecainide, propafenone, dofetilide, sotalol, and amiodarone (Page et al., 2016). These medications require close monitoring for side effects including prolongation of the QT interval.

Another treatment for SVT is an electrophysiologic study and catheter ablation. This procedure involves placing catheters inside the heart, locating the specific electrical mechanism for the SVT, and eliminating it by either heat (radiofrequency) or cooling (cryo) ablation. This procedure can be curative. For patients with AVNRT, catheter ablation has a greater than 95% success rate with less than 1% risk of AV block (Page et al., 2016). For AVRT, cardiac ablation is successful 93% to 95% of the time with about a 3% risk of major complications (Page et al., 2016). Atrial tachycardia ablation is reported to have success rates between 90% and 95% with a complication rate of less than 1% to 2% (Page et al., 2016). Catheter ablation is also the gold standard for therapy for typical atrial flutter as the procedure is around 90% successful (Herzog et al., 2017; Page et al., 2016).

Long-term therapy for atrial fibrillation also includes catheter ablation as well as AV node ablation and pacemaker implantation. Atrial fibrillation ablation success rates are not as high as seen with other types of SVT (El-Harasis et al., 2019). Metanalysis from randomized trials shows freedom from recurrent atrial fibrillation occurance is around 60% and many patients require more than one ablation procedure and the periprocedural complication rate is approximately 5% (Willems et al., 2019). Finally, an AV node ablation and pacemaker implantation can control the ventricular heart rate and improve patient symptoms (January et al., 2014). This option is typically done for elderly patients as the procedure results in pacemaker dependency (January et al., 2014).

CONDUCTION DEFECTS

An interruption or delay in conduction of electrical impulses between the atria and ventricles is called atrioventricular block (AVB). This is classified based on the site of block and severity of conduction abnormality. This includes first-degree AVB, second-degree Mobitz Type I AVB, second-degree Mobitz Type II AVB and third degree AVB. Patients with first degree AVB will have a long PR interval, measuring over 200 milliseconds. This represents a delay in the conduction in the AV node. The prolonged PR interval is constant, and many patients are asymptomatic. Patients with second degree Mobitz Type I AVB have a successive prolonged delay in impulses from the previous impulse resulting in a prolonged PR interval that continues to lengthen in duration until the QRS is dropped (the impulse does not reach the ventricle). This is often seen in active, healthy patients and is usually asymptomatic (Kusumoto et al., 2019). Patients with second degree Mobitz Type II AVB have impulses from the SA node that fail to conduct to the ventricles. The PR interval is constant but then suddenly there is a dropped QRS complex. While less common, this AVB is more serious as it is a precursor to complete heart block, or third degree AVB. Complete heart block, also called third degree heart block, is characterized by absence of electrical impulse conduction from the atria to the ventricle. Instead, the atrial signals do not conduct to the ventricles. If the heart block occurs at the AV node, the ventricular rate will be 40 to 60 beats per minute. If the conduction block occurs at the bundle branches, the ventricular rate will be under 40 beats per minute.

PRESENTING SIGNS AND SYMPTOMS/HISTORY AND PHYSICAL FINDINGS

Symptoms for AV block can vary from asymptomatic to syncope. Patients with first degree AVB and those with second degree Type Mobitz I AVB will often be asymptomatic. However, patients with second degree Mobitz II AVB can present with lightheadedness, fatigue, and hypotension. Patients with third degree AVB usually present with chest pain, dizziness, fatigue, and syncope.

DIFFERENTIAL DIAGNOSIS AND DIAGNOSTIC CONSIDERATIONS

Differential diagnosis for patients with symptoms such as lightheadedness, hypotension, chest pain, and syncope are varied. However, a 12-lead ECG can document conduction abnormalities. Patients with conduction disorders should also be screened and treated for sleep apnea if applicable as it can eliminate the need for pacemaker implantation in many patients (Kusumoto et al., 2019). Other potential transient or reversible causes of AVB include digoxin toxicity, overdoses of antiarrhythmic medications, and Lyme carditis (Kusumoto et al., 2019).

TREATMENT

Patients with conduction defects do not necessarily need treatment. Treatment of reversible causes of AVB is indicated. For patients with first degree AVB or second degree Mobitz Type I AVB, no treatment is necessary. In hemodynamically significant AVB, atropine can be given to enhance AV conduction and temporary transvenous pacing is reasonable (Kusumoto et al., 2019). However, patients with second degree Mobitz Type II and third degree AVB should undergo permanent pacemaker implantation to restore normal AV conduction regardless of symptoms (Kusumoto et al., 2019).

VENTRICULAR DYSRHYTHMIAS

Ventricular dysrhythmias range from a single premature ventricular contraction (PVC) to ventricular fibrillation, that is, a cardiac arrest (Al-Khatib et al., 2018). PVCs are common in the general population (Al-Khatib et al., 2018). VT is defined as a ventricular rate greater than 100 beats per minute with three more PVCs in a row (Al-Khatib et al., 2018). During VT, the atrial rate cannot be determined as the p wave is usually absent or dissociated. The QRS is wide, and the rate is usually between 100 and 250 beats per minute. VT can be sustained or nonsustained and can be monomorphic (QRS complexes are the same) or polymorphic (QRS complexes vary in configuration). VT most often occurs in patients with ischemic or structural heart disease and is a consequence of that disease (Al-Khatib et al., 2018).

PRESENTING SIGNS AND SYMPTOMS/HISTORY AND PHYSICAL FINDINGS

Patients with VT can present with palpitations, dizziness, chest pain, syncope, or even cardiac arrest. The clinical presentation depends on the heart rate, ventricular function, and the presence/absence of cardiac drugs. History should include known heart disease, precipitating factors such as exercise and emotional stress, risk factors for heart disease, current medications, and alcohol or illicit drug use (Al-Khatib et al., 2018). Family history should also be included, especially history of SCD (Al-Khatib et al., 2018). Exam findings can include murmurs, jugular vein distention (JVD), abnormal pulses, edema, and abnormal blood pressure (Al-Khatib et al., 2018).

DIFFERENTIAL DIAGNOSIS AND DIAGNOSTIC CONSIDERATIONS

Patients who present with palpitations, dizziness, chest pain, and syncope may have an arrhythmia. Patients with sustained VT should have a 12-lead ECG done while in the tachycardia (Al-Khatib et al., 2018). Patients with newly diagnosed VT need to be screened for ischemic heart disease. For those with known heart disease, the dysrhythmia can occur due to permanent damage within the myocardium. However, other causes need to be assessed including use of sympathomimetic agents such as inotropes or illicit drugs, systemic diseases that affect the myocardium such as sarcoidosis, and other congenital disorders such as tetralogy of Fallot and ARVC. Labs should also be ordered including chemistry panel, toxicology screening, and cardiac enzymes. An echocardiogram should be done to assess ventricular function and rule out structural heart abnormalities (Al-Khatib et al., 2018).

TREATMENT

Acute treatment focuses on stability. Unstable patients require synchronized cardioversion for those with monomorphic VT or defibrillation for those with polymorphic

VT or those without a pulse. For patients who are stable, an electrophysiology consultation is recommended. Consideration can be given for antiarrhythmic medications (sotalol, amiodarone) as these medications are essential in controlling the dysrhythmia, although there is no evidence that they improve survival when given for primary or secondary prevention of sudden death (Al-Khatib et al., 2018). Long-term treatment will depend on the underlying cause, but can include antiarrhythmic medications, an electrophysiology study and ablation, and/or an implantable cardioverter-defibrillator for those at high risk of recurrent life-threatening dysrhythmias (Al-Khatib et al., 2018).

KEY TAKEAWAYS

- All dysrhythmias can present with similar symptoms.
- Suspected dysrhythmias need to be documented via either a 12-lead ECG or ambulatory monitoring for definitive diagnosis and best treatment.
- In general, treatment options for symptomatic bradycardia involve removing potential causes and if ongoing symptoms, permanent pacemaker implantation.
- Treatment options for most tachycardias include rate control, rhythm control, or electrophysiology study and ablation.

3.12: THROMBOLYTICS/PERCUTANEOUS CORONARY INTERVENTION

Paula S. McCauley

Immediate reperfusion is the hallmark treatment for acute coronary syndrome (ACS) by either fibrinolytic medications or mechanical intervention and must be made within minutes of the presentation of the patient with ACS. Door-to-needle or door-to-balloon time benchmarks have documented outcomes with significant impact and improvement on morbidity and mortality. Historically the initial intervention for ACS was with fibrinolytic therapy. Over time, treatment expanded to include percutaneous coronary intervention (PCI) with angioplasty and intracoronary stenting.

Today PCI is the preferred intervention and healthcare systems have developed programs to provide PCI either within their respective facility or through a collaborative agreement with a tertiary care facility that can provide rapid access to PCI. Fibrinolytic therapy is considered if in a remote location without the ability to provide PCI or if there is a delay in transport to a tertiary center. The decision for the type of intervention will depend on the facility's capabilities where the patient presents. Transfer to a tertiary center is provided with consideration for a pharmaco-invasive approach: angiography and possible PCI. Improved outcomes have been documented with combined therapy as treatment with thrombolytics alone may have persistent reduction

in vascular flow in the infarct-related artery (Danchin et al., 2020; Gregory et al., 2020; Keeley et al., 2003; Levine et al., 2016).

Fibrinolytic Therapy

Fibrinolytic therapy or thrombolysis includes lysis of intracoronary thrombus with "clot busting" medication. Recombinant tissue-type plasminogen activator alteplase (tPA), reteplase (rPA), tenecteplase (TNK-tPA), and early streptokinase (which is no longer available in the United States) are all fibrinolytic drugs that act by stimulating the natural fibrinolytic mechanism.

Current guidelines recommend use of fibrinolytic therapy for ACS if symptoms have begun within 12 hours of presentation and PCI is not available within 120 minutes of first medical contact in patients with no contraindications for thrombolytics (Huynh et al., 2009; Paganini et al., 2017).

The greatest benefit from fibrinolytics is when they are administered within 2 to 3 hours after initial symptoms. Attempts to start therapy should occur within 10 minutes of diagnosis. EMS systems are equipped with prehospital protocols, ability to obtain and transmit ECGs, and for the paramedic to administer the chosen medication under medical control directions (Benham & Fannell, 2017).

Contraindications to fibrinolytics are either absolute or relative and included in Box 3.3.

Percutanous Coronary Intervention

PCI was initially developed in the 1980s. Angioplasty is described as enlargement of the vessel lumen through compression. Early on PCI was accomplished primarily by balloon catheters; advancements in technology now include atherectomy and intracoronary stents which have been used since the early 1990s. Atherectomy devices permit drilling or grinding of the atheroma and calcium. Aspiration thrombectomy extracts thrombus or provides distal embolic protection during PCI (Gregory et al., 2020).

Stents are either bare metal stents (BMSs) or drug eluting stents (DESs). BMSs are used for patients with a high bleeding risk who are unable to be treated with dual antiplatelet therapy (DAPT) or likely to undergo invasive or surgical procedures within the next year. DESs contain a polymer coating with an antiproliferative drug that reduces restenosis. The second-generation DESs are currently used in the United States and have more favorable outcomes with lower need for target vessel revascularization. DAPT therapy is necessary post placement to prevent in-stent restenosis (Gregory et al., 2020).

Intravascular Evaluation

Intravascular ultrasonography or IVUS was developed to provide intraluminal information including level of plaque, degree of luminal narrowing, and vessel wall integrity. It is used to evaluate stent deployment and indeterminate lesion assessment.

BOX 3.3 CONTRAINDICATIONS TO FIBRINOLYTICS

Absolute contraindications to thrombolytics:

- History of intracranial hemorrhage
- Known structural cerebral vascular lesion
- Significant closed-head or facial trauma within 3 months
- Intracranial or intraspinal surgery within 2 months
- Ischemic stroke within 3 months
- Intracranial neoplasm
- Active internal bleeding (e.g., serious GI bleeding) excluding menses
- Suspected aortic dissection
- Severe refractory uncontrolled hypertension
- Streptokinase: Previous treatment within 6 months

Relative contraindications to thrombolytics:

- Recent (within 10 days) puncture of a noncompressible blood vessel
- Poorly controlled hypertension or significant hypertension on presentation (diastolic blood pressure >110 mmHg or systolic blood pressure >180 mmHg)
- Diabetic hemorrhagic retinopathy or hemorrhagic ophthalmic condition
- Oral anticoagulant therapy
- Major surgery within 3 weeks
- Pregnancy, active peptic ulcer, dementia
- Internal bleeding within 2 to 4 weeks
- Traumatic or prolonged (>10 minutes) cardiopulmonary resuscitation (CPR)
- History of nonhemorrhagic cerebrovascular accident (CVA) beyond 3 months

Source: Adapted from Benham, M. D., & Fannell, M. W. (2017). Cardiac emergencies. In C. Stone & R. L. Humphries (Eds.), *Current diagnosis & treatment: Emergency medicine* (8th ed.). McGraw Hill. https://accessmedicine-mhmedical-com.ezproxy.lib.uconn.edu/content.aspx?bookid=2172&sectionid=165064287.

Intracoronary Doppler pressures are utilized to estimate lesion severity. Fractional flow ratio (FFR) is obtained, comparing pressure distal to a lesion, to determine if there is hemodynamic significance. In an angiographically intermediate (40%–70%) stenosis, an FFR lower than 0.80 is consistent with hemodynamic or ischemic significance, indicating higher need for intervention.

Both IVUS and FFR assist in decision-making for non-culprit lesions or staged interventions with multivessel disease (Gregory et al., 2020).

PRESENTING SIGNS AND SYMPTOMS

Patients presenting with acute vascular thrombosis, complete or incomplete, with ST-elevation myocardial infarction (STEMI), non-ST segment elevation myocardial infarction (NSTEMI), or unstable angina may undergo coronary intervention or thrombolysis. Full discussion of ACS is included elsewhere in this chapter. In an asymptomatic or mildly symptomatic patient, objective evidence of a moderate to large area of viable myocardium or moderate to severe ischemia on noninvasive testing is an indication for PCI.

Consideration for intervention will depend on the patient presentation. Those presenting with STEMI are taken for emergent left heart catheterization, those with NSTEMI may be less urgent, and are typically admitted and treated with systemic anticoagulation, guideline-directed medical therapy (GDMT), cardiac enzymes, and to trend ECGs. They may also undergo further investigation within 24 hours of admission. If positive enzymes, a left heart catherization is performed; if negative, a stress test may be considered.

A brief review of symptoms may include pain or discomfort located in the chest, upper extremities, back, neck, or jaw. Anginal equivalents for many patients do not include typical chest pain and they may complain of fatigue, dyspnea on exertion, paresthesia, or fatigue.

HISTORY AND PHYSICAL FINDINGS

The decision for treatment of ACS patients is largely based on the history and physical. The patient's story is the most important factor in decision-making for intervention. Along with diagnostics including ECG and enzymes, the patient's account of their pain and symptoms along with exacerbating and mitigating factors are the most important data utilized in decision-making. A complete review of systems is important as well as social history, family history, lifestyle, and substance and alcohol use/abuse. Onset of symptoms is crucial in decision-making for fibrinolysis.

Risk factors for ACS include age, gender, diabetes, hypertension, dyslipidemia, tobacco abuse, obesity, and sedentary lifestyle.

DIFFERENTIAL DIAGNOSIS AND DIAGNOSTIC CONSIDERATIONS

As discussed in the ACS section of this chapter.

TREATMENT

All patients with ACS regardless of choice of intervention (PCI vs. fibrinolytic) should receive systemic anticoagulation therapy with either heparin or Lovenox, a high intensity statin, and dual antiplatlet therapy (DAPT). Beta blockade should be considered unless contraindicated by bradycardia, heart block, or cardiogenic shock.

Dual Antiplatelet Therapy

DAPT reduces the risk of in-stent restenosis and further ischemic events. Current guideline recommendations are for DAPT for a 1-year duration. ASA 325 mg loading dose followed by 81 mg daily is recommended. A loading dose of a P2Y12 receptor inhibitor should be given before the procedure in patients undergoing PCI unless concerns for multivessel disease, which may require coronary artery bypass grafting (CABG).

Options for P2Y12 receptor inhibitors include:
- Clopidogrel: 300 or 600 mg, followed by 75 mg daily
- Prasugrel: 60 mg followed by 10 mg daily
- Ticagrelor: 180 mg followed by 90 mg twice daily

Benefits with each of these are very similar for long-term therapy, morbidity, and mortality. Specific benefits include ticagrelor's rapid onset and so it is preferred in acute events. It has a shorter half-life of 12 hours and requires a twice daily dose. It can be costly depending on the patient's insurance coverage. Plavix has been widely used and evaluated, including with use of triple therapy which includes aspirin, Plavix, and systemic coagulation in patients with concurrent or paroxysmal atrial fibrillation. Prasugrel has been associated with a higher risk of bleeding and is contraindicated in patients with prior history of CVA (Paganini et al., 2017).

Decisions about duration of DAPT are best made on an individual basis and should integrate clinical judgment, assessment of the benefit/risk ratio, and patient preference as well as prescription drug coverage. Historically, DAPT has been continued for 12 months with BMS and first-generation DES. With the newer second-generation stents, several studies have indicated that a shorter time frame is adequate and consideration for holding or stopping DAPT earlier if bleeding is encountered or if there is need for other interventions with high risk of bleeding (Gregory et al., 2020; Paganini et al., 2017)

For patients requiring CABG there is a required wash out time frame if given antiplatelet therapy, approximately 5 days, to reduce bleeding risk with the surgery. Patients referred for elective procedures including CABG who have been given clopidogrel and ticagrelor should be instructed to discontinue for at least 5 days and prasugrel for at least 7 days before surgery. In patients referred for urgent CABG, clopidogrel and ticagrelor should be discontinued for at least 24 hours to reduce major bleeding (Paganini et al., 2017).

GPIIb/IIIa Inhibitors

GPIIb/IIIa inhibitors such as abciximab, tirofiban, and eptifibatide were used with aspirin prior to P2Y12 inhibitors to prevent thrombotic complications. They inhibit GPIIb/IIIa receptors, which bind fibrinogen and mediate platelet aggregation. Several studies have failed to show a benefit with their use and due to an increased risk of bleeding these agents have largely been removed as standard treatment with PCI. They may be used short term immediately after the procedure if there is a large burden of thrombus, distal occlusion of small vessels, or inadequate P2Y12 loading prior to the procedure (Gregory et al., 2020; Levine et al., 2016)

Multivessel PCI Versus CABG

Historically patients with multivessel disease or left main disease were referred for CABG. In STEMI patients often the culprit lesion was addressed with subsequent referral for CABG. Currently, on the basis of multiple randomized controlled trials findings, the prior recommendation with regard to multivessel primary PCI in hemodynamically stable patients with STEMI has been upgraded and modified to include consideration of multivessel PCI, either at the time of primary PCI or as a planned, staged procedure. The patient's history and comorbidities, especially diabetes, as well as bypass targets or need for concurrent valvular conditions are all considerations for these decisions. Heart teams—multidisciplinary teams that include the primary cardiologist, interventional cardiologist, CV surgeon, and anesthesia provider as well as input from other consultants—are now considered best practice for shared decision-making in these cases (Gregory et al., 2020).

Complications

PCI is a relatively safe procedure, performed multiple times daily in most facilities with highly trained interventional teams. A radial versus femoral approach has significantly reduced the recovery time and restrictions but is not without typical risks. Risks and complications include:

Associated risks:
- Dissection/perforation
- Thrombosis
- Vasospasm
- Restenosis
- In stent thrombosis
- Stroke
- Contrast-induced nephropathy
- Anaphylaxis to contrast

Vascular complications:
- Hemorrhage
- Hematoma
- Pseudoaneurysm
- Ateroventricular fistula
- Dissections
- Thrombosis
- Coronary vasospasm

Fibrinolytic therapy increases risk of bleeding and stroke. Hemorrhage is most frequently associated with GI tract followed by intracerebral hemorrhage (Gregory et al., 2020).

Postprocedure Care

Routine care with PCI recovery is either same day or extended observation overnight. With STEMI/NSTEMI a stay for up to 72 hours is typical.

Postprocedure care includes:
- A baseline ECG following the procedure
- Frequent vital signs and vascular exams
- Evaluation of the access site immediately after completion

Radial Approach

- Initial care with a radial approach usually incorporates a compression device that is applied for up to 2 hours. Gradual reduction in pressure is attained over time with frequent assessment for bleeding.
- The limb is elevated and use restricted for the initial recovery time. Postdischarge the patent is instructed to limit lifting and strain on the extremity for 1 to 2 weeks.

Femoral Approach

- With a femoral approach there are now closure devices that are routinely used versus manual compression. Manual compression is required for a minimum of 30 minutes followed by external compression devices. Intravascular closure devices are standard procedure and require minimal manual compression time.
- Retroperitoneal bleeding is of great concern following a femoral approach; it is difficult to assess due to the potential for large accumulation in the retroperitoneal space without obvious bleeding or hematoma on exam. Hypotension, back pain, and bradycardia are common signs and symptoms that should alert the provider to apply compression and obtain an emergent CT scan of the abdomen and pelvis.
- Other complications include development of a pseudoaneurysm or AV fistula. Here the importance of evaluating the site for a bruit or thrill is vital (Gregory et al., 2020; Levine et al., 2016).

TRANSITION OF CARE

Postprocedure the patient is transferred to the ICU if STEMI presentation, progressive/intermediate care unit for NSTEMI or with an elective procedure. Stay may encompass 48 to 72 hours for STEMI, 24 hours for extended recovery for NSTEMI or elective procedure. Reperfusion arrhythmia, stent thrombosis, and access site complications are immediate concerns that require monitoring.

Discharge Care

Guideline-directed medical therapy (GDMT) is continued upon discharge and should include DAPT, high intensity statin therapy, beta blockade, and ACE-i or ARB. The importance of DAPT must be emphasized with the patient at discharge. Following PCI, vessel wall remodeling occurs, along with it the risk of thrombosis. DAPT must be continued for 1 year with DES and at a minimum 1 month with BMS is necessary.

Physical restrictions discussed previously depend on the access site; limitations with lifting and strenuous exercise may be 1 to 3 weeks.

Referral for cardiac rehabilitation is recommended for patients who experience ACS, providing the patient with progressive recovery and lifestyle coaching in risk factor modification including smoking cessation, heart healthy diet, and exercise (Gregory et al., 2020; Levine et al., 2016).

Follow-up post procedure should include a visit within 1 to 2 weeks for access site evaluation and a comprehensive exam to evaluate for treatment adherence, medication side effects, progression or improvement in post infarct cardiomyopathy or heat failure. Routine follow-up in 3 to 6 months and then annually is standard.

CLINICAL PEARLS

- Fibrinolytic therapy is indicated for ACS if symptoms have begun within 12 hours of presentation and PCI is not available within 120 minutes of first medical contact.
- Clinical contraindications for PCI include intolerance to long-term, antiplatelet therapy.
- Door-to-balloon time of 90 minutes is associated with significant reduction in morbidity and mortality in STEMI patients.
- For patients with NSTEMI or unstable angina, early invasive strategy is recommended.

KEY TAKEAWAYS

- A heart team approach should be used in patients with multivessel disease and diabetes or severe left main disease.
- DAPT for a BMS is a minimum of 4 weeks; DAPT for a drug-eluting stent is a minimum of 12 months
- Regardless of therapy chosen all patients presenting with ACS should initially receive systemic anticoagulation, DAPT, high intensity statin and consideration for beta blockade unless contraindicated.

EVIDENCE-BASED RESOURCES

2011 ACCF/AHA/SCAI Guideline for PCI and the 2013 ACCF/AHA Guideline for the Management of STEMI.

2020 AHA/ACC Key Data Elements and Definitions for Coronary Revascularization: A Report of the ACC/American Heart Association Task Force on Clinical Data Standards (Writing Committee to Develop Clinical Data Standards for Coronary Revascularization).

ACC/AATS/AHA/ASE/ASNC/SCAI/SCCT/STS 2016 Appropriate Use Criteria for Coronary Revascularization in Patients With ACS: A Report of the ACC Appropriate Use Criteria Task Force, American Association for Thoracic Surgery, American Heart Association (AHA), American Society of Echocardiography, American Society of Nuclear Cardiology, Society for Cardiovascular Angiography and Interventions, Society of Cardiovascular CT, and the Society of Thoracic Surgeons.

3.13: VALVULAR HEART DISEASE

Stacey Evans and Lynda Stoodley

Valvular heart disease (VHD) is damage or destruction to any of the four valves of the heart, leading to incompetence (also known as regurgitation), or narrowing (also known as stenosis) of the valve. Major causes of VHD include rheumatic heart disease, endocarditis, congenital heart disease, connective tissue disorders, calcification with aging, heart failure (HF), and ischemia (Centers for Disease Control and Prevention [CDC], 2019). MR and AS are the most common VHD in the community and hospital settings, while rheumatic heart disease is the most common in developing countries (Huntley et al., 2019). About 2.5% of the U.S. population has VHD and about 13% of people born before 1943 have VHD (Otto & Bonow, 2014).

Aortic Valve Disorders

Disorders of the aortic valve include AS and aortic regurgitation (AR). The aortic valve is trileaflet and stenosis is usually caused by degenerative calcification or progressive stenosis of a congenital bicuspid valve (Maganti et al., 2010) as people born with a bicuspid aortic valve are predisposed to develop AS (Shipton & Wahba, 2001). A bicuspid valve has only two leaflets, instead of three. With AS, the orifice of the valve decreases, leading to decreased blood flow through the valve. As AS progresses, changes to the left ventricular (LV) dimensions can occur, further comprising cardiac function.

AR also results from abnormalities of the aortic leaflets, their supporting structures in the aortic root and annulus, or both (Maganti et al., 2010) with rheumatic heart disease being one of the most common causes. With AR, the valve leaflets do not close properly leading to blood flowing back into the LV during systole, which can cause increased stroke volume, systolic blood pressure, and afterload. The left ventricle can dilate and hypertrophy, leading to LV failure.

Mitral Valve Disorders

MR most often is the result of disorders of the valve leaflets themselves or from any of the surrounding structures that comprise the mitral apparatus (Shipton & Wahba, 2001). Mitral valve regurgitation occurs because of valve incompetency leading to the inability of the leaflets to close properly, causing backflow into the left atrium. Chronic MR can be a primary abnormality of the valve structures (leaflets, chordae tendineae, papillary muscles, and/or annulus) or may be secondary to LV dysfunction.

Mitral stenosis (MS) is an obstruction of blood flow through the valve, leading to increased pressure and dilation in the left atrium. Rheumatic fever is the most common cause of MS.

Tricuspid Valve Disorders

The tricuspid valve is the "forgotten valve" and often overlooked by providers (AHA, 2018). Tricuspid regurgitation (TR) is a leakage of blood backward through the tricuspid valve each time the right ventricle contracts resulting in an increased blood volume in the right atrium.

Tricuspid stenosis (TS) is an uncommon valvular abnormality most often found in combination with TR and/or other valvular lesions and rarely an isolated lesion. Rheumatic heart disease is the most common cause of TS.

Pulmonic Valve Disorders

Pulmonic stenosis (PS) is narrowing of the pulmonic valve in which the valve is stiffened causing obstruction of blood flow. This disease is benign and typically congenital, although it can be present in adults and usually is in conjunction with severe cardiac structural diseases (American Heart Association, 2018).

Pulmonary regurgitation (PR) is a "leaky" pulmonary valve, often occurring in healthy and normal hearts. Chronic PR can lead to right ventricular overload resulting in right ventricular remodeling and progressive decline in function (Thomas et al., 2021).

PRESENTING SIGNS AND SYMPTOMS

Often, patients with VHD might not experience symptoms for many years and often are unaware that a valvular problem is present. Patients may be found to have a heart murmur or have incidental findings on noninvasive testing (Otto et al., 2021b). When the diseased valve develops slowly, there may or may not be symptoms until the valve is incompetent and the condition has become quite advanced. Although some patients may deny symptoms, upon further inquiry, they may report decreased activity levels to avoid having symptoms. They may be developing subtle indications of progressive valvular pathology and not realize it, because of their lack of activity (Stoodley & Keller, 2017).

Patient symptoms of acute and chronic VHD can often differ in their presentation. Gradual symptoms may be progressive SOB, chest pain, or presyncope with exertion. Others may present to the hospital in acute systolic HF as their first VHD diagnosis (Stoodley & Keller, 2017). If symptoms of HF, angina, or syncope develop, morbidity is concerning, with current literature documenting that 50% of patients with AS who present with angina, syncope, or HF survive for 5, 3, or 2 years, respectively, without aortic valve replacement (AVR).

HISTORY AND PHYSICAL FINDINGS

Evaluation of patients with VHD must include a comprehensive history and physical exam. If VHD is suspected, correlation with noninvasive testing such as an ECG, chest x-ray, or transthoracic echocardiogram (TTE), should occur (Otto et al., 2021b). An echocardiogram should be obtained to confirm VHD and to evaluate the valve anatomy, the severity of valve dysfunction, and the response of the ventricle and pulmonary circulation (Otto et al., 2021b).

VHD physical findings are consistent with signs of congestive heart failure (CHF). Peripheral edema, abdominal fullness, or jugular venous distention may occur if the ventricles begin to fail from the valvular pathology. If the VHD occurs suddenly as with a chordae rupture with an acute myocardial infarction (MI), sudden onset of symptoms can present as severe chest pain, shortness of breath (SOB), or syncope. Electrolyte abnormalities and elevated B-type natriuretic peptide (BNP) may be present also.

With AS, physical findings vary with the severity of valve calcification, stenosis, and LV function, although the most common is a harsh crescendo/decrescendo systolic ejection murmur that radiates to the neck. The murmur is best heard at the right upper sternum.

Physical findings of AR are a widened pulse pressure and increase in stroke volume, but this may also be seen in other conditions of hyperdynamic circulation (Wang, 2020). A diastolic murmur, best heard at the third left intercostal space radiating along the left sternal border, may be present. In severe cases, head bobbing can occur.

Physical findings of MR vary and are dependent on the degree of decompensation and the severity and chronicity. The apical impulse can be hyperdynamic and the apical pulse may be laterally displaced given the severity of the MR. A harsh holosystolic murmur that may radiate to the axilla may be present on physical exam.

With MS, an apical, low pitched rumbling in mid-diastole, a diastolic murmur best heard at the apex, may be present. A diastolic thrill may also be appreciated.

DIFFERENTIAL DIAGNOSIS AND DIAGNOSTIC CONSIDERATIONS

One of the most common findings in patients with VHD is a murmur, which is turbulent blood flow through the heart. Many murmurs are considered innocent, in which no valvular pathology is found. Innocent heart murmurs are common, with about 10% of adults affected, and are more common in pregnant women (Cash & Gunter, 2021). Innocent murmurs are systolic murmurs, while a diastolic murmur is always pathologic.

Differentiating Diastolic and Systolic Murmurs

Diastolic murmur includes but is not limited to: (a) MS, which is the most common and normally caused by IE and chronic rheumatic heart disease; (b) AR, associated with rheumatic heart disease, or bacterial endocarditis caused by the gradual loss of apposition of the aortic cusps in diastole; and (c) TS includes IE, seen most often in IV drug users, and carcinoid syndrome (Thomas et al., 2021).

Systolic murmurs include: (a) AS, which is the most common valvular pathology in the developed world, and arises from senile calcification or a congenital anomaly, such as a bicuspid aortic valve; (b) TR, also associated with IV drug users as well as carcinoid syndrome; and (c) MR commonly associated with infectious endocarditis (IE), rheumatic heart disease, congenital anomalies, and inferior wall MIs (Thomas et al., 2021).

Patients with IE or thoracic aortic aneurysms may also present with a murmur. Obtaining noninvasive studies such as a TTE or CT scan will help determine the diagnosis.

TREATMENT

American College of Cardiology (ACC)/AHA VHD recommend use of disease stages A, B, C, and D based on symptoms, valve anatomy, the severity of valve dysfunction, and the response of the ventricle and pulmonary circulation (Otto et al., 2021b), which assists with medical management and/or timing of intervention on the diseased valve. This classification system labels the valvular lesion progression, representing patients who are symptomatic and have developed symptoms as a result of VHD (Nishimura et al., 2014). The disease stages consist of Stage A (risk for development of VHD), Stage B (progressive with mild to moderate severity and asymptomatic), Stage C (asymptomatic severe), Stage C1 (asymptomatic, severe without ventricular decompensation), Stage C2 (asymptomatic severe with ventricular decompensation), and Stage D (symptomatic severe; Otto et al., 2021b).

Treatment is based on severity of the valve dysfunction and patient symptomology. If not severe, treatment can consist of medical therapy and is often managed by a clinician that specializes in HF or valvular diseases. If being considered for valve intervention, the patient should be evaluated by a multidisciplinary team (Otto et al., 2021b).

In patients who do not have severe disease or have minimal symptoms, close follow-up and surveillance of the patient's symptoms and valve pathology progression is needed (Stoodley & Keller, 2017). Surveillance monitoring with echocardiography depends on the patient's valve disorder and its effect on the ventricles (Nishimura et al., 2014).

Comorbid disorders such as hypertension, diabetes mellitus, hyperlipidemia, and atrial fibrillation must be treated with standard GDMT (Otto et al., 2021b). "Close BP monitoring is also important because abruptly lowering the BP in someone with AS may cause syncope, whereas an elevated BP may worsen VHD symptoms" (Stoodley & Keller, 2017).

Surgical and transcatheter interventions are performed on patients with severe VHD (Otto et al., 2021b). The type of valve intervention (medical, surgical, or percutaneous) depends on the valve pathology and involvement, the patient's comorbidities, and their preoperative risk and frailty (Nishimura et al., 2014). The timing of a valve intervention needs to be balanced with minimizing risks of the procedure but improving a patient's symptoms (Nishimura et al., 2014). "The purpose of valvular intervention is to improve symptoms, prolong survival, and minimize the risk of VHD-related complications, such as irreversible ventricular dysfunction, pulmonary hypertension, stroke, and atrial fibrillation (AF)" (Otto et al., 2021b).

Valvular Repair Versus Replacement

Surgical repair may be performed as it is generally best to repair a valve and preserve a person's own heart tissue when possible. Valvular repair often includes the separation of the valve flaps (leaflets or cusps) that have fused, replacing the cords that support the valve, and removal of excess valve tissue so that the leaflets or cusps can close tightly. Surgeons may often tighten or reinforce the ring around a valve (annulus) by implanting an artificial ring (Matiasz & Rigolin, 2018).

However, in some conditions if the tissue is too damaged and cannot be repaired, the valve will need to be replaced through open heart surgery. Valvular replacement may be from another human heart, animal (cow or pig), or a manufactured mechanical (biological or tissue) valve. These options include surgical implantation of mechanical valves, which are long-lasting valves made of durable materials, and tissue valves (which may include human or animal donor tissue).

There are newer minimally invasive surgical options which include transcatheter aortic valve implantation (TAVI) and transcatheter aortic valve replacement (TAVR). During this minimally invasive procedure a new valve is inserted and is placed inside the diseased valve without removing the old, damaged valve (Otto et al., 2021a), similar to placing a stent in an artery.

TRANSITION OF CARE

Self-monitoring of symptoms and vital sign measurement should be encouraged. Patients must be advised to report worsening symptoms. In addition, patient education to follow a heart healthy diet, and medication compliance is imperative. Other comorbidities such as diabetes mellitus, hypertension, or hyperlipidemia should be controlled. In addition, influenza and pneumococcal vaccinations should be given to appropriate patient groups with VHD (Nishimura et al., 2014).

If the patient undergoes surgery to repair or replace the diseased valve, education postvalvular surgery is important. In addition, depending on the position of the valve during surgical replacement, patients might need to take blood thinning medication for prevention of blood clots. If so, it is imperative to provide thorough education regarding anticoagulants.

CLINICAL PEARLS

- ACC/AHA guidelines recommend VHD be classified as stages A, B, C, and D based on symptoms, valve anatomy, the severity of valve dysfunction, and the response of the ventricle and pulmonary circulation

(Otto et al., 2021b), which assists with medical management and/or timing of intervention on the diseased valve.
- Treatment is based on severity of the valve dysfunction and patient symptomology.
- Type of valve intervention (medical, surgical, or percutaneous) depends on the valve pathology and involvement, the patient's comorbidities, and their preoperative risk and frailty.
- Diastolic murmurs are always pathologic.

KEY TAKEAWAYS

- If a patient has been identified as having VHD, continual monitoring for progression of the valvular lesion or the development of symptoms is crucial.
- Close follow-up and surveillance of the patient's symptoms and valve pathology progression is crucial (Stoodley & Keller, 2017).

EVIDENCE-BASED RESOURCES

The 2014 AHA/ACC VHD guidelines focus on the management of adult patients with valve disorders.

2020 ACC/AHA Guideline for the Management of Patients with VHD: A Report of the ACC/American Heart Association Joint Committee on Clinical Practice Guidelines

2017 AHA/ACC Focused Update of the 2014 AHA/ACC Guideline for the Management of Patients with VHD: A Report of the ACC/American Heart Association Task Force on Clinical Practice Guidelines

2018 AHA/ACC Guideline for the Management of Adults With Congenital Heart Disease: A Report of the ACC/American Heart Association Task Force on Clinical Practice Guidelines.

2020 New ACC/AHA VHD Guideline Spotlights Less-Invasive Treatments

SPRINGER PUBLISHING CONNECT™

A robust set of instructor resources designed to supplement this text is located at http://connect.springerpub.com/content/reference-book/978-0-8261-6079-9. Qualifying instructors may request access by emailing textbook@springerpub.com.

REFERENCES

Full list of references can be accessed at http://connect.springerpub.com/content/reference-book/978-0-8261-6079-9

CHAPTER 4

CARDIOVASCULAR SURGERY

Lori Dugan Brien, Genevieve MacDonald, Kelly A. Thompson-Brazill, and Catherine C. Tierney

LEARNING OBJECTIVES

- Examine the indications and contraindications for coronary artery bypass graft surgery versus percutaneous coronary intervention.
- Compare and contrast the pre- and postoperative management of patients with infective endocarditis versus those with rheumatic or nonrheumatic valvular heart disease.
- Evaluate which patients would benefit from surgical or hybrid ablation of atrial fibrillation.
- Describe which patients would benefit from pericardial window creation.
- Differentiate the pain management strategies of enhanced recovery after surgery (ERAS) after cardiac surgery from usual postoperative care.
- Describe the indications for using vasopressor and/or inotropic medications after heart surgery.
- Utilize national guidelines to determine which patients would benefit from ventricular assist device (VAD) implantation or extracorporeal membrane oxygenation (ECMO).

INTRODUCTION

Cardiothoracic (CT) surgery is a broad specialty that encompasses surgeries that are performed on the heart, major thoracic blood vessels, and lungs. These procedures include coronary artery bypass graft (CABG), aortic valve replacement, mitral valve repair or replacement, repair of the aortic root and/or ascending aorta, surgical drainage of pericardial effusions (pericardial window), surgical treatment of atrial fibrillation (AF), ventricular assist device (VAD) placement, and cannulation for extracorporeal life support (ELS). Note that cardiac transplantation is discussed in Chapter 23, "Solid Organ Transplantation." Given their complex physiology and unique management needs, CT surgery patients are transferred from the operating room (OR) to the cardiothoracic intensive care unit (CTICU). CTICU clinicians—including adult-gerontology acute care nurse practitioners (AGACNPs),

physician assistants (PAs), cardiac surgeons, and intensivists—work alongside highly skilled nurses and respiratory therapists to provide optimal care for these patients. Astute physical assessment, diagnostic reasoning, critical thinking, and communication skills are essential for providers managing CT surgery patients. This chapter outlines current evidence-based practices in the care of CT surgery patients from admission to the CTICU through hospital discharge.

4.1: PREOPERATIVE ASSESSMENT OF PATIENTS UNDERGOING CARDIAC SURGERY

PREOPERATIVE DIAGNOSTIC TESTING

Standard preoperative laboratory studies include complete blood count (CBC), basic metabolic panel (BMP), thyroid stimulating hormone (TSH), liver function tests (LFTs), prothrombin time (PT), international normalized ratio (INR), activated partial thromboplastin time (aPTT), urinalysis, as well as blood typing and crossmatching for potential transfusions of blood and/or blood products (Bojar, 2021).

Checking hemoglobin A1C and albumin levels helps evaluate pre-operative risk. Patients with hemoglobin A1C <6.5 have decreased rates of ischemia, complications, and sternal wound infections (Engelman et al., 2019). Low prealbumin levels are associated with prolonged mechanical ventilation, length of stay (LOS), increased morbidity, wound complications, and higher readmission rates (Engelman et al., 2019; Wischmeyer et al., 2018). In addition to prealbumin, nutritional scoring systems can help determine which patients would benefit from referral to a dietitian for nutrition optimization prior to surgery. The Pre-Op Nutrition Screening (PONS) tool incorporates the following assessments in determining the need for nutritional intervention: unplanned weight loss >10% of body weight in the last 6 months; body mass index (BMI) <18.5 in patients less 65 years old and BMI <20 in patients more than 65 years old; eating <50% of meals in the week prior; and/or albumin <3.0 (Wischmeyer et al., 2018). Moreover, it is important to assess patients for frailty. In addition to nutritional support, frail patients may benefit from preoperative rehabilitation (i.e., "prehabilitation") with physical (PT) and occupational (OT) therapy prior to surgery (Engelman et al., 2019).

A preoperative electrocardiogram (ECG) is ordered for all adult cardiac surgery patients. The ECG assesses for evidence of new or worsening ischemia and the presence of arrhythmias (Bojar, 2021). Two-view chest radiographs are also performed to evaluate for acute and chronic pulmonary disease (Bojar, 2021). An arterial blood gas (ABG) is recommended in patients with a room air oxygen saturation <90% (Bojar, 2021). In patients with significant smoking histories or those with chronic obstructive pulmonary disease (COPD), pulmonary function testing (PFT) is useful to elucidate the severity of disease (Bojar, 2021). The data are also an important component of preoperative risk stratification. Patients with severely abnormal PFTs (e.g., FEV_1 <50% predicted, FEV_1/FVC <70% predicted, and diffusing capacity of carbon monoxide <50% predicted), and/or room air PaO_2 <60 mmHg, PCO_2 >50 mmHg have an increased risk of postoperative morbidity and mortality (Bojar, 2021).

Preoperative Imaging

Non-contrast computed tomography (CT) scans of the chest are used to evaluate the anatomy of the thoracic cavity, as well assess the ascending aorta for calcific plaques that may preclude aortic cross clamping due to risk of stroke (Bojar, 2021; Panza et al., 2021). Coronary CT scans may be ordered to assess for coronary artery disease (CAD) in patients with low CAD risk factors who are undergoing non-CABG procedures such as valve or aortic surgery (Faroux et al., 2019). Computed tomographic angiography (CTA) is recommended for all patients undergoing minimally invasive, on-pump CABG procedures in order to minimize the risk of aortic dissection from cardiopulmonary bypass (CBP) cannulation (Bonatti et al., 2021). CTA scans of the chest, abdomen, and pelvis are required for all patients under consideration for transcatheter aortic (TAVR) or transcatheter mitral (TMVR) valve replacement to assess dimensions of the vasculature and the height of the left main (LM) coronary artery above the aortic valve (Francone et al., 2020).

Transthoracic echocardiograms (TTEs) are performed to evaluate left ventricular ejection fraction (LVEF), assess valve function, and identify cardiac wall motion abnormalities (Bojar, 2021). Transesophageal echocardiograms (TEEs) are indicated in patients with valvular dysfunction (e.g., mitral regurgitation [MR]) for surgical planning (Bojar, 2021). Carotid ultrasound may be ordered in patient with calcific aortic stenosis (AS), LM disease, carotid bruits, or history of carotid stenosis to determine if carotid endarterectomy is needed before, during, or after the cardiac surgical procedure (Bojar, 2021). Vein mapping studies are ordered to evaluate the location and quality of the greater saphenous veins in patients with arterial or venous insufficiency, varicosities, and prior surgeries such as vein stripping to treat varicose veins (Bojar, 2021). Arterial doppler studies of the palmar arch or digital plethysmography with radial compression are indicated to determine if it is safe to use one of the radial arteries as a conduit (Bojar, 2021).

Lastly, in patients with ischemic cardiomyopathy and severely reduced ejection fractions (EFs), it is important to determine if the heart muscle is stunned, hibernating, or permanently damaged (Khera & Panza, 2017). Stunned myocardium is a systolic dysfunction that results from temporary ischemia, such as an MI with rapid restoration of perfusion (Panza et al., 2021). Hibernating myocardium is a compensatory mechanism that alleviates ischemia by reducing myocardial contractility in areas that are chronically hypoperfused (Panza et al., 2021). Magnetic resonance or nuclear medicine viability studies are ordered to determine if the hypokinetic areas of the myocardium will likely recover with restoration of coronary circulation (Panza et al., 2021). If the areas of viable myocardium are fed by the occluded coronary arteries, then CABG is performed (Panza et al., 2021).

Relative Contraindications for Open Heart Surgery

Cardiac surgeons carefully consider the risk/benefit to each patient prior to scheduling surgery (Khera & Panza, 2017). After a thorough history, physical exam, and review of preoperative test results, surgeons often consult with members of the multidisciplinary heart team to determine if a patient is a suitable operative candidate (Khera & Panza, 2017). Age, itself, is not a contraindication for heart surgery (Khera & Panza, 2017). Ischemic cardiomyopathy with low EF and serious comorbidities may be at high risk of postoperative morbidity and mortality (Khera & Panza, 2017). Patients with advanced alcoholic cirrhosis whose Childs-Turcotte-Pugh (CTP) Classification of Cirrhosis scores are ≥8 are considered CTP class C and have an average operative mortality risk of 52% (Bojar, 2021).

The Society of Thoracic Surgeon's (STS) Adult Cardiac Surgery Risk Score has a superb predictive value for estimating postoperative adverse events (e.g., stroke, prolonged mechanical ventilation, renal failure, deep sternal wound infection [DSWI]) for patients undergoing CABG alone or in combination with mitral or aortic valve surgery (Lawton et al., 2021; STS, 2021a). The STS allows participating hospitals to publicly share their surgical outcome data on the STS website (STS, 2021b). Prior to offering a patient surgery for symptom relief and longevity benefits, the cardiac surgeon will enter the patient's information into the STS short-term risk calculator which predicts the risk of mortality, renal failure, permanent stroke, prolonged mechanical ventilation, DSWI, reoperation, morbidity or mortality, and short/long LOS (STS, 2021c). The surgeon then shares the STS risk with the patient and their family. This is part of the informed consent process and promotes shared decision-making.

4.2: SURGICAL TREATMENT OF MULTIVESSEL CORONARY ARTERY DISEASE

In 2018, 157,704 isolated coronary artery bypass graft (CABG) surgeries were performed at 1,088 Society of Thoracic Surgeons (STS) member sites (Bowdish et al., 2020). There are numerous factors that guide the decision to perform surgical versus percutaneous revascularization in patients with multivessel coronary artery disease (MVCAD). Percutaneous coronary intervention (PCI) or fibrinolytics are the first-line revascularization methods for patients with ST segment elevation myocardial infarctions (STEMI) due to the quick restoration of blood flow to the myocardium. Patients with STEMIs may require CABG if they have complex anatomy that is not amenable to PCI, or if they develop post-myocardial infarction (MI) mechanical complications such as mitral regurgitation (MR) due to acute papillary muscle rupture, ventricular septal defect, or ventricular free wall rupture (Alexander & Smith, 2016).

Although CABG is the standard of care for left main (LM) or MVCAD , the patient should be evaluated by a heart team which includes an interventional cardiologist and cardiothoracic surgeon to determine which option is best for the individual patient (Alexander & Smith, 2016; Shaefi et al., 2019). Lesion severity and lesion complexity are the most important criteria informing the decision to pursue surgical revascularization versus PCI. Severe lesions are those with ≥50% LM coronary artery stenosis and non-LM lesions ≥70% (Lawton et al., 2021). CABG is indicated with severe LM disease and MVCAD with or without LM disease (Lawton et al., 2021). Complex lesions include those located in the coronary ostia (ostial disease), LM, or proximal left anterior descending (LAD) coronary arteries, and that are present at the branching points of two or three coronary arteries (bifurcating and trifurcating, respectively; Lawton et al., 2021).

Other criteria that increase lesion complexity are vessels that are severely tortuous, heavily calcified, those with chronic total occlusion (CTO), and diffuse CAD with significant vessel narrowing distal to the primary lesion (Lawton et al., 2021). Lesions that are thrombotic and those >20 mm in length also raise the level of complexity (Lawton et al., 2021). Patients with CAD (≥70% stenosis) that have persistent angina despite PCI and medical management may benefit from CABG (Alexander & Smith, 2016).

The Synergy Between PCI with TAXUS and Cardiac Surgery (SYNTAX) scoring system was developed to facilitate surgical decision-making by evaluating a patient's coronary artery anatomy and the estimated complexity of performing PCI (Alexander & Smith, 2016; Lawton et al., 2021). SYNTAX scores are grouped into three risk categories: low (≤22), medium (22–32), and high (≥33). The SYNTAX II score also includes clinical variables. Unlike the STS risk score, the SYNTAX II score does not predict post operative adverse events (Lawton et al., 2021). Data from the original SYNTAX trial revealed that patients randomized to CABG had lower composite rates of stroke, repeat revascularization procedures, MIs, and death after 5 years (Alexander & Smith, 2016). Moreover, the risk of incomplete revascularization (IR) is higher in PCI versus CABG patients. In 2021, the Synergy Between PCI with TAXUS and Cardiac Surgery: Extended Survival (SYNTAXES) study found that at 10-years postprocedure, patients with newly diagnosed three-vessel CAD who were randomized to PCI in the SYNTAX study had higher 10-year mortality rates than those assigned to CABG (Takahashi et al., 2021). Interestingly, there were no mortality differences in those with LM CAD who received either PCI or CABG, which may be due to more complete revascularization in the LM PCI group (Mehta, 2021).

CABG is the preferred method of revascularization in patients with diabetes mellitus. The 2021 American College of Cardiology (ACC)/American Heart Association (AHA) guidelines recommend CABG for patients with diabetes mellitus and mitral valve coronary artery disease (MVCAD) unless they are poor operative candidates, in which case the guidelines recommend percutaneous cardiac intervention (PCI; Lawton et al., 2021). Studies such as Future Revascularization Evaluation in Patients with Diabetes Mellitus: Optimal Management of Multivessel Disease (FREEDOM) trial have demonstrated significant decreases in myocardial infarction (MI) and death over a 5-year period in patients randomized to CABG versus PCI (Alexander & Smith, 2016; Lawton et al., 2021). Of note, in the FREEDOM study, the overall risk of stroke was lower in the PCI group. Additional indications for CABG include coronary artery blockages >50% with need for concomitant procedures such as valve operations, septal myectomy, ventricular septal defects, ventricular aneurysms, ascending aortic aneurysms, coronary anomalies, or coronary dissections (Lawton et al., 2021; Neumann et al., 2019).

ON PUMP CORONARY ARTERY BYPASS GRAFTING PROCEDURE

- Laboratory studies; complete blood count (CBC), comprehensive metabolic panel (CMP), C-reactive protein (CRP), erythrocyte sedimentation rate (ESR), coagulation studies, A1C, prealbumin, urinalysis (UA)
  - Evaluate possibility of infection; elevated white blood cell count (WBC)/ESR, evidence of urinary tract infection
  - Determine if nutritional consult required preoperatively
  - Evaluate renal function to determine if a renal consult is needed, and the risk of acute kidney injury (AKI) requiring dialysis postoperatively
  - Consider endocrinology consult for elevated A1C >10: Evidence suggests blood glucose control (<180mL/dL) for 24 hours preoperatively and 48 postoperatively reduces risk of postoperative complications.
  - Treatment of anemia: Determine if further workup is indicated; obtain iron studies and a hematology consult. If occult positive, consider a GI consult for esophagogastroduodenoscopy (EGD) or colonoscopy
  - If evidence of thrombocytopenia, consider heparin-induced thrombocytopenia (HIT) and whether hematology consultation is warranted.

- Echocardiogram: Evaluate wall motion abnormalities, left ventricular function, valvular function.
- Noncontrast CT chest: Evaluate lungs, aorta, and anatomy.
- Carotid ultrasound: Evaluate for carotid stenosis.
- Pulmonary function test and room air arterial blood gas (ABG): If smoking history or pulmonary disease.
- Vein mapping: If indicated for varicose veins, previous interventions, or significant peripheral vascular disease.
- MRI viability study: Consider if significant ischemia/wall motion abnormality that would indicate that revascularization would prove ineffective.
- Panorex to evaluate for periodontal abscesses: Dental extractions if valve surgery planned.
- Discontinuing certain medications prior to surgery.
  - Anticoagulants/platelet aggregators such as clopidogrel, tricagelor, or prasugel, direct oral anticoagulants (DOACs), warfarin, IIa/IIIb inhibitors, and low molecular weight heparin (LMWH).
  - Metformin (held prior to coronary angiography as well): Can increase the risk of metformin associated lactic acidosis.
  - ACE inhibitors and ARBs: Contribute to vasoplegia in the postoperative phase.
  - Immunomodulators: Can impair healing.
  - NSAIDs: Can contribute to bleeding and renal impairment.

CLINICAL PEARLS

- SYNTAX score: Grading system used to evaluate complexity and prognosis of patients undergoing PCI (https://syntaxscore.org/calculator/start.htm)
- STS Risk Calculator: Calculator used to calculate patients' risk of mortality and morbidities for most commonly performed cardiac surgeries (http://riskcalc.sts.org/stswebriskcalc/calculate)

Coronary Artery Bypass Grafting

CABG is most commonly performed through a median sternotomy incision using cardiopulmonary bypass (CPB) under general endotracheal anesthesia (Shaefi et al., 2019). In preparation for the procedure, anesthesia places central vascular access (e.g., introducer sheath or central venous catheter) and monitoring lines (e.g., arterial line, pulmonary artery catheter; Shakhnovich et al., 2019). An indwelling bladder catheter with temperature probe is placed for accurate urine output and core temperature monitoring. Preoperative antibiotics are administered prior to the skin incision.

Once the patient is prepped, draped, and a time-out is performed, the surgeon opens the chest. Conduits, which allow blood to flow around the coronary artery blockages, are made from arteries such as the left internal mammary or thoracic artery (LIMA or LITA), or veins such as the greater saphenous (Alexander & Smith, 2016; Lawton et al., 2021). A heparin bolus of 5,000 units

is given intravenously (Bojar, 2021). The surgeon is responsible for dissecting the LIMA from the left subclavian artery. It is skeletonized and used in situ to bypass the LAD artery (Alexander & Smith, 2016; Lawton et al., 2021). The right internal mammary or thoracic artery (RIMA or RITA) is less commonly used (Alexander & Smith, 2016; Lawton et al., 2021). The first assistant, either an NP, PA, or certified registered nurse first assistant (CRNFA), harvests the peripheral conduit which will become bypass grafts. The greater saphenous vein, either harvested open or endoscopically, is frequently employed as a conduit, but does not maintain patency as well as arterial grafts (Mack et al., 2021). Lesser saphenous veins and gastroepiploic arteries require laparoscopic harvesting and are only used in rare cases when there is no other available conduit (Mack et al., 2021). The 2021 ACC/AHA guidelines recommend using a radial artery graft to the second most important coronary artery that requires bypass (Lawton et al., 2021). Radial grafts have better long-term patency then saphenous vein grafts (SVG) and are associated with increased survival and lower adverse cardiac events (Lawton et al., 2021). Despite arterial graft longevity, multiarterial graft procedures are uncommon as they are technically difficult to perform, associated with a higher risk of DSWI, and have no definitive benefit compared to conventional conduit (Mack et al., 2021). Patients with radial grafts require calcium channel blockers (CCB) for 1-year postop to prevent vasospasm in the graft (Lawton et al., 2021).

Once the conduit is obtained, the surgeon prepares to place the patient on the CPB pump by giving a loading dose of heparin (refer to the section "Cardioplegia, Myocardial Protection, and the Cardiopulmonary Bypass Pump" for more details). Next, the surgeon inserts large bore cannulas into either the central (vena cava and ascending aorta) or peripheral vasculature (axillary, innominate, or femoral arteries) depending on the operative approach (Fiedler et al., 2020). CPB is initiated. The aorta is cross clamped. Then the heart is arrested using cardioplegia solution (Fiedler et al., 2020; Mack et al., 2021). Bypass grafts are performed by suturing conduit from the aorta (proximal anastomosis) to the coronary artery beyond the lesion (distal anastomosis). The LIMA is typically taken in situ with its proximal end branching from the left subclavian (Bojar, 2021). Blood flow in the grafts is measured with flow probes (Bojar, 2021). An intraoperative transesophageal echocardiogram (TEE) performed by anesthesia evaluates the ejection fraction and the presence of new right or left ventricular wall motion abnormalities which may signal graft dysfunction or occlusion (Bojar, 2021). The process for separating the patient from CPB begins (Fiedler et al., 2020).

At the end of the case, mediastinal chest tubes are placed for blood and fluid drainage. The left pleural space is typically opened during the procedure. A pleural chest tube is placed to evacuate air and blood/fluid from the pleural space. The chest tubes are attached to a pleural drainage system set to −20 cm dry suction (Bojar, 2021). Epicardial pacing wires may be placed to allow for temporary pacing in case of postoperative bradycardia or heart block (Bojar, 2021).

Traditionally, surgeons have performed sternal fixation with wire cerclage. Newer studies have shown that rigid sternal fixation with sternal plating systems allows for improved upper extremity mobility and decreases postoperative pain in addition to sternal and wound complications (Engelman et al., 2019). After sternal fixation, the subcutaneous tissues and skin are closed (Bojar, 2021).

Cardioplegia, Myocardial Protection, and the Cardiopulmonary Bypass Pump

CPB allows surgery to be performed on a motionless heart with a bloodless surgical field (James et al., 2020). Prior to inserting CBP cannulas, a 3 mg/kg loading dose of heparin with an activated clotting time (ACT) goal of 400 to 480 seconds, depending on the type of circuit, is administered to prevent clotting when blood comes in contact with the CPB circuit (Bojar, 2021). Heparin resistance due to antithrombin III deficiency is likely if a 5 mg/kg of heparin fails to produce an ACT >480 seconds (Bojar, 2021). ACTs are monitored every 20 to 30 minutes during CPB (Bojar, 2021). Cardioplegia (CP) solution is a hyperkalemic mixture of blood and crystalloid fluid administered by a certified clinical perfusionist (CCP) who runs the CPB pump (Parrino, 2018). The CPB pump regulates flow to the organs as well as blood oxygen and carbon dioxide (CO_2) levels (Parrino, 2018). Traditional "blood" CP contains a higher ratio of blood to crystalloid (e.g., 1:1, 2:1, 4:1, or 8:1; Mack et al., 2021). The del Nido CP strategy (1:4 blood to crystalloid ratio) developed for pediatric cases has been gaining popularity in adult isolated CABG procedures in the last several years (Mack et al., 2021). In addition to causing reversible cardiac arrest, CP protects the myocardium by slowing cellular metabolism and conserving energy, thereby decreasing the risk of perioperative MI and mortality (Mack et al., 2021). Blood temperature is lowered to 34 to 35°C, depending on surgeon preference and type of procedure (Bojar, 2021).

In order to understand how CP is delivered, it is important to understand that cardiac venous drainage occurs via both the greater and lesser systems. The greater system drains 70% of the venous blood into the right atrium (James et al., 2020). The lesser system is comprised of the arteriosinusoidal and Thebesian veins (James et al., 2020). Antegrade (forward flow) CP is administered down the right and left coronary arteries via the aortic root (James et al., 2020). Antegrade CP is initiated with a high potassium solution (20–25 mmol/L) and a high rate (300 mL/min) in order to produce a rapid diastolic cardiac arrest (James et al., 2020; Mack et al., 2021). Retrograde CP is administered via the coronary sinus and comprises 70% of the blood flow through

the coronary sinus and the 30% thru the Thebesian and arteriosinusoidal route (James et al., 2020; Shakhnovich et al., 2019). CP is administered throughout the case to provide myocardial protection, either continuously or intermittently (James et al., 2020). Intermittent CP consists of a lower potassium (7–10 mmol/L) solution given at flow rates of 100 to 150 mL/min every 15 to 20 minutes to maintain cardiac arrest while on CPB (James et al., 2020). Moreover, CP solution contains bicarbonate or phosphate buffers to counteract lactic acid produced during anaerobic metabolism, and also includes a high osmolality component such as mannitol to help decrease intracellular edema (Shakhnovich et al., 2019).

The aorta is cross-clamped just distal to the antegrade cannula. While the aorta is cross-clamped and the heart is arrested, blood drains from the venous cannula (located in the right atrium or the vena cava) and brings it to a venous reservoir and then to the pump. From there blood moves to the heat exchanger which cools the blood, then travels to the membrane oxygenator which oxygenates and removes CO_2 from the blood (Bojar, 2021; Shakhnovich et al., 2019). Blood lost during surgery is suctioned from the surgical field and returned to the cardiotomy reservoir where blood is filtered to remove debris before moving to the venous reservoir (Bojar, 2021; Parrino, 2018). Blood then enters the systemic blood pump (Shakhnovich et al., 2019). Blood from the pump is returned to the patient via the aortic root vent cannula located in the ascending aorta (Parrino, 2018). The root vent consists of two tubes which join into one. One of the tubes is used to administer anterograde CP into the aortic root and down the coronary arteries (Parrino, 2018). The second tube is used to remove air from the left atrium (LA) at the end of procedures where the heart is opened (Parrino, 2018).

Restarting the heart occurs spontaneously after removing the cross-clamp and resuming normal circulation (Shakhnovich et al., 2019). The patient is warmed toward 36°C (96.8°F) prior to weaning from CPB (Bojar, 2021). Decannulation occurs after the patient is separated from CBP (Fiedler et al., 2020). Protamine sulfate is administered for heparin reversal (Bojar, 2021). An antifibrinolytic such as aminocaproic acid or tranexamic acid is administered intravenously to inhibit the breakdown of fibrin clots and decrease postop bleeding (Bojar, 2021). Coagulopathic patients may require administration of desmopressin (DDAVP), platelets, cryoprecipitate, or factor VII, depending on severity (Bojar, 2021). Once hemostasis is obtained, the chest is closed (Bojar, 2021).

Off-Pump Coronary Artery Bypass Graft

CABG surgery may be performed on a beating heart without using a cardiopulmonary bypass pump, or off-pump (OPCAB). Stabilization devices are used to position the heart and minimize movement while sewing the anastomoses (Shaefi et al., 2019). Fewer than 20% of all CABGs are performed as off-pump, with many surgeons reserving this technique for patients with one or two vessel disease, porcelain aorta (severe atheromatous plaquing at or near the site of aortic cross-clamping), and patients at risk for significant postoperative complications including severe pulmonary disease (Shaefi et al., 2019). Keeling and coworkers (2017) demonstrated a 5.5% conversion rate from OPCAB to ONCAB. Common reasons for conversion included need for improved visualization of the surgical field and hemodynamic instability (Keeling et al., 2017).

Minimally Invasive Surgical Revascularization

Minimally invasive procedures are associated with a decreased amount of surgically induced tissue trauma, earlier functionality, and faster postoperative recovery compared to standard median sternotomy incisions (Bonatti et al., 2020; Gobolos et al., 2019; Kitahari et al., 2019). Minimally invasive cardiac surgery (MICS) originated in 1994 and is used for patients requiring minimal grafting such as those with single vessel LAD disease or those with previous or planned PCIs to non-LAD vessels (Bonatti et al., 2020). MICS combined with PCI is referred to as hybrid coronary revascularization (HCR; Kiaii & Teefy, 2019). MICS can occur in conjunction with percutaneous revascularization for those patients deemed high risk for traditional CABG but would benefit from LIMA to LAD bypass (Bojar, 2021; Fuster et al., 2017; Zipes et al., 2019).

MICS encompasses different approaches including minimally invasive direct coronary artery bypass (MIDCAB) which is also called MICS coronary artery bypass graft (MICS-CABG), and totally endoscopic coronary artery bypass grafting (TECAB; Bonatti et al., 2021). MIDCAB procedures are performed via left anterior thoracotomy incision at the 4th intercostal space (ICS), giving the cardiac surgeon a direct view of the heart. They are performed while the patient is intubated and sedated. Historically, these procedures only involved bypassing the LAD with the LIMA in situ, but technological advances now allow the both the LIMA or RIMA to be used in situ or as "Y" grafts (Bonatti et al., 2021). MIDCAB procedures have decreased over the years due to the advent of thoracoscopic and robotic-assisted procedures (Bonatti et al., 2020, 2021).

TECAB surgery requiring the use of robotic technology was introduced in 1998 (Gobolos et al., 2019). Robotics improved visualization and magnification, while allowing the surgical team better camera control and surgical dexterity (Bonatti et al., 2021). In TECAB an incision is made at the 4th ICS at the anterior axillary line, in addition to creating two ports for instrumentation (Bonatti et al., 2021). The robot is used for harvesting the LIMA and grafting it to the LAD. TECAB can be done either off pump or on CPB via femoral cannulation. Triple and quadruple vessel TECAB have been reported but are rare. Studies have demonstrated that robotic-assisted TECAB increases the operative time compared to MIDCAB (Bonatti et al., 2021). In 2018, a proof-of-concept study showed that TECAB could be safely performed endoscopically, without robotic assistance (Gorki et al., 2018). The procedure is now called non-robotic TECAB (nrTECAB) (Bonatti et al., 2021).

Despite the benefits of MICS over traditional median sternotomy CABG, MICS is not without risks. Gobolos and coworkers (2019) published a systematic review of complications associated with TECAB, which included a 4.2% incidence of reoperation due to postoperative hemorrhage (Gobolos et al., 2019). Conversion to open median sternotomy or larger thoracotomy incision in two systematic reviews ranged from 4.3% to 11.5% (Bonatti et al., 2021; Gobolos et al., 2019). Common reasons for conversion include dense adhesions and bleeding (Bonatti et al., 2021; Gobolos et al., 2019).

CLINICAL PEARLS

- Angiotensin converting enzyme (ACE) inhibitors, angiotensin receptor blockers (ARB), and angiotensin receptor neprilysin inhibitors should be discontinued within 48 hours prior to surgery, as these medications are associated with postoperative vasoplegia (Bastopcu et al., 2021).
- If possible, oral P2Y12 antiplatelet agents should be stopped prior to surgery to prevent intraoperative bleeding. It is recommended to hold clopidogrel for 5 days, ticagrelor for 5 days, and prasugrel for 7 days (Bojar, 2021, p. 186).
- Nonsteroidal anti-inflammatory drugs (NSAIDs) are contraindicated in postoperative CABG patients. These medications have an FDA black box warning for early bypass graft closure (Hospira, 2021).

KEY TAKEAWAYS

- Medical therapy directed at modifiable risks can have a significant impact on secondary prevention and disease progression.
- Patients' overall health, age, and functional status are all important factors in determining surgical candidacy.
- All patients with CAD need secondary prevention medications to ameliorate disease progression (Lawton et al., 2021).
- Patients with radial grafts require CCB for 1-year postop to prevent vasospasm in the graft (Lawton et al., 2021).

EVIDENCE-BASED RESOURCES

For the most up to date guidelines, visit the American College of Cardiology's website. https://www.acc.org/guidelines

SYNTAX score: Grading system used to evaluate complexity and prognosis of patients undergoing PCI. https://syntaxscore.org/calculator/start.htm

STS Risk Calculator: Calculator used to calculate patients' risk of mortality and morbidities for most commonly performed cardiac surgeries.
http://riskcalc.sts.org/stswebriskcalc/calculate
Parrino, P. E. (2018). Cardiopulmonary bypass: An introduction. *CTS Net.* https://doi.org/10.25373/ctsnet.7364945.

4.3: SURGICAL TREATMENT OF VALVULAR HEART DISEASE

Proper valve function allows forward inflow through the atria and ventricles and is vital for normal cardiac output (CO). Understanding the various valvular disorders, their clinical presentations, and diagnostic criteria, medical management, and indications for surgical or percutaneous valve repair or replacement are essential for providing quality patient care (Bojar, 2021).

AORTIC STENOSIS

Once the diagnosis of AS is made, valve hemodynamics and symptoms are used to determine the stage of AS to further guide management (Otto et al., 2020). Asymptomatic patients should be followed closely with serial echocardiograms and clinical examinations (Knawar et al., 2018). Unfortunately, no medical treatment halts the progression of the AS once it occurs (Kang et al., 2020). It is important, however, to treat cardiovascular risk factors such as hypertension, hyperlipidemia, and diabetes mellitus with guideline-directed medical therapy (GDMT; Otto et al., 2020). Patients should be advised to maintain a heart-healthy lifestyle by exercising, eating a healthy diet, maintaining a normal body weight, and not smoking. In addition, patients should be educated to maintain optimal oral health to prevent infective endocarditis (IE; Otto et al., 2020).

Progression of AS is measured through serial echocardiograms and evaluation of symptoms. AS progression can vary; however, on average, peak velocity will increase by 0.3 m/sec, mean pressure will increase by 7 mmHg, and valve area will decrease by 0.1cm² annually (Kang et al., 2020). Patients should be educated to report symptoms immediately to their clinician. Patients who progress to severe valvular disease or who develop such symptoms as shortness of breath, heart failure, angina, or syncope should be evaluated by a multidisciplinary team either at a primary or comprehensive heart valve center (Davidson & Davidson, 2021; Otto et al., 2020). Table 4.1 shows potential intra- and postoperative cardiac surgery complications.

Valve Replacement: Mechanical Versus Bioprosthetic

Patients who are referred for surgical valve replacement must consider the type of valve they would prefer to be implanted. There are benefits and risks associated with both mechanical and bioprosthetic valves. A benefit of

TABLE 4.1: Potential Intra- and Postoperative Cardiac Surgery Complications

INTRA-OPERATIVE	EARLY POST-OPERATIVE	LATE POST-OPERATIVE
Aortic injury	Acute renal insufficiency or failure	
	Acute respiratory failure	
Arrhythmias (atrial and ventricular tachyarrhythmias, bradycardia, heart block)	Arrhythmias (atrial and ventricular tachyarrhythmias, bradycardia, heart block)	
Bleeding	Bleeding	Deep sternal wound infection
Brachial plexus injury	Bypass graft failure	Bypass graft failure
	Constipation	
	Delirium, short-term neurocognitive dysfunction	
	Dysphagia	
	Electrolyte abnormalities	
	Hemodynamic instability (e.g., cardiogenic shock, hypovolemia, vasoplegia)	
Mesenteric ischemia	Heparin-induced thrombocytopenia	
	Hypercarbia	
	Hyperglycemia	
	Hypoxia	
	Ileus	
	Pneumonia	
	Pneumothorax	
	Pulmonary edema	
Stroke	Stroke	

Source: Alexander, J. H., & Smith, P. K. (2016). Coronary artery bypass grafting. *The New England Journal of Medicine, 374,* 1954-1964. https://doi.org/10.1056/NEJMra 1406944; Bojar, R. M. (2021). *Manual of perioperative care in adult cardiac surgery* (6th ed.). John Wiley & Sons.

mechanical valves is their durability which decreases the risk of requiring subsequent valve replacement surgery. However, all mechanical heart valves regardless of position, such as aortic or mitral, require lifelong anticoagulant therapy with warfarin (Otto et al., 2020).

If oral anticoagulation (OAC) is held prior to an invasive procedure or surgery, bridging with therapeutic low molecular weight heparin (LMWH) subcutaneously or unfractionated heparin intravenously is indicated to prevent thromboembolism as subtherapeutic warfarin levels can lead to valve thrombosis (Otto et al., 2020).

Bioprosthetic heart valves are derived from bovine or porcine pericardial tissue (Figure 4.1; Joseph et al., 2017). Bioprosthetic valves do not require lifelong anticoagulation. Unfortunately, they have a higher rate of deterioration especially in younger patients, leading to an increased need for subsequent valve replacement (Rimmer et al., 2019). Approximately 50% to 60% of patients will experience bioprosthetic valve failure, such as stenosis or regurgitation, by 15% postprocedure (Davidson & Davidson, 2021). The choice of valve for replacement should occur via shared decision-making, accounting for patient's age, preferences, and values, as well as risks of long-term anticoagulation and potential for valve reintervention (Otto et al., 2020).

Surgical Aortic Valve Replacement

Surgical aortic valve replacements (SAVR) are performed through a full median sternotomy incision or through a minimally invasive incision with an upper sternotomy to the 4th or 5th intercostal space (ICS) or through a right anterior incision of the 2nd or 3rd ICS (Kirmani et al., 2017). All SAVR patients are placed on CPB. Cannulation sites for the CPB pump can be either central or peripheral, depending on the surgical approach. Once on CPB, an aortotomy is carried out to expose the native valve. Then the valve leaflets are removed, and the annulus is debrided. If indicated the aortic root can either be enlarged or replaced. The new valve is then seated and sutured in place (Celik et al., 2020).

Transcatheter Aortic Valve Replacement

Transcatheter aortic valve replacement (TAVR) is a catheter-based procedure in which a new tissue valve is implanted within the diseased native valve at the aortic root using a nonsurgical endovascular approach (Francone et al., 2020). Patients with severe symptomatic AS in either their native aortic valve or in a bioprosthetic AVR may be TAVR candidates (Davidson & Davidson, 2021). TAVR procedures are typically performed in a hybrid room in the cardiac catheterization laboratory. Hybrid rooms have advanced imaging technologies and function as ORs (Hertault et al., 2017). The procedure is performed under conscious sedation or general anesthesia depending on the surgical approach and surgeon preference (Butala et al., 2020). Conscious sedation is growing due to lower mortality rates, lengths of stay, and hospital costs (Butala et al., 2020).

The femoral artery (transfemoral) is the preferred route due to its minimal invasiveness, shorter recovery times, and lower length of hospital stays (Mach et al., 2021).

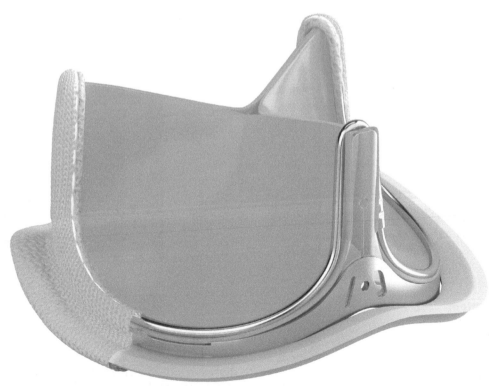

FIGURE 4.1: Inspiris Resilia® bioprosthetic heart valve.
Source: Courtesy of Edwards Lifesciences, LLC, Irvine, CA

Large bore sheaths are used to obtain femoral vascular access. Heavily calcified, tortuous, or small diameter arteries preclude the transfemoral route (Mach et al., 2021). If the patient's anatomy is not suitable for the transfemoral route, TAVR may be alternatively performed via the carotid artery (transcarotid) or through the axillary/subclavian artery (transsubclavian). A newer alternative approach is transcaval, which involves using transcaval introducers and creating a retroperitoneal connection between the inferior vena cava (IVC) and the aorta (Greenbaum et al., 2017). Post TAVR insertion, the transcaval access sites are closed with nitinol occluders (Greenbaum et al., 2017). If the patient's anatomy does not allow for percutaneous insertion, potential surgical approaches include a transapical implantation via a mini sternotomy or transapical through a small thoracotomy (Mach et al., 2021).

Despite the advances in TAVR technology, not everyone is a suitable candidate for the procedure. For example, hemodynamically unstable critically ill patients with severe AS may benefit from percutaneous balloon dilatation to alleviate symptoms and stabilize the patient. This may serve as a bridge to future intervention (Otto et al., 2020). Patients with severe symptomatic AS who are not expected to have significant improvements in quality of life or who have a life expectancy of <12 months post-TAVR may benefit from palliative care consultation (Otto et al., 2020). Palliative consultants meet with patients and their families to outline goals of care as part of the shared decision-making process.

TAVR patients are at risk of developing both asymptomatic and symptomatic valve thrombosis. Symptomatic thrombosis can present in a variety of ways including stroke, The majority of cases are asymptomatic, and are often referred to as subclinical valve thrombosis (Basra et al., 2018). Currently, in patients without an indication for systemic OAC, the AHA/ACC guidelines recommend treatment with lifelong aspirin 75 mg to 100 mg daily in addition to the clopidogrel daily for 3 to 6 months (Otto et al., 2020).

AORTIC REGURGITATION

Aortic regurgitation (AR), also known as aortic insufficiency (AI) occurs when an incompetent aortic valve is unable to close completely during diastole. It can occur acutely or develop over a period of years. If it is chronic, the development of heart failure symptoms may occur over years. In long-standing AR, the reflux of blood into the left ventricle (LV) causes dilatation and can lead to dilated cardiomyopathy (Flint et al., 2019). AR is classified as either primary or secondary, depending on the etiology. Primary causes of AR include degeneration of the valve leaflets themselves, which is common in patients with bicuspid aortic valves (Flint et al., 2019). Secondary causes of AR include abnormalities of the valve's supporting structures such as the aortic root or annulus (Flint et al., 2019). AR is also categorized as acute or chronic AR. The pathophysiology, etiologies, and severity of patient presentations in acute and chronic AR

differ. The indications for and timing of surgery also vary (Flint et al., 2019).

Acute Aortic Regurgitation

New onset acute AR is a life-threatening situation that requires prompt surgical intervention (Bojar, 2021). Acute AR is most often caused by endocarditis or aortic dissection but can also be caused by trauma or an iatrogenic complication from a transcatheter procedure (Flint et al., 2019; Otto et al., 2020). Acute pulmonary edema develops from acute volume overload on the LV and low CO. It causes hemodynamic instability and may lead to cardiogenic shock (Flint et al., 2019). Urgent diagnosis is made via transthoracic echocardiogram (TTE) or transesophageal echocardiogram (TEE). Patients with suspected AR due to a Stanford Type A aortic dissection should undergo immediate CT angiography (CTA). CTA is the gold standard for diagnosing aortic dissection. Acute Type A dissections require blood pressure and heart rate control to prevent aortic rupture, prior to emergent surgical intervention (Rimmer et al., 2019). During the operation to replace the damaged part of the aorta, the cardiac surgeon carefully evaluates the aortic valve (Flint et al., 2019). Depending on the amount of AR and anatomic disruption to the annulus, a valve-sparing ascending aortic repair may be possible instead of an AVR (Rimmer et al., 2019).

Chronic Aortic Regurgitation

Patients with chronic AR may be asymptomatic for years (Otto et al., 2020). The LV of patients with chronic AR responds to the volume overload through compensatory mechanisms to include increasing end-diastolic volume, increasing chamber compliance, and eventual LV hypertrophy. Increased wall thickness provides hemodynamic compensation and ejection fraction (EF) is initially maintained. When the EF becomes reduced from chronic volume and pressure overload, patients subsequently develop LV dysfunction and symptoms typically appear (Amano & Izumi, 2021).

AR management is dependent on the causes of the AR and the staging of the disease based on echocardiogram findings to include valve anatomy, hemodynamics, severity of LV dilation, LV systolic function as well as patient symptoms. Patients are staged from A to D. Stage A patients are at risk of developing AR, while stage D patients have symptomatic AR (Otto et al., 2020). Medical management includes diuresis to decrease pulmonary vascular congestion and improve oxygenation. ACE inhibitors, angiotensin II receptor blockers (ARBs), and nondihydropyridine CCB such as amlodipine (Flint et al., 2019). Beta-blockers are not commonly used to treat hypertension in patients with AR. Beta blockers may worsen AR symptoms since they slow the heart rate and prolong diastole (Flint et al., 2019). Intra-aortic balloon pump (IABP) counter pulsation will worsen AR during balloon inflation during diastole. As a result, IABP use is contraindicated in severe AR (Bojar, 2021).

Indications for Surgical Intervention for Aortic Regurgitation

One of the most important indications for surgical correction of AR is the development of symptoms such as dyspnea, pulmonary edema, and hypotension (Flint et al., 2019). Symptomatic patients are at an increased risk of death from AR (Otto et al., 2020). Worsening left ventricular function in the setting of AR is a class I indication for SAVR (Flint et al., 2019). Those with AR have better outcomes when SAVR is performed before the onset of symptoms (Otto et al., 2020). Patients with moderate to severe AR undergoing other cardiac surgical procedures should be considered for concomitant SAVR to avoid the need for repeat sternotomy and cardiac surgery in the future (Otto et al., 2020). SAVR is preferred over transcatheter AVR (TAVR) for most patients with AR (Otto et al., 2020). In patients with AR, the paucity of calcification of the annulus increases the risk of TAVR migration and paravalvular leak (Flint et al., 2019).

Surgical Aortic Valve Repair and Replacement for Aortic Regurgitation

In AR, SAVR is carried out much in the same manner as described earlier for AS, except for valve debridement (Bojar, 2021). Selected patients with AR may avoid aortic valve (AV) replacement if the valve is suitable for repair (Rimmer et al., 2019). Patients with AR may have concomitant aortic root aneurysms. Aortic root and/or ascending aortic aneurysms require replacement with Dacron tube grafts (Rimmer et al., 2019). Patients with AR and associated proximal aortic aneurysms may be candidates for valve-sparing procedures which ameliorate AR by resuspending the aortic valve (Rimmer et al., 2019).

MITRAL REGURGITATION

MR, also known as mitral insufficiency (MI), can occur from primary or secondary causes. Primary causes of MR involve abnormalities in the mitral valve apparatus to include the leaflets, chordae tendineae, papillary muscles, or the mitral annulus. The most common cause of primary MR is mitral valve prolapse due to degenerative disease (Harb & Griffin, 2017). Primary MR can also be caused by IE, rheumatic heart disease, mitral annular calcification, and other connective tissue disorders. Secondary causes of MR involve disorders that alter the size or function of the LV, which prevents the mitral valve from closing during systole. The treatment of MR depends upon the cause and severity, and whether it is acute or chronic (Harb & Griffin, 2017).

Acute Mitral Regurgitation

Acute MR can occur from IE, chord rupture, or papillary muscle rupture causing an abrupt increase in LV filling pressures and subsequent development of pulmonary edema. There is also a reduction in forward flow leading to cardiogenic shock (Harb & Griffin, 2017). MR is initially medically treated with diuretics, vasodilators, and inotropes (Harb & Griffin, 2017). Some patients benefit from IABP insertion to stabilize hemodynamics prior to urgent surgical intervention (Bojar, 2021).

Chronic Mitral Regurgitation

Chronic MR involves gradual LV and LA remodeling and enlargement from prolonged volume overload. The early compensated stage is followed by a decompensated stage when symptoms develop (Harb & Griffin, 2017). Asymptomatic patients with both primary and secondary chronic MR should have a TTE to assess LV size and function, mechanism of MR, and pulmonary artery pressures (Otto et al., 2020). Patients with secondary chronic MR with reduced EF and heart failure should also be treated medically with goal-directed medical therapy (GDMT) for heart failure. GDMT agents include ACE inhibitors or ARB, beta-blockers, diuretics, and aldosterone antagonists to improve symptoms, reduce LV volume, prevent or reverse myocardial remodeling, and decrease the severity of secondary MR (Baumgartner et al., 2017; Grayburn et al., 2020).

Indications for Surgical Intervention

Primary Mitral Regurgitation

There are several indications for surgical intervention in patients with primary MR. Interventions include surgical mitral valve repair (SMVr), surgical mitral valve replacement (SMVR), transcatheter mitral valve repair (TMVr), or transcatheter mitral valve replacement (TMVR). Mitral valve intervention is recommended in symptomatic patients with severe primary MR regardless of LV systolic function. It is also recommended in asymptomatic patients with severe primary MR and LV systolic dysfunction (LVEF ≤60% or LVESD ≥40 mmHg) and asymptomatic patients with normal systolic function but increasing LV size or decreasing EF by echocardiogram. SMVr is preferred over replacement in patients with severe primary MR from degenerative disease who are surgical candidates (Otto et al., 2020). Patients with severe symptomatic primary MR who have a prohibitive risk for SMVr should be considered for TMVr if the patient has a life expectancy of at least 1 year and they have the appropriate anatomy for the procedure to be successful (Otto et al., 2020).

Secondary Mitral Regurgitation

There are several indications for surgical interventions for patients with secondary MR as well. Mitral valve surgery can be considered in patients with severe secondary MR who are undergoing coronary artery bypass graft (CABG) for coronary artery disease. It is also reasonable in patients with chronic severe secondary MR from atrial annular dilation who have preserved LV systolic function (LVEF ≥50%) or LV systolic dysfunction (LVEF <50%) who have persistent symptoms despite optimal GDMT for heart failure (HF; Otto et al., 2020). Chordal sparing SMVR is preferred over SMVr in patients with CAD and chronic severe secondary MR related to LV systolic dysfunction (LVEF <50%) who are undergoing surgery for persistent symptoms despite optimal GDMT for HF (Otto et al., 2020).

Surgical Mitral Valve Repair or Replacement

Mitral valve surgery can be performed via median sternotomy or can be done through a minimally invasive approach such as partial sternotomy, right parasternal approach, or right anterolateral mini thoracotomy (Del Forno et al., 2021). Patients are placed on cardiopulmonary bypass (CPB). Access to the mitral valve is typically made through a left atriotomy and the mitral valve is inspected once it has been exposed. The surgeon analyzes the leaflets for mobility and chordal elongation or rupture. The subvalvular apparatus and the mitral annulus are also analyzed for degeneration, calcification, and dilation. This guides surgical planning. MVr often involves a prosthetic annuloplasty ring or band to restore the normal shape of the annulus and prevent future dilation. The most common leaflet repair involves resection of P2 as prolapse or flail of P2 is the most frequent cause of degenerative MR. Patients may also have repair of the anterior mitral leaflet or the chords (Del Forno et al., 2021). SMVr is preferable to replacement. However, SMVR is indicated when a satisfactory repair is not possible. Preservation of the chordae tendinae (chordal sparing) during the MVR is preferred, as it improves LV function and minimizes the risk of LV rupture (Bojar, 2021).

Transcatheter Mitral Valve Repair

TMVr, also called transcatheter end to end repair (TEER), is a percutaneous procedure performed with fluoroscopy via a femoral access where leaflets can be clipped together by MitraClip™ (Abbott Laboratories, North Chicago, IL; Abbott Laboratories, 2021; Baumgartner et al., 2017; Otto et al., 2020), which is the only FDA approved device for this purpose (Davidson & Davidson, 2021). It is typically performed in patients who are not candidates for open valve surgery (Davidson & Davidson, 2021; Otto et al., 2020). TMVr is preferred in patient with suitable anatomy for the procedure in patients with chronic severe secondary MR related to systolic function (LVEF <50%) who have persistent symptoms while on optimized GDMT. Patient must have an LVEF between 20% and 50%, pulmonary artery systolic pressure <70 mmHg, and LV end systolic diameter (LVESD) <70 mm to be considered for TMVr (Otto et al., 2020). A recent meta-analysis by Goel and coworkers (2020) demonstrated that TMVr along with medical management decreases hospital readmissions for acute HF compared to medical management alone.

Transcatheter Mitral Valve Replacement

TMVR may offer improved MR reduction in symptomatic patients with suitable anatomy, who are not candidates for SMVR (Hensey et al., 2021). Cardiac CT scans and TEEs are used to evaluate anatomy and assist with surgical planning (Hensey et al., 2021). The procedure is performed transapically or via transseptal puncture (Hensey et al., 2021). Potential complications of TMVR include paravalvular leaks, left ventricular outflow tract (LVOT) obstruction due to the proximity of the mitral and aortic valves, regional wall motion abnormalities due to compression of the left circumflex coronary artery, and pericardial effusions (Hensey et al., 2021). Valve-in-valve TMVR may be done in select patients with failure of a bioprosthetic SMVR (Davidson & Davidson, 2021).

MITRAL STENOSIS

Mitral stenosis (MS) is most commonly caused by rheumatic heart disease from untreated Streptococcus infection. MS from rheumatic heart disease progresses slowly over time. Other less common etiologies of MS include radiation valvulitis, congenital causes, systemic inflammatory disorders, or obstructing lesions such as infectious vegetations or atrial myxoma (Harb & Griffin, 2017). Patients with mild to moderate MS should be followed closely with a yearly physical exam, chest radiograph, and ECG. An echocardiogram should also be performed when any changes are noted (Bojar, 2021). Medical treatment includes diuretics and treatment of atrial fibrillation (AF), should it develop, with rate control agents and anticoagulation with warfarin (Harb & Griffin, 2017). Patients with severe MS, those with mitral valve area (MVA) <1.5 cm², or those with progressive MS with exertional symptoms should be referred to a comprehensive valve center (Otto et al., 2020).

Indications for Mitral Stenosis Intervention

Patients who develop symptoms from MS should have a TTE to establish the diagnosis, assess the hemodynamic severity of the MS, diagnose any concomitant valvular abnormalities, and assess valve morphology for subsequent percutaneous balloon commissurotomy (PMBC) or SMVR (Otto et al., 2021).

Mitral valve repair or replacement is indicated in severely symptomatic patients with severe rheumatic MS (MVA <1.5 cm²). Mitral valve surgery may also be indicated in patients who have failed PMBC or who are undergoing cardiac surgery for another indication (Otto et al., 2021). Severely symptomatic patients with multiple comorbidities who are not surgery candidates should be referred to a comprehensive valve center for consideration of PMBC (Otto et al., 2021).

Percutaneous Mitral Balloon Commissurotomy

PMBC is recommended for symptomatic patients with severe rheumatic MS with appropriate valve morphology, if there is no LA thrombus seen on TEE. PMBC may also be considered in asymptomatic patients with severe MS (MVA <1.5cm²) and in those with elevated pulmonary pressures (PAP) >50 mmHg (Otto et al., 2021). Additionally, patients who have MS but no evidence of MR, who develop new onset AF may be PMBC candidates (Otto et al., 2021). Contraindications to PMBC include mitral valve area (MVA) >1.5 cm², mild MR, severe bicommissural calcification, absence of commissural fusion, severe concomitant valve disease, concomitant coronary artery disease, and the presence of LA or LV thrombus (Wunderlich et al., 2019).

PMBC is performed in the cardiac catheterization lab under conscious sedation. TEE is performed to confirm absence of LA or LV thrombus. Access to the LA is obtained by guiding a catheter through transseptal puncture under fluoroscopy. Once access is obtained, the correct balloon size is determined by patient height, body surface area, and degree of mitral calcification. The balloon tipped catheter is then advanced across the mitral valve and inflated between the two mitral leaflets (Wunderluch et al., 2019). The procedure is considered successful if the MVA is increased to >1.5 cm^2 without complications. Complications include cardiac tamponade from unintentional puncture during the procedure, embolic events from either thromboembolism or air embolism, or development of MR from a commissural tear or rupture of a component of the subvalvular apparatus (Wunderlich et al., 2019).

Surgical Mitral Valve Repair or Replacement

Mitral valve repair or replacement is indicated in severely symptomatic patients with severe rheumatic MS who are not candidates for PMBC, have failed PMBC, or are undergoing cardiac surgery for other reasons (Otto et al., 2020). SMVR or repair is performed with CPB by median sternotomy or lateral thoracotomy. The mitral valve is replaced with either a bioprosthetic or mechanical valve, the latter requiring life-long anticoagulation with warfarin. In some cases, the valve can be repaired by releasing fused chordae, elongating shortened chordae, or implanting an annuloplasty ring, if indicated (Wunderlich et al., 2019). Mitral valve repair has been shown to have fewer complications and all-cause death than mitral valve replacement (Fu et al., 2021). Refer to Table 4.1, Potential Intra- and Postoperative Complications of Cardiac Surgery.

KEY TAKEAWAYS

- Recognition of valvular heart disease prior to the onset of symptoms leads to superior outcomes with intervention.
- Patients with valvular heart disease need to be monitored closely with serial clinical exams which include auscultation of heart tones; changes in heart sounds, functional capacity, or the initiation of symptoms should prompt echocardiography.
- Echocardiography is the standard tool in evaluation of valvular heart disease, providing measurements for grading of severity.
- Patients with symptomatic or severe valvular heart disease should be referred to either a primary or comprehensive valve center for evaluation with a multidisciplinary team.

4.4: INFECTIVE ENDOCARDITIS

Infective endocarditis (IE) is the most fatal form of valvular heart disease, with nearly a 100% mortality if untreated (Pettersson & Hussain, 2019). It can occur in native valves and prosthetic (bioprosthetic or mechanical) valves. In recent years, the rates of IE and the number of surgeries for the treatment of IE have increased due to higher numbers of invasive procedures and medical device implantations, improved survival among patients with congenital cardiac anomalies, and increasing rates of IV drug use. Other IE risk factors include, advanced age, diabetes, and end-stage renal disease requiring dialysis (Jamil et al., 2019; Wang et al., 2018). IE has an in-hospital mortality rate of 15% to 20% and 1-year mortality rate of up to 40% (Pettersson & Hussain, 2019). Due to the high mortality rate and complex presentation of patients with IE, the treatment requires a multidisciplinary team including cardiologists, infectious disease specialists, neurologists, and cardiac surgeons (Pettersson et al., 2017). Together, the endocarditis team can determine whether medical management with or without valve repair or replacement is indicated.

Some organisms are more aggressive and can cause severe valvular regurgitation and heart failure (HF) or embolization; early surgical intervention may be warranted. Less virulent organisms may be treated with IV antibiotics alone without need for surgical intervention. The standard length of treatment with IV antibiotics is 6 weeks (Pettersson & Hussain, 2019).

The valve infected is also an important consideration in the management of the patient with IE. Left-sided IE is an infection of the mitral or aortic valve and it carries a higher incidence of embolism and stroke, therefore early surgical intervention is often warranted. Right-sided IE of the tricuspid or pulmonic valve can often be treated with IV antibiotics alone. The indications for surgical intervention in right-sided IE include septic pulmonary embolism, persistent infection, or severe tricuspid regurgitation (Pettersson & Hussain, 2019).

DIFFERENTIAL DIAGNOSIS AND DIAGNOSTIC CONSIDERATIONS

The diagnosis of IE is made using the Modified Duke Criteria and is discussed in Chapter 3, "Disorders of the Cardiovascular System." The Modified Duke Criteria evaluates major and minor criteria and determines if a patient is definite, possible, or excluded from the diagnosis of endocarditis.

SURGICAL TREATMENT OF ENDOCARDITIS

There are several indications for early surgical intervention for patients with IE. Patients who have signs of heart failure, severe valvular dysfunction, a paravalvular abscess, a large vegetation measuring >10 mm, recurrent systemic embolization, persistent infection despite antibiotics, or prosthetic valve endocarditis (PVE) should be considered for early surgery (Pettersson et al., 2017). In addition, IE from *Staphylococcus aureus*, *Streptococcus bovis*, or fungi increases a patient's risk for embolism in left-sided endocarditis, as does mobile vegetations, a prior history of embolism, and having an anterior mitral valve endocarditis (Yanagawa et al., 2016).

Once there is an indication for surgery, surgeons should proceed with valve repair or replacement without delay. Studies have shown that delaying surgery has the potential to cause patient harm including worsening heart failure, repeat embolic events, and possibly death (Yanagawa et al., 2016). The surgery should be scheduled within days of diagnosis in the absence of stroke with neurological deficits.

Timing of surgery in patients with neurological symptoms is decided between neurologists and cardiac surgeons based on the risk of expanding the stroke or causing hemorrhagic conversion during the surgery. Patients with neurological symptoms should have imaging with CT and MRI to determine the cause, location, and size of the infarct and to look for intracranial bleeding and mycotic aneurysm. Typically, surgery is delayed for 1 to 2 weeks in patients with embolic stroke and 3 to 4 weeks in patients with hemorrhagic stroke as these patients are at higher risk for further intracranial bleeding during surgery (Pettersson & Hussain, 2019).

Prior to surgery, an operative risk assessment should be performed. The Society of Thoracic Surgeons (STS) endocarditis score as well as the DeFeo and colleagues score are two tools that can be used to predict operative mortality risk based on patient comorbidities, the clinical status of the patient, and the experience of the surgeon and operative team among others (De Feo et al., 2012). Patients are at a higher risk of operative mortality when they are on preoperative inotropes, have an intra-aortic balloon pump (IABP), have had prior open-heart surgery, or have end-stage renal disease requiring hemodialysis (Habib et al., 2015; Pettersson et al., 2017). The most common complications of surgery for IE are bleeding, need for transfusion of blood products, cardiac tamponade, reoperation, stroke, acute kidney injury (AKI), pneumonia, and heart block (Habib et al., 2015).

Pre- and Postoperative Management of Patients With Infectious Endocarditis

There are several standards of care for the perioperative management of patients with IE. First, preoperative antibiotics should be continued based on culture and sensitivities. Intraoperatively, all patients should have a transesophageal echocardiogram (TEE) before valvular repair to assess for expansion of the infection and function of the valves. A TEE should also be done intraoperatively post valvular repair or replacement to assess valvular repair or prosthetic valve function and to determine if there is any residual pathology or complication of surgery (Pettersson & Hussain, 2019; Pettersson et al., 2017).

The surgery is performed via open sternotomy using cardiopulmonary bypass (CPB). The surgery involves radical debridement and removal of the infected tissue to prevent residual infection. Repair or replacement of the valve is determined by the valve infected and the degree of infection at the time of surgery. Mitral valve and tricuspid valve repair is preferred over replacement while the aortic valve typically requires replacement with a bioprosthetic or mechanical valve. The choice of type of valve is determined by the patient's age, life expectancy, comorbidities, risk of bleeding with anticoagulation, and anticipated compliance with anticoagulation. Mechanical heart valves should be avoided in patients with intracranial hemorrhage, large strokes, or at high risk for bleeding with anticoagulation. Extension of infection into the surrounding tissue may require additional debridement and surgical reconstruction to include aortic root replacement. All surgical specimens should be sent to the microbiology and pathology labs for testing (Pettersson & Hussain, 2019; Pettersson et al., 2017).

Postoperatively, the standards of care are similar to those for any other valvular surgery. Additionally, all patients with IE should be treated with a prolonged course of IV antibiotics. The typical duration of treatment is 6 weeks, but the choice and duration of antibiotic regimen may be adjusted based on the organism and sensitivity to antibiotics (Habib et al., 2015; Pettersson & Hussain, 2019; Pettersson et al., 2017).

Antiplatelet or anticoagulant therapy is prescribed in all patients who have had valvular repair or replacement. Patients who have bioprosthetic aortic or mitral valves are recommended to have warfarin anticoagulation for 3 months postsurgery followed by lifelong aspirin therapy. Patients who receive mechanical valves should have lifelong warfarin therapy with international normalized ratio (INR) goal of 2.5 for aortic valves and 3.0 for mitral valves. Anticoagulant therapy should be initiated as soon as surgical risk for bleeding is mitigated (Otto et al., 2020).

TRANSITION OF CARE

The transition of care after hospitalization is determined by many patient factors. Patients may be able to transition to home if they have a safe environment to return to with adequate family or social support. Early case management consultation is required in the hospital course to determine what level of care will be needed as the patient transitions out of the hospital system. Patients will require IV antibiotics to complete their full 6-week course. Patients and family require education about the administration of antibiotics and the care of peripherally inserted central venous catheters (PICC). Home health nursing consultation is required. Patients who do not have adequate social support or patients who have a history of IV drug abuse may not be able to transition to home and will require transition to a skilled nursing facility or acute rehabilitation facility after discharge from the hospital (Stoicea et al., 2017). Patients who will be receiving warfarin therapy will need prothrombin time/INR laboratory monitoring for dose adjustments.

KEY TAKEAWAYS

- Endocarditis can occur in native or prosthetic valves.
- The majority of cases of endocarditis are caused by *Staphylococci*, *Streptococci*, or *Enterococcus*.
- A multidisciplinary team involving cardiology, cardiothoracic surgery, neurology, and infectious disease is necessary to properly manage IE.
- Left-sided IE is an infection of the mitral or aortic valve and it carries a higher incidence of embolism and stroke; therefore, early surgical intervention is often warranted.
- Oral anticoagulant (OAC) with warfarin anticoagulation is recommended for 3 months after bioprosthetic surgical aortic valve replacement (SAVR) or mitral valve replacement (MVR) surgery. However, cardiac surgeons may avoid routine OAC in this population due to bleeding risk, unless there is a compelling indication such as postoperative atrial fibrillation (AF).
- Patients who receive mechanical valves require life-long warfarin therapy with INR goal of 2.5 for aortic valves and 3.0 for mitral valves.
- IV antibiotic therapy will be continued at discharge to complete a 6-week course.
- Patients who do not have adequate social support or patients who have a history of IV drug abuse may not be able to transition to home and will require transition to a skilled nursing facility or acute rehabilitation facility after discharge from the hospital.

4.5: PERICARDITIS

INFECTIOUS PERICARDITIS

Viral illness is suspected of causing roughly 80% of idiopathic cases of acute pericarditis, with the majority stemming from adenoviruses, enteroviruses (e.g., Coxsackie viruses), herpesviruses (e.g., cytomegalovirus, human herpes 6 viruses, Epstein-Barr viruses), and parvovirus B19 (Imazio et al., 2015). Conversely, purulent pericarditis is uncommon. This type of acute endocarditis may result from bloodstream infections associated with infectious endocarditis or myocardial abscesses. In other cases, it is caused by direct pathogen spread from pulmonary infections (e.g., empyema or pneumonia) or trauma (Adler et al., 2015; Doctor et al., 2017). Tubercular pericarditis is uncommon in developed countries but may account for up to 70% of cases of acute pericarditis in developing nations. Tubercular pericarditis is very fatal, especially in those with immunosuppression. Patients with HIV have 40% 6-month mortality (Imazio et al., 2015).

Patients with purulent pericarditis often present with a septic picture. They may be febrile, tachycardiac, and/or hypotensive (Adler et al., 2015). This condition has a high mortality rate and immediate treatment of sepsis with fluid resuscitation and broad-spectrum antibiotics, along with consulting cardiology or cardiothoracic surgery for drainage, are paramount for survival (Adler et al., 2015).

Percutaneous or surgical drainage is necessary for patients with hemorrhagic or purulent pericarditis (refer to section 4.6, "Pericardial Effusion/Cardiac Tamponade"). Pericardiectomy is indicated in those with constrictive pericarditis. It is often done as a last resort since it has an associated with a 5% to 10% mortality (Bojar, 2021; Doctor et al., 2017; Imazio et al., 2017). Those at increased risk of death include poor systolic left ventricular (LV) function, elevated pulmonary artery pressures, and those whose condition was caused by radiation therapy (Bojar, 2021). The operation is performed via median sternotomy with cardiopulmonary bypass (CPB) pump standby. The procedure may take several hours depending on the extent of the calcific adhesions. The adhesions that cannot be safely removed are left in place (Bojar, 2021).

4.6: PERICARDIAL EFFUSION/CARDIAC TAMPONADE

Approximately 66% of patients with pericarditis will develop pericardial effusions. The majority of these effusions are small, asymptomatic, and do not require intervention. Hemodynamically insignificant effusions are seen on approximately one out of every 10 transthoracic echocardiograms. Pericardial effusions can result from the same inflammatory and noninflammatory conditions that cause pericarditis (Lekhakul et al., 2018). Iatrogenic effusions occur from trauma during procedures such cardiac device implantation (e.g., pacemakers or internal cardioverter defibrillators), catheter ablation (CA) of arrhythmias, or heart surgery (Horr et al., 2017).

PRESENTING SIGNS AND SYMPTOMS

The presentation of pericardial effusions varies based on how quickly the fluid accumulates in the pericardial sac. Rapid fluid buildup may cause more severe symptoms and be immediately life-threatening, even with relatively low volumes of blood of fluid in the pericardial sac (Vakamudi et al., 2017). Patients with acute tamponade may present with dizziness, lightheadedness, syncope, pre-syncope, hypotension, narrowed pulse pressure, tachycardia, tachypnea, orthopnea, and shortness of breath (Honasoge & Dubbs, 2018). Chronic pericardial effusions may increase in size over time, eventually leading to severe symptoms and risk of death. Dyspnea, fatigue, dysphagia, hoarseness (if recurrent laryngeal nerve compression), hiccups (if phrenic nerve compression), and nausea (if diaphragm compression) may be related to slowly enlarging effusions. Although Beck's Triad is part of the "classic" presentation of cardiac tamponade, not all patients will have these signs

(Honasoge & Dubbs, 2018). Beck's Triad consists of three concomitant physical findings which include muffled heart sounds, jugular venous distention (JVD), and hypotension (York et al., 2018). Hypotension is a late sign of cardiac tamponade due to increased adrenergic compensation (Appleton et al., 2017). Pulsus paradoxus (systolic blood pressure decrease >10 mmHg with inspiration) and hepatojugular reflex may be present (Honasoge & Dubbs, 2018).

As the effusion progresses to cardiac tamponade an obstructive shock picture develops: CO decreases, and systemic vascular resistance (SVR) increases. External compression of the heart increases right atrial pressure (RAP), also known as central venous pressure (CVP), and left atrial pressure (LAP) rise. LAP is commonly referred to as pulmonary artery occlusion pressure (PAOP). Once tamponade occurs, pressures within the right and left heart equalize (RAP = PAOP; Appleton et al., 2017; York et al., 2018).

DIAGNOSTIC FINDINGS

Obtaining an emergent transthoracic echocardiogram helps confirm the presence of pericardial tamponade. Echocardiogram findings include right atrial collapse (Figure 4.2), right ventricular early diastolic collapse, LA collapse, inferior vena cava (IVC) plethora (failure to decrease proximal diameter by 50% or more on inspiration), and significant variation in mitral and tricuspid valve inflow during respiration (Honasoge & Dubbs, 2018; Vakamudi et al., 2017). Other diagnostic studies such as ECG (may see evidence of low voltage and/or electrical alterans which is defined as variation in the QRS complex amplitude with each heartbeat) and chest radiograph (e.g., enlarged pericardial silhouette often called a "water bottle" sign) may indicate potential tamponade, but they are not confirmatory tests (Honasoge & Dubbs, 2018; York et al., 2018).

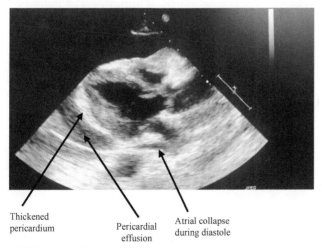

Thickened pericardium

Pericardial effusion

Atrial collapse during diastole

FIGURE 4.2: Cardiac tamponade on echocardiogram.
Source: Courtesy of Kelly A. Thompson-Brazill, DNP, ACNP-BC, FCCM.

CLINICAL PEARLS

- IVC plethora is defined as a diameter >2.1 cm with less than 50% decrease in the IVC diameter with inspiration (Vakamudi et al., 2017).
- Estimated pericardial effusion size is based on the degree of separation of the pericardium and the myocardium at the end of diastole (Vakamudi et al., 2017)
  - Small effusion <10 mm
  - Moderate effusion 10 to 20 mm
  - Large effusion 20 to 25 mm
  - Very large effusion >25 mm

TREATMENT

IV administration of crystalloid fluid and vasopressor medications such as dopamine or norepinephrine may help temporize labile blood pressures until the pericardial fluid is emergently evacuated (Honasoge & Dubbs, 2018; Vakamudi et al., 2017). Supplemental oxygen is often needed to correct hypoxia. Some patients may require intubation and mechanical ventilation (Honasoge & Dubbs, 2018).

Percutaneous Drainage

Pericardiocentesis is the generally preferred emergency drainage procedure since it does not require general anesthesia. It is done using ultrasound or echocardiographic guidance to prevent iatrogenic injury to the right ventricle (Maisch et al., 2017; Vakamudi et al., 2017). A pericardial catheter stays in place for at least 24 hours and remains until the drainage is <100 mL in a 24-hour period and there is resolution of the effusion on echocardiogram (Vakamudi et al., 2017).

Surgical Drainage

Surgical drainage of the pericardial effusion is indicated for located effusions and effusions located where it is not safe to attempt a percutaneous procedure and recurrent pericardial effusions that fail pericardiocentesis (Bojar, 2021). Since these patients are often hemodynamically unstable and at risk for cardiac arrest during anesthesia induction, it is preferrable to perform the surgery in a cardiac OR with a trained cardiac surgery team.

The procedure requires making a subxiphoid incision, entering the pericardium. This allows for drainage of the fluid and excision of a portion of pericardium. A chest tube is inserted and left to drain for a few days until the drainage is minimal and the effusion is completely evacuated (Bojar, 2021). The pericardial fluid is sent for a variety of testing including cell count (white and red blood cells) glucose, lactate dehydrogenase (LDH), protein, fluid pH, and culture. Medical cytology and pericardial biopsy determine if metastatic cancer is the etiology of the pericardial effusion (Vakamudi et al., 2017). See Chapter 5, "Thoracic Surgery," for a full discussion of transudative and exudative effusion fluid analysis and differential diagnoses.

Malignant pericardial effusions are a marker of advanced disease and are associated with a poor prognosis. The majority of cases occur in patients who already have a cancer diagnosis. Unfortunately for some, the cytology from pericardial effusion may be the first time they learn they have cancer (Lekhakul et al., 2018). A recent propensity-matched study by Horr and colleagues (2017) revealed decreased incidence in reaccumulation of pericardial effusions in patients who underwent surgical versus percutaneous drainage (10% vs. 24%, p <0.0001). Patients who developed effusions after cardiac surgery and those who required drainage during cardiac arrest resuscitation were excluded (Horr et al., 2017).

4.7: SURGICAL TREATMENT OF ATRIAL FIBRILLATION

Atrial fibrillation (AF) is the most common chronic cardiac arrhythmia in adult-gerontology patients (Davies et al., 2017; Michaud & Stevenson, 2021). Candidates for cardiac surgery procedures have an increased incidence of both chronic and acute onset AF (Michaud & Stevenson, 2021; Wang et al., 2020). In a recent study, 19% of newly diagnosed AF patients had a major event causing sympathetic nervous system activation prior to the onset of AF (Michaud & Stevenson, 2021; Wang et al., 2020). These triggers include cardiac surgery, myocardial infarction, pericarditis, myocarditis, as well as sepsis, pneumonia, pulmonary embolus, and respiratory failure (Wang et al., 2020). AF significantly increases the risk for embolic stroke and heart failure (HF), as well as doubling the risk of myocardial infarction (MI) and increasing the risk of mortality 40% to 50% (Badhwar et al., 2017).

Patients with AF have a wide variety of symptoms, ranging from asymptomatic to fatigue, palpitations, diminished exercise capacity, hypotension, angina, and/or syncope (Michaud & Stevenson, 2021). Besides focusing on modifying risk factors such as hypertension and diabetes, providers prescribe medications to control heart rate, achieve and maintain normal sinus rhythm, and prevent stroke (Michaud & Stevenson, 2021). Unfortunately, not all patients achieve rate or rhythm control. Patients with severe symptoms or those who do not tolerate atrioventricular (AV) nodal blocking or antiarrhythmic agents, or systemic anticoagulation should consult with an electrophysiologist. These patients may require direct current (DC) cardioversion or more invasive procedures to control rhythm and improve their quality of life (Michaud & Stevenson, 2021). A recent study demonstrated that patients with AF that underwent rhythm-control treatments had significantly lower rates of hospital admissions for acute coronary syndromes (ACS) and HF.

RHYTHM CONTROL PROCEDURES

Catheter-based, surgical, and hybrid rhythm control procedures are commonly employed to restore sinus rhythm and prevent embolic strokes (Davies et al., 2017). Catheter ablation (CA) is typically the first invasive procedure performed (Bisleri & Glover, 2017). If CA is unsuccessful, members of the multidisciplinary heart team (electrophysiologists and cardiac surgeons), may decide to pursue surgical ablation (SA) or a combined CA and SA procedure (Badhwar et al., 2017; Bisleri & Glover, 2017; Davies et al., 2017).

CLINICAL PEARLS

- Decreased symptoms
- Lower incidence of embolic stroke
- Improved quality of life
- Longer survival

Surgical Ablation

Surgical AF ablation targets the triggers (macrocircuits) for paroxysmal atrial fibrillation (PAF) located in or near the four pulmonary veins that return oxygenated blood to the left atrium (LA; Bisleri & Glover, 2017; Michaud & Stevenson, 2021; Ruaengsri et al., 2018). Surgical AF ablation dates back to the early 1980s, but it failed to produce reliable rhythm control until the Cox-maze SA procedure was first performed in 1987 (Davies et al., 2017). Over the years, the operation was refined. SA is now performed via mini thoracotomy in patients undergoing minimally invasive mitral and/or tricuspid valve surgery, in addition to the standard median sternotomy approach used for coronary artery bypass and multivalve surgery (Ruaengsri et al., 2018). The initial Cox-maze was time consuming and technically difficult. It involved creating surgical incisions and hand-suturing them. The current Cox-maze IV utilizes energy-emitting devices (radiofrequency or cryoablation) to create transmural lesions sets in the myocardium (Davies et al., 2017). The surgically created lesions inhibit the transmission of abnormal electrical impulses. The lesions essentially produce a "maze" by limiting the conduction to the "corridors," thereby preventing the signals from reaching large portions of the atrium (Badhwar et al., 2017; Davies et al., 2017). There are several methods for achieving SA. These include biatrial maze, right atrial maze, left atrial maze (most commonly performed with mitral valve surgery), and bilateral pulmonary vein isolation (PVI; Badhwar et al., 2017; Bisleri & Glover, 2017; Davies et al., 2017; Figure 4.3). Bilateral PVI is primarily used in patients with paroxysmal AF. Biatrial maze has higher rates of eradicating AF compared to other types of SA. Unfortunately, it is also associated with increased rates of sinoatrial node dysfunction requiring permanent pacemaker (PPM) insertion (Bojar, 2021).

AF is common in cardiac surgery patients. AF is present in 30% of patients with mitral valve disease, 14% with aortic valve disease, and 6% of those with isolated coronary artery disease (Badhwar et al., 2017). According to the 2017 Society of Thoracic Surgeons guidelines,

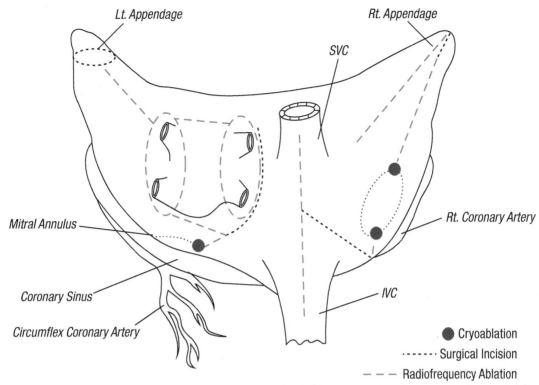

FIGURE 4.3: Cox-maze IV lesion set (median sternotomy approach). Left-sided lesions: 1. right pulmonary vein lesions; 2. left pulmonary vein lesions; 3. superior connecting lesion, left pulmonary vein to right pulmonary vein (roof); 4. inferior connecting lesion, left pulmonary vein to right pulmonary vein (floor); 5. mitral annulus lesion and 6. coronary sinus lesion. Right-sided lesions: 7. SVC to IVC lesions; 8. tricuspid valve lesions (10 o'clock); 9. right atrial free wall lesion and 10. tricuspid valve lesions (2 o'clock).

IVC: inferior vena cava; LAA: left atrial appendage; RF: radiofrequency; SVC: superior vena cava.

Source: Reproduced with permission from Lall, S. C., Melby, S. J., Voeller, R. K., Zierer, A., Bailey, M. S., Guthrie, T. J., Moon, M. R., Moazami, N., Lawton, J. S., & Damiano, R. J., Jr. (2007). The effect of ablation technology on surgical outcomes after the Cox-maze procedure: a propensity analysis. *The Journal of Thoracic and Cardiovascular Surgery, 133*(2), 389–396. https://doi.org/10.1016/j.jtcvs.2006.10.009.

SA performed in conjunction with other cardiac surgical procedures such as valve surgery (e.g., aortic or mitral) and/or coronary artery bypass graft (CABG) is a Class IA recommendation (Badhwar et al., 2017). There are several Class IIA indications for SA in patients who do not need concomitant open heart surgery. These include symptomatic patients who have failed Class I/III antiarrhythmic therapy or CA, patients with longstanding or persistent symptomatic AF. Left atrial ablation during SA is also a Class IIA recommendation (Badhwar et al., 2017).

The left atrial appendage (LAA) is a finger-like outpouching of left atrial tissue. It is comprised of several lobes that may promote arrhythmia generation and contain up to 90% of atrial thrombi (Delgado et al., 2017; Wats et al., 2020). Surgical LAA ligation (LAAL) is typically performed in conjunction with SA or other cardiac surgeries. The appendage cavity is obliterated by either oversewing the entrance with suture or using epicardially applied devices such as the AtriClip® (AtriCure, Mason,

OH, USA) to prevent blood from entering the LAA. Some cardiac surgeons prefer surgically removing (amputation) the LAAL to excluding it (Badhwar et al., 2017).

CLINICAL PEARLS

- Periprocedural anticoagulation (Bojar, 2021):
  - Stop direct acting oral anticoagulant (DOAC) agents 36 to 48 hours prior to surgery.
  - Stop vitamin K agonists (warfarin) 5 days prior to surgery.
    - A heparin bridge is indicated in patients at high risk for embolic stroke (e.g., stroke or embolus within the previous 3 months, CHA_2DS_2-VASc score ≥5, and/or rheumatic MS).

Hybrid Ablation

The convergent procedure (CVP) is a hybrid (combination) of both surgical and catheter-based ablation (Khan et al., 2020). It was first performed by Dr. Andy C. Kiser in 2009 for the treatment of longstanding or persistent AF (Wats et al., 2020). Like stand-alone SA, CVP is a Class IIA indication for symptomatic patients who fail anti-arrhythmic therapy or cardiac ablation (CA; Badhwar et al., 2017). It is performed in a hybrid OR which is typically located in the cardiac catherization laboratory (Bisleri & Glover, 2017). Traditional catheter-based techniques ablate AF triggers within the endocardium, while surgical methods focus on those in the epicardium. The CA and SV procedures may be performed the same day (concurrent) or on different days (staged) 6 to 8 weeks apart (Kahn et al., 2020).

In addition to the standard femoral accesses for CA, CVP utilizes a subxiphoid incision to access the pericardium. Pericardioscopy allows the surgeon to laparoscopically insert a radiofrequency catheter ablation (RFA) catheter from the upper abdomen into the pericardium. This allows the surgeon to directly see the tissue and creates an RFA lesion set on the epicardium of the posterior wall of the heart (Wats et al., 2020). After SA, the electrophysiologist completes the CA portion of the procedure (Bojar, 2021). Potential complications include cardiac tamponade, phrenic nerve palsy, and death (Box 4.1). Not surprisingly, complication rates are higher with CVP compared to CA or SA alone (Wats et al., 2020).

Atrioventricular Nodal Ablation

As a last resort, symptomatic patients who have failed medical therapy and/or CA, SA, or hybrid AF ablation may benefit from AV node ablation. This may be an option for patients with symptomatic AF refractory to medication, particularly those who have episodes of medication-induced bradycardia. AV node ablation is a CA that prevents RVR by inducing complete heart block

---

BOX 4.1 POTENTIAL POSTOPERATIVE COMPLICATIONS OF HYBRID ABLATION

- Cardiac arrest–implement Cardiac Surgical Unit–Advanced Life Support (CSU-ACLS) protocol
  - Goal of re-sternotomy within 2 minutes of arrest
- Cardiac tamponade
- Pneumothorax
- Hemothorax
- Cardiogenic shock
- Renal failure
- Mesenteric ischemia
- Cerebrovascular accident
- Delirium

Source: Data from Wats, K., Kiser, A., Makati, K., Sood, N., DeLurgio, D., Greenberg, Y., & Yang, F. (2020). The convergent atrial fibrillation ablation procedure: Evolution of a multidisciplinary approach to atrial fibrillation management. *Arrhythmia & Electrophysiology Review*, 9(2), 88–96. https://doi.org/10.15420/aer.2019.20

(Michaud & Stevenson, 2021). The downside to this procedure is that it requires permanent pacemaker insertion (Michaud & Stevenson, 2021).

CLINICAL PEARLS

- An ablation is not considered a "failure" unless AF recurs 6 months or more after the procedure (January et al., 2019).

PROCEDURES THAT REMEDY ANTICOAGULATION INTOLERANCE

Not all patients are candidates for oral anticoagulation (OAC) due to the associated bleeding risks. The HAS-BLED (hypertension, abnormal renal function, abnormal liver function [1 point each], stroke, bleeding history or predisposition, labile INR, elderly [age >65 years], drugs/alcohol concomitantly [1 point each]) score was developed to identify patients with high risk of bleeding (Lip et al., 2018). The maximum HAS-BLED score is 9. According to the 2018 CHEST Antithrombotic Therapy for AF guidelines, OAC should not be withheld in patients with an elevated bleeding risk (e.g., HAS-BLED score ≥3) or risk of falls since the benefit may outweigh the risk (Lip et al., 2018). Clinicians should consider alterative stroke prevention strategies in those with a history of major or nonmajor bleeding, and, additionally, the presence of drug interaction and documented nonadherence to OACs. Patients at high risk of bleeding should have more frequent provider follow-up and lab monitoring (Lip et al., 2018).

WATCHMAN FLX™

The WATCHMAN FLX™ (Boston Scientific, Marlborough, MA, USA) is a left atrial appendage closure (LAAC) device approved for use in patients with nonvalvular AF (NVAF; Figures 4.4). It is inserted endovascularly in the cardiac catheterization lab. OAC is recommended for 45 days or until the LAA is completely closed. Once the cavity is closed, OAC is stopped. Patients are prescribed dual antiplatelet therapy (DAPT) with aspirin and clopidogrel for the next 6 months (Boston Scientific, 2021). The first-generation device's efficacy was demonstrated in the PROTECT AF and PREVAIL studies. The PROTECT AF was a multicenter, prospective randomized control trial (RCT) in which patients with NVAF and CHADS$_2$ score ≥1, were randomized to receive either the intervention (device) or the control (long-term warfarin). The results demonstrated the LAAC device was equivalent to warfarin in preventing strokes, but was associated with complications (Reddy et al., 2017). Some of the adverse effects of the procedure may include cardiac perforation, cardiac tamponade device embolization requiring retrieval, bleeding requiring transfusion, and death (Boston Scientific, 2021). Due to the adverse event rate in PROTECT EF, another RCT (PREVAIL) comparing LAAC to warfarin, was conducted (Reddy et al., 2017).

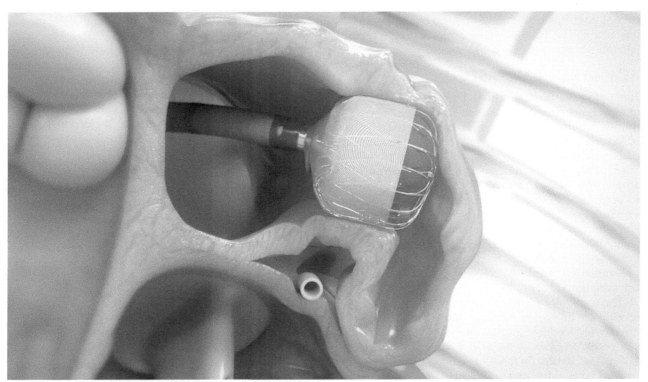

FIGURE 4.4: Watchmen FLX™ device insertion.
Source: ©2022 Boston Scientific Corporation or its affiliates. All rights reserved

PREVAIL's inclusion criteria required a CHADS$_2$ score >2 or one of the CHADS$_2$ criteria (congestive heart failure, hypertension, age >75 years, diabetes mellitus, history of transient ischemia attack or stroke) and another risk factor for stroke (Holmes et al., 2014). Although the PREVAIL trial did not demonstrate LAAC's non-inferiority to warfarin, the combined 5-year-outcomes of the PREVAIL and PROTECT AF trials showed LAAC was non-inferior to warfarin and reduced the incidence of major bleeding, hemorrhagic stroke, and mortality compared to warfarin (Reddy et al., 2017).

Thorascopic Left Atrial Appendage Ligation

LAAL decreases stroke risk by more than 50% in patients with AF (Davies et al., 2017). It is typically done in combination with other open heart surgical procedures such as CABG or valve surgery. However, newer minimally invasive techniques such as video-assisted thorascopic surgery (VATS) have made it possible to perform LAAL on patients who do not need CABG or valve surgery (VATS surgical technique and postoperative care is covered in Chapter 5, "Thoracic Surgery"). Stand-alone LAAL is indicated in patients with contraindications to long-term OAC (e.g., history of or risk for life-threatening bleeding; January et al., 2019). Thorascopic LAAL does not require OAC or DAPT postprocedure as does the WATCHMAN FLX™ device. The WATCHMAN FLX™ device is contraindicated in instances where patients are not candidates for OAC or DAPT due to bleeding risk (Boston Scientific, 2021). In these cases, thorascopic LAAL may be a safer option (January et al., 2019).

CLINICAL PEARLS

■ Patients are generally prescribed antiarrhythmic medication for 60 to 90 days postablation.
■ Patients should wear an event monitor (e.g., Holter) before antiarrhythmics are discontinued (January et al., 2019).

4.8: POSTOPERATIVE CARE OF THE CARDIAC SURGERY PATIENT

Patients are often hemodynamically unstable immediately after cardiac surgery and are therefore admitted to the cardiac thoracic intensive care unit (CTICU). Upon admission to the CTICU, the anesthesia provider (anesthesiologist, certified registered nurse anesthetist, or certified anesthesia assistant) should provide a detailed hand-off at the bedside regarding the priority of surgery (e.g., emergent, urgent, elective), type of procedure (e.g., valve type/size, coronary arteries bypassed), estimated blood loss, urine output, fluid and blood/blood products administered, intraoperative events, such as arrhythmias, coagulopathy, current vasoactive infusions, epicardial pacemaker settings (if applicable), current ventilator settings, and the most recent labs results (Hannan et al., 2020). Potential postoperative complications are summarized in Box 4.1.

HEMODYNAMIC MANAGEMENT

Hemodynamic instability may be related to a number of issues including hypovolemia (blood loss, insensible fluid loss, fluid shifts), vasodilatation (due to sedatives or vasoplegia) which can occur from rapid rewarming, and myocardial stunning (Bojar, 2021). Care of patients after cardiothoracic surgery involves balancing fluid administration and titration of vasoactive medications to optimize CO and blood pressure. Appropriate fluid administration, along with titration of vasopressors and inotropes, is critical in maintaining tissue perfusion. Many complications of cardiac surgery are related to tissue hypoperfusion; therefore, therapy is aimed at preventing an imbalance between oxygen delivery and consumption (Li et al., 2017).

There is a delicate balance between under resuscitation and over resuscitation of IV fluids post operatively. Under-resuscitation can lead to impaired tissue perfusion from hypovolemia-induced hypotension. Over-resuscitation, on the other hand, can lead to volume overload and subsequent pulmonary edema, interstitial edema, and poor wound healing (Simmons et al., 2018). Volume overload is associated with increased morbidity and mortality (Boyd et al., 2011; Marik, 2016; Micek et al., 2013; Silva et al., 2013). One intervention to prevent over- or under-resuscitation is to implement goal-directed therapy (GDT) using algorithms to guide clinicians in their assessment of the need for fluid administration and the response of patients. GDT has been shown to reduce complications and shorten hospital length of stay (LOS) compared to standard therapy in several studies involving cardiac surgical patients (Aya et al., 2013; Giglio et al., 2012; Li, 2018; Osawa et al., 2016).

GDT involves determining fluid responsiveness using hemodynamic measurements such as stroke volume index. If a patient is hypotensive or has a low CO and is determined to be fluid responsive, nurses administer isotonic intravenous fluid to increase CO or blood pressure. If patients are not fluid responsive, vasoactive medications are titrated to support blood pressure or CO. Blood pressure is often supported with vasopressors such as norepinephrine, phenylephrine, and vasopressin. CO is often supported with inotropes such as dobutamine, milrinone, or epinephrine (Brien et al., 2020).

POSTOPERATIVE BLEEDING

Care of the patient immediately after cardiac surgery also requires close monitoring for surgical bleeding. Cardiac surgical patients have chest tubes that are monitored every 15 minutes in the first few hours after surgery. Persistent bleeding (>200 mL in 1 hour or >2 mL/kg x 2 hours) is associated with the need for blood and blood product transfusion. It has also been shown to increase the duration of mechanical ventilation, rates of reoperation, and hospital LOS (Bojar, 2021). The factors that are associated with increased risk of bleeding include male sex, body mass index (BMI), duration of cardiopulmonary bypass (CPB), presence of metabolic acidosis, tachycardia, low platelet count, and elevated INR (Demirci et al., 2017; Pereira et al., 2018). Chest tubes are removed postoperatively once risk of bleeding has subsided and chest tube output is minimal.

VENTILATOR MANAGEMENT

Cardiac surgery patients require full mechanical ventilatory support during surgery and into the CTICU. Lung protective strategies for ventilator settings such as a low tidal volume of 6 mL/kg and positive end expiratory pressure (PEEP) of 10 cm water intraoperative and 5 cm water in the ICU have been shown to reduce pulmonary complications (Engelman et al., 2019; Zamani et al., 2017). The majority of cardiac surgery patients can be safely awakened and liberated from mechanical ventilation within 6 hours of admission to the CTICU (Crawford et al., 2016).

The Society of Thoracic Surgeons (STS) classifies prolonged mechanical ventilation as greater than 24 hours. Patients who require prolonged mechanical ventilation experience higher incidence of sepsis, ventilator-associated pneumonia, renal failure, deep sternal wound infection (DSWI), dysphagia, and posttraumatic-stress disorder (Engelman et al., 2019; Takaki et al., 2015). This increased risk has been shown to begin as early as 12 hours after surgery (Crawford et al., 2016). The STS and the ERAS Society both urge that cardiac surgery programs work toward extubation within 6 hours (Engelman et al., 2019). Systematic ventilator weaning and extubation protocols have been shown to increase success in accomplishing this 6-hour goal, improve outcomes and decrease the trauma of ventilator weaning for patients (Cove et al., 2016; Crawford, et al., 2016; Fitch et al., 2014; Khalafi et al., 2016; Richey et al., 2018; Tierney et al., 2019).

Postoperative cardiac surgery patients who are hemodynamically stable, on minimal ventilator settings, not exhibiting signs of postoperative bleeding and have warmed to 36°C (96.8°F) are candidates for weaning. Hemodynamic stability definitions may vary among programs, but all include normal blood pressure, heart rate, and CO parameters and the requirement of minimal vasoactive and inotropic support (Farooq et al., 2021; Fitch et al., 2014; Richey et al., 2018; Tierney et al., 2019; Zamani et al., 2017).

Extubation protocols all contain similar components which comply with clinical guidelines for ventilator weaning. Once sedation is tapered off, patients must be awake, calm, and able to follow commands in order to proceed to a breathing trial of either pressure support (PS) with or without continuous positive airway pressure (CPAP) or T-piece. If patients can pass a breathing trial for 20 to 30 minutes without hemodynamic instability, an ABG analysis is done and mechanical breathing parameters are measured (Farooq et al., 2021; Fitch et al., 2014; Richey et al., 2018; Tierney et al., 2019; Zamani et al., 2017).

An ABG can be predictive of ventilator weaning failure. Lower PaO_2 and pH and higher $PaCO_2$ values are consistent with failed extubation while normal arterial blood gas (ABG) parameters correlate with successful weaning (Mabrouk et al., 2015). The most reliable predictor of extubation failure is the rapid shallow breathing index (RSBI), calculated by dividing the respiratory rate by the tidal volume. Patients breathing too fast are apt to fatigue, while those breathing shallowly are at increased risk for atelectasis and pneumonia. A RSBI score of 105 or greater correlates with an 89% extubation failure. If a modified RSBI using weight or BMI is used, the prediction accuracy increases to almost 100% (Takaki et al., 2015).

Negative inspiratory force (NIF) or maximum inspiratory pressure (MIP) measures the strength of the diaphragm and can also be used to support safe extubation. A NIF or MIP of −25 to −30 or less has been shown to predict success in weaning while a NIF or MIP of greater than −20 predicts extubation failure (Baptistella et al., 2018; Vahedian-Azimi et al., 2020; Vu et al., 2020).

Patients are normally extubated to nasal cannula oxygen titrated to maintain an SaO_2 of 94% or higher. There is some evidence that postextubation use of noninvasive ventilation (NIV) such as CPAP and bilevel positive airway pressure (BiPAP) can decrease reintubation rates as well as other postoperative pulmonary complications including atelectasis and pneumonia (Liu et al., 2020). High flow nasal cannula (HFNC) oxygen, while useful in preventing reintubation in patients with hypoxic respiratory failure after extubation, has not been found to decrease other pulmonary complications associated with cardiac surgery and is not as effective in preventing reintubation as CPAP and BiPAP (Huang et al., 2018).

Patients unable to be liberated from the ventilator on the day of surgery should have spontaneous awakening trials (SAT) and spontaneous breathing trials (SBT) daily per the ABCDEF bundle which guides patient care in the ICU. Daily SAT and SBT have been demonstrated to decrease sedation, days on the ventilator, hospital LOS, and mortality among ICU patients (Marra et al., 2017).

PULMONARY HYGEINE

Pulmonary complications are a frequent occurrence after surgery. Preoperative pulmonary comorbidities such as smoking, obstructive sleep apnea, and obesity increase patient risk of pulmonary complications as does the type of and length of surgery. Thoracic surgery and placement of a nasogastric tube and endotracheal tube also increase risk. The main pulmonary complications for surgery patients are atelectasis and pneumonia due to pain, anesthesia, and the placement of drainage tubes (Eltorai et al., 2018; Freitas et al., 2012; Strickland et al., 2013; Thompson-Brazill, 2019). Although atelectasis is

more common, pneumonia is associated with higher mortality (Strickland et al., 2013). In cardiac surgery patients, there is an additional risk of pleural effusion (Freitas et al., 2012).

Incentive spirometry (IS) is commonly used after heart surgery to reverse atelectasis. However, there is a paucity of evidence to support the use of IS or airway clearance techniques such as chest physiotherapy in postoperative patients (Eltorai et al., 2018; Freitas et al., 2012; Strickland et al., 2013). Early mobilization is recommended for all surgical patients to minimize postoperative pulmonary complications, assist with airway clearance, and reduce atelectasis (Eltorai et al., 2018; Strickland et al. 2013). Pain management is also important to minimize patient splinting and allow for deep breathing and mobilization (Thompson-Brazill, 2019). In high-risk patients, the use of positive pressure ventilation such as CPAP and BiPAP have been demonstrated to reduce pulmonary complications (Eltorai et al., 2018; Liu et al., 2020).

CHEST TUBE MANAGEMENT

Chest tubes are placed in the mediastinum and pleural space(s) after cardiothoracic surgery to drain blood that is a result of postoperative bleeding (Baribeau et al., 2019). The chest tubes are then placed to a pleural drainage system that has three chambers. One chamber collects the fluid that needs to be drained, the second provides a water seal to prevent air from flowing back into the pleural space, and the third can be used to apply suction to inflate the lung if needed (Venuta et al., 2017).

Postoperative retained blood is associated with an increased risk of atrial fibrillation (AF), acute kideny injury (AKI), and increased LOS so it is important to maintain chest tube patency (Baribeau et al., 2019). Strategies such as milking and stripping chest tubes to keep them patent are not recommended and can be harmful due to the negative pressure on the cardiac structures (Baribeau et al., 2019; Deng et al., 2017). Chest tubes with active tube clearance systems are now available and early studies show them to improve outcomes for patients by reducing postoperative AF, AKI, blood loss, and length of ICU stay (Baribeau et al., 2019). Chest tube removal is safe with serous drainage up to 100 mL in 8 or <300 mL in 24 hours (Bojar, 2021).

4.9: POSTOPERATIVE ATRIAL FIBRILLATION

ETIOLOGIES AND PREVENTION STRATEGIES

Postoperative atrial fibrillation (POAF) is a common postoperative complication that occurs in 25% to 50% of cardiac surgery patients (January et al., 2019). The incidence is approximately 30% in isolated coronary artery bypass graft (CABG) patients, 40% in valve replacement surgery patients, and up to 50% in combination bypass-valve surgeries (O'Brien et al., 2019). AF most often occurs between postoperative days 2 and 4 (O'Brien et al., 2019; Van Gelder et al., 2016). Risks for AF include age; comorbidities such as renal insufficiency, COPD, vascular disease, and obesity; intraoperative factors to include cardiopulmonary bypass (CPB) and valve replacement surgery; and postoperative use of inotropes, and electrolyte imbalances and inflammation (January et al., 2019; Kadric & Osmanovic, 2017). Recent studies have shown that patients who develop POAF are at higher risk for mortality, heart failure, stroke, recurrent AF, and other postoperative complications (Batra et al., 2019; Caldonazo et al., 2021; Hui & Lee, 2017). POAF has also been shown to increase hospital LOS, ICU stay, and hospital readmission rates (Caldonazo et al., 2021; Gillinov et al., 2016).

Beta-blockers, amiodarone, sotalol, and colchicine have been shown to reduce the incidence of AF after open heart surgery when used prophylactically in preoperative patients (January et al., 2014). The use of a statin in the preoperative period has also been correlated with decreased postoperative AF in CABG patients although no such association exists for patients undergoing heart valve replacement (Hui & Lee, 2017; January et al., 2014; Kadric & Osmanovic, 2017). All patients undergoing CABG should receive beta-blockers for at least 24 hours before CABG to reduce the risk of postoperative AF. Starting beta-blockers as soon as possible postoperatively to prevent AF is a Class I recommendation (O'Brien et al., 2019).

TREATMENT OF POSTOPERATIVE ATRIAL FIBRILLATION

Once a patient develops AF after surgery, rate control is the first step in treatment (January et al., 2014). Rate control is defined as management of the heart rate such that it meets a patient's physiologic demands and avoids adverse effects. Since there is no mortality benefit to rhythm control over rate control, resolution of symptoms is the main reason to seek rhythm control in addition to rate control (Van Gelder et al., 2016). If a patient is asymptomatic with their AF, it is not unreasonable to prescribe medications for heart rate control and stroke prophylaxis (January et al., 2014).

Beta-blockers are the first line agents of rate control unless otherwise contraindicated. They control the ventricular rate by interfering with the sympathetic response in the AV node that causes tachycardia (Van Gelder et al., 2016). If beta-blockade is either ineffective or contraindicated, second-line medications such as diltiazem or verapamil which are nondihydropyridine calcium channel blockers (CCBs) may be used (January et al., 2014). These agents provide rate control by depressing the atrioventricular and sinoatrial nodes as well as inhibiting cardiac muscle contractility. CCBs are contraindicated in patients with heart failure due to their effect on the cardiac muscle. Dual therapy may be needed to gain adequate rate control (Van Gelder et al., 2016). Antiarrhythmic agents such as amiodarone are often used to restore and maintain sinus rhythm (SR; January et al., 2014).

In patients who are hemodynamically unstable, synchronized cardioversion is indicated to convert the rhythm to SR, lower heart rate, and improve blood pressure. In cases where AF lasts >48 hours, transesophageal echocardiography (TEE) is needed prior to DC cardioversion to confirm that there is no intracardiac thrombus. Anticoagulation is recommended for 4 weeks after cardioversion, if there is no bleeding risk (January et al., 2014).

Secondary Prevention Measures

To prevent further ischemic cardiovascular events, all postoperative cardiothoracic patients should receive antiplatelet therapy with aspirin. Aspirin has been associated with significant reductions in graft occlusion, morbidity, and mortality in CABG patients (Paquin et al., 2020). Patients with aspirin allergies may benefit from aspirin desensitization therapy or use of an alternative antiplatelet agent such as clopidogrel. Patients with acute myocardial infarctions, with or without ST segment elevation, should be treated with a P2Y12 inhibitor for 1 year postsurgery in addition to aspirin to reduce the risk of future thrombotic complications (Sousa-Ava et al., 2018). Patients undergoing OP CAB, TAVR, and MitraClip® procedures and those with recent drug-eluting stents should receive P2Y12 therapy (Bojar, 2021).

Beta-blockers lower myocardial oxygen demand which is associated with lower risk of adverse cardiovascular events and mortality in patients undergoing CABG (Zhang et al., 2015). All patients having CABG surgery should be prescribed a beta-blocker, unless contraindicated, preoperatively, postoperatively, and at time of discharge (Bojar, 2021).

Statins should be administered to all patients who have had CABG surgery as well. There is substantial evidence that statins improve survival in patients with CAD. In addition to reducing atherosclerosis in native coronary arteries, statins slow the progression of atherosclerosis in vein grafts and reduce adverse cardiovascular events after CABG (Paquin et al., 2020). CABG patients should be prescribed high-intensity statins postoperatively and at discharge. High-intensity statin therapy, which includes atorvastatin 80 mg or rosuvastatin 20 to 40 mg, has been shown to improve outcomes in patients with CAD (Arnett et al., 2019).

Angiotensin converting enzyme inhibitors (ACEI) or ARB are indicated in patients with MI, EF <40%, diabetes, or chronic kidney disease, unless contraindicated (Bojar, 2021).

Oral Anticoagulation

Some cardiothoracic patients require additional anticoagulation with direct acting oral anticoagulants (DOACs) or warfarin. Patients with AF for greater than 48 hours or valve replacement surgery will require anticoagulation therapy in the absence of an absolute contraindication. Patients who have bioprosthetic aortic or mitral valves are recommended to have warfarin anticoagulation for 3 months postsurgery followed by lifelong aspirin therapy. Patients who receive mechanical valves should have lifelong warfarin therapy with an INR goal of 2.5 for aortic valves and 3.0 for mitral valves. Anticoagulant therapy should be initiated as soon as surgical risk for bleeding is mitigated (January et al., 2019; Otto et al., 2020).

4.10: ENHANCED RECOVERY AFTER SURGERY–CARDIAC SURGERY

Enhanced recovery after surgery (ERAS) is an interdisciplinary approach applied to the entire perioperative process, includes preoperative counseling and prehabilitation, intraoperative surgical and anesthesia techniques to reduce pain and hasten recovery from anesthesia, and postoperative care that emphasizes early removal of lines and tubes, early mobilization, goal directed fluid management, minimizing opioids, and avoidance of GI complications (Engelman et al., 2019; Lu et al., 2020; Williams et al., 2018). Although initially developed for colorectal surgery, ERAS after cardiac surgery (ERAS-CS) has successfully applied these principles to the cardiac surgery population (Williams et al., 2018).

PREOPERATIVE STRATEGIES

The prehabilitation phase of ERAS-CS occurs prior to surgery. All patients are advised to cease smoking and minimize alcohol use. Debilitated patients may receive physical and occupational therapy to improve physical function. Those with suspected nutritional deficiencies are referred to dietitians in order optimize their nutritional intake and ideally obtaining normal serum albumin levels (Coleman et al., 2019; Engelman et al., 2019; Hirji et al., 2021). Those with uncontrolled diabetes receive intensive therapy to lower their risk of sternal wound infection and ischemia (Engelman et al., 2019). Moreover, ERAS-CS has altered the traditional preoperative fasting paradigm, by administering a carbohydrate drink, such as Gatorade®, 2 hours before surgery. This prevents hunger, thirst, and insulin resistance. It has also been associated with improved return of bowel function and decreased GI complications (Coleman et al., 2019; Engelman et al., 2019; Lu et al., 2020; Williams et al., 2019).

Clinicians can use this time to set realistic expectations about the surgery and its recovery. Early discussion about pain management strategies and early mobility calms anxieties and promotes patient and family participation (Coleman et al., 2019; Lu et al., 2020; Thompson-Brazill, 2019; Thompson-Brazill et al., 2020; Williams et al., 2019).

INTRAOPERATIVE STRATEGIES

Although, the intraoperative phase of ERAS focuses on the activities of cardiac surgeons, surgical advanced practice providers, and anesthesiology providers, it is important for AGACNPs who do not work in the OR to understand how the phases fit together to optimize patient outcomes. Recommended ERAS-CS anesthesia protocols employ the use of short-acting anesthetics to promote early extubation, avoid hypothermia, facilitate multi-modal pain management, and prevent nausea and vomiting (Engelman et al., 2019; Williams et al., 2019). Surgical practices shown to contribute to improved patient outcomes include the use of antifibrinolytic agents such as epsilon aminocaproic acid and tranexamic acid to prevent the need for blood transfusion, as well as using a rigid sternal fixation device for sternal closure instead of replacement of the traditional sternal wires (Engelman et al., 2019; Lu et al., 2020).

POSTOPERATIVE STRATEGIES

There are many evidence-based components of the postoperative enhanced recovery protocol (ERP) for cardiac surgery. The principles of early extubation, goal directed fluid management and chest tube management have been discussed but are important parts of ERAS-CS and contribute to the improvement of patient outcomes. The ERAS-CS protocol supports the evidence-based recommendations for surgical site infection that are outlined by the Society of Thoracic Surgeons (STS) and supported by the World Health Organization (WHO), Surgical Care Improvement Project (SCIP) and Centers for Disease Control and Prevention (CDC; Engelman et al., 2019; Hirji et al., 2021; Lu et al., 2020). These measures include the use of intranasal mupirocin to prevent or treat staphylococcal colonization prior to surgery; surgical hair clipping; weight-based prophylactic cephalosporin (or other appropriate antibiotics depending on allergies and comorbidities) administration 30 to 60 minutes prior to surgical incision with redosing in operations lasting greater than 4 hours; limiting the duration of postop antibiotic prophylaxis to <48 hours; and removal of surgical dressing at 48 hours after surgery (Engelman et al., 2019).

Other aspects of the ERAS-CS protocol include continuous insulin infusions to maintain blood glucose at less than 180 mg/dL (in both diabetic and nondiabetic patients), maintaining normothermia (36–38°C; 96.8–100.4°F), delirium screening, multimodal pain management (Engelman et al., 2019; Galindo et al., 2018; Lu et al., 2020).

Multimodal Pain Management

The ERAS Cardiac Society embraces the use of a multimodal approach to pain management for the cardiac surgery patient. Using scheduled nonopioid analgesics such as acetaminophen and gabapentin has been shown to improve pain control and reduce opioid use in postoperative cardiac surgery patients by 30% (Williams et al., 2019). It is paramount to note that some traditional opioid-sparing medications are avoided in this population. For example, nonsteroidal anti-inflammatory medications (NSAIDs) have a black box warning for cardiac surgery patients due to risk of bleeding, kidney injury, and thromboembolism (Coleman et al., 2019; Gregory et al., 2020; Lu et al., 2020). Steroids increase the risk for deep sternal infections and have not been found to decrease pain in cardiac surgery patients (Coleman et al., 2019). Special concern must be used to develop pain management protocols that reduce pain and promote recovery while minimizing the risks associated with opioids such as opioid-induced respiratory depression (Gregory et al., 2020; Thompson-Brazill, 2019). While ERAS-CS does not outline a specific protocol, it recommends consideration of the following medications in its guidelines (Engelman et al., 2019; Lu et al., 2020).

Thromboprophylaxis

The decision to use pharmacologic venous thromboembolic (VTE) prophylaxis is not straightforward in the cardiac surgery population. While both hospitalization and cardiac surgery increases risk for VTE due to a prothrombotic state, cardiac surgery patients are also at risk for significant bleeding in the first few days following surgery. A systematic review and meta-analysis conducted by Ho et al. (2015) showed that subcutaneous thromboprophylaxis decreases pulmonary embolisms and deep vein thromboses after cardiac surgery without carrying significant risk for postoperative bleeding or tamponade. The ERAS Cardiac Society recommends mechanical prophylaxis to begin in the operative room and considering pharmacologic thromboprophylaxis beginning postoperative day one (Engel et al., 2019; Lu et al., 2020).

Early Mobilization

The benefits of early mobilization and the ill effects of bed rest are well documented. In cardiac surgery patients where invasive ventilation and monitoring are common, providers have been reluctant to mobilize patients until these devices are removed. A systematic review of the literature shows that despite invasive devices, mobilization remains more beneficial than bed rest. Early mobilization is safe, feasible and leads to improved respiratory function, muscle strength, and overall functional capacity in cardiac surgery patients (Coleman et al., 2019; Santos et al., 2017).

MECHANICAL CIRCULATORY SUPPORT

Mechanical circulatory support (MCS) improves hemodynamics and supports organ perfusion in patients with refractory cardiogenic shock, severe heart failure, and postmyocardial infarction. MCS is also indicated for patients undergoing high-risk percutaneous cardiac intervention (PCI; Zhou et al., 2021).

MCS devices include intra-aortic balloon pumps (IABPs), ventricular assist devices (VADs), veno-arterial extracorporeal membrane oxygenation (VA-ECMO), and total artificial hearts (TAH; Zhou et al., 2021). This chapter discusses VADs and ECMO.

4.11: VENTRICULAR ASSIST DEVICES

Left-ventricular assist devices (LVADs) are use in heart failure (HF) patients with reduced ejection fraction (HFrEF) with stage IIIb to IV symptoms. The VAD removes blood from the left ventricles via its inflow cannula. The blood is brought into the VAD pump. The impeller, which is a magnetically levitated frictionless pump, reintroduces blood into the ascending aorta via the outflow graft (Molina et al., 2021; Zhou et al., 2021). There are two main LVAD categories: temporary and durable. Lower flow temporary LVADs are smaller and percutaneously inserted (Han et al., 2018; Zhou et al., 2021). LVADs with higher flow rates are larger and require surgical cutdowns for insertion (Han et al., 2018; Zhou et al., 2021). Duration of LVAD use depends on the model. The Tandem Heart® (Tandem Life, Pittsburgh, PA) provides short-term support for up to 6 hours (LivaNova, 2020). The Impella® (Abiomed, Danvers, MA) 2.5 and CP are approved for use for up to 4 days. The Impella® devices 5.0 and 5.5 can be used up to 14 days (Abiomed, 2022). The CentriMag (Thoratec, Pleasanton, CA) device has the highest level of continuous flow (up to 10 L/min). It requires surgical implantation via sternotomy or thoracotomy (Sultan et al., 2018). It is approved for use as an LVAD, right ventricular assist device (RVAD), or biventricular assist device (BiVAD). It can stay in place for up to 30 days (Abbott, 2022a).

Durable VADs, such as the Heartmate® II and Heartmate® 3 (Abbott, Abbott Park, IL), are designed to provide long-term support in patients with end-stage left heart failure (NYHA stage D, LV EF <25%) and no contraindications (Figure 4.5; Abbott, 2022b). Durable VADs can be used as either a bridge to recovery, a bridge to decision, a bridge to transplant, or as destination therapy (Han et al., 2018; Papanastasiou et al., 2020; Zhou et al., 2021). LVADs are contraindicated in patients who have hypertrophic cardiomyopathy, limited life expectancy, malignancy, age >80 years, serious comorbidities, and active infection, among others (Han et al., 2018). Since systemic anticoagulation with heparin is required during and after VAD placement, patients who are allergic to or cannot tolerate anticoagulation are not VAD candidates (Han et al., 2018; Sultan et al., 2018). They are surgically implanted via sternotomy or thoracotomy, with the inflow cannula positioned in the apex of the LV and the outflow cannula placed in the ascending aorta (Han et al., 2018; Zhou et al., 2021).

According to the STS Interagency Registry for Mechanically Assisted Circulatory Support (INTERMACS), 27,298 durable MCS devices were implanted in adults >19 years old between 2010 and 2019, with 96% of patients receiving LVADs and 4% requiring BiVAD placement (Molina et al., 2021). In 2019, 77% of 3198 primary LVADs implanted were for destination therapy

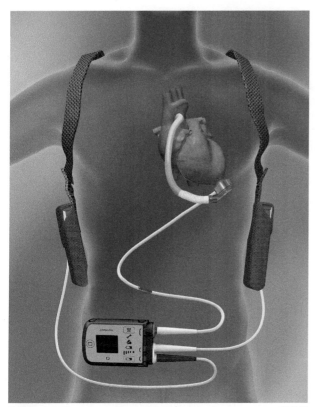

FIGURE 4.5: Heartmate 3® ventricular assist device system: LVAD pump, driveline to controller, and cords to rechargeable batteries. *Source:* Courtesy of Abbott, Abbott Park, IL

(Molina et al., 2021). The 1- to 2-year survival rates for durable LVAD patients were 82.3% and 73.1%, respectively (Molina et al., 2021).

LVAD complications are categorized by the amount of time that has elapsed since LVAD implantation. Early complications occur within 90 days and late complications after 90 days postprocedure (Molina et al., 2021). The common early complications include right heart failure, bleeding, infection, respiratory failure, renal failure, hemolysis, pump thrombosis, and the development of moderate to severe aortic insufficiency (AI)/regurgitation (Han et al., 2018; Molina et al., 2021; Papanastasiou et al., 2020; Xia et al., 2019). Common late complications include pump thrombosis, stroke, neurological dysfunction, driveline infection, and bleeding (Molina et al., 2021; Papanastasiou et al., 2020). Risk of rehospitalization is also higher 90 or more days out from surgery compared to the early postop period (65.9% vs. 37%; Molina et al., 2021). Despite the adverse events associated with LVADs, the survival rate is improving for those whose VADs are destination therapy, with the current survival rate nearing 5 years (Molina et al., 2021).

4.12: EXTRACORPOREAL MEMBRANE OXYGENATION

Unfortunately, not all patients recover as expected after cardiac surgery. Postcardiotomy cardiogenic shock (PCCS) occurs in 0.5% to 6% of cases (McGugan, 2019). Extracorporeal membrane oxygenation (ECMO) is a type of extracorporeal life support that can support either the heart (veno-arterial [VA]) or the lungs (veno-venous [VV]) for prolonged periods of time in order to allow organ recovery or as a bridge to transplantation. It is a technically complex, labor-intensive process that requires specialized training and equipment (Panchal et al., 2019). ECMO is most commonly performed in tertiary or quaternary referral hospitals. ECMO itself is considered when patients have a 50% risk of death (Extracorporeal Life Support Organization, 2017) and is often indicated in patients with a high mortality risk (typically at least 80%; Extracorporeal Life Support Organization, 2017). All patients on ECMO should be intubated and mechanically ventilated. High volume ECMO centers are associated with improved outcomes such as lower mortality and higher survival to hospital discharge (Dalia et al., 2019).

The ECMO circuit contains an oxygenator, centrifugal pump, and heat exchanger similar to that of CPB circuit (Bojar, 2021). The type of ECMO utilized depends on the patient's clinical condition. The two main categories of ECMO are VA and VV. VA ECMO provides both circulatory support and blood oxygenation while bypassing the cardiopulmonary circulation. It drains blood from the cannula in the venous system (femoral vein), removes CO_2 and oxygenates the blood, and returns it to the arterial circulation via a cannula located in either the femoral, axillary, or carotid artery (Bojar, 2021; Lorusso et al., 2021; McGugan, 2019). It is indicated in patients with progressively deteriorating heart failure, refractory cardiogenic shock, PCCS, and cardiac arrest (Bojar, 2021; McGugan, 2019). Extracorporeal cardiopulmonary resuscitation (ECPR) involves placing the patient on ECMO or cardiopulmonary bypass (CPB) during CPR. ECPR provides oxygenation and circulatory support while the resuscitation team searches for reversible causes of cardiac arrest (Panchal et al., 2019). Conversely, VV ECMO does not provide circulatory support: It only oxygenates blood and is used in patients with severe respiratory failure who have preserved cardiac function (Bojar, 2021). A full discussion of possible ECMO management and weaning is beyond the scope of this chapter. Please refer to the section on evidence-based resources for more information.

There are multiple relative contraindications to ECMO. Relative contraindications include conditions that are not compatible with life or a good quality of life if the patient recovers from ECMO (e.g., end-stage cancers, neurologic/mental status impairment, high risk of systemic bleeding with anticoagulation). Others include

TABLE 4.2: Complications of Extracorporeal Membrane Oxygenation

HEMATOLOGIC	CARDIOVASCULAR	OXYGENATION	MULTISYSTEM	MECHANICAL
Bleeding requiring transfusion Bleeding requiring reoperation Coagulopathy Hemolysis Thrombus formation	LV distention (VA-ECMO) LV thrombus due to low cardiac output (VA-ECMO) Limb ischemia Stroke	Pulmonary edema from LV distention Upper body hypoxia (VA-ECMO)	Acute kidney injury (may need dialysis) Infection or sepsis	ECMO pump dysfunction or failure Air in ECMO circuit Clots in ECMO circuit

ECMO, extracorporeal membrane oxygenation; LV, left ventricle; VA-ECMO, veno-arterial extracorporeal membrane oxygenation

Source: Data from Bojar, R. M. (2021). *Manual of perioperative care in adult cardiac surgery* (6th ed.). John Wiley & Sons; McGugan, P. L. (2019). The role of veno-arterial extracorporeal membrane oxygenation in post-cardiotomy cardiogenic shock. *Critical Care Nursing Clinics of North America, 31*(3), 419–436. https://doi.org/10.1016/j.cnc.2019.05.009

age and size of the patient, as well a medical futility (e.g., very ill patients who have been on prolonged conventional therapy or have a fatal diagnosis; Extracorporeal Life Support Organization, 2017). Prior to initiating ECMO, providers should discuss medical futility and indications for stopping ECMO (e.g., devastating neurological injury such as intracranial hemorrhage or brain death, inability to wean from ECMO, no recovery of heart or lung function, and/or not a candidate for VAD implantation or organ transplant; Extracorporeal Life Support Organization, 2017).

In addition to the potential for neurological injury, there are a number of other complications that may occur on ECMO (Table 4.2), one of which is bleeding. ECMO requires systemic anticoagulation to prevent blood clotting in the circuit. Heparinization begins with a heparin bolus 50 to 100 units/kg IV before cannulation is performed, regardless of bleeding (Extracorporeal Life Support Organization, 2017). This is followed by a continuous heparin infusion which is titrated to a goal ACT 1.5 times normal (Extracorporeal Life Support Organization, 2017). In cases where heparin-induced thrombocytopenia is present, an IV direct thrombin inhibitor (e.g., bivalirudin or argatroban) is indicated to prevent thrombotic events. Bleeding may occur (McGugan, 2019). Thromboelastography and other tests such as anti-factor Xa, aPTT, and fibrinogen may help identify coagulopathies. IV antifibrinolytics, blood, or blood product administration may be required to stem severe or life-threatening bleeding (Extracorporeal Life Support Organization, 2017; McGugan, 2019).

KEY TAKEAWAYS

- Durable VADs are primarily used to support left ventricular function in patients with end-stage heart failure as a bridge to transplant or as destination therapy.
- ECMO is indicated in patients with a high risk of mortality from acute cardiac or pulmonary failure.
- There are many factors to consider when deciding if a patient is a candidate for ECMO.

- Discussion of the risks and benefits of ECMO should be discussed with family prior to its initiation.
- Palliative care consultation regarding goals of care and scope of medical treatment should be considered.
- Not all patients on ECMO are candidates for durable MCS such as VADs or transplantation.
- Despite ECMO, patients may experience organ failure, devastating neurological issues, or failure to regain cardiac or pulmonary function, which may necessitate withdrawal of care.

EVIDENCE-BASED RESOURCE

Extracorporeal Life Support Organization. (2017, August). *General guidelines for all ECLS cases*. https://www.elso.org/Portals/0/ELSO%20Guidelines%20General%20All%20ECLS%20Version%201_4.pdf

4.13: DISCHARGE FOLLOWING CARDIAC SURGERY

The criteria for discharge after cardiac surgery includes all chest tubes and wires being removed, the heart has remained in normal sinus rhythm, and the patient is tolerating a regular diet and is having bowel movements. Also, patients should be weaned off supplemental oxygen, have a weight close to baseline, and blood within normal limits (Afflu et al., 2021). Patients can anticipate discharge as early as 3 to 5 days after cardiac surgery. Patients should have someone stay with them after heart surgery for 1 to 2 weeks (Bojar, 2021; Hillis et al., 2011).

Transitions of care from hospital to the community or another facility must be structured and provide for a seamless continuation of care. Readmission after cardiac surgery is reported for almost 20% of Medicare patients. This is attributed to poor preparation of patients and family as well as poor communication with the patient's Primary care provider (PCP) and outpatient providers (Mohanty et al., 2016). Proper discharge planning includes coordination of care with the PCP, teaching that includes the patient's caregivers, as well as patient and provider access to the electronic medical record (EMR;

Mohanty et al., 2016). Home health nursing and physical and occupational therapy can help patients stay in their homes and facilitate recovery (Bojar, 2021).

DISCHARGE INFORMATION

Patients should understand that recovery from open heart surgery is a process that usually takes between 4 weeks and 3 months. Along with incisional pain, it is normal to experience changes to sleep, appetite, and bowel pattern. Many patients have memory issues and trouble concentrating. Others have mood swings or a postoperative depression. Understanding that these symptoms are expected and usually resolve on their own can be comforting for patients. Symptoms that do not improve independently may require treatment (Bojar, 2021). Discharge medications should be outlined for patients in a chart that includes the indication, the dosage, and the times. All incisions should be examined daily for signs of redness, warmth, swelling, and drainage. Patients should shower daily using warm water and a mild soap and pat dry. Tub baths or submerging incisions in water is prohibited until cleared by the surgeon. All ointments, creams, and powders should be avoided. Unless otherwise instructed, incisions are left open to air. Women with large breasts and a sternotomy incision should wear a bra without underwires to prevent pulling on the incision and skin dehiscence.

Walking is an important part of postop recovery. Some patients may benefit from physical and occupational therapy either at home or at an inpatient rehabilitation facility. Following sternotomy, patients must observe sternal precautions for up to 8 to 12 weeks depending on their surgeon's preference. This limits any lifting, pulling, and pushing with the arms to 5 to 10 lbs. Driving should be avoided until cleared by the surgeon, usually 4 to 6 weeks (Adams et al., 2016; Bojar, 2021). Unfortunately, sternal precautions prevent patients from regaining muscle mass in the 6 to 8 weeks after surgery and may limit their independence (Adams et al., 2016). A team at Baylor University Medical Center in Dallas, Texas devised a less-restrictive approach to sternal precautions, called "Keep Your Move in the Tube®" (Adams et al., 2016). Gach and colleagues (2021) data showed patients with "keeping your move in the tube" modified sternal precautions had approximately a 3 times higher rate of being discharged to home compared to those with restrictive sternal precautions. Additionally, cardiac rehabilitation is recommended for cardiac surgery patients beginning 4 to 8 weeks after discharge and is associated with improved functional status (Hillis et al., 2011).

SELF-MONITORING, LIFESTYLE MODIFICATION, AND POSTDISCHARGE FOLLOW-UP

Patients are encouraged to check their pulse, temperature, weight, and incisions daily. A heart healthy diet low in cholesterol and salt is encouraged and diabetics must maintain a normal hemoglobin A1C. Smoking cessation is strongly encouraged and leads to a statistically significant decrease in 10-year mortality after surgery (Hillis et al., 2011). Survival is closely linked to patients' adherence to diabetes, hypertension, and lipid management plans (Bojar, 2021).

FOLLOW-UP APPOINTMENTS

A follow-up appointment should be scheduled with the surgeon for a wound check in 7 to 10 days.

Patients should make an appointment to see their cardiologist and primary care provider within 2 to 3 weeks after discharge (Hillis et al., 2011).

CLINICAL PEARLS

- Ensure patients receive and understand education regarding their medications including reason for taking, adverse effects, and when to call their provider.
- In order to improve medication adherence, AGACNPs should work with patients and social workers to determine if the patients can afford their medications, have transportation to a pharmacy, and if they are able to fill their medication boxes.
- Prior to discharge, the patient should be instructed to call the provider if they experience:
  - Shortness of breath or chest pain that is worsening or unrelieved with rest or pain medications.
  - New or worsening cough.
  - Irregular or unusually fast (>120) or slow (<60) heart rate.
  - Redness, drainage, or dehiscence of incisions.
  - Temperature of 38°C (101°F) with or without chills.
  - Weight increase of more than 2 lbs. (1 kg) per day for 2 days.
  - Dizziness, fainting or severe fatigue (Hillis et al., 2011).

KEY TAKEAWAYS

- Cardiac surgery is a broad field that encompasses many procedures which ameliorate symptoms and improve longevity for patients with coronary artery disease, valvular heart disease, atrial fibrillation, and other disease processes.
- The ACC/AHA guidelines recommend that treatment options for patients should be based on clinical indications and discussed among the multidisciplinary heart team.
- The surgical procedures and the postoperative management are complex.
- It takes a skilled multidisciplinary team comprised of cardiac surgeons, cardiologists, intensivist, anesthesia providers, advanced practice providers, pharmacists, registered nurses, physical and occupational therapists, dietitians, case managers, social workers, and laboratory and diagnostic imaging professionals to achieve excellent patient outcomes.

EVIDENCE-BASED RESOURCES

American Association of Thoracic Surgeons. Journal of Cardiovascular and Thoracic Surgery Previous Issues and Supplements. https://www.jtcvs.org/issues

American College of Cardiology. Guidelines and Documents. https://www.acc.org/guidelines

American Heart Association. Guidelines and Statements. https://professional.heart.org/en/guidelines-and-statements

Heart Rhythm Society. Clinical Resources. https://www.hrsonline.org/guidance/clinical-resources

Society of Critical Care Medicine. Guidelines. https://www.sccm.org/Clinical-Resources/Guidelines

Society of Thoracic Surgeons. Resources. https://www.sts.org/resources

A robust set of instructor resources designed to supplement this text is located at **http://connect.springerpub.com/content/reference-book/978-0-8261-6079-9.** Qualifying instructors may request access by emailing **textbook@springerpub.com.**

REFERENCES

Full list of references can be accessed at http://connect.springerpub.com/content/reference-book/978-0-8261-6079-9

CHAPTER 5

THORACIC SURGERY

Abbye Solis, Kelly A. Thompson-Brazill, and Catherine C. Tierney

---

LEARNING OBJECTIVES

- Recognize the signs and symptoms of pulmonary pathologies that may require surgical intervention.
- Utilize surgical risk assessment tools to determine pulmonary and cardiac risk in a presurgical patient.
- Correlate patient pathology and clinical goals with thoracic surgical approach and therapies.
- Describe proper management of chest tubes to include suction, patency, and safe removal.
- Create an individual, comprehensive multimodal pain management plan for a patient following thoracic surgery
- Discuss important considerations for transition of care for patients after thoracic procedures.

INTRODUCTION

Thoracic surgery includes surgical intervention of any organs of the thorax region, e.g., esophagectomy, gastrectomy, hiatal hernia repair, lung lobe resection, and lung biopsy. For purposes of this chapter, the focus will be evaluation of diseases of the lungs and lung parenchyma requiring thoracic surgery. Diseases of the lung often originate from the presenting symptoms of shortness of breath, acute and chronic cough, hemoptysis, or recurrent infections. However, initial symptoms can also include costal pain or back pain. Pre-existing lung diseases, such as chronic obstructive pulmonary disease (COPD), make nonspecific initial complaints difficult for the provider to interpret. However, it has been estimated that 40% of smokers are symptomatic at the time of emergency presentation (Price & Sikora, 2020). The key is critically thinking about presenting signs and symptoms with an open mind.

5.1: PULMONARY PATHOLOGY REQUIRING THORACIC SURGERY

PRESENTING SIGNS AND SYMPTOMS

Diseases of the lung often originate from the presenting symptoms of shortness of breath, acute and chronic cough, hemoptysis, or recurrent infections. However, initial symptoms can also include costal pain or back pain. Pre-existing lung diseases, such as chronic obstructive pulmonary disease (COPD), make nonspecific initial complaints difficult for the provider to interpret. However, it has been estimated that 40% of smokers are symptomatic at the time of emergency presentation (Price & Sikora, 2020). Depending on the disease state, patients requiring thoracic surgery may present with many different signs and symptoms. The diagnoses for which thoracic surgery is indicated include primary lung cancer, pulmonary abscess or empyema, treatment of blunt and penetrating traumatic injuries including hemothorax, pneumothorax, and surgical treatment of emphysema. Surgery is also performed to provide a tissue sample (e.g., lung parenchyma, lung nodules, thoracic lymph nodes) for biopsy in order to diagnose the underlying pathology.

The following is a list of the most common chief complaints among patients who required thoracic surgery consultation (Araujo et al., 2020; Planchard et al., 2018; Wu et al., 2019):

- Chills
- Fever
- Night sweats
- Weight loss (unintentional)
- Hoarse voice
- Acute shortness of breath
- Dyspnea on exertion
- Chest wall pain
- Pleuritic pain
- Persistent cough
- Productive cough
- Hemoptysis

HISTORY AND PHYSICAL EXAM FINDINGS
Past Medical History

Obtaining a thorough history of present illness, past medical history, and review of systems is an important step in determining differential diagnoses. Lung cancers, empyemas, and pneumothoraces typically require thoracic surgical intervention. Common etiologies of lung cancer include genetics, history of smoking, or toxin exposure. Familial risk of lung cancer has been reported in several registry-based studies after regression analysis excluding other known risk factors such as smoking. Alpha-1 antitrypsin deficiency as well a multitude of genetic variants may increase the risk of developing lung cancer (Tubío-Pérez et al., 2021; Wang et al., 2017).

People may come in contact with chemicals and other materials that are carcinogenic through environmental or occupational exposures. There are multiple environmental factors that may cause lung cancer, including outdoor air pollution, particulate matter in the air, diesel fuel exhaust, radon-222, second-hand smoke, and soot. Work-related carcinogens include carbon biomass from burning household items (fire fighters), welding fumes, coal dust (coal miners), asbestos, silica, and spray application of pesticides, among many others (Markowitz & Dickens, 2020). Those with pleural abscess or empyema often have a history of chronic lung disease and may have a history of lack of gag reflex or poor dentition.

Aspiration, both silent and overt, and poor oral care are often the source of infection in people who present with pleural abscesses (Godfrey et al., 2019). Common situations that lead to aspiration include decreased level of consciousness as in the case of intoxication, seizure, or anesthesia; neurological brainstem dysfunction after cerebrovascular accident or with multiple sclerosis, or amyotrophic lateral sclerosis; oral or laryngeal dysfunction due to surgery or radiation; and esophageal or gastrointestinal dysfunction that leads to reflux of stomach contents (Chan et al., 2019). Patients with alpha-1 antitrypsin deficiency are at risk for infection. Immunocompromised patients may develop complicated pulmonary infections (Witzke & Anikin, 2017). These include patients with human immunodeficiency virus (HIV), diabetes (DM), and those on immunosuppressive therapy such as systemic corticosteroids, biologics, and chemotherapy. Infection is also prevalent in those who have a history of illicit IV drug use and those with significant dental disease (Chan et al., 2019; Witzke & Anikin, 2017).

Patients with primary spontaneous pneumothorax (PSP) may have no past medical history although the etiology appears to be the presence of pleural or subpleural blebs at the apices of the lungs. These patients have no history of trauma or precipitating events, but many will have a recurrence if not surgically treated. Smoking correlates to a 12% risk for pneumothorax in otherwise healthy, young, predominantly male patients between the ages of 10 and 30. The condition is also most often seen in those with a tall, thin build (MacDuff et al., 2010; Wong et al., 2019).

Secondary spontaneous pneumothorax (SSP) is the presence of air in the pleural space as a result of an underlying lung disease which causes the formation of pulmonary bullae. COPD is the primary culprit but interstitial lung disease, tuberculosis (TB), and bronchiectasis are also implicated. Alpha-1 antitrypsin deficiency is a genetic disorder. Those with the disorder lack a protease inhibitor which leads to the overextension of alveoli and premature emphysema can also cause SSP requiring surgical intervention (Jeon et al., 2017).

Physical Exam Findings

Vital signs including respiratory rate and oxygen saturations vary according to the type and severity of the underlying pulmonary disease process. Lung cancer patients may experience tachypnea and low oxygen saturation. Signs of COPD and digital clubbing can be seen in the long-term smoker (Araujo et al., 2020). Breath sounds will range from diminished in the patient with mass or pneumothorax, to wheezing in COPD, to cavernous breath sounds with rales in a patient with pneumonia or effusion. Egophony can be heard in the patient with empyema or pneumonia (Araujo et al., 2020; Witzke & Anikin, 2017; Wong et al., 2019). Reduced excursion of the chest wall is common in a patient presenting with a large pneumothorax (Wong et al., 2019). Percussing the thorax reveals dullness in the presence of a mass, tactile fremitus in patients with pneumonia or abscess, and possible crepitus or hyperresonance in a patient with a pneumothorax (Araujo et al., 2020; Wong et al., 2019). The presence of supraclavicular lymphadenopathy is a sign of metastatic disease (Araujo et al., 2020).

Diagnostic Tests

A posteroanterior and lateral chest radiograph (CXR) can reveal evidence of pneumonia, a mass, pleural effusion, parapneumonic effusion, or pneumothorax. Pleural ultrasound is highly useful in evaluating pleural effusions and may discern patterns that differentiate transudative from exudative effusions. Ultrasound is more effective than CXR in estimating the amount of fluid present. CT is the most comprehensive test. The contrast-enhanced CT can provide evidence of infiltrate, mass, pleural effusion, parapneumonic effusion, pneumothorax, blebs, lymphadenopathy as well as other abnormalities of the chest (Shen et al., 2017).

PREOPERATIVE RISK ASSESSMENT

Pulmonary Risk Assessment

Patients with known pulmonary vascular disease and pulmonary hypertension (HTN) benefit from a pulmonology consult to optimize their pulmonary function prior to thoracic surgery (Fleisher et al., 2014). It is important to weigh both the ventilation and diffusion function of all patients requiring surgical removal of part or all of a lung. Prior to surgery, the patient's lung function, the extent of resection needed, effects on quality of life are evaluated, and the risk of complications and mortality are calculated (Jiang et al., 2019; Roy, 2018).

Assessment of Pulmonary Function Tests

Pulmonary function assessment includes interpreting noninvasive pulmonary function tests (PFT). Forced expiratory volume in 1 second (FEV_1) and diffusion capacity for carbon monoxide (DLCO) are independent predictors of perioperative morbidity and mortality (Jiang et al., 2019; Lederman et al., 2019; Roy, 2018). All thoracic surgery candidates should have preoperative pulmonary function testing (Matheos et al., 2020). Patients are deemed suitable for pneumonectomy if FEV_1 is greater than 2 L and for lobectomy if FEV_1 is greater than 1.5 L (Jiang et al., 2019).

PREDICTED POSTOPERATIVE (PPO) FEV_1 IS CALCULATED USING THE EQUATION:

PPO FEV_1 = Preoperative FEV_1 × (1−y/z), where
y = Segments to be removed and
z = Total number of segments or number of functional segments.
There are 19 lung segments in total: right = RUL-3; RML-2; RLL-5; left =LUL-3, lingula-2; LLL- 4 (Roy, 2018).
An FEV_1 of <60% is associated with increased mortality and pulmonary complications. PPO FEV_1 <40% is considered high risk (Jiang et al., 2019).
PPO DLCO is calculated using the equation:
PPO DLCO = DLCO × (1−y/z)

If both FEV_1 and DLCO are greater than 80% of predicted, no further evaluation is needed, and elective surgery can be planned. If PPO FEV_1 and PPO DLCO are both >60%, the patient will likely tolerate lung resection. If the PPO FEV_1 and PPO DLCO are 30% to 59%, consider a low-level exercise test such as a stair climbing test or shuttle walk test. If PPO FEV_1 and PPO DLCO are <30%, or low-level exercise test is poor, a cardiopulmonary exercise test (CPET) is recommended. If poor, consider subsegmental surgical resection or nonsurgical treatment (Lederman et al., 2019; Roy, 2018).

Cardiac Risk Assessment

Thoracic surgery, regardless of approach, would be defined as a moderate- to high-risk procedure. Patients undergoing thoracic surgery often have associated risk factors and comorbid conditions that increase their risk (Fleisher et al., 2014). The Canadian Cardiovascular Society (CCS) defines a surgery that requires an overnight hospital stay as one that places sufficient stress on a patient to cause a cardiac event (Duceppe et al., 2017). Both the American College of Cardiology/American Heart Association (ACC/AHA) and the CCS recommend assessment of cardiac risk prior to thoracic surgery (Duceppe et al., 2017; Fleisher et al., 2014).

There are certain pre-existing cardiac conditions that require the consultation of a specialist prior to surgery. Patients with greater than moderate valvular stenosis or regurgitation should undergo an echocardiogram prior to surgery if one has not been performed in the last year or their clinical status has changed since the last echocardiogram. Patients with a cardiovascular implantable electronic device (CIED) need an operative plan to be made with the cardiologist and the device technician prior to any surgical intervention (Fleisher et al., 2014).

Studies show that 11.6% of patients over age 50 have an increase in troponin post noncardiac surgery. All patients >50 years old or who have comorbidities such as HTN or DM, which predispose them to cardiac disease, should be evaluated for cardiac risk prior to thoracic surgery. It is recommended that providers use a cardiac risk calculator to determine a patient's odds of a cardiac event during surgery. The Revised Cardiac Risk Index (RCRI) or National Surgical Quality Improvement Program (NSQIP) can be used to assist providers in identifying patients who require further testing. These calculators use the risk of the procedure combined with the patient's comorbidities to calculate risk of major adverse cardiac events (MACE; Duceppe et al., 2017; Fleisher et al., 2014).

Patients with a low cardiac risk having low risk surgeries are not recommended to have preoperative 12-lead ECGs or further testing. A preoperative 12-lead ECG is reasonable prior to thoracic surgery in patients with known arterial vascular disease or history of arrhythmia or heart valve disease and may even be considered in asymptomatic patients without heart disease history prior to the more invasive thoracic surgeries (Fleisher et al., 2014).

An N-terminal fragment of pro-B-type natriuretic peptide (NT-proBNP) or B-type natriuretic peptide (BNP) level is suggested preoperatively in patients older than 65 years of age, or patients between the ages of 45 and 64 with a history of cardiac disease or RCRI score ≥1. These peptides are released from the myocardium during times of stress or myocardial stretch. An elevated level of NT-proBNP or BNP can be predictive of poor outcomes (Duceppe et al., 2017). If a patient is deemed to be at elevated risk, the providers next need to establish the patient's functional capacity (Fleisher et al., 2014).

The Duke Activity Status Index (DASI) or Modified DASI (M-DASI) can be used to calculate functional capacity (Fleisher et al., 2014; Riedel et al., 2021). If a patient scores moderate or better, calculated as ≥4 METs in functional capacity, no further cardiac testing is indicated in an asymptomatic patient. A MET is a metabolic equivalent with one MET equaling the energy required to sit quietly at rest. Moderate activity (3–6 METs) requires the burning of 3 to 6 times the calories of sitting quietly. This includes activities such as climbing stairs, walking around the block and sexual activity (Riedel et al., 2021).

If a patient is unable to exercise at a moderate level, further cardiac testing is warranted if it will impact decision-making and preoperative care. Pharmacologic stress testing can be done with either vasodilators (e.g., adenosine, dipyridamole, regadenoson) or with an inotrope such as dobutamine. Imaging is done at rest then after the stressor to measure the patient's response. A simple ECG can be used but has the lowest sensitivity and specificity for detecting coronary disease. Echocardiography is more sensitive and can reveal wall motion abnormality indicative of ischemia. Nuclear imaging is referred to as myocardial perfusion imaging (MPI) and is the most sensitive and specific for identifying cardiac ischemia. MPI can be done using radioactive isotopes with either single photon emission computed tomography (SPECT) and technetium-99/tetrofosmin-labeled tracer or by positive emission tomography (PET) using $[^{15}O]$ H_2O tracer (Danad et al., 2017). Cardiac magnetic resonance (CMR) imaging can also be used to evaluate myocardial perfusion using gadolinium (Sammut et al., 2018). The presence of a large area of myocardial ischemia is associated with increased risk of perioperative myocardial infarction or death, and a normal study has high negative predictive value. Pharmacologic stress testing that reveals myocardial ischemia may require further workup and treatment depending on the severity (Fleisher et al., 2014). It is important to note that routine intervention for coronary artery disease (CAD) prior to noncardiac surgeries has not been shown to reduce morbidity and mortality (Raghunathan et al., 2020). The Coronary Artery Revascularization Prophylaxis (CARP) trial did not show differences in short-term outcomes or long-term mortality in patients who underwent coronary artery revascularization prior to aortic or infra-renal vascular surgery (Santilli, 2006).

DIFFERENTIAL DIAGNOSIS AND DIAGNOSTIC CONSIDERATIONS

Thoracic surgery is performed to diagnose and/or treat diseases of the lungs and thorax. It is highly invasive and comes with its own risks. Surgical consultation is appropriate after a thorough assessment of the patient has determined that surgical intervention is the best option for both the patient and the disease. A biopsy provides histological (tissue) diagnosis for patients with tumors or disease not diagnosed by traditional bronchoscopy with biopsy, thoracentesis, or percutaneous fine needle aspiration or core biopsy (Planchard et al., 2018).

Surgical resection is the definitive treatment for small cell carcinoma (SCCA) Stage T1-2 N0 (National Comprehensive Cancer Network, 2019) and early stage non-small cell carcinoma (NSCCA): Stages I and II and some locally advanced IIIA. Surgery provides the greatest chance of cure in patients who have a resectable lesion, do not have metastasis, and can tolerate surgery (National Comprehensive Cancer Network, 2020). In SSCA, there is no benefit shown for surgical intervention for more invasive tumors (Barnes et al., 2017).

Surgical resection may also be done to reduce lung volume and improve lung function in select patients with emphysema and hyperinflation on optimal medical therapy (van Geffen et al., 2019). Surgery may also be indicated to treat pleural spaced infections called empyemas. The empyema may develop from infected bronchiectasis, a lung abscess, or from a parapneumonic effusion. A lung abscess is necrosis of the lung parenchyma which leads to formation of a pus-filled cavity. The primary treatment for this is medical therapy which includes broad-spectrum antibiotics and drainage of the infection via thoracentesis or chest tube. Surgical treatment is warranted in the 10% to 15% percent of patients who do not respond to medical therapy alone and can require decortication (Witzke & Anikin, 2017).

Spontaneous pneumothorax is the accumulation of air in the pleural space as a result of the rupture of a pulmonary bleb (primary) or due to underlying lung disease (secondary). Symptomatic or large pneumothoraces require chest tube insertion to remove the air and re-expand the lung. Patients are then observed, and chest tubes removed when there is no evidence of air leak from the damaged lung. Once chest tubes are safely removed patients are discharged home. In patients with a persistent air leak after 4 days surgical intervention is indicated. Surgery is also recommended for prevention of pneumothorax recurrence after a patient's second ipsilateral spontaneous pneumothorax, first contralateral pneumothorax, or synchronous bilateral pneumothorax. Surgery may also be indicated if the patient has increased professional risk, pregnancy, or a spontaneous hemothorax (MacDuff et al., 2010).

5.2: SURGICAL LUNG RESECTION

BULLECTOMY

Bullectomy (also referred to as bleb resection) is the surgical removal of the bullae or blebs in the apex of the lung. When surgical treatment for a primary spontaneous pneumothorax (PSP) is indicated, a three-port video-assisted thoracic surgery (VATS) procedure is preferred. The blebs are resected using a stapler device which leaves a staple line in place as the bleb is cut away. Saline is instilled into the chest to test for air leaks prior to closure (Mithiran et al., 2019). Bullectomy surgery may also include either a chemical or mechanical pleurodesis or both. When combined with a pleurodesis, the rate of pneumothorax recurrence drops from between 10% and 20% to just between 1% and 6% (Mithiran et al., 2019).

Chemical pleurodesis is most often done with talc or tetracycline. The agent is distributed over the visceral and parietal pleura, the diaphragm, and the mediastinum. The toxic chemical causes an inflammatory reaction on both the lung parenchyma and the chest wall so that adhesions form, obliterating the pleural space and preventing future lung collapse (Mithiran et al., 2019). Mechanical pleurodesis is done via abrasion of the parietal pleura with a scratch pad, brush, or pleurectomy, which separates the parietal pleura from the endothoracic fascia of the chest wall (Mithiran et al., 2019). A chest tube is then placed through one of the ports into the apex of the lung for re-expansion. The tube is placed to a closed drainage collection and placed to low continuous suction at 10 to 20 cm H_2O (Mithiran et al., 2019).

Management of Secondary Spontaneous Pneumothorax

Bullectomy is indicated in patients with advanced emphysema, with recurrent spontaneous pneumothoraces, and bullous emphysema noted on CT of the chest (Sampson & Meyers, 2016). The surgery is often done thoracoscopically (VATS) but may need conversion to open thoracotomy if significant adhesions are present. During the procedure, the thoracic surgeon excises either one large bulla or multiple bullae by stapling off the affected lung tissue from healthier areas of lung parenchyma and removing from the chest (Sampson & Meyers, 2016). Persistent air leaks from the lung parenchyma are very common after bullectomy. If the air leaks do not seal with conservative measures (e.g., altering degrees of negative pressure suction, blood patches, optimizing nutrition), interventional pulmonology may elect to place endobronchial valves (EBV; Terry & Traystman, 2016). Please refer to the section on surgical treatment of emphysema and EBV placement for endoscopic lung volume reduction (ELVR) for more details.

SEGMENTECTOMY

A segmentectomy or surgical removal of one or more segments of the lung is technically more challenging than removing a lobe.

Performing a segmentectomy over lobectomy is controversial and although oncologic outcomes have been found to be similar, studies have failed to prove superior long-term lung function benefits of segmentectomy over lobectomy either in early stage tumors or in patients with poor lung function (Charloux & Quoix, 2017; Ko et al., 2019; Nakazawa et al., 2017; Sui et al., 2019). A segmentectomy is described as either a typical segmentectomy involving the left upper lobe, the lingula, the superior segments, and the basilar segments. An atypical segmentectomy involves the resection of individual segments or combined segments. The surgical resection can also be described based on the shape of the intersegmental planes: linear, V-shaped, or three-dimensional (Nakazawa et al., 2017).

Segmentectomy may be considered for several reasons: (a) pulmonary preservation in patients with small tumors <2 cm; (b) in patients with metastatic disease, segmentectomy allows for the possibility of future resections; and (c) in patients who do not meet criteria for lobectomy due to poor lung function (Charloux & Quoix, 2017; Nakazawa et al., 2017; Sui et al., 2019).

Segmentectomy is most often performed using a VATS procedure, although more robotic anatomic segmentectomies (RATS) are now being performed and atypical segmentectomies may require an open thoracotomy. The surgical approach depends on the anatomy of the lobe being segmented, with each approach requiring division of the segmental arteries and bronchus and mobilization of the segmental veins (Ko et al., 2019). Preoperative planning

with 3D imaging is needed to map out the bronchovascular anatomy and ensure adequate margins will be achieved (Nakazawa et al., 2017). A margin at least equal to the diameter of the tumor is considered best practice (Nakazawa et al., 2017). Sharp dissection with scissors followed by electrocautery and fibrin sealant has been found to be superior to stapler use in preserving lung function and prevention of postoperative air leaks (Nakazawa et al., 2017).

LOBECTOMY

A pulmonary lobectomy refers to the removal of a complete anatomic lobar portion of the lung. The surgical approach is via thoracotomy or thoracoscopy either by VATS or by RATS. The less invasive approach has been shown to be associated with shorter lengths of stay, decreased incidence of perioperative complications, increased discharge to home, and even improved survival. Lobectomy is the most common treatment for nonsmall cell lung cancer but can also be used to treat TB, lung abscess, bronchiectasis, nonmalignant tumors, fungal infections, and congenital anomalies (Nwogu et al., 2015). The operative technique utilizes the standard surgical procedure with dissection of the vein, arteries, and airway for the lobe performed and hilar structures ligated using an endovascular stapler (Ko et al., 2019). Lymph nodes are taken for biopsy from the mediastinum in all approaches. Chest tubes are left in place at the end of the procedure via the camera port in the case of a thoracoscopic approach (Gonfiotti et al., 2018).

PNEUMONECTOMY

Pneumonectomy is the complete removal of one of the lungs. This is a high-risk procedure with mortality within 30 days observed at 5% to 13% (Slinger & Campos, 2020). With the trend toward less invasive surgery, pneumonectomy is reserved for patients with central NSCCA malignancies, not resectable via lobectomy, and lungs irrevocably damaged by TB, bronchiectasis, aspergillosis, or radiation pneumonitis (Janet-Vendroux et al., 2015). Pneumonectomies are usually done via a posterolateral thoracotomy, although some centers are performing them via VATS. During the procedure, all vessels and bronchi are secured with a stapler device. The bronchial stump may be covered with adjacent tissue and reconstructed to prevent air leak and collection of secretions. A test for air leak is done prior to chest closure. The management of the empty thoracic space left behind varies based on surgeon training: 750 to 1500 mL of air may be initially removed to stabilize the mediastinum after surgery. Some thoracic surgeons leave no tube in place while others leave a catheter through which to remove air should there be a significant mediastinal shift. Still others may place a drain to balance the mediastinum. A postoperative CXR should be done and repeated daily to observe for mediastinal shift (Slinger & Campos, 2020). A highly invasive extrapleural pneumonectomy may be performed for the treatment of metastatic pleural mesothelioma. This involves resection of the lung, parietal pleura, diaphragm, lymph nodes, and chest wall (Slinger & Campos, 2020).

SLEEVE RESECTION

In patients with cancerous lesions, trauma, or stricture limited to one of the mainstem pulmonary bronchi, a mainstem bronchial sleeve resection may be performed. A sleeve resection is preferred to pneumonectomy for eligible tumors as significant lung function can be preserved. This procedure is usually done via posterolateral thoracotomy to allow access to the trachea and hilum as each is freed prior to the procedure to avoid tension on the anastomosis. Minimally invasive techniques such VATS and RATS are increasingly common (Abdelsattar et al., 2017). Sleeve resection surgery involves removing the offending piece of the mainstem bronchus, then reattaching the unaffected lung to the healthy proximal margin. The anastomosis site is reinforced with vascularized pleura, pericardium, or muscle flap to reduce risk of bronchopleural fistula and promote healing. If performed for carcinoma, the distal and proximal resection sites are examined histologically. If the distal site is positive, an upper lobectomy is performed. If proximal malignancy is found and further resection is not possible, radiation postoperatively is recommended. The objective of bronchial sleeve resection is preservation of healthy lung tissue and normal lung function in a distinct population of patients who would otherwise require pneumonectomy (Abdelsattar et al., 2017; Bolukbas et al., 2019).

KEY TAKEAWAYS

- Thoracic surgery can be a tool to diagnose, treat and palliate conditions of the chest and lung.
- Surgical consultation is made once it has been determined that surgery is appropriate for both the patient and their condition.
- A thorough preoperative evaluation is important to prevent adverse outcomes and optimize recovery. Pulmonary and cardiac risk assessments predict if a patient will tolerate surgery and have adequate quality of life afterward.
- Choice of surgical approach is determined by the underlying pathology and surgeon skill level.
- Minimally invasive surgical approaches such as VATS and RATS are associated with shorter hospital stays and less discomfort.

5.3: LUNG CANCER

PRESENTING SIGNS AND SYMPTOMS

History and Physical Findings

Patients presenting with any complaints of the thoracic region should have a comprehensive past medical history, including exposure to tobacco (primary or secondary exposure), heavy metals, environmental toxins, and asbestos as all of these predispose adults to pulmonary diseases (Markowitz & Dickens, 2020). The largest risk factor for developing lung cancer exposure to carcinogens is most specifically cigarette smoking (Stein & Luebbers, 2019). Detailed information about onset of symptoms, quality of symptoms, and associated symptoms should be prioritized.

Physical exam findings for those with diseases of the lung requiring surgical intervention are broad. The provider should utilize all examination skills, such as inspection, auscultation, percussion, and palpation, to identify abnormalities. Inspection can diagnose thoracic wall irregularities, tracheal positioning, and work of breathing, such as use of accessory muscles. Auscultation can distinguish between normal and abnormal lung sounds. While lung percussion only has a sensitivity of 10% to 20%, the specificity of dullness to percussion is 85% to 99% in identifying a consolidation or pleural effusion—both of which require further diagnostic testing. Palpation of the thorax identifies areas of tenderness, potentially large lymph nodes in the axillary and supraclavicular regions, and checks for any obvious masses not previously known to the patient (Chesnutt et al., 2021). Additionally, the provider should assess for nonpulmonary signs of a disease state, such as nail clubbing, cyanosis, peripheral edema, and elevated jugular venous distention (Chesnutt et al., 2021).

DIFFERENTIAL DIAGNOSIS AND DIAGNOSTIC CONSIDERATIONS

CXR are the initial step for evaluating pulmonary and thoracic abnormalities. Pulmonary nodules are incidentally found on less than 0.5% of routine chest imaging in nonsmokers. Detection rates increase to 9% in high-risk smokers. Moreover, when routine lung cancer screenings involving low-dose chest CT are performed, the incidence of solitary pulmonary nodules rises to 33% (Khan et al., 2019).

Unfortunately, not all patients undergo routine lung cancer screening. Most patients have already progressed to advanced and/or incurable disease when diagnosed (Jonas et al., 2021). Distant metastasis is present in approximately 56% of patients at initial diagnosis, 22% have regional spread, and only 15% of lung cancers are localized in the lungs at time of diagnosis (Pass et al., 2018). The median time from onset of symptoms to diagnosis of an oncologic process is 4 months (Price & Sikora, 2020). Given this short time interval, the U.S. Preventive Services Task Force published 2021 guidelines, suggesting annual CT screening for those at high risk of an oncologic process, defined as adults aged 50 to 80 years old who currently smoke or have quit within the last 15 years with at least a 20-year pack year history (Jonas et al., 2021).

Fleischner's Criteria

Guidelines for the management of solid pulmonary nodules were first published by The Fleischner's Society in 2005, with subsolid nodule guidelines published thereafter in 2013 (MacMahon et al., 2017). These guidelines, also referred to as Fleischner's criteria, are accepted as the gold standard for interval evaluation and risk stratification for incidentally found pulmonary nodules. However, these guidelines exclude immunocompromised patients, those already diagnosed with cancer, and those under the age of 35 years old (Khan et al., 2019). Additionally, pulmonary nodules (both solid and subsolid) must be at least 6 mm in size (Khan et al., 2019; MacMahon et al., 2017). See Figures 5.1 and 5.2 for solid versus subsolid recommendations for follow-up.

International Association for the Study of Lung Cancer Staging Criteria

Standard nomenclature for the staging of lung cancer provides consistent language about the anatomic disease burden of lung cancer. The International Association for the Study of Lung Cancer (IASLC) is the largest multidisciplinary global organization that publishes this standard taxonomy, allowing for consistent and reliable communication when classifying lung tumors. This nomenclature is accepted worldwide. The three central components of IASLC are: *T* for extent of

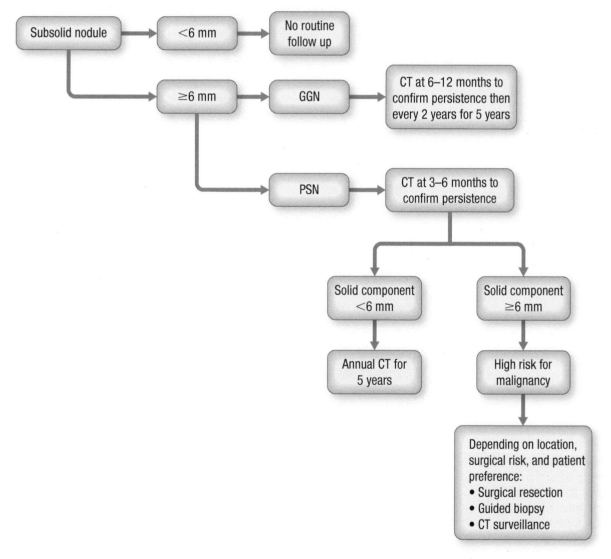

FIGURE 5.1: Management of a patient with a subsolid solitary pulmonary nodule.
GGN, ground glass nodule; PSN, partially solid nodule.

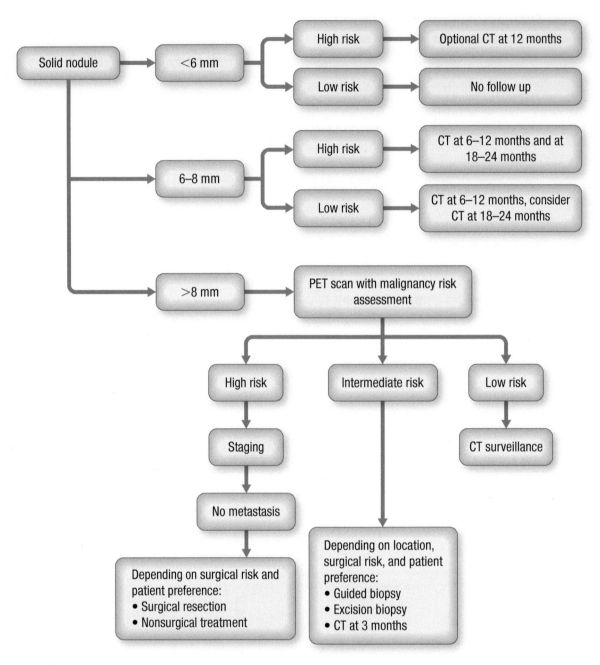

FIGURE 5.2: Suggested management of a patient with a solid solitary pulmonary nodule.

primary tumor, *N* for lymph node involvement, and *M* for distant metastases (Detterbeck et al., 2017). The tumor, or *T*, category describes size and invasion of the tumor into adjacent thoracic structures. The *N* indicates lymph node involvement. Distant metastases, or *M*, specifies intra-thoracic versus extra-thoracic lesions. The T, N, and M components are then subdivided into descriptors (e.g., T3 or N2) differentiating characteristics within each component (Detterbeck et al., 2017).

5.4: SURGICAL TREATMENT OF EMPHYSEMA

More than 30 million people in the United States have chronic obstructive pulmonary disease (COPD; Riley & Sciurba, 2019). Despite significant advances in drug therapy over the last 20 years, patients may develop severe disease refractory to medical management (Mirza et al., 2018;

Riley & Sciurba, 2019; Terry & Dhand, 2020). Alveolar destruction results in airflow obstruction and impaired gas exchange. Over time, air trapping and lung hyperinflation occur (Shah et al., 2017). As emphysema progresses, large (>1 cm), thin-walled air spaces called blebs may develop in the lungs. Blebs refer to lesions <1 to 2 cm. Lesions that are >2 cm are called bullae (van Berkel et al., 2010). These terms are often used interchangeably. Bullae can compress functional lung tissue leading to symptoms such as increased shortness of breath. The bullae are prone to rupture causing secondary (resulting from an underlying disease) spontaneous pneumothoraces (van Berkel et al., 2010). Surgical interventions may improve symptoms in carefully selected patients with upper lobe predominant bullous emphysema (van Agteren et al., 2016).

LUNG VOLUME REDUCTION SURGERY

Lung volume reduction surgery (LVRS) was first performed in 1957 for patients with severe COPD (Shah et al., 2017). The procedure improves the function of healthy areas of lung parenchyma, gas exchange, expiratory air flow and quality of life (Palamidas et al., 2017; Shah et al., 2017). However, it is not commonly performed due to the risk of morbidity and mortality and the paucity of dominant upper lobe heterogeneous emphysema (Sciurba et al., 2010, 2016). During LVRS, the thoracic surgeon removes the diseased upper lobe lung tissue. Excising damaged lung tissue decreases ventilation perfusion (VQ) mismatch by redistributing blood flow to functional lung units, thereby augmenting gas exchange (Lim et al., 2020; Mortensen & Berg, 2019; Shah et al., 2017). There are numerous contraindications to this procedure (Table 5.1). To qualify for this procedure, patients must have symptoms refractory to optimal medical management, abstain from tobacco for at least 6 months, and successfully complete pulmonary rehabilitation (Shah et al., 2017). Additionally, candidates must have a moderate to severe impairment in the diffusing capacity of the lungs for carbon monoxide (DLCO) <50%, significant airflow obstruction, lung hyperinflation, and heterogeneous emphysema (combination of damaged and preserved lung tissue) noted on high-resolution chest CT (HRCT), and VQ mismatch to various areas of the lungs (Mortensen & Berg, 2019; Shah et al., 2017). VQ mismatch is assessed using pulmonary scintigraphy. Scintigraphy is a nuclear imaging study that identifies heterogeneous areas of lung ventilation and perfusion. It correlates with the degree of emphysema and patient-reported symptoms better than high-resolution CT (Mortensen & Berg, 2019).

Postoperative complications of LVRS are similar to those associated with other thoracic surgeries. According to the Cochrane Database of Systematic Reviews, LVRS was associated with higher short-term mortality than medical management (van Agteren et al., 2016). This is similar to a higher 90-day mortality noted in subjects who underwent LVRS versus those in the control

TABLE 5.1: Contraindications to Lung Volume Reduction Surgery

Patient specific	Ongoing tobacco use
	Unable to complete pulmonary rehabilitation
	Extremes of body weight
	Significant comorbidities
	Previous thoracotomy or pleurodesis
Imaging findings	Bronchiectasis
	Homogeneous emphysema
	No preserved lung tissue
	No surgical targets
	Chest wall abnormalities that prevent surgery
Physiologic findings	DLCO <10%
	$PaCO_2$ >60 mmHg
	PA mean pressure >35 mmHg
	PA systolic pressure >45 mmHg
	Left ventricular ejection fraction <40%

Source: Data from Koster, T. D., & Slebos, D. J. (2016). The fissure: Interlobar collateral ventilation and implications for endoscopic therapy in emphysema. *International Journal of Chronic Obstructive Pulmonary Disease, 11*, 765–773. https://doi.org/10.2147/COPD.S103807; Mortensen, J., & Berg, R. M. G. (2019). Lung scintigraphy in COPD. *Seminars in Nuclear Medicine, 49*(1), 16–21. https://doi.org/10.1053/j.semnuclmed.2018.10.010; Sciurba, F. C., Criner, G. J., Strange, C., Shah, P. L., Michaud, G., Connolly, T. A., Deslee, G., Tillis, W. P., Delange, A., Marquette, C. H., Krishna, G., Kalhan, R., Ferguson, J. S., Jantz, M., Maldonado, F., McKenna, R., Majid, A., Rai, N., Gay, S., … Slebos, D. J. (2016). Effect of endobronchial coils versus usual care on exercise tolerance in patients with severe emphysema: The RENEW randomized clinical trial. *JAMA, 315*(20), 2178–2189; Shah, P. L., Herth, F. J., van Geffen, W. H., Deslee, G., & Slebos, D. J. (2017). Lung volume reduction for emphysema. *The Lancet Respiratory Medicine, 5*(2), 147–156. https://doi.org/10.1016/S2213-2600(16)30221-1

group during the original National Emphysema Treatment Trial (NETT; Fishman et al., 2003). LVRS improves dyspnea, but studies vary regarding which patients achieve postoperative LVRS symptom reduction. In NETT, only those participants with upper-lobe predominant emphysema and poor baseline exercise tolerance benefited from LVRS (Fishman et al., 2003). Despite a recent longitudinal data analysis of the NETT which demonstrated a significant reduction of dyspnea up to 5 years after LVRS, it did not increase long-term survival (Lim et al., 2020).

ENDOBRONCHIAL LUNG VOLUME REDUCTION

Endobronchial lung volume reduction (ELVR) is an emerging alterative to LVRS for decreasing lung hyperinflation caused by emphysema (Mortensen & Berg, 2019). ELVR is suitable for patients with less parenchymal destruction than those who qualify for LVRS (Shah et al., 2017). ELVR is performed during bronchoscopy by interventional pulmonologists. The procedure consists of inserting one-way endobronchial valves (EBV) into all the bronchi in the targeted lobe. The EBV prevent air flow into those sections of the lung. Endobronchial "exclusion" of the lobe leads to "reabsorption" atelectasis, which diminishes the extraneous lung volume. The goal is complete lobar atelectasis (Koster & Slebos, 2016; Shah et al., 2017).

In 2010, Sciurba and coworkers published the results of the Endobronchial Valve for Emphysema Palliation Trial (VENT). This study evaluated the effects of EBV placement ($n = 220$) versus standard medical management ($n = 101$). The experimental group demonstrated moderate improvements in forced expiratory volume over 1 second (FEV_1) and exercise capacity but had higher rates of hemoptysis and hospitalization for acute exacerbation of COPD (AECOPD; Sciurba et al., 2010). Earlier trials demonstrated the development of pneumonia distal to the EBV and pneumothoraces were the most common complications (Sciurba et al., 2010).

Despite these encouraging data, not all patients respond to treatment. One hypothesis is the presence of collateral ventilation (CV) (Koster & Slebos, 2016). Air flow through the lungs generally follows a standard pattern: Air enters the trachea, moves into the mainstem bronchus, travels into segmental bronchi (right and left mainstem bronchi) then to subsegmental bronchi, and lastly, through terminal bronchioles to alveoli (Rhoades & Bell, 2018). CV describes air flow through partially open (incomplete) fissures or channels to parts of the lung, instead of via the expected anatomic route (Terry & Traystman, 2016). Intralobar collateral ventilation (ICV) is common due to variations in human anatomic structure during fetal development (Koster & Slebos, 2016). Interestingly, there is more air flow through these incomplete fissures in patients with emphysema compared to those with normal lung (Koster & Slebos, 2016).

High resolution CT are indirect tests used to detect incomplete fissures associated with CV (Koster & Slebos, 2016; Sciurba et al., 2010). The Chartis System® (PulmonX Inc., Redwood City, CA, USA) is a newer diagnostic modality which directly provides data on expiratory flow, pressure, and resistance to determine the presence of CV (Koster & Slebos, 2016). During bronchoscopy, a balloon-tip catheter is inserted in the chosen airway and inflated. If the expiratory airflow (measured in mL/min) decreases when the balloon is occluding the airway, the test result is negative. A negative Chartis rules out CV (Koster & Slebos, 2016). Conversely, if there is no reduction in expiratory airflow, the test result is positive. A positive Chartis signifies the presence of CV (Koster & Slebos, 2016).

ALTERNATIVE THERAPY NOT AVAILABLE IN THE UNITED STATES

Endobronchial coiling is approved in Europe for endoscopically treating emphysema and severe lung hyperinflation by inducing atelectasis (Deslee et al., 2016; Klooster et al., 2015; Palamidas et al., 2017). During bronchoscopy, small nitinol wires (coils) are inserted under into subsegmental airways of one lung using fluoroscopic guidance. Once coils are deployed, they return to their original shape. Unlike EBV, the coils do not block air flow. The coils compress areas of emphysema, which improves elastic recoil of nearby lung tissue. Small studies showed positive effects on quality of life, pulmonary function, and exercise tolerance, but those benefits came at a high financial cost (Deslee et al., 2016; Klooster et al., 2015; Palamidas et al., 2017). Other studies have demonstrated less benefit (Sciurba et al., 2016). The U.S. Food and Drug Administration (FDA) has rejected applications for endobronchial coiling products due to the high risk of complications (e.g., hemoptysis, pneumothorax, pneumonia) versus usual care (FDA, 2018).

KEY TAKEAWAYS

- All patients with severe emphysema should be medically optimized and complete a pulmonary rehabilitation program, prior to consideration of surgical or endovascular lung volume reduction.
- LVRS improves symptoms and quality of life in selected patients, but it is associated with complications compared to medical management.
- ELVR is a less invasive approach to lung volume reduction. It is associated with decreased morbidity and mortality compared to surgical lung volume reduction. Alternative treatment for emphysema is available in Europe. It is not currently FDA approved due to the higher incidence of complications versus usual care.

POSTOPERATIVE CARE

Chest Tube Management

Thoracostomy or chest tube management is determined by many factors including the type of surgery performed and if the tube is needed to drain fluid, air, or both (Box 5.1). Systematic reviews have found that placing one 28F chest tube after thoracoscopic lobectomy is safe and effective and also decreases cost, hospital stay, and risk for transcutaneous infection. The placement of two chest tubes prolongs hospitalization without benefit of reducing need for thoracentesis (Deng et al., 2017; Gao et al., 2017; Kheir, 2108). If there is no air leak, a 19F Blake drain can be as effective as a 28F chest tubeat fluid removal with less discomfort to the patient (Deng et al., 2017).

Stripping

Routinely stripping chest tubes after thoracic surgery to maintain patency and promote drainage does not improve patient outcomes (Deng et al., 2017; Gao, et al., 2017; Kheir, 2018; Pompili et al., 2017). Chest tube stripping should only occur when the tubes are occluded or if cardiac tamponade is suspected (Loughran, 2019).

BOX 5.1 CHEST TUBES FOLLOWING LUNG RESECTION VIA THORACOSCOPY

A chest tube may be unnecessary after lung resection surgery via thoracoscopy if the following conditions are met:

- No air leak evident during the intraoperative test.
- Patient has no emphysematous bullae.
- No pleural adhesions were found upon entering the pleural space.
- There has been no prolonged pleural effusion

Source: Data from Deng, B., Qian, K., Zhou, J. H., Tan, Q. Y., & Wang, R. W. (2017). Optimization of chest tube management to expedite rehabilitation of lung cancer patients after video-assisted thoracic surgery: A meta-analysis and systematic review. *World Journal of Surgery*, 41(8), 2039–2045. https://doi.org/10.1007/s00268-017-3975-x.

Suction

Placement of a postoperative chest tube to suction or to water seal is a controversial topic. Review of the studies comparing suction versus no suction reveals no clear guideline for practice. While suctioning up to 20 cm H_2O improved pleura to pleural adherence and obliteration of the pleural space, prolonged suction at high levels has been shown to prolong air leak by pulling air through the chest tube. Suction has also been associated with increased drainage (Batchelor et al., 2019; Deng et al., 2017; Pompili et al., 2017). Water seal alone has been found to be effective for sealing small air leaks and encourages early mobilization as the patient is not limited due to a connection to wall suction, but it is insufficient to seal moderate to large air leaks (Batchelor et al., 2019; Pompili et al., 2017).

Current practice reflects these data with most routine use of suction avoided, 8 to 20 cm H_2O suction for 12 to 48 hours postoperatively for pleura-pleural adherence, if needed, then removing the chest tube if no air leak is present and drainage allows (Batchelor et al., 2019; Pompili et al., 2017). If an air leak persists, suction may be decreased or removed at this time to lessen the pull of air through the tube and seal the leak (Pompili et al., 2017). Electronic drainage systems have been developed to measure a patient's intrapleural pressure while the tube is in place. A pressure is set and maintained via varying levels of suction applied to the tube. More widespread use of these drainage systems may reveal improved knowledge of the optimum suction needed (Batchelor et al., 2019; Deng et al., 2017; Pompili et al., 2017).

Removal

A systematic review of studies published between 2000 and 2015 found that chest tubes can safely be removed with drainage up to 450 mL in 24 hours if the fluid is not bloody, infected, or chylous (Batchelor et al., 2019; Gao et al., 2017; Haywood et al., 2020; Kheir, 2018). Of note, patients who had chest tubes removed with 450 mL of drainage had a higher incidence of post-chest tube removal thoracentesis. Based on these data, a lower output limit may be a more reasonable goal. Some providers recommend using 300 mL in 24 hours as a conservative guide (Gao et al., 2017; Kheir, 2018). Removal of chest tubes on postoperative day (POD) 2 regardless of drainage is thought to be safe practice (Deng et al., 2017) The fluid profile of pleural fluid (PF) to blood protein ratio <0.5 can corroborate the decision to remove tubes (Gao et al., 2017). Removal of chest tubes is equally safe both at the end of inspiration and the end of expiration at preventing post removal pneumothorax (Gao et al., 2017; Kheir, 2018). The process of removal requires coordination with the patient to perform a Valsalva maneuver while the chest tubes are rapidly pulled in one swift movement (Kheir, 2018).

Perioperative Pain Management

As with all surgeries, postoperative pain is expected after thoracic surgery. The level of pain patients experience depends on the surgical approach, the organs or tissues involved (skin, subcutaneous fat, muscles), and the degree of the tissue disruption (Thompson-Brazill, 2019). Thoracotomy, for example, is one of the most painful surgeries based on standardized pain scales, such as visual analogue score. Thoracotomy involves incising muscles, intentionally fracturing ribs, and retracting tissues to gain exposure. Thoracotomy, thorascopic, and robotic approaches also cause pain due to lung resection and the chest tube placement (Thompson-Brazill, 2019). A population-based cohort study appraised the incidence of persistent pain in older adults after major (e.g., cardiac, thoracic, abdominal, pelvic) surgery. Thoracic patients were 2.58 times more likely to have prolonged opioid use than those who had nonthoracic procedures (Clarke et al., 2014).

Although minimally invasive procedures (e.g., VATS and RATS) result in less postoperative pain than traditional thoracotomies, all of these surgical approaches are associated with splinting and decreased respiratory effort leading to postoperative atelectasis, poor airway clearance, pulmonary shunting, alveolar collapse, and hypoxemia. Acute pain management is important as untreated postoperative pain can lead to a chronic condition called postthoracotomy pain syndrome (Lederman et al., 2019; Marshall & McLaughlin, 2020).

Intraoperative Pain Management Strategies

Thoracic Epidural Anesthesia

Thoracic epidural anesthesia (TEA) is s the traditional gold standard for patients undergoing a thoracotomy. It provides excellent pain management with lower opioid use and less need for rescue analgesia. The limiting side effects include hypotension, bradycardia, urinary retention, paresthesia, or spinal injury due to epidural hematoma, failed or partial block (Batchelor et al., 2019; Lederman et al., 2019).

Paravertebral Nerve Blocks

Paravertebral nerve blocks (PVB) involve infiltrating local anesthetic near the somatic and sympathetic nerves in the paravertebral space. Although PVBs have a 10% failure rate, studies have demonstrated PVBs deliver similar pain control to that of TEA without the accompanying risks (Batchelor et al., 2019; Lederman et al., 2019).

Intercostal Nerve Blocks

Intercostal nerve blocks (ICNB) are performed by injecting a long-acting local anesthetic agent such as extended-release bupivacaine (Exparel™) at the time of surgery or continuous bupivacaine infused by a catheter placed by the surgeon upon wound closure (Batchelor et al., 2019; Lederman et al., 2019).

Postoperative Multimodal Pain Management

Enhanced Recovery after Thoracic Surgery (ERATS) has taken the ERAS model and applied it to the thoracic surgery population. ERATS recommends a multimodal pain management protocol that emphasizes opioid sparing practices. Opioids are associated with increased nausea and vomiting, decreased mobilization, and prolonged return to a normal diet. Adjuvant therapies that potentiate analgesia while minimizing side effects are recommended (Batchelor et al., 2019; van Haren et al., 2018).

Acetaminophen

Acetaminophen is a low-risk medication that has been shown to reduce the use of opioid medication by 20%; it should be prescribed around the clock to patients without contraindications (Marshall & McLaughlin, 2020; van Haren et al., 2018).

Nonsteroidal Anti-inflammatory Drugs

Nonsteroidal anti-inflammatory drugs (NSAIDs) when combined with acetaminophen have better pain-relieving effects than either medication alone. Caution must be taken in hypovolemia and the elderly as there is risk for kidney injury (Marshall & McLaughlin, 2020; van Haren et al., 2018).

N-Methyl-D-Aspartate Antagonists

IV ketamine infusions have an equal analgesic effect compared to TEA. Ketamine is associated with reduced postoperative opioid use and should be considered in some patients, particularly those who have high preoperative opioid use (Marshall & McLaughlin, 2020).

Gabapentin

Gabapentin has been found to decrease postoperative nausea and vomiting in thoracic surgery patients and is an effective adjunctive therapy (Marshall & McLaughlin, 2020; van Haren et al., 2018).

Glucocorticoids

A one-time dose of dexamethasone 10 to 14 mg has been associated with decreased postoperative nausea and pain with mobility without increasing complications (Marshall & McLaughlin, 2020; van Haren et al., 2018).

Opioids

Opioids should be used sparingly. Their benefits must be balanced with risk of side effects and complications such as opioid-induced respiratory depression (Batchelor et al., 2019; Gupta et al., 2018). Recommendations are to start with tramadol if the preceding agents are ineffective then add opioids for pain greater than 4/10 as needed (van Haren et al., 2018). Patient-controlled analgesia (PCA) allows patients to give themselves IV opioid medication such as morphine or hydromorphone with the push of a button, improves patient satisfaction, and reduces the need for rescue analgesia. It should be used as needed and it has less risk of oversedation than parenteral opioid use (Lederman et al., 2019).

Postoperative Atrial Fibrillation

The risk of atrial fibrillation after thoracic surgery is greater than 15% for patients undergoing lobectomy or significant lung resection and can increase complications and length of stay. Atrial fibrillation risk increases with invasiveness of surgical approach and extent of resection with VATS seems to be somewhat protective with pneumonectomy carrying the greatest risk (Batchelor et al., 2019; Frendl et al., 2014: Haywood et al., 2020). The guidelines of the American Association for Thoracic Surgery (AATS, 2014) recommend avoidance of beta blocker withdrawal in thoracic surgery patients by continuing beta-blockers in patients who are on them prior to surgery. They also support maintaining a magnesium level >2.0 which can be preventive as well as therapeutic. Atrial fibrillation prophylaxis with diltiazem or amiodarone may be reasonable in high-risk patients but does not show improved patient outcomes (Frendl et al., 2014; Haywood et al., 2020).

Enhanced Recovery After Thoracic Surgery

Enhanced recovery after surgery (ERAS) protocols are evidenced-based, fast-track guidelines applied across the entire perioperative course. They have been shown to decrease complications and length of stay in colorectal surgery patients (Batchelor et al., 2019). These principles are now applied to the thoracic surgery population in the ERATS guidelines. These guidelines include preparing a patient preoperatively through nutritional assessments, smoking cessation, limited fasting, and beginning pain management. During the procedure, minimally invasive techniques, local anesthesia, judicious fluid management, and limitation of tube and line insertion are practiced as well as nausea and pain management. In the postoperative phase, the focus moves toward early mobilization, deep vein thrombosis (DVT) prevention, and early removal of invasive tubes. The multimodal pain management previously discussed is followed in an attempt to prevent prolonged pain (Batchelor et al., 2019; Haywood et al., 2020; van Haren et al., 2018).

TRANSITION OF CARE

Patients undergoing thoracic surgery are at increased risk for readmission (10%–17%) and for increased mortality if they are readmitted (19%). These data prompt providers to improve discharge coordination and ensure patient safety as they transition away from inpatient and into outpatient care (Shargall et al., 2016). Communication with the patient's primary care provider and pulmonary and oncology specialists is imperative to ensure a smooth transition across the care continuum (Thompson-Brazill et al., 2020).

Discharge Considerations

Inpatient discharge planning begins upon admission to the hospital and includes input from physical therapy, occupational therapy, nursing, medicine, and pharmacy. Dietary, speech and language pathology, and respiratory therapy are also consulted, if necessary. The care coordinator must then create a discharge plan with the patient and the family that integrates all the recommendations. Home care services are ordered based on this assessment (Shargall et al., 2016).

Home nursing care is not routinely needed for thoracic surgery patients unless the patient has other comorbidities. High-risk patients (e.g., altered mental status, syncope or near syncope, falls, shortness of breath, generalized weakness, and/or failure to thrive) may benefit from home health nursing visits and telehealth follow-up (Ouslander et al., 2020). Some may require temporary admission to a skilled nursing facility (SNF; Ouslander et al., 2020). All patients need education for surgical site care (minimal care is required) and signs and symptoms of infection. Surgical site infections (SSI) occur in approximately 11% of patients undergoing lung resection and are associated with diabetes mellitus, steroid use, and chemotherapy. Wound care consultation is indicated if surgical wound healing is impaired (Imperatori et al., 2017).

A small subset of patients will be discharged home with a chest tube. Patients with persistent air leak after pulmonary resection can be managed at home with chest tubes attached to a portable device. The simplest and least expensive of these devices is called a Heimlich valve. There are other devices that also provide the ability to collect pleural drainage. Each device has a one-way valve that allows air to flow out of the chest but will not allow air to flow back into the chest. Patients are then followed up in an outpatient clinic weekly to evaluate the leak and lung expansion. Prior to discharge, patients and their caregivers need education to properly care for the tubes and prevent infection. This information sharing can occur via in-person teaching, reviewing videos, and/or reading printed information (Thompson-Brazill et al., 2020) The vast majority of these tubes can be discontinued at the first visit (Toth et al., 2019). The largest risk of discharge with a chest tube is development of an empyema which may lead to readmission and need for additional procedures (Piccolo et al., 2015; Reinersman et al., 2018; Toth et al., 2019).

Patients undergoing thoracic surgery to treat an empyema may require home IV antibiotics. Current guidelines advise 3 weeks of antimicrobial therapy following surgical drainage. This will require placement of a peripherally inserted central catheter (PICC) line and in-home nursing to teach patients and families administration of antibiotics and care of the line (Birkenkamp et al., 2016). A follow-up appointment with the thoracic surgeon will be scheduled for 1 to 2 weeks post-surgery. This may include a CXR to determine if the infected fluid has been adequately evacuated and to determine if the chest tube should be removed (Toth et al., 2019). Surgical pathology and cultures that were not available while the patient was in the hospital will be reviewed with the patient. If necessary, patients may receive an oncology consultation.

KEY TAKEAWAYS

- Placement of chest tubes is common after thoracic surgery but limiting the number of tubes and the time they are in place improve outcomes.
- Pain management is imperative as thoracic surgery patients are at risk for prolonged pain syndromes. A multimodal approach to pain is recommended.
- Discharge planning for the thoracic surgery patient requires guidance from the interdisciplinary care team to prevent readmission. The need for home services is often dictated by the cause for surgery and patient comorbidities.

CLINICAL PEARLS

- Removal of chest tubes is equally safe at the end of inspiration and the end of expiration.
- Stripping chest tubes does *not* improve patient outcomes.
- Waterseal is often adequate to seal small air leaks and promotes early mobility.
- Avoid beta-blocker withdrawal to prevent postoperative atrial fibrillation.
- Acetaminophen scheduled around the clock decreases opioid use by 20%.

5.5: PLEURAL EFFUSIONS

Pleural fluid lubricates the pleura and allows the layers to move freely. The fluid is produced by the parietal pleura and absorbed by the pleural lymph system.

BOX 5.2 PLEURAL FLUID ANALYSIS BIOMARKERS FOR COMMON CAUSES OF PLEURAL EFFUSIONS

- **Hemothorax:** Hematocrit PF/serum = >0.5
- **Chylothorax:** Presence of chylomicrons in PF
- **Pseudochylothorax:** Presence of cholesterol crystals or cholesterol/triglyceride level >1
- **Malignant pleural effusion:** Cytology showing malignant cells
- **Urinothorax:** Creatinine PF/serum = >1 with pH <7.30
- **Pancreatitis:** PF amylase > 110 U/L

Source: Data from Mercer, R. M., Corcoran, J. P., Porcel, J. M., Rahman, N. M., & Psallidas, I. (2019). Interpreting pleural fluid results. *Clinical Medicine*, 19(3), 213–217. https://doi.org/10.7861/clinmedicine.19-3-213.

Pleural effusions represent an imbalance between the systems of production and absorption (Ferreiro et al., 2019; Mercer et al., 2019). The mechanisms by which increased fluid builds up in the pleural layers causing an effusion include increased hydrostatic pressure, decreased oncotic pressure, trauma to a thoracic duct or blood vessel, leakage from the abdominal cavity, and obstruction of lymphatic drainage. Differential diagnostic findings associated with pleural fluid analysis are included in Box 5.2.

PRESENTING SIGNS AND SYMPTOMS

- Shortness of breath, dyspnea, or breathlessness
- Activity intolerance
- Chest pain
- Cough
- Fever (Asciak & Rahman, 2018; Ferreiro et al., 2019; Mercer et al., 2019)

HISTORY AND PHYSICAL EXAM FINDINGS

History

Although there are many reasons for the development of a pleural effusion, three quarters of pleural effusions are due to one of four causes: heart failure, malignancy, tuberculosis, or pneumonia (Ferreiro et al., 2019; Mercer et al., 2019). A known history of these conditions will guide the diagnostic process. Other chronic conditions that can lead to pleural effusion include renal and liver failure and recent trauma or surgery to the chest (Ferreiro et al., 2019). Breathlessness is the most commonly reported symptom of pleural effusions (Muruganandan et al., 2020).

Physical Examination

Regardless of the type of pleural effusion, the pulmonary exam will have similar findings. The examiner will find diminished movement of the chest and decreased vocal fremitus on the side of the effusion. Breath sounds over the fluid collection will be decreased as will vocal resonance. A stony dullness will be noted with percussion over the effusion. In patients with a malignant pleural effusion (MPE), other signs of cancer such as palpable masses or lymphadenopathy may be present depending on the primary cancer (Asciak & Rahman, 2018).

DIFFERENTIAL DIAGNOSIS AND DIAGNOSTIC CONSIDERATIONS

The primary step in diagnosing the etiology of a pleural effusion is determining if the fluid is transudative or exudative. Transudate effusions develop when there is an alteration in the hydrostatic or oncotic pressure. These effusions have higher levels of fluid compared to protein, so they are not usually related to a pleural pathology. Exudate occurs from either increased capillary permeability or inability of lymphatics to drain. Exudative effusions are caused by a pleural-based disease, either infection or neoplasm (Ferreiro et al., 2019; Mercer et al., 2019). Light's criteria (Box 5.3) can determine if the effusion is transudative or exudative. Determining if the effusion is unilateral or bilateral may also aid in diagnosis.

Transudative Pleural Effusions

Heart Failure

The most common transudative pleural effusions are due to heart failure and these are diagnosed by CXR. Pleural effusions due to heart failure are generally bilateral. A pleural fluid sample is not needed unless the patient fails treatment with diuretics. An elevated N-terminal pro-brain natriuretic peptide (NT-pro-BNP) is highly sensitive (94%) and specific (91%) for diagnosing heart failure. A low NP-pro-BNP would indicate the etiology of the effusion is not heart failure (Ferreiro et al., 2019; Mercer et al., 2019).

BOX 5.3 LIGHT'S CRITERIA

Protein: Pleural/serum = >0.5 LDH:
Pleural/serum = >0.6 or PF LDH > ⅔ serum LDH in upper limits of normal
Any one of these criteria can diagnose an exudate.

Source: Data from Ferreiro, L., Toubes, M. E., San Jose, M. E., Suarez-Antelo, J., Golpe, A., & Valdes, L. (2019). Advances in pleural effusion diagnostics. *Expert Review of Respiratory Medicine*, 14(1), 51–66. https://doi.org/10.1080/17476348.2020.1684266; Mercer, R. M., Corcoran, J. P., Porcel, J. M., Rahman, N. M., & Psallidas, I. (2019). Interpreting pleural fluid results. *Clinical Medicine*, 19(3), 213–217. https://doi.org/10.7861/clinmedicine.19-3-213.

Hepatic Hydrothorax

The second most common cause of a transudative pleural effusion is due to portal hypertension and ascites. The fluid in the abdomen moves into the pleural space due to the negative pressure gradient. Defects in the diaphragm can also cause this condition (Ferreiro et al., 2019).

Trapped Lung

A "trapped lung" occurs as the result sequelae of untreated pulmonary inflammation. The inflammatory response causes the formation of a fibrinous rind that traps the lung in place and prevents full lung expansion. After the inflammation is treated, if the lung is still unable to expand, transudative fluid will fill the pleural space (Ferreiro et al, 2019).

Exudative Pleural Effusion

Infectious pleural effusions (IPE) are usually the result of a bacterial pneumonia but can also be the result of a ruptured esophagus or a lung abscess due to bronchiectasis, tuberculosis, or tumor. IPEs are classified as noncomplicated, complicated, and empyema. The earlier the presence of an IPE is discovered, the more likely the patient can achieve resolution without an invasive procedure. In all cases of IPE, identification of the appropriate antibiotic is the key to successful treatment. Microbiology and cytology specimens can be diagnostic (Ferreiro et al., 2019; Mercer et al., 2019).

A pleural fluid sample is indicated in all patients with suspected IPE. The pleural fluid should be sent for culture, cytology, and fluid analysis. In a noncomplicated pleural effusion, the lab values are as follows: pH >7.20; LDH <1000; glucose >60. In the presence of a pH <7.20, the effusion is considered complicated and drainage is indicated. Empyemas are staged according to the viscosity of the fluid in the space. In Stage I, the fluid is free moving; in Stage II, there is thick, nonmobile fluid which may be septated; and in Stage III, the fluid is nonmoving and fibrin deposition has occurred to form a pleural rind that can trap the lung (Mercer et al., 2019; Shen et al., 2017).

Malignant Pleural Effusion

MPE is the second most common form of exudative pleural effusion. The source is most often from malignancy of the breast, lung, or lymph but can also be due to mesothelioma. Nonmetastatic causes of paramalignant pleural effusion can result from etiologies such as pulmonary embolism, secondary effects of radiation treatment, and obstructive pneumonitis (Asciak & Rahman, 2018; Ferreiro et al., 2019). It is important to note that pleural effusion cytology is not reliable for diagnosing MPE. It has an average sensitivity of approximately 60% (Ali et al., 2019; Ferreiro et al., 2019). Cytology sensitivity is higher for adenocarcinoma (79%) and very low for mesothelioma (6%;Ferreiro et al., 2019). There is no evidence that successive fluid samples improve diagnostic accuracy (Ali et al., 2019; Ferreiro et al., 2019).

Tuberculous Pleural Effusion

Tuberculosis (TB) is a highly infectious disease that causes pleural effusion by both increasing capillary permeability and impairment of lymphatic drainage. The Mantoux skin test is negative in approximately 30% of patients with tuberculous PE. Diagnosis of a tuberculous pleural effusion (TB is confirmed by Ziehl-Neelsen staining or a positive culture of pleural fluid but this is only moderately sensitive). Measuring pleural fluid adenosine deaminase (ADA), a lymphocyte immune reactant, can be helpful. But understand that a false positive ADA can occur in the setting of IPE, rheumatoid effusion, and MPE. Often, it is difficult to get a diagnosis in these patients by pleural fluid alone and a tissue sample or positive sputum culture is required (Ferreiro et al., 2019: Mercer et al., 2019).

Diagnostic Procedures: Biopsy

Closed Pleural Biopsy

Closed pleural biopsy (CPB) is potentially indicated when a diagnosis is not found with pleural fluid analysis, a procedural attempt at tissue biopsy may be made prior to surgical consultation. CPB or "needle biopsy" uses a beveled needle and either CT or ultrasound guidance to obtain a piece of abnormal pleural tissue to examine. Radiographically guided CPB increases the diagnostic yield to up to 85% if abnormal tissue is visualized. Avoid performing the procedure if there are no visible abnormal sites to biopsy (Ali et al., 2019).

Pleuroscopy for Biopsy

Pleuroscopy is done under thoracic ultrasound. Utilizing local anesthesia, an incision is made at the 5th or 6th intercostal space where the lung is seen to move freely. A thoracoscope is used to examine the pleura and multiple biopsies are taken with forceps. A small-bore chest tube is placed to expand the lung. The pleuroscopy and CPB have similar diagnostic success for MPE and tuberculous PE (Ali et al., 2019).

Diagnostic Procedures: Imaging

Chest Radiograph

The presence of bilateral effusions and cardiomegaly is diagnostic of heart failure (Ferreiro et al., 2019). A single-sided effusion that is very large is suspicious for malignancy (Asciak & Rahman, 2018). A minimum of 175 to 200 mL is required to blunt the costophrenic angles and reveal a free-flowing pleural effusion. Traditionally, if a lateral decubitus x-ray showed an effusion measuring 1 cm, a pleural fluid sample would be indicated. Many effusions are complex, non-free-flowing, and have septations that are not easily seen by a standard chest x-ray (CXR). A non-gravity dependent pleural effusion can indicate septation or loculation revealing an IPE (Asciak & Rahman 2018; Ferreiro et al., 2019; Shen et al., 2017).

Pleural Ultrasound

Pleural ultrasound (US) is recommended along with CXR when evaluating a pleural space infection. It is better than a CXR at identifying small effusions and estimating volume. The portability of US at the bedside has made it an invaluable tool for critical care and emergency department providers (Shen et al., 2017). Pleural US recognizes septations and enhanced echogenicity which are identified as patterns of infection (Ferreiro et al., 2019; Shen et al., 2017). It identifies pleural thickening, pleural nodules, and diaphragm thickening which are indications of malignant effusion (Ferreiro et al., 2019). It is recommended that pleural US be used to guide all pleural interventions as it improves results and reduces risk (Asciak & Rahman, 2018; Ferreiro et al., 2019; Shen et al., 2017).

Computed Tomography

CT of the chest enhanced by IV contrast is useful in evaluating exudative effusions. CT criteria for malignancy includes circumferential pleural thickening, nodular pleural thickening, parietal pleural thickening of greater than 1 cm, and mediastinal pleural involvement (Ferreiro et al., 2019). For infections in the pleural space, CT may identify a cause such as a mass, foreign body, or rupture in the esophagus (Shen et al., 2017). The split pleura sign of thickening and increased enhancement of the visceral and parietal pleura is indicative of an empyema and is enhancement of the chest wall adipose tissue. CT can distinguish free fluid from loculated, identify air bubbles, and reveal a comprehensive picture of the lungs and other structures of the thorax (Ferreiro et al., 2019; Shen et al., 2017).

Magnetic Resonance Imaging

Magnetic resonance imaging (MRI) of the chest is helpful in identifying tumors of the chest wall, soft tissue mediastinum and diaphragm although poor resolution due to lung movement may impact findings. MRI can differentiate transudates from exudates using diffusion weight and dynamic enhanced contrast (Ferreiro et al., 2019; Shen et al., 2017).

Positron Emission Tomography

Fluorine 18 (^{18}F)-fluorodeoxyglucose (FDG) positron emission tomography (PET/CT) can identify hypermetabolic tissue that may be a primary malignancy or metastatic spread. The areas of hypermetabolic uptake of FDG are called "PET avid." Unfortunately, areas of infection and inflammation are often PET avid. In these cases, other imaging modalities are more appropriate (Ferreiro et al., 2019; Shen et al., 2017).

PLEURAL EFFUSION TREATMENT

Thoracentesis

Thoracentesis or removal of pleural fluid with a large bore needle under ultrasound guidance is the first line treatment to obtain pleural fluid for diagnosis and to drain the pleural space. Thoracentesis can provide important information about the pleural effusion beyond provision of fluid for analysis. Once drained, reassess

the patient for symptomatic improvement. If dyspnea does not improve, there may be another underlying etiology. A recent study showed improvements in dyspnea, 6-minute walk test, heart rate, and respiratory rate, and statistically significant improvements in FEV_1 (P <0.001) and FVC (p <0.001; Muruganandan et al., 2020.) Also, once the fluid is removed, a CXR should be obtained to look for the re-expansion of the lung into the space that the fluid occupied. Lack of expansion may indicate the presence of a trapped lung (Ali et al., 2019). In an MPE, this could guide further treatment. Lack of symptom response to fluid removal may indicate that further treatment would be unhelpful. Poor lung expansion precludes the use of pleurodesis and the provider should consider use of an intrapleural catheter (IPC) should the fluid reaccumulate (Ali et al., 2019). In an IPE, inability to fully drain the effusion or expand the lung indicates need for a more invasive treatment (Shen et al., 2017).

Tube Thoracostomy

Tube thoracoscopy, or chest tube insertion, is indicated to drain fluid or air from a pleural cavity. A tube is placed for pleural fluid in the presence of a large or persistent pleural effusion, a parapneumonic effusion, a complicated IPE, a hemothorax, or a chylothorax. Chest tubes are placed under strict sterile technique at the bedside, in the radiology department, or in a pulmonary lab. Ultrasound guidance should be used to best target the fluid collection and minimize risk of complications. Recent studies have shown that small bore catheters such as 8F pigtail catheters are as effective as traditional large bore catheters (24–32F) at draining pleural effusions and are associated with less pain (Hamad & Alfeky, 2021; Porcel, 2018).

Thrombolytic Therapy

When a chest tube does not adequately drain a complicated parapneumonic effusion or empyema, intrapleural fibrinolytic agents are often inserted in the pleural space via the chest tube to break up the effusion and enable drainage. A 2019 Cochrane review established that fibrinolytics are useful in draining the pleural space and decrease the need for surgery in patients with empyema (Altmann et al., 2019). The combination of tissue plasminogen activator (tPA) and deoxyribonuclease (DNASE) once daily through the thoracostomy tube in a multinational study (MIST2) resulted in 92.3% of patients having resolution of their sepsis and drainage of their effusion without surgical consultation. The complication rate was less than a 4% risk of nonfatal bleeding. These results have led to the use of fibrinolytic therapy as the first line of treatment for complicated empyemas over surgical drainage (Piccolo et al., 2015; Porcel, 2018).

Pleuroscopy and Medical Thoracoscopy

Pleuroscopy is done under thoracic ultrasound in an interventional radiology or pulmonology suite. Utilizing local anesthesia, an incision is made at the 5th or 6th intercostal space much like would be done to insert a chest tube. A thoracoscope is used to examine the pleura then forceps can be used to obtain a biopsy, as described previously, or to treat an empyema through the lysis of adhesions and loculations that are not amenable to fibrinolytic agents or DNASE (Ali et al., 2019). A small-bore chest tube is left in place. Also called a medical thoracoscopy, this is a procedure that straddles the line between tube thoracostomy and video-assisted thoracoscopic surgery (VATS). It is more cost-effective as it is done under local anesthesia and may be better tolerated by frail patients. Recent studies have shown it is safe and effective in Stage I and II empyemas and can reduce the length of stay when compared with intrapulmonary fibrinolytic therapy (Asciak & Rahman, 2018; Kheir et al., 2020; Sumalani et al., 2018).

Surgical Drainage of Empyema and Decortication

An empyema is a complex collection of infectious fluid in the pleural space. Drainage is necessary to evacuate the empyema and allow for lung re-expansion. In addition to treating the patient with broad-spectrum antibiotics, a chest tube is inserted, and pleural fluid is sent for culture and sensitivity, along with the other pleural fluid diagnostics mentioned this chapter (Godfrey et al., 2019). tPA/DNASE may be instilled in the pleural space via the chest tube to facilitate purulent fluid removal (Godfrey et al., 2019). Surgery may be necessary to evacuate empyemas that do not improve with instillation of tPA/DNASE (Godfrey et al., 2019; Shen et al., 2017). The goals of surgical intervention include completely evacuating the infectious material and achieving full lung expansion. Although VATS is recommended as the first line of approach, conversion to an open thoracotomy may be necessary to successfully decorticate the lung (Godfrey et al., 2019; Shen et al., 2017).

Decortication involves entering the thoracic cavity, evacuating the loculated effusion then carefully dissecting the pleural peel away from the lung parenchyma including the fissures. The lung is then re-inflated to observe expansion and check for air leaks. All leaks must be sutured prior to closure. One or two chest tubes are then left in place to aid lung expansion and fully evacuate the infectious material (Godfrey et al., 2019). The basilar empyema tube may be left in place and removed gradually to avoid a residual collection of fluid and promote full lung expansion (Shen et al., 2017).

Pleurodesis

Chemical pleurodesis can be performed either during surgical thoracoscopy or via a thoracostomy tube. The preferred agent is talc or silicate-based, asbestos-free powder which, when put into the pleural space, causes an inflammatory response that leads to pleural adhesion formation eliminating the pleural space, not allowing pleural fluid to reaccumulate. This procedure can be up to 75% effective. It is contraindicated in patients with a

"trapped" lung. Talc is inserted via a chest tube or at the time of a medical thoracoscopy. After insertion of the talc, the chest tube is placed to low suction and removed once the fluid is completely drained. Patients generally tolerate the procedure well but may experience pain, fever, and, rarely, infection at the tube site (Asciak & Rahman, 2018; Guinde et al., 2018).

Intrapleural Catheter

Intrapleural catheter (IPC) insertion is a viable option for all patients with recurrent MPE. A small 15.5F silicone catheter is placed into the pleural fluid under local anesthesia. The patient or their caregiver can then drain the fluid at home as needed, decreasing the need for hospitalization and medical visits. Almost 50% of patients will eventually have a spontaneous pleurodesis and the catheter can be removed. Complications are rare and include pneumothorax, tube displacement or obstruction, and infection (Asciak & Rahman, 2018; Guinde et al., 2018).

Palliative Treatments

For patients with MPE, it is often necessary to mitigate the symptoms of persistent or recurrent pleural effusion when the etiology cannot be removed. If initial drainage of a MPE provides relief of breathlessness, and the patient has a prognosis of survival of greater than 1 month, the option for chemical pleurodesis or placement of an IPC should be offered (Asciak & Rahman, 2018).

TRANSITION OF CARE

Length of hospital stay and discharge disposition are linked to the etiology of the pleural effusion and the method of treatment chosen. IPEs often require longer hospital stays as full treatment of the sepsis, drainage of the effusion, and full expansion of the lung is required before discharge. A stepwise process of chest tube placement, fibrinolytic therapy, then ultimately invasive procedures can lead to a prolonged inpatient stay. Early medical and surgical thoracoscopy has been shown to decrease length of stay. Treatment during this process includes continued antibiotic therapy, pain management, mobilization and pulmonary hygiene as well as serial CXRs to monitor progress. Chest tubes are usually removed prior to discharge although occasionally an empyema tube will be left in place and slowly removed as an outpatient (Shen et al., 2017).

Treatment of MPE focuses on transitioning patients out of the hospital and keeping them at home. Length of hospital stay is often dependent on the difficulty in making a diagnosis. Pleurodesis and chest tube management can also prolong inpatient hospitalization. Postprocedure care includes pain management if treatment included chest tube insertion or chemical pleurodesis, pulmonary hygiene, mobilization, thrombosis prophylaxis, and symptom management (Ali et al., 2019; Porcel, 2019).

KEY TAKEAWAYS

- Clinically significant pleural effusions require that the etiology be discovered.
- Light's criteria (Box 5.3) can determine if the effusion is transudative or exudative.
- Other pleural fluid tests can help narrow down potential causes of effusions.
- It is more difficult to determine the etiologies and treat exudative compared to transudative effusions.

CLINICAL PEARLS

- Bilateral pleural effusions are often heart failure and do not require a pleural fluid sample before treating.
- Large unilateral pleural effusions are suspicious for malignancy.
- Effusions with septations and gas are infectious.

EVIDENCE-BASED RESOURCES

American Cancer Society (n.d.). *Lung cancer screening guidelines.* https://www.cancer.org/health-care
-professionals/american-cancer-society-prevention
-early-detection-guidelines/lung-cancer-screening
-guidelines.html

American College of Chest Physicians. (2013). *Diagnosis and management of lung cancer* (3rd ed.). American College of Chest Physicians Evidence-Based Clinical Practice Guidelines

Global Initiative for Chronic Obstructive Lung Disease. (2019). *2020 Strategy for prevention, diagnosis, and management of COPD.* https://goldcopd.org/wp-content/
uploads/2019/12/GOLD-2020-FINAL
-ver1.2-03Dec19_WMV.pdf

A robust set of instructor resources designed to supplement this text is located at http://connect.springerpub.com/content/reference-book/978-0-8261-6079-9. Qualifying instructors may request access by emailing **textbook@springerpub.com.**

REFERENCES

*Full list of references can be accessed at http://connect
.springerpub.com/content/reference-book/978-0-8261-6079-9*

CHAPTER 6

VASCULAR DISORDERS

Amy Elliott, Ann Eschelbach, Valerie J. Fuller, Clare Harris, and Ann Luciano

LEARNING OBJECTIVES

- Identify aneurysms and dissections, treatment guidelines, and risk factor modifications for patients with aortic aneurysms.
- Describe guideline-based care for the patient with carotid artery stenosis.
- Recognize signs and symptoms of venous thromboembolism (VTE) and potential treatment options
- Differentiate between an arteriovenous fistula and an arteriovenous graft and their complications
- Apply guideline-based recommendations for treatment of patients with peripheral arterial disease (PAD).
- Differentiate common symptoms of acute versus chronic mesenteric ischemia.

INTRODUCTION

Vascular disease includes any disease that affects the arteries and/or veins and is a leading cause of morbidity and mortality worldwide. This chapter provides the reader with an overview of the diagnosis and treatment of aneurysmal disease, venous thromboembolism (VTE), extracranial carotid disease, peripheral arterial disease (PAD), mesenteric ischemia, and dialysis access. Care of patients with these conditions can be complex and often requires a multimodal and team-based approach.

6.1: ANEURYSMS

An aneurysm is an abnormal dilatation of a blood vessel, typically defined as >50% of the diameter of normal adjacent vessels. Aortic aneurysms can occur in either the thoracic or abdominal aorta and up to 25% of patients may have coexisting thoracic and aortic aneurysmal disease (Braverman & Schermerhorn, 2022). Thoracic aortic aneurysms (TAAs) involve the ascending and descending aorta and abdominal aortic aneurysms (AAAs) involve the infrarenal aorta (Guo et al., 2006). Aneurysms are most commonly located in the infrarenal aorta followed by the ascending thoracic aorta and can be either fusiform (symmetrically dilated) or saccular (focal outpouching; Braverman & Schermerhorn, 2022; Guo et al., 2006). See Figure 6.1. TAAs are caused by a degenerative process whereas AAAs are most commonly associated with atherosclerosis.

PRESENTING SIGNS AND SYMPTOMS

Most aortic aneurysms are asymptomatic until disruption or dissection occurs. Often, they are found incidentally on imaging studies such as echocardiogram, x-ray, CT scan, or ultrasound.

Thoracic Aortic Aneurysms

If symptomatic, presenting signs and symptoms may include persistent cough, wheezing, shortness of breath, dysphagia, or hoarseness from laryngeal nerve compression (Erbel et al., 2014). TAA rupture often presents with sudden, severe chest or back pain, hypotension, hematemesis, or hemoptysis (Braverman & Schermerhorn, 2022).

Abdominal Aortic Aneurysms

If symptomatic, presenting signs and symptoms may include chest, abdominal, low back, and/or scrotal pain with a pulsatile abdominal mass. AAA rupture often results in sudden severe abdominal pain, hypotension, and syncope (Braverman & Schermerhorn, 2022).

HISTORY AND PHYSICAL FINDINGS

A thorough medical, family, and social history should be obtained. Relevant patient history includes increased age, other atherosclerotic diseases, smoking history, and hypertension. A smoking history is significantly associated with aneurysmal disease—more than 90% of patients with an AAA have smoked cigarettes at some point in their lifetime and persistent tobacco use leads to ongoing aneurysm growth (Chaikof et al., 2018). Males are at greater risk as are individuals with a family history of aneurysmal disease.

Thoracic Aortic Aneurysms

Physical exam findings are typically limited but may include aortic murmur. There are several genetic defects associated with TAA (Table 6.1).

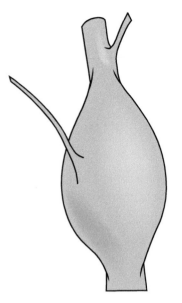

(A) Fusiform (symmetrically dilated)

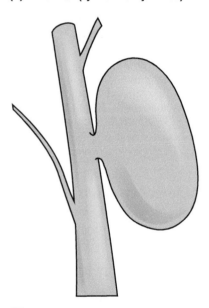

(B) Saccular (focal outpouching)

FIGURE 6.1: (A) Fusiform (symmetrically dilated); and (B), saccular (focal outpouching) aneurysms.

Abdominal Aortic Aneurysms

Physical exam findings in asymptomatic disease may include palpation of a pulsatile abdominal mass but physical exam has been shown to be only moderately sensitive for detecting AAA (Chaikof et al., 2018). There may also be associated iliac or popliteal aneurysms on exam (coexisting disease can be seen in over 60% of patients).

Given the association with tobacco use, the U.S. Preventive Services Task Force (USPSTF) recommends a one-time screening for AAA with ultrasonography in males aged 65 to 75 years who have ever smoked (https://www.uspreventiveservicestaskforce.org/uspstf/recommendation/abdominal-aortic-aneurysm-screening).

DIFFERENTIAL DIAGNOSIS AND DIAGNOSTIC CONSIDERATIONS

- Differentials for TAA include myocardial infarction, pulmonary embolism (PE), pericarditis, or aortic dissection.
- Differentials for AAA include pancreatitis, mesenteric ischemia, ruptured gastric ulcer, appendicitis, cholelithiasis, nephrolithiasis, or diverticulitis.
- Diagnostic considerations: Imaging should be completed with ECG-gated contrast CT scan (if possible) to decrease motion artifact. Centerline reconstruction should be completed by radiology for the most accurate measurements as axial images may overestimate dimensions given the tortuosity of the aorta (Hiratzka et al., 2010a; Ihara et al., 2013).

TREATMENT

Thoracic Aortic Aneurysms

Treatment is recommended for all symptomatic TAAs (Erbel et al., 2014; Hiratzka et al., 2010b). For asymptomatic patients, repair depends on the disease present, size, type (genetic conditions, degenerative, etc.), comorbid conditions, and expansion rate. Surgical treatment can be open surgical repair (OSR) or thoracic endovascular aortic repair (TEVAR).

Abdominal Aortic Aneurysms

Elective repair of asymptomatic AAAs involves a careful determination of comorbid medical conditions, life expectancy, rupture risk, repair risk, aneurysm size, and expansion rate. Risk of rupture within 5 years of diagnosis is increased for AAAs larger than 5 cm (McGloughlin & Doyle, 2010). Repair is recommended when the diameter exceeds 5.4 cm or when there is rapid expansion (>1 cm/year), young age, and in females (repair in females should be considered closer to 5 cm; Braverman & Schermerhorn, 2022). Symptomatic nonruptured aneurysms should be treated urgently. Ruptured AAAs represent a true surgical emergency and are associated with significant mortality, more than 50% of patients die before hospitalization and another 30% to 40% die after reaching the hospital but before treatment (Braverman & Schermerhorn, 2022; Chaikof et al., 2018). Surgical treatment can be OSR or endovascular aortic repair (EVAR).

TABLE 6.1: Genetic Defects Associated With Thoracic Aneurysm

DISORDERS WITH KNOWN AFFECT AORTA INCREASED RISK RUPTURE	GENOTYPES	PHENOTYPE	SURGICAL INDICATION
Marfan syndrome	*FBN1*	Lanky stature, scoliosis, dural ectasia, stretch marks hypermobile joints, lens dislocation, pectus deformity	4.5 or greater
Loeys-Dietz	*TGFB1, TGFB2*	Scoliosis, pectus deformity, translucent skin, bruise easily, flat feet, stretch marks, bifid uvula	4.5
Ehlers-Danlos vascular	*COl.3A1*	Hypermobile joints, difficulty with wound healing, loose skin, intestinal perforations	4.5
Familial thoracic aneurysms	*ACTA2, SMAD3, MYH11*	N/A	5.0

KEY TAKEAWAYS

- Blood pressure control
- Smoking cessation is essential to slow aneurysm growth
- First degree relatives should also be screened for aneurysmal disease
- Serial imaging to evaluate growth
- Consider genetic counseling for younger patients with aortic aneurysms
- Aneurysms are not always surgical but require continued evaluation.

EVIDENCE-BASED RESOURCES

2010 ACCF/AHA/AATS/ACR/ASA/SCA/SCAI/SIR/STS/SVM guidelines for the diagnosis and management of patients with thoracic aortic disease: A report of the American College of Cardiology Foundation/American Heart Association Task Force on Practice Guidelines, American Association for Thoracic Surgery, American College of Radiology, American Stroke Association, Society of Cardiovascular Anesthesiologists, Society for Cardiovascular Angiography and Interventions, Society of Interventional Radiology, Society of Thoracic Surgeons, and Society for Vascular Medicine.

2014 ESC guidelines on the diagnosis and treatment of aortic disease: Document covering acute and chronic aortic disease of the thoracic and abdominal aorta of the adult. The Task Force for the Diagnosis and Treatment of Aortic Disease of the European Society of Cardiology (ESC).

6.2: AORTIC DISSECTIONS/RUPTURE

Aortic dissection is defined as disruption in the media layer of the aortic wall leading to separation of the wall thereby creating true and false lumens (Figure 6.2; Hiratzka et al., 2010a). These may be classified as acute (within 2 weeks), or chronic (more than 3 months) as defined by DeBakey et al. (1982).

In the DeBakey classification of aortic dissection (Figure 6.3):
- Type I involves the ascending aorta, arch, and descending thoracic aorta and may progress to involve the abdominal aorta.
- Type II is confined to the ascending aorta.
- Type IIIa involves the descending thoracic aorta distal to the left subclavian artery and proximal to the celiac artery.
- Type IIIb dissection involves the thoracic and abdominal aorta distal to the left subclavian artery.

In the Stanford classification of aortic dissection (Figure 6.3):
- Type A involves the ascending aorta and may progress to involve the arch and thoracoabdominal aorta.
- Type B involves the descending thoracic or thoracoabdominal aorta distal to the left subclavian artery without involvement of ascending aorta.

Risk factors for aortic dissection include hypertension, atherosclerosis, stimulant use (cocaine or methamphetamines), weightlifting, trauma, genetic or congenital disorders, or inflammatory/infectious diseases (Braverman & Schermerhorn, 2022; Hiratzka et al., 2010a).

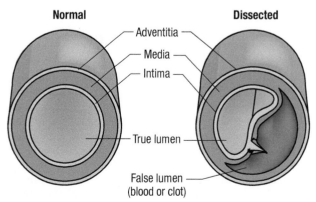

FIGURE 6.2: Aortic dissection. Aortic dissection is a tear in the innermost layer, the intima, which then allows blood to flow in a true and false lumen over a length of the vessel.

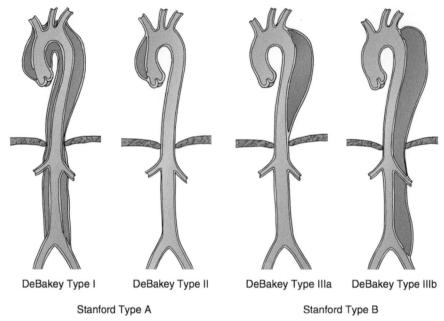

DeBakey Type I   DeBakey Type II   DeBakey Type IIIa   DeBakey Type IIIb

Stanford Type A   Stanford Type B

FIGURE 6.3: Classification of aortic dissections: DeBakey and Stanford types.
Source: Reproduced with permission from Alfson, D. B., & Ham, S. W. (2017). Type B aortic dissections. *Cardiology Clinics, 35*(3), 387–410. https://doi.org/10.1016/j.ccl.2017.03.007.

PRESENTING SIGNS AND SYMPTOMS

The most common presentation of aortic dissection is the sudden onset of severe chest, back, or abdominal pain. Pain quality may be described as ripping, tearing, sharp, or stabbing. Pain the neck, throat, or jaw suggests involvement of the ascending aorta and pain in the back, abdomen, or lower extremities suggests involvement of the descending aorta (Braverman & Schermerhorn, 2022). Other complications such as end-organ ischemia, myocardial infarction, cardiac tamponade, heart failure, or stroke may also be seen. Hypotension and shock are associated with higher mortality, as well as concomitant ischemia, myocardial infarction, and death in 55% of patients (Evangelista et al., 2018).

HISTORY AND PHYSICAL FINDINGS

Physical findings can be highly variable and depend on the type and extent of dissection. Pain is common and hypertension is present in 80% of type B dissections and 30% of type A dissections (Braverman & Schermerhorn, 2022). Type A dissections will more commonly present with chest pain, while type B dissections are more likely to present with back pain (Hiratzka et al., 2010a). Other exam findings may include syncope, aortic murmur, cardiac tamponade, pericardial effusion, congestive heart failure, acute renal failure, stroke, mesenteric ischemia, upper or lower extremity ischemia, hypotension, or shock (Braverman & Schermerhorn, 2022; Hiratzka et al., 2010a).

Diagnostic imaging for aortic dissections includes echocardiogram (transthoracic echocardiogram [TTE]/transesophageal echocardiogram [TEE]), MRI, or CT angiography (CTA; Braverman & Schermerhorn, 2022).

DIFFERENTIAL DIAGNOSIS AND DIAGNOSTIC CONSIDERATIONS

- Abdominal dissection: Pancreatitis, mesenteric ischemia, ruptured gastric ulcer, appendicitis, cholelithiasis, nephrolithiasis, or diverticulitis.
- Thoracic dissection: Myocardial infarction, pulmonary embolism, pneumonia, pericarditis.

TREATMENT

Surgical consultation should be obtained for all dissections. Initial management includes blood pressure, heart rate, and pain control. A systolic blood pressure of 100 to 120 and heart rate of less than 60 is recommended using IV beta-blockers such as labetalol, metoprolol, or esmolol (nondihydropyridine calcium channel antagonists can be used if beta-blockers are contraindicated; Hiratzka et al., 2010b). Hypotension should be treated with IV fluids. Vasopressors may be added if there is refractory hypotension, but these have the potential to extend the luminal dissection. Surgical management depends on the location of the dissection but remains the treatment of choice for type A aortic dissections (Braverman & Schermerhorn, 2022). Uncomplicated type B aortic dissections are most commonly treated with blood pressure, pulse, and pain control. Complicated type B dissections are those associated with malperfusion, refractory hypertension, rapid increase in aortic diameter, or recurrent symptoms and should be fixed surgically with thoracic endovascular aortic repair (TEVAR; Braverman & Schermerhorn, 2022).

TRANSITION OF CARE

Urgent consult with vascular or cardiothoracic surgery for operative management if indicated. Cardiology consultation is also recommended.

KEY TAKEAWAYS

- Type A dissection is a surgical emergency.
- Uncomplicated type B dissections are treated medically. Complicated type B dissections should be surgically repaired with TEVAR.
- Early identification improves the rate of successful treatment.

EVIDENCE-BASED RESOURCES

2010 ACCF/AHA/AATS/ACR/ASA/SCA/SCAI/SIR/ STS/SVM guidelines for the diagnosis and management of patients with thoracic aortic disease. A report of the American College of Cardiology Foundation/American Heart Association Task Force on Practice Guidelines, American Association for Thoracic Surgery, American College of Radiology, American Stroke Association, Society of Cardiovascular Anesthesiologists, Society for Cardiovascular Angiography and Interventions, Society of Interventional Radiology, Society of Thoracic Surgeons, and Society for Vascular Medicine https://www.ahajournals.org/doi/10.1161/CIR.0b013e3181d4739e?url_ver=Z39.88-2003&r-fr_id=ori:rid:crossref.org&rfr_dat=cr_pub%20%200pubmed.

6.3: CAROTID ARTERY DISEASE

Atherosclerosis is a systemic disease affecting all vascular beds. Carotid stenosis, which is attributed to atherosclerosis, is a ≥50% stenosis of the internal carotid artery (ICA; Aboyans et al., 2018). The incidence of carotid stenosis, as with other atherosclerotic disease, increases with age (Aday & Beckman, 2017). Males are diagnosed with carotid stenosis more frequently than females, and non-Hispanic, White and American Indians are at higher risk than other racial groups (Aday & Beckman, 2017). Carotid stenosis is the cause for approximately 10% to 20% of all strokes and is a risk factor for future cardiovascular complications (Aday & Beckman, 2017; Mortimer et al., 2018). Asymptomatic patients with carotid stenosis have a 3% increased risk of stroke in the next year, while patients with transient ischemic attack (TIA)

have a 25% risk of stoke within 14 days of the TIA (Aboyans et al., 2018; Gaba et al., 2018). The European Society of Cardiology guidelines recommend that treatment for carotid stenosis includes risk factor modification as well as antiplatelet and statin use for all patients (Aboyans et al., 2018). Carotid endarterectomy (CEA) and stenting are available treatment options for patients with stroke and carotid artery stenosis.

PRESENTING SIGNS AND SYMPTOMS

Patients with carotid stenosis can present in one of two ways. Asymptomatic patients present with abnormal duplex testing, a new carotid bruit or concern for systemic vascular disease. Asymptomatic means that no prior symptoms can be identified or that symptoms occurred greater than 6 months ago (Aboyans et al., 2018).

Symptomatic patients describe symptoms attributable to the carotid stenosis within the preceding 6 months (Aboyans et al., 2018). Symptoms can include sudden unilateral weakness, numbness/tingling, trouble speaking, amaurosis fugax (a temporary loss of vision that is often described as a curtain or a shade that comes down over the eye), confusion or memory problems, headache without other known cause, and difficulty walking or lack of coordination. Patients with symptoms indicative of a possible stroke should be immediately evaluated in the emergency department for more aggressive management.

HISTORY AND PHYSICAL FINDINGS

A careful assessment of the history of the patient's symptoms is an important first step in diagnosing carotid stenosis. A history of a sudden onset and recovery of dysarthria, unilateral weakness, ataxia, and/or amaurosis fugax, are concerning symptoms for carotid artery stenosis. TIAs are stroke symptoms that resolve within minutes to a few hours and are fully resolved within 24 hours. A stroke has symptoms that are longer lasting and often produce disability (Mortimer et al., 2018). In addition to symptoms, lifestyle habits, physical activity, and diet should be assessed (Aboyans et al., 2018). Assessment for symptoms of disease in other vascular beds (cardiac, renal, and peripheral arterial system) should be completed. A review of vital signs is important, bilateral blood pressure asymmetry (>15 mmHg) is a marker for increased cardiovascular risk (Aboyans et al., 2018). The carotid, abdominal, and femoral arteries should be assessed for bruits. Table 6.2 includes associated and differential diagnoses for carotid stenosis.

DIFFERENTIAL DIAGNOSIS AND DIAGNOSTIC CONSIDERATIONS

Carotid imaging by duplex is the most common and least expensive diagnostic test to assess for carotid stenosis (Class 1 recommendation: meaning the treatment

TABLE 6.2: Differential and Associated Diagnoses of Carotid Stenosis

DIFFERENTIAL DIAGNOSIS	MOST COMMON AGE OF ONSET	SYMPTOMS	PREFERRED IMAGING
Vertebral artery stenosis	Age >50 years	Dizziness, visual disturbance, sudden falls, confusion	Duplex, CTA, MRA
Carotid dissection	Age 40–50 years	Headache, cervical pain, dizziness, trauma to neck	Duplex, CTA, MRI
Fibromuscular dysplasia	Middle-aged females	Headaches, pulsatile tinnitus, MI, TIA, stroke	Duplex, CT, MRI cerebral angiogram,
Takayasu's arteritis	Young Asian females (15–40 years old)	Headache, posterior neck pain, carotidynia (pain at site of carotid artery), positional lightheadedness	Bloodwork, CTA, MRA
Giant cell arteritis	Older patients ≥50 years (mean age 75)	Headache, jaw claudication, visual symptoms, blindness	Bloodwork, CTA, MRI
Valvular heart disease	50–70 years old	Syncope, fatigue, dyspnea, decreased exercise tolerance	Echocardiography

Source: Data from Aboyans, V., Ricco, J. B., Bartelink, M. E. L., Björck, M., Brodmann, M., Cohnert, T., Collet, J. P., Czerny, M., De Carlo, M., Debus, S., Espinola-Klein, C., Kahan, T., Kownator, S., Mazzolai L, Naylor AR, Roffi M, Röther J, Sprynger M, Tendera M, … ESC Scientific Document Group. (2018, March 1). 2017 ESC guidelines on the diagnosis and treatment of peripheral arterial diseases, in collaboration with the European Society for Vascular Surgery (ESVS): Document covering atherosclerotic disease of extracranial carotid and vertebral, mesenteric, renal, upper and lower extremity arteries endorsed by: The European Stroke Organization (ESO), the Task Force for the Diagnosis and Treatment of Peripheral Arterial Diseases of the European Society of Cardiology (ESC) and of the European Society for Vascular Surgery (ESVS). *European Heart Journal, 39*(9), 763–816. https://doi.org/10.1093/eurheartj/ehx095; Martinelli, O., Venosi, S., BenHamida, J., Malaj, A., Belli, C., Irace, F. G., Gattuso, R., Frati, G., Gossetti, B., & Irace, L. (2017, May). Therapeutical options in the management of carotid dissection. *Annals of Vascular Surgery, 41*, 69–76. https://doi.org/10.1016/j.avsg.2016.07.087; Michailidou 2020, Mrsic 2017; Narula, N., Kadian-Dodov, D., & Olin, J. W. (2018). Fibromuscular dysplasia: Contemporary concepts and future directions. *Progress in Cardiovascular Diseases, 60*(6), 580–585. https://doi.org/10.1016/j.pcad.2018.03.001

is beneficial or effective; Aboyans et al., 2018; Aday & Beckman, 2017). Patients with carotid duplex results that are concerning for significant stenosis (≥70%) should undergo a head/neck CTA to more fully evaluate the carotid stenosis (Class I recommendation; Mortimer et al., 2018). CTA or MRA is useful because it can assess circulation from the aortic arch up to the brain parenchyma. CTA can be used to determine ischemic versus hemorrhagic stroke, but MRA is better at assessing tissue ischemia (Aboyans et al., 2018). MRA can be used for patients who have renal dysfunction, which prohibits the use of iodinated contrast mediums, although it may overestimate stenosis due to calcification (Aboyans et al., 2018). Carotid angiogram can be considered but it has a higher peri-procedural risk of stroke given introduction of catheters into the carotid vessel. Carotid angiogram is typically reserved for patients with renal insufficiency; those who are obese or have devices exclude the patient from MRA or CTA or when carotid stenting is planned (Aboyans et al., 2018).

TREATMENT

Conservative Management

Current literature suggests that management of stroke risk factors is important to reduce the risk of stroke and decrease progression of systemic atherosclerosis that can cause cardiovascular complications in patients with carotid artery stenosis. Patients on optimal medical management to minimize cardiovascular risk factors have an annual TIA risk of 1.78% and an annual stroke risk of 0.34% (Aday & Beckman, 2017). Close monitoring of risk factors and adjustments in treatment regimens are recommended to assess patient compliance and response to the suggested treatment regimens (Cheng & Brown, 2017).

Management of carotid artery stenosis with lifestyle management is essential to reduce stroke risk and other cardiovascular complications. A heart healthy diet (high in fruits and vegetables, decreased sodium intake) as well as an exercise program (30–40 minutes of moderate to intense activity 3–4 times/week) is recommended (Class I recommendation). Patients who are obese have a higher risk of developing diabetes and hypertension (Cheng & Brown, 2017), which are both risk factors for stroke. A weight loss program leading to a body mass index (BMI) <25 is recommended to decrease cardiovascular risk factors (Aboyans et al., 2018; Aday & Beckman, 2017). Significant alcohol consumption (greater then 60 g/day or 4–6 drinks/day) has been shown to increase the risk of stroke (although in the same study, light alcohol use (24 g/day or 1–2 drinks/day) was associated with a decreased stroke risk; Cheng & Brown, 2017).

Smoking cessation is of utmost importance to reduce the risk of stroke, further cardiovascular events, and worsening systemic atherosclerosis (Class I recommendation). Patients who smoke any type of tobacco have a 50% increase in relative risk for ischemic stroke (Cheng & Brown, 2017). Complete smoking cessation should be advised with a discussion of nicotine replacement medications and participation in a smoking cessation program for assistance. Management of diabetes (HgbA1c <7.0%) is recommended to prevent microvascular complications of atherosclerosis (Class I recommendation; Aday & Beckman, 2017).

Pharmacologic Management

Antiplatelet

Antiplatelet therapy with long-term aspirin use (81 mg/day) is a Class I recommendation for all patients with carotid artery stenosis who are asymptomatic (Class I recommendation; Aboyans et al., 2018). Patients who do not tolerate aspirin should be prescribed clopidogrel 75 mg/day (Gaba et al., 2018). Dual antiplatelet therapy (DAPT), aspirin with clopidogrel, or aspirin with dipyridamole is recommended for all patients who are symptomatic or who undergo carotid revascularization (Class I recommendation; Aboyans et al., 2018; Cheng & Brown, 2017). In the acute setting, no benefit was found in preventing recurrent strokes with unfractionated heparin, low molecular weight heparin, or warfarin (Cheng & Brown, 2017).

Statins

Management of hyperlipidemia with a high intensity statin use (atorvastatin 40 mg or 80 mg/day or rosuvastatin 10–20 mg/day as primary agents) with reduction of low density lipoprotein (LDL) levels by 50% (if LDL is 70–135 mg/dL) is a Class I recommendation (Aboyans et al., 2018). In several trials, use of a statin was shown to reduce the risk of future stroke by 33% (Cheng & Brown, 2017). The risk of myopathy related to statin use is concerning for some patients and should be discussed with the patient to promote statin compliance.

Hypertension Management

Management of hypertension with a target blood pressure less than 140/80 mmHg (less than 130/80 mmHg for patients with diabetes mellitus or prior stroke) is important to prevent future stroke risk. The medication regimen prescribed should be individualized for the patient (Gaba et al., 2018). The guidelines suggest that any pharmacologic agent that reaches the target blood pressure is more important than the specific agent used (Class I recommendation; Gaba et al., 2018).

Management of Asymptomatic Patients

There are differing opinions for management of the asymptomatic patient with carotid stenosis (Aday & Beckman, 2017). Most of the large trials evaluating carotid stenosis were completed in eras without a defined optimal regimen for risk factor modification. Newer trials have shown there is a 60% to 80% reduction in stroke risk with optimum medical therapy including medical management. It is important not to forget lifestyle modification, as well as treatment of risk factors (Cheng & Brown, 2017), in the management of carotid stenosis.

Revascularization Techniques

Revascularization for Asymptomatic Patients

There has been significant debate about treating asymptomatic patients with revascularization procedures to reduce stroke risk (Mortimer et al., 2018). Current guidelines do not recommend treating asymptomatic patients with less than 60% carotid stenosis (Class III recommendation: Treatment is not effective and may be harmful) (Aboyans et al., 2018). Treatment recommendations for asymptomatic patients with 60% to 99% stenosis are less clear (Aboyans et al., 2018). The guidelines suggest revascularization for asymptomatic patients with 60% to 99% stenosis and who have imaging features such as stenosis progression, contralateral TIA/stroke, and/or plaque appearance that represents an increased stroke risk despite optimum medical management (Class IIb recommendation: Usefulness is less established; Aboyans et al., 2018). The CREST-2 trial is ongoing evaluating current optimum medical therapy alone (Gaba et al., 2018) compared to optimum medical therapy plus revascularization. Study results provide additional information on the current best treatment regimen for patients with carotid stenosis who are asymptomatic (Aboyans et al., 2018).

Management of Symptomatic Patients

Revascularization is recommended for patients with symptoms of a stroke or TIA in the last 6 months and in whom a carotid duplex showed 60% to 99% lesion in the ipsilateral (same side) carotid artery (Class I recommendation) (Aboyans et al., 2018; Mortimer et al., 2018). The North American Symptomatic Carotid Endarterectomy Trial (NASCET) suggested that there is greater benefit when the revascularization procedure is completed within 14 days of symptom onset (Class I recommendation; Mortimer et al., 2018). The Asymptomatic Carotid Stenosis Trial (ACT-1) and the Carotid Revascularization for Primary Prevention of Stroke Trial (CREST) compared patients treated with CEA with those treated with stenting. They showed similar rates of complications (stroke, myocardial infarction [MI], death) in long term follow-up in both groups (Aday & Beckman, 2017). CEA is recommended for patients with a carotid artery stenosis of 70% to 99% when the procedure morbidity and mortality rate is less than 6% (Class I recommendation; Aboyans et al., 2018). Carotid artery stenting (CAS) is generally recommended for patients who are at high surgical risk, have had previous neck radiation or surgery, or have had recurrent stenosis after CEA (Class IIa recommendation: Evidence in favor of usefulness; Gaba et al., 2018).

CLINICAL PEARLS

- Carotid duplex is the imaging test of choice in patients who have concerning symptoms.
- Medical therapy (antithrombotic drugs, statin therapy, smoking cessation, weight loss, diabetes control, and other lifestyle modifications) is recommended for all patients with asymptomatic or symptomatic carotid artery stenosis.

KEY TAKEAWAYS

- In "average surgical risk" patients with an asymptomatic 60% to 99% stenosis, carotid endarterectomy (CEA) should be considered in the presence of clinical and/or more imaging characteristics that may be associated with an increased risk of late ipsilateral stroke, provided documented perioperative stroke/death rates are <3% and the patient's life expectancy is >5 years (Aboyans et al., 2018).
- Surgery is recommended in symptomatic patients with 70–99% carotid stenosis, provided the documented procedural death/stroke rate is <6%. CEA should be considered in symptomatic patients with 50–69% carotid stenosis, provided the documented procedural death/stroke rate is <6% (Aboyans et al., 2018)
- There is no indication for revascularization in complete carotid occlusion

EVIDENCE-BASED RESOURCES

Aboyans, V., Ricco, J. B., Bartelink, M. E. L., Björck, M., Brodmann, M., Cohnert, T., Collet, J. P., Czerny, M., De Carlo, M., Debus, S., Espinola-Klein, C., Kahan, T., Kownator, S., Mazzolai L, Naylor AR, Roffi M, Röther J, Sprynger M, Tendera M, ... ESC Scientific Document Group. (2018, March 1). 2017 ESC guidelines on the diagnosis and rreatment of peripheral arterial diseases, in collaboration with the European Society for Vascular Surgery (ESVS): Document covering atherosclerotic disease of extracranial carotid and vertebral, mesenteric, renal, upper and lower extremity arteries Endorsed by: The European Stroke Organization (ESO) The Task Force for the Diagnosis and Treatment of Peripheral Arterial Diseases of the European Society of Cardiology (ESC) and of the European Society for Vascular Surgery (ESVS). *European Heart Journal, 39*(9), 763–816. https://doi.org/10.1093/eurheartj/ehx095.

Patnode, C. D., Henderson, J. T., Thompson, J. H., Senger, C. A., Fortmann, S. P., & Whitlock, E. P. (2015). *Behavioral counseling and pharmacotherapy interventions for tobacco cessation in adults, including pregnant women: A review of reviews for the U.S. Preventive Services Task Force.* Agency for Healthcare Research and Quality (US). http://www.ncbi.nlm.nih.gov/books/NBK321744/.

6.4: VENOUS THROMBOEMBOLISM

Venous throboembolism (VTE) includes both deep vein thrombosis (DVT) and pulmonary embolism (PE) and is a common clinical problem for both inpatient and outpatient populations. DVT accounts for most cases of PE and is most common in the legs. Upper extremity venous thrombosis accounts for only 5% to 10% of all DVTs. VTE is the third most common vascular disease in the United States behind heart attack and stroke (Weitz & Chan, 2020). VTE can be fatal in its acute phase or lead to chronic illness and disability that can range from leg pain and swelling to chest pain, shortness of breath, and pulmonary hypertension. VTE also tends to recur, with a recurrence rate as high as 30% within 5 years of stopping anticoagulation (Imberti et al., 2018).

Rapid diagnosis and management of VTE is vital to prevent extension and embolization along with disease-related morbidity and mortality (Tritschler et al., 2018). Anticoagulation is the mainstay of therapy for VTE. The emergence of new anticoagulants has made treatment more convenient for both patients and providers, in addition to lowering hospital length of stay and treatment costs (Imberti et al., 2018).

PRESENTING SIGNS AND SYMPTOMS

Diagnosis of VTE can be challenging and cannot be made on signs and symptoms alone. The symptoms of both DVT and PE are nonspecific and often overlap with symptoms of other serious health conditions. VTE diagnosis is confirmed in less than 20% of suspected cases (Chopard et al., 2020). It is therefore not ideal to perform testing in all suspected cases. Formal criteria, or decision rules, such as the Wells score can accurately rule out VTE and thus avoid unnecessary testing, treatment, and the associated risks (Wells et al., 1997). The diagnosis of DVT or PE should be made in a sequence of steps including assessment of the patient's history and symptoms, clinical decision rules to evaluate probability, and, finally, imaging for those patients in whom VTE cannot be ruled out.

Symptoms of DVT
- Swelling
- Pain
- Warmth or redness
- Nearly always unilateral

Symptoms of PE
- Shortness of breath
- Chest pain
- Cough or hemoptysis
- Apprehension

HISTORY AND PHYSICAL FINDINGS

Virchow's triad explains the pathogenesis of thrombosis as a result of stasis, endothelial injury, and hypercoagulability (Bagot & Arya, 2008). Triggers frequently involve more than one part of the triad.

History

Selective history of predisposing factors in VTE:
1) Stasis
   a. Prolonged bedrest or hospitalization
   b. Immobilization (e.g., stroke or paralysis)
   c. Compression of vein (e.g., tumor, anatomical, pregnancy)
   d. Congestive heart failure
   e. Prolonged travel (>6 hours)
2) Endothelial injury
   a. Surgery
   b. Trauma
   c. Previous DVT
   d. Indwelling catheters or wires
   e. IV drug abuse
3) Hypercoagulability
   a. Family history of VTE
   b. Inherited blood clotting disorder
   c. Systemic disease that increases risk (malignancy, inflammatory bowel disease (IBD), nephrotic syndrome, vasculitis)
   d. Estrogen therapy (oral contraceptives or hormone replacement)
   e. Pregnancy or postpartum status
4) Characteristics
   a. Age >50 years
   b. Obesity
   c. Cigarette smoking

Physical Examination

Physical examination in VTE:
DVT
- Unilateral limb swelling, pain, redness, warmth
- One calf larger in circumference than the other
- Dilated superficial veins
- Pain and tenderness over surrounding veins
- Discoloration of the limb

PE
- Tachypnea
- Tachycardia
- Evidence of lower extremity DVT
- Hypotension
- Fever
- Crackles
- Hypoxia: O_2 saturation <95% on room air
- Syncope
- Hemodynamic instability (systolic blood pressure <90 mmHg, O_2 saturation ≤90%)

DIFFERENTIAL DIAGNOSIS AND DIAGNOSTIC CONSIDERATIONS

DVT
- Cellulitis
- Muscle injury/trauma
- Ruptured Baker's cyst
- Venous insufficiency
- Superficial thrombophlebitis
- Lymphedema
- Edema, fluid overload

PE
- Acute coronary syndrome
- Chronic obstructive pulmonary disease (COPD) exacerbation
- Acute congestive heart failure
- Pneumonia

Diagnostic Considerations

Once the diagnosis of DVT and PE is suspected, the AGACNP should quantify the clinical probability using decision rules prior to ordering laboratory tests or imaging studies. Multiple risk assessment tools are available and used to quantify the probability of VTE. Their use can reduce the need for widespread advanced imaging (Freund et al., 2018). For DVT, the Wells score is the most known and commonly used (Table 6.3; Serhal & Barnes, 2019). The Wells score and Pulmonary Embolism Rule-out Criteria (PERC) are common models used for PE diagnosis (Table 6.4; Freund et al., 2018).

If pretest probability with the Wells score or PERC is high, proceed with imaging. Patients with suspicion of

TABLE 6.3: Pretest Probability for Deep Vein Thromboembolism (Modified Wells Score)

Paralysis or recent orthopedic casting of lower extremity	**1**
Recent bedridden >3 days, or surgery in last 4 weeks	**1**
Localized tenderness in the deep vein system	**1**
Symptomatic calf 3 cm larger than the other	**1**
Pitting edema greater in affected leg	**1**
Collateral (nonvaricosed) visible superficial veins	**1**
Active cancer or cancer in last 6 months	**1**
Alternate diagnosis more likely than DVT	**−2**
Prior DVT	**1**
Score ≥2 DVT is likely Score ≤1 DVT is unlikely	

Source: Adapted from Wells, P. S., Anderson, D. R., Bormanis, J., Guy, F., Mitchell, M., Gray, L., Clement, C., Robinson, K. S., & Lewandowski, B. (1997). Value of assessment of pretest probability of deep vein thrombosis in clinical management. *Lancet, 350,* 1795–1798. https://doi.org/10.1016/S0140-6736(97)08140-3.

TABLE 6.4: Models for Pulmonary Embolism Diagnosis

PRETEST PROBABILITY OF PULMONARY EMBOLISM (WELLS SCORE)	
Clinical signs and symptoms of DVT	3
PE is the #1 diagnosis or equally likely	3
Heart rate >100 bpm	1.5
Immobilization × 3 days or surgery in last 4 weeks	1.5
Prior PE or DVT	1.5
Hemoptysis	1
Malignancy within 6 months	1
Score >6 points high probability of PE Score >2 to <6 moderate probability of PE Score <2 low probability of PE	

PULMONARY EMBOLISM RULE-OUT CRITERIA (PERC)
Age ≥50 years
Heart rate ≥100 bpm
Oxygen saturation ≤95% on room air
Unilateral leg swelling
Hemoptysis
Surgery or trauma with general anesthesia within 4 weeks
Prior DVT or PE
Estrogen-containing hormone use
Presence of any PERC element suggests further evaluation is needed

Source: Data from Freund, Y., Cachanado, M., Aubry, A., Orsini, C., Raynal, P. A., Féral-Pierssens, A. L., Charpentier, S., Dumas, F., Baarir, N., Truchot, J., Desmettre, T., Tazarourte, K., Beaune, S., Leleu, A., Khellaf, M., Wargon, M., Bloom, B., Rousseau, A., Simon, T., ... PROPER Investigator Group. (2018, February 13). Effect of the pulmonary embolism rule-out criteria on subsequent thromboembolic events among low-risk emergency department patients: The PROPER randomized clinical trial. *JAMA, 319*(6), 559–566. https://doi.org/10.1001/jama.2017.21904.

VTE *and* underlying malignancy go directly to imaging as probability is already high.

If pretest probability is low or moderate, consider drawing an age-adjusted D-dimer. D-dimer is a sensitive marker for VTE, and a negative result excludes the diagnosis without the need for further testing in most cases. If the D-dimer is positive, it does not confirm diagnosis of acute thrombosis, as it is not specific to VTE, but it does indicate the need for further testing. Compression ultrasound with Doppler of the extremity is the most common modality for diagnosing DVT (Liederman et al., 2020). Venography can be used if ultrasound is not possible. CT pulmonary angiography (CTPA) is the gold standard for the diagnosis of PE in clinical practice. The

ventilation/perfusion (VQ) scan is an option for those with contraindication to CT scan. Clinicians faced with the diagnosis of VTE must organize testing to strike the best balance between diagnostic power, resource stewardship, and the best outcomes for their patient (Figure 6.4; Liederman et al., 2020).

TREATMENT

Once the diagnosis of VTE is made, anticoagulation is the mainstay of treatment in most cases. Prompt initiation of anticoagulation is key as the goal of treatment is to prevent extension and embolization of clot and thus reduce morbidity and mortality (Tritschler et al., 2018). The location of a DVT significantly affects the chances of embolization. A proximal DVT in the popliteal, femoral, or iliac veins is far more likely to embolize when compared to a distal DVT that is confined to the calf veins (peroneal, posterior, anterior tibial, and muscular veins; Kabashneh et al., 2020). Not all patients who have acute VTE need to be admitted to the hospital for treatment. Numerous clinical studies have demonstrated that most patients with uncomplicated VTE can be safely and effectively treated as outpatients. Outpatient treatment has advantages of lower cost and greater comfort for patients, while inpatient treatment provides closer monitoring and quicker response to clinical changes. The American College of Chest Physicians (ACCP) recommends home treatment whenever feasible (Grade 1B; Kearon et al., 2016). Other treatment options for specific circumstances include catheter directed therapies, surveillance, and placement of inferior vena cava filters.

Anticoagulation

The initial phase of anticoagulation encompasses the first 5 to 10 days of treatment and historically represents the time patients were on parenteral anticoagulation. Management of unfractionated heparin often resulted in extended hospital stays. Since low-molecular weight heparin (LMWH) usage has become standard, complications of anticoagulation have decreased. The emergence of new oral agents (direct oral anticoagulants [DOACs]) has further streamlined treatment of VTE and eliminated the need for parenteral anticoagulation in many patients. Evidence based clinical practice guidelines recommend DOACs as the preferred choice in most patients with noncancer related VTE (Grade 2B; Kearon et al., 2012). These agents have several advantages over warfarin, including rapid onset of action, fewer diet and drug interactions, and predictable pharmacokinetic profile, which allow for simplified drug administration of a standard dose without need for lab monitoring and dose adjustment (Tritschler et al., 2018). In addition, DOACs have lower rates of major bleeding than warfarin (Chopard et al., 2020). Selection of an initial agent is not specified in the American College of Clinical Pharmacy (ACCP) guidelines, so is most often guided by experience,

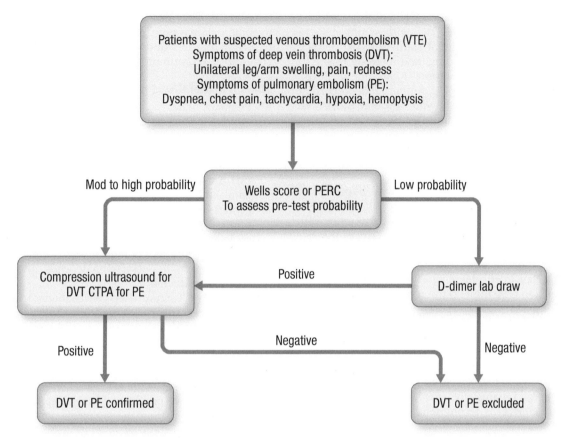

FIGURE 6.4: Diagnosis of venous thromboembolism.

convenience, and patient specific factors. Cost is an important factor as it can impact medication adherence.

Options for initial management include immediate treatment with a DOAC, initial parenteral anticoagulation followed by a DOAC or direct thrombin inhibitor, or parenteral anticoagulation overlapped with vitamin K agonist until that drug reaches therapeutic levels. Despite the lack of direct reversal agents for DOACs, the risk of death due to major bleeding was far less for DOACs than for vitamin K agonists in thousands of patients in the original clinical trials for DOAC use in VTE and atrial fibrillation (Tritschler et al., 2018).

Long-term anticoagulation (3 months) is recommended for patients with proximal VTE. (Grade 1B; Kearon et al., 2016). Extended anticoagulation (>3 months) is determined with the patient and primary care provider or specialist based on ongoing risk of recurrent VTE. Determining how long to continue anticoagulation remains one of the most important decisions in the management of VTE (Serhal & Barnes, 2019).

For each patient, the decision to anticoagulate must weigh the risk of morbidity and mortality without anticoagulation against the risk of bleeding with anticoagulation. Absolute contraindications to anticoagulation include active bleeding; severe bleeding diathesis; recent, planned or emergency high bleeding-risk surgery/procedure; major trauma; and acute intracranial hemorrhage (ICH). Relative contraindications to anticoagulation include recurrent gastrointestinal bleeding, intracranial or spinal tumors, large abdominal aortic aneurysm with uncontrolled hypertension, recent, planned, or emergent low bleeding-risk surgery/procedure (Kearon et al., 2016).

Catheter-Directed Therapies: Thrombolysis and Suction Thrombectomy

Deep Vein Thrombosis

ACCP guidelines state that anticoagulation therapy alone is acceptable in all patients with acute proximal DVT who do not have impending venous gangrene (Grade 2C; Kearon et al., 2016). This recommendation has not changed despite multiple studies investigating endovenous catheter-directed venous thrombolysis for acute iliofemoral DVT. Thrombolysis has been associated with higher bleeding risk and no improvement in VTE recurrence or quality of life scores beyond 6 months (Tritschler et al., 2018). Patients who may benefit from thrombolysis are those with threatened limb loss (venous gangrene or phlegmasia [massive VTE]) or those with all of the following: iliofemoral DVT with symptoms <14 days duration, good functional status, life expectancy of >1 year, low risk of bleeding, and a strong desire to prevent postthrombotic syndrome (Kearon et al., 2016). Patients with iliofemoral DVT experience more recurrent VTE and more postthrombotic syndrome than those with more distal DVT, and they should be reassessed for more aggressive therapy if symptoms do not improve with anticoagulation alone (Thukral & Vedantham, 2020).

Pulmonary Embolism

In patients with acute PE associated with hypotension or evidence of shock and who have a low bleeding risk, systemic thrombolysis is recommended (Grade 2B). Systemic thrombolysis for massive PE reduces mortality, decreases the incidence of chronic thromboembolic pulmonary hypertension, and improves quality of life (Weitz & Chan, 2020). Massive PE is defined a systemic hypotension (<90 mmHg) for greater than 15 minutes or requiring inotropic support, pulselessness, or persistent bradycardia. Submassive PE is acute PE without systemic hypotension but evidence of right ventricular dysfunction or myocardial necrosis (Malik et al., 2016).

In patients with acute PE who have a high bleeding risk, who have failed systemic thrombolysis, or who become hemodynamically unstable, catheter-assisted thrombus removal is recommended if the appropriate expertise and resources are available (Grade 2C; Kearon et al., 2012).

Vena Cava Filters

The inferior vena cava (IVC) filter is placed in the inferior vena cava to prevent thrombi from traveling to the lungs. They are indicated in patients with proximal acute venous thromboembolism (VTE) who have an absolute contraindication to anticoagulation or in whom anticoagulation has failed. IVC filter placement is not recommended for a patient who is on anticoagulation (Grade 1B; Kearon et al., 2012). If a filter is placed, anticoagulation should be started as soon as it is safe to do so and the filter then removed. Timely filter removal (if possible) is important as complications associated with the indwelling filter increase over time (Chopard et al., 2020).

Surveillance

For asymptomatic patients with DVT limited to the calf veins and no risk factors for extension, serial duplex ultrasound imaging is preferred over anticoagulation. If no extension is noted after 1 week (some studies suggest 2 weeks), anticoagulation is not needed (Serhal & Barnes, 2019).

Compression Stockings

Elastic compression stockings have not been shown to reduce the development of postthrombotic syndrome, so they are not routinely recommended for that purpose (Grade 2B). They are helpful in reducing leg swelling in some patients with DVT, so should be considered to reduce symptoms and enhance function and mobility (Thukral & Vedantham, 2020).

Special Populations

■ Pregnant patients: LMWH is recommended as the initial and long-term anticoagulant of choice rather than other agents (Grade 2C).

■ Phlegmasia: For patients with massive iliofemoral DVT or phlegmasia cerulea dolens (massive DVT that causes marked swelling of the extremity with pain and cyanosis), with symptoms for <14 days and good functional status, systemic or catheter-directed thrombolytic therapy and/or clot removal (e.g., catheter extraction, catheter fragmentation, surgical thrombectomy) is recommended.(Grade 2C). The most appropriate intervention depends upon the institution's expertise.

■ Proximal (<5 cm from deep vein confluence) or extensive (>5 cm) superficial vein thrombosis: Treatment of thrombophlebitis (thrombosis of the superficial veins) includes symptomatic care to reduce pain and inflammation with warm compresses, nonsteroidal anti-inflammatory drugs (NSAIDs), and compression therapy. Patients with superficial vein thrombosis that is in close proximity to the deep venous system (3 to 5 cm from the saphenofemoral or saphenopopliteal junction) or is an extensive thrombosis (≥5 cm in length) are at higher risk for extension to DVT, and prophylactic dose anticoagulation is recommended for 45 days (Grade 2C). For prophylaxis, fondaparinux, low-molecular-weight heparin and DOACs appear to be equally effective (Kearon et al., 2016).

■ Those with COVID-19 virus infection: The inflammatory response in patients with COVID-19 infection can lead to a hypercoagulable state. Early VTE prophylaxis should be provided for all patients admitted to the hospital with COVID-19 infection (Obi et al., 2021).

TRANSITION OF CARE

Treatment of VTE is divided into three segments: initial (diagnosis to 5–10 days), long term (3 months), and extended therapy (beyond 3 months). Prompt initial treatment is critical to prevent long-term morbidity. The recurrence rate of VTE is high, however. A patient with initial unprovoked VTE has a risk of recurrence: 10% at 1 year, 30% at 5 years, after stopping anticoagulation (Tritschler et al., 2018). Treatment, therefore, must also involve secondary prevention and prophylaxis. Ensuring the patient has appropriate follow up with a primary care provider or a specialist remains important to make the decision of if and when to stop anticoagulation.

Periprocedural management of patients on anticoagulation is a common clinical scenario. It is recommended that patients do not interrupt anticoagulation for 3 months after an acute episode of VTE unless it is an emergency (Kearon et al., 2016). After 3 months, if anticoagulation will be continued, it is generally reasonable to interrupt anticoagulation for short periods for needed procedures. This is another arena that is easier for both patients and providers to navigate when using short-acting DOACs versus warfarin.

6.5: ACUTE THROMBOEMBOLIC EVENTS

Thromboembolism is the formation of a blood clot in one region of the body that breaks off and travels to a secondary location. This can occur in both the arterial and the venous systems and will result in a broad range of clinical scenarios. The morbidity and mortality of thromboembolism depends on the location and extent of the embolus. Many clinical diagnoses associated with acute thromboembolism are described in detail in other sections of this text and include stroke, myocardial infarction, pulmonary embolism, and mesenteric ischemia.

For patients with acute embolic events, treatment involves managing the acute insult, identifying the source of emboli, and preventing recurrence. Acute management of the thromboembolic event is specific to the site of embolism and is too broad to be discussed here. Once the initial insult is managed, evaluation should focus on identifying the source of embolus. A thorough history can reveal predisposing factors to thrombosis. Risks for thrombosis are factors that result in stasis, endothelial injury or an acquired or inherited hypercoagulable state (Virchow's triad; Bagot & Arya, 2008). Identifying the source of embolism allows for focused secondary prevention. Sources of venous thromboembolism (VTE) are discussed in the preceding section on VTE.

HISTORY AND PHYSICAL FINDINGS

Selective history in arterial embolism
1) Stasis
   - Atrial fibrillation/arrhythmia
   - Valvular heart disease
   - Cardiomyopathy with low ejection fraction
   - Aneurysm
   - Paradoxical from lower extremity deep vein thrombosis (DVT) via patent foramen ovale
2) Endothelial injury
   - Unstable plaque rupture
   - Instrumentation (angiogram, stent placement)
   - Open aortic or cardiac surgery
   - Trauma
3) Hypercoagulability
   - Malignancy
   - Inherited blood clotting disorder
   - Acquired antiphospholipid antibody syndrome, heparin-induced thrombocytopenia
   - Endocarditis/infection

DIFFERENTIAL DIAGNOSIS

- Lymphedema
- Hematoma or abscess
- Muscle strain or tear
- Ruptured Baker's cyst
- Superficial thrombophlebitis
- Arterial insufficiency

TREATMENT

Treatment of thromboembolism is focused on eliminating or controlling the provoking factors and is thus quite varied. Many lifestyle-related risk factors for arterial and venous thrombosis overlap including advancing age, obesity, and smoking. Patients should be educated regarding lifestyle characteristics and modifiable risk factors. Secondary prevention of arterial and venous embolism differs significantly, however. Anticoagulation is the mainstay of treatment for VTE (Imberti et al., 2018). Platelets play a significant role in the development of arterial thrombosis compared to venous thrombosis. Arterial thrombosis typically starts with the accumulation of lipid plaques in the arterial wall, provoking inflammatory cells and platelet activation (Vandvik et al., 2012). Antiplatelet agents are therefore recommended over anticoagulation for secondary prevention of most arterial thromboembolic events (Vandvik et al., 2012).

KEY TAKEAWAYS

- VTE symptoms are nonspecific, and diagnosis is confirmed in <20% of suspected cases.
- Clinicians faced with diagnosing VTE must strike the balance between diagnostic power, resource stewardship, and adverse effects for the patient.

CLINICAL PEARLS

- VTE includes DVT and PE
- Anticoagulation is the mainstay of treatment for VTE. DOACs have streamlined the initial treatment of VTE and made outpatient treatment a viable option.
- DVT prophylaxis should be considered in all acutely ill hospitalized patients using either drugs (i.e., SC heparin) or mechanical methods (pneumatic devices).

6.6: VASCULAR ACCESS

Procedures involving dialysis access are the most common vascular surgical procedures performed in the United States (Rasmussen et al., 2008). Arterial venous fistulas are the preferred access for most hemodialysis patients because they have been closely associated with improved clinical outcomes including cost savings, lower infection rates, decreased hospitalization, decreased interventional procedures, improved patency, and survival benefits (Halinski & Koncicki, 2018). Management of vascular access requires a multidisciplinary approach including the patient, nephrologist, surgeon, dialysis nurse and technician, interventionalist, diabetes specialist, nutritionist, and social worker. There are three main types of vascular access used for hemodialysis: arteriovenous fistula, arteriovenous graft, and central venous catheter. An arteriovenous fistula is created by connecting an artery to a vein; an arteriovenous graft is created with a prosthetic graft used as a bridge between an artery and vein, and central venous access is a central line placed either in the internal jugular vein or the subclavian vein. The internal jugular vein is preferable to the subclavian for the site of access, as chronic subclavian vein catheterization is associated with thrombosis and/or stenosis with risk of dysfunctional hemodialysis access in the upper extremity (Rasmussen et al., 2008).

HISTORY AND PHYSICAL EXAM

Review medical history, determine which is the dominant hand (access generally placed in the nondominant hand), ask about prior chest or upper extremity surgery, if a pacemaker is present, if there has been any prior central line placement or prior fistula/grafts and, if so, the location. The exam should include assessment of pulses in bilateral arms, presence of edema, surgical scars, skin temperature, condition of skin, blood pressure in both arms, and if there is prominent venous collateral. After access has been created, signs or symptoms that can indicate a problem include a weak or diminished thrill, significant arm swelling, prolonged bleeding after needles are removed, poor flow during dialysis, an inadequate hemodialysis run, or difficult cannulation. Consider ordering a duplex ultrasound or fistulogram to evaluate for stenosis, thrombosis or other problems if there are issues with the arteriovenous fistula or graft.

TREATMENT

An angiogram may be needed with angioplasty if the duplex ultrasound or fistulogram show evidence of stenosis of the fistula or graft or of the native artery or vein. Surgical intervention may be required to revise the graft or to create a new fistula or graft.

TRANSITION OF CARE

Once the vascular access is created the vascular surgeon will turn over care to the nephrologist and remains available for surgical intervention if required.

CLINICAL PEARLS

- After an arteriovenous fistula the recommendation is to allow 2 to 3 months before use to allow for maturation of the fistula and 4 weeks for an arteriovenous graft.
- Patients should check for a thrill every day and notify their healthcare provider as soon as they note a difference.

KEY TAKEAWAYS

- Fistula first, catheter last.
- Bleeding, swelling, infection, cold hands, and loss of thrill should be reported immediately by patients and dialysis nurse to the healthcare provider.
- Prompt reporting of abnormalities can help save a deteriorating access site.

6.7: PERIPHERAL ARTERIAL DISEASE

Peripheral arterial disease (PAD) is atherosclerosis in the noncoronary arteries affecting 12% to 20% of patients over 65 and increasing to 50% of patients 85 years or older (Firnhaber & Powell, 2019). Males and females are equally affected, and African Americans have a higher incidence of PAD and associated mortality when compared to non-Hispanic White patients (Berti-Hearn & Elliott, 2018; Shu & Santulli, 2018). Patients who are at risk for PAD include those over age 65 with risk factors for atherosclerosis, patients with known vascular disease in another vascular bed (carotid, cardiac, renal, abdominal), and smokers (Firnhaber & Powell, 2019). Patients who have PAD are more likely to have a cardiovascular event (myocardial infarction and/or stroke, and/or an amputation), and have a decreased quality of life when compared to patients without PAD (Gerhard-Herman et al., 2016). Patients with PAD can present with one or more symptoms depending upon the severity of the disease.

PRESENTING SIGNS AND SYMPTOMS

The patient is initially seen for symptoms of claudication (leg pain with exercise) causing a decreased exercise tolerance, absent/diminished pulses, or development of a new foot wounds/tissue loss. A complete history of the patient's symptoms should be obtained. It is important to review the onset, duration, severity, and advancement of symptoms. Assessment of limitations at home, at work, or during recreational activity is valuable in determining the severity of the patient's disease (Berti-Hearn & Elliott, 2018). Lifestyle habits, physical activity, and diet should be reviewed (Aboyans et al., 2018). Determining the severity and location of the leg symptoms and whether the discomfort is present with activity or rest, is essential while distinguishing PAD during differential diagnoses of leg pain. The differential diagnosis of a patient with leg pain upon exercise is listed in Table 6.5.

Asymptomatic patients compromise 50% of patients with a diagnosis of PAD. These patients may have decreased pedal pulses and abnormal arterial testing without any limitations to their ability to exercise (Shishehbor & Jaff, 2016). Approximately 15% of patients with PAD have classic claudication symptoms (Thomas et al.,

2019). Claudication is typically described as a pain, heaviness, weakness, fatigue, or cramping with exercise that resolves within 10 minutes of rest. Claudication is classically described in the calves, hips, and buttocks (Firnhaber & Powell, 2019). Claudication occurs during exercise because blockages in the artery limit the blood flow to muscle causing anaerobic muscle metabolism (Thomas et al., 2019). Once the patient stops exercising,

TABLE 6.5: Differential and Associated Diagnosis of Patient With Leg Pain upon Exercise

	CLINICAL FEATURES	SYMPTOM RESOLUTION	DIAGNOSIS
Peripheral arterial disease	Cramping pain with exercise (claudication)	Typically relieved within 10 minutes of rest	ABIs
Spinal canal stenosis: Neurogenic claudication	Low back pain, numbness/tingling in feet, weakness in legs	Less pain when leaning forward or sitting	Exercise ABIs, ultrasound, x-ray, MRI
Peripheral neuropathy	Numbness, tingling, pain, burning, shooting pain	Rubbing feet, putting pressure on feet	Bloodwork, electromyograph, nerve conduction study, nerve biopsy
Nerve root compression: Herniated disc, sciatica pain	Radiating pain, loss of sensation and weakness, reduction, or loss of reflexes	Improved with lying in bed	X-ray, CT, MRI, myelogram
Osteoarthritis of hip or knee	Pain in groin that can travel to the thigh, worse when rising from a seated position or in the morning	Improves with rest	X-ray, MRI
Venous claudication	Usually unilateral leg tightness and pain with exercise	Takes 20–30 minutes to resolve, improves with leg elevation	Exercise ABIs, venous reflux
Restless legs syndrome	Uncontrolled urge to move legs while sitting or lying down, more frequent in evening or at night	Moving temporarily eases symptoms	Symptom history, bloodwork, sleep study
Nocturnal leg cramping	Cramping in legs usually occurring when in bed	Stretching and leg massage will improve	Symptom history
Gout	Significant pain, erythema, swelling in joints	Improves with anti-inflammatory management	X-ray, bloodwork, joint fluid examination
Deep vein thrombosis	Cramping, swelling, warm or discolored skin	Typically unilateral	Venous duplex ultrasound
Symptomatic Baker's cyst	Tightness, stiffness, swelling, pain behind the knee	Worsening with walking or standing	Ultrasound, x-ray, MRI
Blue toe syndrome	Sudden painful blue discoloration of toes	Usually occurs in one leg (rarely both legs)	ABIs, CTA,
Chronic or exercise induced compartment syndrome	Pain in the front of the leg (shin) with exercise; pain is reproducible	Quickly relieved with rest; typically seen in young endurance athletes	Measurement of compartment pressures
Myositis	Deep aching, flu-like muscle pain	Sometimes occurs with statin therapy, improves with stopping statin	Bloodwork

ABI, ankle-brachial indices; CTA, CT angiogram.

Source: Modified from Conte, S. M., & Vale, P. R. (2018, April). Peripheral arterial disease. *Heart, Lung and Circulation, 27*(4), 427–432. https://doi.org/10.1016/j.hlc.2017.10.014; Gerhard-Herman, M. D., Gornik, H. L., Barrett, C., Barshes, N. R., Corriere, M. A., Drachman, D. E., Fleisher, L. A., Fowkes, F. G., Hamburg, N. M., Kinlay, S., Lookstein, R., Misra, S., Mureebe, L., Olin, J. W., Patel, R. A., Regensteiner, J. G., Schanzer, A., Shishehbor, M. H., Stewart, K. J., ... Walsh, M. E. (2016). AHA/ACC guideline on the management of patients with lower extremity peripheral artery disease: A report of the American College of Cardiology/American Heart Association Task Force on Clinical Practice guidelines. *Circulation, 135*(12), e726–e779. https://doi.org/10.1161/CIR.0000000000000471

the muscle no longer needs increased blood flow, and the symptoms resolve. Thirty percent of patients presenting with PAD have atypical symptoms (symptoms not consistent with claudication) with abnormal studies (Patel, Sakhuja, & White, 2020). Patients with more severe disease describe ischemic rest pain (2%–3% of patients with PAD). With more obstruction to blood flow in the legs, patients may report constant pain localized to their toes or distal foot (Sutton et al., 2018). Patients can also have pain at night while lying flat in bed that wakes them from sleep (rest pain). This pain may be relieved by hanging their leg off the bed at night or by sleeping with their feet dependent in a chair (Berti-Hearn & Elliott, 2018). The most severe symptom for PAD is a poorly healing ulcer on the foot (Patel, Sakhuja, & White, 2020). Wounds can occur due to injury or trauma to the foot or can occur spontaneously in areas (typically the toes or heel) with decreased blood flow (Berti-Hearn & Elliott, 2018). Chronic limb ischemia (CLI) is identified as rest pain ≥2 weeks, along with poorly healing ulcerations or gangrene on the feet (Shu & Santulli, 2018). Patients with rest pain and/or poorly healing ulcerations are at high risk of amputation and have a high mortality rate (26% at 1 year and 56% at 5 years) (Patel, Sakhuja, & White, 2020; Thomas et al., 2019).

Acute limb ischemia (ALI) is the sudden onset of the "6 Ps": Pain, Pallor, Pulselessness, Poikilothermia (cold sensation), Parathesias (numbness/tingling), and Paralysis (Patel, Sakhuja, & White, 2020). Based on the degree of symptoms, patients can be assigned a limb category: viable (limb not immediately threatened), threatened, and irreversible (Gerhard-Herman et al., 2016). The patient will have absent pulses, and studies will demonstrate absent or low ankle brachial index (ABI) or toe brachial index (TBI) values. Often the cause is trauma, thrombosis, or embolus to a distal artery in the leg or foot. In patients with ALI without known trauma, testing for a cardiovascular cause of thromboembolism can be helpful (Gerhard-Herman et al., 2016). ALI is a medical emergency and patients should be directed to a local emergency department for urgent evaluation and treatment (Firnhaber & Powell, 2019).

HISTORY AND PHYSICAL FINDINGS

Physical Exam

A full vascular exam should be done for the patient (including heart sounds and assessment for carotid and abdominal bruits) given the increased risk of cardiovascular outcomes for patients with PAD (Class I recommendation: Treatment is useful and effective; Gerhard-Herman et al., 2016). On assessment of the legs and feet (shoes and socks should be off for the exam; Patel, Sakhuja, & White, 2020), you may find lower extremity hair loss, shiny skin, muscle atrophy, atrophic nails (thick with

ridges), decreased capillary refill, and cyanotic or mottled skin (Berti-Hearn & Elliott, 2018). Dependent rubor, a reddening of the skin secondary to impaired autoregulation of arterioles, may also be present (Firnhaber & Powell, 2019). All pulses should be examined (femoral, popliteal, dorsalis pedis, and posterior tibial), comparing both legs for presence and strength of the pulses. Presence of a femoral bruit is a marker for future ischemia cardiac events (Aboyans et al., 2018). Assess for skin ulcerations in between and underneath the toes and in the heel area. Arterial wounds have a "punched out" appearance with minimal drainage and a pale wound bed and often cause significant pain for the patient unless severe neuropathy is present (Berti-Hearn & Elliott, 2018).

DIFFERENTIAL DIAGNOSIS AND DIAGNOSTIC CONSIDERATIONS

Further testing is recommended for patients who are at risk for PAD and have symptoms or positive physical exam findings. (Berti-Hearn & Elliott, 2018). The initial diagnostic test to establish a diagnosis of PAD is the ABI (Class I recommendation; Gerhard-Herman et al., 2016). The ABI is a noninvasive and highly sensitive and specific test for the diagnosis of PAD (Berti-Hearn & Elliott, 2018). ABI values of less than 0.9 are considered diagnostic for PAD. See Table 6.6 for interpretation of ABI results. Exercise ABIs can be considered in patients who describe symptoms consistent with PAD and have normal ABIs at rest. Exercise ABIs can differentiate arterial claudication from neurogenic or venous claudication (Class I recommendation; Thomas et al., 2019). TBI are done for patients who have noncompressible vessels due to increased calcification in the arterial wall (Class I recommendation). A toe brachial index of over 30 and a skin perfusion pressure of over 40 are predictors of enough blood flow to support wound healing in patients with PAD (Donohue et al., 2020).

In patients with noncompressible ABIs, it may be helpful to order an arterial duplex (Gerhard-Herman et al., 2016), which may show an approximate level of stenosis in the leg arteries or early re-stenosis of a bypass graft or stent by velocity criteria (Class I recommendation; Aboyans et al., 2018). The 6-minute walk test can be done in a clinic or inpatient setting and is useful to trend walking distance over time. Decreased walking distance has been shown to correlate with the patient's quality of life (Sutton et al., 2018). Transcutaneous oximetry $TcPO_2$ is useful to determine healing potential for wounds or amputation sites. A $TcPO_2$ reading of less than 40 mmHg or a toe reading of less than 30 mmHg indicates poor healing potential (Donohue et al., 2020).

Advanced imaging for patients with PAD is important when they have significant symptoms or poorly heal-

TABLE 6.6: Interpretation of Ankle- and Toe-Brachial Indices Results

ANKLE-BRACHIAL INDEX (ABI)	RESULTS	TYPICAL SYMPTOMS
1.0 to 1.3	Normal	
0.9 to 1.0	Borderline PAD	Often none
0.7 to 0.9	Mild PAD	Claudication
0.4–0.7	Moderate PAD	Claudication
Less than 0.4	Severe PAD	Ischemic rest pain and/or tissue loss
Greater then 1.3	Non-compressible (calcified) vessels	
TOE BRACHIAL INDEX (USED WHEN ABI IS NONCOMPRESSIBLE)		
0.7 or greater	Normal	
0.4–0.7	Mild to moderate	Claudication
Less than 0.4	Severe	Ischemic rest pain or tissue loss

PAD, peripheral arterial disease.

Source: Data from Firnhaber, J. M., & Powell, C. S. (2019, March 15). Lower extremity peripheral artery disease: Diagnosis and treatment. *American Family Physician, 99*(6), 362–369; Gerhard-Herman, M. D., Gornik, H. L., Barrett, C., Barshes, N. R., Corriere, M. A., Drachman, D. E., Fleisher, L. A., Fowkes, F. G., Hamburg, N. M., Kinlay, S., Lookstein, R., Misra, S., Mureebe, L., Olin, J. W., Patel, R. A., Regensteiner, J. G., Schanzer, A., Shishehbor, M. H., Stewart, K. J., ... Walsh, M. E. (2016). AHA/ACC guideline on the management of patients with lower extremity peripheral artery disease: A report of the American College of Cardiology/American Heart Association Task Force on Clinical Practice guidelines. *Circulation, 135*(12), e726–e779. https://doi.org/10.1161/CIR.0000000000000471; Shu, J., & Santulli, G. (2018, August). Update on peripheral artery disease: Epidemiology and evidence-based facts. *Atherosclerosis, 275*, 379–381. https://doi.org/10.1016/j.atherosclerosis.2018.05.033

ing wounds, and revascularization is being considered (Class I recommendation; Gerhard-Herman et al., 2016). CT angiogram with runoff gives detailed images of the vessels (lesion location and type, level of calcification, degree of stenosis; Aboyans et al., 2018). Due to use of iodinated contrast, nephrotoxicity is a concern. Adequate hydration prior to the exam should be encouraged to reduce the risk of contrast-induced nephropathy (CIN; Aboyans et al., 2018). Patients with abnormal creatinine (≥1.5 mg/dL) or a history of renal transplant may need pre-hydration for renal protection prior to contrast use. Lower extremity angiogram is the gold standard to fully evaluate the blood flow in the leg arteries, and the patient can be treated with angioplasty or stenting during the same procedure. Contrast use can be more carefully managed in patients with renal disease during an angiogram to avoid contrast nephropathy.

TREATMENT

Atherosclerosis is a systemic disease, and patients who have stenosis in one vascular bed are at higher risk for cardiovascular mortality and morbidity (such as myocardial infarction or stroke; Aboyans et al., 2018). Patients with PAD have decreased functional status due to their symptoms and decreased quality of life measurements when compared to patients without PAD. Unfortunate-

ly, patients with PAD often remain undertreated with respect to guideline-based management (Patel, Sakhuja, & White, 2020). The management of PAD should be undertaken by a multidisciplinary team with primary care and vascular specialists (Class I recommendation). PAD is a chronic disease and regular visits to care providers is important to monitor for complications and possible progression of the disease (Berti-Hearn & Elliott, 2018; Donohue et al., 2020; Sutton et al., 2018).

All patients with PAD should be managed with guideline-based therapy (Patel, Sakhuja, & White, 2020). Treatment for PAD can be conservative with lifestyle modifications alone or with pharmacologic or procedural interventions. The goal of treatment is to manage risk factor reduction, disease progression, and increase the patient's ability to walk longer distances thus improving their quality of life (Gerhard-Herman et al., 2016).

Risk Factor Management

Diabetes

PAD patients with diabetes have a 10-fold increased risk of amputation due to microvascular disease in the feet (Sutton et al., 2018). Management of A1C (target of less than 7%) is important to decrease the risk of vascular complications from diabetes mellitus (Class I recommendation). Given the incidence of decreased sensation in the feet and neuropathy, the importance of good foot care should be discussed with any patient who has abnormal ABI/TBIs to minimize tissue loss (Class I recommendation; Gerhard-Herman et al., 2016). This includes daily inspection of the feet, wearing properly-fitting shoes, and prompt attention to any wounds that develop. Wound infections should be evaluated and treated to prevent tissue loss (Gerhard-Herman et al., 2016).

Hypertension

Management of hypertension is recommended to decrease the risk of heart failure, myocardial infarction, stroke, and death in patients with vascular disease (Class I recommendation; Gerhard-Herman et al., 2016). The goal blood pressure for patients with PAD is <130/80 (Whelton et al., 2017). No trial has found one group of antihypertensive medications to be superior for treating PAD, and beta-blockers do not worsen claudication or walking distance in patients with PAD as previously suspected (Patel, Sakhuja, & White, 2020). Angiotensin-converting enzyme (ACE) inhibitors and angiotensin-receptor blockers (ARBs) have been found to reduce cardiovascular events in patients with PAD (Class IIa recommendation: Evidence in favor of usefulness; Firnhaber & Powell, 2019).

Smoking Cessation

Patients who smoke have a 2.2-fold higher prevalence of developing symptoms consistent with PAD. Ongoing tobacco use is well known to accelerate the progression of symptoms of PAD (Firnhaber & Powell, 2019). In addition, patients who continue to smoke after a revascularization procedure have lower long-term patency rates than nonsmokers or those that are able to quit prior to their procedure (Firnhaber & Powell, 2019). Smoking cessation should be encouraged for current smokers with PAD (Class I recommendation). It is recommended that providers use the 5A's model as the approach for treating tobacco use: Ask, Advise, Assess, Assist, and Arrange follow-up (Patnode et al., 2015). Multifactorial medication management (varenicline, buproprion, or nicotine replacement therapy [NRT]) and referral to a smoking cessation program or behavioral counseling have been shown to be most successful with smoking cessation (Patnode et al., 2015). Many patients who are able to quit smoking notice an improvement in their claudication walking distance (Gerhard-Herman et al., 2016). Exposure to secondhand smoke should also be assessed and avoided (Aboyans et al., 2018).

Exercise

Exercise therapy should be discussed with every patient who has PAD (Berti-Hearn & Elliott, 2018). This is a life-long Class I recommendation for the patient regardless of symptoms and revascularization procedures. Exercise therapy is thought to work by muscle training for hypoxic environments and collateral vessel growth (Gerhard-Herman et al., 2016). It also has beneficial effects of improving the patient's glycemic index, blood pressure, weight, and cholesterol, which decreases future cardiovascular risk. The best exercise program is detailed in Table 6.7. Patients are instructed to walk to moderate or severe pain, stop and rest as needed, and then continue walking. This cycle is repeated for the duration of the exercise period (Thomas et al., 2019). Exercise programs are more successful if done in a supervised setting, but many patients can succeed doing the program at home. While walking was found to be the most effective management for PAD, patients also benefit from

TABLE 6.7: Supervised Program for Peripheral Arterial Disease

EXERCISE PROGRAM INSTRUCTIONS	
Frequency	At least 3 sessions per week
Duration	30–45 minutes of exercise/session for at least 12 weeks (6 months is preferred)
Exercise type	Walking is the best studied (treadmill, track, sidewalk)
Distance	Walk until claudication symptoms are 3 to 4 (moderate to severe) before stopping to rest
Time to improvement	Patients often notice symptom improvement in 4–6 weeks
Results	100%–150% improvement in walking distance

Source: Data from Conte, S. M., & Vale, P. R. (2018, April). Peripheral arterial disease. *Heart, Lung and Circulation, 27*(4), 427–432. https://doi.org/10.1016/j.hlc.2017.10.014; Gerhard-Herman, M. D., Gornik, H. L., Barrett, C., Barshes, N. R., Corriere, M. A., Drachman, D. E., Fleisher, L. A., Fowkes, F. G., Hamburg, N. M., Kinlay, S., Lookstein, R., Misra, S., Mureebe, L., Olin, J. W., Patel, R. A., Regensteiner, J. G., Schanzer, A., Shishehbor, M. H., Stewart, K. J., ... Walsh, M. E. (2016). AHA/ACC guideline on the management of patients with lower extremity peripheral artery disease: A report of the American College of Cardiology/American Heart Association Task Force on Clinical Practice guidelines. *Circulation, 135*(12), e726–e779. https://doi.org/10.1161/CIR.0000000000000471; Novakovic, M., Jug, B., & Lenasi, H. (2017, August). Clinical impact of exercise in patients with peripheral arterial disease. *Vascular, 25*(4), 412–422. https://doi.org/10.1177/1708538116678752; Thomas, S. G., Marzolini, S., Lin, E., Nguyen, C. H., & Oh, P. (2019 November). Peripheral arterial disease: Supervised exercise therapy through cardiac rehabilitation. *Clinics in Geriatric Medicine, 35*(4), 527–537. https://doi.org/10.1016/j.cger.2019.07.009

other forms of exercise (biking, elliptical, low-intensity walking) if they have difficulty walking (Gerhard-Herman et al., 2016). A regular exercise program is part of lifelong management of PAD symptoms (Patel, Sakhuja, & White, 2020).

Wound Management

Patients with PAD and poorly healing wounds on their feet have a higher incidence of amputation and cardiovascular mortality if not aggressively treated (Donohue et al., 2020). The most common causes of poorly healing foot ulcers are arterial disease, venous disease, neuropathy, and a history of diabetes mellitus. Often patients have mixed etiology ulcers when two or more comorbidities are present. TBIs can help with differential diagnosis as patients with poorly healing foot wounds and normal TBIs (>0.7) with triphasic waveforms generally have greater wound healing with aggressive wound management than those with abnormal TBIs and waveforms (Donohue et al., 2020). Referral to a wound specialist is important for the initiation of aggressive wound management to prevent or minimize amputation (Class II recommendation).

Pharmacologic Management

Antiplatelet

Antiplatelet therapy can help reduce the risk of cardiovascular adverse events and prevent platelet aggregation at the site of stenosis. Aspirin (81 mg daily) is a Class I recommendation for all patients with PAD due to their high risk of cardiovascular events (Berti-Hearn & Elliott, 2018). Clopidogrel (Plavix) is used for patients who have undergone revascularization procedures or who do not tolerate aspirin. Dual antiplatelet therapy (aspirin plus Plavix) does not show a beneficial effect in patients that have not had a revascularization procedure and is associated with increased bleeding risk (Firnhaber & Powell, 2019). Data from the COMPASS trial suggest that low dose rivaroxaban (Xarelto; 2.5 mg BID) in addition to aspirin (100 mg daily) reduces the risk for future cardiovascular and limb events in patients with PAD. Consider low dose Xarelto plus aspirin for patients with PAD who are young, current smokers who decline smoking cessation, or have aggressive systemic atherosclerosis (Koutsoumpelis et al., 2018).

Statins

There is significant evidence that treating hyperlipidemia will reduce the progression of atherosclerosis and limb complications with PAD (Class I recommendation; Corrado et al., 2020). Studies suggest that lipid lowering treatment improves walking distances (160 meters) in patients with PAD. It is recommended that a diagnosis of PAD is a marker for systemic atherosclerosis and should be treated with lower LDL goal targets (Corrado et al., 2020). Patients who are concerned about statin-related myopathy should be reassured that the minor

risk of the myopathy symptoms is greatly outweighed by the benefits of statin treatment (Corrado et al., 2020). The ACC/AHA PAD guidelines recommend high dose atorvastatin (40 mg or 80 mg daily; Gerhard-Herman et al., 2016). For patients who cannot tolerate a high-dose statin medication or are truly statin intolerant, a nonstatin cholesterol medication (ezetimibe) can be considered (Gerhard-Herman et al., 2016). The role of the newer PCSK9 inhibitors in LDL management is evolving for patients with PAD (Aboyans et al., 2018).

Cilostazol

Cilostazol (Pletal) is a phosphodiesterase III inhibitor that acts as a vasodilator and inhibits platelet aggregation (Gerhard-Herman et al., 2016). When given to patients with PAD a significant improvement in walking distance can be seen after 4–6 weeks of medication. Cilostazol is the only pharmacologic therapy that is effective in increasing walking distance in PAD (Patel, Sakhuja, & White, 2020). Cilostazol is contraindicated in patients with heart failure of any severity and an echocardiogram should be considered prior to the initiation of therapy. Diarrhea, leg swelling, and palpitations are the most common reasons patients do not tolerate the drug (Gerhard-Herman et al., 2016).

Revascularization

The ACC/AHA PAD guidelines recommend an individualized approach to revascularization (Gerhard-Herman et al., 2016). The choice of revascularization techniques (endovascular, surgical, or a combination of both) depends upon the location and degree of stenosis as well as the experience of the team treating the patient (Berti-Hearn & Elliott, 2018). Patients with claudication generally have inflow (iliac) or femoral-popliteal disease, while patients with rest pain often have multilevel and tibial disease (Shishehbor & Jaff, 2016).

Claudication

Conservative management with an exercise program and/or Pletal should be attempted by the patient with lifestyle limiting claudication before they are offered a revascularization procedure. No trials show a benefit in revascularization for patients with PAD who are asymptomatic (Class IIa recommendation; Gerhard-Herman et al., 2016). The CLEVER trial (Claudication: Exercise Versus Endoluminal Revascularization) showed that exercise and endovascular revascularization complement each other: exercise by improving strength and walking distance for the patient and endovascular procedure by decreasing pain and increasing quality of life (Shishehbor & Jaff, 2016). Endovascular techniques are appropriate for patients with lifestyle-limiting claudication who have inflow (aortic and iliac) disease (Class 1 recommendation) and femoral-popliteal disease (Class II recommendation). Surgical options are recommended for patients with lifestyle-limiting claudication who have common femoral or long femoral-popliteal stenosis. Bypass to distal vessels (below the knee) should not be done for patients with claudication (Class III recommendation: Harmful; Gerhard-Herman et al., 2016).

Chronic Limb Ischemia

Patients with CLI are at higher risk for mortality and morbidity (amputation) than patients with claudication alone (Gerhard-Herman et al., 2016). Patients should be offered a revascularization procedure as management for their symptoms with the goals of wound healing and symptom improvement (Class I recommendation). Patients who have short segment stenosis of the inflow arteries (disease in the iliac or common femoral) or femoral-popliteal disease should be considered for endovascular angioplasty and stenting procedures. Studies are ongoing to determine the effectiveness of endovascular procedures in the tibial (below the knee) vessels (Shishehbor & Jaff, 2016). Surgical revascularization (endarterectomy or bypass surgery) should be considered for long femoral-popliteal lesions or below the knee stenosis. Recommendations are for bypass with autogenous vein rather than prosthetic when available. A wound care team should be involved to maximize wound healing potential along with revascularization (Class I recommendation; Gerhard-Herman et al., 2016).

Long-Term Follow-Up

PAD is a chronic condition without a known cure. Patients are best managed by conservative therapy, with revascularization as needed and periodic follow-up clinical evaluations (Gerhard-Herman et al., 2016). Compliance with risk factor reduction, medical management, exercise therapy and smoking cessation should be assessed at regular intervals. Foot care by podiatry should be recommended. Patients who have undergone limb revascularization should be followed to ensure patency of the procedure. Early identification of complications can prevent worsening of symptoms and occlusion of previously placed stents and bypasses (Gerhard-Herman et al., 2016).

CLINICAL PEARLS

- Patients who have leg pain symptoms that are improved when using a shopping cart or a walker to lean on and have normal ABIs: Consider spinal stenosis as a diagnosis.
- Patients who describe rest pain-type symptoms (pain, numbness/tingling) with ABIs greater than 0.4: Consider other causes of symptoms (neuropathy, spinal stenosis).
- Patients who describe cramping at night that forces them to get out of bed or put weight on their feet: Consider nocturnal leg cramping as a diagnosis.

KEY TAKEAWAYS

- All patients with PAD, regardless of symptoms, should be treated with aspirin (81 mg daily) and atorvastatin (40 mg or 80 mg daily) for risk factor reduction, smoking cessation, and an aggressive walking program.
- Cilostazol can be considered for patients with lifestyle-limiting claudication, rest pain, or poorly healing ulcerations.
- Revascularization can be considered for patients with claudication who fail both cilostazol (Pletal) and an aggressive exercise program.
- Patients with rest pain or poorly healing ulcerations should be treated with conservative management while undergoing evaluation for revascularization.

EVIDENCE-BASED RESOURCES

Gerhard-Herman, M. D., Gornik, H. L., Barrett, C., Barshes, N. R., Corriere, M. A., Drachman, D. E., Fleisher, L. A., Fowkes, F. G., Hamburg, N. M., Kinlay, S., Lookstein, R., Misra, S., Mureebe, L., Olin, J. W., Patel, R. A., Regensteiner, J. G., Schanzer, A., Shishehbor, M. H., Stewart, K. J., . . . Walsh, M. E. (2016). AHA/ACC guideline on the management of patients with lower extremity peripheral artery disease: A report of the American College of Cardiology/American Heart Association Task Force on Clinical Practice guidelines. *Circulation*, 135(12), e726–e779. https://doi.org/10.1161/CIR.0000000000000471

Aboyans, V., Ricco, J. B., Bartelink, M. E. L., Björck, M., Brodmann, M., Cohnert, T., Collet, J. P., Czerny, M., De Carlo, M., Debus, S., Espinola-Klein, C., Kahan, T., Kownator, S., Mazzolai L, Naylor AR, Roffi M, Röther J, Sprynger M, Tendera M, … ESC Scientific Document Group. (2018, March 1). 2017 ESC Guidelines on the Diagnosis and Treatment of Peripheral Arterial Diseases, in collaboration with the European Society for Vascular Surgery (ESVS): Document covering atherosclerotic disease of extracranial carotid and vertebral, mesenteric, renal, upper and lower extremity arteries Endorsed by: The European Stroke Organization (ESO) The Task Force for the Diagnosis and Treatment of Peripheral Arterial Diseases of the European Society of Cardiology (ESC) and of the European Society for Vascular Surgery (ESVS). *European Heart Journal*, 39(9), 763–816. https://doi.org/10.1093/eurheartj/ehx095

Patnode, C. D., Henderson, J. T., Thompson, J. H., Senger, C. A., Fortmann, S. P., & Whitlock, E. P. (2015). *Behavioral counseling and pharmacotherapy interventions for tobacco cessation in adults, including pregnant women: A review of reviews for the U.S. Preventive Services Task Force*. Agency for Healthcare Research and Quality (US). http://www.ncbi.nlm.nih.gov/books/NBK321744/

Whelton, P. K., Carey, R. M., Aronow, W. S., Casey, D. E., Jr., Collins, K. J., Himmelfarb, C. D., DePalma, S. M., Gidding, S., Jamerson, K. A., Jones, D. W., MacLaughlin, E. J., Muntner, P., Ovbiagele, B., Smith, S. C., Jr., Spencer,

C. C., Stafford, R. S., Taler, S. J., Thomas, R. J., Williams, K. A., Sr., . . . Jackson, T. (2018). 2017 ACC/AHA/AAPA/ABC/ACPM/AGS/APhA/ASH/ASPC/NMA/PCNA Guideline for the Prevention, Detection, Evaluation, and Management of High Blood Pressure in Adults: A Report of the American College of Cardiology/American Heart Association Task Force on Clinical Practice Guidelines. *Hypertension*, 71, e13–e115. https://doi.org/10.1161/HYP.0000000000000065

6.8: MESENTERIC ISCHEMIA

Mesenteric ischemia is a manifestation of peripheral vascular disease, where the blood supply is insufficient to meet the demands of the visceral organs and is classified as either acute or chronic. Mesenteric ischemia is an uncommon cause of abdominal pain, accounting for less than one of every 1000 hospital admissions; however, an inaccurate or delayed diagnosis can result in catastrophic complications: Mortality among patients in whom this condition is acute is 60% to 80% (Clair & Beach, 2016). The mesenteric arterial circulation compromises three principal branches of the abdominal aorta, namely the celiac axis (CA), superior mesenteric artery (SMA), and inferior mesenteric artery (IMA) (Gnanapandithan & Feuerstadt, 2020). After eating a meal, the blood flow through these arteries increases within 60 minutes due to an increased demand of the intestine. Diffuse atherosclerosis, usually occurring at the origin of these vessels, is the primary mechanism and accounts for 95% of chronic mesenteric ischemia (Patel, Waheed, & Costanza, 2020). Chronic occlusion of a single vessel allows collateral blood flow to compensate thus symptoms do not typically present until at least two primary vessels are occluded (Patel, Waheed, & Costanza, 2020). Acute mesenteric ischemia develops primarily due to one of four pathophysiology mechanisms: (a) acute arterial embolism (40%–50%); (b) acute arterial thrombosis (20%–30%); (c) nonocclusive mesenteric ischemia (25%); and (d) mesenteric venous thrombosis (5%–15%; Lim et al., 2019). Arterial embolism and arterial thrombosis are the two major causes of acute mesenteric arterial occlusion.

PRESENTING SIGNS AND SYMPTOMS

- Acute: Sudden severe onset of periumbilical pain which is out of proportion to the exam; nausea, and vomiting; can be critically ill.
- Chronic: Chronic abdominal pain, significant unintentional weight loss, food phobia (food fear), food aversion, abdominal bloating, diarrhea, postprandial pain in epigastrium (dull ache, crampy, or colicky) occurring 30 to 60 minutes after eating a meal which can persists for a few hours and can be worse after a heavy or fatty meal.

HISTORY AND PHYSICAL FINDINGS

- Acute: Abdominal pain out of proportion to the exam findings, diffuse abdominal tenderness, rebound tenderness and guarding, absent bowel sounds, atrial fibrillation, possible abdominal distention with progression to grossly distended abdomen, occult blood in stool, signs of dehydration and shock (which indicate a deteriorating clinic course). History of prior embolic event, recent myocardial infarction, heart failure, hemodialysis (causes a low flow state), vasoconstrictive medications, use of cocaine, use of ergotamines.
- Chronic: Active bowel sounds, epigastric abdominal bruit, malnourished, cachectic, no rebound tenderness or guarding, and postprandial abdominal pain. History of coronary artery disease, peripheral artery disease, tobacco use, hypertension, hyperlipidemia, or carotid artery disease. Key questions to ask: Do you have abdominal pain after eating and have you had a significant weight loss?

DIFFERENTIAL DIGANOSIS AND DIAGNOSTIC CONSIDERATIONS

- Acute: Vasculitis, ruptured abdominal aortic aneurysm, aortic dissection, perforated bowel, acute small bowel obstruction, and any acute surgical abdomen
- Chronic: Malignancy, median arcuate ligament syndrome, volvulus, intussusception, ascites, upper GI bleed, fibromuscular dysplasia, chronic pancreatitis, peptic ulcer disease, bowel disorder, eating disorder, vasculitis, chronic cholecystitis

TREATMENT

- Acute: *Initial management*—NPO, gastric decompression, fluid resuscitation, hemodynamic monitoring, correct electrolyte abnormalities, pain control, anticoagulate (heparin drip) under most circumstances and begin broad spectrum antibiotics (Tendler & Lamont, 2020).
  - *Order labs*—Complete blood count (CBC; evaluating for leukocytosis), comprehensive metabolic panel (CMP; evaluating for metabolic acidosis), amylase, lipase, phosphorus, D-dimer (possible indicator of thrombus), occult blood test, lactic acid.
  - *Imaging studies*—ECG, CT angiogram (preferred due to readily available and lower cost) or MRA.
  - Consult vascular surgery, general surgery, or interventional radiology promptly (depending on what service is available at your institution); prepare patient for possible emergent surgery for revascularization, thrombolysis with endovascular angioplasty, and/or stenting. Palliative medicine may need to be consulted for poor surgical candidates.

- **Chronic:** Evaluate nutrition status, CMP, CBC, lipid panel. Mesenteric artery duplex scan, ECG (arrhythmia), Echocardiogram (valve disease or decreased ejection fraction), review medications that may Cause vasoconstriction. Obtain CT angiogram if duplex scan is inconclusive, may need angiogram with angioplasty +/– stenting, consider use of pre and post TPN, mesenteric revascularization grafting or endarterectomy. Management of cardiovascular risk factors- smoking cessation, HTN management, statins, antiplatelet and anticoagulate (short or long term).

TRANSITION OF CARE

- **Acute:** Sign off to ICU, surgical or IR team for ongoing management of care.
- **Chronic:** medical management of cardiovascular risk factors with antiplatelet, antihypertensive medication and statin. Enroll/counsel in smoking cessation program. Refer to Vascular surgery/vascular medicine for ongoing follow up.

CLINICAL PEARLS

- Risk factors for mesenteric ischemia include any condition that reduces perfusion of the intestines or predisposes one to mesenteric arterial embolism, arterial thrombosis, venous thrombosis, or vasoconstriction.
- The classic clinical description for acute mesenteric ischemia is abdominal pain out of proportion to the physical exam.
- Mesenteric ischemia can be acute or chronic and arterial or venous

KEY TAKEAWAYS

- Any patient with acute abdominal pain with metabolic acidosis has mesenteric ischemia until proven otherwise.
- A thorough medical history can assist with the early diagnosis of mesenteric ischemia as the physical exam may be normal initially.
- Survival outcomes are worse with arterial causes.

A robust set of instructor resources designed to supplement this text is located at **http://connect.springerpub.com/content/ reference-book/978-0-8261-6079-9.** Qualifying instructors may request access by emailing **textbook@springerpub.com.**

REFERENCES

Full list of references can be accessed at http://connect .springerpub.com/content/reference-book/978-0-8261-6079-9

CHAPTER 7

PULMONARY DISORDERS

LEARNING OBJECTIVES

- Demonstrate comprehension of common chronic lung diseases (CLDs) and disorders.
- Utilize the appropriate skills and assessment techniques to identify and diagnose common CLDs and disorders.
- Implement treatment when appropriate for CLDs following the current evidence-based clinical guidelines.
- Provide education and initiate health promotion strategies in the care of the patient with CLD.
- Identify and initiate appropriate referrals to the pulmonary specialist.
- Describe the pathophysiology of respiratory failure.
- Define the four types of respiratory failure and describe the derangements, causes, and management for each type.
- Differentiate transudative and exudative etiologies of pleural effusions.
- Develop an evidence-based management and treatment plan for a patient with pleural effusion.
- Analyze objective clinical findings to determine level of risk associated with pulmonary embolism (PE).
- Develop an evidence-based management and treatment plan for a patient with PE.

INTRODUCTION

Disorders of the pulmonary system refer to the lower respiratory tract that is made up of the large and small airways, lung tissue, and pleural space. Acute disorders of the airways, lung tissue, and pleural space are often caused by episodic events such as trauma, infection, exacerbation of chronic disease, or thromboembolism, whereas chronic disorders are often caused by the chronic exposure of behavioral or environmental factors leading to obstructive or restrictive lung disease and progressive dysfunction (American Lung Association, n.d.). The American Lung Association also reports that more than 35 million cases of chronic lung diseases (CLD) can be prevented in the United States including asthma, chronic obstructive pulmonary disease (COPD), and interstitial lung diseases. This chapter discusses the acute and chronic lung disorders the AGACNP must be skilled in diagnosing and managing.

7.1: ACUTE LUNG INJURY AND ACUTE RESPIRATORY DISTRESS SYNDROME

Leanne H. Fowler

Acute respiratory distress syndrome (ARDS) is a life-threatening acute inflammatory lung disease causing hypoxemic respiratory failure; it is a severe type of acute lung injury (ALI) characterized by refractory hypoxemia and bilateral non-cardiogenic pulmonary edema (NCPE; American Thoracic Society, European Society of Critical Care Medicine, & Society of Critical Care Medicine [ATS/ESICM/SCCM], 2017). Definitions for ALI and ARDS involve the acute onset of illness, bilateral and patchy infiltrates visualized on chest radiograph, and poor systemic oxygenation in the presence of normal left atrial or end-diastolic left ventricular pressures. The Adult Gerontology Acute Care Nurse Practitioner (AGACNP) can use the PaO_2/FiO_2 ratio to differentiate ALI (ratio <300) from ARDS (ratio <200). A patient diagnosed with ARDS can also have the illness defined by a validated assessment tool called the Lung Injury Score (LIS; Murray et al., 1988). The LIS uses the (a) PaO_2/FiO_2 ratio, (b) total respiratory compliance, (c) the level of positive end-expiratory pressure (PEEP), and (d) the severity of bilateral radiographic infiltrates consistent with pulmonary edema that is scored on a 0.0 to 4.0 scale. A score of 2.5 or greater is congruent with severe disease (Reilly & Christie, 2015). Clinicians also use the Berlin Definition of ARDS (2012) terminology defined as mild (ratio 201–300), moderate (ratio 101–200), or severe (ratio ≤100) with the other clinical features presented but without use of the ALI term (Thompson et al., 2017). This section will use the terminology from the Berlin Definition of ARDS and 2017 ARDS guideline that classifies the severity of ARDS by the degree of hypoxemia the patient is experiencing (ATS/ESICM/SCCM, 2017; Force et al., 2012).

The incidence of ARDS is often underrecognized yet is associated with higher mortality rate (50%) than all cancers except lung cancer (Thompson et al., 2017). The most common cause of death for patients diagnosed with ARDS is due to the severity of the underlying insult or a subsequent nosocomial lung infection or sepsis. Patient with ARDS rarely die from progressive hypoxia and respiratory failure (Reilly & Christie, 2015). The underuse of lung protective practices and underrecognition lead to undertreatment and increased morbidity and mortality in patients with

TABLE 7.1: Direct and Indirect Causes of Acute Respiratory Distress Syndrome

DIRECT LUNG INJURIES	INDIRECT OR SYSTEMIC CAUSES
Aspiration pneumonitis	Acute pancreatitis
Bacterial pneumonia, multifocal	Blood transfusion
Chest trauma with lung contusion	Fat-emboli syndrome
Legionnaires' disease	Graft failure, lung transplant
Near drowning	Sepsis
Pneumocystis carinii	Shock syndromes
Thermal or chemical inhalations	Systemic inflammatory response
Viral pneumonia	syndrome

confluent opacities and a narrow cardiothoracic silhouette (Thompson et al., 2017). Precipitating causes of ARDS are listed in Table 7.1.

CLINICAL PEARLS

- Identify patients at high risk for developing ARDS to improve patient outcomes.
- Trend the patient's PaO_2:FiO_2 ratio to monitor severity of lung injury while hospitalized.

Pathogenesis of Acute Respiratory Distress Syndrome

The lung's first response to injury, known as the exudative phase of ARDS, is characterized by the accumulation of protein-rich edema within the interstitium and alveolus causing capillary congestion and intra-alveolar hemorrhage. The exudative phase involves early (first 48 hours) and late (several days after injury) immune and inflammatory responses to the injury that can make the lung tissue more susceptible to damage with mechanical stretch (Thompson et al., 2017). Late immune and inflammatory responses during the exudative phase are associated with extensive necrosis of type I alveolar epithelial cells causing diffuse alveolar damage (Reilly & Christie, 2015). The second phase of ARDS, known as the proliferative phase, initiates repair processes of the epithelium that are vital for the host's survival and for recovery of the architecture and function of the lung. The latest phase (fibrotic or fibroproliferative phase) is not experienced by all patients diagnosed with ARDS but is characterized by pulmonary hypertension (PH), further decline in lung compliance, and an increase in minute ventilation and dead-space fraction (Reilly & Christie, 2015). The fibrotic phase is associated with prolonged mechanical ventilation and increased mortality (Thompson et al., 2017).

Transfusion-Related Acute Lung Injury

A less common but possible cause of ALI is related to the transfusion of blood products and is known as transfusion-related acute lung injury (TRALI). Approximately 6 hours post transfusion, patients that received a blood product transfusion can develop hypoxemia and bilateral pulmonary infiltrates on chest radiograph due to TRALI. The clinical findings are generally reversible in the first 1 to 3 days after cessation for most cases. The pathogenesis of TRALI is most associated with the transfusion of red blood cell products causing the proliferation of leucoagglutination antibodies. Patients recover well with supportive therapy and TRALI occurs less with restrictive transfusion practices (Carson et al., 2017).

COVID 19-Associated Acute Respiratory Distress Syndrome

A distinct and atypical form of virus-induced ARDS, known as CARDS, was identified during the COVID-19 pandemic with pathophysiological mechanisms and the development of comorbidities that varied from what was traditionally known about ARDS (Pfortmueller et al., 2020). After studying the pathology and histology of lung tissue from cadavers who succumbed to COVID-19 during the pandemic, CARDS involved severe pulmonary edema, impaired alveolar homeostasis, pulmonary remodeling that led to fibrosis, and endotheliitis that led to vascular thrombosis and immune cell activation (Ackermann et al., 2020; Ehre, 2020). Patients who recovered from CARDS reported residual dyspnea during various levels of exertion and required broncho-dilating or corticosteroid inhalers that were not required pre-CARDS diagnosis (Pfortmueller et al., 2020).

PRESENTING SIGNS AND SYMPTOMS

Approximately 12 to 72 hours after a predisposing lung injuring event, a patient can develop rapid onset and/or progressive respiratory distress. Patients also present with varying degrees of anxiety, agitation, hypoxia associated with SpO_2 readings less than 85%, and labored breathing. The hallmark finding for patients presenting with signs and symptoms of ARDS is hypoxemia that is refractory to supplemental oxygen administration.

HISTORY AND PHYSICAL FINDINGS

Patient History

Patients presenting with signs and symptoms of ARDS are most associated with an insulting lung injury (see Table 7.1). Patients at the greatest risk for developing ARDS after an insulting lung injury include those with a history of obesity, chronic alcohol misuse, protein malnutrition, and severe lung injury from trauma, bacterial pneumonia, or a viral pneumonia associated with influenza or severe acute respiratory syndrome (SARS). Patients of advanced age also have an increased incidence of developing ARDS (Reilly & Christie, 2015).

Vaping and E-Cigarette Use

Patients with a history of vaping or e-cigarette use have been found to have a degree of ALI. In a small multicenter cohort retrospective study of CT images, patterns of parenchymal organizing pneumonia, regional or diffuse ground-glass opacity, and consolidation were found in patients with a vaping and/or e-cigarette history of use (Klipathogenan et al., 2021). The younger the patients, the more injury appreciated. Additionally, patients that admitted to vaping tetrahydrocannabinol (THC), nicotine, or both were most commonly found with lung injury patterns (Klipathogenan et al., 2021). Establishing a relationship with the patient to facilitate the collection of an honest social history can assist the AGACNP in a more accurate risk assessment of patients for ALI and ARDS.

Physical Examination

The general appearance of a patient with ARDS is ill-appearing and uncomfortable. Patients suspected to have ARDS can have vital signs indicating fever, tachycardia, and hypoxia. Patients can also present with hypotension or significant hemodynamic instability depending on the underlying illness; peripheral pulses may be weak and thready. The AGACNP may observe an anxious, agitated, or restless mood and pale skin with diaphoresis. Patients' lung examinations may include labored breathing, diffuse crackles, and cyanosis. Heart sounds can be regular or rapid, and hypoxia can increase the patient's risk for arrhythmias.

DIFFERENTIAL DIAGNOSIS AND DIAGNOSTIC CONSIDERATIONS

The diagnosis of ARDS is identifying a syndrome of events that are nonspecific to the primary lung insult. Therefore, evaluating the patient's entire case is necessary to identify the causative lung insult.

Differential Diagnoses

The differential diagnoses associated with patients with acute hypoxemic respiratory failure should include ARDS, acute cardiogenic pulmonary edema (ACPE), pneumonia, and rheumatologic disorders that can cause diffuse alveolar hemorrhage. The differential diagnoses associated with patients with known ARDS should consider the predisposing etiologies such as sepsis, pneumonia, trauma, TRALI, CARDS, or gastric aspiration. Further evaluation with serum laboratory and imaging diagnostic tests is necessary to confirm suspicions of the patient's severe hypoxemic illness.

Evidence-based assessment tools such as the LIS and Lung Injury Prediction Score (LIPS) should be used to help define the patient ARDS (Reilly & Christie, 2015). The Berlin Definitions of ARDS can also be used to diagnose ARDS and standardize the recognition of severe illness (Force et al., 2012; Thompson et al., 2017). Most of the assessment tools require data that can only be obtained from serum and imaging tests.

Diagnostic Tests

Evaluation of the patient suspected to have ARDS should include obtaining a chest radiograph, arterial blood gases (ABGs), a serum chemistry panel, and complete blood count (CBC). Consider a serum lactic acid level and sputum, urine, and blood cultures in patients who are suspected to have ARDS secondary to sepsis or another severe infection.

A serum lactic acid level can be included in the primary workup of patients without the suspicion of sepsis because of its utility to indicate the severity of impaired tissue perfusion. Other serum laboratory tests that should be considered in the primary workup include cardiac enzymes to evaluate the patient for demand ischemia of myocardial cells. Cardiac enzyme levels should be collected with a 12-lead EKG to also aid in the evaluation of the patient for ischemic myocardial complications of ARDS. Additionally, a serum brain natriuretic peptide (BNP) level can be useful in differentiating cardiogenic from noncardiogenic acute pulmonary edema.

Chest Radiograph

The characteristic radiographic features of ARDS include bilateral, patchy, alveolar infiltrates that are consistent with pulmonary edema but without the cardiovascular features of a widened vascular pedicle and enlarged cardiac silhouette. In the early phases of ARDS, the infiltrates are variable and can be described as mild interstitial or alveolar infiltrates, or patchy or confluent infiltrates. The AGACNP should know that the radiographic findings of ARDS do not correlate reliably to the severity of hypoxemia. It is also important to recognize that asymmetrical bilateral, patchy infiltrates can be interpreted as a lobar pneumonia or segmental atelectasis. Nevertheless, the presence of bilateral, patchy infiltrates and moderate to severe hypoxemia should increase the AGACNP's index of suspicion for ARDS (Reilly & Christie, 2015). Patients who do not show improvement or persistent decline in lung function and worsening radiographic findings might benefit from the segmental lung imaging that CT provides.

CLINICAL PEARLS

- Differentiate cardiogenic from noncardiogenic pulmonary edema (NCPE) during the physical exam.
- Recognize hemodynamic patterns with ARDS: Pulmonary artery (PA) occlusive pressure (PAOP) <18 mmHg; pulmonary vascular resistance (PVR) >300 mmHg.
- Recognize radiographic patterns of ARDS: Diffuse (bilateral) patchy infiltrates.

Bronchoscopy Procedures

Patients with an unclear etiology for ARDS may benefit from bronchoscopy with bronchoalveolar lavage (BAL). For example, patients with diffuse alveolar hemorrhage secondary to a systemic lupus erythematosus (SLE) exacerbation or granulomatosis with polyangiitis can be identified. Another example of the benefit a BAL can provide includes the patient with acute eosinophilic pneumonia who would have characteristic eosinophilic infiltrates visualized in the lungs. Furthermore, the analysis of fluid obtained during BAL can be measured for the eosinophil count. Performance of a BAL for patients with severe ARDS can be performed safely in the patient without severe hypoxemia. Lung biopsy is not routinely performed for patients diagnosed with ARDS but may be necessary as a last resort measure to determine the patient's diagnosis. Lung biopsy is an option for patients with poor recovery and an unclear etiology of the disease (Reilly & Christie, 2015).

Invasive Monitoring

Hemodynamic monitoring of the patient with ARDS can be helpful to trend volume status with a central venous pressure (CVP) and to trend arterial blood pressures. Therefore, the AGACNP should determine when central venous catheter or arterial catheter placement is indicated and necessary for the efficient evaluation of the patient. Arterial catheter placement can also facilitate the timely collection of arterial blood gases (ABGs). Pulmonary artery (PA) catheter monitoring and documentation of a normal pulmonary capillary wedge pressure (PCWP) of less than 20 mmHg is the definitive differential for ARDS versus cardiogenic pulmonary edema. PA catheters increase the risk for pulmonary infarct and cardiac arrhythmias in patients with ARDS, and therefore should be utilized only when other diagnostics have not provided adequate information for further treatment.

TREATMENT

The primary goal of treatment for the patient with ARDS is to support oxygenation and to minimize or eliminate the cause of lung injury. Additional goals of treatment include lung-protective ventilation, conservative fluid resuscitation, and hemodynamic management. Treatment plans are largely supportive unless the underlying etiology is known. When the underlying lung insult is known (e.g., sepsis, pancreatitis, shock), treatment goals also include eliminating or minimizing the cause of injury to the lung (Thompson et al., 2017). Patients with ARDS are usually cared for in the critical care unit until their condition is deemed stable.

Oxygenation

Refractory hypoxemia is a hallmark feature of ARDS and should be prioritized to reverse. Oxygenation is improved with alveolar recruitment and is not improved with the administration of supplemental oxygen alone in moderate to severe ARDS cases. High levels of FiO_2 may be necessary in the treatment of ARDS but can be toxic to the endothelial layers of lung tissue. Therefore, in combination with supplemental oxygen, the administration of positive end expiratory pressure (PEEP) is used via mechanical ventilation to improve alveolar diffusion of oxygen into the blood. Because of the pathogenesis of ARDS, supportive treatment with mechanical ventilation is a cornerstone of care. However, mechanical ventilation itself can also cause tissue trauma that is known as ventilator-induced lung injury (VILI). Therefore, when intubation and mechanical ventilation are required, goal-directed or protocolized management has demonstrated superior outcomes over nonprotocolized management (ATS/ESICM/SCCM, 2017). A summary of the mechanical ventilation protocol is provided in Table 7.2.

Lung-Protective Mechanical Ventilation

The goal of lung-protective ventilation is to prevent VILI (also known as barotrauma) from the overdistention of alveoli. Patients diagnosed with ARDS who require mechanical ventilation will benefit more from intubation and mechanical ventilation than noninvasive positive pressure ventilation (NIPPV). Patients with mild to moderate ARDS may start with NIPPV when they are fully awake and alert. There is little evidence to support the use of NIPPV as a primary treatment strategy for patients diagnosed with severe ARDS. Patients with severe ARDS and established palliative care plans may benefit from the use of NIPPV as a strategy to improve oxygenation (ATS/ESICM/SCCM, 2017; Thompson et al., 2017).

When invasive mechanical ventilation is required, lung-protective mechanisms include maintaining tidal volumes (V_T) between 4 and 6 mL/kg of predicted body weight (PBW) when peak plateau pressures (Pplat) exceed 30 mmHg (ATS/ESICM/SCCM, 2017). Lower tidal volumes in assist control ventilator modes aim to reduce more harm to the injured lung from overdistention and to prevent injury to the residual healthy lung.

Low tidal volumes (or lung-protective ventilation strategies) are supplemented with PEEP of at least 5 cm of water (ATS/ESICM/SCCM, 2017). The AGACNP should monitor the patient's oxygenation and hemodynamic status and incrementally titrate PEEP up toward the oxygenation goal and per the patient's tolerance to higher levels of PEEP. As oxygenation improves, the AGACNP should titrate FiO_2 levels down before reducing PEEP levels to maintain alveolar gas exchange.

Pressure Control Ventilation

Lung protective mechanical ventilation strategies also include the use of pressure control ventilation (PCV) settings instead of volume control settings. PCV is useful in patients with severe ARDS and decreased lung compliance. The use of PCV settings offers patients with severe ARDS reduced peak airway and end-inspiratory pressures. Pressure control settings can also use inverse ratio ventilation (IRV) providing a benefit of lengthening the inspiratory time in the inspiratory-to-expiratory (I:E >1) ratio in an effort to reduce peak plateau pressures. The drawbacks of using PCV with IRV settings include limited expiratory time and the potential to underestimate levels of PEEP. The PCV with IRV settings should

TABLE 7.2: Mechanical Ventilation Management Protocol Summary

PROTOCOL	SUMMARY
Inclusion criteria	Acute onset of: – PaO_2/FiO_2 ≤300 (corrected for altitude) – Bilateral, patchy, diffuse infiltrates (consistent with pulmonary edema) – No clinical evidence of LA hypertension

Initial set-up and follow-up management	Calculate the PBW for any ventilator mode
	– Women = 45.5. + 2.3 (height [in inches] – 60)
	– Men = 50 + 2.3 (height [in inches]– 60)
	Set an initial V_T = 8 mL/kg PBW
	– Reduce V_T by 1 mL/kg ≤ 2 hr until V_T = 6 mL/kg PBW
	Set an initial rate to the estimated baseline minute ventilation but not ≥35 bpm
	Adjust V_T and rate to achieve the goals below:
	– Oxygenation goal = PaO_2 55–80 mmHg or SpO_2 88%–95%
	  o Initial PEEP of 5 cmH_2O, then incremental titrations of FiO_2 and PEEP combinations
	– Pplat goal = ≤30 cmH_2O
	  o Check Pplat during 0.5 sec inspiratory pause Q4h and post changes to PEEP or V_T
	  o For Pplat ≥30 cmH_2O, reduce V_T 1 mL/kg to minimum of 4 mL/kg
	  o For Pplat <25 cmH_2O and V_T <6 mL/kg, increase V_T 1 mL/kg to Pplat >25 cmH_2O or V_T = 6 mL/kg
	  o If Pplat <30 with breath stacking or dyssynchrony, increase V_T in 1 mL/kg increments to 7–8 mL/kg if Pplat remains ≤30 cmH_2O
	– pH goal = 7.30 to 7.45
	  o Acidosis management
	    ■ If pH 7.15–7.30, increase rate to pH >7.30 or $PaCO_2$ <25 (maximum rate of 35 bpm)
	    ■ If pH <7.15, increase V_T 1 mL/kg to pH >7.15
	      • Pplat >30 can be exceeded
	      • $NaHCO_3$ can be administered
	  o Alkalosis management
	    ■ If pH >7.45, reduce rate when possible
	– I:E ratio goal = Maintain duration of I <E

Weaning	Daily SBT criteria
	– FiO_2 ≤0.40 and PEEP ≤8 OR FiO_2 ≤0.5 and PEEP ≤5
	– PEEP and FiO_2 ≤values of previous day
	– If patient with acceptable SBT efforts, reduce rate by 50% for 5 min to evaluate efforts
	– SBP ≥90 mmHg without vasopressor support
	– No NMB administration
	Conduct SBT when all criteria are met for at least 12 hr, initiate trial for 120 min with FiO_2 ≤0.50 and PEEP ≤5 cmH_2O
	– Place on T-piece, trach collar, or CPAP ≤5 and PS ≤5 cmH_2O
	– Evaluate patient tolerance, up to 2 hr
	  o SpO_2 ≥90% and/or PaO_2 ≥60 mmHg
	  o Spontaneous V_T ≤4 mL/kg PBW
	  o Rate ≤35 bpm
	  o pH ≥7.3
	  o No respiratory distress (cannot have ≥2 of following):
	    ■ HR ≥120% of baseline
	    ■ Marked respiratory labor
	    ■ Marked dyspnea
	    ■ Abdominal paradox
	    ■ Diaphoresis
	– If patient can tolerate ≥30 min, can be extubated
	– If patient cannot tolerate ≥30 min, resume pre-wean ventilator settings

HR, heart rate; I:E ratio, inspiration to expiration ratio; LA, left atrial; NMB, neuromuscular blockage; PBW, predicted body weight; Pplat, plateau pressure; Q4h, every 4 hr; SBP, systolic blood pressure; SBT, spontaneous breathing trial; V_T, tidal volume.

Sources: Data from American Thoracic Society, European Society of Critical Care Medicine, & Society of Critical Care Medicine. (2017). An official American Thoracic Society/European Society of Critical Care Medicine/Society of Critical Care Medicine clinical practice guideline: Mechanical ventilation in adult patients with acute respiratory distress syndrome. *American Journal of Respiratory Critical Care Medicine, 195*(9), 1253–1263. https://doi.org/10.1164/rccm.201703-0548ST; National Heart Lung & Blood Institute ARDS Network. (2008). *NIH NHLBI ARDS clinical network mechanical ventilation protocol summary*. http://www.ardsnet.org/files/ventilator_protocol_2008-07.pdf

be used as a salvage or rescue ventilation strategy for the patient with severe ARDS (Thompson et al., 2017). The 2017 ARDS guidelines recommend against IRV (ATS/ESICM/SCCM, 2017).

Prone Positioning

Placing patients in the prone position to improve hypoxemia can be performed whether they are mechanically ventilated or can ventilate spontaneously. Patients with severe ARDS improve oxygenation after being placed in or instructed to lie in the prone position for at least 12 hours at a time for 10 days or more (ATS/ESICM/SCCM, 2017; Reilly & Christie, 2015). Proning is another oxygenation and recruitment strategy found to increase functional residual capacity (FRC), enhance regional diaphragmatic motion, enhance the distribution of perfusion, and improve the clearance of secretions. The AGACNP should ensure the patient's skin and eye safety is maintained, and all lines, tubes, and drains remain in place during the proning period (Reilly & Christie, 2015).

Fluid Management

Conservative fluid management involves a goal-directed strategy to limit lung edema in the patient with ARDS without shock. Conservative fluid management goals involve maintaining the four parameters listed in Box 7.1. Conservative fluid management protocols include the use of furosemide, fluid replacement as needed, and reassessment time frames when patients meet or exceed the recommended goals (Grissom et al., 2015). The AGACNP should recognize the challenge in maintaining the balance of needs between the lungs and the cardiovascular system. In conditions with a systemic inflammatory response (e.g., sepsis, acute severe pancreatitis,

---

BOX 7.1: CONSERVATIVE FLUID MANAGEMENT GOALS IN ACUTE RESPIRATORY DISTRESS SYNDROME WITHOUT SHOCK

MAP >60 mmHg
UO >0.5 ml/kg PBW/hr
CVP >4 to 8 mmHg
Effective circulation (CI ≥2.5)

CI, cardiac index; CVP, central venous pressure; MAP, mean arterial pressure; PBW, predicted body weight; UO, urine output.

Source: Data from Grissom, C. K., Hirshberg, E. L., Dickerson, J. B., Brown, S. M., Lanspa, M. J., Liu, K. D., Schoenfeld, D., Tidswell, M., Hite, R. D., Rock, P., Miller, R. R., Morris, A. H., & Morris, A. H. (2015). Fluid management with a simplified conservative protocol for the acute respiratory distress syndrome. Critical Care Medicine, 43(2), 288–295. https://doi.org/10.1097/CCM.0000000000000715

---

shock syndromes), intravascular volume depletion is a part of the pathogenesis and may require more aggressive fluid management strategies. The patient with ARDS can have worse outcomes with aggressive fluid management strategies. Therefore, evidence-based recommendations for patients experiencing shock syndromes and ARDS include fluid replacement with crystalloids and the use of vasopressor infusions to achieve tissue perfusion (Grissom et al., 2015).

Extracorporeal Life Support

Extracorporeal life support (ECLS) is used to provide gas exchange and systemic perfusion in patients with heart and lung failure secondary to severe illness or use during cardiopulmonary bypass surgery. The mechanism of bypassing the lungs for oxygenation to the ECLS system is thought to reduce VILI in patients diagnosed with severe ARDS. However, the benefit to survival to patients with ARDS and use of ECLS remain under investigation (Reilly & Christie, 2015).

Pharmacotherapies

There is little to no evidence available to indicate a specific pharmacotherapeutic regimen for patients diagnosed with ARDS. The reason there may be little evidence is because of the nonspecific etiologies for the disease. The pharmacotherapies studied the most included inhaled nitric oxide, glucocorticosteroids, and neuromuscular blocking (NMB) agents and did not demonstrate improvement in short-term or long-term mortality (Thompson et al., 2017).

Inhaled Nitric Oxide

Inhaled nitric oxide selectively vasodilates pulmonary capillaries and arterioles and can improve oxygenation and long-term lung function in the patient diagnosed with ARDS. However, use of the gas does not reduce mortality rates and is associated with increased acute kidney injury (Reilly & Christie, 2015; Thompson et al., 2017).

Glucocorticosteroids

Although ARDS is a severe inflammatory lung disease causing acute hypoxemic respiratory failure, glucocorticosteroids have demonstrated varying survival benefits. These drugs are also associated with worsened outcomes if started after 14 days of the onset of ARDS. The short-term benefits of glucocorticosteroids in demonstrating improved oxygenation and airway pressures in patients with pneumonia did not demonstrate improved survival (Thompson et al., 2017). The benefit of early glucocorticosteroid use in early or mild ARDS, or to prevent nosocomial ARDS in the critically ill, is still under investigation (Thompson et al., 2017).

Neuromuscular Blockade

NMB agents are frequently used in patients with severe respiratory failure in an effort to improve oxygenation by minimizing ventilator dyssynchrony and oxygen demand. Prolonged use of NMB agents is associated with prolonged neuromuscular weakness among critically ill populations (Reilly & Christie, 2015). For this reason, the short-term use of NMB agents for patients with ventilator dyssynchrony secondary to severe ARDS remains under investigation (National Heart, Lung, & Blood Institute PETAL Clinical Trials Network, 2019).

TRANSITION OF CARE

The clinical course of patients diagnosed with ARDS varies in severity of illness and duration of illness. Patients diagnosed with ARDS secondary to a direct lung insult (e.g., opioid overdose, gastric aspiration, blunt trauma) can have short durations of illness, whereas patients with systemic inflammatory responses can have prolonged duration of illness, ventilator days, critical care unit stays, and recovery which may last months after the initial onset of illness. Unfortunately, patients can die at any point in the prolonged severe illness or prolonged recovery stages (Reilly & Christie, 2015).

Survivors of severe ARDS may have long-term sequelae such as a reduced quality of life or residual organ system dysfunction. The AGACNP should evaluate survivors of ARDS for impaired lung, heart, brain (including cognitive and psychosocial effects), and musculoskeletal complications to treat and/or refer appropriately for specialized care (Reilly & Christie, 2015).

KEY TAKEAWAYS

- ALI is an acute inflammatory condition of the interstitial lung tissue caused by blunt trauma, lung infection, or severe inflammation of nearby organs or systemic inflammatory syndrome.
- ALI is also known as NCPE that can be focal or diffuse.
- ARDS is a more severe type of ALI that is characterized by refractory hypoxemia and bilateral lung involvement.
- Alveolar recruitment strategies improve diffusion capacity and oxygenation.
- There is no specific pharmacotherapeutic regimen recommended to treat ARDS or ALI.

EVIDENCE-BASED RESOURCES

National Heart, Lung, and Blood Institute ARDS Network. (2008). *NIH NHLBI ARDS clinical network mechanical ventilation protocol summary*. http://www .ardsnet.org/files/ventilator_protocol_2008-07.pdf
Pfortmueller, C. A., Spinetti, T., Urman, R. D., Luedi, M. M., & Schefold, J. C. (2020). COVID-19-associated acute respiratory distress syndrome (CARDS): Current knowledge on pathophysiology and ICU treatment – a narrative review. *Best Practice & Research Clinical Anesthesiology, 35*(3), 351–368. https://doi.org/10.1016/j .bpa.2020.12.011

7.2: ACUTE PULMONARY EDEMA

Leanne H. Fowler

Pulmonary edema is the movement of intravascular fluid into the interstitial and alveolar spaces of the lung. Acute pulmonary edema can occur secondary to multiple acute etiologies including cardiac pathologies such as left ventricular heart failure or valvular dysfunction; acute inflammatory responses from lung infection; chemical (e.g., inhalation injury, aspiration) or mechanical traumatic lung injury; or systemic inflammatory diseases (McCance et al., 2019); experiencing high altitudes for long periods of time (Zafren et al., 2021); or a postictal phase after convulsive seizures (Seyal et al., 2013). The underlying pathophysiology of all pulmonary edema results from a combination of multiple mechanisms such as altered capillary permeability, increased capillary pressure, decreased capillary oncotic pressures, increased negative interstitial pressure, or lympatic insufficiency (Woods & Mazor, 2020). Acute pulmonary edema can be categorized as cardiogenic (increased capillary pressure and permeability) or noncardiogenic (decreased capillary oncotic pressures, impaired capillary permeability, and increased negative interstitial pressure). This chapter describes acute pulmonary edema as acute cardiogenic pulmonary edema (ACPE) or noncardiogenic pulmonary edema (NCPE).

PRESENTING SIGNS AND SYMPTOMS

Patient presentations of acute pulmonary edema are similar whether it is cardiogenic or noncardiogenic. Patients often complain of sudden onset or progressively worsening dyspnea at rest or worsening with exertion. Acute dyspnea is a hallmark symptom that can be accompanied by orthopnea, nonproductive cough that can progress to frothy pink sputum production, diaphoresis, wheezing (often called cardiac asthma), or cyanotic discoloration of their fingers, toes, or lips.

HISTORY AND PHYSICAL FINDINGS

The history and physical examination of the patient with acute pulmonary edema is critical to develop appropriate and timely differential diagnoses. It is important for the AGACNP to focus questions and the physical examination to systems that will allow timely differentiation of the etiologies of acute pulmonary edema.

History

Patients should be asked about the sequence of symptoms and associated events causing symptoms to improve or worsen. For instance, the patient with ACPE can have precipitating symptoms of heart failure such as bilateral lower extremity dependent edema, right upper quadrant pain, chest pain, dyspnea on exertion, orthopnea, and PND. Patients with acute NCPE may describe symptoms of a preceding infectious or systemic inflammatory illness or having experienced blunt trauma, recent mountain climbing (achieving altitudes greater than 2,500 meters/8,200 feet), or convulsive seizures. The AGACNP should be sure to ask questions related to the multiple etiologies of acute pulmonary edema.

The patient's past medical history, family history, surgical history, and home medications are all important data to obtain that can inform the AGACNP of the patient's risk for acute pulmonary edema. For instance, if the patient has a history of hypertension that is managed with a home regimen of antihypertensive medications, medication adherence should be explored. A patient with a medical history of an autoimmune disease predisposes the patient to severe infectious illness and vulnerability to severe pneumonia and lung injury. Occupational hazards from chemicals or gases within the environment can predispose patients to inhalation injuries. A history of cardiothoracic surgeries can increase a patient's risk for direct lung injury, systemic inflammatory conditions postoperatively, or cardiac valve dysfunction that could result in acute pulmonary edema.

Physical Examination Findings

A patient's general appearance during the presentation of acute pulmonary edema is associated with acute respiratory distress, labored and tachypenic respirations, and some degree of anxiety. Patients may be hypertensive or hypotensive and are often hypoxic during severe distress. Febrile patients should be examined for sources of infection, systemic inflammation, or neurogenic conditions that can cause or be complicated by acute pulmonary edema. The lung exam will reveal bilateral pulmonary rales and/or decreased breath sounds. In NCPE, lung sounds are often associated with diffuse pulmonary rales during auscultation, whereas ACPE is more often bibasilar or within dependent areas of the lung fields. Examination of the cardiac system can reveal jugular vein distention, a positive hepatojugular reflex, or an S3 or S4 gallop that is especially associated with ACPE. Another finding associated with ACPE is dependent peripheral edema and ascites. Pink frothy sputum in patients with high-altitude pulmonary edema (HAPE) should be considered an ominous sign and is often associated with altered mental status and significant respiratory distress (Zafren et al., 2021)

DIFFERENTIAL DIAGNOSIS AND DIAGNOSTIC CONSIDERATIONS

The differential diagnoses associated with acute pulmonary edema are consistent with the varying etiologies for the condition. The AGACNP should consider metabolic, inflammatory, infectious, or toxic etiologies (Table 7.3).

Diagnostic Tests

It can be difficult to differentiate ACPE from NCPE from the history and physical examination alone. Diagnostic tests should be ordered to confirm or exclude the

TABLE 7.3: Differential Diagnoses for Acute Pulmonary Edema

ACUTE PULMONARY EDEMA TYPE	DIFFERENTIAL DIAGNOSIS
Cardiogenic	Acute myocardial infarction Acute decompensating heart failure Acute cardiac valve dysfunction Renal insufficiency
Noncardiogenic	Aspiration pneumonitis Blunt pulmonary trauma High altitude pulmonary edema (HAPE) Inhalation injury (e.g., chemical, gas, thermal) Pneumonia Sarcoidosis Viral pneumonitis

BOX 7.2: INITIAL DIAGNOSTIC WORKUP FOR PULMONARY EDEMA

General Laboratory Evaluation
Arterial blood gases
Brain natriuretic peptide (BNP)
Complete blood count
Comprehensive metabolic panel
Serum and urine toxicology screen
Thyroid stimulating hormone (heart failure)

Imaging Study Modalities
Chest radiograph
CT (complex lung disease)
Echocardiogram (ACPE)
Point-of-care ultrasound of lung

Risk Stratification for Cardiovascular Disease
Fasting lipid profile
HgA1c
Thyroid stimulating hormone (if not already collected)

highest suspicions for acute pulmonary edema, to evaluate the patient's severity of illness, and to help guide the patient's individualized treatment plan (Box 7.2). Laboratory and imaging studies are most often used to evaluate the patient's condition upon initial presentation of illness and for follow-up evaluation. Invasive or noninvasive hemodynamic measurements can also be obtained to evaluate patients for increased intracardiac pressures associated with ACPE (Ingbar & Thiele, 2018). Invasive hemodynamic monitoring obtained from vascular access devices (e.g., central venous catheter, pulmonary artery [PA] catheter) should be carefully considered weighing the patient's risk for complications such as infection, bleeding, and pulmonary infarction.

Laboratory Tests

Arterial blood gases (ABGs)s can be used to evaluate the patents oxygenation and acid-base status. A serum brain natriuretic peptic (BNP) level can be used to evaluate the degree of severity of the patient's fluid overload status; to establish a baseline level for trending subsequent levels to when re-evaluating the patient for improvement or demise; and, when accompanied with goal-directed medical therapy for ACPE, to prevent heart failure (Yancy et al., 2017). Cardiac biomarkers, such as a troponin level, are used to evaluate the patient for myocardial infarction. Metabolic panels help to evaluate the patient's organ function and for electrolyte imbalances, and to guide diuresis in the patient with fluid overload. Toxicology panels are used to evaluate the patient for drugs that can lead to the etiologies (e.g., acute myocardial infarction, seizures, aspiration) of acute pulmonary edema. A complete blood count (CBC) can be used to evaluate the patient for anemia, infection, or other inflammatory illnesses that may be contributing to the patient's illness, or trend the progress of the patient's illness. Patient presentations lending concern for acute decompensated heart failure-related pulmonary edema should have a thyroid stimulating hormone (TSH) level drawn during the initial evaluation of the patient. With consideration to the prevalence of hypertension and cardiovascular disease in the United States, it may be beneficial to order studies facilitating the patient's risk stratification of cardiovascular disease such as a lipid panel, TSH, and HgA1c (Yesodhara & Afari, 2021).

Imaging Studies

There are a few different imaging modalities to consider for the initial evaluation of the patient with pulmonary edema. Practitioners must evaluate the patient's severity of illness and medical history in order to determine the most appropriate first-line imaging modality. Point-of-care ultrasound (POCUS) applications can be useful for almost all patients for the rapid bedside evaluation of a patient with pulmonary edema. However, the AGACNP should determine whether the patient should have a chest radiograph or CT imaging of the chest before ordering the study. Chest radiographs are most commonly used to evaluate patients with or suspected to have cardiogenic or NCPE. However, for patients with a known complex medical history (e.g., persistent pneumonia, multifocal lung consolidations found during the physical examination, known lung masses, acute respiratory distress with hemoptysis), or severe thoracic trauma, initial chest imaging with CT imaging may be more useful to the timely diagnosis and management of the patient (Smith & Farrell, 2019). Patients suspected to have ACPE can also benefit from an echocardiogram to distinguish valvular dysfunction from myocardial dysfunction, and a 12-lead EKG to evaluate patients for ischemic, arrhythmic, or other cardiac causes of pulmonary edema (Yesodhara & Afari, 2021).

Point-of-Care Ultrasound

There are sonographic patterns used to differentiate ACPE from NCPE (Table 7.4). Water in the lung produces a sonographic image with "B-lines" similar to the "Kerley B-lines" visualized with a chest radiograph. The AGACNP can use POCUS lung applications to identify the patterns of B-lines at the bedside during the patient's initial evaluation. The patterns differentiating NCPE from ACPE are related to the amount of water in the lung, the distribution of water in the lung, the presence of lung sliding at the pleural line, and the presence of pleural effusions (Brown et al., 2015).

Echocardiography

A diagnostic echocardiogram (performed by a sonographer) is useful in noninvasively measuring intracardiac pressures and visualizing the function of cardiac valves and the myocardium. This imaging modality helps the AGACNP to differentiate ACPE from NCPE (Smith & Farrell, 2019). An echocardiogram cannot evaluate for a primary lung injury as the insult responsible for ARDS, but it can inform the practitioner if poor cardiac function is contributing to the severity of the patient's illness.

Chest Radiograph

There are radiographic patterns used to differentiate ACPE from NCPE (Table 7.5). Radiographic patterns of pulmonary edema depend on the amount of fluid in the lung (or severity of illness) and the distribution of the fluid from the pulmonary vasculature (early phase of illness) out to the peripheral interstitial lung tissue (described as Kerley B-lines), alveoli, and increased accumulation in the pleural spaces (late phase of illness). Cardiogenic causes of acute pulmonary edema are described as bilateral and symmetric findings that start with the cephalad redistribution of perihilar vasculature engorgement that develops into peribronchial cuffing,

TABLE 7.4: Point-of-Care Ultrasound Characteristics of Pulmonary Edema

PULMONARY EDEMA TYPE	POINT-OF-CARE ULTRASOUND FINDING
Noncardiogenic	Diffuse, nonhomogeneous distribution of B-lines Increased frequency of B-lines, 3 mm apart (alveolar edema) Reduced lung sliding May or may not have a pleural effusion presence
Cardiogenic	Diffuse, homogeneous distribution of B-lines Variable frequency of B-lines, depends on severity of edema Present lung sliding Often associated with pleural effusion presence

Source: Data from Brown, S. M., Blaivas, M., Hirshberg, E. L., Kasal, J., & Pustavoitau, A. (2015). *Comprehensive critical care ultrasound*. The Society of Critical Care Medicine.

TABLE 7.5: Chest Radiograph Characteristics of Pulmonary Edema

PULMONARY EDEMA TYPE	CHEST RADIOGRAPH FINDING
Noncardiogenic	Focal or diffuse, asymmetric, and patchy airspace disease May resolve over weeks
Cardiogenic	Early stages of pulmonary edema • Perihilar vascular congestion • Peribronchial cuffing Later stages of pulmonary edema • Batwing or diffuse, gravitational interstitial edema • Airspace disease (alveolar edema) • Bilateral pleural effusions Widened vascular pedicle; may resolve over days

Source: Data from Smith, W. L., & Farrell, T. A. (2019). *Radiology 101: The basics and fundamentals of imaging* (5th ed.). Wolters Kluwer Health.

and then progress to bilateral gravitational (dependent) peripheral interstitial edema. The vascular pedicle width on chest radiograph can also be used to evaluate patients for intravascular volume overload secondary to left ventricular dysfunction. Serial chest radiograph images can be obtained to evaluate the improvement or progression of disease. The AGACNP can anticipate the resolution of ACPE radiographic findings to occur over a period of days (Smith & Farrell, 2019).

Noncardiogenic causes (e.g., acute respiratory distress syndrome [ARDS], inhalation injury, blunt trauma, high altitude) of acute pulmonary edema are associated with asymmetric radiographic findings that are described as patchy alveolar edema without interstitial infiltrates or perihilar vascular engorgement. The radiographic findings are either in the area of lung injury or seen as a diffuse ground glass appearance. During the serial re-evaluation of chest radiograph findings in patients with NCPE, the AGACNP can anticipate the resolution of findings to occur over a period of weeks (Smith & Farrell, 2019).

TREATMENT

The treatment of patients with acute pulmonary edema should be based on the specific etiology and supportive therapies needed for oxygenation and ventilation. Specific goal-directed therapies aimed to support cardiac function and oxygenation are prescribed for patients with ACPE and can be put in categories to reduce preload, reduce afterload, or increase contractility, whereas the treatment regimens for NCPE are more supportive and related to either the elimination or the reduction of the lung's exposure to the cause of injury.

Supportive Therapies

Supplemental oxygen should be used to maintain oxygen saturation levels above 92%. Patients who have a poor response to supplemental oxygen often need

positive pressure ventilation to facilitate the recruitment of alveoli and increase gas exchange. Noninvasive positive pressure ventilation (NIPPV) is helpful to rest the respiratory muscles and reduce the work of breathing in awake patients. Mechanical ventilation with PEEP is indicated for patients who do not improve with NIPPV, who are not awake and alert, or who have severe hypoxemia and pulmonary edema. Mechanical ventilation can be beneficial to patients by facilitating the movement of the alveolar edema into the extra-alveolar space, decreasing preload (venous return) to the heart, and by increasing lung volumes and reducing atelectasis.

Acute Cardiogenic Pulmonary Edema

The reduction of preload and afterload can be accomplished by reducing venous return arterial blood pressure, and intravascular volume management. Loop diuretics are prescribed to reduce intravascular volume by increasing diuresis for patients with preserved left ventricular ejection fraction (Yancy et al., 2017). Venodilators, nitrates, renal replacement therapy, or ultrafiltration is indicated for patients with renal insufficiency and refractory volume overload (Yancy et al., 2017).

Afterload reduction can also be accomplished with diuresis and nitrates. Additionally, in the absence of acute kidney injury, the prescription of angiotensin-converting enzyme (ACE) inhibitors reduces afterload with the reduction of blood pressure. Patients with severe illness, those experiencing cardiogenic shock, or those refractory to medical therapies may require afterload reduction through the use of mechanical circulatory devices such as an intra-aortic balloon pump or a percutaneously placed circulatory device.

Inotropic and inodilator medications are used to enhance myocardial contractility in patients with ACPE secondary to cardiogenic shock. Inotropic agents (e.g., dobutamine, digitalis) are used to increase myocardial contractile force while inodilator agents (e.g., milrinone) act to increase myocardial contractile force while increasing peripheral and pulmonary vasodilation. Inotropic agents improve ACPE by improving contractility and the forward flow of blood volume through the heart and lungs.

Noncardiogenic Pulmonary Edema

Supportive therapies with the specific aim to reduce the pulmonary insult associated with NCPE depends on the cause of the insult. For example, the patient diagnosed with sepsis may develop ARDS secondary to the circulating infectious endotoxin and systemic inflammatory response. Therefore, eliminating the source of systemic infection with IV antibiotics, cautious volume resuscitation with crystalloids or blood products, mechanical ventilation with proning, and (in the setting of refractory shock) IV hydrocortisone treat the lung injury (Rhodes et al., 2017). Another example is the patient diagnosed with HAPE should immediately descend with little exertion and can be considered for hyperbaric therapy when available. Phosphodiesterase-5 inhibitors or nifedipine can be used as PA pressure reduction agents in addition to the patient's immediate descent (Zafren et al., 2021). Other therapies in addition to the support therapies mentioned earlier should be guided by the underlying cause of the lung injury causing NCPE.

CLINICAL PEARLS

- Late findings of ACPE include pink, frothy sputum and cyanosis.
- Early finding of ACPE is progressively worsening dyspnea on exertion and a nonproductive cough.
- Pink frothy sputum in the patient with HAPE is an ominous sign and the patient should be returned to lower altitudes urgently.
- Avoid premature closure during the differential diagnosis process.
- Consider cardiac and extracardiac etiologies for each complaint to help avoid anchoring to a diagnosis.
- POCUS lung applications can enhance the physical exam with timely visualization of interstitial lung fluid at the bedside.
- Ultrasound imaging is more sensitive to visualizing lung fluid than radiographs.

KEY TAKEAWAYS

- There are different physiologic mechanisms associated with cardiogenic and NCPE.
- A prudent history and physical examination can help differentiate patients with cardiogenic from NCPE.
- HAPE can be life-threatening and is treated by returning the patient to lower altitudes.
- Radiographic patterns of patients with cardiogenic pulmonary edema can have a central or bibasilar presentation, and response is faster than NCPE.
- Left ventricular function can be supported by fluid management, afterload reduction, inotropic supportive agents, and mechanical assist devices.

7.3: ACUTE RESPIRATORY FAILURE

Donna Lynch-Smith

Acute respiratory failure is one of the most common causes for intensive care unit admissions. Seventy-five percent of patients with acute respiratory failure will require mechanical ventilation. Causes of acute respiratory failure may be of primary pulmonology pathology or secondary to nonpulmonary pathology such as cardiac, metabolic, neurologic, infection, and systemic disorders.

Respiratory failure is categorized according to pathophysiologic derangements in respiratory function. Respiratory failure can be categorized into four types: Respiratory Failure Type I, Type II, Type III, and Type IV.

RESPIRATORY FAILURE TYPE I–ACUTE HYPOXIC RESPIRATORY FAILURE

Acute hypoxic respiratory failure is the most common type of respiratory failure defined as severe arterial hypoxemia refractory to supplemental oxygen with partial pressure of arterial oxygen (PaO_2) less than 60 mmHg or arterial oxygen saturation (SaO_2) less than 90%. The physiology of this type of respiratory failure is due to alveolar flooding and intrapulmonary shunting (Levitsky, 2018).

Pathophysiologic derangements in respiratory function are:

- Low inspired oxygen partial pressure
- Alveolar hypoventilation
- Diffusion impairment
- Ventilation-perfusion mismatch
- Right to left shunt

PRESENTING SIGNS AND SYMPTOMS

Signs and symptoms of acute respiratory failure include those of the underlying disease combined with hypoxia, or low blood oxygen. Type I respiratory failures are accompanied by hypercapnia—excessive CO_2 in the bloodstream—with arterial pH less than 7.25. Signs and symptoms of Type I respiratory failure include those of the underlying disease combined with hypercapnia (Table 7.6).

TABLE 7.6: Signs and Symptoms of Hypoxia and Hypercapnia

HYPOXIA (LOW BLOOD O_2)	HYPERCAPNIA (HIGH BLOOD CO_2)
Anxiety	Asterixis
Arrhythmias	Dyspnea
Bradycardia or tachycardia	Headache
Confusion increasing to somnolence	Hypertension
Cyanosis	Impaired consciousness
Dyspnea	Papilledema
Hypocapnia (initially)	Peripheral and conjunctival hyperemia
Restlessness	Tachycardia
Tachypnea	Tachypnea
Tremor	

Source: Data from Sorge, R., & DeBlieux, P. (2020). Acute exacerbations of chronic obstructive pulmonary disease: A primer for emergency physicians. *Journal of Emergency Medicine, 59*(5), 643–659. https://doi.org/10.1016/j.jemermed.2020.07.001

HISTORY AND PHYSICAL FINDINGS

Acute onset respiratory symptoms of less than 1 week from initial insult are reported. Chest x-ray (CXR) imaging reflects bilateral opacities that are not caused by cardiac failure or fluid overload. Shunt physiology is the underlying process for acute hypoxic respiratory failure. Clinical settings for acute hypoxic respiratory failure are listed under differential diagnoses.

DIFFERENTIAL DIAGNOSIS AND DIAGNOSTIC CONSIDERATIONS

Differential Diagnoses

The differential diagnoses for respiratory failure Type I are summarized in Table 7.7.

Diagnostic Considerations

Diagnostic tests for underlying etiology should include:
- Arterial blood gases (ABGs)s including evaluation of the A-a gradient.
- CXR or CT to evaluate patients for infectious, inflammatory, or neoplastic disease. For example, severe community acquired pneumonia (CAP; bacterial or viral) can be visualized by radiographic tests. Radiographic tests can help to confirm diagnostic suspicions and can facilitate an appropriate treatment plan.
- Complete blood count (CBC) with differential to evaluate for infection/inflammatory conditions.
- Cultures including blood, sputum, and urine, SARS–CoV2 testing and serology. Serum chemistries including bicarbonate and electrolytes, inflammatory markers—lactic acid level, C-reactive protein (CRP), creatine phosphokinase, and procalcitonin.
- EKG and echocardiogram to evaluate for cardiogenic etiologies.
- Bronchoscopy may be utilized for diagnostic purposes through biopsy or cultures.
- Pulmonary function studies (PFTs) to evaluate overall lung function.

TREATMENT

Initial evaluation includes assessment of airway, breathing, and circulation. Treatment will focus on reversal of the underlying cause of respiratory failure.

Oxygenation

Supplemental oxygen or high flow nasal cannula or mask is initially utilized, moving to noninvasive mechanical ventilation, and invasive mechanical ventilation if refractory hypoxia is encountered. Goals of oxygenation include correction of hypoxemia and arterial oxygen (PaO_2) of 60 mmHg or arterial oxygen saturation greater than 90%. Administer humidified high flow nasal cannula escalating to noninvasive positive-pressure ventilation (NIPPV) such as continuous positive airway pressure (CPAP) to prevent alveolar collapse during expiration starting at 5 cmH_2O up to 15 cmH_2O, and bi-level positive airway pressure that supports both inspiration and expiration with an inspiratory pressure of 5 to 10 cmH_2O and an expiratory pressure of 5 cmH_2O. Lastly, perform invasive mechanical ventilation.

Indications for mechanical ventilation include apnea, respiratory arrest, hemodynamic instability, failure of supplemental oxygen to increase PaO_2 to 55 to 60 mmHg, and unresponsive and hemodynamically unstable patients.

Mechanical ventilation may be conventional as in volume-controlled ventilation or nonconventional as in pressure-controlled ventilation, airway pressure release ventilation (APRV) and high frequency oscillatory ventilation (HFOV). Ventilatory strategies may include partial liquid ventilation (PLV) and extracorporeal membrane oxygenation (ECMO).

Supportive Care

Nutrition is crucial with acute respiratory failure. Enteral feedings are preferred if possible. Parenteral nutrition should be utilized if unable to administer enteral feedings. Avoid overfeeding to prevent an increase in CO_2 production. Correct hypokalemia and hypophosphatemia to prevent worsening of hypoventilation. Meticulous titration of sedatives-hypnotics and opioid according to the sedation scale to prevent over sedation and prolongation of intubation. Provide stress ulcer prophylaxis with sucralfate, histamine H_2-receptor antagonists, or proton pump inhibitors and VTE prophylaxis.

TABLE 7.7: Differential Diagnoses for Type I Acute Respiratory Failure

SYSTEM	DIFFERENTIAL DIAGNOSES
Pulmonary	• Acute respiratory distress syndrome (ARDS) • Alveolar hemorrhage • Asthma • Chronic obstructive pulmonary disease (COPD) • Interstitial fibrosis • Lung injury • Pneumonia • Pneumothorax • Pulmonary edema • Pulmonary embolism • Pulmonary hypertension • Severe acute respiratory syndrome coronavirus 2 (SARS-CoV-2)
Nonpulmonary	• Blood transfusions • Gastric aspiration • Heart failure • Intravascular volume overload • Near-drowning • Pancreatitis

Source: Data from Chesnutt, A., Chesnutt, M., Prendergast, N., & Prendergast, M. (2021). Acute respiratory failure. In M. Papadakis & S. McPhee. *Current medical diagnosis & treatment* (60th ed.). McGraw-Hill.

TYPE II RESPIRATORY FAILURE–HYPERCAPNIC RESPIRATORY FAILURE

Hypercapnic respiratory failure is defined as partial carbon dioxide ($PaCO_2$) greater than 45 mmHg producing respiratory acidosis with a pH less than 7.35 and in the absence of chronic CO_2 retention. Hypercapnic respiratory failure is a result of alveolar hypoventilation resulting in the inability to effectively eliminate CO_2. Causes of hypoventilation include:

1. Impaired central nervous system (CNS) resulting in impaired ventilatory drive (due to drug overdose, brainstem injury, sleep apnea, or severe untreated hypothyroidism).
2. Impaired strength with resultant failure of neuromuscular function in the respiratory system (due to respiratory weakness secondary to fatigue, electrolyte imbalances, or decreased muscle strength) due to neuromuscular diseases such as amyotrophic lateral sclerosis (ALS), Guillain-Barré syndrome (GBS), and myasthenia gravis (MG).
3. Increased loads on the respiratory system such as resistive loads due to bronchospasm, reduced lung compliance due to atelectasis, alveolar edema, intrinsic PEEP, reduced chest wall compliance due to pleural effusion, pneumothorax, and abdominal distention increased minute ventilation due to pulmonary embolism (PE) and sepsis.

PRESENTING SIGNS AND SYMPTOMS

- Mild to moderate: Mild dyspnea, headache, sluggishness, and hypersomnolence
- Moderate to severe: Change in level of consciousness, delirium, confusion, coma, asterixis, seizures, papilledema, warm skin, and dilated superficial veins.

HISTORY AND PHYSICAL FINDINGS

Risks of hypercapnic respiratory failure include use or abuse of sedative drugs, medications such as tricyclic antidepressants, long-term steroid use, malnutrition, chest wall deformities such as kyphoscoliosis, trauma to airways, conditions such as COPD, interstitial lung disease, severe sepsis, and neuromuscular diseases.

DIFFERENTIAL DIAGNOSIS AND DIAGNOSTIC CONSIDERATIONS

Differential Diagnoses

The differential diagnoses for Type II acute respiratory failure include:

- Cardiogenic shock
- Cor pulmonale
- Cyanosis
- Diaphragmatic paralysis
- Dilated cardiomyopathy
- Emphysema
- Myocardial infarction
- Noninvasive ventilation
- Obstructive sleep apnea
- PE

Diagnostic Testing

- ABG: Acute hypercapnic respiratory failure $PaCO_2$ greater than 45 mmHg with a pH of less than 7.35. Assess the alveolar arterial (A-a) gradient. Global hypoventilation reflects a normal (A-a) gradient with hypercapnia. Lung disease reflects a wide (A-a) gradient with hypercapnia.
- CBC with differential evaluating for infections/inflammation.
- Serum chemistries to evaluate for magnesium and phosphorous deficiencies, and bicarbonate evaluating to evaluate for acid base disorders such as chronic COPD.
- Drug/toxicology screening.
- Thyroid function.

Other diagnostic tests include bronchoscopy, echocardiogram, and pulmonary function tests. Diagnostic imaging can be used to rule out pathology. For example, a CXR may identify COPD findings such as blebs, hyperinflation, and flattened diaphragm, or interstitial lung disease, pneumonia, and thoracic cage abnormalities. A CT of the thorax can be used to identify emphysematous changes or PE, while a CT of the head and spinal cord can evaluate for cerebrovascular accident, tumors, and spinal cord injuries.

TREATMENT

Treatment is aimed at reversing the underlying cause of respiratory failure.

- Supplemental oxygen is provided for patients with concomitant hypoxic respiratory failure. Assess the patient's baseline PaO_2 and $PaCO_2$. Achieve a pulse oxygen saturation of 90% to 93% or a PaO_2 of 60 to 70. In severe cases achieve a pulse oxygen saturation of equal or greater to than 88% or a PaO_2 of 55 to 60. Noninvasive mask ventilation in patients who are hemodynamically stable, and able to protect their airway. Bilevel positive airway pressure (BIPAP) supports both inspiration and expiration utilizing an inspiratory pressure of 8 to 12 cmH_2O and an expiratory pressure of 3 to 5 cmH_2O. Invasive mechanical ventilation is used for the unresponsive and hemodynamically unstable patient. Mechanical ventilation may be conventional as in volume-controlled ventilation or nonconventional as in PCV, APRV and HFOV. Ventilatory strategies may include ECMO and extracorporeal carbon dioxide removal ($ECCO_2R$).

TYPE III RESPIRATORY FAILURE–PERIOPERATIVE RESPIRATORY FAILURE

Perioperative respiratory failure is due to atelectasis from a decrease in functional residual capacity (FRC) causing dependent lung units to collapse. Causes of decreased FRC are:

1. General anesthesia
2. Surgery (chest and abdominal)
3. Obesity

PRESENTING SIGNS AND SYMPTOMS

Presenting signs and symptoms of Type III respiratory failure include dyspnea, tachypnea, and hypoxemia.

TREATMENT

Treatment includes elevation of head of bed, frequent position changes, control of incisional discomfort, chest physiotherapy, and NIPPV.

TYPE IV RESPIRATORY FAILURE– HYPOPERFUSION OF RESPIRATORY MUSCLES IN SHOCK STATES

In a normal state, respiratory muscles will consume up to 5% of cardiac output. In shock states, respiratory muscles consume up to 40% of cardiac output. Causes of hypoperfusion are cardiogenic shock, septic shock, and hypovolemic shock.

PRESENTING SIGNS AND SYMPTOMS

Signs and symptoms of Type IV respiratory failure are related to the type of shock causing hypoperfusion.

TREATMENT

Treatment for Type IV respiratory failure includes intubation and mechanical ventilation and treatment of shock states.

CLINICAL PEARLS

- High flow oxygen therapy improves the respiratory status in acute hypoxic respiratory failure without hypercapnia.
- Noninvasive ventilation is an option in the management of acute hypercapnic respiratory failure.
- Supplemental oxygen, frequent position changes, head of bed elevation along with chest physiotherapy are management options for acute respiratory failure due to perioperative atelectasis.
- Intubation and invasive mechanical ventilation are used in the management of acute respiratory failure due to hypoperfusion of respiratory patients who are in shock.

KEY TAKEAWAYS

- Respiratory failure is categorized according to pathophysiologic derangements in respiratory function. Respiratory failure can be categorized into four types: Respiratory Failure Type I, Type II, Type III, and Type IV.

7.4: AIR-LEAK SYNDROMES

Leanne H. Fowler

An air-leak syndrome involves the escape of air into a cavity that does not normally contain air. Pleural diseases resulting in pneumothorax or pneumomediastinum account for more than 35,000 hospitalizations per year in the United States affecting men more than women and adults older than 45 years more than other adult age groups (Mummadi et al., 2021; Wang et al., 2020). The air-leak syndromes discussed in this chapter include pneumothorax and pneumomediastinum and involve syndromes associated with pleural disease and acute respiratory distress.

Pneumothorax

A pneumothorax is the presence of gases that are normally exchanged by the alveoli being leaked into the pleural space from ruptured lung tissue. A pneumothorax can occur spontaneously (primary), secondary to underlying lung disease, due to barotrauma with mechanical ventilation, or because of penetrating or blunt chest trauma.

Spontaneous Pneumothorax

A spontaneous pneumothorax occurs in the absence of trauma and most often occurs due to the rupture of pleural blebs (Wang et al., 2020). A pleural bleb is a blister-like, air-filled structure within the visceral layer of the upper lobes and apices of the lung that can occur from chronic tobacco use in adults or congenitally in young and often thin adolescents or adults. The prevalence of pulmonary blebs is unknown within the general population but is known to be a significant etiological factor in the pathology of spontaneous pneumothorax (de Bakker et al., 2020).

Recent research during the severe acute respiratory syndrome (SARS) coronavirus 2019 (COVID-19) found a higher incidence of spontaneous pneumothorax than the general population (Miro et al., 2021). Other researchers have also found patients with rare but specific genetic mutations have a higher prevalence of recurrent spontaneous pneumothorax (Sattler et al., 2020).

Secondary Pneumothorax

A secondary pneumothorax occurs as a complication of acute and chronic lung disease (Wang et al., 2020). For example, patients living with emphysema can develop pneumothorax secondary to the condition of the lungs and variation in lung pressures with coughing, sneezing, or acute illness. Patients experiencing a secondary pneumothorax have higher morbidity and mortality rates (Wang et al., 2020).

Traumatic Pneumothorax

An air-leak syndrome caused by a traumatic pneumothorax can occur with blunt or penetrating trauma to the thoracic cavity. Patients can experience a combination hemopneumothorax where the therapeutic intervention would require draining of the air and the blood collecting in the pleural space. During the performance of invasive thoracic procedures (e.g., central venous catheter placement, needle thoracostomy), iatrogenic traumatic pneumothorax can occur.

Tension Pneumothorax

A tension pneumothorax is a medical emergency that most often occurs secondary to mechanical ventilation in patients with high inspiratory peak pressures or during the cardiopulmonary resuscitative efforts provided to patients. Patients experiencing a tension pneumothorax develop severe cardiovascular compromise and obstructive shock due to the increased intrapulmonary pressures upon the mediastinal space.

Pneumomediastinum

A pneumomediastinum is the leaking of pulmonary gases into the mediastinal space. The primary causes of this air-leak syndrome are related to perforation of the esophagus, trachea, or main bronchi; rupture of alveolar units with leakage directly into the mediastinal space; or rupture of air-filled structures within the neck or abdomen and leaks into the mediastinal space. This chapter focuses on the rupture of alveoli into the mediastinal space.

PRESENTING SIGNS AND SYMPTOMS

Patients who experience an air-leak syndrome of the lung can develop mild to severe respiratory distress presenting as a syndrome of signs, symptoms, or complications. The signs and symptoms associated with an air-leak syndrome occur acutely on a spectrum from a mild sharp pleuritic chest pain with or without dyspnea to severe pleuritic or midsternal chest pain and severe respiratory distress. Patients experiencing a pneumothorax most often complain of a focal, sharp pleuritic chest pain and dyspnea. Patients experiencing a pneumomediastinum most often complain of severe midsternal chest pain and dyspnea (Light, 2018a).

HISTORY AND PHYSICAL FINDINGS

A thorough history and physical examination of patients who have experienced an air-leak syndrome can be useful in assessing the patient's risk for recurrent events. The patient with no prior history of an air-leak syndrome may need further investigation to identify if there is undiagnosed lung disease or other risk factors for pneumothorax or pneumomediastinum. A thorough history and physical examination can provide the AGACNP with clues about the cause of the air-leak syndrome and potentially the patient's risk for complications or a recurrent event.

History

Patients with a medical history of chronic lung disease have the greatest risk for developing a life-threatening air-leak syndrome, especially a pneumothorax (Wang et al., 2020). Collecting a thorough history from the patient, near-by witnesses, or family can help the AGACNP understand the mechanism of injury in events causing a traumatic pneumothorax. Other data to collect during the history are the patient's exposure to tobacco smoke or other inhaled toxins, blunt or penetrating thoracic trauma, mechanical ventilation, and cardiopulmonary resuscitation. A review of home medications can inform the practitioner if anticoagulant or antiplatelet medications are taken regularly and thus place the patient at increased risk for bleeding if invasive procedures are needed. Also, a thorough family history to identify if there are relatives with recurrent spontaneous pneumothorax can help the practitioner identify the need for genetic evaluation (Sattler et al., 2020).

A postmortem study reported that a third of individuals in the general population who have no history of lung disease were found to have the presence of small pulmonary blebs (de Bakker et al., 2020). The researchers' findings suggest that a third of the general population without a history of lung disease could be at risk for pneumothorax. Therefore, the AGACNP should be aware of the general population who are at some degree of risk for spontaneous pneumothorax in the absence of underlying lung disease.

Physical Examination

The physical examination of patients with an air-leak syndrome should focus on the inspection, palpation, and auscultation of the neck, thorax, and abdomen. Tracheal shift can be present with muffled heart sounds in the patient with a tension pneumothorax but are otherwise per the patient's baseline heart sounds. Lung sounds are absent over the area of a moderate to large pneumothorax of any kind. If the patient has a pneumothorax that leaks air into the subcutaneous space, asymmetrical skin regions can be inspected, and crepitus can be palpated in the affected area. Patients in respiratory distress may be positioned in an upright or tripod position and have accessory muscle usage, intercostal muscle retractions or bulging, and cyanosis.

Pneumomediastinum

The physical examination of patients with pneumomediastinum involves palpation for subcutaneous emphysema, or crepitus, in the area of the suprasternal notch and lower neck. Another examination finding specifically associated with this problem is Hamman's sign. Hamman's sign is the crunchy noise heard over the precordium with each heartbeat (Light, 2018a).

DIFFERENTIAL DIAGNOSIS AND DIAGNOSTIC CONSIDERATIONS

The differential diagnoses associated with air-leak syndromes are listed in Box 7.3. Diagnostic considerations for the patient presenting with an air-leak syndrome focus on identifying the patient's oxygenation status with the use of bedside pulse oximetry, arterial blood gases (ABGs), and the use of lung imaging to identify the size and location of the air leak.

BOX 7.3: DIFFERENTIAL DIAGNOSES OF AIR-LEAK SYNDROMES

- Bacterial pneumonia
- Empyema
- Pleural effusion
- Pneumomediastinum
- Pneumothorax
  - o Spontaneous
  - o Secondary
  - o Traumatic
  - o Tension

Diagnostic Lung Imaging

Point-of-care ultrasound (POCUS) imaging can be performed by the AGACNP to quickly evaluate the patient suspected to have pneumothorax. The absence of lung sliding can be visualized by the practitioner during the initial physical examination (Smith & Farrell, 2019). The portable anteroposterior and lateral views for chest radiographic imaging are useful in diagnosing pneumothorax from pneumomediastinum. Radiologists or other skilled bedside practitioners can also use the chest radiograph to estimate the size of the pneumothorax in determining a management plan. CT is more sensitive to visualizing and measuring pneumothorax (Smith & Farrell, 2019).

TREATMENT

Treatment plans vary for air-leak syndromes and can depend on the severity of patient symptoms, illness, and bleeding risk. Patients who develop secondary pneumothoraces often develop more life-threatening conditions requiring hospitalization and urgent-to-emergent intervention when compared to those without a medical history of chronic lung disease (Wang et al., 2020). Patients diagnosed with a tension pneumothorax require emergent intervention to prevent death. Routine care includes telemetry to intensive care unit level of care, supplemental oxygen, and decompression of the lung with tube thoracostomy. Supportive therapies to treat acute pain and anxiety may also be needed for patients being cared for with an air-leak syndrome.

Patients diagnosed with a pneumomediastinum do not commonly require surgical intervention. High concentrations of inspired supplemental oxygen, analgesia as needed for pain, and watchful waiting is the standard treatment course. Needle aspiration is reserved for patients who present with compression of the heart and/or great vessels.

Tube Thoracostomy

A small pneumothorax is likely to heal without intervention and follow-up management can be provided outpatient in patients who are asymptomatic and without significant risk for decline. Indications for tube thoracostomy insertion (also known as chest tube placement)

include moderate to large pneumothorax in patients who are symptomatic, clinically unstable, mechanically ventilated, and/or have underlying lung disease (e.g., pneumothorax, mechanical ventilation, hemodynamic instability, chest trauma, status post needle decompression for tension pneumothorax) that places them at risk for further decline (Dev et al., 2007). Patients with a history of antiplatelet therapy use are at risk for postprocedure bleeding complications such as hemothorax, hematoma, or other serious hemorrhage (Dangers et al., 2020).

Complications

Serious complications can occur secondary to thoracostomy tube placement such as tube blockage, pleural space infections, bleeding, tension pneumothorax, and right ventricle decompression leading to subsequent cardiogenic shock. The AGACNP should have a plan for the rapid management of all possible complications a patient can experience after chest tube placement.

Needle Decompression

Needle decompression is performed for patients with a tension pneumothorax or persistent pneumomediastinum in the presence of cardiovascular tamponade (Light, 2018a, 2018b). For patients with a tension pneumothorax, the procedure is performed emergently after the clinical diagnosis is made without the use of radiographic chest imaging in most cases (Light, 2018b).

Recurrent Pneumothorax Prophylaxis

Patients with the greatest risk for recurrent secondary pneumothorax are those with underlying lung disease and a limited cardiopulmonary reserve. Patients with spontaneous pneumothorax and known pulmonary blebs are at risk for recurrence as well. Therefore, after the first occurrence, chest-tube placement guidelines recommend that prophylactic measures are taken to prevent recurrence during the same hospitalization as the first occurrence (Wang et al., 2020). Prophylactic strategies include pleurodesis or blebectomy that can be performed with or without video-assisted thorascopic surgery (VATS). Prophylactic procedures with VATS are preferred due to improved outcomes and a lower occurrence of complications (Wang et al., 2020).

CLINICAL PEARLS

- Air-leak syndromes can be caused by air leaking from the lung or GI tract.
- Performing a thorough history and physical exam should focus on narrowing down the cause of the air-leak syndrome.
- A tension pneumothorax is diagnosed clinically with the patient's presentation, limited history, and examination.
- Rapid recognition and intervention of a tension pneumothorax improves morbidity and mortality rates.

KEY TAKEAWAYS

- Air leak syndromes can occur from air leaking from the lung or GI tract.
- Air leak syndromes can occur spontaneously.
- Spontaneous pneumothoraces are often associated with a history of pulmonary blebs.
- A tension pneumothorax is a medical emergency.
- A tension pneumothorax is diagnosed clinically and often managed without chest radiography.
- A pneumomediastinum is most often managed with supplemental oxygen.
- A tube thoracotomy is reserved for moderate to large pneumothoraces in symptomatic patients.

7.5: ASTHMA

Leanne H. Fowler

Asthma is a chronic inflammatory disease of the airways effecting millions of Americans yearly and is one of the most common chronic childhood illnesses. After puberty, persons who identify as female are affected more than those identifying as male across all socioeconomic categories and race/ethnicities (Centers for Disease Control and Prevention [CDC], 2021). The chronic disease is characterized by recurring symptoms, bronchial hyperresponsiveness, airflow obstruction, and underlying inflammatory response (National Heart, Lung, and Blood Institute [NHLBI], 2007). Therefore, patients can have varying presentations of asthma on a spectrum from controlled disease to severe, persistent disease or status asthmaticus. Status asthmaticus occurs infrequently but can be life-threatening. Persons affected with uncontrolled asthma can have decreased quality of life without adequate chronic management of the disease.

There are several etiological factors involved in the chronic disease of asthma such as genetic predisposition, allergens (e.g., dust mites, pet dander), and environmental exposures. Patients with a history of atopy (a predisposition to allergy), are associated with a genetic predisposition for the development of asthma. Additionally, viral respiratory infections are also associated with the development of chronic asthmatic disease or acute exacerbations of known asthmatic disease (NHLBI, 2007).

The pathology of asthma involves the infiltration of bronchial tissue with inflammatory cells (e.g., neutrophils, eosinophils, lymphocytes, mast cells) and inflammatory mediators (e.g., chemokines, cytokines, nitric oxide, immunoglobulin E) that cause epithelial injury and subsequent bronchial spasm and mucus secretion. Consequently, airflow obstruction occurs and, in some patients, structural changes of the airways occur, causing the progressive loss of lung function (NHLBI, 2007). The scope of this section focuses on the evaluation and management of persons 13 years and older with acute and complex chronic asthma.

PRESENTING SIGNS AND SYMPTOMS

Uncontrolled or acute exacerbations of asthma symptoms are characterized by progressive or persistent wheezing, a nonproductive cough (initially), and dyspnea. Acute severe asthma presentations can also include chest tightness, hypoxemia, and respiratory failure refractory to inhaled bronchodilator therapy (status asthmaticus). Patients may endorse symptoms that are worse at night and may be awakened with symptoms in the early morning hours. Prior to the development of an acute asthma exacerbation (also known as an asthma attack), patients can report the sensation of itching skin, difficulty taking a deep breath, and anxiety. If symptoms are not reversed with therapy, patients report the initial nonproductive cough progressing to a productive cough of thick, clear to pale yellow sputum. Patients presenting with an acute asthma exacerbation secondary to a respiratory infection may have fever, chills, myalgias, arthralgias, signs of an upper or lower respiratory illness, increased cough or dyspnea above their baseline, and purulent sputum production (Ray et al., 2016).

Patients with chronic asthma are most associated with chronic allergies and recurrent exacerbations related to worsening seasonal allergies or infections. Patients can present with the symptoms of chronic rhinitis, rhinosinusitis, or chronic skin allergies that worsen with exposure to cold temperature, pets, or other triggers.

HISTORY AND PHYSICAL FINDINGS

Patient History

When collecting a history, it is important to assess the patient's severity and control of symptoms. Inquiring about the patient's baseline of symptoms with adherence to chronic management therapies can inform the AGACNP's future management plan. Patients experiencing status asthmaticus or other forms of uncontrolled severe asthma are most often those who were not adherent or not well-controlled by their treatment plans (Dharmage et al., 2020). Furthermore, patients with poor social determinants of health are at the greatest risk for recurrent severe exacerbations and episodes of status asthmaticus. The patient with a personal medical history and a first-generation family history of atopy, rhinitis, and chronic rhinosinusitis are prone to also have asthma. Patients with a history of gastroesophageal reflux disease (GERD) can also present with symptoms of asthma that can be caused by silent GERD. Therefore, patients with a history of obesity and/or high caffeine or other stimulant intake should be considered as having lifestyle or comorbidity factors contributing to a reactive airway disease like asthma. Adults presenting with an acute asthma exacerbation should be assessed for a history of chronic asthma that was not previously diagnosed or for the new development of disease during adulthood (Barnes, 2018).

Asthma can be triggered by environmental and behavioral lifestyle factors. Therefore, it is important to ask patients about their exposure to tobacco, pet dander, and other inhaled allergens or toxins in the home and/or within work environments. A thorough environmental history will also include asking patients about how much carpet, window curtains, or other materials are in the home that dust, pet dander, mold, or other triggers can accumulate (Dharmage et al., 2020; NHLBI, 2007).

Behavioral or lifestyle factors known to trigger asthma are most often associated with the inhalation of smoke or chemicals. Patients reporting a personal history of smoking should be evaluated for the amount of tobacco use and their readiness to quit. Patients who do not have a personal smoking history should be asked if anyone in the home smokes where the patient would have second-hand exposure. An occupational or other household history focused on the use of or exposure to chemicals can be helpful in identifying if the patient had an allergic or reactive episode of asthma. Other lifestyle factors to ask about include if cold air or exercise triggers wheezing in the patient (Dharmage et al., 2020; NHLBI, 2007).

Physical Examination Findings

The general appearance, upper respiratory tract, neck, skin, thorax, and lungs are the primary focus of the physical examination of a patient with asthma. Patients with acute asthma may have an uncomfortable and distressed general appearance, whereas the patient with chronic asthma may have an expected general appearance for a person who is generally healthy and without acute illness. Because the cells and mucosa of the upper respiratory tract are very similar to those of the lower respiratory tract, signs of allergy, inflammation, or infection should be evaluated. Inspecting the neck and thorax for rash or labored respirations is useful in evaluating the patient's severity of illness or signs of atopy or other exanthems (Barnes, 2018; NHLBI, 2007).

Lung sounds in the patient with acute asthma can include wheezes and rhonchi. Patients may also demonstrate a prolonged phase of forced exhalation (because of the obstructive nature of the disease). Focal wheezing may be associated with peribronchial mass or a focal pneumonia, whereas a patient with left ventricular failure may have bibasilar rales and wheezes. In a patient with controlled chronic asthma, lung sounds are without adventitious sounds.

DIFFERENTIAL DIAGNOSIS AND DIAGNOSTIC CONSIDERATIONS

Common differential diagnoses the AGACNP should consider for adult patients with asthma include upper or lower respiratory infection, bronchial mass (benign or malignant), toxic inhalation, acute heart failure, or GERD. When evaluating the patient with acute or chronic asthma, diagnostic tests should be ordered with the most likely cause first.

Diagnostic Tests

Evaluation of Acute Asthma

Patients with chronic asthma can identify an emerging asthma exacerbation if daily peak flow monitoring is performed with the chronic management plan. Peak flow measurements are not diagnostic but can be used to assess if the patient's asthma control is declining.

A two-view chest radiograph is the most common diagnostic test ordered for patients with acute asthma. Although the radiograph is often unrevealing and results in no acute cardiac or pulmonary disease processes appreciated, they should be obtained to exclude more severe lung illness. The chest radiograph should be ordered to evaluate patients for findings of pneumonia or if a bronchial mass is present to help practitioners differentiate etiological or contributing factors to the patient's asthma presentation. Patients with chronic asthma may have hyperexpanded lungs visualized by radiograph. CT imaging of the chest is not commonly indicated for patients with asthma unless a mass or nodule is suspected or found on plain film radiograph. CT imaging may also be indicated if the patient has a complex and/or atypical presentation of pneumonia.

Patients with signs of systemic or severe illness should be evaluated with a complete blood count and chemistry panel to evaluate for infectious, inflammatory processes or eosinophilia. However, patients with acute asthma exacerbations are not frequently evaluated with serum laboratory tests. The physical examination and lung imaging are usually all that are needed in the episodic evaluation of acute asthma.

Status Asthmaticus

Patients suspected to have status asthmaticus and impending respiratory failure should have their airway secured and ventilation stabilized. When stabilized, these patients' arterial blood gases (ABGs) should also be evaluated in addition to the other diagnostic tests mentioned earlier. The patient's age and comorbidities should be considered during the risk stratification for their decline and need for evaluation for other diagnostic tests (e.g., CT for altered mental status, lactic acid level for sepsis).

Diagnosing Asthma

The approach to the diagnosis of asthma includes (a) identifying the trigger; (b) identifying comorbid conditions that contribute to asthma episodes and/or disease; and (c) assessing disease severity of symptoms and quality of life impairment (Box 7.4).

Spirometry

A definitive diagnosis of asthma can be obtained by lung spirometry during nonacute phases of asthma. Pulmonary

BOX 7.4: SYMPTOM ASSESSMENT OF ASTHMA SEVERITY

- Ability to engage in normal activities of daily living or desired activities
- Missed work or school days
- Need for short-acting beta agonist (SABA)
- Night-time awakening
- Quality of life

function tests (discussed in a later section of the chapter) are used to diagnose chronic asthma when reversibility of airflow obstruction is measured after an inhaled short-acting beta agonist (SABA) is administered during testing. Alveolar gas diffusion is usually normal. Other factors used to establish a diagnosis with asthma include a history of repeated episodes of airflow obstruction symptoms or airway hyperresponsiveness; if present, other alternative diagnoses can be excluded (Barnes, 2018; NHLBI, 2007).

Patients with an allergic etiology of asthma can be evaluated with skin testing to identify the trigger(s) associated with the disease. Skin testing results help the patient and practitioner control exposure to triggers when possible. However, skin testing is not specific or sensitive for diagnosing asthma.

Other tests that can be helpful during the diagnosis of asthma are serum immunoglobulin E (radioallergosorbent testing [RAST]) levels (total levels and those specific to inhaled allergens) and fractional exhaled nitric oxide (FeNO). The RAST tests are not specific to asthmatic disease but can also help in identifying triggers in an effort to control the patient's exposure to them. The FeNO testing is ordered to evaluate the patient for eosinophilic airway inflammation as a contributing factor to the pathology of the patient's asthmatic disease and is more useful in diagnosing asthma than it is for chronic obstructive pulmonary disease (COPD; Miskoff et al., 2019).

TREATMENT

The general approach to treating patients with asthma includes (a) reducing environmental triggers; (b) reducing comorbidities associated with exacerbating asthma (e.g., rhinitis, rhinosinusitis, GERD); and (c) classifying asthma by disease severity, impairment, and risk for poor outcomes. Patients with asthma require a multifaceted approach to improve quality of life and reduce impairment. Treatment regimens are guided by symptom control (NHLBI, 2007, 2020).

Behavioral or Lifestyle Management

Reducing environmental triggers for asthma is first-line treatment and should be emphasized throughout all phases of care. In-home pets should be avoided when possible—especially sleeping in the same bed as the person with asthma. Other interventions include reducing the amount of carpet, curtains, or other fabrics in the home that contribute to accumulated dust and other allergens. Additionally, the use of dust-mite covers on mattresses and pillows are recommended to reduce nighttime allergy triggers. Smoking cessation or tobacco smoke avoidance is highly recommended to reduce episodes of asthma exacerbations in adolescents and adults.

Pharmacotherapy

Drug classes for asthma management can be categorized into bronchodilators and inflammation controllers (Table 7.8). Bronchodilators (beta agonists are the most effective) increase airflow by relaxing the smooth muscle of the bronchi and increasing the diameter of the airway. Inflammation controllers treat asthma by inhibiting inflammatory processes responsible for tissue swelling and mucus secretion. Selecting pharmacotherapies used to treat asthma involves a stepwise approach (Table 7.9) focused on symptom control for patients 12 years and older.

TABLE 7.8: Pharmacotherapies for Asthma

CATEGORY	DRUGS

Bronchodilators	Beta agonists
	    Albuterol (SABA)
	    Terbutaline (SABA)
	    Salmeterol (LABA)
	    Formoterol (LABA)
	Anticholinergics (muscarinic receptor antagonist)
	    Ipratropium bromide (SAMA)
	    Tiotropium bromide (LAMA)
	Theophylline

Inflammation Controllers	Inhaled corticosteroids (ICS)
	Systemic corticosteroids
	    Hydrocortisone
	    Methylprednisolone
	Antileukotrienes
	Cromones (used more in childhood asthma)
	Immunomodulators
	    Azathioprine
	    Cyclosporine A
	    Methotrexate
	    Gold
	    IV gamma globulin
	Anti-IgE
	    Omalizumab
	Anti-interleukin-5
	Immunotherapy

LAMA, long-acting muscarinic antagonist; SAMA, short-acting muscarinic antagonist.

Source: Data from Cloutier, M. M., Dixon, A. E., Krishnan, J. A., Lemanske, R. F., Pace, W., & Schatz, M. (2020). Managing asthma in adolescents and adults. 2020 asthma guideline update from the National Asthma Education and Prevention Program. Journal of the American Medical Association, 324(22), 2301–2317. https://doi.org/10.1001/jama.2020.21974

TABLE 7.9: Stepwise Approach to Asthma Management

STEP	MILD INTERMITTENT	MILD PERSISTENT	MODERATE PERSISTENT	SEVERE PERSISTENT	VERY SEVERE PERSISTENT
1	SABA PRN symptom relief				
2		Low-dose ICS		High-dose ICS	
3			LABA		
4				LABA	
5					Oral steroid

ICS, inhaled corticosteroid; LABA, long-acting beta agonist; PRN, as needed; SABA, short-acting beta agonist.

Source: Adapted from https://www.nhlbi.nih.gov/sites/default/files/publications/AsthmaCliniciansGuideDesign-508.pdf

Bronchodilators

Bronchodilators have subcategories of short-acting and long-acting agents and are the most effective type of drug in this category. SABAs are most useful for rapid onset symptom relief and have a duration of action between 3 and 6 hours. Patients can also use SABAs just before physical exertion to prevent exercise-induced asthma. Long-acting beta agonists (LABAs) have the same mechanism of action with a slower onset but longer duration of action. The longer duration of action aids patients in medication adherence and prevents mid-day disruptions in routine life activities. All patients with a diagnosis of asthma should at least have a SABA prescribed as needed. All patients should be educated about the purpose of bronchodilators. Patient should understand SABAs should remain on-hand for urgent or emergent symptom relief, and to notify their primary care provider when they are needed more than twice weekly (suggesting poor control of asthma).

Anticholinergic agents are also known as antimuscarinic antagonists and act to bronchodilate and reduce secretions within the airways. These drugs are often used in combination with beta agonists to synergize the effects of bronchodilation. Theophylline is used the least in adults requiring asthma management because of its side-effect profile and adults' predisposition to comorbid heart and lung disease.

Inflammation Controllers

Drugs used to control the inflammatory processes of asthma aim to reduce the hyperactive response to triggers and to improve the quality of life of patients with mild to severe persistent disease. Patients with mild to moderate asthmatic disease are most often treated with low-dose inhaled corticosteroids (ICS) with or without an oral antileukotriene for control of symptoms. Antileukotrienes (e.g., montelukast or zafirlukast) act to prevent eosinophilic inflammation of the airways but to a lesser degree than ICS. Patients with persistent severe disease can be treated with short tapers of oral corticosteroids to gain control of acute exacerbations. Immunologic therapies (e.g., anti-interleukin-5 and anti-immunoglobulin-E

agents, methotrexate, cyclosporine A, azathioprine) can also be prescribed for patients with severe to very severe persistent disease. Immunologic therapies benefit patients by reducing the need for ICS or short steroid tapers for asthma control. However, the side effect profile is greater than that of recommended steroid use.

ASTHMA OVERLAPPING WITH CHRONIC OBSTRUCTIVE PULMONARY DISEASE

Patients diagnosed with chronic asthma can develop overlapping COPD and vice versa. There are more patients with asthma that also have features of COPD than the other way around. It is also true that both conditions can occur concurrently. As mentioned, the FeNO is specific to differentiating asthma from COPD and is useful in planning the patient's management plan (Miskoff et al., 2019).

7.6: CHRONIC LUNG DISEASE

Latanja L. Divens

Chronic lung diseases (CLDs) are common disorders that impact the global population. There are numerous conditions that are included in CLD, which often result in disability, mortality, and increased healthcare costs. The most common CLD is chronic obstructive pulmonary disease (COPD) which includes chronic bronchitis (CB) and emphysema. These conditions often have similar presenting features such as dyspnea and coughing. It is necessary for providers to possess a firm comprehension of the CLDs to assist in diagnosing, treating, managing, and educating patients and families about these conditions. In addition, providers must be educated in evidence-based practice guidelines to support the care that is provided.

CHRONIC OBSTRUCTIVE PULMONARY DISEASE

COPD is the fourth leading cause of death in the United States and affects approximately 32 million individuals in the United States. COPD is a term used to describe two related diseases: CB and emphysema (Global Initiative for Chronic Obstructive Lung Disease [GOLD], 2020). COPD is defined as an obstructive, partially reversible condition of the lungs that affects the airways and alveoli. It is characterized by limited airflow, obstruction, and persistent, prolonged respiratory symptoms such as dyspnea, cough, and fatigue. The condition is often triggered by tobacco use or environmental stimuli such as poor air quality, occupational exposure, and bronchitis (Rakel & Rakel, 2016).

Pathophysiology

Pathologic changes occur in both the central and peripheral bronchioles, and the lung parenchyma. This often results secondary to noxious stimuli, with the most common insulting agent being tobacco products. Pathologic changes in the airways result in an augmented response in individuals at risk for COPD development. These pathogenic mechanisms cannot be stabilized effectively by antiproteases, resulting in destruction of the lung (Goroll & Mulley, 2014).

PRESENTING SIGNS AND SYMPTOMS

Presenting signs and symptoms of COPD include dyspnea, chronic cough, chronic sputum production, and recurrent lower respiratory tract infections. Dyspnea is characterized by feelings of breathlessness, increased work of breathing, and chest tightness. Dyspnea is often a common presenting symptom and individuals often report feelings of suffocation and air hunger. Coughs are considered chronic when lasting for 3 or more months; coughs may be productive or nonproductive and may result in wheezing. Chronic sputum production results from irritation of the airways. Sputum is typically clear but may change to yellow or green if an infection is present. Recurrent lower respiratory tract infections develop due to an inability to release secretions trapped in the lower airways; COPD often leads to pneumonia. Females with COPD often present with sputum production and a chronic productive cough, whereas males present with dyspnea and wheezing (Han et al., 2021).

HISTORY AND PHYSICAL FINDINGS

The history should include a detailed evaluation of risk factors and characteristics of dyspnea. Any history of recurrent or prolonged respiratory infections that required treatment with an antibiotic should be investigated. A childhood history of recurrent bronchitis, respiratory tract infections, recurrent sinus infections, nasal polyps, or history of asthma should be explored. The family history must also be considered including allergies, tuberculosis, cystic fibrosis, and COPD. An occupational history including exposure to noxious inhalants or fumes must be obtained (GOLD, 2020).

Most patients with COPD present with worsening symptoms because they have acclimated to living with common symptoms. The most common presenting symptoms are dyspnea, chronic cough, and progressive exercise intolerance. The physical exam of individuals with mild to moderate symptoms may not provide significant information. In more severe cases, the physical exam often reveals tachypnea and respiratory distress. The respiratory rate normally increases in proportion to the severity of the disease. Individuals may use accessory respiratory muscles and demonstrate paradoxical breathing (Hoover's sign). Findings from the thoracic exam include hyperinflation (barrel chest), purse-lip breathing, wheezing, prolonged expiration, hyperresonance with percussion, and diffusely decreased breath sounds. Additionally, auscultation may demonstrate course crackles on inspiration (Rakel & Rakel, 2016).

DIFFERENTIAL DIAGNOSIS AND DIAGNOSTIC CONSIDERATIONS

It is important to distinguish COPD from other causes of chronic cough or dyspnea and is necessary for initial diagnosis. Chronic cough may be a side effect of certain medications, allergy-based conditions, and many common conditions including chronic rhinitis, mitral stenosis, and GERD (GOLD, 2020).

Differential diagnoses may be related to signs of a chronic cough or dyspnea (Table 7.10).

Diagnostics

A clinical diagnosis of COPD should be considered in all individuals with dyspnea, a chronic cough, sputum production, and a history of exposure to risk factors including tobacco use and occupational and environmental exposures. The gold standard for diagnosis and assessment for COPD is spirometry testing. Although spirometry is the most sensitive method of diagnosis, it should not be the only method for diagnosis because of its low specificity (GOLD, 2020). The following investigations may also be considered: chest radiograph, CT (not recommended, but useful in ruling out other causes of dyspnea), lung volume and diffusing capacities, oximetry, arterial blood gases (ABG) measurement, and exercise testing. Recognizing that COPD goes beyond dyspnea,

TABLE 7.10: Chronic Obstructive Pulmonary Disease Differential Diagnoses

CHRONIC COUGH	DYSPNEA
• Asthma • Cardiac disease (congestive heart failure, mitral stenosis, congenital heart disease) • Chronic sinusitis • Gastroesophageal reflux disease (GERD) • Interstitial lung disease • Neoplasm	• Asthma • Cystic fibrosis • Hyperthyroidism • Neuromuscular disease • Obesity • Pulmonary embolism • Pulmonary hypertension

Source: Data from Global Initiative for Chronic Obstructive Lung Disease. (2020). Pocket guide to COPD: Diagnosis, management, and prevention. A guide for health care professionals. https://goldcopd.org/wp-content/uploads/2020/03/GOLD-2020-POCKET-GUIDE-ver1.0_FINAL-WMV.pdf

it is now recommended that a comprehensive assessment of symptoms be completed. Several measures exist including the COPD Assessment Test (CAT) and the COPD Control Questionnaire (CCQ; GOLD, 2020).

In addition to spirometry and pulse oximetry, diagnostics should include both imaging and laboratory testing. Laboratory testing should include complete blood count (CBC) with differential, an ABG, and alpha-1 antitrypsin. The CBC will be used to determine anemia, infection, or allergic components. Alpha-1 antitrypsin testing should be conducted to determine any deficiency which may contribute to a diagnosis of COPD. The final diagnosis of COPD is made with spirometry, indicating a decreased ratio of forced expiratory volume in 1 second over forced vital capacity (FEV_1/FVC; GOLD, 2020).

TREATMENT

Smoking Cessation

Smoking cessation has a significant influence on the natural progression of COPD. All individuals who are diagnosed with COPD and use tobacco products should be counseled on smoking cessation. The five As of smoking cessation is one method that has been used successfully; these are ask, advise, assess, assist, and arrange. Providers can use the five As of smoking cessation to encourage individuals to discontinue the use of tobacco products (Rakel & Rakel, 2016)

Medications for Stable Chronic Obstructive Pulmonary Disease

The goal of treatment for COPD is focused on reducing both disability, mortality, and improving quality of life. Several of the medications used are focused on improving potentially reversible causes of air flow obstruction. Most of the medications used in the treatment of COPD are focused on reversing the effects of the following mechanisms of airflow limitation: bronchial smooth muscle contraction, bronchial mucosal congestion, airway inflammation, and increased airway secretions. The following medication classes are used for treatment and management of the disease: bronchodilators, beta-2 agonists, and cholinergic/muscarinic agonists (Table 7.11):

- Bronchodilators are central to the management COPD. Individuals with COPD often use one or more of these medications as part of their treatment plan.
- Antimuscarinics inhibit acetylcholine at parasympathetic sites in bronchial smooth muscle causing bronchodilation.
- Methylxanthines work by increasing the amount of cAMP in smooth muscle tissues which ultimately results in bronchodilation.
- Combination bronchodilator therapy is utilized to treat bronchospasms associated with COPD in individuals requiring more than one bronchodilator.

TABLE 7.11: Chronic Obstructive Pulmonary Disease Medications

MEDICATION CLASS	MEDICATION EXAMPLES
Bronchodilators	• *Short-acting (SABA):* Fenoterol, levalbuterol, albuterol • *Long-acting (LABA):* Arformoterol, formoterol, indacaterol
Antimuscarinic drugs	• *Short-acting (SAMA):* Ipratropium bromide, oxitropium bromide • *Long-acting (LAMA):* Aclidinium bromide, glycopyrronium bromide, tiotropium
Methylxanthines	• Aminophylline • Theophylline
Combination bronchodilator therapy	• *Short-acting (SABA/SAMA):* Fenoterol/ipratropium, salbutamol/ipratropium • *Long-acting (LABA/LAMA):* Formoterol/aclidinium, formoterol/glycopyrronium, indacaterol/glycopyrronium
Anti-inflammatory agents	• Inhaled corticosteroids • Oral glucocorticoids • Triple inhaled therapy • Phosphodiesterase-4 inhibitors • Antibiotics

Source: Data from Global Initiative for Chronic Obstructive Lung Disease. (2020). *Pocket guide to COPD: Diagnosis, management, and prevention. A guide for health care professionals.* https://goldcopd.org/wp-content/uploads/2020/03/GOLD-2020-POCKET-GUIDE-ver1.0_FINAL-WMV.pdf

- Anti-inflammatory agents include corticosteroids, oral glucocorticoids, and phosphodiesterase-4 inhibitors. These medications are available in several forms including metered dose inhalers, dry powder inhalers, nebulizer solution, tablets, and liquids.

Vaccinations

All individuals who are diagnosed with COPD should receive the influenza vaccine yearly and the 23–valent pneumococcal polysaccharide vaccine (GOLD, 2020).

Complications

Acute exacerbations of COPD (AECOPD) are key indicators of disease progression. The most common signs and symptoms of an oncoming exacerbation are:

- Increased coughing, wheezing, or dyspnea
- Changes in the color, thickness, or amount of mucus
- Fatigue for more than one day
- Edema of the legs or ankles
- Difficulty sleeping
- Feeling the need for increased oxygen (Ko et al., 2016)

AECOPD can treated by the administration of bronchodilators, systemic corticosteroids, antibiotics, supplemental oxygen, mucolytics, vaccinations, long term

BOX 7.5: FACTORS IN ACUTE EXACERBATIONS OF CHRONIC OBSTRUCTIVE PULMONARY DISEASE THAT MAY REQUIRE HOSPITALIZATION

- Acute respiratory failure
- Onset of cyanosis
- Presence of serious comorbidities
- Severe symptoms such as worsening dyspnea and tachypnea

Source: Data from Sorge, R., & DeBlieux, P. (2020). Acute exacerbations of chronic obstructive pulmonary disease: A primer for emergency physicians. *Journal of Emergency Medicine, 59*(5), 643–659. https://doi.org/10.1016/j.jemermed.2020.07.001

macrolides, and noninvasive ventilation. Life-threatening cases such as extreme hypoxemia or hypercapnia of AECOPD may require hospitalization (Box 7.5).

TRANSITION OF CARE

Following an acute exacerbation of COPD, patients may require long-term supportive services. These services may include pulmonary rehabilitation, symptom control management education, oxygen therapy, ventilatory support, or surgical interventions. Surgical interventions might include lung volume reduction surgery or lung transplantation. Palliative care should be an early component of care of the COPD patient.

CLINICAL PEARLS

- All patients who present with dyspnea should be evaluated for both pulmonary and cardiac disease.
- Tobacco use is the most common cause of COPD.

KEY TAKEAWAYS

- Presenting signs and symptoms include dyspnea, chronic cough, chronic sputum production, and recurrent lower respiratory tract infections.
- Most patients with COPD present with worsening symptoms because they have become acclimated to living with common symptoms (Miskoff et al., 2019).
- A clinical diagnosis of COPD should be considered in all individuals with dyspnea, a chronic cough, sputum production, and a history of exposure to risk factors including tobacco use, occupational and environmental exposures.
- The gold standard for diagnosis and assessment for COPD is spirometry testing.
- Acute exacerbations of COPD are key indicators of disease progression.

EVIDENCE-BASED RESOURCE

GOLD Pocket Guide to COPD Diagnosis, Management, and Prevention 2020. https://goldcopd.org/

CHRONIC BRONCHITIS AND EMPHYSEMA

CB is classified as an obstructive airway disease. CB is a common lung condition that occurs secondary to inflammation of the bronchial tubes and the air passages that extend from the trachea into the small airways and alveoli. CB is a common condition among smokers which often is the initiating source of inflammation. The histologic hallmark of CB is mucus gland hyperplasia. The condition also results in structural changes in the airways, abnormalities in the ciliary bodies, smooth muscle hyperplasia, and thickening of the bronchial walls. These changes, in addition to loss of alveolar attachments, result in airflow limitation (Rakel & Rakel, 2016).

Emphysema is the permanent enlargement of distal air spaces to the terminal bronchioles. This enlargement results in a significant decline in alveolar surface area. The loss of alveoli results in a limitation in air flow from two mechanisms that include decreased elastic recoil in the alveolar walls and a loss of airway supporting structures. Emphysema has three morphologic patterns: centriacinar, panacinar, and distal acinar. Both CB and emphysema are primarily caused by tobacco use or exposure (Rakel & Rakel, 2016).

According to the GOLD, the current guidelines do not distinguish between CB and emphysema. These diseases are considered to be chronic air flow obstructive diseases contained within COPD (GOLD, 2020).

CLINICAL PEARLS

- The histologic hallmark of CB is mucus gland hyperplasia.
- Emphysema is the permanent enlargement of distal air spaces to the terminal bronchioles.
- Both CB and emphysema are primarily caused by tobacco use or exposure.

KEY TAKEAWAYS

- According to the GOLD, the current guidelines do not distinguish between CB and emphysema.
- These diseases are considered to be chronic air flow obstructive diseases contained within COPD.

EVIDENCE-BASED RESOURCE

GOLD Pocket Guide to COPD Diagnosis, Management, and Prevention 2020. https://goldcopd.org/

IDIOPATHIC PULMONARY FIBROSIS

Idiopathic pulmonary fibrosis (IPF) is a chronic, progressive, interstitial, fibrosing pneumonia. The condition is found in older adults and has a poor prognosis (Godfrey & Ouellette, 2019).

Pathophysiology

IPF was previously thought to be caused by inflammation which progressed to widespread parenchymal fibrosis. After treatment trials of anti-inflammatory agents and immunomodulatory demonstrated a reduced response, this hypothesis was proven to be inaccurate. The new proposed thought of the pathogenesis of IPF is that the condition is an epithelial-fibroblastic disease that results from exposure to noxious agents such as tobacco, viral infections, environmental pollutants, gastroesophageal reflux, and chronic aspiration. This new thinking suggests that any of these inciting agents may result in damage to the alveolar epithelium. After injury, it is believed that atypical activation of alveolar epithelial cells stimulates the migration, production, and activation of mesenchymal cells resulting in irreversible destruction of the parenchyma of the lung (Godfrey & Ouellette, 2019).

Etiology

As stated in the title of the disease, the exact cause of IPF is unknown. The following conditions have been proposed as causes:

- History of tobacco use
- Occupational exposures to fumes
- Older age
- Male sex
- Genetics or a family history (Godfrey & Ouellette, 2019)

PRESENTING SIGNS AND SYMPTOMS

Individuals typically present with symptoms of dyspnea or a chronic, nonproductive cough after 6 months of living with the condition. IPF causes scarring of the lungs which eventually results in reduced oxygen intake. Individuals may not present with any symptoms. There is currently no effective treatment besides lung transplantation. It is believed that a cascade of epithelial inflammation triggers the condition. The onset of dyspnea is often gradual and worsens with time. Systematic symptoms may also occur including low grade fever, weight loss, fatigue, arthralgias, and myalgias (Vega-Olivio & Criner, 2018).

HISTORY AND PHYSICAL FINDINGS

History

A detailed medical history which includes past medical, family, social, occupational, medications, environmental, and risk factors for human immunodeficiency virus (HIV) should be completed. The history should include a detailed evaluation of risk factors and characteristics of interstitial lung disease. Current use of drugs including amiodarone, bleomycin, and nitrofurantoin should be noted as they have the potential to cause pulmonary fibrosis. Any history of obstructive sleep apnea should also be investigated (Godfrey & Ouellette, 2019).

Physical Findings

Velcro (bibasilar inspiratory) crackles are a common finding in IPF. Clubbing of the hands is also seen in approximately 25% to 50% of individuals. Signs of pulmonary hypertension may be present. The condition may result in murmurs including a loud pulmonary component of the second heart sound, a fixed split S2, or a holosystolic tricuspid regurgitation murmur. IPF may also result in right ventricular hypertrophy. Edema of the legs may also be present (Vega-Olivio & Criner, 2018).

DIFFERENTIAL DIAGNOSIS AND DIAGNOSTIC CONSIDERATIONS

An important part of diagnosing IPF requires that heart disease is ruled out in regard to exertional dyspnea. Heart failure can be ruled out by obtaining echocardiography, a chest radiograph, or CT. Differential diagnoses may include but are not limited to the conditions noted in Box 7.6.

Diagnostics

A clinical diagnosis of IPF should be considered in all individuals with any risk factors including a nonproductive cough of 6 months or more, a history of tobacco use, or exertional dyspnea. The diagnostic workup should include laboratory studies, imaging, and procedures.

BOX 7.6: DIFFERENTIAL DIAGNOSES FOR IDIOPATHIC PULMONARY FIBROSIS

- Asbestosis
- Bacterial pneumonia
- Cardiogenic pulmonary edema
- Chemical workers' lung
- Farmer's lung
- Heart failure
- Histoplasmosis
- Lung cancer
- Nonspecific interstitial pneumonia
- Recurrent pulmonary edema
- Sarcoidosis
- Viral pneumonia

Source: Godfrey, A., & Ouellette, D. (2019, July 15). Idiopathic pulmonary fibrosis. *Medscape*. https://emedicine.medscape.com/article/301226-overview

Laboratory Studies

- Antinuclear antibodies (ANA) or rheumatoid factor
- C- reactive protein (CRP)
- Erythrocyte sedimentation rate

Imaging

- Chest radiography
- High resolution chest CT

Additional Testing

- Pulmonary function testing
- 6-minute walk testing
- Bronchoalveolar lavage
- Transthoracic echocardiography

Procedures

- Bronchoscopy
- Lung biopsy

The diagnosis of IPF requires an integration of all components of the diagnostic workup (Godfrey & Ouellette, 2019).

TREATMENT

Lung transplantation is the most therapeutic intervention for patients with IPF. With no known cure and few supportive therapeutic options, the treatment for IPF must focus on controlling the risks and disease progression of comorbid conditions. Common comorbidities of IPF include but are not limited to COPD, obstructive sleep apnea, gastroesophageal reflux, and coronary artery disease.

Medical treatment should include smoking cessation and supplemental oxygen for individuals with hypoxemia (PaO_2 <55 mmHg or a pulse oximetry <88% at rest). Individuals should also receive vaccinations for influenza and pneumococcal infection. At present, two medications are approved by the Food and Drug Administration for the treatment of IPF— nintedanib and pirfenidone. Both drugs are classified as antifibrotic agents. These drugs can help reduce additional lung scarring. Additional medications including N-acetylcysteine (NAC), prednisone, and azathioprine, given in conjunction with each other, have been shown to slow the progression of IPF (Vega-Olivio & Criner, 2018).

Complications

Acute Exacerbations

Acute exacerbation of IPF is defined as an acute deterioration of the respiratory system. Individuals often experience a rapid worsening of breathing typically within 30 days, the identification of abnormalities on high resolution CT, and no obvious signs of infection or heart failure. Supportive management is provided including the use of corticosteroids and supplemental oxygen. Mechanical ventilation in patients with progressive IPF disease must consider the patients functional lung status and counseling about the possibility weaning could be very difficult. The decision to mechanically ventilate should be the patient's choice with consideration of the patient's end-of-life goals and plan (Collard et al., 2016).

TRANSITION OF CARE

Transitions of care for IPF patients must include multidisciplinary teams that include pulmonologists, radiologists, and pathologists experienced with the treatment of IPF. Communication among these specialists is necessary to promote and support the health of patients with IPF (Vega-Olivio & Criner, 2018).

CLINICAL PEARLS

- There is currently no effective treatment for IPF besides lung transplantation.
- The diagnosis of IPF requires an integration of all components of the diagnostic workup.

KEY TAKEAWAYS

- Individuals typically present with symptoms of dyspnea or a chronic, nonproductive cough after 6 months of living with the condition.
- The history should include a detailed evaluation of risk factors and characteristics of interstitial lung disease and HIV.
- A clinical diagnosis of IPF should be considered in all individuals with any risk factors including a nonproductive cough of 6 months or more, a history of tobacco use, or exertional dyspnea.
- With no known cures and few treatment options, the treatment for IPF must consider any comorbid conditions.

EVIDENCE-BASED RESOURCES

American Thoracic Society, European Respiratory Society, Japanese Respiratory Society, and Latin American Thoracic Society
Idiopathic Pulmonary Fibrosis Clinical Practice Guidelines. (2018).

7.7: EMPYEMA

Adrienne Markiewicz and Alyssa Profita

Empyema is defined as pus in the pleural space resulting from translocation of bacteria. It most commonly develops as a complication of bacterial pneumonia and parapneumonic effusion. Of the 1 million patients hospitalized for pneumonia in the United States, 32,000 develop empyema as a subsequent complication (Shen et al., 2017). Additional etiologies include chest trauma, esophageal rupture, mediastinitis, infected congenital cyst of the airways and/or esophagus, bronchogenic carcinoma, and postsurgical complications.

PRESENTING SIGNS AND SYMPTOMS

As empyema is most commonly a complication of bacterial pneumonia, patients with empyema will likely have symptoms of pneumonia including fever, cough, shortness of breath, and pleuritic chest pain. Empyema should always be considered in patients with known pneumonia who have not clinically improved, have associated pleural effusion, or have clinically decompensated. Patients will demonstrate increasing oxygen requirement, persistent fevers, ongoing leukocytosis, and may develop shock if source control is not achieved.

HISTORY AND PHYSICAL EXAM FINDINGS

A history of fevers, chills, cough, shortness of breath, and exposure to sick persons are suggestive of pneumonia. On physical exam patients may be tachypneic or have shallow breathing with or without sputum production. On auscultation, rales and rhonchi will be present and the patient may have egophony and increased tactile fremitus over the affected lobes.

DIFFERENTIAL DIAGNOSIS AND DIAGNOSTIC CONSIDERATIONS

The diagnosis of empyema lies first in establishing the history and confirmation via imaging. Chest x-ray (CXR) is the first step in evaluating the patient for pneumonia. A CXR can demonstrate a focal infiltrate or consolidation. Patients with empyema will also have an associated parapneumonic effusion visible by chest radiograph. The effusion can be further qualified by ultrasound or CT scan. MRI is not recommended (Shen et al., 2017).

Not all parapneumonic effusions represent empyema. Once an effusion has been identified, drainage and subsequent analysis of the fluid through thoracentesis is essential to confirm the diagnosis. Analysis of pleural fluid to exclude exudative effusion is completed using Light's criteria (Light et al., 1972). Table 7.12 describes Light's criteria. Pleural fluid obtained from the thoracentesis should be sent to the lab for cell count, glucose, protein, LDH, pH, and gram stain. Serum LDH and total protein should also be measured. Table 7.13 lists the classification and diagnostic criteria for parapneumonic effusions and empyema. Patients with confirmed or suspected empyema should have a pigtail or other small-bore chest tube left in place at the time of thoracentesis for continued drainage and potential administration of fibrinolytic therapy. Other than causes of pneumonia (e.g., bacterial, turberculosis, fungal) differential diagnoses for empyema should also include other causes for exudative pleural effusions such as a malignant etiology.

TREATMENT

Antibiotic Selection

Antimicrobial selection is dependent on the patient's clinical history and risk factors, as well as the local antimicrobial resistance patterns (Shen et al., 2017).

TABLE 7.12: Light's Criteria

PLEURAL FLUID	PLEURAL FLUID/SERUM PROTEIN RATIO	PLEURAL FLUID/SERUM LDH RATIO
Transudative	<0.5	<0.6
Exudative	> or equal to 0.5	> or equal to 0.6

Source: Light, R. W., Macgregor, M. I., Luchsinger, P. C., & Ball, W. C. (1972). Pleural effusions: The diagnostic separation of transudates and exudates. *Annals of Internal Medicine, 77*(4), 507–513. https://doi.org/10.7326/0003-4819-77-4-507

TABLE 7.13: Classification of Parapneumonic Effusions

UNCOMPLICATED PARAPNEUMONIC EFFUSION	COMPLICATED PARAPNEUMONIC EFFUSION	EMPYEMA
Pneumonia present	Pneumonia present	Pneumonia present
Exudative by Light's criteria	Exudative by Light's criteria	Exudative by Light's criteria
Gram stain is culture negative	Gram stain is culture negative	Gram stain is culture positive
Glucose >60	Glucose <60	Glucose <60
PH >7.2	PH <7.2	PH <7.2
		Pus drained from pleural space

Source: Data from Light, R. W., Macgregor, M. I., Luchsinger, P. C., & Ball, W. C. (1972). Pleural effusions: The diagnostic separation of transudates and exudates. *Annals of Internal Medicine, 77*(4), 507–513. https://doi.org/10.7326/0003-4819-77-4-507; Shen, K. R., Bribriesco, A., Crabtree, T., Denlinger, C., Eby, J., Eiken, P., Jones, D. R., Keshavjee, S., Maldonado, F., Paul, S., & Kozower, B. (2017). The American Association for Thoracic Surgery consensus guidelines for the management of empyema. *Journal of Thoracic and Cardiovascular Surgery, 153*(6), e129–e146. https://doi.org/10.1016/j.jtcvs.2017.01.030

A second- or third-generation cephalosporin along with metronidazole or aminopenicillin with beta-lactamase inhibitor is recommended for patients with community-acquired pneumonia (CAP). In patients who have hospital acquired or surgical complications causing empyema, methicillin resistant *Staphylococcus aureus* (MRSA) and *Pseudomonas aeruginosa* coverage should be added. MRSA antimicrobial selection includes vancomycin or linezolid while cefepime or piperacillin/tazobactam are generally effective for *Pseudomonas*. Antimicrobial therapy should be adjusted once culture data have resulted. The duration of therapy is determined by the organism identified, clinical response, and ability to achieve source control (Shen et al., 2017).

Pleural Drainage

Complicated parapneumonic effusions or empyema should be drained via small bore chest tube. In the case of multiple loculated fluid collections or adhesions, fibrinolytic therapy can be utilized (Shen et al., 2017). Dornase alpha and tissue plasminogen activator (TPA) are the two most used agents for this purpose and should be instilled, allowed to dwell within the pleural space, and then drained. If the patient is able, the efficacy of fibrinolytic therapy can be enhanced by postural drainage. Fibrinolytic therapy is continued for 3 days. In one randomized control trial, 92.7% of patients were successfully managed with fibrinolytic therapy alone, eliminating the need for surgical intervention (Mehta et al., 2016). The major risk of this therapy, though rare, is hemorrhage into the pleural space and patients should be closely monitored for this complication.

Surgical Intervention

Empyema that does not resolve with antimicrobials, drainage, and fibrinolytics may require surgical intervention. Video-assisted thoracoscopic surgery (VATS) allows complete drainage of infected fluid from the pleural space and allows the lung to re-expand (Shen et al., 2017). VATS is the preferred surgical intervention for empyema compared to open thoracotomy as research has found that patients have better postoperative pain control, shorter lengths of stay, decreased blood loss, and reduction in postoperative reduced respiratory decompensation, and decreased cost (Shen et al., 2017).

CLINICAL PEARLS

- Empyema is a common complication of bacterial pneumonia.
- Pleural fluid analysis is required to diagnose.
- Treatment includes source control and antimicrobial coverage for appropriate organisms.
- Surgical intervention is required to obtain source control.

7.8: HEMOPTYSIS

Leanne H. Fowler

Hemoptysis is most often a sign or symptom of pulmonary or pulmonary vascular disease but can also occur secondary to a variety of organ-specific or systemic diseases. It is defined as the coughing up of blood from the respiratory tract (Ittrich et al., 2017). It can come from multiple areas within the respiratory tract from the glottis or to the alveoli. Bleeding most commonly comes from the arterial supply of vessels within the bronchi or mid-sized airways; the vascular involvement of hemotypsis can make stopping the bleeding more difficult (Almeida et al., 2020; Ittrich et al., 2017).

Etiological factors associated with hemoptysis include infection by viral, bacterial, fungal, or mycobacterial pathogens. The condition can also occur from inflammatory (e.g., inhalation injuries, autoimmune disease), malignant (e.g., cancer of the lung, bronchi, esophagus), vascular (e.g., pulmonary embolism, vasculitis), or traumatic (e.g., foreign body aspiration, puncture from invasive procedures) etiologies. The most common etiologies of hemoptysis are infectious and malignant.

PRESENTING SIGNS AND SYMPTOMS

Patient with hemoptysis often complain of coughing up blood that can be described as blood-tinged sputum, coughing up bright red blood or dark red blood clots. In addition to the onset, duration, and alleviating/aggravating factors, patients should be asked about the amount and the severity of bleeding involved to help discern the patient's risk for hemorrhage, instability, and death. Patients do not often die from severe hemorrhage but can die from asphyxiation of blood filling the gas-exchanging alveoli units of the lung.

The patient's presentation of illness is directly related to the underlying disease causing the hemoptysis. For instance, patients with an underlying infectious disease of the lower respiratory system can include a review of systems describing fever, chills, generalized myalgia and/or arthralgia, cough with hemoptysis, and dyspnea, whereas patients with an underlying lung cancer may report a review of systems that is positive for unintentional weight loss, dysphagia, odynophagia, chest pain, and/or dyspnea.

HISTORY AND PHYSICAL FINDINGS
Patient History

The past medical history is necessary to identify risk factors for or an actual history of infection, autoimmune disease, bleeding disorders, liver disease, cancer, and/or trauma. The patient's surgical history is also important to identify the patient's recent history for tracheal intubation or bronchoscopy that could be responsible for the hemoptysis. Home medications should be reviewed to evaluate patients for the use of antiplatelet or anticoagulating agents that can contribute to bleeding. Regular use of nonsteroidal anti-inflammatory drugs (NSAIDs) can also increase a patient's propensity to bleed.

Patients should be asked to quantify the amount of hemoptysis experienced using the reference of teaspoons (5 mL), tablespoons (15 mL), or cups (about 237 mL). Massive hemoptysis is considered to be blood loss related to 400 mL or more in a 24-hour period or 100 to 150 mL coughed up at one time (Brady & Kritek, 2018).

Physical Examination

The general physical examination should focus on evaluating the patient's general appearance for respiratory distress and vital signs for hemodynamic stability. The mucous membranes of the nose and mouth, and skin should be evaluated for signs of bleeding. The practitioner should also inspect the sputum when possible to evaluate the character and amount of bleeding. A focused examination looking for signs and symptoms associated with the patient's underlying disease (e.g., pneumonia, cancer, trauma) should be performed.

Patients with an acute inflammatory or infectious etiology may present with pharyngitis or other findings associated with upper or lower respiratory pulmonary infection. Patients with malignant etiology may present with evidence of significant weight loss, a palpable and nontender mass of the neck, and difficulty breathing if the airway is compromised. Patients with chronic lung disease or chronic inflammatory diseases can have clubbing of the fingers. Patients with bleeding disorders may have petechiae, telangiectasias, and/or ecchymosis of the skin or mucous membranes.

DIFFERENTIAL DIAGNOSIS AND DIAGNOSTIC CONSIDERATIONS

The history and physical examination should help the AGACNP differentiate if the blood is coming from the respiratory tract or the gastrointestinal tract. Other differential diagnoses should be inclusive of the amount of hemoptysis and conditions associated with the etiologies of hemoptysis. Nonmassive hemoptysis is seen most commonly. Nonmassive hemoptysis presentations in patients without risk factors for cancer are usually related to an acute infectious etiology. Massive hemoptysis is seen less commonly and most often associated with bronchial artery or diffuse alveolar hemorrhage. Box 7.7 includes a list of common differential diagnoses for patients presenting with hemoptysis.

Diagnostic Tests

Diagnostic testing should focus on identifying the underlying cause of hemoptysis. Patients should have serum laboratory tests ordered to evaluate the patient for infection, blood loss, organ function, and bleeding disorders. Practitioners with a high index of suspicion for a

---

BOX 7.7: DIFFERENTIAL DIAGNOSES FOR PATIENTS PRESENTING WITH HEMOPTYSIS

- Pneumonia
  - Active tuberculosis
  - Aspergillosis
  - Viral
  - Community-acquired bacterial
- Bronchiectasis
- Bronchial artery hemorrhage
- Cancer
  - Lung cancer
  - Bronchial cancer
- Cystic fibrosis (most common in children and adolescents)
- Goodpasture syndrome (diffuse pulmonary hemorrhage)
  - Systemic lupus erythematous
  - Glomerulonephritis with pulmonary hemorrhage
- Pulmonary embolus

---

malignant etiology can include a more extensive evaluation of the patient by evaluating biomarkers for cancer.

Chest Imaging

Imaging modalities of the lung will include chest radiograph or CT of the chest. Chest radiograph images are ordered to evaluate the lungs for evidence of infection or bronchogenic or lung masses. Evaluating the patient with IV contrast-enhanced CT imaging is useful when vascular etiologies are suspected. A noncontrast study of the chest with CT is reasonable for evaluating sectional images of the soft tissue of the lung and chest cavity, such as in patients with diffuse alveolar hemorrhage. Patients with high risk factors for a malignant etiology may benefit from CT imaging of the head, abdomen, and pelvis.

Bronchoscopy

Patients at high risk for malignancy should be evaluated by a flexible bronchoscopy to exclude a bronchogenic neoplasm as the cause for hemoptysis. Bronchoscopy should be performed following evaluation of the lung and chest by CT imaging. If a bronchogenic mass is identified by CT and accessible for biopsy without bronchoscopy, bronchoscopy can be deferred to a later time, if needed (Brady & Kritek, 2018).

TREATMENT

The treatment goals for patients diagnosed with hemoptysis are categorized for patients with nonmassive hemoptysis and those with massive hemoptysis. Treatment for nonmassive hemoptysis is dependent upon the underlying condition causing the hemoptysis. For example, the patient with an infectious etiology is treated with antimicrobial agents to eradicate the pathogen or provided therapies to allow the infection to run its course but support full recovery of health. Patients with pulmonary emboli are treated with anticoagulation and therapies aimed at maintaining adequate oxygenation. Patients with active and persistent bleeding should have anticoagulant or antiplatelet therapies held until bleeding is controlled.

Specialty Consultation

Consultation with a pulmonologist, interventional pulmonologist, or thoracic surgeon may be indicated for outpatient or inpatient evaluation and management. Patients with an unclear etiology of hemoptysis should be referred to a pulmonologist for further evaluation and management. Patients with massive hemoptysis or indications for surgical intervention should be referred to an interventional pulmonologist or thoracic surgeon for further evaluation and management.

Massive Hemoptysis

The treatment goals for patients with massive hemoptysis focus on protecting the nonbleeding lung, locating the site and source of bleeding, and controlling the bleed (Brady & Kritek, 2018). Asphyxiation from massive pulmonary hemorrhage can occur quickly, thereby necessitating the need for rapid intervention aimed to preventing further lung injury and facilitate adequate oxygenation.

Interventions

In an effort to protect the nonbleeding lung, position the patient with the bleeding lung down when the location of the bleeding is known. Other interventions to protect the nonbleeding lung are to avoid tracheal intubation when possible, to allow the cough reflex to expel blood clots. If intubation is necessary, one-lung intubation and ventilation can provide some protection of the nonbleeding side (Brady & Kritek, 2018).

Localizing the source of bleeding is difficult in most patients without angiography. Controlling the bleeding is most effective through surgical interventions such as bronchial artery embolization, resection of the involved airway and vessel, or tamponading the bleed with the insertion of a balloon catheter through the airway (Almeida et al., 2020; Ittrich et al., 2017). Rebleeding can occur if the underlying cause has not been adequately treated.

7.9: MECHANICAL VENTILATION

Leanne H. Fowler and Donna Lynch-Smith

Mechanical ventilation is a life-saving intervention used to assist the patient in maintaining adequate gas exchange. Current mechanical ventilation technologies use positive-pressure ventilation noninvasively via a mask or invasively via tracheal intubation. Indications for mechanical ventilation include respiratory failure

> **BOX 7.8 INDICATIONS FOR MECHANICAL VENTILATION**
>
> 1. **Apnea**
>   a. Central nervous system catastrophic event
> 2. **Acute ventilatory failure**
>   a. pH ≤7.30 with $PaCO_2$ >50 mmHg
>   b. Clinical signs: Altered respiratory mechanics
> 3. **Acute respiratory failure**
>   a. Hypoxic respiratory failure (mechanisms)
>   1) Hypoventilation: Diffusion limitation: Right-to-left shunt: VQ mismatch: Low inspired PO_2: High altitudes
>   b. Hypercapneic respiratory failure (mechanisms)
>   1) Inadequate respiratory muscle function: Impaired neural transmission: Excessive ventilatory demand: Decreased ventilatory drive
> 4. **Impending respiratory failure**
>   Deterioration of patient's status that is refractory to maximum therapy
> 5. **Severe oxygenation deficit**

secondary to acute systemic illness, acute or chronic lung disease (CLD), drug overdose, severe brain injury (e.g., anoxic or traumatic), or chronic or progressive neuromuscular disease (Box 7.8). The use of general anesthesia is also an indication for mechanical ventilation to support the patient during surgical procedures. The ultimate goal of using mechanical ventilation is to support the patient's need for effective gas exchange, effective delivery of oxygen, decreased work of breathing, and recovery to lung function that does not require mechanical ventilator support.

FUNDAMENTAL PRINCIPLES OF MECHANICAL VENTILATION

Mechanical ventilators are designed to support the mechanics of ventilation and to facilitate the diffusion of the gases exchanged by augmenting the frequency of breaths per minute and manipulating the breath sequence, targeting scheme, and control variables of ventilation (i.e., pressure, volume, and flow) during different phases of a mechanical breath (Esan et al., 2018).

The breath sequence is how breaths are delivered by the mechanical ventilator. Breaths can be delivered spontaneously, intermittently mandatory, or continuously mandatory. Spontaneous breaths are initiated and cycled (ended) by the patient whereas mandatory breaths are initiated and cycled by the ventilator. Mechanical ventilatory support occurs on a spectrum from unassisted spontaneous breathing to complete mandatory breathing. The mechanical ventilator can be set for patterns of control that are triggered at present intervals to assist the patient's rate, tidal volume, and airway pressures when an alteration in the patient's breathing is sensed (Esan et al., 2018).

The targeting scheme is the settings and programming that provide the mechanical ventilator feedback of the patient's lung compliance, airway resistance, and respiratory effort. Targeting schemes reflect the relationship between the patient and the mechanical device. The mechanical ventilator senses patient factors so that delivered breaths are responsive to the patient's rate, tidal volume, flow, and airway pressures (Esan et al., 2018).

Ventilation Terminology

The AGACNP must not only understand the terminology associated with managing patients with mechanical ventilation, but must also use the terms appropriately. Communicating with the healthcare team is most effective when all parties are speaking the same language with the same meaning. Table 7.14 summarizes terms and definitions associated with mechanical ventilation.

Phases of Mechanical Ventilator Breaths

There are four phases to each breath, or each ventilator cycle: (a) The trigger variable, (b) limit variable, (c) cycle variable, and (d) baseline variable. The trigger variable refers to how the breath is initiated. The breath is either patient-triggered (based upon airway pressures and flow) or ventilator-triggered (based upon timing per minute). The limit variable refers to the maximum preset limits to the amount of pressure, volume, or flow that can be reached and maintained before inhalation ends. The cycle variable refers to the preset amount of pressure, volume, flow, or time in which the ventilator delivers its support that ends inhalation and begins

exhalation. The baseline variables are pressure, volume, or flow settings to support sustained opening of airways and alveoli during exhalation (Esan et al., 2018).

MODES OF MECHANICAL VENTILATION

Modes of mechanical ventilation are the settings that specify the control variables, the breath sequence, and targeting scheme. Conventional modes of mechanical ventilation refer to the traditional modes of assist control ventilation (ACV) or continual mandatory ventilation (CMV), intermittent mandatory ventilation (IMV) or synchronized intermittent mandatory ventilation (SIMV), and pressure support ventilation (PSV). Alternative modes of ventilation are hinged upon newer technologies within the mechanical ventilator such as microprocessors. These technologies allow for more complex settings that can provide dual control modes discussed more below (Esan et al., 2018). Table 7.15 includes brief descriptions of the modes of ventilation.

Conventional Modes

Continuous Mandatory and Assist-Control Ventilation

The CMV mode provides mandatory breaths at a set rate, or frequency, which are triggered (initiated), limited, and cycled (ended) by the ventilator. The ventilator controls the breath sequence by tidal volume (volume controlled) or pressure targets (pressure controlled). Patients who are able to initiate and cycle their own breaths can interfere with the settings of CMV mode. Therefore, patients will either require deep sedation or paralysis to tolerate CMV mode, or ACV mode should be used (Esan et al., 2018).

TABLE 7.14: Terms and Definitions Associated With Mechanical Ventilation

TERM	DEFINITION
Baseline variables	The pressure, volume, or flow settings to support sustained opening of airways and alveoli during exhalation
Breath rate or frequency	The number of breaths per minute
Control variables	The volume or pressure settings used to deliver mandatory breaths
Cycle variables	The preset amount of pressure, volume, flow, or time in which the ventilator delivers its support that ends inhalation and begins exhalation
Limit variables	Maximum preset limits to the amount of pressure, volume, or flow that can be reached and maintained before inhalation ends
Mechanical ventilation	Using a mechanical device to support the respiratory mechanics necessary for adequate gas exchange
Minute ventilation	The volume of air inhaled and exhaled per minute
Peak inspiratory pressure	The highest pressure achieved during inhalation
Plateau pressure	The highest pressure achieved at the end of inhalation or during the no-flow period
Trigger variables	How the breath is initiated–patient-triggered or ventilator-triggered
Target schemes	Patient factors the ventilator can sense related to the patient's rate, tidal volume, flow, and airway pressures
Tidal volume	The amount of air inhaled and exhaled with each respiratory cycle
Ventilator mode	The settings used to determine the pressure or volume control variables

TABLE 7.15: Descriptions of Modes of Ventilation

MODE	DESCRIPTION
Assist-control ventilation (ACV)	• The ventilator senses patient-triggered breaths. All breaths (patient- or ventilator-triggered) receive a set tidal volume or pressure target and rate.
Continuous mandatory ventilation (CMV)	All breaths are controlled by the ventilator. Patient triggered breaths are not allowed. Pharmacologic agents such as sedation and neuromuscular blockade will nullify patient-initiated breaths. • **Volume Controlled:** Ventilator will deliver set tidal volume at a set breath rate to control minute ventilation. • **Pressure Controlled:** Ventilator will deliver set pressure at a set breath rate. Tidal volume and minute ventilation will vary.
Dual-modes	**Volume-assured pressure support (VAPS):** Each breath supported with pressure and volume to maintain the preset tidal volume as sensed by volume targets. **Volume-support ventilation (VSV):** Each breath supported with varying levels of pressure to maintain the present tidal volume as sensed by pressure targets. **Pressure regulated volumn control (PRVC):** Breath-to-breath support to maintain the minimal peak inspiratory pressure to maintain the present tidal volume as sensed by volume targets. The minimal pressure delivered adjusts between breaths as needed by the patient. **Auto-Mode:** Breath-to-breath support that switches between pressure and volume support to pressure or volume control settings to maintain the preset tidal volume. This mode can sense if spontaneous efforts fail and switch to mandatory breaths when needed.
Pressure support ventilation (PSV)	A preset level of inspiratory pressure on the ventilator. Respiratory rate, inspiratory time, and tidal volume are controlled by the patient. Can be used to support spontaneous breaths on IMV mode or for weaning patients from mechanical ventilation.
Synchronized intermittent mandatory ventilation (SIMV)	Breaths are mostly patient-triggered and cycled. The ventilator will deliver set tidal volume at a set breath rate. Spontaneous breaths between or above the mandatory breath rate will not receive the set tidal volume but may receive pressure support.

The primary difference between ACV and CMV is that the trigger depends on patient effort and the ventilator's sensitivity to the patient's effort. Otherwise, ACV also provides the same support as CMV. Many brands of mechanical ventilators now use CMV and ACV interchangeably. However, it is an important distinction the AGACNP must be aware of because in patients with a high respiratory drive, respiratory alkalosis can occur with ACV. Consequently, the patient's work of breathing increases, the ventilator's sensitivity to the patient's effort becomes inadequate, and patient-ventilator dyssynchrony occurs (Esan et al., 2018). The CMV/ACV modes provide the highest level of ventilatory support and are often required for severe critical illness or patients requiring general anesthesia.

VOLUME CONTROL VENTILATION

VCV is the most commonly used control variable within the CMV/ACV or SIMV modes. This control variable provides a fixed minute ventilation during mandatory breaths but requires the practitioner to set the inspiratory flow and time. This control variable is most supportive to the patient with compliant lung disease as airway pressures increase in patients with noncompliant or restrictive lung disease. Increased airway pressures or ventilator-patient dyssynchrony can cause ventilator-induced lung injury (VILI).

PRESSURE CONTROL VENTILATION

PCV is used for patients with noncompliant or restrictive lung diseases and are at high risk for VILI. The ventilator sets the inspiratory flow variables to maintain low airway pressures. However, the patient will have varying tidal volumes and minute ventilation.

Synchronized Intermittent Mandatory Ventilation

The SIMV, or IMV, mode of mechanical ventilation is a middle-level support for patients who are able to trigger and cycle their own breaths spontaneously in between or above the mandatory ventilator breaths triggered, limited, and cycled. Therefore, at least the set rate of breaths are mandatory and breaths taken above the set rate are spontaneous. Additionally, the ventilator synchronizes the mandatory breath with the patient-triggered breath to deliver a set tidal volume and breath frequency. If the ventilator does not sense an inspiratory breath, a mandatory breath will be initiated at the scheduled time. For example, if the ventilator is set to deliver a 400 cc tidal volume for 12 breaths per minute (or every 5 seconds), then the mandatory settings will try to synchronize with the patient-triggered breath to provide the set ventilation support each minute. Spontaneous breaths will not receive a set tidal volume, but most are supported by pressure support (PS) to augment the spontaneous tidal volume (Esan et al., 2018).

Pressure Support Ventilation

PSV is the lowest-level mode of ventilator support or it can be a supplemental setting to support airway pressures during the IMV mode. The patient has to trigger, limit, and cycle all of their own breaths. Some ventilators label this mode as CPAP and is often the mode used for weaning patients from mechanical ventilator support. Low levels of PS (5–10 cmH$_2$O) nullify the resistance of the endotracheal tube and ventilator tubing for mandatory and spontaneous breaths. Low levels of PS are generally used for ventilator liberation. Higher levels of PS (10–20 cmH$_2$0) are used to augment tidal volume.

The PSV mode should not be confused with PCV. Tidal volume and rate are not set during PSV. Therefore, a patient must be able to generate (with or without airway PS) an adequate spontaneous tidal volume and rate for adequate gas exchange. The ventilator assists spontaneous breaths with a set inspiratory pressure level that is limited by the patient's peak inspiratory flow rate (Esan et al., 2018). The patient's work of breathing should be monitored closely during PSV. The PSV mode is contraindicated in patients with an impaired respiratory drive (e.g., spinal cord injury, brain injury, progressive neuromuscular disease).

CLINICAL PEARLS

- Conventional modes are most commonly used for initial ventilator settings.
- Pulmonary specialist consultation should be initiated for patients requiring alternative and nonconventional modes of ventilation.

Alternative Modes

Alternative modes of ventilator support have emerged with the production of modern devices. These modes allow for more complex delivery of ventilatory support by sensing inspiratory pressures or tidal volumes of the patient. Alternative modes include dual-control modes and nonconventional modes such as APRV, proportional assist ventilation (PAV), adaptive support ventilation (ASV), high-frequency ventilation (HFV), and HFOV, to name a few. This section focuses on dual control modes of ventilation.

Dual Control Modes

Dual control modes involve the ventilator being able to deliver and regulate pressure or volume within one breath or from breath-to-breath. To deliver dual control modes, the ventilator must be able to sense the intrapulmonary mechanics of the patient and use it as feedback communication to the ventilator in an effort to adjust its settings from breath-to-breath or within each breath. The pressure and volume settings alternate automatically to maintain the practitioner-set tidal volume (Esan et al., 2018).

VOLUME-ASSURED PRESSURE SUPPORT

The VAPS mode is also known as pressure augmentation. This mode uses dual control of preset pressure and volume limits within one breath. The breath can be patient- or ventilator-triggered and senses when a tidal volume is not reached within the breath to switch from a pressure-limited to a volume-limited breath. This mode aims to reach the pre-set tidal volume during each breath (Esan et al., 2018).

VOLUME SUPPORT VENTILATION

This mode allows for varying levels of PS for each breath. All breaths are patient-triggered but are pressure-limited and flow-cycled by the ventilator to maintain a steady tidal volume from breath-to-breath (Esan et al., 2018).

PRESSURE-REGULATED VOLUME CONTROL

This mode is similar to VCV except that it senses the tidal volume as the feedback communication variable to adjust pressure limits from breath-to-breath. The PRVC mode tests the patient's spontaneous inspiratory pressures in an effort to maintain the lowest deliverable peak inspiratory pressure (PIP) within the set inspiratory time to maintain the practitioner-set tidal volume. As the patient's spontaneous efforts increase, this mode adjusts the delivered pressure from breath-to-breath (Esan et al., 2018).

AUTO-MODE VENTILATION

This mode combines PRVC with VSV functions to control breath-to-breath time cycled breaths. This mode works for patient- or ventilator-triggered or cycled breaths. Furthermore, this mode can switch between pressure and volume support to pressure or volume control settings if the patient's spontaneous breaths fail and mandatory breaths are needed (Esan et al., 2018).

CLINICAL PEARLS

- Control modes deliver mandatory breaths at predetermined settings.
- Mandatory breaths can be delivered in the CMV/ACV or SIMV modes.

ADJUNCTIVE STRATEGIES TO MECHANICAL VENTILATION

Venovenous Extracorporeal Membrane Oxygenation

Venovenous ECMO is used to support the respiratory system by removing blood from a large vein such as the femoral vein and returning it to another large vein that is contralateral such as the femoral or superior vena cava. The blood passes through an artificial lung membrane which oxygenates the removed carbon dioxide and oxygenates the blood. The native lungs still participate in this process depending on the disease process and blood that is diverted to the artificial lung membrane (Extracorporeal Life Support Organization [ELSO], 2017). More research is needed to provide highly appraised research evidence recommending ECMO use in patients with severe acute respiratory distress syndrome (ARDS) (Hoegl & Zwissler, 2017). See the indications for ECMO in Box 7.9.

NONINVASIVE POSITIVE PRESSURE VENTILATION

NIPPV refers to the delivery of positive or negative airway pressure without an invasive tracheal airway.

BOX 7.9: INDICATIONS FOR EXTRACORPOREAL MEMBRANE OXYGENATION

- Consider in hypoxic respiratory failure with risk of mortality ≥50%
- Indicated in hypoxic respiratory failure with risk of mortality ≥90%
- CO_2 retention with a plateau pressure ≥ 30 cmH$_2$O
- Severe air leak syndrome
- Intubation needed on lung transplant patient
- Immediate cardiac or respiratory collapse (pulmonary embolism, blocked airway, or unresponsive to optimal care)

BOX 7.10: INDICATIONS FOR NONINVASIVE POSITIVE PRESSURE VENTILATION

- Acute exacerbation of COPD
- Severe acute exacerbation of asthma
- Acute respiratory failure
  - Hypercapneic, secondary to acute exacerbation of COPD
  - Hypoxemic
  - Postoperative
- Acute cardiogenic pulmonary edema
- Palliative care in the setting of COPD and acute heart failure

BOX 7.11: CONTRAINDICATIONS FOR NONINVASIVE POSITIVE PRESSURE VENTILATION

- Imminent risk for respiratory arrest
- Hemodynamic instability
- Uncooperative or agitated patient
- Increased secretions warranting frequent suctioning
- Facial trauma
- PaO$_2$:FiO$_2$ ratio less than 200
- Multiorgan failure

Noninvasive mechanical ventilation can deliver positive airway pressures during inspiratory (CPAP) and expiratory phases (bi-level positive airway pressure, or Bi-PAP) of spontaneous ventilation. Providing BiPAP ventilation allows alveolar units of the patient's lungs to remain open during expiration thereby improving gas exchange. The most common modes of NIPPV used are CPAP and BiPAP.

The indications for NIPPV are listed in Box 7.10. Patients who cannot maintain awakeness or their own airway protection are not good candidates for NIPPV. Other contraindications are noted in Box 7.11.

The advantages of NIPPV include avoiding the complications associated with tracheal intubation and mechanical ventilation, NIPPV does not usually require sedation, and it is less costly when compared to invasive mechanical ventilation (Esan et al., 2018).

CLINICAL PEARLS

- Patients with acute COPD exacerbation and ACPE benefit from NIPPV.
- NIPPV should be a first-intervention in awake patients with acute COPD exacerbation and ACPE.

HISTORY AND PHYSICAL FINDINGS

A thorough history and physical examination are important in differentiating the etiologies associated with the need for mechanical ventilation support. Asking questions focused on differentiating metabolic, infectious, drug toxicity, thrombotic, or mechanisms of traumatic injuries are important for gaining insight into the factors contributing to illness that the practitioner cannot observe or measure. Likewise, performing a physical examination focused on collecting evidence to support the history and affirm or deny the practitioner's suspicions contributes to appropriate and prioritized differential diagnoses.

History

An expanded problem-focused or comprehensive review of systems should be performed initially to evaluate the patient for pulmonary and extrapulmonary disease; and to evaluate the patient for the source of illness. Patients with a past medical history of CLD are at high risk for prolonged mechanical ventilation, failure to wean, and/or complications associated with mechanical ventilation. When a history of chronic restrictive lung disease is present, the practitioner should anticipate monitoring the patient for increased PIPs or plateau pressures in an effort to reduce the patient's risk for barotrauma and pneumothorax.

The Ventilator-Dependent Patient

Patients could be dependent upon noninvasive or invasive types of mechanical ventilation. Patients requiring mechanical ventilation at home have been shown to improve their symptoms, health status, overall mortality, and need for hospital readmission (Wijkstra & Duiverman, 2020). Patients with a history of COPD, obesity hypoventilation syndrome, and obstructive sleep apnea are often treated with NIPPV strategies at home. Patients with a history of chronic and/or progressive neuromuscular disease are often ventilator-dependent via tracheostomy secondary to varying degrees of respiratory muscle dysfunction (Wijkstra & Duiverman, 2020). Patients living with neuromuscular dysfunction can also often have impaired protective cough and gag reflexes thereby placing them at risk for aspiration and/or poor clearance of airway secretions.

Patients living with ventilator-dependent conditions may have a history of and can be at risk for recurrent lung infections and mucus plugging. Acute lung infections may cause the patient to require increased or modified mechanical ventilator support. Progressive neuromuscular diseases may also cause the patient to require increased needs of mechanical ventilator support. The AGACNP should be sure to collect a history focused on the patient's medical history, progression of acute illness, baseline ventilator settings, and baseline need for supplemental oxygen. Not all patients living with ventilator-dependent conditions require supplemental oxygen.

Physical Examination

The initial physical examination of a patient requiring mechanical ventilation should also be problem focused or comprehensive to complement and be congruent with the history collected. The follow-up exam of patients being mechanically ventilated should focus on examining the patient's hemodynamic status, work of breathing, oxygenation, amount of secretions, and overall progression or improvement of illness. The follow up exam of patients should also be vigilant in recognizing complications associated with mechanical ventilation such as the new production of purulent sputum, worsening breath sounds, and palpation of crepitus within the skin of the thorax.

DIFFERENTIAL DIAGNOSIS AND DIAGNOSTIC CONSIDERATIONS

Patients requiring mechanical ventilation have respiratory distress and/or impending respiratory failure, or need to support ventilation during a surgical procedure requiring general anesthesia. Diagnoses associated with NIPPV and mechanical ventilation via tracheal intubation are noted in Table 7.16.

TABLE 7.16: Differential Diagnoses for Conditions Requiring Mechanical Ventilation

TYPES OF MECHANICAL VENTILATION	DIFFERENTIAL DIAGNOSES
Noninvasive positive pressure ventilation (only for the awake patient)	Acute exacerbation of severe COPD Acute or chronic respiratory failure Obstructive sleep apnea Acute respiratory distress syndrome

Mechanical ventilation with intubation	Acute respiratory failure
	    Hypoxemic and/or hypercapneic
	    Acute respiratory distress syndrome
	    Postcardiopulmonary resuscitation
	    Status asthmaticus
	    Neuromuscular disease
	Drug overdose
	Anoxic brain injury
	Severe head trauma or traumatic brain injury

Diagnostic Tests

The diagnostic tests associated with the management of patients requiring mechanical ventilation are those necessary to evaluate and manage the causes of respiratory failure (see Section 7.3, Acute Respiratory Failure). A chest radiograph should be obtained immediately after intubation and daily during the follow-up evaluation of patients being mechanically ventilated to confirm tube placement and trend the progression or improvement of lung disease.

TREATMENT

The management of patients requiring mechanical ventilation includes understanding the basic principles of ventilation and phases of ventilator breaths, the types of positive pressure ventilation, the modes of ventilation, and the timely weaning of mechanical ventilation. Managing patients requiring mechanical ventilation also requires the ability to prevent, identify, and manage the complications associated with mechanical ventilation. Consulting a pulmonary specialist to manage patients with mechanical ventilation has the best safety and quality outcomes for these patients. However, the AGACNP practicing within a critical care or hospital medicine service must know when to initiate, modify, and discontinue mechanical ventilatory support, and minimize the patient's risk for complications.

Initial Mechanical Ventilation Management

Respiratory failure is the primary indication for mechanical ventilation. The AGACNP must recognize if the patient has acute or chronic respiratory failure and the underlying etiology when determining the kind of mechanical ventilation to initiate. For example, the patient with a history of COPD presenting with an acute exacerbation and respiratory failure should be closely evaluated for chronic respiratory failure and the potential benefit of NIPPV at home. On the other hand, a patient presenting with altered mental status and hemodynamic instability should be prepared for intubation and mechanical ventilation. Verifying the patient's indications and contraindications for mechanical ventilation are necessary before initiating the life-saving intervention.

Initiating Mechanical Ventilation via Tracheal Intubation

Patients requiring the initiation of mechanical ventilation should be managed in critical care units or step-down critical care units by a pulmonary specialist. Although some patients may have mechanical ventilation initiated in the emergency department, they should be admitted to the unit with the most appropriate nursing competency levels for care. Some hospitals may or may not have step-down units.

The principles of airway management are not discussed in this chapter. However, basic and difficult airway management knowledge and competency (e.g., patient assessment, techniques, use of equipment) are necessary in contributing to the comprehensive management of patients requiring mechanical ventilation. The AGACNP must be able to recognize and trouble-shoot when a patient has tube migration, unintentional extubation, or other complications associated with the endotracheal tube (e.g., cuff leak) and initiate interventions to correct the problem in a timely manner.

Initial Ventilator Settings

The mode, rate, tidal volume, inspiration/expiration (I/E) ratio, supplemental PS, and supplemental oxygen are the basic settings to consider when initiating mechanical ventilation via endotracheal intubation. Patient conditions should greatly influence the initial settings (Table 7.17). Patients requiring invasive mechanical ventilation are generally critically ill and should be started with volume- or pressure-controlled mandatory breath settings. Patients with ventilator dyssynchrony may require sedation or neuromuscular paralysis to improve oxygenation by reducing oxygen consumption and demand when controlled settings are employed.

RESPIRATORY RATE AND TIDAL VOLUME

Setting the initial rate and tidal volume of mechanical ventilation should consider the patients $PaCO_2$ level. An initial respiratory rate of 8 to 12 breaths per minute is standard. Patients with hypercapnia can benefit from induced hyperventilation via mechanical ventilation but should be monitored closely to ensure alkalosis does not develop. An initial tidal volume should range from 5 to 8 mL/kg. Tidal volumes can be set per a weight-based formula for the body weight of males and females to achieve a goal of 4 to 8 mL/kg of predicted or ideal body weight. Lung-protective strategies tidal volumes (4 to 6 mL/kg) are initiated for patients at risk for VILI.

SUPPLEMENTAL OXYGEN

Patients with a PaO_2 less than 60 mmHg should have an initial FiO_2 set to achieve oxygen saturation greater than 90%. Patients with a history of COPD may need to start at lower FiO_2 levels. The PaO_2 level should be reevaluated within 15 to 30 minutes of mechanical ventilator initiation to titrate the FiO_2 level and reconsider the need for increased alveolar recruitment with PEEP or positioning techniques. Maintaining FiO_2 levels less than 0.4 are not associated with lung injury.

INSPIRATION/EXPIRATION RATIO

The normal I/E ratio is 1:2 and this is a standard initial setting for patients without CLD. Patients with a history of COPD should have a reduced I/E ratio set to 1:4 or 1:5 to prevent breath stacking and further air-trapping. An inverse I/E ratio (2:1) can be useful in patients with restrictive lung disease or ARDS.

SUPPLEMENTAL PRESSURE SUPPORT

Low amounts of PS (+8 to +10 cmH_2O) can be used to supplement mandatory breaths delivered in the IMV mode. Supplemental PS helps to overcome dead space and improve minute ventilation. The use of supplemental PS should not be confused with the PSV mode of ventilation.

POSITIVE-END EXPIRATORY PRESSURE

PEEP is another supplemental setting used to augment airway pressures during the expiratory phase in an effort to recruit functional alveoli by preventing collapse during

TABLE 7.17: Initial Ventilator Settings for Critical Patient Conditions

LUNG CONDITION	MODE	V_T (cmH$_2$O)	RATE (BPM)	I:E RATIO	PEEP
Healthy lungs	PC or VC	6–8	8–12	1:2	3–5
COPD*	PC or VC	6–8	8–12	1:4–5	025
Chronic restrictive disease	PC or VC	4–6	15–30		5
ARDS	VC	4–6	Up to 35	1:1.5–2	**
Neuromuscular disease	PC or VC	6–8	10–15	1:2	5
Head trauma	PC or VC	6–8	15–20	1:2	5
Hypovolemia	PC or VC	6–8	10–12	1:2	0

*Consider NIPPV early. **Per FiO_2/PEEP combination oxygenation goals.

ARDS, acute respiratory distress syndrome; bpm, breaths per minute; COPD, chronic obstructive pulmonary disease; I:E, inspiration: expiration; PC, pressure control; PEEP, positive end expiratory pressure; VC, volume control; V$_T$, tital volume

Source: Adapted from Esan, A., Khusid, F., & Raoof, S. (2018). Ventilator technology and management. In J. M. Oropello, S. M. Pastores, & V. Kvetan (Eds.), *Critical care*. McGraw Hill; National Heart Lung & Blood Institute ARDS Network. (2008). *NIH NHLBI ARDS clinical network mechanical ventilation protocol summary*. http://www.ardsnet.org/files/ventilator_protocol_2008-07.pdf

expiration, and to reduce the need for high amounts of supplemental oxygen that can injure functional alveolar units. Initial PEEP settings of +3 to +5 cmH$_2$O are standardly used to prevent decreases in FRC in mechanically ventilated patients. Another benefit to using PEEP is in the setting of patients with pulmonary edema to shift alveolar water back into the interstitial space. Furthermore, the use of PEEP increases intrathoracic pressures and thereby reduces venous return to the right heart in patients with cardiogenic pulmonary edema.

Patients with ARDS have scattered injured and healthy alveoli across all lung fields. The use of higher settings of PEEP ($\geq$ +5 cmH$_2$O) in patients with ARDS helps to improve diffusion of oxygen within the healthy and injured alveolar units. However, higher settings of PEEP can cause traumatic injury to the healthy alveolar units and worsen injury to the ARDS-injured units. Therefore, the use of PEEP in combination with low tidal volumes is recommended as a lung-protective strategy to prevent further lung injury.

Lung-Protective Mechanical Ventilation Prevention Strategies

Lung-protective mechanical ventilation strategies can be used individually or in combination. Primary lung-protective strategies include the use of low tidal volumes (4–8 mL/kg of predicted or ideal body weight) and maintaining plateau pressures below 30 cmH$_2$O. Prone positioning for 12 hours or more per day has strong recommendations for use in patients with severe ARDS. Additionally, higher levels of PEEP along with alveolar recruitment maneuvers, are beneficial to patients with moderate to severe ARDS (Hoegl & Zwissler, 2017). Patients should be monitored for hypotension and general intolerance to these strategies. More and more research supports the use of lung-protective mechanical ventilation strategies for initial settings for all lung conditions (Esan et al., 2018; Fernando et al., 2021; NHLBI, 2008).

Initiating Noninvasive Positive Pressure Ventilation

After verifying the patient's indications and contraindications for NIPPV, selection of the most appropriate mask interface should be performed. A mask that is comfortable and maintains an adequate seal to the nose and/or mouth is most appropriate. Patient comfort and preference for a nose, mouth, or face mask should be a priority in the selection process to facilitate adherence to its use (in both inpatient and outpatient use of NIPPV).

Selecting the NIPPV modes can be performed during or just after the other steps with consideration of the patient's underlying problem. For instance, patients with cardiogenic pulmonary edema or acute exacerbation of COPD may benefit the most from initial BiPAP settings, whereas patients with suspected obstructive sleep apnea could benefit more from initial CPAP settings. The AGACNP initiating NIPPV should monitor the patient's tolerance, work of breathing, and overall response to this intervention. Evaluate the patient for the need to increase, decrease, or modify the mode of NIPPV settings before leaving the bedside.

Initial Settings

The standard of care for initiating NIPPV start with low inspiratory and/or expiratory pressures. For instance, initial CPAP settings may start at +8 to +10 cmH$_2$O and if BiPAP is initiated, initial expiratory pressures may start with +4 to +5 cmH$_2$O. When ordering NIPPV, orders with only an inspiratory pressure is CPAP and those written with an inspiratory pressure over an expiratory pressure (+8/+4) is BiPAP. Supplemental oxygen is titrated into the NIPPV tubing or mask to maintain oxygen saturation at or above the patient's goal.

Noninvasive Positive Pressure Ventilation Failure

The AGACNP must recognize when the patient fails NIPPV. Patients without improvement after 2 hours of NIPPV initiation should be stopped and escalated up to mechanical ventilation via tracheal intubation. Signs of NIPPV failure include poor improvement of oxygenation status upon ABG evaluation, persistent or worsened work of breathing, patient/ventilator dyssynchrony, or patient intolerance and desire to stop its use.

FOLLOW-UP MECHANICAL VENTILATION MANAGEMENT AND MONITORING

The follow-up management of patients being mechanically ventilated should focus on evaluating the patients' oxygenation status, work of breathing, and hemodynamic stability. Additionally, peak inspiratory and plateau pressures should also be monitored regularly to evaluate the patients' airway resistance and lung compliance. Increased PIP ($\geq$35 cmH$_2$O) suggests increased airway resistance. Patients sustaining increased PIP should be evaluated for increased dead space caused by ventilator tubing or the need for suctioning due to increased secretions or a mucus plug. Increased plateau pressures ($\geq$35 cmH$_2$O) reflects decreased lung compliance. Patients with increased plateau pressures should be evaluated for restrictive lung disease and alternative ventilation modes that help to reduce the risk for VILI (Hoegl & Zwissler, 2017).

Patients experiencing ventilator dyssynchrony can develop increased inspiratory pressures. If modifying the ventilator's settings does not help to facilitate patient/ventilator synchrony, sedation or paralysis should be considered. Plateau pressures should be kept below 30 cmH$_2$O to avoid VILI (Hoegl & Zwissler, 2017).

Noninvasive Positive Pressure Ventilation Monitoring

In addition to monitoring the patient's oxygenation status, work of breathing, and hemodynamic stability, patient synchrony with the NIPPV device should be monitored. Additionally, dysfunction of the device and patient tolerance should be reevaluated with follow-up encounters. Patients demonstrating improved ventilation and oxygenation should be evaluated for liberation from NIPPV support.

Complications

Ventilator-induced or -associated complications are considered iatrogenic injuries. Iatrogenic injuries are unintentional, healthcare-associated harm to patients that are not always preventable but can significantly increase patient morbidity and mortality. Complications associated with mechanical ventilation are listed in Box 7.12. The prevention of ventilator-associated complications hinges upon appropriate use of mechanical ventilatory support and the timely liberation from mechanical ventilation.

Ventilator-Induced Lung Injury

All patients requiring mechanical ventilation are at risk for VILI. VILI can be caused by increased volumes, increased pressures, or prolonged exposure to increased levels of supplemental oxygen. The mechanisms of injury can involve tissue rupture (pneumothorax), overdistention of lung tissue, respiratory muscle weakness (including diaphragm dysfunction), and/or an acute inflammatory response.

Dysphagia

The presence of dysphagia is an independent prognostic indicator for death in critically ill patients (Zuercher et al., 2020). Prolonged duration of invasive mechanical ventilation increases the patient's risk for dysphagia postextubation. Patients who experienced prolonged ventilator days may benefit from being screened for dysphagia before hospital discharge (Zuercher et al., 2020).

BOX 7.12: COMPLICATIONS ASSOCIATED WITH MECHANICAL VENTILATION

- Aspiration pneumonitis or pneumonia
- Cardiovascular compromise
- Critical illness polyneuropathy
- Gastrointestinal effects
  - Dysphagia
  - Stress-related ulcer
- Oxygen toxicity
- Patient/ventilator dyssynchrony
- Pulmonary trauma
  - Barotrauma (increased pulmonary pressure causes rupture)
  - Biotrauma (biological inflammatory response to disease)
  - Volutrauma (overdistention of alveoli)
- Tracheal/esophageal fistula
- Ventilator-associated pneumonia
- Ventilator-induced diaphragm dysfunction

Diaphragm Dysfunction

The development of diaphragm dysfunction is prevalent among mechanically ventilated patients and some researchers question if it is not more prevalent than critical illness polyneuropathy (Supinski et al., 2018). The clinical findings associated with this complication include abdominal paradox (inward sucking motion of the abdominal wall during inspiration), poor weaning despite clinical improvement of acute illness, the combination of good lung mechanics but an increased rapid shallow breathing index (RSBI), and unilateral or bilateral hemidiaphragm elevation visualized by chest radiograph. Additionally, patients presenting with hypercapneic respiratory failure and a clear chest radiograph should be evaluated for neuromuscular etiologies for diaphragm dysfunction that may or may not be related to mechanical ventilation (Supinski et al., 2018).

Mechanical ventilation and sedatives causing deep sedation are associated with the development of ventilator-induced diaphragm dysfunction (VIDD). Reducing sedatives, allowing spontaneous inspiratory efforts as early as possible, early mobility, and gradual liberation from mechanical ventilation contribute to full recovery of the diaphragm's function within hours. prolonged mechanical ventilation reduces the diaphragm's ability to recover rapidly and contributes to the reasons some patients are difficult to liberate from mechanical ventilation (Supinski et al., 2018).

DIAPHRAGM ULTRASOUND

Assessing the function of the diaphragm can be performed within seconds to minutes at the bedside with point-of-care ultrasound (POCUS). Diaphragm ultrasound is performed to predict successful liberation from mechanical ventilation or to assess for its dysfunction contributing to poor liberation efforts. The use of diaphragm ultrasound and RSBI together are more reliable predictors for successful liberation than either method alone (Kilaru et al., 2021).

Pharmacotherapeutic Considerations

Sedation and Neuromuscular Paralysis

Sedatives and neuromuscular blocking agents (NMB) agents should be considered for patients with ventilator dyssynchrony and to reduce the increased oxygen consumption associated with an increased work of breathing. When sedatives do not effectively lower the respiratory drive, NMB agents are required. Patients with multiorgan dysfunction or older adults should be recognized as having a higher risk for poor medication clearance, prolonged induced paralysis, and neuromuscular weakness post critical illness.

Dexmedetomidine is a superior sedative to propofol and benzodiazepines by having less association with drug-induced delirium, oversedation, or prolonged ventilator days. When benzodiazepines are needed, doses should be symptom-triggered using a validated agitation-sedation assessment tool. Patients receiving sedative infusions should be assessed for levels of agitation and sedation using validated tools such as the Richmond Agitation-Sedation Score (RASS). Deep sedation (RASS score of −3 or below) within the first 48 hours of mechanical ventilation were found to have delayed extubation times, prolonged need for mechanical ventilation and for tracheostomy placement, and higher mortality rates (Marra et al., 2017).

Pain Management

Pain management among the mechanically ventilated critically ill population is necessary to reduce physiologic and emotional stress. The assessment, prevention, and management of pain is particularly important for patients experiencing common surgical procedures (e.g., chest tube placement or removal, wound drain removal, vascular access device placement) or for patients who are recovering postoperatively.

Application of the ABCDEF Bundle

The ABCDEF Bundle (Table 7.18) is an evidence-based guideline recommending multiple interventions for the safe and effective management of patients with complex critical illness. The bundle recommends interventions for the assessment, prevention, and management of pain and delirium; assessment of patients ready for liberation from the mechanical ventilator; selection of sedatives; early mobility; and family engagement specifically for critically ill patient populations (Marra et al., 2017). Use of this bundle is indicated for patients who are mechanically ventilated and facilitates improved quality and safety outcomes when used effectively.

Liberation From Mechanical Ventilation

Liberating patients from mechanical ventilation should be an early management goal. The term "liberation" can be used synonymously with weaning or discontinuing mechanical ventilation. Prolonged mechanical ventilation is associated with multiple short- and long-term complications. Once the disease process begins to improve, liberation planning should begin. The practitioner should assess the patient's readiness for liberation by performing daily spontaneous awakening trials (SAT) and spontaneous breathing trials (SBTs). Before performing the trials, the patient must demonstrate readiness for spontaneous breathing (see Box 7.13; Esan et al., 2018).

Spontaneous Awakening Trial

Performing a SAT involves stopping the use of narcotics (when pain is controlled) and sedatives to improve spontaneous inspiratory effort. If the medications have to be restarted, they should be resumed at half of the dose or the dose required to maintain light sedation and adequate pain control. The SAT should be performed daily and before the SBT is attempted. Daily interruption of sedation is associated with the prevention of oversedation and prolonged mechanical ventilation (Marra et al., 2017). A collaborative effort is achieved between the critical care nurse, respiratory therapist, and pulmonary specialist to coordinate and communicate the patient's needs and performance.

Spontaneous Breathing Trial

Performing a SBT should be performed after all indications for SBT noted in Box 7.13 are achieved and after the

TABLE 7.18: Brief Descriptions of the ABCDEF Bundle

A	**A**ssess, Prevent, and Manage Pain	*Assess* with a validated tool *Prevent* with preprocedural dosing or regional anesthesia *Manage* with appropriate opioid, nonopioid, and nonpharmacologic methods
B	**B**oth Spontaneous Awakening (SAT) and Breathing Trials (SBT)	SAT: Stop narcotics and sedatives if pain is managed, daily SBT: Perform daily after SAT
C	**C**hoice of Analgesia and Sedation	Measure agitation and sedation with validated tools Dexmedetomidine was superior to benzodiazepines Use a symptom-triggered approach to sedation
D	**D**elirium: Assess, Prevent, and Manage	*Assess* with a validated tool *Prevent* with risk stratification, reduce benzodiazepine use, improve sleep hygiene, and mobilize early *Manage* with prophylactic strategies and cautious use of haloperidol
E	**E**arly Mobility	Increase physical activity during ICU stay with physical therapy, occupational therapy, getting out of bed, and ambulation. Better outcomes when combined with SAT
F	**F**amily Engagement	Incorporate family wishes, concerns, questions, and participation during rounds, palliative care meetings, and resuscitative efforts

Source: Marra, A., Ely, E. W., Pandharipande, P. P., & Patel, M. B. (2017). The ABCEDF bundle in critical care. *Critical Care Clinics, 33*(2), 225–243. https://doi.org/10.1016/j.ccc.2016.12.005

BOX 7.13: INDICATIONS FOR SPONTANEOUS BREATHING TRIAL

- Partial or complete recovery of the lung disease process
- Adequate oxygenation with PEEP ≤8 cmH$_2$O and FiO$_2$ ≤0.5
- PaO$_2$:FiO$_2$ ratio greater than 200
- pH ≥7.25
- Hemodynamic stability with minimal vasopressor support
- Presence of spontaneous inspiratory effort

BOX 7.14: SIGNS OF SPONTANEOUS BREATHING TRIAL FAILURE

- Sustained respiratory rate ≥35 breaths per minute
- Decreased oxygen saturation ≤90%
- Increased systolic blood pressure ≥180 mmHg
- Increased heart rate ≥140 beats per minute
- Increased anxiety or diaphoresis

SAT (Esan et al., 2018; Marra et al., 2017). Additionally, patients that are acutely hospitalized and mechanically ventilated more than 24 hours can have SBT performed. Ventilator liberation guidelines recommend a SBT be performed with 5 to 8 cmH$_2$O of inspiratory PS in the setting of minimal to no sedation use and early mobility rehabilitation protocols. The guidelines also recommend extubation to NIPPV for patients who passed the SBT but remain high risk for extubation failure. The use of a ventilator liberation protocol is recommended for standardized and goal-directed care of all mechanically ventilated patients (Schmidt et al., 2017).

SPONTANEOUS BREATHING TRIAL FAILURE

Patients that fail the SBT can be returned to the previously tolerated level of ventilator support and retried daily. Signs of SBT failure are listed in Box 7.14. Patients that persistently fail SBTs should be evaluated for tracheostomy placement for prolonged mechanical ventilation and gradual liberation strategies with rehabilitative interventions. Patients with orotracheal intubation longer than 21 days are at high risk for tracheal and esophageal complications (Esan et al., 2018).

Extubation Failure

Some patients may fail extubation despite passing the SBT. Extubation failure often occurs within the first 24 to 72 hours postextubation secondary to upper airway obstruction or the inability of patients to protect their own airway postextubation. Upper airway obstruction can occur with postextubation stridor or poor cough effort and ineffective clearance of secretions. A cuff leak test can help to assess the patient's airway patency and risk for postextubation upper airway obstruction. The suc-

cessful completion of a SBT, a patent upper airway, and the patient's ability to protect their own airway are good predictors of extubation success (Esan et al., 2018).

KEY TAKEAWAYS

- Respiratory failure is the primary indication for mechanical ventilation.
- NIPPV should be initiated early in patients with COPD or cardiogenic pulmonary edema and acute respiratory distress.
- NIPPV should not be initiated in the patient with an altered mental status or inability to protect their own airway.
- Mechanical ventilators can control the triggers, limits, and termination of breaths with and without synchronizing to the patient's spontaneous efforts.
- Mechanical ventilators can synchronize mandatory breaths to the patient's inspiratory efforts to help avoid patient/ventilator dyssynchrony.
- Lung protective strategies benefit all lung conditions requiring mechanical ventilation.
- Prevent and monitor patients for the development of ventilator-associated complications.
- The ABCDEF bundle has multiple evidence-based interventions proven to improve the outcomes of mechanically ventilated patients.
- Nonpulmonary specialty practice requires the knowledge and skills needed for the initiation and basic management of invasive and noninvasive mechanical ventilation.

EVIDENCE-BASED RESOURCES

Schmidt, G. A., Girard, T. D., Kress, J. P., Morris, P. E., Ouellette, D. R., Alhazzani, W., Burns, S. M., Epstein, S. K., Esteban, A., Fan, E., Ferrer, M., Fraser, G. L., Gong, M. N., Hough, C. L., Mehta, S., Nanchal, R., Patel, S., Pawlik, A. J., Schweickert, W. D., … Truwit, J. D. (2017). Libertation from mechanical ventilation in critically ill adults: Executive summary of an official American College of Chest Physicians/American Thoracic Society clinical practice guideline. *Chest, 151*(1), 160–165. http://doi.org/10.1016/j.chest.2016.10.037

National Heart, Lung, and Blood Institute ARDS Network. (2008). *NIH NHLBI ARDS clinical network mechanical ventilation protocol summary.* http://www.ardsnet.org/files/ventilator_protocol_2008-07.pdf

7.10: PULMONARY FUNCTION TESTS

Whitney Haley

Pulmonary function tests (PFTs) are a diagnostic modality utilized to identify various underlying disorders of the lung. Clinicians may request PFTs to be performed on patients that present with respiratory symptoms such as dyspnea, cough, hypoxia, wheezing, or with abnormal CXR findings. PFTs can be utilized to diagnose underlying restrictive or obstructive lung disease and are often used to trend disease progression and response to initiated therapies. Additionally, PFTs are a method to monitor patients who are receiving medications with a risk of pulmonary toxicity or as a screening method prior to surgery. Testing is composed of three testing modalities: spirometry, body plethysmygography, and diffusing capacity of carbon monoxide. These three phases of testing provide quantitative information regarding air flow and volume of air at various phases of the respiratory cycle. Figure 7.1 demonstrates the various volumes obtained during a set of PFTs, and these volumes will be discussed throughout this text.

Spirometry

Spirometry provides information regarding flow in and out of the lung over time. It can be utilized alone to diagnose obstructive lung disease and can suggest patterns of restrictive disease as well. Tidal volume (TV), forced vital capacity (FVC), and forced expiratory volume (FEV_1) can be obtained with spirometry alone. TV is the amount of air the lung takes in and out with normal respiration. FVC is the amount of air forced out of the lung with maximum forceful exhalation. FEV_1 is the amount of air exhaled from the lung in the first second during a forced exhalation. Each of these volumes may be altered from the expected normal range with lung disease. Healthy individuals release 75% of the air from the lung over the first second during a forced exhalation (Corbridge, 2019). FEV_1/FVC ratios less than 0.7 are indicative of an obstructive lung disease. Clinicians can provide a diagnosis of COPD when $FEV_{1/F}VC$ ratios remain <0.7 after administration of a bronchodilator. Reversibility of obstruction after administration of a bronchodilator is diagnostic for asthma, although with well-controlled asthma, FEV_1/FVC ratios may be normal (Corbridge, 2019). A normal FEV_1/FVC ratio with a low FVC is suggestive of restriction such as interstitial lung diseases or neuromuscular disease. This can be explained by the inability of the lung to fully expand.

Spirometry will provide two visual grafts plotting patient results: flow-volume loop and volume-time curve. A flow-volume loop is created by plotting a maximum inhalation effort followed by maximum exhalation effort. Knowledge of a normal loop appearance aids in determining where issues arise within a respiratory cycle (Ranu et al., 2011). Abnormalities during inhalation phase of the loop may suggest upper airway pathologies such as tumor or obstruction. Exhalation abnormalities may suggest obstructive or restrictive disease processes.

Figures 7.2 and 7.3 demonstrate the exhalation phase of normal, obstructive, and restrictive lung diseases.

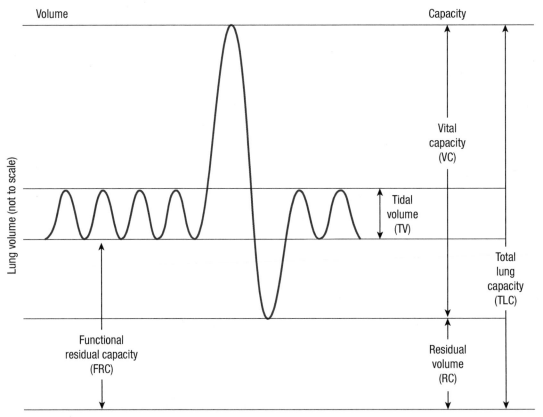

FIGURE 7.1: Diagram of lung volumes and capacities.

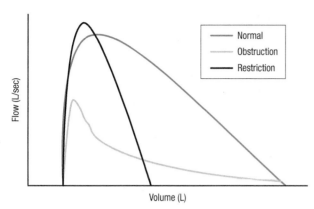

FIGURE 7.2: Exhalation phase of normal, obstructive, and restrictive lung diseases.

Noted in the obstruction tracing is the slowed rate of flow in addition to the increased lung volume as a result of air trapping compared to higher flow rates in a healthy lung. Obstructive pattern tracings appear to have a concave appearance due to slowed flow rates. The restrictive disease tracing, however, has adequate flow rates but lower lung volumes both during inhalation and exhalation. Tracings of restrictive lung disease often appear narrower and peaked.

Volume/time curves are also valuable data derived from spirometry. Again, knowledge of a normal appearing curve pattern aids in identifying where abnormalities arise, and a clinician may more easily identify potential diagnoses. Figure 7.4 demonstrates a normal respiratory tracing in which the largest volume of air is exhaled within the first second. Due to obstructive airflow, COPD and asthma will have a sloping or ramp appearance on the volume/time curve. Restrictive lung disease patterns will follow the pattern of normal flow; however, once again decreased volumes will be noted.

Body Plethysmography

Body plethysmography is performed in an air-tight box and provides information about static lung volumes. Alternatively, helium dilution and nitrogen washout methods can provide these values when body plethysmography is unavailable (Ranu et al., 2011). Residual volume (RV), total lung capacity (TLC), vital capacity (VC), and functional residual capacity (FRC) are values obtained by this method. RV is the amount of air left in the lungs after maximal exhalation. Abnormally elevated RV and TLC are helpful in identifying obstructive lung disease and contrary, low volumes are associated with restrictive disorders. Patients with obstructive disease may have an increased RV due to decreased ability of air to be removed from the lung. FRC is the remaining air in the lung after a normal exhalation. As previously noted, in a patient with well-controlled asthma, spirometry results may have normal FEV_1 and FVC values. RV becomes helpful in diagnosis of asthma in these scenarios as results will be higher than the predicted volumes. Ad-

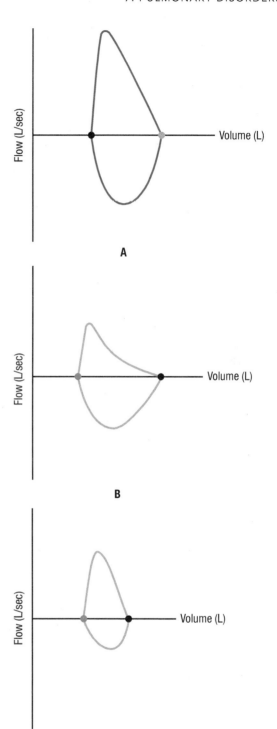

FIGURE 7.3: Exhalation phase of normal (A), obstructed (B), and restricted (C) airflow volume.

ditionally, RV is important in preventing complete lung collapse after exhalation. TLC is the total amount of air in the lungs after maximal inhalation and will often be low in restrictive disease processes due to the inability

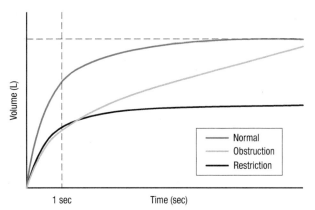

FIGURE 7.4: Respiratory tracing in which the largest volume of air is exhaled within the first second.

of the lungs to fill appropriately. Contrarily, obstructive diseases will present with increased TLC secondary to the increased amount of air trapping. Vital capacity (VC) is the difference in volume between TLC and RV.

Diffusion Capacity

Diffusion capacity of carbon monoxide (DLCO) provides information regarding alveolar membrane integrity and alveolar membrane surface area (Ranu et al., 2011). Alterations in DLCO may arise as a result of diseases affecting the alveoli themselves, such as emphysema and interstitial lung disease (due to increased interstitial thickness, or secondary to diseases that affect the pulmonary vascular bed such as pulonary hypertension [PH] due to capillary volume loss). DLCO is measured by having a patient inhale a concentration of helium and carbon monoxide (CO) and exhale after 10 seconds. At that time the remaining CO is measured providing data regarding the diffusion of CO across the membrane. Conditions that weaken the integrity of alveoli or pulmonary vascular bed will impede the ability of CO to diffuse across the membrane. CO has a high affinity for hemoglobin, and in healthy individuals should be up taken with inhalation. Because of this high affinity, underlying anemia may present as a low DLCO on PFT testing. A decreased DLCO will be seen in conditions such as interstitial lung disease, emphysema, pulmonary vascular disease, or anemia. Less commonly, DLCO may also be increased in conditions that increase the availability of hemoglobin at the alveolar bed such as polycythemia.

7.11: PLEURAL EFFUSION

Sherry Rivera

PRESENTING SIGNS AND SYMPTOMS

More than 1.5 million people experience pleural effusions annually in the United States. The presentation of pleural effusions varies depending on the severity and etiology of disease. Congestive heart failure, malignancy, and bacterial pneumonia are the most common causes of pleural effusions (Kosowsky & Kimberly, 2018). Presenting symptoms can range from being asymptomatic to severe respiratory distress. Patients commonly experience dull or pleuritic chest pain, dyspnea, or nonproductive cough. Other signs and symptoms specific to the underlying disease may be present.

HISTORY AND PHYSICAL FINDINGS

Obtaining the patient's history is an important aspect of narrowing down the list of potential etiologies. Identifying risk factors associated with malignancy, infections, and trauma should be included. A thorough evaluation of symptoms and physical exam findings associated with competing diagnoses is also important. The physical exam should focus on the identification of the pleural effusion, determining potential etiology for development of pleural effusion and elimination of potential competing diagnoses. A thorough exam of the chest should be conducted. Bulging in the intercostal spaces or contralateral shift of the trachea may be identified upon inspection of the chest and neck. Dullness to percussion and reduced tactile fremitus may be present with large effusions. Crackles, decreased or absent breath sounds may be noted over the location of the effusion. Other physical exam findings are dependent upon underlying etiology. Respiratory assessment should be determined upon presentation and following any interventional procedures.

DIFFERENTIAL DIAGNOSIS AND DIAGNOSTIC CONSIDERATIONS

Pleural effusions can be caused by a wide variety of benign and life-threatening conditions. A thorough history and physical exam is especially important to evaluate when differentiating among potential competing diagnoses. Congestive heart failure, cirrhosis, hypothyroidism, hypoalbuminemia, nephrotic syndrome, pulmonary embolism (PE), connective tissue diseases, inflammatory diseases, metastatic disease, infections, and metastatic lesions should be included in the list of potential differential diagnoses. Confirmation of diagnosis should prompt identification of etiology. The main categories of etiologies include transudative, exudative, parapneumonic, malignant, hemothorax, and medication induced. Medications that are associated with the development of pleural effusions include cytotoxic agents, nitrofurantoin, and antimigraine medications.

Diagnostic Testing

Chest radiography, ultrasound, or CT should be completed when a pleural effusion is suspected. Visualization on chest radiography depends on the position of the patient, volume, and the location of the effusion. Small fluid collections may escape detection on an erect PA chest radiograph (Verschakelen et al., 2021). Classic findings include blunting of the costophrenic angle and occurs as the effusion increases in size (200–500 mL; Kosowsky & Kimberly, 2018). Chest CT is helpful when determining etiology, identifying loculated effusions, and differentiating between pleural thickening and effusions. Detection of small pleural effusions is best identified using CT. Thoracic ultrasound is a more sensitive diagnostic tool and is useful for identifying size, location, septations, adhesions, and guidance for thoracentesis.

Thoracentesis is used for diagnostic purposes, symptomatic relief for large volume effusions, and in the presence of cardiac and/or respiratory decompensation due to pleural effusion. Small volume thoracentesis of 50 to 100 mL is indicated to facilitate identification of etiology. A small volume aspiration is indicated if the etiology of a pleural effusion has not been identified previously and the effusion is larger than 1 cm on a decubitus view of a chest radiograph. Thoracentesis is not indicated if a patient has transudative pleural effusions bilaterally unless atypical features are present or unresponsive to treatment (Saguil et al., 2014). In the presence of pneumonia, a pleural effusion larger than 5 cm on a lateral chest radiograph is an indication for further treatment such as chest thoracotomy tube placement, fluid analysis, and IV antimicroabial therapy (Saguil et al., 2014).

Fluid aspirate should be sent for protein, lactate dehydrogenase levels (LDH), Gram staining, cultures, cytology, pH levels, and glucose levels. Cell counts demonstrating lymphocytosis suggest tuberculosis, lymphoma, malignancy, or PE. Cell counts with a predominance of neutrophils suggest bacterial infection and occasionally malignancy. Fluid aspirate cultures that are positive can assist with selecting antimicrobial treatment. Effusions due to parapneumonic causes, malignancies, rheumatoid, acidosis, and tuberculosis commonly have a pH less than 7.3. A pH less than 7.0 is suggestive of empyema or esophageal rupture (Kosowsky & Kimberly, 2018). Light's criteria can be useful to differentiate transudative and exudative effusions (Table 7.19). Light's criteria is the gold standard for classifying pleural effusions (Beaudoin & Gonzalez, 2018) Transudative pleural effusions have a pleural to serum LDH ratio of less than 0.6 or a total protein ratio less than 0.5. Exudative pleural effusions have a pleural to serum LDH ratio greater than or equal to 0.6 or a total protein ratio greater than or equal to 0.5. Elevated amylase levels can occur with diseases of the pancreas, malignancy, and esophageal rupture. Tumor, traumatic injury, or infarction should be considered if gross blood is present (Saguil et al., 2014).

TREATMENT

Treatment is dependent upon etiology and severity of symptoms. Treatment of the underlying condition is an important component of management. Treatment options can include thoracentesis, tube thoracostomy, indwelling tunneled catheter, pleurodesis, and pharma-

TABLE 7.19: Transudative Versus Exudative Effusions

TRANSUDATIVE	EXUDATIVE
Cirrhosis	Asbestosis
Congestive heart failure	Chylothorax
Constrictive pericarditis	Esophageal perforation
Fluid overload	Infection
Glomerulonephritis	Lung cancer
Hypoalbuminemia	Lymphoma
Myxedema	Mesothelioma
Nephrotic syndrome	Pancreatitis
Peritoneal dialysis	Pulmonary embolism
Pulmonary embolism	Radiation
	Rheumatoid arthritis
	Sarcoidosis
	Status postcoronary artery bypass graft
	Systemic lupus erythematosus
	Trauma
	Uremia
	Wegener's granulomatosis

Source: Light, R. W., Macgregor, M. I., Luchsinger, P. C., & Ball, W. C. (1972). Pleural effusions: The diagnostic separation of transudates and exudates. *Annals of Internal Medicine, 77*(4), 507–513. https://doi.org/10.7326/0003-4819-77-4-507

cotherapeutics. The benefits and risks associated with thoracentesis should be evaluated on an individual basis. Thoracentesis should be considered for new or unexplained pleural effusions with at least a 10-mm layer of fluid present on radiograph findings (Murthy, 2021; Verschakelen et al., 2021). Contraindications to thoracentesis include adhesions, coagulopathy, and bleeding disorders (Kosowsky & Kimberly, 2018). Therapeutic thoracentesis is utilized in the presence of acute respiratory or cardiovascular distress (Murthy, 2021).

Parapneumonic effusions and empyema should be treated empirically with antibiotics (Murthy, 2021). Antibiotic treatment decisions should be determined based on the patient's age, underlying comorbid conditions, probable organisms and sensitivities commonly identified within a given community while culture results are pending (Murthy, 2021). Complicated parapneumonic effusions within the hospital setting should be treated with IV antibiotics until the patient is afebrile and clinical status is improved (Murthy, 2021; Verschakelen et al., 2021). Chest radiographs should be evaluated postthoracentesis to evaluate for complications. Referral to pulmonology should be considered if the workup is inconclusive or if thoracentesis is ineffective.

TRANSITION OF CARE

Interactions with patients with pleural effusions can occur in the emergent, inpatient, and outpatient settings. Patients may present to the emergency department due to an acute onset of symptoms related to pleural effusion or due to progression of a chronic condition. Diagnostic workup findings should be communicated with all providers to ensure consistency of management and treatment. Some patients may transition home with a chest tube and should receive extensive education regarding self-management, troubleshooting, and when to seek medical attention.

CLINICAL PEARLS

- Point-of-care ultrasound is an effective method to identify and visualize pleural effusions.
- Patients should be informed of risks associated with pleural effusions and associated with treatment.

KEY TAKEAWAYS

- Congestive heart failure, malignancy, and bacterial pneumonia are the most common causes of pleural effusions.
- The presence of a pleural effusion should prompt an investigation to determine the underlying etiology.
- Thoracentesis can be used for diagnostic purposes and to alleviate symptoms.

EVIDENCE-BASED RESOURCES

British Thoracic Society. (2010). BTS pleural disease guideline 2010. *Journal of the British Thoracic Society, 65*(Suppl. 2), ii1–ii76.

Feller-Kopman, D. J., Reddy, C. B., DeCamp, M. M., Diekemper, R. L., Gould, M. K., Henry, T., Iyer, N. P., Lee, G., Lewis, S. Z., Maskell, N. A., Rahman, N. M., Sterman, D. H., Wahidi, M. M., & Balekian, A. A. (2018). Management of malignant pleural effusions. *American Thoracic Society, 198*(7), 839–849.

7.12: PULMONARY ARTERIAL HYPERTENSION

Cathy McAtee

Pulmonary arterial hypertension (PAH) is an umbrella term used to describe a group of pathologies that emanate from multiple etiologies. Regardless of the underlying cause, all types of PAH have elevated pulmonary artery pressures and flow restrictions secondary to pathological narrowing of the lumen of the arteries. This results in a reduced cross-section of vascular area for blood flow (Humbert et al., 2014). These etiologies can range from idiopathic, genetic mutations, congenital heart disease (CHD), connective tissue disease, drugs, toxins, or the sequelae of infectious diseases. PAH is classified by the World Health Organization (WHO) and currently, PAH is classified as group 1 of the five distinct types of pulmonary hypertension in WHO's clinical classification system (Simonneau et al., 2019, p. 1).

The inflammatory cascade promotes remodeling, endothelial proliferation, and vasoconstriction of the distal pulmonary arteries. Pulmonary arterial hypertension (PAH) is progressive over time and if untreated usually results in right ventricular heart failure and death (Nickel et al., 2012), making diagnosis and treatment a high clinical priority.

Data from all major global PAH registries indicate that prevalence and incidence vary significantly across the world with schistosomiasis being the primary cause of PAH in endemic regions affecting 230 million persons of which 5% may progress to develop schistosomiasis-associated PAH (Sch-PAH). In North America idiopathic PAH (I-PAH) accounts for more than 50% of all cases of PAH. Although Sch-PAH and I-PAH share similar features, Sch-PAH related disease has better hemodynamic profiles and life expectancy (Knafl et al., 2020, p. 2). In the United States the REVEAL (Registry to Evaluate Early and Long-Term PA Disease Management) trial would indicate a mean survival of 2.8 years in idiopathic/heritable PAH and 7 years for other types of PAH (McGoon et al., 2013, p. D53). Women were predominantly affected (79.8%) and 32.5% had a BMI >30 and were older (44.9 years) at the time of diagnosis.

Consideration of newer evidence-based guidelines can assist the AGACNP in proper PH classification, diagnostic workup, referral to specialty centers for targeted PAH therapy, and multidisciplinary approach to management. A better understanding of PAH criteria should ultimately reduce the incidence of over- and under-treatment of PAH (Simonneau et al., 2019, p. 4).

PATHOGENESIS

Congenital Heart Disease

There is a strong correlation between congenital heart disease (CHD) defect size and development of PAH pathophysiology secondary to vasoconstriction, intimal proliferation fibrosis, remodeling of the vascular bed with deposition of smooth muscle in the periphery of pulmonary arteries, medial wall hypertrophy, ventricular hypertrophy, and ventricular fibrosis. Eisenmenger syndrome is a long-term complication of CHD with some improvement in PAH after surgical correction of the congenital defect. Approximately 6% of CHD-PAH patients will have concurrent mutations in the bone morphogenetic protein receptor type II (*BMPR2*) gene (Pascall & Tulloh, 2018).

Idiopathic Pulmonary Hypertension

Although the underlying etiology of I-PAH is unknown, the natural progression of the disease relates to endothelial damage, smooth muscle hypertrophy, vasoconstriction, local hypercoagulability, plexiform remodeling, and endothelial injury related to inflammatory cytokines. This vascular damage interferes with nitric oxide synthesis promoting further vasoconstriction in the vessel. Of the serum biomarkers present in I-PAH such as tumor necrosis factor-alpha, interferon-gamma, and interleukin 6, interleukin 6 levels corresponded to increased mortality (Radchenko et al., 2020). This panvasculopathy occurs affecting all layers of the PA to include intimal hyperplasia, medial hypertrophy, and proliferation of the adventitia in small arterioles (Goldman & Schafer, 2012).

Heritable Pulmonary Artery Hypertension

A genetic predisposition has been recognized as an important factor in PAH and felt to be related to the *BMPR2* gene in over 70% of cases of heritable PAH (H-PAH; Goldman & Schafer, 2012). This genetic mutation shows autosomal dominance, variable expressivity, reduced penetrance with female dominance noted (Chew et al., 2017) There are multiple other mutations with an activin receptor like kinase 1 (*ALK-1*) and endoglin (*ENG*) that are seen concomitantly with PAH accompanied by hemorrhagic telangiectasia (Humbert et al., 2014).

Drug-Toxin Induced Pulmonary Arterial Hypertension

WHO has recognized 16 compounds that have been associated with an acquired form of PAH after drug exposure. This list is not inclusive of FDA-approved medications but also includes illicit recreational stimulants. The pathology of drug-toxin induced PAH (D-PAH) is similar to other PAH etiologies, and it responds accordingly to the palliative effects of PAH pharmacologic and supportive care strategies aimed at slowing progression and improving symptoms. The first drug clearly linked to D-PAH was taken off the market in 1973, but other anorexinogens used for weight loss followed. Drugs and substances that induce D-PAH are aminorex, fenfluramine, dexfenfluramine, benfluorex, and some SSRIs. Illicit drugs that are classified as likely or possible are cocaine, methamphetamine, amphetamines, phenylpropanolamine, interferon alpha and beta, L-tryptophan, dasatanib, and St. John's wort (Orcholoski et al., 2018).

Schistosomiasis-Related Pulmonary Arterial Hypertension

Schistosomiasis-related PAH (SCH-PAH) is caused by parasitic flat worms common in tropical climates and is a complication of hepato-splenic schistosomiasis (Knafl et al., 2020). These blood flukes can penetrate the skin of mammals causing both acute and chronic disease that primarily affects the liver and lungs of the host. Humans can become infected by three Schistosoma species, but *S. mansoni* has been implicated in most cases of human SCH-PAH disease. Eggs of flukes are embolized to the pulmonary artery by portosystemic shunts causing both mechanical obstruction and inflammation which contribute to vascular remodeling through inflammatory cytokines and other mediators (Sibomana et al., 2020).

Connective Tissue Disease

Connective tissue disease-related PAH (CTD-PAH) commonly referred to as systemic sclerosis (SSc-PAH) is a group of diseases such as scleroderma, rheumatoid arthritis, systemic lupus erythematosus (SLE), and mixed connective tissue diseases that are the result of the changes of the pulmonary vasculature and parenchyma related to the underlying autoimmune pathology. These CTDs are a major cause of group 1 PAH and comprise 25% of the total PAH population. The treatment algorithm for SSc-PAH is similar to that of I-PAH (Vonk et al., 2020).

Human Immunodeficiency Viral Infections Pulmonary Arterial Hypertension

Human immunodeficiency viral infections PAH (HIV-PAH) promotes an increase in growth factor expression in T-cell lymphocytes that contributes to HIV-PAH vasculopathy by increasing endothelial proliferation (Ascerl et al., 1999). Treatment of HIV-PH is like other forms of PAH (Goldman & Schafer, 2012).

Portal hypertension-PAH in the setting of portal hypertension is referred to as POPH-PAH and is indistinguishable from other types of PAH pathologically. Palliative treatment is identical to other forms of PAH, but also includes liver transplant (Thomas et al., 2020). The POPH-PAH syndrome occurs in 5% to 10% of patients awaiting liver transplant, and coincidentally 2% to 6% of patients with portal hypertension progress to concurrent PAH (Goldman & Schafer, 2012).

PRESENTING SIGNS AND SYMPTOMS

Regardless of PAH etiology the most common patient complaint is dyspnea with exertion which may progress to dyspnea at rest over time. PAH patients also report angina, hemoptysis, exercise intolerance, syncope, lightheadedness, palpitations, edema, and fatigue (Goldman & Schafer, 2012; Pascall & Tulloh, 2018).

HISTORY AND PHYSICAL FINDINGS

PAH patients generally complain of symptoms such as dyspnea, fatigue, and weight gain that have worsened over time. Sch-PAH patients may report remote travel with occupational, domestic, or recreational use of schistosomiasis-contaminated bodies of water in tropical areas (Sibomana et al., 2020). Obese clients may report previous use of anorexinogens for weight loss. Patients or caregivers may report congenital heart defects and CV surgery as an infant.

Physical exam findings can be described as either early or late (Table 7.20). Late physical findings would be consistent with symptoms of right ventricular heart failure (Goldman & Schafer, 2012; Pascall & Tulloh, 2018).

TABLE 7.20: Physical Exam Findings in Pulmonary Artery Hypertension

EARLY ASSESSMENT FINDINGS	LATE ASSESSMENT FINDINGS
Loud S2 Pansystolic murmur (tricuspid valve) Parasternal lift S4 (right ventricle) Tachypnea	Ascites Clubbing of the nail Cool extremities Diminished pulse pressure Hepatomegaly Jugular venous distention Labored breathing Low SaO$_2$ Nail bed cyanosis Peripheral edema S3 (right ventricle)

DIFFERENTIAL DIAGNOSIS AND DIAGNOSTIC CONSIDERATIONS

Normally the pulmonary artery pressures have 1/10 the resistance to flow when compared with the systemic vascular system (Goldman & Schafer, 2012). Historically a mean pulmonary artery pressure above 25 mmHg at rest has long been considered diagnostic of pulmonary hypertension, but current recommendations from the World Symposium on Pulmonary Hypertension suggest that 20 mmHg at rest in a patient who is supine is diagnostic for pulmonary hypertension. A series of other hemodynamic parameters from right heart catherization and a mandatory cardiac output (CO) are recommended to exclude left heart causes of elevated pulmonary artery pressures such as pulmonary artery wedge pressure (PAWP) <15 and PVR >3 Woods units (WU; Sibomana et al., 2020; Simonneau et al., 2019).

Diagnostic Tests

A diagnostic workup would proceed with a least invasive to highest invasive procedures in a progressive manner. Expertise is needed in the assessment of suspected CHD-PAH in a center of excellence with a multidisciplinary approach to include cardiothoracic surgery (Table 7.21).

Laboratory Tests

There are multiple laboratory tests that may help the AGACNP further classify the PAH type. If there is a high degree of suspicion for Sch-PAH, a stool for ova and parasites would be indicated (Sibomana et al., 2020). For patients exhibiting signs and symptoms consistent with a connective tissue disease such as skin changes, sclerodactyly, hair loss, Raynaud's phenomena, dysphagia, and acid reflux, an antinuclear antibody test would be the first screening test for autoimmune diseases. An NT-proBNP would be assessed on all patients who have symptoms of heart failure (Goldman & Schafer, 2012).

TABLE 7.21: Diagnostic Tests for Pulmonary Arterial Hypertension

DIAGNOSTIC TEST	INDICATION	ASSESSMENT RATIONALE
EKG	All forms of suspected PAH	Right axis deviation RV enlargement RV strain pattern
Chest x-ray	All forms of suspected PAH	Enlarged proximal pulmonary arteries Peripheral tapering of pulmonary vasculature Reduction in retrosternal air space
Full pulmonary function test with diffusions	All forms of suspected PAH	Exclude other etiologies and establish a baseline
Echocardiogram	All forms of suspected PAH	Rule out left heart disease Flattening of intraventricular septum Estimated RV pressures
Overnight oximetry	All forms of suspected PAH	Rule out obstructive sleep apnea
6-minute walk	All forms of suspected PAH	Establish a baseline
Genetic testing	CTD-PAH, PPHN	Positive ANA Positive mutation
HIV, ANA, LFT	Suspected HIV-PAH, CTD-PAH, Sch-PAH	Positive ANA Elevated LFT Positive HIV
Ultrasound abdomen	Sch-PAH	Hepatomegaly Splenomegaly Peri-portal fibrosis Left lobe enlargement
High resolution CT	CTD-PAH, CHD-PAH	PA measurements PA: aorta ratio
Cardiac MRI	CHD-PAH	Clarify anatomy Extracardiac communications Severity of impairment
Right heart catheterization	High suspicion of PAH	Gold standard for definitive diagnosis for all forms of PAH

ANA, antinuclear antibodies; CHD, congenital heart disease; CTD, connective tissue disorder; LFT, liver function test; PA, pulmonary artery; PAH, pulmonary arterial hypertension; PPHN, persistent pulmonary hypertension in the neonate; RV, right ventricle; Sch, schistosomiasis-associated arterial hypertension.

Source: Data from Goldman, L., & Schafer, A. I. (2012). *Goldman's Cecil medicine* (24th ed.). Elsevier Saunders; Pascall, E., & Tulloh, R. M. (2018, May 24). Pulmonary hypertension in congenital heart disease. *Future Cardiology, 14,* 343–353. https://doi.org/10.2217/fca-2017-0065

TREATMENT

Treatment for PAH is not curative but has a significant impact on slowing the progression of disease. These medications are typically focused on intervening in the four major pathways implicated in the pathophysiology of the disease. These pathways include the nitric oxide cyclic guanosine monophosphate signaling pathway (NO-cG-MP), endothelin signaling pathway (ET), calcium channel signaling pathway, and prostacyclin (PGI_2) pathway. NO-cGMP targeted therapies all increase cGMP that relax smooth muscle and have been shown to improve symptoms, functional status, and hemodynamic profiles. Examples of NO-cGMP include inhaled nitric oxide, cGMP agonists (riociguat), phosphodiesterase (PDE5) inhibitors (sildenafil and tadalafil), ET-1 receptor antagonists (Bosentan and ambrisentan) and also show significant improvement in symptoms. Calcium channel blockers (CCB) are used to treat the calcium channel pathway with long-acting nifedipine, and diltiazem preferred over verapamil secondary to verapamil's negative inotropic effects. PGI_2 and its analogs are effective in promoting dilation of the pulmonary arteries in idiopathic PAH and may have other disease modifying properties. Multiple drugs are available globally. These drugs include epoprostenol (synthetic PGI_2), treprostinil, beraprost and iloprost (PHI_2 analogs), and an I prostanoid receptor antagonist (selexapag). These drugs are available in multiple formulations of IV, SC, inhaled, and oral drugs that can inhibit the proliferation of smooth muscle and platelet aggregation delaying progression of symptoms (Woodcock & Chen, 2019). The treatment of PPHN is pulmonary vasodilators such as inhaled nitric oxide and ECMO (Distefano & Sciacca, 2015).

Supportive Therapies

Therapies such as salt restriction, supplemental oxygen to maintain oxygen saturation >90%, and exercise significantly improve quality of life. Vaccines for influenza and pneumococcal pneumonia should be administered to prevent concomitant disease.

Women with PAH are strongly encouraged to use contraception, as pregnancy is related to substantial increases in mortality. Diuretics can improve symptoms for right ventricular failure through diuresis. Digoxin improves right ventricular contractility and symptoms of right heart failure. If anticoagulation is warranted warfarin is preferred in I-PAH and H-PAH with target INR levels of 1.5 to 2.5 (Thenappan et al., 2018).

CLINICAL PEARLS

- Although etiologies for PAH differ, vasodilator and supportive care therapies will help in all cases except for PPHN organic type.

KEY TAKEAWAYS

- Pulmonary hypertension is a disease that requires a highly specialized multidisciplinary approach for disease management.
- AGACNPs should use a stepwise approach in testing and refer patients early in the disease process to specialty centers for targeted PAH therapy.

7.13: PULMONARY EMBOLISM

Sherry Rivera

PRESENTING SIGNS AND SYMPTOMS

Presentation of venous thromboembolism is dependent upon severity, level of acuity, and location affected. Pulmonary embolism (PE) can mimic many conditions making diagnosis challenging at times. Patient symptoms may range in severity from incidental findings and asymptomatic to vague, nonspecific complaints or fulminant cardiogenic shock with a high risk for death. Classic presenting symptoms of PE include unexplained dyspnea, chest pain, hypotension, and cyanosis. Hemoptysis, syncope, or pre-syncopal episodes should also prompt consideration of PE. Acute onset, severe dyspnea associated with anginal chest pain is indicative of central PE. Mild short duration dyspnea is often associated with peripheral PE. Patients with a prior history of congestive heart failure or chronic pulmonary disease may note dyspnea that is worse than usual baseline symptoms.

HISTORY AND PHYSICAL FINDINGS

Time is of the essence to reduce the risk of death when determining if a patient is presenting with a PE. Assessment of risk should include two components. The first is to identify individual risk factors such as genetic or acquired causes which can be patient- and/or environmental-specific factors that predispose a patient to development of a PE. A patient's risk is heightened with recent severe traumatic injury and abdominal, neurologic, or major orthopedic surgery. Malignancy, infections, blood transfusions, spinal cord injury, erythropoietin-stimulating agents, and oral contraceptives are also associated with increased risk. When compared to the general population, individuals with malignancy have a fourfold heightened risk for the development of venous thromboembolic disease and higher risk of mortality. Additional risk factors are listed in Box 7.15.

The other component of risk assessment focuses on determining the triggering cause and level of risk for mortality. Acute high-risk PE is associated with hemodynamic instability and has a high risk for mortality during hospitalization or within 30days. Hemodynamic instability is characterized by cardiac arrest, persistent hypotension unrelated to hypovolemia, sepsis, or new onset arrhythmia, and obstructive shock with a systolic blood pressure less than 90 mmHg which is difficult to maintain despite the use of pressors and presence of end organ hypoperfusion (European Society of Cardiology, 2019).

DIFFERENTIAL DIAGNOSIS AND DIAGNOSTIC CONSIDERATIONS

Conditions that should be considered as competing diagnoses include pneumonia, asthma, chronic obstructive pulmonary disease (COPD), congestive heart failure,

BOX 7.15: RISK FACTORS FOR PULMONARY EMBOLISM

- Atherosclerosis
- Atrial dysrhythmias
- Autoimmune diseases
- Bed rest >3 days
- Central venous catheters
- Chemotherapeutics
- Diabetes
- Genetic factors
- Heart failure
- Hospitalization
- Hypertension
- Immobility
- Increased age
- Infections
- Inflammatory bowel disease
- IV catheters
- Laparoscopic surgery
- Major abdominal surgery
- Malignancy
- Myocardial infarction within last 3 months
- Neurosurgery
- Obesity
- Oral contraceptives especially third generation
- Pregnancy and postpartum period
- Prolonged immobility (including travel)
- Smoking
- Stroke
- Thrombophilia
- Trauma
- Varicose veins

TABLE 7.22: Revised Geneva Rule

CLINICAL FINDINGS	CLINICAL DECISION-MAKING POINTS
Prior pulmonary embolism or deep vein thrombosis	1
Heart rate 75–94 bpm	1
Heart rate 95 bpm or higher	2
Surgery or fracture within last month	1
Hemoptysis	1
Active malignancy	1
Unilateral lower extremity pain	1
Pain with deep palpation of lower extremity venous system and unilateral edema	1
Age 65 years or older	1
CLINICAL PROBABILITY	
Three Level Score	
Low	0–1
Intermediate	2–4
High	5 or greater
Two-Level Score	
Pulmonary embolism likely	3 or greater
Pulmonary embolism unlikely	0–2

Source: Adapted from European Society of Cardiology. (2019). ESC guidelines for the diagnosis and management of acute pulmonary embolism developed in collaboration with the European Respiratory Society: The task force for the diagnosis and management of acute pulmonary embolism of the European Society of Cardiology (ESC). *European Heart Journal, 41*, 543–603. https://doi.org/10.1093/eurheart/ehz405

pericarditis, cardiac tamponade, aortic dissection, acute valve dysfunction, acute coronary syndrome (ACS), anxiety, pneumothorax, hypovolemia, and pericarditis. Prior to conducting diagnostic testing, prediction tools such as the revised Geneva Rule and the Wells Score can be used to classify patients into low, intermediate, and high clinical probability based on assessment of risk factors and evaluation of clinical findings. Table 7.22 is an example of the revised Geneva Rule. A cumulative score of 3 or higher heightens the likelihood of PE.

Diagnostic Testing

The Pulmonary Embolism Rule-Out Criteria (PERC) can be utilized in the emergency department to facilitate decision-making to identify patients that have a higher likelihood of PE and should have additional diagnostic workup. According to PERC, the likelihood of PE is less if the patient is younger than 50 years old, heart rate less than 100 beats per minute, oxygen saturation higher than 94%, no hemoptysis, and lack of risk factors such as recent trauma or surgery, oral contraceptive use, history of venous thromboembolism, or unilateral lower extremity edema.

D-Dimer Assay

The quantitative plasma D-dimer enzyme-linked immunosorbent assay (ELISA) when elevated demonstrates fibrin breakdown by plasma. The D-dimer assay test has a 95% sensitivity for PE but is not specific. The presence of an elevated D-dimer assay test in the presence of clinical findings suggestive of PE should prompt additional workup with diagnostic imaging. Acute systemic illnesses with similar presenting symptoms and clinical findings can also cause elevated D-dimer assay levels making diagnosis more challenging.

Cardiac Biomarkers

Cardiac markers such as troponin and brain natriuretic peptide can be elevated due to the myocardial stretch and microinfarction that can occur as the result of PE.

TABLE 7.23: S1Q3T3 Sign EKG Findings

Lead I	S wave
Lead III	Q wave and inverted T wave
Leads V1–V4	T wave inversion

Electrocardiogram

The S1Q3T3 sign is a common EKG finding in the presence of PE (Table 7.23). Inverted T waves in leads V1–V4 are the most common abnormality seen on EKG results due to right ventricular strain or ischemia.

CT Pulmonary Angiography

CT pulmonary angiography (CTPA) is the primary method for diagnosis of PE. The presence of right ventricular enlargement is indicative of a higher risk for death within 30 days of development of PE. Chest CT with IV contrast dye can also be utilized to differentiate among common causes of acute onset chest pain such as PE, ACS, and acute aortic syndrome.

Lung Scintigraphy

The planar ventilation perfusion (V/Q) scan is considered a second line diagnostic test. V/Q lung scintigraphy can be useful when the use of IV contrast dye is contraindicated.

Pulmonary Angiography

Pulmonary angiography was once considered the gold standard but has been widely replaced by the use of CTPA.

Echocardiography

Transthoracic echocardiography can be useful for determining if findings suggestive of PE are present. The use of echocardiography for the sole diagnosis of PE is not recommended. A pulmonary ejection acceleration time less than 60 msec and a peak systolic tricuspid valve gradient of less than 60 mmHg or decreased contractility of the right ventricular wall is suggestive of PE. Echocardiography is primarily used for identification of competing differential diagnoses such as acute myocardial infarction, pericardial tamponade, or aortic dissection.

TREATMENT

Assessment of risk, physical exam findings, and presence of hemodynamic instability drives treatment decisions. Tachycardia, hypotension, respiratory insufficiency, and syncope are associated with poorer prognosis. The presence of hemodynamic instability, increased severity, presence of right ventricular dysfunction, and elevated troponin levels heighten the risk for death during hospitalization or within 30 days.

Anticoagulation options for treatment of PE include low molecular weight heparin, fondaparinux, unfractionated heparin, non-vitamin K antagonist oral anticoagulants, vitamin K antagonists, and thrombolytic therapies. Treatment choices are made depending on the patient's hemodynamic stability, presence of pulmonary obstruction, comorbid conditions, risk for bleeding, and potential for developing heparin-induced thrombocytopenia. If pulmonary obstruction is present, reperfusion with IV recombinant tissue-type plasminogen activator (rtPA) 100 mg over 2 hours should be administered unless contraindicated. An infusion of heparin can be administered during rtPA infusion.

Treatment also includes hemodynamic and respiratory support, anticoagulation, and reperfusion treatment. Oxygen saturations less than 90% require delivery of supplemental oxygen via nasal cannulation or mechanical ventilation as needed. Vasopressors and inotropes can be utilized to improve hemodynamic stability. Norepinephrine 0.2 to 1.0 µg/kg/min can be used to increase right ventricular inotropy and systemic blood pressure and restore the coronary perfusion gradient. Dobutamine 2 to 20 µg/kg/min also increases right ventricular inotropy and lowers filling pressures but should not be used without administration of a vasopressor because arterial hypotension may be exacerbated. Percutaneous catheter-directed reperfusion treatments have been utilized to fragment, aspirate, or deliver thrombolytic medications at a reduced dose, however data are limited. Surgical embolectomy has also been used in cases with high-risk PE or cardiac arrest.

Treatment Decision-Making

Anticoagulation should be initiated in the presence of suspected PE. A patient's hemodynamic stability and level of risk should be determined. A transthoracic echocardiogram should be conducted to determine if right ventricular dysfunction is present or evaluate CTPA if available. Assessment of clinical probability for PE should be evaluated either utilizing a clinical prediction tool or with clinical judgment for patients with suspected PE but without the presence of hemodynamic instability. If the likelihood of PE is low or intermediate, evaluate a D-dimer test and if positive conduct CTPA testing. Positive CTPA test results should prompt initiation of treatment. If the likelihood of PE is high, conduct CTPA testing and initiate treatment if positive.

Patients who are determined to be low risk without hemodynamic instability, right ventricular dysfunction, adequate family or social support, no other reason for hospitalization, and easy access to medical care can be considered for early discharge to home for continued treatment. Patients with serious comorbid conditions, clinical signs of PE, and PE Severity Index Class greater than 1 should have troponin levels checked. If troponin levels are negative, the patient should be considered intermediate to low risk. If troponin levels are positive and right ventricular dysfunction is present, a patient should be considered intermediate to high risk, hospitalized, monitored, and consider reperfusion. If the patient is hemodynamically unstable and of high risk, reperfusion treatment and hemodynamic support should be initiated.

If the probability for PE is high, anticoagulation treatment with heparin should be initiated as soon as possible even if diagnostic test results are pending. Decisions regarding whether to use low molecular weight heparin, fondaparinux, or unfractionated heparin are determined with consideration of a patient's individualized risk for bleeding, presence of renal dysfunction, and hemodynamic stability. Non-vitamin K antagonist oral anticoagulants offer consistent dosing without the need for routine lab monitoring and with less interactions than vitamin K antagonists. Vitamin K antagonists are considered the gold standard for oral anticoagulation. Vitamin K antagonists should be utilized in conjunction with heparin for a minimum of 5 days and until the international normalized ratio (INR) value is between 2.0 and 3.0 for 2 consecutive days.

TRANSITION OF CARE

The criteria for discharge to home include a low risk for serious complications or death related to PE, no serious comorbid condition or condition that would require hospitalization, and appropriate outpatient care and treatment. Transition of care decisions should include consideration of a patient's level of compliance and conversion from parenteral to oral anticoagulant therapy. Patients should be informed of outpatient INR monitoring, potential food and drug interactions, and schedule for follow-up. Vena cava filter placement may be considered in the presence of recurrent PE, high risk of venous thromboembolism, and contraindication for anticoagulant therapy.

CLINICAL PEARLS

- Risk assessment should include evaluation of individual risk factors and identification of triggering cause
- A patient's level of risk and hemodynamic stability drive treatment decisions.

KEY TAKEAWAYS

- Transthoracic echocardiography provides a quick method to differentiate among acute life-threatening conditions that may present similarly.
- Anticoagulation therapy should be initiated immediately (unless contraindicated) while results of diagnostic workup are pending
- Determine the best treatment options given the patient's level of risk, individual risk factors, comorbid conditions, and resources available.
- Weigh the benefits and risks of continued anticoagulant therapy following discharge.
- Ensure adequate follow-up and monitoring following discharge.

EVIDENCE-BASED RESOURCES

European Society of Cardiology. (2019). ESC guidelines for the diagnosis and management of acute pulmonary embolism developed in collaboration with the European Respiratory Society: The task force for the diagnosis and management of acute pulmonary embolism of the European Society of Cardiology (ESC). *European Heart Journal, 41*, 543–603. https://doi.org/10.1093/eurheart/ehz405

7.14: PULMONARY INFECTIONS

Leanne H. Fowler

Lung infections involve the pulmonary parenchyma and can cause irreversible damage if not recognized and treated appropriately. Differentiating acute from chronic disease, upper from lower respiratory infections, and the pathogens causing the infection is a necessary skill the AGACNP should use when initiating the patient's management plan. Bacterial infections of the lower respiratory system can be associated with long-term sequelae when not recognized and treated appropriately. Viral infections of the lungs often present with symptoms of systemic illness and exacerbated chronic lung disease (CLD) that can increase the patient's risk for greater morbidity and mortality. Fungal infections of the lungs are insidious, are rare among patients with intact immune systems, are typically complex, and can be more challenging to treat than the other pathogens. This section focuses on the lung infections manifesting common clinical presentations and caused by some of the most common pathogens.

Community-Acquired Pneumonia

Community-acquired pneumonia (CAP) is an acute or subacute clinical syndrome defined by clinical criteria (Box 7.16) and involving the transmission of a bacterial or viral pathogen outside of the hospital and without the use of mechanical ventilation. As more Americans are being inoculated against pneumococcal pneumonia, presentations of CAP can be viral, bacterial, or a mixture of both pathogens (Table 7.24). Because the viruses and bacteria that cause CAP coexist, treatment recommendations include empiric treatment against common bacterial pathogens or coinfection (Metlay et al., 2019).

Patients at high risk for CAP include those living with alcohol abuse, asthma, immunosuppression, institutionalization, and those older than 70 years. The physiologic factors of aging, CLD, and/or immunodeficiency such as decreased cough and gag reflexes, and decrease immune responses (e.g., reduced antibody and T-cell response) to pathogen invasion are susceptible to pneumonia as well. The very old patient with compounding factors of aging, CLD, and/or immunocompromising illness (e.g.,

BOX 7.16: DEFINING CLINICAL CRITERIA FOR COMMUNITY ACQUIRED PNEUMONIA

Minor Clinical Criteria
- Respiratory rate ≥30 bpm
- Temperature ≤ 36°C
- Hypotension requiring volume resuscitation
- Confusion or disorientation
- Multilobar infiltrates
- PaO_2:FiO_2 ratio <250
- Thrombocytopenia (platelet count <100,000/uL)
- Leukopenia (white blood cells ≤4,000 cells/uL; not associated with chemotherapy)
- Uremia (blood urea nitrogen ≥20 mg/dL)

Major Clinical Criteria
- Respiratory failure requiring mechanical ventilation
- Septic shock requiring vasopressors

Positive clinical findings for CAP include having either one major criterion or three or more minor criterion.

TABLE 7.24: Pathogenic Pathogens Causing Community Acquired Pneumonia

ETIOLOGY	PATHOGEN
Bacterial	*Streptococcus pneumoniae* (most common) *Haemophilus influenzae* *Mycoplasma pneumoniae* *Chlamydia pneumoniae* Community-acquired methicillin-resistant *Staphylococcus aureus* (CA-MRSA)

Viral	Respiratory viruses
	     Influenza A and B
	     Adenovirus
	     Respiratory syncytial viruses (RSV)
	     Parainfluenza viruses
	     Metapneumoviruses
	         Coronaviruses (responsible for SARS and MERS)

MERS, Middle East respiratory syndrome; SARS, severe acute respiratory syndrome.

HIV, cancer, uncontrolled diabetes) are among the most vulnerable individuals to experience a severe case of CAP and the complications associated with severe CAP.

A severe case of CAP can include hospitalization, intensive-care unit admission, mechanical ventilation, septic shock, and multi-organ failure. Complications of severe CAP include respiratory failure, septic shock, multi-organ dysfunction syndrome, lung abscess, complex pleural effusion, the need for hemodialysis, endocarditis, exacerbation and worsening of other chronic illnesses (especially lung disease), and death. Recovery from severe CAP and its complications can be prolonged by the patient's delay in seeking care, the medical provider's delay in initiating appropriate treatment, poor health literacy, poor posthospitalization follow-up, poor social/family support, or poor social determinants of health in general.

Respiratory Viruses Causing Pneumonia

Respiratory viruses (Table 7.24) are the leading cause of acute lower respiratory tract infections and can cause lung infections that often have airborne and/or droplet transmission from coughing, sneezing, or contact with individuals with a viral respiratory illness. Such illnesses are often seasonal when individuals tend to spend more time indoors, such as the cold weather months. Although uncommon, respiratory viruses can prevail among communities outside of the routine seasons for illness.

Viral infection of the lungs can cause significant morbidity and mortality. Severe viral lung infections can require hospitalization, supplemental oxygen, and/or mechanical ventilation. Severe viral lung infections can also worsen CLD, exacerbate underlying chronic illness, and increase the patient's risks for complications. The complications associated with severe viral lung infections include co-infections with bacterial pathogens or other respiratory viruses, postviral MRSA pneumonia, respiratory failure, and worsened lung function (Crowe, 2018).

Healthcare Communities Associated With Pneumonia

Patients within congregant communities that develop pneumonia were formerly classified to have a healthcare associated pneumonia (HCAP). The HCAP terminology was retired due to the overuse of broader spectrum antibiotics contributing to drug resistance and antibiotic associated complications such as *Clostridium difficile* colitis (Kalil et al., 2016; Metlay et al., 2019). A prudent history should account for patients who were cared for in congregant communities such as nursing homes, skilled nursing facilities, intensive care units, and hospitals in weeks prior to the development of pneumonia. These patients are at risk for acquiring more virulent and multidrug resistant (MDR) infections from pathogens that are not commonly found in congregant communities.

Hospital-Acquired Pneumonia

Hospital-acquired pneumonia (HAP), also known as nosocomial pneumonia or a hospital-acquired infection, is associated with an acute lung infection caused by the transmission of pathogens (sometimes drug-resistant pathogens) common to hospital environments. Although HAP is considered less serious than ventilator-association pneumonia (VAP), it is a serious complication to hospitalization for nonintubated patients (Mandell & Wunderink, 2018). The pathogens associated with HAP can be any of those associated with CAP but are more similar to those responsible for VAP (Table 7.25). MDR pathogens pose the most harm to patients and the AGACNP must identify patients at the most risk for MDR infections during the evaluation

TABLE 7.25: Pathogens Causing Hospital-Acquired Pneumonia and Ventilator-Association Pneumonia

PATHOGENS USUALLY SENSITIVE TO ANTIBIOTICS	MULTIDRUG RESISTANT PATHOGENS
Methicillin-sensitive *Staphylococcus aureus* *Streptococcal* species *Enterobacteriaceae* 　*Escherichia coli* 　*Klebsiella pneumoniae* 　*Proteus* species 　*Enterobacter* species 　*Serratia marcescens*	Methicillin-resistant *Staphylococcus aureus* *Pseudomonas aeruginosa* *Acinetobacter* species *Legionella pneumophila* *Aspergillus* species *Burkholderia cepacia* *Enterobacteriaceae* 　Extended-spectrum beta lactamase (ESBL) strains 　Carbapenem-resistant strains

BOX 7.17: RISK FACTORS FOR VENTILATOR-ASSOCIATION PNEUMONIA (VAP) SECONDARY TO MULTIDRUG RESISTANT PATHOGENS

- Prior use of IV antibiotics within 90 days
- Diagnosed with septic shock at the time of VAP diagnosis
- Diagnosed with acute respiratory distress syndrome (ARDS) at the time of VAP diagnosis
- Hospitalization for 5 days or more prior to VAP diagnosis
- The need for acute hemodialysis before the onset of VAP

Source: Data from Kalil, A. C., Metersky, M. L., Klompas, M., Muscedere, J., Sweeney, D. A., Palmer, L. B., Napolitano, L. M., O'Grady, N. P., Bartlett, J. G., Carratalà, J., El Solh, A. A., Ewig, S., Fey, P. D., File, T. M., Restrepo, M. I., Roberts, J. A., Waterer, G. W., Cruse, P., Knight, S. L., & Brozek, J. L. (2016). Management of adults with hospital-acquired and ventilator-associated pneumonia: 2016 clinical practice guidelines by the Infectious Diseases Society of America and the American Thoracic Society. *Clinical Infectious Diseases*, *63*(5), e61–e111. https://doi.org/10.1093/cid/ciw353

and management of patients suspected to have HAP (Kalil et al., 2016).

Ventilator-Associated Pneumonia

Ventilator-associated pneumonia (VAP) is a type of acute lung infection specifically associated with tracheal intubation. Pathogens responsible for causing VAP are the same as those responsible for HAP (see Table 7.25). Fungal and viral pathogens are less commonly associated with VAP. Immunocompromised patients that develop VAP have the most risk for developing fungal lung infections (Kalil et al., 2016; Mandell & Wunderink, 2018).

Although there are many similarities to HAP, VAP is considered a more serious type of lung infection because of the direct access of pathogens to the lower respiratory system. Airway devices and increased colonization of pathogens that cannot be expectorated are the primary differences between the development of HAP and VAP (Mandell & Wunderink, 2018). Another reason VAP is considered to be more serious than HAP is because of the patient's structural defenses (e.g., epiglottis, cough reflex, gag reflex) to foreign pathogens entering the lungs are obstructed by airway devices. Multidrug resistant pathogens pose the highest risk for increased morbidity and mortality. Risk factors for patients to develop VAP secondary to MDR pathogens are noted in Box 7.17 (Kalil et al., 2016).

Aspiration Pneumonia and Pneumonitis

Aspiration pneumonia occurs after the aspiration of bacteria from the gastrointestinal tract and should be differentiated from other clinical syndromes of aspiration. Aspiration pneumonia involves the development of an acute lung infection in addition to the local inflammatory response that occurs from a chemical pneumonitis caused by aspirating the acidic fluids of the stomach. Aspiration pneumonitis can occur without a pneumonia

developing. Aspiration of foreign bodies can also occur without pneumonia developing (Surana & Kasper, 2018). Adults at high risk for aspiration pneumonia include those with a poor gag reflex, those with a decreased level of consciousness, and those with oral or nasal tracheal intubation for mechanical ventilation. Differentiating aspiration pneumonia from the other noninfectious causes of aspiration pneumonitis is important in developing an appropriate management plan.

Empyema and Parapneumonic Effusion

The term "empyema" is associated with a patient having a pleural space infection or frank pus in the pleural space. The term "parapneumonic" effusion refers to an exudative effusion associated with an underlying pneumonia. A parapneumonic effusion is associated with higher mortality than empyema if not drained and treated appropriately in a timely manner. Mortality is higher among patients with HAP than CAP when diagnosed with a parapneumonic effusion. Geriatric patients can have atypical presentations (e.g., anemia, failure to thrive, fatigue) and should be evaluated for empyema or parapneumonic effusion with every presentation of CAP or HAP (Feller-Kopman & Light, 2018).

Parapneumonic effusions and empyema are acute or subacute infections that are most often caused by bacteria or the local microbiotia responsible for CAP (see Table 7.24), HAP, or VAP (see Table 7.25). Pleural space infections with Streptococcal species and anaerobes are more associated with patients diagnosed with CAP. Pleural space infections with MRSA or gram-negative bacteria are more associated with patients diagnosed with HAP or VAP. Timely treatment of appropriately selected antibiotics are the cornerstone of treatment for patients with empyema or parapneumonic effusion (Feller-Kopman & Light, 2018).

Tuberculosis

Tuberculosis (TB) is one of the oldest infectious diseases among humans worldwide that is caused by the bacteria *Mycobacterium tuberculosis*. *M. tuberculosis* is a slow-growing bacteria transmitted by inhaling the respiratory droplets coughed or sneezed out by infectious bystanders. Upon transmission, it disseminates to the lungs and other organs through the lymphatic vessels and develops granulomas or tubercles. The infectious bacilli can lie latent (noninfectious but active) in oxygen-rich tissue such as the apices of the lung. In oxygen-poor areas, the infectious bacilli cannot grow, or it dies within the necrotic cells and tissue of the tubercle and later calcifies. Host response to TB infection plays a major role in the degree of infection and how the TB forms into chronic infection. Adults can have latent TB for years that later reactivates when their immune responses diminish and allows mycobacterial growth (Raviglione, 2018). This section focuses on pulmonary TB infection of the airways, lung, or pleura.

PRESENTING SIGNS AND SYMPTOMS

Patients with lung infections can have variable presentations that depend on the pathogen, the location of the infection, and the host's response to infection. Patients present to clinics and emergency departments with chief complaints of fever, cough, pleuritic chest pain, and dyspnea. The patient's age and existing comorbidities can blunt immune responses to infection and may limit the patient's ability to develop fever.

Tuberculosis

Patients infected with latent TB are often asymptomatic. Latent TB might be found incidentally with radiograph imaging or during a physical exam as one or more granulomas. Patients with active TB complain of fatigue, night sweats, weight loss, and a productive cough of "rust-colored" sputum occurring over weeks to months.

HISTORY AND PHYSICAL FINDINGS

Obtaining a thorough history of the patient's presenting illness can yield valuable information about the etiology of disease. Typical and atypical lung infections have different patterns in presentation of illness (Table 7.26). A thorough history can also inform the AGACNP of the patient's risk for a complex lung infection or complications associated with lung infections. Coupling historical findings with prudent physical examination findings can facilitate the development of prioritized differential diagnoses.

History

The onset, duration, severity, and characteristics of the patient's signs and symptoms can help differentiate types of lung infection. Cough, fever, and acute dyspnea are the most common complaints patients with lung infections present with. Onset, frequency, and the characteristics of sputum (if any can be expectorated) can also help the AGACNP narrow down etiologies of disease and the patient's severity of illness. Patients who report hemoptysis should be asked about the amount of blood observed to discern if the patient is experiencing active bleeding.

A review of systems often includes signs of systemic illness such as fever, malaise, arthralgias, and myalgias.

TABLE 7.26: Typical and Atypical Pneumonia Presentations

PATHOGEN	HISTORY	PHYSICAL EXAM	DIAGNOSTIC FINDINGS

Typical
S. pneumonia
H. influenzae
*S. aureus**
*K. pneumonia**
*P. aeruginosa**
	Fever, chills
	Cough, productive
	Dyspnea
	Progressive onset over days
		Toxic or ill appearance
		Focal wheezing, rales, or consolidation
		Pleural friction rub
		Purulent sputum
			Chest radiograph
			    Focal pneumonia
			    Pneumatoceles
			    Lung abscess

Aytpical
M. pneumonia
C. pneumonia
Legionella sp.
Respiratory viruses**
	Preceding URI
	Fever or afebrile
	Chills, malaise
	Myalgias, arthralgias
	Nonproductive cough
		Toxic or ill appearance
		Clear, diminished BBS
		Frequent, dry cough
			Chest radiograph
			    Diffuse interstitial prominence –or-
			    Multilobar pneumonia

Tuberculosis	Fever, chills, night sweats, weight loss
	Cough, productive
	Rusty-colored sputum
		Ill appearance
		Generally weak
		Redundant skin
		Skin rash – erythema nodosum
			Chest radiograph
			    Upper lobe cavitary lesion (active)
			    Lower low granulomas (latent)

*More associated with recent hospitalization or history of MDR infections.
**Can involve co-infection with bacteria.
BBS, blateral breath sounds; URI, upper respiratory illness.

Patients with respiratory viral illnesses can also experience gastrointestinal symptoms like nausea, vomiting, or diarrhea. Extrapulmonary signs and symptoms should increase the AGACNP's suspicion for exacerbation or complication of pre-existing chronic illnesses. For example, patients with a history of atherosclerotic cardiovascular or cardiac disease should be evaluated for complaints of chest pain, palpitations, syncope, or dependent edema when acutely ill with pneumonia, especially if hypoxia is present.

Obtaining a medical, surgical, and social history can help the AGACNP stratify the patient's risks for complex lung infection and/or complications associated with lung infection. Patients with a history of irradiation therapy for cancer can present with radiation pneumonitis. A travel history of a recent stay in a hotel or on a ship should increase the AGACNP's suspicion for Legionella infection.

When reviewing the patient's home medications, it is important to specifically ask the patient and/or family the last time antibiotics were taken. Antibiotic use in the prior 90 days to the presenting illness increases the patient's risk for *Enterobacteriaceae* and MDR infections (Mandell & Wunderink, 2018).

Physical Findings

The vital signs of patients with a lung infection should be evaluated for fever, hypoxia, and hemodynamic instability. The patient with respiratory distress may initially need a problem-focused or expanded problem-focused exam inclusive of the patient's general appearance, ENT, neck, lungs, heart, and peripheral vascular system. Patients with pneumonia may reveal focal wheezing or rales, or diminished airflow in the affected area. Increased or decreased tactile fremitus can suggest consolidated lung or pleural effusion. Other examination findings include auscultating a pleural friction rub and/or appreciating flat or dull percussion notes in the presence of pleural disease. A comprehensive exam should be performed for all patients requiring hospitalization after the patient is deemed stable to evaluate the patient for complications associated with lung infections.

DIFFERENTIAL DIAGNOSIS AND DIAGNOSTIC CONSIDERATIONS

Differential diagnoses should be considered for the patient's severity of illness and each presenting complaint (Box 7.18). When there is a high suspicion of index for pneumonia, the etiology suspected should be differentiated and prioritized to appropriately guide empiric antimicrobial treatment or supportive treatment.

Patients complaining of lung infections may have preceding or co-existing upper respiratory illness and/or underlying CLD. Acute dyspnea should also always be considered an angina equivalent and atypical presentation of ACS that can occur concurrently with lung infection.

BOX 7.18: DIFFERENTIAL DIAGNOSES FOR LUNG INFECTIONS

Cough
  Upper respiratory illness with pharyngitis (infectious, allergic, or inflammatory)
  Pneumonia—viral versus bacterial
    Community-acquired
    Hospital- or ventilator-associated
    Aspiration (including pneumonitis)
  Bronchogenic mass—benign or malignant
  Lung mass—benign or malignant
  Noninfectious pneumonitis
  Heart failure
Dyspnea
  Asthma exacerbation
  COPD exacerbation
  Pneumonia
  Pleural effusion
  Noninfectious pneumonitis
  Heart failure
  Acute coronary syndrome
  Pulmonary embolism
Fever
  Pneumonia
  Empyema or parapneumonic effusion
  Sepsis
  Malignancy
Pleuritic chest pain
  Pneumonia
  Pulmonary embolism
  Pleural disease
    Effusion
    Empyema or parapneumonic effusion
    Mass
  Musculoskeletal pain

Source: Data from Crowe, J. E., Jr. (2018). Common viral respiratory infections. In J. Jameson, A. S. Fauci, D. L. Kasper, S. L. Hauser, D. L. Longo, & J. Loscalzo (Eds.), *Harrison's principles of internal medicine* (20th ed.). McGraw Hill

---

Diagnostic Tests

Diagnostic tests should focus on confirming the suspicion of an infectious lung illness or the etiology for the patient's presentation. Stable and generally healthy patients who can be managed outpatient may benefit from available rapid antigen, antibody, or polymerase chain reaction (PCR) tests for suspected viral infections. Sputum cultures, blood cultures, or serum laboratory tests are not routinely needed for the patient's therapeutic management plan. Patients requiring hospital admission should have basic serum laboratory tests for medical screening (e.g., CBC, CMP), sputum collection for gram stain and culture (acid-fast Bacilli staining if TB is suspected), urine antigen test for Legionella if being admitted to the ICU, and two sets of blood cultures if the patient has fever, radiographic evidence of pneumonia, or is hemodynamically unstable. Procalcitonin and CRP levels are used as inflammatory markers to trend the patient's improvement with antibiotic or antiviral therapies in patients with severe illness (Kalil et al., 2016; Metlay et al., 2019).

Tuberculosis Testing

Screening patients at risk for TB can start with skin testing. Patients can have a false-positive reaction and may require chest radiograph screening to evaluate the patient for an upper lobe cavitary lesion. Patients with known TB disease or at high risk for active TB disease (e.g., HIV, autoimmune diseases treated with immune modulating therapies) may need a more sensitive and specific test for active disease, the serum quantiferon gold assay.

Diagnostic Imaging

A two-view chest radiograph provides a timely and thorough imaging modality that can inform the AGACNP if the patient has focal, multifocal, diffuse, or pleuritic pathology with good sensitivity and specificity for acute cardiopulmonary disease. Follow up radiography of the chest is recommended for hospitalized patients with hypoxia, fever, and/or tracheal intubation with mechanical ventilation (Mandell & Wunderick, 2018).

CT of the chest is generally reserved for patients with existing or suspected lung masses, cavitary lesions (common with TB, MRSA, and fungal lung infections), or a lung infection that is not improving with rendered care. Patients infected with S. aureus can develop pneumatoceles with multilobar involvement. Patients infected with active TB can present with an upper-lobe cavitating lesion (Mandell & Wunderick, 2018).

POCUS is another imaging modality that can be performed by the AGACNP to enhance the bedside exam and evaluate the patient for pleural effusion, lung consolidates, or pneumothorax. Lung applications for POCUS are not diagnostic radiographic images but can aid the AGACNP in the timely diagnosis and management of acute lung pathology (Smith & Farrell, 2019).

TREATMENT

Initial management for the patient with acute lung infection should be guided by the patient's severity of illness, local antibiogram, suspected pathogen, risk for decline or complications, and history of recent antibiotic use. Severity of illness should be considered to determine whether the patient should be hospitalized or not. The Pulmonary severity index for CAP (PSI/PORT) estimates mortality for adults and can assist the practitioner's medical decision making when considering the patient's risk for decline.. Severe illness is associated with hypoxia, hemodynamic instability, acute end-organ dysfunction, or a suspicion for sepsis. Patients with multiple co-morbid conditions placing them at risk

for decline or a history of MDR infections should also be considered for hospitalization. The CURB 65 score is another validated tool that can be used to guide whether an older adult with CAP would benefit from hospitalization (Metlay et al., 2019). This section focuses on the treatment of lung infections and not the conditions complicating the patient's care (e.g., ACS, sepsis).

Bacterial Pneumonia

The cornerstone of adequate eradication of bacterial infection is when empiric antimicrobial therapy is guided by the hospital's local antibiogram. Drug resistance patterns aid the prescriber in evaluating patients for failed outpatient treatment, in preventing antibiotic overuse, and reducing the patient's risk for later developing drug resistant infections from inappropriate antibiotic selection.

The outpatient management of bacterial pneumonia involves empiric antibiotic treatment for CAP and supportive therapies for fatigue, cough, and fever. Generally healthy patients who are antibiotic naïve for at least 3 months can be treated with oral macrolides (e.g., clarithromycin, azithromycin) or doxycycline. Patients with two or more co-morbidities or risk for MDR infection can be treated with a respiratory fluoroquinolone, a beta-lactam, or cefuroxime plus a macrolide. Follow-up evaluation by the patient's primary care provider within a few days to a week should be provided to ensure improvement of illness and complications of CAP have not developed (Metlay et al., 2019).

The inpatient management of patients with CAP or HAP involves determining the acuity level of the patient for hospital unit placement, follow-up serum labs and radiographic imaging, sputum culture, blood cultures, adequate nutrition and activity, venous thromboembolism prevention, fall prevention, need for supplemental oxygen, and improvement of the infectious illness. Intravenous antibiotics with broad spectrum coverage should be prescribed empirically initially and then deescalated when the pathogen and its susceptibility is identified. Empiric treatment should consider the patient's risk for drug resistance. Patients with recent hospitalization or use of antibiotics should be considered at risk for drug resistant infections and a different antibiotic used than previously if possible.

Critical care management is reserved for patients with severe hypoxia, respiratory distress, and hemodynamic instability (Kalil et al., 2016; Metlay et al., 2019). Patients with drug-resistant pathogens require isolation and combination antimicrobial therapies. An Infectious Diseases specialist should be consulted for patients with MDR infections and those with critical illness (Kalil et al., 2016).

Aspiration Pneumonia

Aspiration pneumonia is associated with an anaerobic bacterial infection requiring broad spectrum antibiotic coverage for anaerobic and gram-negative pathogens most associated with the gastrointestinal tract. Management of the underlying cause for aspiration should be initiated during hospitalization. For instance, patients with dysphagia require speech pathology consultation for inpatient evaluation and initial management. Patients that experienced overdose and subsequent aspiration should have a swallowing evaluation to exclude mechanical dysfunction and then referral to outpatient therapy for management of the cause of overdose. Because of the higher incidence of empyema and parapneumonic effusion with aspiration events, patients should be re-evaluated before and after discharge for this complication (Mandell & Wunderick, 2018).

Empyema and Parapneumonic Effusion

The management of patients with empyema or parapneumonic effusion is similar. Empiric antibiotic therapy should be initiated intravenously until the pathogen and susceptibility is identified. A pulmonary specialty consultation should be considered for the evaluation and management of this complex infection. Drainage of the pleural space is often required if improvement is not achieved with antibiotic therapy or if an abscess develops. The timely diagnosis and management of patients with an empyema or a parapneumonic effusion improves morbidity and mortality rates. Patients should be re-evaluated after discharge for resolution or recurrence by the pulmonary specialist and primary care provider (Feller-Kopman & Light, 2018).

Tuberculosis

The management of active TB infection is often outpatient and by an infectious disease specialist due to the risk for drug resistant TB (Nahid et al., 2019). A combination of therapies are used for 9 months to a year to treat the infection and the patient will require intermittent organ function monitoring and sputum cultures for susceptibility testing during follow up.

Acutely ill patients with active TB require hospital admission to a negative pressure isolation room with droplet and contact precautions. An infectious diseases consult for intravenous antimicrobial therapy should be initiated if the pulmonary specialist has limited experience with long-term management and prevention of drug-resistant

TB (Nahid et al., 2019). A pulmonary consult should be considered for patients requiring bronchoscopy or positive pressure ventilation. Follow-up management post-discharge is required to ensure successful TB treatment.

Viral Pneumonia

Patients presenting with viral lower respiratory infections can be managed outpatient with supportive therapies in the absence of hypoxia, hemodynamic instability, high risk for decline, or the inability to safely care for oneself or be cared for. Antiviral therapies (e.g., oseltamir, redesivir) and monoclonal antibody therapies can be prescribed within the first 48 to 72 hours of the onset of illness to reduce the patient's severity of illness. Supportive therapies to reduce cough, fever, body aches, and nasal congestion are also helpful in relieving bothersome symptoms. Patients should be re-evaluated within a week to reassess the patient for postviral bacterial infection, improvement of initial illness, and complications of viral pneumonia have not developed.

Severe viral lung infections can involve fever, hypoxia, respiratory failure, ARDS, and/or exacerbation of underlying CLD. Patients often require critical care admission until their oxygenation status is stable. Antiviral therapies can be beneficial to this population despite the onset of illness and is often guided by an infectious disease specialist. Antibacterial therapies are also initiated empirically for atypical pathogens since acute viral illness can include a bacterial co-infection. All patients recovering from a viral respiratory illness should be reevaluated for postviral bacterial infection, especially if hospitalized and at risk for developing a MRSA infection.

A robust set of instructor resources designed to supplement this text is located at http://connect.springerpub.com/content/reference-book/978-0-8261-6079-9. Qualifying instructors may request access by emailing textbook@springerpub.com.

REFERENCES

Full list of references can be accessed at http://connect.springerpub.com/content/reference-book/978-0-8261-6079-9

ENDOCRINE DISORDERS

INTRODUCTION

Endocrine disorders are commonly encountered by AGACNPs, presenting either as the primary etiology or as a secondary disorder due to acute illness as well as therapeutics or treatment. This chapter provides an overview of common endocrine disorders including pathophysiology, signs and symptoms, diagnostics, and evidence-based treatments.

8.1: ADDISON'S DISEASE

Richard Pembridge

Primary adrenal insufficiency (Addison's disease) is an alteration in the functionality of the adrenal cortices. Secondary adrenal insufficiency, a related disorder, is a result of insufficient adrenocorticotropic hormone (ACTH) secretion by the pituitary gland. Addison's disease is an uncommon disorder characterized by inadequate production of cortisol and aldosterone by the adrenal cortex. Adrenal crisis is considered a life-threatening state and therefore a medical emergency. When a reduction in corticosteroids or mineralocorticoid steroids occurs, the patient will develop symptomatology of adrenal insufficiency and possibly adrenal crisis.

PRESENTING SIGNS AND SYMPTOMS

Primary adrenal insufficiency most commonly presents with weakness and fatigue. Associated symptoms include headache, nausea, vomiting, abdominal pain, and diarrhea. The skin may be hyperpigmented from a lack of cortisol and axillary hair is sparse. Weight loss and arthralgias are often reported and the patient may report intake of high sodium foods.

HISTORY AND PHYSICAL FINDINGS

Fatigue and vague abdominal complaints are typically reported. Physical findings may include weight loss, hypotension (often postural), hyperpigmented or pale skin, altered mental status, and tachycardia.

Diagnostic Findings

- Hyponatremia
- Hyperkalemia
- Hypoglycemia
- Increased erythrocyte sedimentation rate (ESR)
- Neutropenia
- Eosinophilia
- Lymphocytosis
- Hypercalcemia
- Reduced plasma cortisol level
- Elevated blood urea nitrogen (BUN)
- Metabolic acidosis

DIFFERENTIAL DIAGNOSIS AND DIAGNOSTIC CONSIDERATIONS

Differential Diagnoses

- Primary adrenal insufficiency (Addison's disease)
- Secondary adrenal insufficiency
- Adrenal crisis

Diagnostic Considerations

- Abdominal CT scan to evaluate the adrenal glands
- Head CT to evaluate the pituitary if secondary adrenal insufficiency is a consideration
- C (Cortrosyn) ACTH stimulation test
- Pan culture to rule out infectious source of adrenal insufficiency
- Cosyntropin stimulation or intravenously test:
  - Synthetic cosyntropin 0.25 mg is given intramuscularly or intravenously. Serum cortisol is obtained within 60 minutes.
  - Normally, cortisol rises to ≥20 mcg/dL; less than 20 mcg/dL is suggestive of adrenal insufficiency.
  - For patients taking corticosteroids, hydrocortisone must not be given for at least 8 hr before test. Other corticosteroids (e.g., prednisone, dexamethasone) do not interfere with specific assays for cortisol and should be administered while awaiting the results of the stimulation test in an unstable patient.

TREATMENT

Acute Treatment

- Volume resuscitation with IV 0.9% normal saline (NS) or dextrose 5% with normal saline (D5NS)
- IV hydrocortisone provides adrenal and mineralocorticoid

- Electrolyte replacement
- Monitor for decompensation
- IV antibiotics if indicated

TRANSITION OF CARE

- Hydrocortisone daily
- Florinef daily, if needed
- Education of signs and symptoms of adrenal crisis

KEY TAKEAWAYS

- Treatment must include aggressive fluids for hypovolemia and hypotension
- Hydrocortisone for corticosteroid replacement
- Florinef for mineralocorticoid replacement
- Patient education on signs and symptoms

8.2: CUSHING'S SYNDROME

Deborah Astemborski

Cushing's syndrome is a metabolic disorder characterized by the presence of hypercortisolemia. Causes of Cushing's syndrome are varied, with the top three causes being iatrogenic from exogenous glucocorticoid use, pituitary corticotropin tumors (ACTH-dependent tumors resulting in Cushing's disease), and ectopic ACTH-secretion from tumors outside of the pituitary gland. Less commonly, adrenal carcinoma and some pulmonary tumors can result in Cushing's syndrome. The diagnosis of Cushing's syndrome can be challenging and requires multiple confirmatory diagnostic tests once clinical suspicion exists. It often requires a multidisciplinary, stepwise approach for biochemical confirmation and to determine the underlying cause of the syndrome quickly and accurately. Due to the presence of significant systemic pathology resulting in diminished quality of life, increased morbidity and mortality associated with Cushing's syndrome, normalization of cortisol levels and treatment of the underlying cause are essential (Nieman, 2015).

Clinical findings associated with Cushing's syndrome should prompt diagnostic biochemical evaluation for hypercortisolemia. Cushing's syndrome is rare, though iatrogenic disease is likely underreported. In the United States, the annual incidence of Cushing's syndrome in individuals less than 65 years old was nearly 49 cases per 1 million persons (Broder et al., 2015). While florid Cushing's syndrome is usually unmistakable, mild Cushing's symptoms may be missed. Early recognition and connection of certain disease processes to hypercortisolemia may not be obvious and can lead to delays in diagnosis. Additionally, several common associated diseases are not pathognomonic for Cushing's disease, so early involvement of an expert provider, such as an endocrinologist, is imperative to ensure a rapid and accurate diagnosis. Once biochemical confirmation of the diagnosis is made, an algorithmic approach for expedient treatment of the disease may limit the potential life-long impact of pathologic hypercortisolemia (Nieman, 2015).

PRESENTING SIGNS AND SYMPTOMS

Since the signs and symptoms of Cushing's syndrome are a direct result of chronic and systemic glucocorticoid exposure, they can be varied and make diagnosis difficult. Many of what are considered historically to be obvious signs and symptoms can be related to other pathologic processes or lifestyle behaviors, such as obesity, hypertension, or diabetes. The signs and symptoms can also present on a spectrum of severity depending on duration and extent of exposure, the source of secretion, or the co-presence of excess androgen (Nieman et al., 2015). One important clinical presentation that can be more indicative of Cushing's syndrome is synchronous development and severity of onset of signs and symptoms. A summary of common and less common signs and symptoms is listed in Table 8.1 (Nieman, 2015).

HISTORY AND PHYSICAL FINDINGS

The systemic impact of hypercortisolemia leading to Cushing's syndrome results in varied presentations. Clinical clues may be ascertained by the provider when the constellation of signs or symptoms of Cushing's disease present simultaneously and with increasing severity; however, this is not always the case. Since the natural history of the disease is progressive, early assessments for certain diagnoses may eventually accumulate to more obvious signs of the disease. As such, patients may present to any

number of specialties with seemingly unconnected concerns, and a provider may not link the specific presentation to the causative factor of excess glucocorticoid until further pathology exists (Nieman, 2015).

Reproductive Impact

Abnormal menstruation in women, including variable cycles, amenorrhea, oligomenorrhea, or excess menses occur in 80% of patients with newly diagnosed Cushing's syndrome. Hypercortisolemia appears to suppress gonadotropin-releasing hormone, resulting in low levels of luteinizing hormone and follicle-stimulating hormone (Lado-Abeal et al., 1998). If there is also the presence of excess adrenal production of androgen, which can be present in women, the diagnosis of adrenal carcinoma should be considered. Women with excess androgen production may present with hirsutism, virilization, and excessively oily skin with facial and body acne; these are not symptoms associated with hypercortisolemia alone (Hutter et al., 1966).

Integumentary Impact

Multiple integumentary system changes are associated with Cushing's syndrome (Box 8.1). Patients may find they bruise more easily due to the loss of subcutaneous tissue integrity from the catabolic effect of excess glucocorticoid. Dark red-to-purple striae, particularly on the flank and abdomen, result from rapid weight gain and venous blood collecting under the thinning and atrophied dermis. Cutaneous fungal infections on the trunk or fingernails may be present, usually due to tinea versicolor. Hyperpigmentation may also present due to excessive adrenocorticotropic hormone (ACTH), rather than hypercortisolemia (Lado-Abeal et al., 1998; Nieman et al., 2008).

Cardiovascular Impact

A variety of pathologic cardiovascular system processes arise in the patient with Cushing's syndrome. Diagnosis based only on the cardiovascular findings is rare, given the prevalence of cardiovascular disease in the general population. Additionally, treatment and risk stratification does not differ significantly even in the presence of hypercortisolemia. Following biochemical remission of hypercortisolemia, these comorbidities may or may not require ongoing monitoring and treatment. Table 8.2 lists common cardiovascular diseases and correlative pathophysiology in Cushing's syndrome (Nieman et al., 2015).

TABLE 8.1: Signs and Symptoms of Cushing's Syndrome

MORE COMMON	LESS COMMON
Abnormal glucose tolerance	Abdominal pain
Decreased libido	Acne
Ecchymoses	Backache
Hirsutism	Edema
Hypertension	EKG abnormalities or atherosclerosis
Lethargy, depression	Female balding
Menstrual changes	Headache
Obesity/weight gain	Osteopenia or fracture
Plethora	Proximal muscle weakness
Round face	Recurrent infections
	Striae

Source: Reproduced with permission from Nieman, L. K. (2015). Cushing's syndrome: Update on signs, symptoms and biochemical screening. *European Journal of Endocrinology, 173,* M33

> ## BOX 8.1: INTEGUMENTARY FINDINGS IN CUSHING'S SYNDROME
>
> - Cutaneous fungal infections
> - Dark red-to-purple striae
> - Easy bruisability
> - Hyperpigmentation

TABLE 8.2: Common Cardiovascular Diseases and Correlative Pathophysiology in Cushing's Syndrome

COMMON CARDIOVASCULAR DISEASES IN CUSHING'S SYNDROME	POSSIBLE CAUSES OF DISEASE AS A CONDITION OF EXCESS GLUCOCORTICOID
• Hypertension	• Increased peripheral vascular sensitivity, increased hepatic production of angiotensinogen, activation of renal mineralocorticoid receptors
• Thromboembolic events	• Glucocorticoid-induced increases in plasma concentrations of clotting factors, elevated serum homocysteine, obesity, surgery
• Heart failure	• Mechanism unclear
• Dilated cardiomyopathy	• Cell hypertrophy, myocardial fibrosis

Musculoskeletal Impact

Patients with Cushing's syndrome may present with osteoporosis secondary to decreased intestinal calcium absorption, decreased bone formation, increased bone resorption, and decreased renal calcium reabsorption. As with any underlying cause of osteoporosis, patients may present with pathologic fractures, including vertebral compression fractures, rib fractures, foot and long bone fractures. Patients may also develop avascular necrosis of the femoral or humeral heads, resulting in significant pain and decreased quality of life. Proximal muscle wasting in the presence of obesity also contributes to pain, weakness, and loss of mobility (Nieman, 2015; Tauchmanovà et al., 2006).

Neuropsychiatric Impact

More than 50% of patients with Cushing's syndrome are diagnosed with one or more neuropsychiatric diseases, including depression, irritability, emotional lability and mood disorders, insomnia, anxiety, panic attacks, paranoia, mania, or insomnia. It is difficult to determine whether these disorders arise secondary to the development of physiologic symptoms, frustration in lack of obtaining a diagnosis, or are directly related to elevated glucocorticoid; however, it is imperative that the patient be screened and treated for the presence of a neuropsychiatric disorder. Resolution of these disorders following successful treatment of Cushing's syndrome is variable and requires ongoing surveillance (Starkman, 2013).

Metabolic and Immunologic Impact

Significant endocrinopathy can result from the presence of chronically elevated glucocorticoid. Glucose intolerance and the development of type 2 diabetes mellitus should be evaluated for and treated aggressively. Progressive obesity, particularly centripetal, is common; however, some patients maintain a normal body mass index and others do not demonstrate the proximal limb wasting commonly associated with Cushing's syndrome. Patients often subsequently develop obesity-related diseases, such as sleep apnea, joint pain, epidural lipomatosis resulting in spinal stenosis, dyslipidemia, and increased intraocular pressure (Dekkers et al., 2013; Nieman, 2015).

Patients are also at increased risk of infection due to immunosuppression from excess glucocorticoid, though the exact mechanism is poorly understood. Glucocorticoids inhibit synthesis of cytokines, contributing to a decrease in the inflammatory action of tumor necrosis factor. Additionally, it may cause a fall in CD4 cells and decrease in natural killer cell activity. Likely, contributions include frequent hospitalizations with potential exposure to bacterial infection, surgical intervention, diabetes or glucose tolerance, and disruption of the normal pituitary-hypothalamic-adrenal axis. Since these patients may be chronically immunosuppressed, normal presentation of severe infection may be blunted so empiric antibiotic choice should be dictated by the potential for opportunistic infections (Dekkers et al., 2013).

DIFFERENTIAL DIAGNOSIS AND DIAGNOSTIC CONSIDERATIONS

Delays in diagnosis of Cushing's syndrome increase morbidity and mortality in these patients; therefore, any clinical suspicion should be evaluated for biochemical confirmation (Nieman, 2015). Depending on the expertise of the clinician, referral to an endocrinologist is appropriate with initial clinical concern for the disease. The first step in diagnosing Cushing's syndrome is to ascertain whether there is an exogenous or iatrogenic source of excess glucocorticoid exposure. If there is exogenous exposure, risks and benefits of continued use or alternative treatments should be considered. Prolonged exposure may result in adrenal insufficiency and require long-term supplementation or carefully monitored weaning (Dekkers et al., 2013; Nieman, 2015).

Current guidelines for diagnosing Cushing's disease require at least two of three positive confirmatory tests, given the potential for diurnal variations in cortisol production based on individual behavior and lifestyle patterns. Serum and salivary cortisol reach a nadir just after sleep in individuals with normal sleep/wake cycles; it can therefore be abnormal in individuals with night shift work schedules, insomnia, or other circadian disruptions. Additionally, the presence of physiologic causes of hypercortisolism (e.g., pregnancy, diabetes, morbid obesity, alcohol dependence) must be taken into consideration when initial laboratory results are interpreted (Dekkers et al., 2013; Nieman, 2015). Also, current medications that may impact the metabolism or laboratory response may need to be discontinued prior to testing, such as oral estrogens or other cytochrome P450 medication interactions (Flockhart, 2007). The following tests should be administered to evaluate for exogenous hypercortisolemia: 24-hour urine free cortisol (UFC), overnight 1 mg dexamethasone suppression test (DST), and late-night salivary cortisol (Nieman, 2015). Individual assays may demonstrate interfacility range variations and should be interpreted as such. Another factor influencing test selection and interpretation is pre-test probability of the disease based on clinical features (Nieman et al., 2008). Figure 8.1 demonstrates biochemical confirmation testing for Cushing's syndrome.

24-Hour Urine Free Cortisol

The 24-hour UFC measures cortisol secretion which is not bound to cortisol-binding globulin over a 24-hour period and has been utilized for several decades in the diagnosis of Cushing's syndrome. This test is unique compared to others as it measures tissue exposure to cortisol over a period of 24 hours versus a singular point of evaluation. There is a degree of inconvenience related to this test, with factors such as under- or overcollection impacting outcome reliability. For this reason, urine volume and creatinine should also be measured; the UFC

can be falsely elevated with a volume greater than 5 liters and falsely low with the glomerular filtration rate (GFR) less than 60 mL/min. Assays vary considerably, though typically 3.5 mcg to 45 mcg is considered normal; however, it is recommended that if the creatinine and volume are within normal limits, the upper limit of normal should be considered a positive test for Cushing's. The test should also be performed at least twice and interpreted along with other relevant individual information (Dekkers et al., 2013; Nieman, 2015).

Dexamethasone Suppression Test

The 1 mg overnight DST determines whether the glucocorticoid negative feedback cycle is normal. Patients are given 1 mg oral dexamethasone to be taken between 2300 and 0000 hr, with a serum cortisol level to be drawn between 0800 and 0900 the following morning. If it is greater than 1.8 mcg/dL, is considered elevated and may be indicative of Cushing's syndrome, but should be interpreted with the other confirmatory tests and patient factors. In some patients, a 2 mg DST over 48 hours is recommended if the results are inconclusive or if the patient has renal or liver failure (Nieman et al., 2015).

Late-Night Salivary Cortisol Test

Serum and salivary cortisol that are biologically active reach a nadir around midnight in individuals with stable, normal sleep/wake cycles. There is subsequently a rise

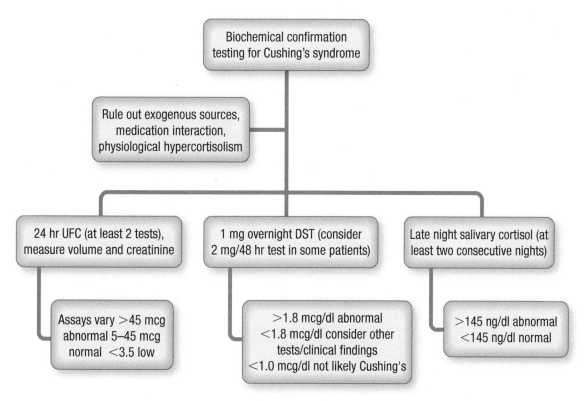

FIGURE 8.1: Biochemical confirmation testing for Cushing's syndrome.

in both levels around 0300 to 0400 and a peak between 0700 and 0900; levels then drop throughout the day depending on stress level, illness, and other factors. Using a salivette to collect a midnight salivary cortisol level for two consecutive nights determines if a patient has biochemically active cortisol without a nadir (<145 ng/dL depending on the assay), which is indicative of Cushing's syndrome. The sample is stable at room temperature and easy to collect, so is often the first screening test completed to determine the presence of hypercortisolemia (Nieman, 2015; Nieman et al., 2015).

Further Testing Options

If these tests are confirmatory or equivocal for hypercortisolemia, further testing should be done by a specialist. If the tests are all within normal range, but the pretest probability is high, re-testing in 6 months should be considered. Any or all of the preceding tests can be repeated if clinical symptoms persist or progress. A dexamethasone-suppressed corticotropin-releasing hormone test, midnight serum cortisol, random serum cortisol or ACTH levels, urinary 17-ketosteroids, insulin tolerance test, loperamide test, adrenal or pituitary imaging, or inferior petrosal sinus sampling are all in the armamentarium of the multidisciplinary specialist when necessary to further confirm the diagnosis of Cushing's syndrome (Nieman et al., 2015).

TREATMENT
ACTH-Dependent Cushing's Syndrome

Once biochemical confirmation of Cushing's syndrome has been completed, specialized care is necessary to optimize patient outcomes. The patient should be evaluated and treated for any comorbid conditions, which may include further specialist referrals and care coordination. If it is determined that the Cushing's syndrome is secondary to elevated ACTH secretion, next steps involve determining if it is ectopic ACTH secretion (EAS) or Cushing's disease (ACTH-secreting tumor of the pituitary gland). Imaging should be performed to look for an ectopic tumor or a pituitary tumor. Surgical resection of the mass is first line treatment in most cases, though patients with multiple comorbidities may represent high-risk surgical candidates. Figure 8.2 represents the current guidelines in an algorithm for treatment of Cushing's syndrome (Nieman et al., 2015).

The patient will likely require surveillance monitoring by an endocrinology provider with expertise in Cushing's syndrome. Recurrence is possible in some patients, which may prompt other therapies such as repeat surgery, radiation treatment, or medication management. Some patients require lifelong exogenous glucocorticoid due to the development of adrenal insufficiency from prolonged hypercortisolemia; additionally, panhypopituitarism may require supplementation following surgery or radiation, including thyroid-stimulating hormone, desmopressin, prolactin, growth hormone, or testosterone. Table 8.3 lists medical treatment options for patients with Cushing's syndrome for whom surgical or other therapies are not an option, or if there is recurrence or failed biochemical remission (Nieman et al., 2015).

ACTH-Independent Cushing's Syndrome

Patients with ACTH-independent Cushing's syndrome will need to undergo adrenal imaging, with referral to general surgery for unilateral or bilateral adrenalectomy depending on findings. This generally results in remission, though the patient will require long-term glucocorticoid supplementation with stress-dose steroid treatment when appropriate. If pathology is indicative of carcinoma, the patient should undergo evaluation and surveillance of possible metastatic disease. Patients who are not surgical candidates may require medication management as outlined in Table 8.3 (Nieman et al., 2015).

TRANSITION OF CARE

The significant quality of life factors and risk for recurrence and ongoing comorbid conditions require persistent continuity of care. The patient will likely require endocrinological monitoring and management, even if early biochemical remission is achieved. Initial postoperative management should be short interval coordinated-care visits with the surgeon and endocrinology teams available to limit patient inconvenience. Patients may require fertility specialists, regular ophthalmologic screening, and even psychiatric care depending on the goals, severity of disease, and specific system impact of Cushing's syndrome in the individual (Nieman, 2015).

KEY TAKEAWAYS

- Cushing's syndrome is a metabolic disorder characterized by the presence of hypercortisolemia.
- Excess glucocorticoid can cause a variety of systemic comorbidities, the severity of which depend on the amount and duration of hypercortisolemia.
- Clinical suspicion of Cushing's syndrome should prompt early biochemical confirmation and specialist referral.
- Comorbid conditions should be treated concurrently during evaluation and ongoing treatment of Cushing's syndrome.
- Surgical resection of a pituitary, ectopic, or adrenal mass is generally first-line treatment once Cushing's syndrome has been confirmed.
- Long-term care will include a multidisciplinary approach for support, surveillance, and diligent coordination of care.

EVIDENCE-BASED RESOURCES

Cushing's Support and Resource Foundation, https://csrf.net/

Pituitary Network Foundation https://pituitary.org/

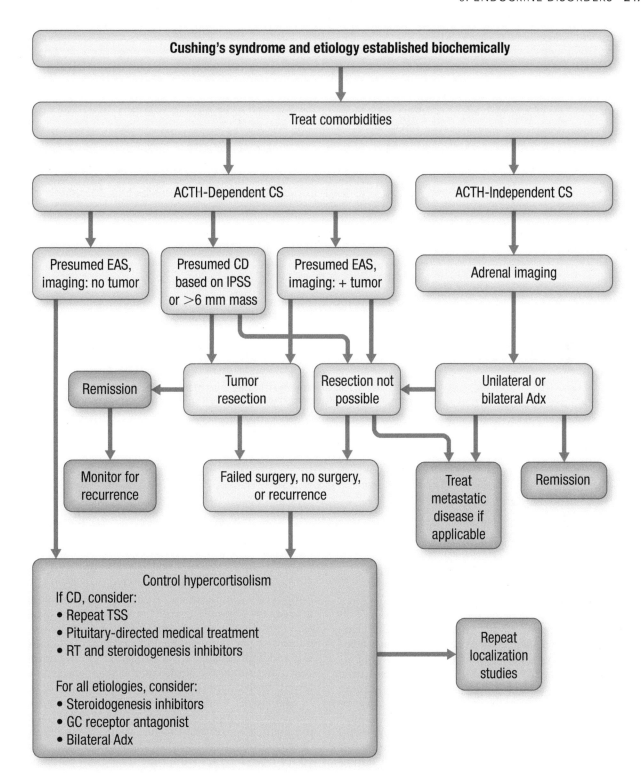

FIGURE 8.2: An algorithm for the treatment of Cushing's syndrome.

ACTH, adrenocorticotropic hormone; Adx, adrenalectomy; CS, Cushing's syndrome; EAS, ectopic ACS secretion; GC, glucocorticoid; IPSS, inferior petrosal sinus sampling; RT, radiation therapy; TSS, transsphenoidal surgery.

Source: Reproduced with permission from Nieman, L. K., Biller, B. M., Finding, J. W., Newell-Price, J., Savage, M. O., Stewart, P. M., & Montori, V. M. (2008). The diagnosis of Cushing's syndrome: An Endocrine Society Clinical Practice Guideline. *Journal of Clinical Endocrinology and Metabolism, 93*, 1526–1540

TABLE 8.3: Medical Treatment of Cushing's Syndrome

DRUG	PROS	CONS	DOS[E]
Steroidogenesis inhibitors			
Ketoconazole[b]	Quick onset of action	Adverse effects: GI, hepatic dyscrasia (death), male hypogonadism; requires acid for biological activity; DDIs	400–1600 mg/day; every 6–8 hr dosing
Metyrapone[b]	Quick onset of action	Adverse effects: GI, hirsutism, HT, hypokalemia; accessibility variable across countries	500 mg/d to 6 g/day; every 6–8 hr dosing
Mitotane[c]	Adrenolytic, approved for adrenal cancer	Slow onset of action; lipophilic/long half-life, teratogenic; adverse effects: GI, CNS, gynecomastia, low WBC and T_4 ↑ LFTs; ↑ CBG, DDIs	Starting dose, 250 mg; 500 mg/day to 8 g/dday
Etomidate	IV, quick onset of action	Requires monitoring in ICU	Bolus and titrate
Pituitary-directed			
Cabergoline		Adverse effects: asthenia, GI, dizziness	1–7 mg/week
Paseriotide[d]		Most successful when UFC <2-fold normal; SC administration; adevrse effects: diarrhea, nausea, cholelithiasis, hyperglycemia, transient ↑ LFTs, ↑QTc	600–900 mcg twice weekly
Glucocorticoid receptor-directed			
Mifepristone[e]		Difficult to titrate (no biomarker); abortifacient; adverse effects: fatigue nausea, vomiting, arthralgias, headache, hypertension, hypokalemia, edema, endometrial thickening	300–1200 mg/day

[a]Except as noted, the lowest dose may be used initially, unless the patient has severe hypercortisolism (UFC more than five times normal), in which case the starting dose may be doubled.
[b]Ketoconazole and metyrapone are approved by the European Medicines Agency for the treatment of Cushing's syndrome.
[c]Mitotane has FDA approval for treatment of adrenal cancer.
[d]Pasireotide has FDA approval for treatment of patients with Cushing's disease who are not surgical candidates or have failed surgery. The agent is also approved in Europe.
[e]Mifepristone has FDA approval for treatment of patients with Cushing's syndrome and diabetes or glucose intolerance who are not surgical candidates or have failed surgery
CBG, corticosteroid binding globulin; CNS, central nervous system; DDI, drug–drug interactions; GI, gastrointestinal; HT, hypertension; ICU, intensive care unit; LFTs, liver function tests; QTc, corrected QT interval; WBC, white blood cell count.
Source: Reproduced with permission from Nieman, L. K., Biller, B. M., Finding, J. W., Newell-Price, J., Savage, M. O., Stewart, P. M., & Montori, V. M. (2008). The diagnosis of Cushing's syndrome: An Endocrine Society Clinical Practice Guideline. *Journal of Clinical Endocrinology and Metabolism, 93,* 1526–1540.

8.3: DIABETES MELLITUS

Dorota Pawlak

Diabetes mellitus is a chronic, metabolic disorder characterized by increased glucose levels resulting from defects in insulin secretion, insulin action, or both. Persistent hyperglycemia can lead to diabetic ketoacidosis (DKA) and/or hyperosmolar hyperglycemic syndrome (HHS). Long-term hyperglycemia is a leading cause of microvascular and macrovascular complications (American Diabetes Association [ADA], 2021; King et al., 1999).

Diabetes mellitus was first described as "too great emptying of urine" in an Egyptian manuscript dating back to 1500 AD. It is now known to be a chronic metabolic disorder characterized by an increased glucose level. Its prevalence has been increasing steadily not only in the United States but globally (Centers for Disease Control and Prevention [CDC], 2020; Kristofi et al., 2021). The rate and progression of diabetes complications vary among individuals and between types of diabetes. Short-term complications include hyperglycemia,

hypoglycemia, DKA (see Section 8.2) and hyperosmolar hyperglycemic syndrome (HHS; see Section 8.3). Long-term complications resulting from prolonged, inadequate glycemic control most commonly manifest as microvascular and macrovascular impediments. The microvascular problems include retinopathy, neuropathy, and nephropathy. Myocardial infarction, peripheral vascular disease, and stroke are the macrovascular long-term complications (Chatterjee et al., 2017).

The largest diabetes study to date is known as the United Kingdom Progressive Diabetes Study (UKPDS); the publication of study results changed the paradigm of diabetes treatment worldwide. UKPDS was conducted for over 20 years with more than 5,000 participants, and it concluded that, in broad terms, there is a reduction of about 25% in macrovascular risk factors for every 1% fall in HbA1C level regardless of the type of diabetes. Improvement in HgA1C to ideal target of <7% with decrease in blood pressure to <140/90 mmHg reduced the risk of major diabetes related eye disorders by one quarter, early kidney disease by one third, stroke by one third, and death from diabetes related causes by one third (King et al., 1999). Current ADA guidelines underscore individualized treatment of diabetes but with an HbA1C target goal of 7% or less.

Types 1 and 2 are the most common diabetes types, but gestational diabetes and diabetes of other causes (drug-induced, HIV-, or cystic fibrosis-related) are also recognized (ADA, 2021; Lovic et al., 2020; Pippitt et al., 2016; Powers et al., 2021). Type 1 diabetes is due to autoimmune destruction of beta-cells which usually leads to absolute insulin deficiency and requires lifelong insulin therapy. Although predominately diagnosed at a young age, the traditional paradigm of type 1 diabetes as exclusively a childhood disease is no longer accurate. Type 1 diabetes can occur at any age. The underlying causes of type 1 diabetes are not yet fully understood. Genetic factors explain part of the autoimmune beta-cells destruction, but environmental factors, such as enterovirus infection, has been recognized and studied worldwide. Persons with type 1 diabetes are prone to other autoimmune disorders such as celiac disease, Hashimoto thyroiditis, Graves' disease (see Section 8.11), Addison's disease (see Section 8.1), and others (ADA, 2021; Mayer-Davis et al., 2018).

Type 2 diabetes, previously referred to as "non-insulin-dependent diabetes," is by far the most common type of diabetes. It is characterized by progressive loss of beta-cells, insulin resistance, and/or both. The term "prediabetes" describes individuals whose glucose levels do not meet diagnostic criteria for type 2 diabetes but are too high to be considered normal: HgA1C of 5.7% to 6.4 %, fasting plasma glucose (FPG) of 100–125 mg/dL or oral glucose tolerance test (OGTT) of 140–199 mg/dL (ADA, 2021; Garber et al., 2020; Gruss et al., 2019).

Genetic predisposition (much stronger than in type 1 diabetes) and environmental factors are identified as common causes of type 2 diabetes. The majority of patients with type 2 diabetes have first- or second-degree relatives with this disorder. Obesity and overweight are common characteristics of patients with type 2 diabetes, as is lack of exercise, which contributes to insulin resistance by decreased absorption of available insulin. The risk of developing type 2 diabetes increases with age, obesity, and lack of physical exercise. Women with polycystic ovarian syndrome, prior gestational diabetes, hypertension, and hyperlipidemia are more prone to developing diabetes than their peers without these characteristics. Type 2 diabetes is also more common among certain racial/ethnic subgroups such as African American, American Indian, Hispanic/Latino, and Asian American (Bellou et al., 2018; Kolb & Martin, 2017).

PRESENTING SIGNS AND SYMPTOMS

Type 1 Diabetes

Children with type 1 diabetes classically present with polyuria, polydipsia, polyphagia, and weight loss. About one third of newly diagnosed children present in DKA, a leading cause of morbidity and mortality. DKA is a result of a relative or absolute lack of insulin combined with elevated levels of insulin counterregulatory hormones such as cortisol, glucagon, catecholamine, and growth hormone. The resulting imbalance manifests as hyperglycemia, hyperosmolarity, ketosis, and acidosis. Osmotic diuresis, (a result of hyperglycemia and circulating ketone bodies) promotes net loss of electrolytes such as sodium, potassium, calcium, magnesium, phosphate, and chloride. Clearance of glucose and ketone bodies is diminished as progressive volume depletion decreases glomerular filtration rate (GFR; Alois & Rizzolo, 2017; Cashen & Peterson, 2019).

Cerebral edema is a major complication and a leading cause of death in children and adults with DKA. The presenting symptom for cerebral edema is often headache, followed by irritability, bradycardia, lethargy, increased blood pressure, papilledema, and hypoxemia. The exact pathophysiology of the cerebral edema is not fully understood, but research suggests that it is due to overaggressive fluid therapy to correct hyperglycemia (Alois & Rizzolo, 2017).

In recent years, a new phenomenon of euglycemic DKA had been observed among patients with both types of diabetes, but more commonly with type 2 diabetes. A relatively new hypoglycemic drug called sodium-glucose contra-transporter 2 inhibitors (SGLT2) appears to be responsible for this type of DKA. The SGLT2 inhibitors increase urinary glucose excretion which lowers blood glucose levels, consequently decreasing insulin secretion from pancreatic beta-cells. Several studies suggested that SGLT2 inhibitors induce ketoacidosis by the decreased amount of circulating insulin which stimulates fatty acid production and its conversion to ketone bodies. Additionally, administration of SGLT2 inhibitors accelerates production of glucagon leading to overproduction of ketone bodies (French et al., 2019; Ogawa & Sakaguchi, 2016; Zhang & Tamilia, 2018).

Type 2 Diabetes

In an outpatient setting, type 2 diabetes can go unrecognized for many years since hyperglycemia develops gradually without causing many of the symptoms. In acute settings, patients with an existing diagnosis or with new onset type 2 diabetes may present with HHS. These patients will report a history of several weeks of polyuria, weight loss, and diminished oral intake that often leads to confusion, lethargy, and even coma. They will have profound hyperglycemia (often much higher than in those with DKA) but ketones level will be low or absent despite the insulinopenic state. The ADA (2021) consensus statement suggests diagnostic criteria for HHS as blood glucose level of at least 600 mg/dL and hyperosmolarity of >320 mOsm/kg. Severe dehydration will be characteristic among those individuals secondary to the chronic nature of hyperglycemia (Dhatariya & Vellanki, 2017).

HHS is often precipitated by other concurrent disease such as stroke or myocardial infarction. Serious infections such as pneumonia, UTI (particularly in older populations), sepsis can also be a contributing factor in the development of HHS. Additionally, previous conditions such as dementia, stroke, or social situation (e.g., living alone), and poor or compromised water intake can also impact the development of HHS.

HISTORY AND PHYSICAL FINDINGS

When taking a patient history, it is important to identify diabetes risk factors which can aid in differentiation among the types of diabetes. Although the majority of younger patients who present with new onset of type 1 diabetes are lean, type 1 diabetes should not be excluded in overweight individuals. Genetic predisposition, age, ethnic/race, overweight/obesity, high carbohydrate diet, lack of physical activity, inadequate blood pressure and cholesterol control are the leading characteristics of type 2 diabetes which may facilitate the differential diagnosis.

Physical Findings

Kussmaul respiration with a fruity odor to the breath, poor skin turgor (a sign of dehydration), and tachycardia are typical physical findings in individuals presenting in DKA. Patients in severe DKA may be hypotensive with progression to hypovolemic shock, and may present with altered consciousness. Mental status can vary depending on severity of disease, from fully alert to profoundly lethargic and even comatose. Abdominal pain, nausea, and vomiting may also be present, and these findings usually correlate with severe acidosis. Hypothermia caused by peripheral vasoconstriction secondary to dehydration may be found on physical exam. Although infection is often a precipitating factor of DKA in patients already diagnosed with type 1 diabetes, fever is seldom present. Hematemesis due to gastritis has also been reported (Nyenwe & Kitabchi, 2016).

Physical findings in the outpatient setting for individuals with type 2 diabetes are often absent or minimal during the initial presentation. With chronic hyperglycemia patients may appear depressed, experience fatigue, may have unhealed wounds, particularly on their lower extremities. Acanthosis nigricans, a dark line on the back of the neck, is often found in individuals who suffer from chronic hyperglycemia.

Patients presenting in HHS will be characterized by severe dehydration and hyperosmolarity manifested on physical assessment as hypotension, tachycardia, and altered mental status. In contrast to patients in DKA, this population exhibits no Kussmal respiration on physical exam and nausea, vomiting and abdominal pain are typically absent (Combs et al., 2015).

DIFFERENTIAL DIAGNOSIS AND DIAGNOSTIC CONSIDERATIONS

Presence of ketones distinguishes DKA from simple hyperglycemia. The major diagnostic criteria for DKA include blood glucose level of 250 to 600 mg/dL, venous pH <7.3 or serum bicarbonate <15 mmol/L, ketonemia greater than 31 mg/dL, or ketonuria greater than 80 mg/dL. DKA is considered mild with pH <7.3 and serum bicarbonate <15 mmol/L, moderate DKA has pH <7.2 and bicarbonate is <10 mmol/L, severe DKA has pH <7.1 and bicarbonate <5 mmol/L. In comparison, HHS has a much higher glucose level of 600 to 1200 mg/dL, venous pH is >7.3, serum bicarbonate is >18 mmol/L, minimal or no plasma ketones, and osmolality is 330 to 380 mmol/kg (Dhatariya, 2019).

Differential diagnoses of DKA can include starvation ketosis, alcoholic ketoacidosis, and other forms of increased anion gap acidosis. However, differential diagnoses for patients with classical symptoms of polyuria, polydipsia, and weight loss, are rather limited to type 1 diabetes and in some instances include type 2 diabetes and/or diabetes due to specific cause. Abdominal pain and nausea and vomiting may be confused with acute abdomen if DKA is not severe. Diagnosis of type 1 diabetes is confirmed by presence of autoimmune markers such as islet cell autoantibodies and autoantibodies to GAD (GAD65), insulin, the tyrosine phosphatases, and zinc transporter (ADA, 2021; Pasquel et al., 2021).

Outside of a critical setting, diagnosis of diabetes requires two abnormal diagnostic test results. These diagnostic tests include FPG value (>126 mg/dL), 2-hr plasma glucose (2-hr PG) value (>200 mg/dL) during a 75-g OGTT and/or HgA1C result greater than 6.5%. The tests can be combined, or the same test can be repeated next day to confirm diagnosis (ADA, 2021). Differentiation between type 1 and type 2 is critical in terms of treatment plan, regardless of whether in the outpatient or hospital setting.

TREATMENT

In nonhospital settings, most children/adolescents with newly diagnosed with type 1 diabetes are referred to a pediatric diabetes clinic for a multidisciplinary team approach and treatment plan. With absolute deficiency of insulin, injection of exogenous insulin is mandated simply to sustain life. There are many modalities via which insulin can be injected, such as insulin syringes, insulin pens, and/or insulin pumps. Continuous glucose monitoring that conveys interstitial glucose level results to the insulin pump are routine. Management of type 1 diabetes is very complex, and it affects not only the individual but the entire family. The continuous need for insulin and constant adjustments of life's normal activities to prevent hypoglycemia may take a toll on physical, psychological, and social well-being. Depression among individuals with type 1 diabetes is common. Without question, diabetes technology has improved the lives of people with type 1 diabetes, but neither a cure nor prevention has been found.

Management of type 2 diabetes had been a great challenge to primary healthcare providers due to increased prevalence and complications. Primary prevention, or at least delaying the onset of type 2 diabetes with the life-style modifications of healthy diet, increased activities, administration of metformin, and screening of high-risk populations has been advocated by various health organizations for years (Aroda et al., 2017; Gruss et al., 2019; Lovic et al., 2020; Moin et al., 2018; Weisman et al., 2018).

Secondary prevention for persons with diabetes aims at achieving an individualized HbA1C target goal. The addition of pharmacologic agents, including insulin, to lifestyle modification is often a necessity. In its annual Standards of Medical Care in Diabetes, the ADA outlines evidence-based treatment recommendations for all types of diabetes. Although the target goal for HgA1C level is recommended to be <7%, the ADA underscores individualized target goals to minimize hypoglycemia. As per ADA (2021) guidelines, patients with established cardiovascular disease, apart from lifestyle modification and metformin, should be prescribed a glucagon-like peptide 1 receptor agonist (GLP-1 RA) or sodium-glucose cotransporter 2 inhibitor (SGLT2i). If still not at target goal for HgA1C, dipeptidyl peptidase 4 inhibitors (DPP-4), basal insulin, thiazolidinediones (TZD), or sulfonylureas (SU) should be considered. Current recommendations for most patients with type 2 diabetes include one agent from either SGLT2i or GLP-1 RA then DPP-4 and/or basal insulin. Patients with diabetes and heart failure should avoid TZDs. An essential part of secondary prevention includes treatment of blood pressure (individualized but <130/80 mmHg) and cholesterol (triglycerides <150 mg/dl, HDL cholesterol >40 mg/dL for males >50 mg/dl for females).

Inpatient Hyperglycemia

In hospitalized patients with diabetes, hyperglycemia is associated with adverse outcomes such as longer hospital stays, increased rate of infection, and mortality (Lansang & Umpierrez, 2016). There are several recommendations for glycemic target control in hospitalized patients by different medical organizations, but general consensus is that hyperglycemia starts at 140 mg/dL and that random blood sugar levels should not be higher than 180 mg/dL. Most hospitals implement their own diabetes protocols based on the ADA and/or the American Association of Endocrinologist guidelines with treatment goals for pre-meal glucose levels of 140 to 180 mg/dL. Higher blood glucose targets may be acceptable for older adults particularly in those with terminal illness and severe comorbidities (Gosmanov et al., 2020). More stringent goals (110–140 mg/dL) are acceptable for selected populations, such as postsurgical patients, but care needs to be taken to avoid hypoglycemia.

In critical care settings, insulin infusions are typically started in clients with persistent blood glucose levels over 180 mg/dL. An integral part of diabetes management in the hospital setting is frequent blood glucose monitoring to prevent hypoglycemia (every 30 minutes to 1 hour). Outside of critical care units, hyperglycemia

of above 180 mg/dL is managed with SC basal and prandial insulins administrations. The use of a sliding insulin scale as a mean of hyperglycemia management is strongly discouraged (ADA, 2021; Dhatariya et al., 2020).

The ADA (2021) recommends that patients with type 1 diabetes who undergo surgery or who are seriously ill should continue their basal insulin infusion either via insulin pump, IV, or as SC injection. Short-acting insulin alone is inadequate and may result in insulin deficiency leading to DKA (e.g., with delayed surgery). Patients with type 2 diabetes on insulin undergoing surgery should have their long-acting insulin reduced by 20% to 50% depending on the clinical setting. Oral antidiabetic drugs should be discontinued upon admission and are generally not recommended in the hospital setting due to a slow onset of action and potential risk for kidney injury with use of radiographic dye (lactic acidosis with metformin). Once clinically stable, oral antidiabetic drugs may be resumed in anticipation of discharge.

Treatment for DKA is discussed in Section 8.4 of this chapter; treatment for hyperglycemic hyperosmolar syndrome is discussed in Section 8.5.

Hypoglycemia

Hypoglycemia is a common side effect of treatment of all types of diabetes. Fear of hypoglycemia is a major barrier to satisfactory long-term glycemic control. Hypoglycemia is a result of an imbalance between glucose supply, glucose utilization, and current insulin levels. It is often defined as blood glucose level <70 mg/dL; severe hypoglycemia is defined as blood glucose level of <40 mg/dL (ADA, 2021). Hypoglycemia symptoms are related to sympathetic activation (palpitation, sweating, tremor, anxiety, and hunger) as well as to brain dysfunction secondary to a decreased level of glucose (difficulty with concentration, irritability, confusion, focal impairment, coma, and death; Iqbal & Heller, 2018). Treatment therapy for hypoglycemia is administration of glucose; depending on the situation and presentation it can be in form of glucose supplements, glucose-elevating agents (glucagon, intranasal glucagon) or IV glucose infusion. Prevention of hypoglycemia in the hospital setting can be accomplished with frequent monitoring of blood glucose level and appropriate adjustment of insulin dose (Iqbal & Heller, 2018).

TRANSITION OF CARE

Diabetes management requires a multidisciplinary approach, but self-management of diabetes is core to diabetes control. Upon discharge patients should be referred to an endocrinology clinic, diabetes educator, dietician, fitness center, and social services to aid in this transition. Diabetes education should be initiated during the patient's admission and if type 1 they must be discharged home with orders for diabetes supplies: insulin, syringes, insulin pens, glucose meter, strips, lancets, glucose tablets, and glucagon.

CLINICAL PEARLS

- Patients with type 2 diabetes may present with no symptoms; therefore, screening for diabetes among individuals with increased risk factors such as obesity and sedentary lifestyle is an important preventive measure.
- More than half of patients with type 1 diabetes have classic symptoms of polyuria, polydipsia, and weight loss on presentation; one third of this population will present in DKA.
- There are set criteria to differentiate DKA and HHS which are critical for treatment purposes.

KEY TAKEAWAYS

- There are four identifiable types of diabetes with type 2 diabetes being the most common (90%–95%).
- Differentiation between type 1 and type 2 diabetes is critical in terms of treatment therapy: Type 2 can be managed with lifestyle modification and pharmaceutical agents; type 1 diabetes requires lifelong insulin therapy to sustain life.
- DKA is most common with type 1 diabetes while HHS is specific to type 2 diabetes. Presenting symptoms and lab values help in differential diagnosis and consequent treatment which varies for each condition.
- Hypoglycemia is the most common and feared side effect of diabetes treatment.
- ADA annually outlines evidence-based diabetes care guidelines for outpatient and hospital settings which are a reference point not only for clinicians in the United States but worldwide.

EVIDENCE-BASED RESOURCES

2021 American Diabetes Association Standards of Medical Care in Diabetes.

2020 Consensus Statement by the American Association of Clinical Endocrinologists and American College of Endocrinology on the Comprehensive Type 2 Diabetes management Algorithm.

2018 International Society for Pediatric and Adolescent Diabetes Clinical Practice Consensus Guidelines 2018: definition, epidemiology, and classification of diabetes in children and adolescents.

8.4: DIABETIC KETOACIDOSIS

Jacqueline Ferdowsali

PRESENTING SIGNS AND SYMPTOMS

The onset of symptoms associated with diabetic ketoacidosis (DKA) is typically within 24-hours after an initiating event and often less than a few hours. The observed and reported signs and symptoms are associated with metabolic derangements including acidosis, hyperglycemia, and a catabolic state. While the classic symptoms of polyuria, polydipsia, and polyphagia are cited frequently in the literature, several studies have demonstrated the frequency of vomiting, abdominal pain, and altered mental state as key presenting signs and symptoms (Ahuja et al., 2019). Box 8.2 lists the commonly encountered presenting signs and symptoms (Fayfman et al., 2017; Nyenwe & Kitabchi, 2016; Umpierrez & Korytkowski, 2016).

HISTORY AND PHYSICAL FINDINGS

An important consideration in the management of DKA is evaluation for a precipitating cause. Commonly encountered causes are infection (14%–16%), new diagnosis of diabetes (17.2%–23.8%), inadequate insulin administration—either intentional or from mechanical failure of an insulin pump (41%–59.6%), physiologic stressful events (4%) such as noninfectious illness, myocardial infarction, alcohol use, pancreatitis, or cerebrovascular events, or use of certain drugs (Box 8.3; Fayfman et al., 2017; Umpierrez & Korytkowski, 2016). The history evaluation should seek information about recent illnesses and medications both prescribed and illicit. The metabolic changes associated with dehydration and

BOX 8.2: DIABETIC KETOACIDOSIS PRESENTING SIGNS AND SYMPTOMS

- Dehydration
- Diffuse abdominal pain
- Fever
- Mental status changes (e.g., confusion, loss of consciousness)
- Nausea/vomiting
- Polyuria
- Polyphagia
- Weight loss
- Weakness

BOX 8.3: DRUGS ASSOCIATED WITH DIABETIC KETOACIDOSIS

- Antipsychotic agents (e.g., clozapine, olanzapine, risperidone)
- Corticosteroids
- Beta-blockers
- Diuretics
- Glucagon
- Illicit drugs and alcohol (e.g., cocaine, cannabis)
- Interferon
- Pentamide
- Sodium glucose cotransporter 2 inhibitors (SGLT2)
- Sympathomimetics
- Thiazide diuretics

a hyperosmolar state lead to the physical exam findings of poor skin turgor, dry mucous membranes, Kussmaul respirations, tachycardia, and hypotension. Patients may be hyperthermic, normothermic, or hypothermic. The development of metabolic acidosis leads to the respiratory compensation of Kussmaul respirations. A fruity acetone odor when the patient is exhaling may be present.

DIFFERENTIAL DIAGNOSIS AND DIAGNOSTIC CONSIDERATIONS

Differential Diagnoses

A main clinical feature of DKA is a high anion gap metabolic acidosis, a differential diagnosis for which includes ingestion of glycols, aspirin, methanol or oxoproline, lactate, and renal failure. There are a few important considerations that impact clinical reasoning. In general, severely altered mental status is often not encountered until the effective osmolality is >320 mOsm/L and with acidemia. Additionally, abdominal pain frequency increases as the severity of DKA increases. In those patients with severe abdominal pain and mild DKA, an alternative etiology of abdominal pain should be investigated (Altkorn, 2020).

Diagnostic Workup

The key admission biochemical evaluation should include a metabolic evaluation. These tests are summarized in Box 8.4. Recommendations have shifted to the use of beta-hydroxybutyrate as the preferred test for evaluation of ketones over measurement of acetoacetate (Nyenwe & Kitabchi, 2016).

Diagnostic Criteria

Elevated ketones are the key diagnostic criteria for DKA. DKA can range from mild (pH 7.25–7.30), moderate (pH 7.00 to less than 7.24), to severe (pH less than 7.0; Kitabchi et al., 2009). The elevation of hyperglycemia should not be used to evaluate the severity of disease as some patients present with only mild elevation of glucose (euglycemic DKA).

BOX 8.4: SUMMARY OF DIAGNOSTIC TESTS FOR DIABETIC KETOACIDOSIS

- 3-hydroxybutyrate or urine or blood acetoacetate
- Anion gap
- Arterial or venous pH
- Bicarbonate
- Blood urea nitrogen (BUN)
- Creatinine
- Glucose
- Potassium
- Serum osmolality
- Sodium
- White blood cell count

TREATMENT

See hyperosmolar hyperglycemic syndrome (HHS) treatment, Section 8.5 of this chapter.

TRANSITION OF CARE

The main transition for a patient with DKA is changing from IV insulin to SC insulin. The main trigger point is the resolution of ketoacidosis which is determined by a blood glucose less than 200 mg/dL, a serum bicarbonate level >15 mEq/L, a venous pH >7.3, and a calculated anion gap less than or equal to 12 mEq/L (Nyenwe & Kitabchi, 2016). Once ready for SC insulin a home regimen may be resumed if well controlled previously or starting a multidose regimen at 0.5–0.8 U/kg/day. A key piece to a successful transition is continuing the insulin IV infusion until 2 hours after the SC insulin has been administered.

KEY TAKEAWAY

- DKA is a rapidly progressive complication of diabetes that requires close monitoring of fluid and electrolytes.

8.5: HYPERGLYCEMIC HYPEROSMOLAR STATE

Jacqueline Ferdowsali

PRESENTING SIGNS AND SYMPTOMS

The onset of symptoms associated with hyperosmolar hyperglycemic syndrome (HHS) can develop over several days to weeks (Kitabchi et al., 2009). The classic symptoms are similar to that of diabetic ketoacidosis (DKA) and include polyuria, polydipsia, weight loss, vomiting, weakness, and mental status changes. Patients with HHS may also develop focal neurologic findings such as hemianopia as well as seizures and blurred vision.

HISTORY AND PHYSICAL FINDINGS

Investigating the main cause of HHS is an important piece of history gathering. Infection, especially urinary tract infection and pneumonia, remains the leading precipitating event (30%–60% of patients) but other important considerations include medication noncompliance or other illnesses such as trauma, myocardial infarction, or cerebrovascular events (Fayfman et al., 2017; Umpierrez & Korytkowski, 2016). A review of current medications is also important as some medications may alter carbohydrate metabolism and lead to HHS (Box 8.5). The metabolic changes associated with dehydration and hyperosmolar state lead to the physical exam findings of poor skin turgor, dry mucous membranes, tachycardia, and hypotension.

BOX 8.5; DRUGS ASSOCIATED WITH DIABETIC KETOACIDOSIS AND HYPERGLYCEMIC HYPEROSMOLAR STATE

- Antipsychotic agents (e.g., clozapine, olanzapine, risperidone)*
- Beta-blockers*
- Corticosteroids*
- Diuretics
- Glucagon
- Illicit drugs and alcohol (e.g., cocaine, cannabis)
- Interferon
- Pentamide
- Sodium glucose cotransporter 2 inhibitors (SGLT2)
- Sympathomimetic
- Thiazide diuretics*

*Indicates medications also associated with the development of hyperosmolar hyperglycemic syndrome.

BOX 8.6: ADMISSION BIOCHEMICAL EVALUATION FOR HYPERGLYCEMIC HYPEROSMOLAR STATE

- Anion gap
- Arterial or venous pH
- Bicarbonate
- Blood urea nitrogen (BUN)
- Chest x-ray
- Complete blood count
- Creatinine
- Electrocardiogram
- Glucose
- Potassium
- Sodium
- Serum and urine ketones
- Serum osmolality
- Urinalysis
- Urine, sputum, or blood cultures

DIFFERENTIAL DIAGNOSIS AND DIAGNOSTIC CONSIDERATIONS

Differential Diagnoses

The main differential diagnosis for HHS is DKA. The key difference being absence of ketoacidosis in HHS. Additionally, the elevation of serum glucose is much higher in HHS. Consideration for other potential causes of elevated serum osmolality may be helpful. These include diabetes insipidus, hypernatremia, as well as alcohol ingestion.

Diagnostic Workup

The key admission biochemical evaluation should include a metabolic evaluation. These and other important tests are summarized in Box 8.6.

Diagnostic Criteria

The diagnostic criteria for HHS include a plasma glucose over 600 mg/dL, effective serum osmolality greater than 320 mOsm/kg, arterial pH greater than 7.30, serum bicarbonate greater than 18, small urine ketones and serum ketones, variable anion gap, and mental status of stupor (Kitabchi et al., 2009). While absence of ketosis is a key finding, in some individuals with HHS it is possible that there may be a high anion gap metabolic acidosis due to ketoacidosis and/or increased serum lactate levels (Umpierrez & Korytkowski, 2016).

TREATMENT

Management of DKA and HHS follow a hyperglycemia treatment approach. The three critical interventions for initial management involve fluid resuscitation, insulin administration, and potassium monitoring and replacement if indicated. The first step begins with fluid replacement. Calculation of the water deficit is helpful to guide fluid resuscitation. Each component is discussed further in more detail. Additionally, depending on the severity of illness, DKA may be treated in the emergency department without admission to the hospital, in a step-down unit if uncomplicated or in the ICU.

Fluids

Isotonic saline should be initially administered at a rate of 15 to 20 mL/kg body weight per hour over the first hour. After this period, the fluid selected should be based on sodium level and degree of volume depletion. If high or normal serum sodium, then 0.45% NaCl at 250 to 500 mL/hr or 0.9% NaCl if low serum sodium at 250 to 500 mL/hr depending on hydration status. Once the serum glucose reaches 200 mg/dL, then the addition of 5% dextrose with 0.45% NaCl should be made. The infusion rate can also be decreased to 150 to 250 mL/hr (Kitabchi et al., 2009). Recent investigation into a two-bag approach to dextrose administration in DKA have demonstrated varying results. While further studies are needed to demonstrate a significant benefit over the traditional one-bag approach, the two-bag approach does not appear to be an inferior treatment strategy (Cho et al., 2021; Haas et al., 2018). Bicarbonate should be administered in patients when the pH is less than 6.9 and until the pH rises above 7.0.

Insulin

Two decision points in treating DKA and HHS involve the administration of IV or SC insulin and whether a bolus dose of insulin should be ordered. Recent research has demonstrated the ability to safely manage uncomplicated mild to moderate DKA with rapid-acting insulin analogues (Nyenwe & Kitabchi, 2016; Umpierrez & Korytkowski, 2016). This strategy involves the hourly administration of a rapid-acting insulin SC until the DKA has resolved. In any patient with severe DKA, HHS, or complications such as anasarca, shock, or mental obtundation an IV insulin approach should be used. Recommendations include the option for either administering a bolus dose of regular insulin followed by a continuous infusion or not giving the bolus dose. Evidence has not supported the benefit of a bolus and some authors advocate avoiding administering a bolus (Brown et al., 2018; Nyenwe & Kitabchi, 2016). To prevent development of cerebral edema the glucose level in HHS should not fall below 200 mg/dL until any encephalopathy has resolved and in DKA below 150 mg/dL until the ketoacidosis resolves. IV insulin should be administered until the DKA or HHS has resolved as evidenced by correction of hyperglycemia and ketoacidosis and the patient is transitioned to a SC insulin administration route.

Potassium

Electrolyte abnormalities are common in DKA and HHS. Careful monitoring and evaluation of serum potassium should be done. Part of this evaluation is monitoring renal function and ensuring that urine output is around 50 mL/hr. The goal for serum potassium is between 4 and 5 mEq/L. Based on the observed potassium level, potassium may need to be added and the insulin held until a safe level is achieved. Phosphate may be depleted in patients with DKA. Cautious replacement should be considered, as overtreatment of hypophosphatemia could cause hypocalcemia. It is generally recommended to only replace phosphate if there are signs of hypophosphatemia (Lee & Rickard, 2018).

TRANSITION OF CARE

Resolution of HHS is achieved once the serum osmolality and mental status normalize. Once ready for SC insulin a home regimen may be resumed if well controlled previously or if starting a multidose regimen at 0.5 to 0.8 U/kg/day. A key piece to a successful transition is continuing the insulin IV infusion until 2 hours after the SC insulin has been administered.

> ### KEY TAKEAWAYS
> - Precipitating causes of DKA and HHS should be investigated through the history and physical exam.
> - Metabolic acidosis may be present in HHS and does not exclude its diagnosis.
> - Fluid administration is a key strategy in managing both DKA and HHS.

8.6: HYPOTHYROIDISM

Jacqueline Ferdowsali

PRESENTING SIGNS AND SYMPTOMS

There are no signs or symptoms that are sensitive or specific to arrive at a diagnosis of hypothyroidism. Typically, younger individuals present with more symptoms, but the number of signs or symptoms does not predict the severity of hypothyroidism (Carlé et al., 2016). Symptom presentation can range from asymptomatic to severely symptomatic as in the case of myxedema coma. While it is rare to encounter a patient with myxedema coma, the identification of myxedema coma (altered mental status, hypothermia, lethargy, bradycardia, organ system dysfunction) should not be delayed as it can lead to death (Chaker et al., 2017). Table 8.4 provides a summary of the signs and symptoms associated with hypothyroidism.

HISTORY AND PHYSICAL FINDINGS

The most common causes of hypothyroidism are classified as primary and are due to a thyroid hormone deficiency. The causes of primary hypothyroidism are summarized in Box 8.7 (Chaker et al., 2017). Important history questions to consider include previous history of autoimmune disease, previous head or neck surgery or history of head trauma, medications associated with hypothyroidism (more common ones include iodine, amiodarone, lithium), recent or current infections and a genetic history of Down or Turner syndrome. The assessment of the thyroid gland is imperative during the physical examination. Findings such as gland enlargement, presence of nodes, firm texture, and tenderness can be helpful in the evaluation for hypothyroidism. Since the thyroid gland has systemic actions, assessment of other systems is also important. This includes a cardiovascular exam for bradycardia and heart failure, skin and hair for hair loss, dryness or periorbital edema, the nervous system for hypoactive reflexes, and a mental status examination.

DIFFERENTIAL DIAGNOSIS AND DIAGNOSTIC CONSIDERATIONS

Differential Diagnoses

The classic symptoms associated with hypothyroidism of fatigue, constipation, and cold intolerance all lack sensitivity and specificity for the diagnosis of hypothyroidism. Potential differential diagnoses for each of these symptoms should be considered. These include anemia, pregnancy, other causes of alterations in thyroid stimulating hormone (TSH) levels, and nonthyroidal illness syndrome. In addition to evaluation of the general symptoms a differential diagnosis of either primary (due to thyroid deficiency), central which includes secondary (due to TSH deficiency from either pituitary), tertiary (a hypothalamic process due to thyrotropin-releasing hormone deficiency), or peripheral (extra-thyroidal) causes of hypothyroidism should be considered (Chaker et al., 2017).

Diagnostic Testing

The thyroid gland is part of the hypothalamic-pituitary-thyroid axis. The gland works through a negative feedback mechanism. Initial testing of thyroid function is done through TSH measurement. In hypothyroidism

TABLE 8.4: Clinical Presentation and Implications of Hypothyroidism

SYSTEM	SYMPTOM	SIGNS
General	Weight gain, cold intolerance, fatigue	Increase in body mass index, myxedema,* hypothermia*
Cardiovascular	Fatigue on exertion, shortness of breath	Dyslipidemia, bradycardia, hypertension, endothelial dysfunction or increased intima-media thickness,* diastolic dysfunction,* pericardial effusion,* hyperhomocysteinemia,* EKG changes*
Neurosensory	Hoarseness of voice, decreased taste, vision, or hearing	Neuropathy, cochlear dysfunction, decreased olfactory and gustatory sensitivity
Neurologic and psychiatric	Impaired memory, paresthesia, mood impairment	Impaired cognitive function, delayed relaxation of tendon reflexes, depression,* dementia,* ataxia,* carpal tunnel syndrome and other nerve entrapment syndromes, myxedema coma*
Gastrointestinal	Constipation	Reduced esophageal motility, nonalcoholic fatty liver disease,* ascites (very rare)
Endocrine	Infertility and subfertility, menstrual disturbance, galactorrhoea	Goiter, glucose metabolism dysregulation, infertility, sexual dysfunction, increased prolactin, pituitary hyperplasia*
Musculoskeletal	Muscle weakness, muscle cramps, arthralgia	Creatine phosphokinase elevation, Hoffman's syndrome,* osteoporotic fracture* (most probably caused by overtreatment)
Hematologic	Bleeding, fatigue	Mild anemia, acquired von Willebrand disease,* decreased protein culture and sensitivity,* increased red cell distribution width,* increased mean platelet volume*
Skin and Hair	Dry skin, hair loss	Coarse skin, loss of lateral eyebrows,* yellow palms of the hand,* alopecia areata*
Electrolytes and Kidney Function		Decreased estimated glomerular filtration rate, hyponatremia*

*Indicates an uncommon presentation.

Source: Reproduced with permission from Chaker, L., Bianco, A. C., Jonklaas, J., & Peeters, R. P. (2017). Hypothyroidism. *Lancet, 390*(10101), 1550–1562. https://doi.org/10.1016/S0140-6736(17)30703-1

BOX 8.7: CAUSES OF PRIMARY HYPOTHYROIDISM

- Chronic autoimmune thyroiditis (Hashimoto's)
- Drugs (amiodarone, lithium, tyrosine kinase inhibitors, interferon-alfa, thalidomide, monoclonal antibodies, antiepileptic drugs, second-line treatment drugs for tuberculosis)
- Genetics
- Iatrogenic (radiotherapy or surgery in the head or neck, radioiodine treatment)
- Iodine deficiency and excess
- Thyroid gland infiltration (infectious, malignant, autoimmune, inflammatory)
- Transient thyroiditis (viral, post-partum, silent, destructive)

the TSH is high, often greater than 10 mU/L. If elevated, free thyroxine (FT4), which is unbound thyroid hormone, should be assessed. Overt hypothyroidism is diagnosed when the FT4 is low. While rare, TSH may be low or normal in cases of central hypothyroidism as there is a problem within either the pituitary or hypothalamus. Additional consideration should be paid to testing in critically ill patients. There may be a significant reduction in TSH levels due to critical illness rather than thyroid pathology and results should be interpreted cautiously. In general, testing in critically ill patients is not recommended unless there is strong clinical suspicion. Clinically, measurement of triiodothyronine (T3) or reverse T3 are not helpful in the diagnosis of hypothyroidism (Garber et al., 2012). If concerned about Hashimoto's thyroiditis, the measurement of thyroid peroxidase antibody and thyroglobulin antibody is helpful. The Choosing Wisely® initiative recommends against routinely imaging the thyroid in hypothyroidism unless there are nodules or a large goiter present (American Board of Internal Medicine Foundation, 2018).

Subclinical hypothyroidism is diagnosed when the TSH is elevated but the FT4 is normal (Biondi et al., 2019). Euthyroid sick is a condition in acutely ill patients in which the FT4 is low as well as a low or normal TSH. No treatment is indicated for this condition.

TREATMENT

Replacement with L-thyroxine is the cornerstone of therapy for hypothyroidism (Jonklaas et al., 2014). Dosing should be based on age, weight, and sex. In general, a dose of 1.6 mcg/kg (ideal body weight) per day is recommended. Older adults should be started on lower doses and titrated at a slower rate due to decreased replacement requirement. Oral administration is generally recommended unless the patient is unable to take enteral supplement. IV preparations are available and should be administered at 75% of the required oral dose. Patient education needs to include the importance of taking the medication on an empty stomach, between 30 and 60 minutes prior to eating breakfast or 3 hours after the evening meal at bedtime. Typically, dosage adjustments are done every 4 to 8 weeks after repeat testing. The goals of treatment are achieving an euthyroid state and normalization of TSH and thyroid hormones.

Treatment of subclinical hypothyroidism is controversial. If treated, the dose of L-thyroxine is lower, around 25 to 75 mcg daily. Patients with TSH levels over 10 mU/L should be treated. There is limited evidence of benefit in treating levels between 7.0 and 9.9 mU/L. Levels of less than 7.0 mU/L are rarely treated unless symptom management is a consideration (Biondi et al., 2019).

8.7: HYPOTHYROIDISM–MYXEDEMA COMA

Alnee Gadberry

Myxedema coma is a rare but severe form of hypothyroidism. A profound lack of thyroid hormone leads to decompensation with a variety of symptoms. It is considered a medical emergency that may lead to death, with an estimated mortality rate of more than 50% without early identification and intervention (Cho et al., 2019; Eledrisi, 2020; Mathew et al., 2011; Wall, 2000).

The name "myxedema coma" is somewhat deceptive, in that the patient rarely presents in a comatose state. It is likely that the patient will present with delirium and a history of hypothyroidism, and it is not uncommon for this to be the initial presentation of hypothyroidism.

Any person with hypothyroidism can develop myxedema coma; however, older women are most affected, with increased occurrence in the winter months (Cho et al., 2019; Mathew et al., 2011; Wall, 2000). Infection, surgery, burns, medications, or cold exposure are all acute events that may precipitate the event, but infection and septicemia seem to be the leading causes (Eledrisi, 2020; Mathew et al., 2011).

Another factor to consider is the discontinuation of thyroid supplementations. This may be overlooked due to critical illness or the use of other medications during critical illness such as amiodarone or certain sedatives (Mathew et al., 2011).

PRESENTING SIGNS AND SYMPTOMS

The hallmark sign of myxedema coma is altered mentation and hypothermia (Cho et al., 2019). Other common findings including bradycardia, hypotension, hypoventilation, hyponatremia, hypoglycemia, and nonpitting generalized edema (Cho et al., 2019; Eledrisi, 2020; Mathew et al., 2011; Wall, 2000). A thyroidectomy scar with other signs of hypothyroidism already mentioned may give clues to help formulate the diagnosis.

HISTORY AND PHYSICAL FINDINGS

Hypoventilation may be severe enough to lead to hypercapnia and need for mechanical ventilation (Wall, 2000). Pleural effusions and pericardial effusions may be present, but these patients tend to be coagulopathic, so drainage is only done if necessary (Mathew et al., 2011). It is common that poor adherence contributes to the diagnosis but as mentioned before it may be the initial presentation in the undiagnosed patient.

DIFFERENTIAL DIAGNOSIS AND DIAGNOSTIC CONSIDERATIONS

A diagnosis is suspected after a thorough history and physical exam are completed and thyroid function test are used to confirm the diagnosis. A thyroid stimulating hormone (TSH), free T4, and cortisol levels should all be drawn (Eledrisi, 2020; Mathew et al., 2011) which will help identify pan hypopituitary or adrenal insufficiency concerns. With primary hypothyrodisim the serum T4 is usually low and TSH may be high (primary hypothyroidism), normal, or low (central hypothyroidism) (Eledrisi, 2020; Mathew et al., 2011).

The cortisol level should be extremely low or extremely high for a diagnosis to be confirmed; if inconclusive an ACTH stimulation test must be completed to assess adrenal function (Eledrisi, 2020; Mathew et al., 2011).

TREATMENT

If myxedema coma is suspected, treatment should not be delayed while awaiting laboratory results (Eledrisi, 2020). The high mortality associated with the condition warrants aggressive therapy of thyroid hormone, steroids, and supportive management (Mathew et al., 2011). The patient should be admitted to the ICU for close monitoring. Mechanical ventilation may be necessary, as well as frequent electrolyte replacement, glucose management, and rewarming.

IV thyroid hormone replacement of levothyroxine 300 to 600 mcg loading dose, followed by 50 to 100 mcg daily dose until oral medications may be resumed (Eledrisi, 2020; Mathew et al., 2011); at the same time, liothyronine 5 to 20 mcg, followed by 2.5 to 10 mcg every 8 hours (Eledrisi, 2020). Lower doses are generally preferred with close monitoring due to the possibility of arrhythmia or myocardial infarction (Eledrisi, 2020).

In most cases, steroids are given until adrenal insufficiency has been ruled out. This is done with hydrocortisone 50 to 100 mg every 8 hours (Eledrisi, 2020; Mathew et al., 2011). Dexamethasone may be used at dose 2 to 4 mg every 12 hours (Eledrisi, 2020; Mathew et al., 2011). Dexamethasone will not affect the serum cortisol or the ACTH stimulation test. If these are proven to be normal, steroids may be discontinued (Eledrisi, 2020; Mathew et al., 2011).

8.8: HYPERTHYROIDISM

Richard Pembridge

Thyroid disease has an impact on the physiological function of many body systems. Hyperthyroidism is characterized by excessive production of thyroxine and triiodothyronine which can result from multiple conditions. Hyperthyroidism can be from a toxic nodular goiter, hyperactivity of the thyroid gland, or toxic adenomas. The thyroid stimulating hormone (TSH) is suppressed because of the excessive response from thyroxine and triiodothyronine. Certain clinical conditions can cause hyperthyroidism such as pregnancy and Hashimoto's thyroiditis. The crisis for hyperthyroidism is called "thyroid storm" which often lands a patient in the hospital setting for symptom management. Definitive treatment is either radioactive iodine (RAI) treatment or a thyroidectomy.

PRESENTING SIGNS AND SYMPTOMS

Patients with hyperthyroidism will complain of heat intolerance and excessive sweating, irritability and dysphoria, and rapid weight loss. Patients will also have symptoms of palpitations, weakness, and fatigue. Signs experienced later into hyperthyroidism may include diarrhea, excessive urination, and women will experience oligomenorrhea. The family member of a patient with hyperthyroidism will often say the patient has periods of confusion, restlessness, irritability, and manic behavior.

HISTORY AND PHYSICAL FINDINGS

As previously mentioned, the patient will have a varying degree of complaints related to hyperactivity. On examination, a provider will assess that the patient has exertional dyspnea, low-grade temperature, increased appetite with profound weight loss, and fine motor tremors. The patient will be tachycardic and possibly experience atrial fibrillation. The deep tendon reflexes will exhibit hyperreflexia. The patient will have a palpable goiter or nodule and an eyelid lag (the eyelid lag is from exophthalmos from prolonged hyperthyroidism) and fine, thinning hair as well as hair loss. If the patient is experiencing thyrotoxicosis, they will exhibit delirium, extreme agitation, possible psychosis, and a stupor state.

Depending on the patient's condition, they may be managed in the outpatient setting versus admitted to control symptoms and hyperthyroidism effects. Findings include the following:

- Low TSH
- Elevated serum T3, T4, thyroid resin uptake, and free thyroixine index
- Hyperglycemia
- Increased erythrocyte sedimentation rate (ESR)
- Elevated serum antinuclear antibody (ANA)
- Hypercalcemia

DIFFERENTIAL DIAGNOSIS AND DIAGNOSTIC CONSIDERATIONS

Differential Diagnoses

- Graves' disease
- Hyperthyroidism
- Hyperactive thyroid nodule
- Graves' ophthalmopathy
- Thyroid storm (thyrotoxicosis)

Diagnostic Considerations

- RAI uptake scan
- MRI of the orbits to assess ophthalmopathy

TREATMENT

Symptom Relief

- Beta-blocker therapy (often propranolol or metoprolol) for tachycardia
- Antithyroid medication methimazole or propylthiouracil (PTH) if not performing a radioactive thyroid uptake scan
- Radioactive I^{131}
- Thyroid surgery

Thyrotoxicosis Treatment

- IV beta blockade
- IV antithyroid agents
- Antipyretics
- IV hydrocortisone
- Supportive physiologic function until euthyroid and surgery or RAI can be administered

TRANSITION OF CARE

- Endocrine follow-up for RAI treatment
- Monitor thyroid function tests periodically watching for euthyroid versus resultant hypothyroidism requiring thyroid hormone replacement

KEY TAKEAWAYS

- Aggressive assessment of the thyroid gland
- Avoid agents that block thyroid hormones unless the patient is severely symptomatic.
- Control symptoms with beta blockers
- Patient education on signs and symptoms and treatment plan

8.9: HYPERPARATHYROIDISM

Matthew Buesking

Hyperparathyroidism (HPT) is a condition caused by oversecretion of the parathyroid hormone. Excess secretion is often a result of parathyroid hyperplasia or adenomas, which cause elevated parathyroid hormone levels (PTH) which then precipitate hypercalcemia, the typical finding of primary HPT (Dulfer et al., 2017). HPT typically presents asymptomatically with elevated serum calcium levels and elevated PTH, where a normal physiologic response to elevated serum calcium should result in suppression of PTH (Insogna, 2018; Wilhelm et al., 2016). Associated with chronic kidney disease (CKD), secondary and tertiary HPT is a result of different physiologic processes. Secondary and tertiary HPT is observed in CKD or end-stage renal disease (ESRD) and postrenal transplant, respectively. Secondary HPT follows chronic hypocalcemia and hyperphosphatemia of CKD, causing hyperplasia of the parathyroid glands and resultant elevation in parathyroid hormone (PTH). Tertiary HPT occurs following chronic dysregulation of the parathyroid-bone-kidney feedback loop that fails to regulate following renal transplantation, causing severe hypercalcemia, hyperphosphatemia, and elevated PTH (Dulfer et al., 2017; van der Plas et al., 2020). Management strategies vary based on form and symptomatology, with well-defined criteria differentiating those that are candidates for medical versus surgical management.

PRESENTING SIGNS AND SYMPTOMS

HPT often presents asymptomatically, usually as an incidental laboratory finding of hypercalcemia, which prompts further evaluation. Primary HPT effects are manifested in skeletal and renal changes, including increased cortical bone loss, fragility fractures, as well as nephrolithiasis or nephrocalcinosis (Insogna, 2018). In well-developed countries, less than 20% of patients with primary HPT present with symptoms such as a fracture or nephrolithiasis (Insogna, 2018). Most commonly, incidental laboratory findings of hypercalcemia on routine laboratory studies prompt further evaluation to include parathyroid hormone testing (Silverberg et al., 2013). Women are disproportionately affected at a ratio of 3:1, typically occurring in the first decade after the onset of menopause (Bilezikian et al., 2018; Insogna, 2018; Silverberg et al., 2013). Rarely, signs of severe hypercalcemia such as neuromuscular weakness or obtundation precede diagnosis; however, this may be observed with large PTH adenomas or carcinomas (Insogna, 2018). Evaluation of constipation from moderate to severe hypercalcemia can also lead to a diagnosis of HPT (Insogna, 2018). With symptomatic HPT, as a result of prolonged hypercalcemia, presenting symptoms include pathologic fractures, renal calculi, pruritus,

muscle weakness, memory loss, depression, and concentration difficulties (van der Plas et al., 2020).

Secondary and tertiary HPT occurs in patients with CKD and ESRD or post kidney transplant. The effect of hypocalcemia and phosphate retention in CKD results in hyperplasia of parathyroid glands, leading to elevated PTH levels, leading to secondary HPT with typical findings of hypocalcemia, hyperphosphatemia, and elevated PTH (Dulfer et al., 2017). The effects of hypercalcemia may be more pronounced in tertiary hypercalcemia where characteristic laboratory findings of hypercalcemia, hyperphosphatemia, and elevated PTH levels result from a chronic irreversible alteration in the parathyroid-bone-kidney feedback loop (van der Plas et al., 2020). Differentiation is made where hypocalcemia is characteristic in secondary HPT while hypercalcemia is characteristic of tertiary HPT, which can be severe (Lou et al., 2015; van der Plas et al., 2020).

HISTORY AND PHYSICAL FINDINGS

Given that HPT is often asymptomatic, a complete history and review of systems may help uncover symptoms that suggest the need to evaluate for HPT. History significant for hyperthyroidism may reveal past nephrolithiasis, fragility fractures, or osteoporosis. Often, symptoms may be insidious with a history that positive for subjective cognitive, musculoskeletal, gastrointestinal, or neuropsychiatric symptoms (Wilhelm et al., 2016). While skeletal and renal symptoms remain the hallmark disease manifestations, additional effects are described including depression, anxiety, memory, and concentration deficits, as well as observations of hypertension and increased morbidity and mortality from cardiovascular causes (Insogna, 2018).

Physical exam findings are often noncontributory given the typical asymptomatic presentation. Less than twenty percent of patients have physical findings as a result of end organ effects such as fractures, renal colic, where effects of hypercalcemia may present with altered mentation, muscle weakness, constipation, or nausea (Bilezikian et al., 2018; Insogna, 2018).

DIFFERENTIAL DIAGNOSIS AND DIAGNOSTIC CONSIDERATIONS

Differential Diagnoses

The differential diagnosis of HPT is similar to that of hypercalcemia, which includes malignancy, primary HPT, tertiary HPT, medication induced (lithium, thiazide diuretics), or vitamin A and vitamin D intoxication, hyperthyroidism, Addison crisis, granulomatous disease, milk-alkali syndrome, chronic renal failure, and Paget's disease. Concurrent elevation of PTH along with hypercalcemia helps differentiate those causes most specific to HPT. Differential diagnosis with both PTH elevation and hypercalcemia includes familial hypocalciuric hypercalcemia (HCC), lithium use, or tertiary HPT (Arrangoiz et al., 2019).

BOX 8.8: CALCULATION FOR CORRECTED SERUM CALCIUM

Corrected calcium = Measured total serum calcium mg/dL + 0.8 (4.0 − serum albumin g/dL)

Diagnosis

Diagnosis of HPT is made when elevation of both calcium and PTH is apparent. Few conditions present with both elevated. HPT can present as normocalcemic with normal total or ionized calcium levels, where secondary causes of elevated PTH including vitamin D deficiency, CKD with estimated glomerular filtration rate (GFR) <60 mL/min, or from medications that increase PTH, including thiazide diuretics, bisphosphonates, denosumab, and lithium use which must be ruled out (Eastell et al., 2009). Ionized calcium or corrected total serum calcium is recommended to establish the degree of hypercalcemia. When ionized calcium cannot be obtained, corrected serum calcium should be calculated to account for albumin alterations with the formula in Box 8.8 (Bilezikian et al., 2014; Eastell et al., 2009). When normocalcemic HPT is suspected, elevated levels of PTH in the setting of normocalcemia should be confirmed on two separate occasions over 3 to 6 months prior to establishing diagnosis (Eastell et al., 2009). Once a HPT diagnosis is established, additional laboratory testing should include vitamin D levels and phosphorous levels (Silverberg et al., 2014). Primary HPT is felt to be more active with greater end organ effects with vitamin D (25(OH)D) levels <20 ng/mL (Bilezikian et al., 2014). Following the determination that HPT is present, the effects of HPT on end organs require evaluation, which guide treatment.

Renal evaluation is necessary to guide treatment course where calciuria and nephrocalcinosis are the most likely end organ effects of HPT (Silverberg et al., 2014). Creatinine clearance should be calculated following diagnosis of HPT, with a level <60 cc/min being an indication for surgical referral. When urinalysis identifies hypercilciuria, a 24-hour urine collection to evaluate calcium and creatinine levels should be collected. Imaging to detect nephrocalcinosis or nephrolithiasis, with x-ray, ultrasound, or CT is also necessary (Bilezikian et al., 2014; Wilhelm et al., 2016). Imaging helps establish the presence of subclinical renal stone disease, which is a decision point on treatment (Silverberg et al., 2014).

Skeletal effects of HPT should also be examined following diagnosis of HPT. The gold standard and the standard of care for examination of skeletal effects and bone marrow density is dual-energy x-ray absorptiometry (DXA; Silverberg et al., 2014). DXA examination of the hips, spine, and distal radius is recommended, with the distal radius being of increased interest due to primary HPT effects on cortical bone, where the distal radius is the most probable site to observe bone loss

and is a common site for fragility fractures (Silverberg et al., 2014; Wilhelm et al., 2016). Fractures or DXA results showing bone loss or osteoporosis is an additional decision point for surgical versus medical treatment recommendations.

Parathyroid imaging is another consideration following diagnosis of HPT. Aberrant secretion of PTH is a result of either adenoma, hyperplasia, or carcinoma of the parathyroid glands where one or more glands may be affected. Multiglandular HPT is seen in approximately 15% of patients (Wilhelm et al., 2016). Parathyroid imaging should not be performed to confirm or exclude a diagnosis of HPT and, often, parathyroid imaging can be reserved for surgical specialists, where imaging is primarily obtained to assist with surgical guidance. Ultrasonography is the most cost-effective imaging technique and when combined with sestamibi imaging, the sensitivity for identification of multiglandular disease increases (Wilhelm et al., 2016).

TREATMENT

Definitive treatment of HPT is surgical with a parathyrodoidectomy (Insogna, 2018). Surgical indications are well described, and surgery is indicated if any criteria in Box 8.9 are met. Surgical management represents the most effective treatment and is less costly than prolonged medical management and monitoring (Wilhelm et al., 2016). Intraoperative monitoring of PTH during parathyroidecromy is able to show normalization of PTH levels within 15 minutes of excision of the diseased parathyroid tissue, enabling high success rates of surgery (Bilezikian et al., 2014). Following parathyroidecromy, bone density improves, fracture incidence is reduced, renal stone incidence is reduced, and neurocognitive symptoms may also improve (Bilezikian et al., 2014).

Medical management is indicated for asymptomatic patients who do not meet surgical criteria, refuse surgery, or are poor candidates for surgery due to serious comorbidities. Ongoing monitoring includes yearly serum calcium and vitamin D levels. Bone density or DXA

BOX 8.9: INDICATION FOR PARATHYROIDECTOMY AND SURGICAL REFERRAL

- Age <50 at diagnosis
- Serum calcium >1 mg/dL above upper end normal
- Fracture/spinal fracture
- T-score of −2.5 or less of lumbar, hip, or distal 1/3 radius
- Creatinine clearance <60 cc/min
- Nephrocalcinosis, nephrolithiasis, or marked calciuria on 24-hr urine
- Neurocognitive or neuropsychiatric symptoms

imaging should be repeated every 1 to 2 years in addition to spinal x-rays to monitor for vertebral fractures. Annual renal studies including 24-hour urine measurement, creatinine clearance, with kidney imaging to evaluate for stone formation are also recommended. Changes of any of these monitoring parameters would be seen with a symptomatic disease transformation, which would then warrant surgical consideration (Insogna, 2018; Silverberg et al., 2014).

In nonsurgical patients, medication management helps with minimizing the effects of hypercalcemia, bone, and kidney disease. Dietary intake of calcium should not be restricted and optimal dietary intake of 1000 to 1200 mg of calcium per day should be maintained. Normal calcium intake does not lead to increased secretion of PTH, whereas calcium restriction may lead to increased PTH levels. Vitamin D levels should be maintained in the 20 to 30 mcg/mL range, with supplementation as needed. The use of Calcinet reduces elevated levels of PTH and calcium; however, it has no effect on bone loss. Thiazide diuretics can also be helpful in reducing nephrolithiasis risk, with added benefit of reducing PTH levels. Antiresorptive therapy or bisphosphonates can increase bone mass; however, they do not have an appreciable effect on hypercalcemia (Bilezikian et al., 2018; Insogna, 2018).

Treatment strategies of secondary HPT favor medical management. Calcinet is used in secondary HPT, which suppresses PTH production by increasing the sensitivity of the calcium receptors of the parathyroid gland (Dulfer et al., 2017). Additional strategies include supplementation of vitamin D, where low vitamin D levels are prevalent in patients with ESRD. Supplementation decreases PTH levels, proteinuria, and bone turnover. Hyperphosphatemia is treated with a low phosphorous diet and phosphate binders. Surgically, kidney transplantation eliminates HPT in approximately 60% of patients with secondary HPT (van der Plas et al., 2020). Tertiary HPT is treated similarly with medication; however, parathyroidecromy is indicated when medication management fails (van der Plas et al., 2020).

TRANSITION OF CARE

All patients having at least one indication for surgery should be referred to a well-qualified surgeon with experience in performing parathyroidecromy. Consider endocrinology referral for patients not meeting surgical criteria or who are not candidates for surgery.

CLINICAL PEARLS

- HPT presents with hypercalcemia and elevated PTH, often asymptomatic.
- End-organ targets of HPT include increased fragility of bone and formation of nephrolithiasis.
- Parathyroidectomy is definitive management, with near universal cure rates.

KEY TAKEAWAYS

- HPT often presents asymptomatically with an incidental finding of hypercalcemia, prompting further evaluation.
- Hypercalcemia and elevated PTH and decreased vitamin D are pathognomonic for HPT.
- Referral to a qualified surgeon for a parathyroidecromy is highly curative.
- Asymptomatic medication management is useful for minimizing risk for fractures and nephrolithiasis.

EVIDENCE-BASED RESOURCES

Bilezikian, J. P., Brandi, M. L., Eastell, R., Silverberg, S. J., Udelsman, R., Marcocci, C., & Potts, J. T. (2014). Guidelines for the management of asymptomatic primary hyperparathyroidism: Summary statement from the fourth international workshop. *The Journal of Clinical Endocrinology and Metabolism, 99*(10), 3561–3569. https://doi.org/10.1210/jc.2014-1413

Insogna, K. L. (2018). Primary hyperparathyroidism. *The New England Journal of Medicine, 379*(11), 1050–1059. https://doi.org/10.1056/NEJMcp1714213

Silverberg, S. J., Clarke, B. L., Peacock, M., Bandeira, F., Boutroy, S., Cusano, N. E., Dempster, D., Lewiecki, E. M., Liu, J.-M., Minisola, S., Rejnmark, L., Silva, B. C., Walker, M. D., & Bilezikian, J. P. (2014). Current issues in the presentation of asymptomatic primary hyperparathyroidism: Proceedings of the fourth international workshop. *The Journal of Clinical Endocrinology and Metabolism, 99*(10), 3580–3594. https://doi.org/10.1210/jc.2014-1415

Wilhelm, S. M., Wang, T. S., Ruan, D. T., Lee, J. A., Asa, S. L., Duh, Q., Doherty, G. M., Herrera, M. F., Pasieka, J. L., Perrier, N. D., Silverberg, S. J., Solórzano, C. C., Sturgeon, C., Tublin, M. E., Udelsman, R., & Carty, S. E. (2016). The American Association of Endocrine Surgeons guidelines for definitive management of primary hyperparathyroidism. *JAMA Surgery, 151*(10), 959–968. doi:10.1001/jamasurg.2016.2310

8.10: PHEOCHROMOCYTOMA

Aaron M. Sebach

Pheochromocytomas are rare adrenal gland tumors that develop in the chromaffin cells of the adrenal medulla. Men and women are equally affected, most commonly in their 40s or 50s. The tumors secrete catecholamines and symptomatic patients present with palpitations, tremors, elevated blood pressure, sweating, pallor, and generalized weakness. However, most patients are asymptomatic and the pheochromcytomas are identified incidentally through abdominal imaging studies. Plasma free metanephrines or a 24-hour urine for fractionated metanephrines are best practice initial diagnostic studies.

Radiologic studies should only be considered after plasma or urine metanephrines are positive. First-line imaging is an abdominal CT scan. Patients with pheochromocytomas should be referred to a general surgeon for adrenalectomy. Genetic testing is recommended for patients with multiple endocrine neoplasia type 2A or 2B, neurofibromatosis, von Hippel-Lindau disease, or a family history of pheochromocytoma.

PRESENTING SIGNS AND SYMPTOMS

Approximately 50% of patients with pheochromocytoma are symptomatic with paroxysmal hypertension reported as the most common presenting symptom (Neumann et al., 2019). The classic triad of symptoms are tachycardia, sweating, and headache, although most patients do not present with all three symptoms. Symptomatic patients commonly present with palpitations, diaphoresis, headaches, pallor, dyspnea, generalized weakness, and tremors due to excessive catecholamine secretion (Neumann et al., 2019).

HISTORY AND PHYSICAL FINDINGS

History

Patients with a history of multiple endocrine neoplasia type 2A or 2B, neurofibromatosis, von Hippel-Lindau disease, or a family history of pheochromocytoma are at risk for pheochromocytomas (Martucci & Pacak, 2014). Pheochromocytomas are identified equally in men and women in their fourth or fifth decade (Guerrero et al., 2009). Most tumors are discovered as incidental findings during abdominal CTs or MRIs (Davidson et al., 2018). Approximately 500 to 1,600 cases are identified each year (Martucci & Pacak, 2014).

Physical Findings

Symptomatic patients will present with headache, generalized sweating, paroxysmal hypertension, pallor, dyspnea, generalized weakness, tremors, and palpitations. Due to the location of pheochromocytomas, there are no specific physical findings.

DIFFERENTIAL DIAGNOSIS AND DIAGNOSTIC CONSIDERATIONS

Differential Diagnoses

- Hyperthyroidism
- Alcohol withdrawal
- Hypertension
- Illicit drug use (e.g., cocaine, phencyclidine, lysergic acid diethylamide)
- Insulinoma
- Anxiety

Diagnostic Considerations

1. **Laboratory Studies** (Lenders et al., 2014)
   a. Plasma-free metanephrines
      i. Patient should be in a supine position during venipuncture to prevent false positives
   b. 24-Hour for urine fractionated metanephrines
      i. Measure urine creatinine concurrently

   c. Stress, ethanol, and prescription medications (e.g., beta blockers, levodopa, buspirone, amphetamines, tricyclic antidepressants) may cause false positives
2. **Radiology Studies** (Lenders et al., 2014)
   a. Radiologic studies should only be considered after plasma or urine metanephrines have confirmed the diagnosis
   b. Abdominal CT scan: First line
   c. Abdominal MRI: Recommended with children and pregnant or lactating women
   d. Scintigraphy: Consider if plasma or urine metanephrines have confirmed the diagnosis and CT or MRI are inconclusive
   e. PET scan: Consider if concern for occult pheochromocytoma
3. **Genetic Testing**
   a. Consider genetic testing in patients with multiple endocrine neoplasia type 2A or 2B, neurofibromatosis, von Hippel-Lindau disease, or a family history of pheochromocytoma

TREATMENT

Surgical Considerations

Adrenalectomy is the standard of care for pheochromocytomas (Brandai et al., 2014). Laparoscopic versus open resection decisions are determined based on the size of the tumor. Blood glucose, heart rate, and blood pressure should be monitored closely during the perioperative period. Plasma free metanephrines should be measured 2 weeks postoperatively and then annually for 10 years (Plouin et al., 2016). Results within the reference range indicate complete resection.

Pharmacologic Considerations

Pharmacologic therapy to block catecholamine production is indicated in patients with hypertensive crisis and during the perioperative period. For the immediate management of hypertensive crisis, phentolamine, a potent alpha-2 blocker is recommended. Chemical sympathectomy can be established with phenoxybenzamine 7 days prior to adrenalectomy.

TRANSITION OF CARE

Patients diagnosed with pheochromoctyoma should be referred to a general surgeon for adrenalectomy. Genetic testing is recommended for patients with multiple endocrine neoplasia type 2A or 2B, neurofibromatosis, von Hippel-Lindau disease, or a family history of pheochromocytoma.

CLINICAL PEARLS

- Most pheochromocytomas are incidental findings.
- Paroxysmal hypertension is the most common sign of a pheochromocytoma.
- Adrenalectomy is the gold standard for treatment.

KEY TAKEAWAYS

- Radiologic studies should be considered only after laboratory studies have confirmed a diagnosis.
- Refer patients with multiple endocrine neoplasia type 2A or 2B, neurofibromatosis, von Hippel-Lindau disease, or a family history of pheochromocytoma for genetic testing.

EVIDENCE-BASED RESOURCES

National Comprehensive Cancer Network Clinical Practice Guidelines in Oncology: Neuroendocrine and Adrenal Tumors (2019).

Endocrine Society Pheochromocytoma and Paraglanglioma Clinical Practice Guideline (2014).

North American Neuroendocrine Tumor Society Consensus for the Management and Treatment of Neuroendocrine Tumors (2013).

Towards Optimized to Practice Program Laboratory Testing Guidelines: Pheochromocytoma (2008).

8.11: SYNDROME OF INAPPROPRIATE ANTIDIURETIC HORMONE

Mary Alt

Syndrome of inappropriate antidiuretic hormone (SIADH) is a disorder of impaired water excretion caused by the inability to suppress the secretion of antidiuretic hormone (ADH). If water intake exceeds the reduced urine output, the ensuing water retention leads to the development of hyponatremia (Kounatidis et al., 2019). SIADH most commonly occurs secondary to another disease process but the elderly may be particularly affected. Any abnormality in the central nervous system (CNS) can increase ADH release from the pituitary gland, leading to SIADH. Malignancies can cause increased ADH production, with small cell lung cancer being the most common. Several medications can lead to SIADH, as well as surgery, pulmonary disease, hormone deficiency or administration, HIV, and genetic predisposition (Yasir & Mechanic, 2020).

Excess ADH also leads to retention of free water by the kidney, resulting in expansion of the intravascular space and hyponatremia. Most patients appear to have disordered regulation of ADH in response to hypoosmolality. The elderly may be at increased risk, and other causes of hyponatremia should be excluded. The treatment of SIADH depends on the causes or contributing factors. SIADH is characterized by serum sodium <135 mEq/L, serum osmolality <275 mOsm/kg, urine sodium >40 mEq/L, and urine osmolality >100 mOsm/kg (Kounatidis et al., 2019). Box 8.10 summarizes important measurements for SIADH. This section explores topic areas by defining SIADH through clinical presentation and lab findings that may help distinguish it from

BOX 8.10: SYNDROME OF INAPPROPRIATE ANTIDIURETIC HORMONE DIAGNOSTIC CRITERIA

- Serum Na <135 mmol/l
- Plasma osmolarity <275 mOsm/kg
- Urine osmolarity >100 mOsm/kg
- Hypotonic hyponatremia with clinical euvolemia
- Absence of signs of hypovolemia (normal eye pressure values, normal venous pressure, no orthostatism)
- Absence of signs of hypervolemia (ascites, edemas)
- Urinary Na >40 mmol/l (in the presence of dietary sodium)
- No hypothyroidism, no adrenal insufficiency (hypocortisolism) or renal failure
- No recent diuretic intake
- Absence of physiological stimuli for AVP secretion (recent surgery, severe pain AVP secretion stimulating drugs...)

Source: Reproduced from De las Peñas, R., Escobar, Y., Henao, F., Blasco, A., & Rodríguez, C. A. (2014). Spanish Society for Medical Oncology. SEOM guidelines on hydroelectrolytic disorders. *Clinical and Translational Oncology, 16*(12), 1051–1059. https://doi.org/10.1007/s12094-014-1234-2

other conditions. The challenges in the evaluation and treatment will be addressed, in particular for the elderly population. A diagnostic approach will be discussed.

PRESENTING SIGNS AND SYMPTOMS

Symptoms of SIADH occur most often when the sodium level is less than 120 mEq/L or with a rapid drop in serum sodium. When hyponatremia is detected in a patient with normal cardiac, renal, hepatic, adrenal, and thyroid functions without diuretic therapy or other factors known to stimulate ADH such as hypotension, severe pain, nausea, and stress, SIADH should be considered (Kounatidis et al., 2019). The severity of hyponatremia determines the signs and symptoms as well the degree of cerebral edema. Nausea and malaise are usually the earliest manifestation, as well as vomiting, difficulty concentrating, headache, lethargy, and eventually obtundation and seizures. If serum levels fall below 115 to 120 mEq/L, coma and respiratory arrest can occur (Yasir & Mechanic, 2020).

HISTORY AND PHYSICAL FINDINGS

The most common presenting symptoms of SIADH are nausea, vomiting, headache, difficulty concentrating, delirium, and muscle cramping. Lab evaluation including serum and urinary testing should be performed. If at all possible, it should be determined if hyponatremia is acute or chronic, as the latter is generally asymptomatic or produces mild symptoms. Concurrent exam with a focus on clinical euvolemia will assist in diagnosis. Evaluation of orthostatic readings, such as a drop of systolic pressure greater than 10 to 20 mmHg or an increase in heart rate greater than 15 beats/min after 3 minutes of standing suggests orthostatic hypotension, and maybe a sign of hypovolemia (Filippatos et al., 2017).

A review of the medication history may also identify causative factors. Given that the syndrome can be seen in a wide variety of clinical states (e.g., drugs, malignancies, pulmonary and neuropsychiatric diseases), a clinically driven and thorough approach may help to identify the cause. Geriatric consideration with hyponatremia include age-related impaired water-excretory capacity, frequent exposure to medications, and diseases associated with hyponatremia (Filippatos et al., 2017). Additionally, nonhypovolemic orthostatic hypotension may be encountered in the elderly due to autonomic dysfunction which can cause postural changes, without the increase of heart rate.

DIFFERENTIAL DIAGNOSIS AND DIAGNOSTIC CONSIDERATIONS

Differential Diagnoses

Other conditions can cause hypotonic hyponatremia. The most frequent cause of SIADH in oncologic patients is a paraneoplastic syndrome that can occur in many tumor types, most frequently seen in small cell lung cancer. Pseudohyponatremia is noted in patients with hyperproteinemia that may be seen in multiple myeloma and other monoclonal gammopathies or with IV immunoglobulin administration and in severe hyperlipidemia. When hyperglycemia is present, the level of serum glucose should be factored. Corrected serum sodium is calculated by adding to measured serum sodium 1.6 mm/L for every 100 mg/dL (5.55 mmol/L) increment of serum glucose above normal up to 400 mg/dL and by adding to measured serum sodium 2.4 mm/L when serum glucose concentrations are higher than 400 mg/dL (22.2 mmol/L; Filippatos et al., 2017).

Hypothyroidism-induced hyponatremia, although rare, should be considered, especially in the euvolemic hypothyroid elderly patient. Idiopathic SIADH may be a possible diagnosis if normal sodium levels are not achieved after thyroid hormone replacement. Urine osmolality (Uosm) is helpful in evaluating hyponatremic patients to establish diagnosis of psychogenic polydipsia (Siddiqui et al., 2018).

Hyponatremia with reduced Uosm has also been reported in ill-nourished heavy drinkers (beer potomania syndrome), and in reset osmostat syndrome (e.g., patients with quadriplegia, malignant disorders, or malnutrition chronic states; Feder et al., 2019). A rare genetic-related condition called nephrogenic syndrome of inappropriate antidiuresis (NSIAD) results from activating mutations in the arginine vasopressin receptor type 2 (AVPR2). In some cases, it should be considered in the investigation of unexplained hyponatremia, with implications for management and targeted gene testing.

Cerebral salt wasting (CSW) is a potential cause of hyponatremia in the setting of disorders of the CNS. CSW is characterized by hyponatremia with elevated urine sodium and hypovolemia. Patients with SIADH and CSW share almost identical clinical presentations, making early recognition extremely difficult. Symptoms do not usually appear unless the serum sodium is less than 120 mEq/L and are nonspecific. Initial symptoms may include headache, lethargy, inattention, nausea, muscle cramps and weakness and may progress to confusion, hallucinations, psychosis, and dysarthria with worsening hyponatremia. The one difference in clinical presentation is the patient's fluid volume status (FVS). Patients with SIADH are typically euvolemic whereas patients with CSW are hypovolemic and may appear dehydrated. Determination of the patient's FVS has been the gold standard in identifying one condition over the other, as clinically diagnosing a patient based upon presentation can be almost impossible. Several reviews on whether CSW is a distinct condition or a special form of SIADH have been considered (Rudolph & Gantioque, 2018). It is important to distinguish between CSW and SIADH as the two are treated with opposite treatment strategies. Both conditions will have a sodium level less than 135 mEq/L, a serum osmolality less than 275 mOsm/kg, a normal or elevated urinary sodium and osmolality level, a urinary specific gravity of >1.010, a decreased urine output, and initially an elevated fractional excretion of uric acid (FeUA >10). The key difference is that once hyponatremia is corrected and returns to baseline, the FeUA in SIADH will return to baseline (<10), but with CSW, the FeUA will continue to stay elevated (Rudolph & Gantioque, 2018). For CSW the patient is given fluids and sodium supplementation, while for SIADH, the patient is fluid restricted (Nakajima et al., 2017).

Diagnostic Considerations

Renal function and a random serum glucose test should be performed to ensure that hyperglycemia and uremia are not causing pseudohyponatremia. Laboratory tests for SIADH include serum osmolality and serum sodium, urine sodium and osmolality. A thyroid profile, serum cortisol, potassium, chloride, blood-urea nitrogen (BUN) and creatinine with ratio, FeUA, fasting lipid profile and LFTs also should be performed. Patients with a long smoking history, weight loss, or pulmonary symptoms must have a chest x-ray and CT scan to look for small cell lung cancer (Yasir & Mechanic, 2020). Glucocorticoid deficiency should be excluded by proper tests.

Drugs Causing Hyponatremia

There are certain drugs that can affect sodium levels. The first group are drugs affecting sodium and water homeostasis such as diuretics. Diuretics are the most common cause of community-developed hyponatremia. Diuretic-induced hyponatremia is caused almost exclusively by thiazide or thiazide-like agents or loop diuretics, which inhibit sodium chloride reabsorption in the ascending limb loop of Henle and reduce the osmolarity of the medullary interstitium. Loop diuretics rarely are associated with hyponatremia because they impair both the renal concentrating and diluting mechanisms. Conversely, thiazide diuretics act solely in the distal tubules and do not interfere with urinary concentration and the ability of ADH to promote water retention, which is the critical point for the development of hyponatremia.

The next class of medications can increase ADH secretion centrally by potentiating the effect of endogenous ADH at the renal medulla and reset the osmostat, thus lowering the threshold for ADH secretion. Offending agents are drugs that increase ADH secretion centrally such as psychotropic agents which have been implicated as the cause of hyponatremia and include antidepressants (tricyclics, selective serotonin reuptake inhibitors [SSRIs], monoamine oxidase inhibitors [MAOIs]) and antipsychotic drugs (phenothiazines and butyrophenones). However, it should be emphasized that low serum sodium levels in emotionally disturbed or psychotic patients may not be a direct consequence of these medications. Among the most frequent causes of hyponatremia in this population are the underlying psychosis itself and the compulsive water drinking. The causality between psychotropic agents and hyponatremia was shown more persuasively with antidepressants and mainly with SSRIs, which cause hyponatremia more frequently than other antidepressant drugs (Siddiqui et al., 2018). Older age and concomitant use of diuretics are the most important risk factors for the development of hyponatremia associated with SSRIs.

Finally, consideration of drugs that create potentiation of ADH effect such as antiepileptic drugs like carbamazepine can cause hyponatremia by increasing ADH release from the neurohypophysis (Woodward et al., 2018).

TREATMENT

Treatment depends on the severity of symptoms; however, restriction of oral water remains the mainstay of treatment. Additionally, oral salt tablets or IV saline are also considered. Loop diuretics can help to decrease the urine concentration as well as increase water excretion. For treatment, 3% hypertonic saline can be given and should not exceed more than 8 mEq/L per 24 hours. Rapid correction can result in osmotic demyelination of the CNS leading to complications such as "locked-in" syndrome causing quadriplegia (Yasir & Mechanic, 2020). Tolvaptan is a selective vasopressin V2-receptor antagonist indicated for the treatment of clinically significant hypervolemic and euvolemic hyponatremia (serum sodium <125 mEq/L) or less marked hyponatremia that is symptomatic and resisted correction with fluid restriction and must be given while hospitalized due to the need to evaluate a therapeutic response and monitor labs (Humayun & Cranston, 2017). Addressing the underlying primary condition causing SIADH is the goal in treatment. An endocrinology consult should always be considered.

CLINICAL PEARLS

- SIADH is often a diagnosis of exclusion and the absence of other potential causes of hypo-osmolarity must always be verified.
- Causes of SIADH can be corrected if caused by self-limited disease, or through cessation of drugs that cause SIADH. A thorough clinical evaluation with medical and drug history is critical.
- Special attention is needed in the elderly population to exclude endocrinopathies as a cause of hyponatremia, and in particular polypharmacy with offending drugs.
- Treatment is focused on correction of serum sodium levels after identifying the underlying cause, careful clinical review of volume status, duration of hyponatremia, and the presence of symptoms.

KEY TAKEAWAYS

- SIADH is often a diagnosis of exclusion and the absence of other potential causes of hypo-osmolarity must always be verified. Some causes of SIADH can be corrected and a thorough clinical evaluation, including a review of the medical and drug history, is essential.

EVIDENCE-BASED RESOURCE

Humayun, M. A., & Cranston, I. C. (2017). In-patient Tolvaptan use in SIADH: Care audit, therapy observation and outcome analysis. *BMC Endocrine Disorders, 17*(1), 69. https://doi.org/10.1186/s12902-017-0214-2

8.12: THYROID CANCER

Camille Brockett-Walker

Thyroid cancer is a malignant tumor or growth originating within the thyroid gland. It is the most common type of endocrine cancer and the fifth most common cancer seen in women in the United States (Cabanillas et al., 2016). According to data from the American Cancer Society, it is estimated that there were about 44,280 new cases of thyroid cancer in the United States in the year 2021, as compared to 52,890 cases in 2020 (American Cancer Society [ACS], 2021). Thyroid cancer is diagnosed in all stages of life from young children through seniors,;however, most individuals are diagnosed between the ages of 20 and 55. Thyroid cancers can display an expansive clinical picture, ranging from tumors with low mortality, which is most common, to more aggressive malignancies. Although highly treatable, the challenge that clinicians face is balancing the therapeutic approach in a disease with such a broad clinical range (Cabanillas et al., 2016).

There are four types of thyroid cancer: papillary, follicular, anaplastic, and medullary. Papillary and follicular thyroid cancers are commonly called differentiated thyroid cancer (DTC). These types of cancer cells appear and act like normal thyroid cells (American Thyroid Association [ATA], 2020). Papillary and follicular thyroid cancers grow at a slow rate and account for more than 90% of all thyroid cancers (ATA, 2020). Anaplastic thyroid cancer is also referred to as undifferentiated thyroid cancer. Unlike differentiated cells, undifferentiated cancer cells do not resemble or behave like normal thyroid cells. This is the rarest and most aggressive type of thyroid cancer, accounting for only 1% to 2% of all thyroid cancers (Cabanillas et al., 2016). It is difficult to control and can spread rapidly within the neck and to other parts of the body (Cabanillas et al., 2016). Medullary thyroid carcinoma (MTC) accounts for 3% to 4% of all thyroid cancers and originates in the parafollicular neuroendocrine cells of the thyroid (Cabanillas et al., 2016). There is a strong genetic component in MTC and 25% of all MTCs are seen in families (ATA, 2020).

Treatment for thyroid cancer includes surgery, radioactive iodine (RAI) treatment, and chemotherapy. The prognosis for any individual with thyroid cancer depends on several factors, but overall it is very good. According to the ATA, the 10-year survival rate for DTC is 100%; however, the recurrence can be up to 30% (ATA, 2020). Therefore, it is important that patients get regular follow-up examinations to detect whether the cancer has re-emerged.

PRESENTING SIGNS AND SYMPTOMS

In its early stages, thyroid cancer rarely causes symptoms. However, some symptoms that could appear are pain in the neck, jaw, or ear (ACS, 2021). Some patients experience compression to the esophagus which may cause dysphagia (ACS, 2021). Patients can also have complaints of dyspnea and even less commonly, dysphonia which can be caused if a thyroid cancer invades the vagus nerve (ACS, 2021). Individuals can also experience lymphadenopathy. Despite these symptoms, unless there is a large neck mass that can be easily seen on exam, the discovery of a thyroid nodule is usually by chance, found by the patient or during a routine physical exam or incidentally found on imaging done for other disorders. Research suggests that thyroid nodules that were unlikely to be diagnosed in the past are now being found at higher frequencies due to the growing use of diagnostic imaging (Cabanillas et al., 2016). Thyroid function tests, such as the thyroidstimulating hormone (TSH) used to identify underlying thyroid dysfunction, are usually normal and do not assist in identifying thyroid cancer.

HISTORY AND PHYSICAL FINDINGS

History

If a patient presents with possible signs and symptoms suggestive of thyroid cancer, taking a history to identify risk factors is very important. Risk factors include radiation exposure, genetic conditions and family history (ATA, 2020). The origin of radiation exposure includes certain medical treatments and radiation fallout from power plant accidents or nuclear weapons (ATA, 2020). For example, children who lived near Chernobyl, the site of a 1986 nuclear plant accident that exposed millions to radioactivity, or adults involved with the clean-up after the accident, and those who lived near the plant have had higher rates of thyroid cancer (ATA, 2020). Other examples include children who were treated with radiation for things such as fungal infections or enlarged tonsils or adenoids before the 1960s (ACS, 2021). Higher rates of thyroid cancer can also occur among people with uncommon genetic conditions such as familial adenomatous polyposis (FAP), Cowden disease, Carney complex, type I and familial nonmedullary thyroid carcinoma.

Physical Findings

There are many physical examination techniques for examination of the thyroid. However, combining the examination and the presence of risk factors and associated signs and symptoms discussed during patient history taking strengthens the accuracy of the thyroid examination. Palpable nodules are present on physical examination in approximately 5% of the population, and thyroid cancer occurs in 7% to 15% of thyroid nodules (Wong et al., 2018). Nodules increase in frequency with age and are four times more likely to occur in women than in men. On examination of the thyroid, firmness, lack of mobility, size of the nodule(s), adherence to surrounding structures, and lymphadenopathy are important clues indicating an increased probability of carcinoma (Wong et al., 2018). However, these features lack specificity for malignancy.

DIFFERENTIAL DIAGNOSIS AND DIAGNOSTIC CONSIDERATIONS

Thyroid nodules are very common, and most are benign. Performing an ultrasound-guided fine needle aspiration (FNA) is the gold standard diagnostic test. The ATA released guidelines in 2015 endorsing a risk-stratified approach in the use of FNA biopsy of thyroid nodules, in which nodules less than 1 cm in size should not be biopsied (Roman et al., 2017). According to the Bethesda System for Reporting Thyroid Cytology, the sensitivity of thyroid FNA for malignant cases is 57.89% and specificity 88.10% (Erkinuresin & Demirci, 2019). Usually, the results will fall into one of four categories: benign (up to 80% of cases), malignant (5%), inconclusive (up to 20%), and unsatisfactory (<5%) (ATA, 2020). If the diagnosis is not clear after an FNA biopsy, a core biopsy using a larger needle, or a surgical "open" biopsy to remove the nodule, are other options. If the results of the biopsy do not show malignancy, other differentials to consider in the assessment of thyroid nodules are thyroiditis, colloid nodules, hyperplastic nodules, or fluid-filled cyst nodules.

TREATMENT

Thyroid cancer treatment aims to remove all or most of the cancer and help prevent the disease from recurring or spreading. Treatments include surgery, RAI treatment, and chemotherapy.

Surgery

Surgery is generally the first and most common treatment for thyroid cancer. The scope of surgery for DTC depends on the size of the tumor and whether the tumor is restricted to the thyroid (ATA, 2020). Surgical options include a lobectomy or total thyroidectomy. For small cancers measuring less than 1 cm that are confined to the thyroid without signs of lymph node involvement, a simple lobectomy is an acceptable treatment (ATA, 2020). Recent studies even suggest that small tumors, called micropapillary thyroid cancers, may be subject to low intensity treatment options and observed without surgery depending on their location in the thyroid (Tuttle, 2018). A total thyroidectomy is warranted if it is determined that the cancer has spread into surrounding areas or there is cervical lymph node involvement. Often, thyroid cancer is cured by surgery alone; however, if the cancer is large, has metastasized to the lymph nodes, or if there is high risk for recurrence, RAI may be used after the initial surgical intervention (ATA, 2020).

Radioactive Iodine

RAI is an adjuvant treatment, performed with the goal of destroying occult microscopic foci of neoplastic cells within the thyroid remnant (Cabanillas et al., 2016). Thyroid cells and most DTCs absorb and concentrate iodine which is why RAI is used to eliminate all remaining normal thyroid tissue after thyroidectomy (ATA, 2020). This is referred to as radioactive remnant ablation (RRA). RRA differs from RAI in that RAI is usually recommended for patients with known postoperative residual disease, patients with distant metastases, or patients with locally invasive lesions (ATA, 2020). Effective and safe use of RAI treatment requires appropriate patient preparation. This involves increasing the patient's TSH above the normal range via the administration of recombinant TSH or the temporary holding of thyroid hormone administration to stimulate thyroid cell uptake of RAI (ATA, 2020).

Chemotherapy

Systemic treatments such as chemotherapy can be used for advanced DTC that do not respond to other treatments, as well as for anaplastic thyroid cancer and medullary thyroid cancer (ATA, 2020). Chemotherapy agents that have shown potential in the treatment of other advanced cancers are becoming more widely available for treatment of thyroid cancer (ATA, 2020). These drugs can possibly slow down or partially reverse the growth of the cancer. Although systemic cytotoxic chemotherapy has produced disappointing results there has been some promise shown with the use of tyrosine kinase inhibitors (TKIs) used in phase II clinical trials. These medications include sunitinib, sorafenib, and pazopanib. Clinical trials have not demonstrated a statistically significant difference in overall survival; however, expert consensus favors the selective use of TKIs in treating patients facing imminent threat to life (Cabanillas et al., 2016).

TRANSITION OF CARE

After surgical intervention, the management of thyroid cancer is usually done in the outpatient setting. The overall prognosis of DTC is good; however, follow-up examinations are essential because of possibility of recurrence or persistent disease. Routine ultrasounds of the neck are useful to look for nodules, lumps, or cancerous lymph nodes that might indicate recurrence (ATA, 2020). Most patients who have had a thyroidectomy for cancer require thyroid hormone replacement with levothyroxine. During the first year after treatment, blood tests are done to help titrate dosages of thyroid replacement therapy but also to help monitor for persistent or recurrent cancer. Thyroglobulin (Tg) is a common "cancer marker" that is followed. After treatment with surgery and RAI, the Tg level should be low to undetectable. A positive serum Tg level indicates that thyroid cells, either normal or cancerous, are still present and the patient may need closer monitoring (Cabanillas et al., 2016).

KEY TAKEAWAYS

- Papillary and follicular thyroid cancers are referred to as DTC and account for more than 90% of all thyroid cancers.
- DTC (papillary and follicular) have a very high long-term survival rate, especially when diagnosed early.
- Unless there is an obvious neck mass that can be seen, most nodules are detected by chance during a routine physical examination.
- FNA is the most reliable way to determine whether a nodule is benign or malignant.
- The initial surgery is the most important part of treatment.
- If the thyroid was removed surgically, the patient will be on lifelong thyroid hormone replacement therapy.

EVIDENCE-BASED RESOURCES

American Cancer Association: https://www.cancer.org/cancer/thyroid-cancer.html
American Thyroid Association: https://www.thyroid.org

8.13: THYROID STORM

Melissa Diehl Weidner

Thyroid storm or severe thyrotoxicosis is a medical emergency that must be quickly identified in patients with systemic decompensation (Ross et al., 2016). With appropriate treatment, mortality rates can be between 10% and 30%. Without treatment the mortality rate can be over 90% (Schreiber, 2017). Due to high potential mortality, thyroid storm must be managed aggressively in an intensive care unit (Ylli et al., 2019). Thyroid storm is most often seen in women between 30 and 50 years of age who have a medical history of thyroid or autoimmune disorders, (specifically Graves' disease) but there are many other possible etiologies as well (Schreiber, 2017; Sharp et al., 2016). There are no laboratory studies or objective evidence to make the diagnosis. Diagnosis is primarily based on patient history and clinical presentation; however, use of the Burch-Wartfsky Point Scale for the diagnosis of thyroid storm can also be helpful (Ross et al., 2016; Schreiber, 2017). Treatment focuses on blocking hormone excretion or production (e.g., thionamides or cholestyramine), treatment of any precipitating causes (such as infection), strategies to combat systemic decompensation (e.g., IV fluids and glucocorticoids), remedies to treat symptoms (e.g., beta-blockers and acetaminophen) ,and definitive treatment for the hyperthyroidism (Chiha, 2015; Ross et al., 2016)

PRESENTING SIGNS AND SYMPTOMS

Patients present with usual signs of hyperthyroidism including tachycardia, tremors, weight loss, goiter, brisk reflexes, and proptosis (Ylli et al., 2019). However, when the state of thyroid storm has been reached signs and symptoms are much more intense and variable. They include hyperpyrexia, tachycardia with heart rate commonly over 130, arrhythmias, in particular atrial fibrillation, complaints of palpitations, heat intolerance, dyspnea, restlessness, irritability, nausea, and vomiting (Schreiber, 2017; Sharp et al., 2016; Ylli et al., 2019). Patients may also have hypertension with a widened pulse pressure, hypotension if shock is present, dehydration, changes in mental status, abdominal discomfort, cachexia, and multiorgan failure (Schreiber, 2017; Sharp et al., 2016; Ylli et al., 2019). It is important to note that not all patients will have all these symptoms; they may only have two or three and present to a clinician with other complaints. Thyroid storm is also less common in older adults and symptoms tend to be less intense (Ross et al., 2016; Sharp et al., 2016).

HISTORY AND PHYSICAL FINDINGS

Patients typically present with the signs and symptoms outlined in the previous section. Friends or family may report a change in mental status or signs of central nervous system (CNS) dysfunction over the days prior to presentation (Sharp et al., 2016). On physical examination they may appear jittery, diaphoretic, and manic. There may be diaphoresis, erythema of the skin, and edema of the extremities (Sharp et al., 2016). Vital signs will likely show a fever, tachycardia, hypertension, and rapid shallow breaths (Schreiber, 2017; Sharp et al., 2016; Ylli et al., 2019).

DIFFERENTIAL DIAGNOSIS AND DIAGNOSTIC CONSIDERATIONS

Differential Diagnoses

The definite pathology of thyroid storm is not clearly understood (Chiha et al., 2015). However, is it apparent that when simple thyrotoxicosis converts to the life-threatening thyroid storm, there is usually a precipitating event (Chiha et al., 2015; Schreiber, 2017). A history of Graves' disease is the most common cause, but patients with undiagnosed thyrotoxicosis often have a recent history of nonthyroid surgery, pregnancy, infection, major trauma, amiodarone use, or iodine exposure from radiocontrast dye (Chiha et al., 2015; Schreiber, 2017). Other etiologies include stress, thyroid tumor, goiter, genetics, withdrawal or change in medication regimen, molar pregnancy, myocardial infarction, hypoglycemia, and DKA (Chiha et al., 2015; Schreiber, 2017). While there are many possible precipitating factors, the cause remains unknown in 25% to 43% of patients admitted to the inpatient setting (Chiha et al., 2015).

Distinguishing Features

A complete blood count (CBC) may show a mild anemia and leukocytosis with a left shift (Ylli et al., 2019). Signs of dehydration or hemoconcentration, hypercalcemia, and hyperglycemia are also likely present (Ylli et al., 2019). Electrolytes are usually normal; if hyponatremia, hyperkalemia, or hypercalcemia is present, the possibility of concomitant adrenal insufficiency must be considered. Serum thyroid hormones ordinarily show elevated T3 and T4 with a suppressed thyroid stimulating hormone (TSH) (Schreiber, 2017). Other helpful diagnostic modalities include radioactive iodine (RAI) uptake study, thyroid ultrasound, and aspirate biopsy (Ross et al., 2016; Schreiber, 2017). Use of these modalities will depend on patient stability and the level of suspicion for thyroid storm.

The Burch-Wartofsky Score is widely accepted as a tool to aid in the diagnosis of thyroid storm. As shown in Figure 8.3, it assigns a numerical value to precipitating event, body system dysfunction, and thermoregulation (Schreiber, 2017; Ylli et al., 2019). A score of 45 or greater is very suspicious for thyroid storm; a score of 25 to 44 is suggestive of an impending thyroid storm; less than 25 does not likely represent thyroid storm (Chiha et al., 2015; Ross et al., 2016; Ylli et al., 2019). Scoring systems should be used only as an aid in the diagnosis of thyroid storm and treatment should not be delayed as it is mainly a clinical diagnosis (Chiha et al., 2015; Ylli et al., 2019).

Thermoregulatory dysfunction
Temperature (8°F)
99.0–99.95   0
100.0–100.9   10
101.0–101.9   15
102.0–102.9   20
103.0–103.9   25
>104.0   30
Cardiovascular
Tachycardia (beats per minute)
100–109   5
110–119   10
120–129   15
130–139   20
>140   25
Atrial fibrillation
Absent   0
Present   10
Congestive heart failure
Absent   0
Mild   5
Moderate   10
Severe   20

Gastrointestinal-hepatic dysfunction
Manifestation
Absent 0
Moderate (diarrhea, abdominal pain, nausea/vomiting) 10
Severe (jaundice) 20

Central nervous system disturbance
Manifestation
Absent 0
Mild (agitation) 10
Moderate (delirium, psychosis, extreme lethargy) 20
Severe (seizure, coma) 30

Precipitant history
Status
Positive   0
Negative 10

Scores totaled
>45 Thyroid storm
25–44 Impending storm
<25 Storm unlikely

FIGURE 8.3: Burch-Wartofsky Point Scale for the diagnosis of thyroid storm.

Source: Reproduced with permission from Feingold, K. R., Anawalt, B., Boyce, A., Chrousos, G., de Herder, W. W., Dhatariya, K., Dungan, K., Hershman, J. M., Hofland, J., Kalra, S., Kaltsas, G., Koch, C., Kopp, P., Korbonits, M., Kovacs, C. S., Kuohung, W., Laferrère, B., Levy, M., McGee, E. A., … Wilson, D. P. (2000). *Point scale for the diagnosis of thyroid storm*. https://www.ncbi.nlm.nih.gov/books/NBK278927/figure/thyroid-storm.F1/

TREATMENT

The approach to treating thyroid storm should be comprehensive to halt thyroid hormone synthesis and secretion, treat thyroid hormones already in peripheral circulation, determine precipitating event or cause, support systemic decompensation, and initiate treatment (Ylli et al., 2019). Initial therapies should focus on airway management, careful fluid resuscitation, treatment of the precipitating event, and cooling of the body temperature with cooling blankets and acetaminophen (Sharp et al., 2016). Clinicians should avoid adminstering salicylates in this patient population because they can raise free hormone levels by lowering binding capacity to T4-binding globulin, intensifying thyroid storm (Chiha et al., 2015; Sharp et al., 2016). Should agitation be an issue, sedation with benzodiazepines or typical antipsychotics is recommended (Ross et al., 2016; Sharp et al., 2016). If the patient has persistent hypotension, vasopressors should be started as well (Chiha et al., 2015). Additionally, corticosteroids are started with a 300 mg loading dose of hydrocortisone IV, followed by 100 mg every 8 hours. Steroids serve the dual purpose of preventing adrenal insufficiency and decreasing the peripheral rate of conversion of T4 to T3 (Chiha et al., 2015; Ross et al., 2016).

Parathyroid hormone (PTH) is started to combat new thyroid hormone production. It is given orally with a loading dose of 500 mg to 1000 mg followed by 250 mg every 4 hours (Chiha et al., 2015). PTH is insoluble at physiologic pH and cannot be given IV. Therefore, if not able to give the medication orally, it may be given via nasogastric tube or rectally (Chiha et al., 2015). If given rectally, the dose is 400 mg to 600 mg every 6 hours (Chiha et al., 2015; Ylli et al., 2019). To inhibit thyroid hormone release into circulation, sodium iodide can be started at a dose of 0.5 mg IV every 12 hours or lithium can be used orally with a dose of 300 mg every 6 to 8 hours (Chiha et al., 2015).

Additionally, to block the systemic effects of the circulating thyroid hormone, beta-adrenergic blockage is essential. Propranolol is most commonly used because it is a non selective beta-adrenergic receptor antagonist (or beta-blocker) and has the ability to decrease the conversion of T4 to T3 (Chiha et al., 2015). If beta-blockade is needed more rapidly for decompensation or arrhythmia, esmolol can also be used via a bolus dose of 0.25 mg/kg to 0.5 mg/kg, followed by a continuous drip of 0.05 mg to 0.1 mg/kg/min (Chiha et al., 2015; Ylli et al., 2019). In patients who have a contraindication to beta-blockers, calcium antagonists such as verapamil or diltiazem can be used (Chiha et al., 2015). If unresponsive to these treatments, providers can also consider plasmapheresis or emergency subtotal or total thyroidectomy (Chiha et al., 2015; Ross et al., 2016).

TRANSITION OF CARE

After discharge from acute care, initial treatments should be weaned over the next 1 to 2 weeks. The patient will need close monitoring during taper given the long half-life of T4 (Chiha et al., 2015; Ylli et al., 2019). Once this has occurred, definitive treatment for hyperthyroidism is required. Treatment options depend on the triggering event (Chiha et al., 2015). One option is continuing therapy with PTH. However, if nonadherence with the medication regimen is an issue, iodine ablation or surgical intervention should be considered (Chiha et al., 2015; Ylli et al., 2019).

CLINICAL PEARLS

- If thyroid storm is suspected, start treatment as soon as possible given the high mortality.
- Identify and treat precipitating cause.
- Once resolved, it requires definitive treatment

EVIDENCE-BASED RESOURCES

Chiha, M., Samarasinghe, S., & Kabaker, A. S. (2015). Thyroid storm: An updated review. *Journal of Intensive Care Medicine*, 30(3), 131–140. https://doi.org/10.1177/0885066613498053

Ross, D. S., Burch, H. B., Cooper, D. S., Greenlee, M. C., Laurberg, P., Maia, A. L., Rivkees, S. A., Samuels, M., Sosa, J. A., Stan, M. N., & Walter, M. A. (2016). 2016 American Thyroid Association guidelines for diagnosis and treatment of hyperthyroid and other causes of thyrotoxicosis. *Thyroid*, 26(10), 1343–1421. http://doi.org/10.1089/thy.2016.0229

A robust set of instructor resources designed to supplement this text is located at **http://connect.springerpub.com/content/reference-book/978-0-8261-6079-9.** Qualifying instructors may request access by emailing **textbook@springerpub.com.**

REFERENCES

Full list of references can be accessed at http://connect.springerpub.com/content/reference-book/978-0-8261-6079-9

CHAPTER 9

HEMATOLOGIC AND ONCOLOGIC DISORDERS

Jamie L. Oliva and Elizabeth Palermo

LEARNING OBJECTIVES

- Compare and contrast the common anemias in acute and critical care.
- Summarize the major inherited and acquired disorders of bleeding and clotting.
- Compare and contrast the diagnosis and treatment of various oncologic disorders.
- Give examples of oncologic emergencies encountered in acute and critical care.
- Describe roles and responsibilities of the AGACNP in diagnosing and treating patients with hematologic and oncologic disorders.

INTRODUCTION

The specialties of hematology and oncology include a broad variety of acute and chronic problems and impact multiple body systems. Patients may enter acute and critical care settings with these problems; they may develop these problems as a consequence of acute and critical illness; or they may be diagnosed during an illness episode. Furthermore, the fields of hematology and oncology are growing, with new understanding of disease processes and newer therapies to manage them.

Adult Gerontology Acute Care Nurse Practitioners (AGACNPs) may manage patients with these problems in all these contexts. In this chapter, we build on the AGACNP's foundation in advanced physiology and pathophysiology with an overview of the more common blood disorders and malignancies encountered in acute and critical care to support rapid identification of these problems and provision of evidence-based care to patients with these disorders.

9.1: ANEMIA

By definition, anemia is the condition of having reduced circulating red blood cell (RBC) mass, which may be due to a deficiency in the number, size, or function of RBCs, resulting in the decreased transport of oxygen from lungs to tissue (Bunn, 2017). According to the World Health Organization (WHO, 2011), anemia is diagnosed when the hemoglobin level is less than 13.0 g/dL in males and less than 12.0 g/dL in females, with normal variations due to age, pregnancy, residence in elevation above sea level, and smoking.

Anemia is a common blood disorder. Approximately one third of the world's population is affected by some type of anemia, with iron deficiency anemia being the predominant type (Kassebaum et al., 2014). In the United States, approximately 6% of the population meets the criterion for anemia, with increased prevalence in adults over age 65 (Le, 2016). The increased prevalence in the older adult population, which may range from 10% to 24%, is not due to the aging process alone; rather, gastrointestinal diseases, inflammatory problems, poor nutrition, and use of multiple medications that impair clotting may contribute (Stauder et al., 2018). With the broad variety of anemia etiologies the differential diagnostic approach should focus on acute versus chronic, inherited or acquired; with the underlying morphology of blood loss, inadequate production or cell destruction. Regardless of etiology, it is important for the AGACNP to consider anemia not as a disease, but rather a manifestation of a disease or problem requiring further assessment. Furthermore, anemia is associated with increased risk of many problems, including cognitive impairment, functional impairment, falls, fractures, and prolonged hospitalization (Stauder et al., 2018). Therefore, AGACNPs must know possible causes, diagnostic strategies, and implications for management at the time acute care is sought. Upon determining that there is an anemia diagnosis, care should be taken to determine if it is a new problem or a known problem by interviewing the patient and carefully reviewing the medical record. If the problem appears new, a thorough medical history, current exam, and laboratory work will often yield the diagnosis, and specialty consultation may be necessary.

There are many diverse anemia diagnoses; the types, findings, and laboratory tests are summarized by red cell morphology in Table 9.1. The major anemias are further reviewed in this chapter.

TABLE 9.1: Anemia Types, Findings, and Laboratory Tests by Red Cell Morphology

	HB	HCT	MCV	MCHC	RDW	PERIPHERAL SMEAR	RETIC	IRON	TIBC	T_{sat}	FERRITIN	B_{12}	FOLIC
MICROCYTIC													
Iron deficiency	↓	↓	↓	↓	↑	Anisocytosis, poikilocytosis	↑	↓	↑	↓	↓		
Thalassemias	↓	↓	↓	↓	N/↑	Basophilic stipling, target cells	↑	N/↑	N	N	N/↑		
Sideroblastic anemia	↓	↓	N/↓	↓	↑	Dimorphic, anisocytosis, poikilocytosis, target, siderocytes	N/↓	↑	↓	↑	N/↑		
MACROCYTIC													
B_{12} deficiency			↑	↑		Macro-ovulocytes anisocytosis, poikilocytosis				↑MMA ↑Homocysteine		↓	
Folic acid deficiency			↑	↑		Macro-ovulocytes anisocytosis, poikilocytosis				N MMA ↑Homocysteine			↓
Alcohol use			↑	↑		Round, target						N/↓	N/↓
NORMOCYTIC													
Chronic diseases/ inflammation	↓	↓	N	N	N	Relatively normal or r/t disease	N/↓	↓	↓	↓	N/↑		
Sickle Cell Anemia	↓	↓	N	N		Sickled	↑				↑		

Hb, hemoglobin; HCT, hematocrit; iron, circulating; iMCV, mean corpuscular volume; N, normal; RDW, red cell distribution width; retic, reticulocyte count: circulating; circulating immature RBCs; up arrow = elevated; down arrow = decreased.

iron, circulating iron; TIBC, total iron binding capacity: available iron binding sites on transferrin; T_{sat}, transferrin saturation: ratio of iron to TIBC, estimates occupied transferrin iron binding sites; ferritin, main iron storage protein; B_{12}, vitamin B_{12} level; folate, folic acid level

Source: Adapted from Bottomley, S. (2021). Sideroblastic anemias: Diagnosis and management. UpToDate. https://www.uptodate.com/contents/sideroblastic-anemias-diagnosis-and-management#H2262170328; Camaschella, C., & Weiss, G. (2021). Anemia of chronic disease/anemia of inflammation. UpToDate. https://www.uptodate.com/contents/anemia-of-chronic-disease-anemia-of-inflammation; Means, R. T. (2021). Hematologic complications of alcohol use. UpToDate. https://www.uptodate.com/contents/hematologic-complications-of-alcohol-use; Verhovsek, M., & McFarlane, A. (2017). Abnormalities in red blood cells. In S. C. McKean, J. J. Ross, D. D. Dressler, & D. B. Scheurer (Eds.), Principles and practice of hospital medicine (2nd ed.). McGraw-Hill. https://accessmedicine.mhmedical.com/content.aspx?bookid=1872&sectionid=146983235

IRON DEFICIENCY ANEMIA

Iron is essential for normal erythropoiesis; iron deficiency anemia occurs when low iron levels result in decreased hemoglobin, characterized by microcytic hypochromic RBC (Camaschella, 2015). Iron deficiency may occur due to inadequate dietary iron intake. In a recent study, the rising prevalence of iron deficiency anemia in the United States was shown likely to be due to reduced red meat consumption and decreasing amounts of iron in agricultural products (Sun & Weaver, 2021). Iron deficiency may also occur due to blood loss. For example, adolescent girls and young adult females may be susceptible from menorrhagia (Camaschella, 2015). Adults and older adults may experience chronic blood loss secondary to gastrointestinal bleeding from ulcers or malignancy (Stauder et al., 2018). Finally, iron deficiency can occur when iron is not properly absorbed and may be seen with patients who have had gastrectomy, gastric bypass, or bariatric surgery, or those who have *Helicobacter pylori* infection or celiac disease impairing absorption (Camaschella, 2015).

PRESENTING SIGNS AND SYMPTOMS

Patients may present with no symptoms, and it is possible that the AGACNP may detect iron deficiency as an incidental finding on the CBC. Like other anemias, symptoms develop as the anemia progresses due to decreased oxygen delivery to tissue, including weakness, fatigue, poor concentration, palpitations, chest pain, and dyspnea (Camaschella, 2015; Holcomb, 2005). Unique to iron deficiency, patients may experience pica, ice craving, or restless legs syndrome (Auerbach, 2021a).

HISTORY AND PHYSICAL FINDINGS

Due to the relationship of IDA and dietary intake, the AGACNP should ask the patient about diet and consumption of foods with iron. The medical and surgical history should be reviewed with the patient for possible reasons for iron absorption or iron loss problems. The AGACNP should ask about any evidence of blood loss from the gastrointestinal, gynecologic, or urologic systems. Asking about stool color and character is important as blood loss from upper gastrointestinal bleed is characteristically black and tarry (Holcomb, 2005). A detailed medication review is essential to identify agents that may contribute to blood loss, including antiplatelet agents, anticoagulants, glucocorticoids, and nonsteroidal anti-inflammatory agents (NSAIDs; Stauder et al., 2018).

The patient without symptoms from iron deficiency anemia may not have any obvious physical exam findings. With more advancing anemia, the patient may appear pale and the cardiovascular exam may reveal tachycardia, a systolic flow murmur, and pale nailbeds (Bunn, 2017). A rectal examination should be performed to assess the stool and collect for occult blood testing (Holcomb, 2005).

DIFFERENTIAL DIAGNOSIS AND DIAGNOSTIC CONSIDERATIONS

When an anemia is suspected from the complete blood count (CBC) results, further laboratory testing is necessary to distinguish iron deficiency from other potential causes. In iron deficiency anemia, the serum iron level will be low and serum ferritin level (which reflects iron stores) will also be low; when the ferritin level is less than 15 ng/L, iron deficiency anemia can be diagnosed (Peng & Uprichard, 2017).

Once the diagnosis of iron deficiency anemia is made, the etiology should be pursued. The patient's history should elicit if the origin is due to inadequate dietary intake or malabsorption of iron. If the problem is believed to be due to blood loss, the source should be identified. If not clear from the patient's history, consideration for more testing should be considered. For example, evaluation with upper endoscopy or colonoscopy should be pursued to evaluate for gastrointestinal sources of blood loss (Stauder et al., 2018).

TREATMENT

The primary treatment for iron deficiency is iron replacement. Oral iron supplements may be prescribed for once daily or every other day administration, with vitamin C added to improve absorption. Side effects with oral iron supplements are common and include nausea, vomiting, or constipation, which may impact the patient's tolerance and compliance with the oral regimen. When oral iron supplements are not tolerated or when the problem is due to poor iron absorption, IV iron infusions may be ordered. With iron infusions, patients will not experience the gastrointestinal side effects and the problem of malabsorption can be overcome. The regimen depends on the agent that is ordered (Camaschella, 2015).

When the etiology of iron deficiency anemia is blood loss, the source of the blood loss should be identified and treated. RBC transfusion should be reserved for those patients who suffer from active bleeding, hemodynamic instability, or evidence of tissue ischemia, such as chest pain (Auerbach, 2021b). Iron supplementation does not work quickly enough for the unstable patient but should still be considered as the iron content in the transfused product may not be enough to increase the patient's depleted stores (Auerbach, 2021b).

ANEMIA OF CHRONIC DISEASE

Anemia of chronic disease is a result of impaired synthesis of RBC secondary to other entities such as chronic inflammatory states, malignancy, chronic renal disease, chronic liver disease, and endocrine disorders including hypothyroidism (Bunn, 2017).

Chronic inflammatory states include chronic infections, such as subacute bacterial endocarditis and osteomyelitis or tuberculosis; autoimmune inflammatory disorders, such as rheumatoid arthritis and lupus (Bunn, 2017). In the setting of infection and active inflammation, cytokines increase hepcidin, which causes serum iron to decrease from impaired iron absorption in the gastrointestinal tract, while activated macrophages consume RBCs and hold onto iron; in addition, the bone marrow produces more white blood cells (WBCs) at the expense of RBC production (Ganz, 2019). Decreased RBC production and shortened lifespan of RBCs results in the anemia.

Malignancy can be associated with chronic anemia when the treatment causes myelosuppression; however, even without treatment, cancer causes inflammation from inflammatory factors associated with the malignancy itself, tumor necrosis, invasion of bone marrow, or damage to surrounding tissue by tumor, resulting in anemia of chronic disease (Bunn, 2017).

In chronic renal disease, loss of renal function is accompanied by decreased erythropoietin production required to stimulate bone marrow RBC production. The degree of anemia is proportional to the degree of functional loss. (Bunn, 2017).

Chronic liver disease may result in anemia due to changes in the synthesis of the RBC membrane that leads to a decreased lifespan for the RBC (Bunn, 2017). The anemia associated with liver disease is further exacerbated when alcohol is the cause of the liver disease. Alcohol suppresses marrow production of all blood cell types, resulting in pancytopenia (Bunn, 2017). In addition, patients with heavy alcohol use may also have anemia due to poor nutritional intake and impaired processing of folic acid and vitamin B_{12} (Bunn, 2017), leading to a mixed picture when interpreting blood work.

PRESENTING SIGNS AND SYMPTOMS

As with most acquired anemias, patients may be asymptomatic. Symptoms, such as fatigue, weakness, dyspnea, or palpitations, are evidence of decreased oxygen delivery to tissue from advancing anemia. When the etiology of the anemia is due to infection or an inflammatory disorder, symptoms reported may be more consistent with the primary problem and not the anemia. The AGACNP must obtain more information to distinguish the etiology of the symptoms.

HISTORY AND PHYSICAL FINDINGS

Due to the relationship of this anemia to other conditions, it is important for the AGACNP to elicit from the patient a detailed history of prior diagnoses that may be responsible. Medical histories and symptoms consistent with chronic infections, inflammatory disorders, liver or renal dysfunction, or malignancy should be reviewed with the

patient. When anemia is more severe or not well tolerated by the patient, the physical exam may be notable for tachycardia, pallor, and pale nailbeds (Bunn, 2017). Otherwise, the physical exam should be performed with a focus on searching for findings that might support the cause of this anemia, such as cirrhosis or splenomegaly (as with liver disease), facial edema or hair loss (as with hypothyroidism), or joint pain and deformities (as with rheumatoid arthritis).

DIFFERENTIAL DIAGNOSIS AND DIAGNOSTIC CONSIDERATIONS

The diagnosis of anemia of chronic disease is made by evaluating laboratory studies. The CBC will show decreased hemoglobin with normocytic/normochromic RBCs. Iron studies will show a decrease in serum iron and increased ferritin, or storage iron, and a decreased reticulocyte count (Ganz, 2019). The timing of these findings may lag behind the onset of the inciting problem by weeks or months due to the lifespan of RBCs; however, critically ill patients may show the changes associated with anemia of chronic disease as early as 1 week into the critical care course (Ganz, 2019). In addition, indicators of inflammation, such as WBC count, erythrocyte sedimentation rate, and C-reactive protein, may be checked to identify or monitor inflammatory activity (Ganz, 2019).

While the finding of normocytic/normochromic cells with elevated ferritin suggests anemia of chronic disease, it is important to note that the patient must have a chronic disease or inflammation to have anemia of chronic disease. If the patient does not have a diagnosis that could cause anemia of chronic disease, the AGACNP should embark on further evaluation to identify the underlying cause of this anemia.

TREATMENT

Treatment of anemia of chronic disease is first directed toward improved management of the underlying disease that has caused this anemia, with improvement in the hemoglobin level seen in as few as 2 weeks (Ganz, 2019). When primary illness treatment is not successful or possible (as with chronic kidney disease), the AGACNP can consider ordering synthetic erythropoietin when the hemoglobin level is <10 mg/dL (Ganz, 2019). True anemia of chronic disease due to inflammation should not require iron supplementation: Although the serum iron level is low, this is due to sequestering of iron by macrophages and not true iron deficiency (Ganz, 2019). However, in the case of renal disease or when there is co-existing iron deficiency, patients do need iron supplementation for erythropoietin to be effective. Transfusion with RBCs can be considered in cases where the anemia and symptoms are severe; however, the AGACNP should weigh the risks and benefits of transfusion against those of the anemia when making a treatment decision for an individual patient.

ANEMIA DUE TO HEMOLYSIS

Hemolysis, or the premature destruction of RBCs, is one explanation for normocytic, normochromic anemia (Marin, 2013). When the rate of RBC destruction outpaces erythropoiesis, symptoms and clinical signs of anemia become evident (Dhaliwal et al., 2004). Conditions resulting in hemolysis may be acquired or inherited and due to processes intrinsic or extrinsic to RBCs (Luzzatto, 2018; Phillips & Henderson, 2018).

PRESENTING SIGNS AND SYMPTOMS

Presenting signs and symptoms among individuals with hemolytic anemia are like those of anemia irrespective of etiology. Symptoms may be vague, particularly in the initial stages of red cell hemolysis. Individuals with induced, mild, or chronic hemolysis present with fatigue, back pain, palpitations, and hematuria (Means & Brodsky, 2021). These and the symptoms of weakness, dizziness, dyspnea, activity intolerance, and jaundice have been reported.

HISTORY AND PHYSICAL FINDINGS

In addition to the anemia symptoms listed, the history of present illness may be significant for ingestion of or exposure to foods, drugs, or toxins known to be associated with hemolysis (Al-Nouri et al., 2015). A recent or current infection may be reported (Means & Brodsky, 2021). The health history could be significant for prosthetic heart valve surgery, thermal injury, physical injury, and blood product transfusion (Lichtman et al., 2003).

Capturing a history of anemia or familial blood disorders is optimal (Ma, 2021).

Objective exam findings are varied. Vital sign findings may include fever, tachycardia, and low oxygen saturation (Cascio & De Loughery, 2017). In addition, the physical examination can reveal mental status changes; conjunctival, mucosal, or skin pallor; scleral icterus; jaundice; heart murmur; hepatomegaly; splenomegaly; and dark-colored urine.

Blood count analysis may reveal a decreased hematocrit and hemoglobin (Hgb; Brodsky, 2021). In addition, schistocytes (RBC fragments), and occasionally Heinz bodies (denatured Hgb) and bite cells are present on the peripheral blood smear. Other laboratory tests that support hemolysis include a decreased haptoglobin; elevated lactate dehydrogenase (LDH); unconjugated hyperbilirubinemia; a newly positive direct antiglobulin test (DAT); reticulocytosis; and hemoglobinuria (Brodsky, 2021; Ma, 2021).

DIFFERENTIAL DIAGNOSIS

Common diagnoses of anemia due to hemolysis are included in Table 9.2.

MANAGEMENT

The management of hemolytic anemia is highly dependent on the etiology and severity of the hemolysis. Mild induced or chronic hemolysis is self-limited and the need for transfusion support is rare, whereas identification and cessation of the precipitating event and education about foods, medications, and drugs that contribute to induced or chronic hemolysis comprise the primary interventions (Brodsky, 2021). While possible, massive hemolysis is rare, and it is more common that morbidity and mortality following massive hemolysis is due to the underlying medical problem or its sequelae.

TABLE 9.2: Common Diagnoses of Anemia Due to Hemolysis

DIAGNOSES	EXAMPLES
Food, drug, toxin, or chemical-induced hemolytic anemia	Favism, penicillin, rifampin, salicylates, sulfonamides, nitrofurans, dapsone, phenazopyridine, nalidixic acid, methylene blue, amyl nitrate, spider venom, and formaldehyde
Hemolytic anemia due to infection	Streptococcus and Parvovirus B19
Hemolytic uremic syndrome	Familial hemolytic uremic syndrome
Hemolytic anemia due to red cell enzymopathies	Inherited G6PD deficiency
Traumatic hemolytic anemia	Microangiopathies, thermal injury, and near drowning
Autoimmune or immune-mediated hemolytic anemia	Warm- and cold-reacting antibodies, and hemolytic transfusion reactions
Inherited hemoglobinopathies	Thalassemia and sickle cell disease

Source: From Lichtman, M. A., Beutler, E., Kipps, T. J., & Williams, W. J. (2003). *Williams' manual of hematology* (6th ed.). McGraw-Hill.

SICKLE CELL DISEASE

Sickle cell disease (SCD) refers to a group of inherited defects in the hemoglobin molecule, resulting in the hemoglobin S variant of normal hemoglobin. When sickle cell hemoglobin is deoxygenated, long chains (polymers) form, causing the RBCs to become rigid and crescent shaped. The deformed RBCs adhere to each other and to vessel walls, blocking flow through small vessels and activating inflammation, resulting in tissue ischemia, acute and chronic pain, and ultimately organ damage (Bunn, 2017). Patients who are homozygous for the gene (*HbSS*) have the most severe form of the disease—red cells with hemoglobin S, hemolytic anemia, and acutely painful vaso-occlusive episodes (VOEs)—resulting in multisystem complications. Patients who are heterozygous for the gene are said to have the sickle cell trait and are less likely to exhibit the severe manifestations than the homozygous patients. Approximately 300,000 infants around the world are born with SCD each year, primarily from sub-Saharan Africa, the Mediterranean basin, the Middle East, and India (Piel et al., 2017). There are an estimated 100,000 people with SCD in the United States; it is most common in patients who are African American, but also occurs in patients of Hispanic, Arabic, and Asian Indian descent (Piel et al., 2017).

SCD affects all body systems. At baseline, patients with SCD have chronic hemolytic anemia due to the shortened lifespan of the RBCs. Over time, patients with SCD may develop chronic complications due to recurrent vaso-occlusion and tissue hypoxia, including pulmonary hypertension, heart failure with preserved ejection fraction, retinopathy, functional hyposplenism, avascular necrosis, skin ulceration, kidney disease, iron overload, and chronic pain (Piel et al., 2017). Acute presentations include painful VOE, priapism, acute chest syndrome, acute anemia, stroke, and sepsis (Verhovsek & McFarlane, 2017).

Patients with this disorder present very early in life. AGACNPs are rarely involved in the diagnosis of SCD because newborns in the United States are screened at birth for this disorder; if positive, the child will manifest symptoms consistent with SCD long before adulthood. With advances in treatment strategies and infection prevention, SCD is no longer just a childhood disease. Patients with SCD now typically survive well into adulthood (Verhovsek & McFarlane, 2017); therefore, AGACNPs need to be prepared to care for patients with SCD who may present to acute and critical care with acute VOEs or with exacerbations of the chronic complications of the disease.

PRESENTING SIGNS AND SYMPTOMS

VOEs (formerly known as "crises") are the most common reason for hospital admission (Verhovsek & McFarlane, 2017). VOEs are characterized by the acute onset of severe pain, particularly but not limited to the back, lower extremities, and chest (Bunn, 2017). Patients with SCC often describe the pain as being characteristic of their typical VOE, which may be helpful in distinguishing the pain from other possible causes (Bunn, 2017). When the pain is too severe for the patient to manage with the outpatient pain plan or there are other accompanying symptoms, evaluation and management require an emergency department visit and hospital inpatient admission (Verhovsek & McFarlane, 2017).

HISTORY AND PHYSICAL FINDINGS

The primary presenting complaint will be acute, severe pain. Because viral or bacterial infections are often triggers for VOEs, patients may also report symptoms of respiratory, urinary, or other infections prior to onset of acute pain (Bunn, 2017). Other triggers for VOEs include pregnancy, dehydration, extreme temperature changes, stress, and surgery, although in most cases there is no identifiable trigger (Vacca & Blank, 2017). The AGACNP should perform a thorough pain assessment to distinguish between typical VOE pain and that which may indicate another pathology. Medication reconciliation should be performed to determine what is the patient's baseline pain management regimen and to continue essential therapeutic agents in the patient's care. The AGACNP should also ask the patient about the baseline hemoglobin/hematocrit and transfusion history to determine the severity of the patient's anemia.

On examination, patients with VOEs appear with varying degrees of discomfort. Normal vital signs and/or appearance do not reflect the degree of pain experienced by the patient; however, abnormal vital signs may indicate an underlying pathology related or not related to the VOE and warrant further evaluation. Abnormal physical findings may not be seen on the examination for VOE; however, features, such as scleral icterus from hemolysis, may point the AGACNP toward complications present in the patient. There is no specific laboratory test for VOEs, although the reticulocyte count and/or the WBC may be elevated (Verhovsek & McFarlane, 2017).

DIFFERENTIAL DIAGNOSIS AND DIAGNOSTIC CONSIDERATIONS

The diagnostic priority is to determine if the acute pain is due to a cause other than an uncomplicated VOE (National Heart, Lung, and Blood Institute [NHLBI], 2014). An infectious workup should be pursued, particularly if the patient complains of symptoms or fever. Of particular concern in the patient with SCD is acute chest syndrome, which is VOE in the pulmonary vasculature, characterized by acute chest pain, fever, respiratory symptoms, and pulmonary infiltrate on x-ray (Bunn, 2017). If undetected, the patient with acute chest syndrome may progress to respiratory failure or even death

(Verhovsek & McFarlane, 2017). Otherwise, laboratory testing and imaging should be ordered specific to the alternative diagnoses being considered.

TREATMENT

The patient with VOE should be cautiously given IV fluids to rehydrate and reduce viscosity without exacerbating underlying heart or kidney failure. The acute pain of VOE is treated with a multimodal strategy, including IV opiates, NSAIDs, acetaminophen, and nonpharmacologic adjuncts (Bunn, 2017). Exchange transfusion, in which a patient's sickled cells are drawn off and replaced with donor red cells, can be considered with unrelieved, ongoing VOE with worsening anemia (Verhovsek & McFarlane, 2017).

For complicated VOE cases that do not respond to standard care, the AGACNP should consult hematology or pain management specialists for assistance.

TRANSITION OF CARE

Patients with SCD can experience many barriers to care, including consistent primary care, access to SCD specialists, and maintenance/preventive medications. In addition, there are many new therapies available to reduce VOEs and hospitalizations that can improve the quality of life for the patient with SCD (Bunn, 2017). Inpatient care may provide an opportunity for the AGACNP to use therapeutic communication to engender trust and assist with referrals to help reduce barriers and improve the care of patients with SCD.

Patients with SCD with multiple complications may be followed by several providers and specialists. The AGACNP supports continuity of care across care settings through direct communication with the patient's providers and with accurate, up-to-date documentation in the electronic medical record. The AGACNP coordinates care for the patient at discharge, ensuring that follow-up is arranged, and therapies are continued.

CLINICAL PEARLS

- Patient presentations and laboratory values often do not fall into discrete categories due to multiple pathologies (such as malignancies or combined iron deficiency and anemia of chronic disease). Use laboratory testing but also consider the whole clinical picture when making an anemia diagnosis.
- In acute and critical care, it is easy to be satisfied with a hemoglobin of 8 to 10 g/dL. This is not normal! This patient is anemic. When noting the patient's low hemoglobin level, the AGACNP should also note an anemia diagnosis in the record. If there is not one, the AGACNP should investigate the patient's baseline and define the etiology for the anemia.
- To have an anemia of chronic disease, the patient must have a chronic disease.

9.2: INHERITED BLEEDING DISORDERS

Inherited bleeding disorders include hemophilia A, hemophilia B, and von Willebrand disease (VWD). Hemophilia A and B are caused by mutations in genes that code for clotting factors, usually inherited in an X-linked recessive pattern and primarily expressed in males (Online Mendelian Inheritance in Man [OMIM], 2021a, 2021b). While hemophilia A and B are phenotypically similar, gene mutations produce insufficiency of Factors VIII and IX, respectively (Hemophilia of Georgia, 2021). Hemophilia is rare; that is, the prevalence of the clinical disorder for Type A is 1 in 5,000 and Type B is 1 in 30,000 live births (OMIM, 2021a, 2021b). Females are often carriers of the genes associated with hemophilia even in the absence of the disorder itself and prenatal genetic testing is often sought (National Heart, Lung, and Blood Institute [NHLBI], 2019).

A more common inherited bleeding disorder, VWD results from a gene mutation that impacts the synthesis of sufficient and effective clotting factor called von Willebrand factor (VWF) (OMIM, 2021c). In contrast to the sex-linked inheritance pattern of hemophilia, the VWD inheritance pattern varies and both males and females can be affected (OMIM, 2021c). The Centers for Disease Control and Prevention (CDC, 2021d) estimates that 1% of the U.S. population or 3.2 million people have VWD. In both diseases, patients suffer from abnormal bleeding, although there are variations in severity (Bunn & Furie, 2017a).

PRESENTING SIGNS AND SYMPTOMS

The timing of a hemophilia diagnosis depends on its severity. The more severe cases will present in childhood, with reports of excessive bleeding and bruising with walking and crawling, while more mild cases may not present until adulthood, when the patient experiences a trauma or bleeds after a surgery (Arruda & High, 2018). Throughout their lives, patients with severe hemophilia experience hemarthroses or bleeding into major joints that cause pain and reduce range of motion (Arruda & High, 2018). In acute situations, the AGACNP may care for patients who have bleeding into tighter spaces, such as the brain, and need emergency evaluation and treatment due to the risks of compression.

Like hemophilia A and B, time to diagnosis is related to the severity of the VWF deficit. Mild forms are apparent only when abnormal bleeding occurs, such as after surgery or a severe injury (Goodeve, 2017). In contrast, severe forms have been diagnosed earlier, usually following an assessment for heavy bleeding that occurred after minor trauma or in the absence of injury (spontaneous bleeding).

HISTORY AND PHYSICAL FINDINGS

Regardless of the etiology of an inherited bleeding disorder, patients will report bleeding. Bleeding ranges from superficial to hemorrhage, due to physical trauma, or occurs spontaneously (Ma, 2021). Patients with bleeding disorders have reported frequent or long-lasting gingival bleeding and epistaxis; prolonged or excessive bleeding with minimal injury or after surgery or dental work; superficial bruising to deep hematoma; heavy or prolonged menses; hematuria;, hemorrhoidal bleeding to melena; and tight or painful joints (Ma, 2021).

DIFFERENTIAL DIAGNOSIS AND DIAGNOSTIC CONSIDERATIONS

Because there are many causes of bleeding, pertinent positives and negatives from a thorough health history and physical exam will facilitate an organized diagnostic strategy. The differential for VWD includes mild hemophilia A, inherited platelet disorders, and the possibility that there is no bleeding disorder (Rick, 2022). Furthermore, blood count abnormalities and coagulopathies are often absent; however, VWD screening tests are available to inform other laboratory tests having low and high yield within given case scenarios (Hayward & Moffat, 2013; Hayward et al., 2012). Establishing an individual's pre-test probability for diagnoses in the differential prior to selecting additional tests is optimal (Hayward, 2018).

MANAGEMENT

The management of hemophilia A or B involves supplementation of the absent or inadequate clotting factor to prevent and control bleeding. Patients with mild hemophilia A and most symptomatic carriers receive genetic counseling and education, including a plan to treat bleeding events (Konkle et al., 2017a). A general hemostasis plan for bleeding in hemophilia A is administration of IV or nasal desmopressin (DDAVP, or 1-deamino-8-D-arginine vasopressin) or Factor VIII concentrate within 1 hour of the onset of bleeding. As an extension of the treatment plan for a mild disorder, severe hemophilia A requires the use of prophylactic infusions of Factor VIII several times a week in addition to a hemostasis plan.

Patients with mild hemophilia B receive genetic counseling and education, including a plan to treat bleeding events. A general hemostasis plan for bleeding in hemophilia B is administration of recombinant or plasma-derived Factor IX concentrate within 1 hour of the onset of bleeding (Konkle et al., 2017b). Furthermore, severe hemophilia B can be managed with prophylactic infusions of Factor IX concentrate several times a week in addition to a hemostasis plan.

In either type of hemophilia, vitamin K administration is ineffective for hemostasis. The rationale is that vitamin K impacts the coagulation deficit along the extrinsic pathway of the coagulation cascade where prolonged prothrombin time (PT) occurs (Palta et al., 2014). In hemophilia, there are deficiencies of Factors VIII and IX which are along the intrinsic pathway of the coagulation cascade (Bunn & Furie, 2017a). A prolonged partial thromboplastin time (PTT) occurs with intrinsic pathway factor deficiencies.

The management of bleeding due to VWD commonly involves the stimulation of VWF with DDAVP or factor replacement with genetically engineered proteins from human plasma, depending on VWD type and severity of bleeding (Rick, 2022). Topical thrombin has been effective to achieve hemostasis for superficial bleeding and aminocaproic acid has been utilized to stabilize platelet plugs established after surgery.

9.3: ACQUIRED BLEEDING DISORDERS

Acquired bleeding disorders are more common than the inherited bleeding disorders. There are multiple possible causes of acquired causes of abnormal hemostasis, including but not limited to kidney disease, liver disease, acute coagulopathies, acquired coagulation factor inhibitors, and platelet disorders (Hurwitz et al., 2017).

PLATELET DISORDERS: THROMBOCYTOPENIAS

Platelet problems result from an inadequate number of platelets (i.e., quantitative) or platelets rendered nonfunctional (i.e., qualitative). Platelets may be adequate in number but do not effectively function in the settings of uremia or drugs (e.g., aspirin, NSAIDs, thienopyridines; Bunn & Furie, 2017b). The rest of this section focuses on the quantitative platelet disorders, or thrombocytopenias.

Thrombocytopenia, defined as platelet count <150,000/mcL, may be identified when a patient presents with evidence of bleeding while being followed for a chronic illness (such as liver disease), or may be an incidental finding on a complete blood count ordered for another reason (VanDruff, 2019). Thrombocytopenia can be further defined as mild (platelet count 100,000–150,000/mcL), moderate (50,000–99,000/micLr), or severe (<50,000/mcL; Arnold & Cuker, 2021). It is reasonable to associate a low platelet count with bleeding; however, there are also conditions in which a low platelet count is associated with excessive clotting (Warkentin, 2019).

Thrombocytopenia can be classified by the underlying etiology: decreased production (as with bone marrow suppression), increased platelet destruction (as with immune system attacks on platelets), and distribution changes (such as splenic sequestration) (Lambing, 2007). Given the complexities of these disorders, the AGACNP should consider consultation with the hematology service, particularly if the presentation is not consistent with objective data, if there is bleeding, or if advanced treatment is needed.

PRESENTING SIGNS AND SYMPTOMS

Patients with thrombocytopenias may present with no signs or symptoms, particularly when the decreased platelet count is incidentally detected. Otherwise, patients may present with symptoms that prompt a complete blood count when the thrombocytopenia is discovered. These symptoms can include gingival bleeding, epistaxis, hematuria, hematochezia, or menorrhagia (VanDruff, 2019). Patients may have petechiae, which are small, reddish-purple macules that do not blanch with pressure (Bunn & Furie, 2017b). Unlike the inherited bleeding disorders, which present with deep bleeding and hematomas, patients with thrombocytopenia present with more superficial bleeding, such as petechiae and purpura (Bunn & Furie, 2017b).

HISTORY AND PHYSICAL FINDINGS

The patient may report the signs and symptoms already presented, along with increased purpura or complaint of bruising very easily. In collecting the history, the timing of symptoms is important in distinguishing the etiology. Because the lifespan of platelets is 7 to 10 days, thrombocytopenia will become apparent after a week or so. If the problem is due to platelet consumption or destruction, the thrombocytopenia will manifest much more quickly—in hours to a few days (Bunn & Furie, 2017b). The patient's past medical history should be reviewed for chronic diseases and any history of transfusion (Lambing, 2007). The AGACNP should ask the patient about any new medications because some have been implicated in both marrow production, platelet dysfunction, and immune destruction of platelets. Alcohol use and liver disease may cause thrombocytopenia, so the patient's history with alcohol should be carefully explored. The patient's personal and family histories should be reviewed for autoimmune, bleeding, and clotting disorders (Lambing, 2007).

Physical examination should be performed with special attention to skin for the appearance of petechiae, purpura, and ecchymoses. Lymph nodes should be checked for lymphadenopathy consistent with lymphoproliferative disorders. Assess the abdomen for hepatomegaly and/or splenomegaly. The peripheral vascular assessment is conducted to evaluate for evidence of arterial or venous thromboses or distal limb ischemia (Warkentin, 2019).

DIFFERENTIAL DIAGNOSIS AND DIAGNOSTIC CONSIDERATIONS

The CBC is done to trend the direction and quantity of the platelet count and to evaluate for the presence of anemia, with further attention to the red cell indices to better define the anemia, if present. A peripheral blood smear should be obtained to evaluate the character of the platelets, evidence of hemolysis, or the presence of blasts (indicating bone marrow disease; VanDruff, 2019). Additional testing may be ordered depending on the index of suspicion for a pathology.

Immune Thrombocytopenia

In immune thrombocytopenia (ITP; once referred to as immune thrombocytopenia purpura), the patient's immune system attacks receptors on the platelet membrane, leading to platelet destruction and depletion (VanDruff, 2019). This immune attack may be primary or secondary to another underlying syndrome, such as autoimmune disorders, viral illnesses, or pregnancy (VanDruff, 2019). In children, ITP often occurs after a viral illness and typically resolves over time; in adults, ITP occurs insidiously, with no viral prodrome, and becomes a chronic condition over the lifetime (Bunn & Furie, 2017b).

DIFFERENTIAL DIAGNOSIS AND DIAGNOSTIC CONSIDERATIONS

In ITP, the patient may or may not have purpura or bleeding, and the spleen and lymph nodes are normal (Bunn & Furie, 2017b). In addition, the peripheral smear, white blood cell count (WBC) and differential, and the hemoglobin/hematocrit levels are all normal, unless there has been recent bleeding (Bunn & Furie, 2017b). If the ITP is suspected to be secondary to another autoimmune or lymphoproliferative disease, then an autoimmune laboratory workup or bone marrow biopsy should be pursued.

TREATMENT

The first-line treatment for ITP is corticosteroids over several weeks (VanDruff, 2019). Patients are known to relapse and may need to remain on steroids for long periods. If there is no improvement in the platelet count or if the side effects of steroids cannot be tolerated, rituximab may be attempted. Thrombopoietin receptor agonists (TPORAs), immunosuppression, or chemotherapeutic agents may be required for refractory cases. Finally, because the spleen is a site of platelet destruction and antiplatelet antibody production, splenectomy can be considered if pharmacologic treatment is not successful (VanDruff, 2019).

When ITP is accompanied by bleeding and anemia, intravenous immunoglobuling (IVIG) can be given along with the steroids (VanDruff, 2019). Platelet transfusion is reserved only for those patients who have severe hemorrhage—although transfusion will quickly correct the platelet count, the donor platelets are susceptible to the same antibody response and destruction as the native platelets, so transfusions are not a long-term or routine treatment for ITP (VanDruff, 2019).

Thrombotic Thrombocytopenic Purpura

TTP is a thrombotic microangiopathy; that is, due to an immune reaction, thrombocytopenia and hemolysis occur, with the formation of microclots blocking capillaries resulting in organ damage (Warkentin, 2019). The patient develops autoantibodies to ADAMTS13, a protease that ordinarily cleaves large VWF protein chains. When antibodies inhibit this protease, the large VWF strands cause platelet consumption and aggregation, leading to thrombocytopenia and the diffuse microclots that occlude small vessels (VanDruff, 2019). The resulting tissue ischemia causes organ failure, most commonly in the brain and the kidneys; in addition, the microclots force shearing of the blood flow in the vessels, leading to the hemolysis and anemia that are characteristic of this syndrome (VanDruff, 2019). TTP is not common, but carries with it a high mortality rate, so recognition of this syndrome is essential (Hurwitz et al., 2017).

HISTORY AND PHYSICAL FINDINGS

The history may be notable for a recent viral syndrome. Patients present to care with malaise and viral symptoms. They may have neurologic symptoms ranging from headache to altered mental status to seizures (Bunn & Furie, 2017b). Physical examination may reveal petechiae, purpura, and mucocutaneous bleeding but no overt hemorrhage (VanDruff, 2019). In TTP, the CBC will show severe thrombocytopenia. Laboratory findings are notable for evidence of hemolysis: anemia from the hemolysis, elevated lactate dehydrogenase (LDH), elevated indirect bilirubin, and low haptoglobin. The peripheral blood smear in TTP will show schistocytes, a manifestation of hemolysis. Blood-urea-nitrogen (BUN) and creatinine should be checked for evidence of kidney failure; the urinalysis may show hemoglobinuria and proteinuria (evidence of hemolysis and kidney injury) and an elevated lactic acid level suggests tissue ischemia (VanDruff, 2019). The PT/INR and PTT are normal, which differentiates TTP from disseminated intravascular coagulopathy (DIC; Bunn & Furie, 2017b). Once TTP becomes the primary diagnosis, an ADAMTS13 level can be checked to confirm but should not delay treatment (VanDruff, 2019).

The first line treatment for TTP is therapeutic plasma exchange, in which the patient's blood is run through a pheresis machine, the components separated, the plasma removed, and donor plasma added. This procedure decreases the ADAMTS13 antibody and returns normal VWF back to the patient (Bunn & Furie, 2017b). Corticosteroids are also used to suppress ADAMTS antibodies (VanDruff, 2019). Rituximab can be added if there is not an adequate response (VanDruff, 2019). Platelet transfusion in TTP is contraindicated as the addition of platelets will "fuel the fire" of microthrombi formation (VanDruff, 2019). Caplacizumab is a newer drug that blocks the aggregation of platelets to the massive VWF protein chains; when used with plasma exchange and for 30 days after the exchange, caplacizumab can reduce the time to normal platelet count and reduce recurrence of TTP (Scully et al., 2019).

Heparin-Induced Thrombocytopenia

Heparin-induced thrombocytopenia (HIT) is caused by the development of antibodies against complexes of heparin and platelet factor 4 (PF4) in patients receiving unfractionated heparin (UFH) or low molecular weight heparin (LMWH; Hurwitz et al., 2017). Type I HIT is caused by the direct effect of heparin on the platelet, causing a nonimmune platelet aggregation, which consumes the platelet supply and causes thrombocytopenia but not thrombosis (Crowther, 2021a). This is considered a mild form of HIT, with resolution occurring from the discontinuation of the heparin product (Crowther, 2021a). In Type II HIT, immunoglobulin G (IgG) antibodies bind to the heparin-PF4 complex, leading to the formation of immune complexes that activate platelets; these platelets then aggregate, which leads to their consumption and the deposition of thrombi in arteries and veins (Crowther, 2021a; Hurwitz et al., 2017). This thrombotic aspect causes more morbidity and mortality than the thrombocytopenia aspect or bleeding (VanDruff, 2019).

Patients at most risk for HIT tend to be female, major surgical or trauma patients who received therapeutic heparin, although any patient receiving a heparin product is at risk. In addition, there is greater risk with UFH than there is with LMWH (VanDruff, 2019). Suspicion for HIT should be raised when there is a sudden, unexpected decrease in the platelet count (to <150,000 or a relative decrease of 50% or more from the patient's baseline), particularly when the patient is hospitalized or has recently been hospitalized and treated with heparin products for anticoagulation or venous thromboembolism (VTE) prophylaxis (Hurwitz et al., 2017).

On examination, the patient may have no abnormal findings, or there may be evidence of peripheral arterial and/or venous thrombosis and sequelae: skin necrosis at injection sites, limb ischemia, and organ ischemia/infarction (Crowther, 2021a). Frank bleeding is not common.

Timing of HIT onset varies depending on the patient's history of exposure to heparin; without prior exposure to heparin, the thrombocytopenia may manifest 5 to 10 days after the exposure. When the patient has prior exposure, more rapid onset of thrombocytopenia is seen (Hurwitz et al., 2017). Once HIT is suspected, the AGACNP should calculate the pretest probability of HIT using the 4Ts score (Cuker et al., 2012; Table 9.3). If the probability of HIT is low, then the AGACNP should continue to evaluate the cause of the thrombocytopenia; if the probability of HIT is intermediate or high, the AGACNP should stop all heparin-containing products, start a nonheparin anticoagulant (other than warfarin, which may make gangrene worse when used early in HIT), and order HIT antibody testing (Crowther, 2021a).

There are two types of diagnostic tests for HIT: HIT ELISA, an immunoassay to detect antibodies to the PF4-heparin complex, and functional assays, such as the serotonin release assay (SRA) and the heparin-induced platelet activation assay (HIPA; Crowther, 2021a). The SRA measures serotonin released from aggregated platelets when exposed to HIT antibodies and is currently considered the gold standard for HIT diagnosis due to its high sensitivity and specificity. In the HIPA test, patient plasma with the HIT antibody is mixed with platelet-rich plasma; the test is positive for HIT when the platelets are activated by the patient's serum (Crowther, 2021a).

TABLE 9.3: The 4Ts Pretest Clinical Scoring System for Heparin-Induced Thrombocytopenia Evaluation

4Ts	2 POINTS	1 POINT	0 POINTS
Thrombocytopenia	Platelet count falls >50% and platelet nadir ≥20	Platelet count 30%–50% or platelet nadir 10–19	Platelet count falls <30% or platelet nadir <10
Timing of platelet count fall	Clear onset days 5–10 or platelet fall ≤1 day (prior heparin exposure within 30 days)	Consistent with days 5–10 fall, but not clear (missing platelet counts); onset after day 10; or fall ≤1 day (prior heparin exposure 30–100 days ago)	Platelet count ≤4 days without recent exposure
Thrombosis or other sequelae	New thrombosis (confirmed); skin necrosis; acute systemic reaction after IV unfractionated heparin bolus	Progressive or recurrent thrombosis; non necrotizing (erythematous) skin lesions; suspected thrombosis (not proven)	None
Other causes of thrombocytopenia	None apparent	Possible	Definite
Scoring	1–3: Low probability of HIT 4–5: Intermediate probability of HIT 6–8: High probability of HIT		

Source: Adapted from Cuker, A., Gimotty, P. A., Crowther, M. A., & Warkentin, T. E. (2012). Predictive value of the 4Ts scoring system for heparin-induced thrombocytopenia: A systematic review and meta-analysis. *Blood, 120*(20), 4160–4167. https://doi.org/10.1182%2Fblood-2012-07-443051

Note that treatment should be initiated immediately, without waiting for results of the HIT antibody test so as to not further permit activation of platelets and development of clotting (Crowther, 2021a).

Treatment should begin when there is moderate or high suspicion of HIT, before the diagnosis is confirmed, to reduce the risk of thrombosis. Treatment goals are two-fold: first, to stop the platelet activation process and second, to reduce the risk of thrombosis (Crowther, 2021b). To stop platelet activation, all heparin products should be stopped; this includes VTE prophylaxis, anticoagulation, and use of heparin to maintain line patency, such as with hemodialysis catheters and circuits. In addition, treatment-dose anticoagulation with a nonheparin product should be initiated. Options include argatroban and bivalrudin, which are IV direct thrombin inhibitors; they are short-acting but require ongoing monitoring with coagulation testing and dose titration and are most appropriate for urgent anticoagulation in inpatient settings (Crowther, 2021b). Fondaparinux is a parenteral option that is given SC, so is appropriate for outpatient use. The direct oral anticoagulants (DOAC) may also be ordered; these include apixaban, dabigatran, and rivaroxaban. Warfarin should be avoided at initiation as it increases the risk of gangrene associated with thrombosis; however, once the thrombocytopenia subsides, warfarin may be started if overlapped with other anticoagulants for at least 5 days and if the platelet count has recovered (Crowther, 2021b). The choice of anticoagulation depends on concomitant bleeding or presence of clot, the patient's renal and/or hepatic function, indication (e.g., if the patient with HIT also has a prosthetic heart valve, then DOACs are contraindicated and warfarin is used), and cost (Crowther, 2021b). The AGACNP should monitor the platelet count with anticoagulation to ensure that it is recovering.

If the antibody testing is negative, the AGACNP may consider resuming heparin products, if indicated. If HIT is confirmed, the anticoagulation should be continued for at least 4 weeks, and longer if the patient has a confirmed thrombus (Crowther, 2021b). In addition, the AGACNP should document the HIT diagnosis in the medical record and the patient's allergy/adverse reaction list to ensure that other providers do not put the patient at risk by ordering heparin products in the future.

DISSEMINATED INTRAVASCULAR COAGULOPATHY

Disseminated intrvascular coagulopathy (DIC) or consumptive coagulopathy is the complex pathological activation of the coagulation system due to an underlying insult, such as sepsis, trauma, obstetrical emergencies, and serious malignancies, overwhelming regulatory mechanisms causing systemic bleeding and clotting (Bunn & Furie, 2017a). Tissue factor release triggered by injured tissue, endotoxin release, cancer procoagulants and others activate the coagulation cascade to consume massive amounts of platelets and coagulation factors; with clot deposition throughout the vasculature (Bunn & Furie, 2017a). In addition, the fibrinolytic system is activated, breaking down clots and causing bleeding without adequate replacement of coagulation factors and platelets to compensate (Bunn & Furie, 2017a). These patients are often critically ill or become critically ill very quickly.

HISTORY AND PHYSICAL FINDINGS

On physical examination, the AGACNP will note skin with petechiae, purpura, ecchymosis, gangrene, or bleeding from venipuncture, line, and surgical sites; the AGACNP may also observe hematuria or hematochezia

(Hurwitz et al., 2017). Vital signs may demonstrate hemodynamic instability if there is ongoing blood loss.

DIFFERENTIAL DIAGNOSIS AND DIAGNOSTIC CONSIDERATIONS

There is not a single test to diagnose DIC. Rather, the AGACNP will need to evaluate several lab values. The CBC will reveal anemia from blood loss and severe thrombocytopenia as platelets are depleted, and the peripheral smear will show schistocytes and large platelets (Warkentin, 2019). Coagulation studies are notable for prolonged PT/INR, prolonged PTT, decreased fibrinogen, and variable fibrin degradation products (one of which, d-Dimer, will be elevated due to presence of clotting; Bunn & Furie, 2017a). Chemistry studies may show renal dysfunction.

The AGACNP may also use viscoelastic testing such as thromboelastography to monitor coagulation, assess for coagulopathy, determine need for transfusion, and assess responses to interventions (Kutcher & Cohen, 2021). Thromboelastography is a point of care test that allows the AGACNP to assess clot initiation, clot strength, and fibrinolysis using multiple coagulation measures (Kutcher & Cohen, 2021). The test, with results provided in tracing patterns that are associated with different functions and deficiencies, can be used to assess coagulation and guide management in DIC and other clinical situations with massive bleeding, such as cardiac surgery, massive trauma, or liver transplantation (Kutcher & Cohen, 2021).

TREATMENT

The primary management strategy of DIC is to manage the underlying pathology that caused it (Bunn & Furie, 2017a). The AGACNP also needs to manage hemodynamics, hypoxia, and venous access to stabilize the patient. Bleeding control can be attempted with transfusion of platelets, fresh frozen plasma, cryoprecipitate, and packed RBCs; if clotting exceeds bleeding, a low dose heparin infusion can be attempted to prevent and/or control thrombosis (Hurwitz et al., 2017).

TRANSFUSION THERAPY

Approximately 10.7 million blood transfusions are administered in the United States each year, with most of the blood used for trauma, critical care, surgery, inpatient medical care, and cancer care (Elflein, 2021). Blood products have saved many lives; however, there are several risks associated with transfusions, including infections, immune system reactions, and volume overload. AGACNPs can be good stewards of the blood supply and prevent complications by carefully selecting candidates, following guidelines for transfusion, and implementing blood management strategies. Examples of blood products, indications, and relevant guidelines are in Table 9.4.

INDICATIONS

Red Blood Cell Transfusion

Red blood cells (RBCs) are transfused when patients need increased oxygen-carrying capacity of the blood (Bunn & Kaufman, 2017). Current guidelines recommend considering the hemoglobin level, the patient's overall condition, patient preferences, and alternative therapies when deciding on transfusion therapy. Signs and symptoms that may indicate need for transfusion include decreased intravascular volume, shortness of breath, reduced exercise tolerance, lightheadedness, cardiac-related chest pain, hypotension, or tachycardia unresponsive to fluid challenge (Carson et al., 2016).

In the setting of anemia with hypovolemia, such as with trauma, major surgery, or gastrointestinal hemorrhage, RBCs will increase oxygen carrying capacity and blood volume, which are both desirable in these situations. Good quality evidence demonstrates that use of a restrictive transfusion threshold of hemoglobin <7 g/dL (for hemodynamically stable hospitalized adults and critically ill patients) or hemoglobin <8 g/dL (for patients undergoing orthopedic or cardiac surgery and for those with underlying cardiovascular disease) results in a lower 30-day mortality, reduced blood use, reduced expense, and fewer serious adverse events compared with a more liberal transfusion strategy (Carson et al., 2016). Although these guidelines do not include patients with acute coronary syndromes, oncology, or chronic-transfusion dependent anemia, routine transfusion for anemias based only on a hemoglobin threshold is not recommended when patients do not have symptoms or other treatments can be used (Carson et al., 2016).

Platelet Transfusion

Platelet transfusion is indicated for prevention or treatment of bleeding due to low platelet count or dysfunctional platelets (Kaufman et al., 2017). Transfusion is generally reserved for situations in which the platelet count is low, and bleeding is possible, as with interventional or surgical procedures. Goal-directed transfusion to a parameter to reduce the risk of spontaneous bleeding is typically reserved for patients receiving chemotherapy or stem cell transplant (American Red Cross, 2021). Prophylactic platelet transfusion is generally avoided in immune-mediated thrombocytopenia due to the potential (albeit low) risk of thrombosis, although if the patient is actively bleeding, it is recommended that platelets not be withheld (American Red Cross, 2021).

Plasma Transfusion

Plasma contains albumin and multiple clotting factors; AGACNPs may order transfusion with plasma for patients who have clotting factor deficiencies as with liver disease, patients with supratherapeutic INR from warfarin, DIC, and massive transfusion protocols (Bunn & Kaufman, 2017). There is a need for stronger evidence on

TABLE 9.4: Blood Products, Indications, and Guidelines

PRODUCT	CONTENTS	INDICATIONS	PERTINENT GUIDELINES
Packed red blood cells (PRBCs)	Red cells with plasma removed	Increase oxygen carrying capacity for symptomatic anemia, active bleeding	Not indicated until the hemoglobin level is 7 g/dL for hospitalized adult patients who are hemodynamically stable, including critically ill patients; threshold 8 g/dL recommended for patients undergoing orthopedic surgery, cardiac surgery, and those with preexisting cardiovascular disease; does not apply to patients with acute coronary syndrome, severe thrombocytopenia, and chronic transfusion dependent anemia (Carson et al., 2016)
Platelets	Pooled from multiple donors, single donor, or human leukocyte antigen (HLA) matched	Active bleeding, replacement for marrow aplasia, acquired or inherited platelet dysfunction	Prophylaxis for spontaneous bleeding for therapy-induced hypoproliferative thrombocytopenia, elective central venous catheter placement with count <20K, elective lumbar puncture with count <50K, major elective non-neuraxial surgery with count <50K; treat bleeding with cardiopulmonary bypass with perioperative bleeding and thrombocytopenia and/or evidence of platelet dysfunction (Kaufman et al., 2015)
Fresh frozen plasma	All clotting factors, fibrinogen, plasma proteins, electrolytes, protein C/S, antithrombin	Documented Factor V/XI deficiency, warfarin reversal when prothrombin complex concentrate not available, DIC, massive transfusion, TTP treatment, therapeutic plasma exchange	Use in massive transfusion, INR reversal in warfarin-related intracranial hemorrhage; surgical intervention in individuals with bleeding and deficiencies of multiple coagulation factors (Roback et al., 2010) Use of prophylactic FFP prior to procedures in nonbleeding patients with abnormal clotting tests is not supported by good quality evidence (Carson et al., 2021)
Cryoprecipitate	Fibrinogen, Factor VIII, along with von Willebrand factor	DIC, massive transfusion, third line prescription for von Willibrand disease, alternate Factor VIII for hemophilia	Routine use of cryoprecipitate as an alternative treatment for congenital fibrinogen deficiency, dysfibrinogenemia, Factor XIII deficiency, hemophilia A, or von Willebrand disease is not recommended and should be considered only when there is risk of loss of life or limb and the specific factor concentrate is not available. Use of this component may be considered for uremic bleeding after other modalities have failed (American Red Cross, 2021)
Whole blood	Red cells, plasma, and platelets	Autologous donation, massive transfusion	Military and civilian trauma only; generally not indicated
Leukocytes	Pooled granulocytes	Alternate to neutrophil growth factors with severe neutropenia and severe sepsis	Very limited indications

Source: Adapted from Bunn, H. F., & Kaufman, R. (2017). Blood transfusion. In J. C. Aster & H. F. Bunn (Eds.), *Pathophysiology of blood disorders* (2nd ed.). McGraw-Hill. https://accessmedicine.mhmedical.com/content.aspx?bookid=1900&sectionid=137395856; DeLoughery, T. G. (2018). Transfusion medicine. *MD Edge Hematology and Oncology, 13*(5), 30–44; Raval, J. S., Griggs, J. R., & Fleg, A. (2020). Blood product transfusion in adults: Indications, adverse reactions, and modifications. *American Family Physician, 102*(1), 30–38

which to base transfusion practices (Roback et al., 2010); however, there is growing evidence that some plasma practices may not be necessary. For example, a recent randomized controlled trial evaluated the practice of giving plasma prior to procedures in patients with cirrhosis with mildly elevated INR, defined as 1.5 to 2.5. The investigators found no differences in postprocedure hemoglobin levels between groups and only minimal change in INR in the treatment group (Carson et al., 2021).

Massive Transfusion

Massive transfusion, traditionally defined as requiring more than 10 units of packed RBCs in 24 hours, (Committee on Trauma of the American College of Surgeons, 2015) may be required to achieve hemodynamic stability (Bunn & Kaufman, 2017). Patients with massive blood loss due to trauma, surgery, or gastrointestinal hemorrhage require transfusion with multiple blood products, with better outcomes when using a 1:1:1 ratio of plasma, RBCs, and platelets to replicate the content of whole blood (Evert et al., 2017). Facilities may have massive transfusion protocols developed with input from the emergency department, critical care services, anesthesiology, and the blood bank; these protocols streamline processes to reduce delays and have been shown to improve survival and decrease use and waste of blood products (Passerini, 2019).

RISKS AND REACTIONS

Risks with blood product transfusion can be divided into three types: infectious, immune-related, and nonimmune-related (Raval et al., 2020). Risks associated with immune system reactions to blood products pose greater risks to recipients than do infectious diseases, with transfusion-related acute lung injury (TRALI) being the most common cause of transfusion-related mortality (Bunn &

TABLE 9.5: Transfusion Reactions

REACTION	ETIOLOGY	FEATURES	INTERVENTIONS
INFECTIOUS			
HIV, hepatitis B and C, West Nile virus	Bloodborne organisms transmission via donated blood	• Disease transmission	Prevention strategies: • Donor screening for risks • Blood bank testing for infectious agents
IMMUNE MEDIATED			

Febrile nonhemolytic transfusion reaction	• Recipient antibodies bind to white blood cells (WBCs) in the blood product; proinflammatory cytokines produced within the product or generated by recipient reaction
	• Occurs within 4 h of transfusion
		• Fever
		• May be accompanied by
		  o Chills
		  o Rigors
		  o Hypertension
		  o Tachycardia
		  o Tachypnea
			• Stop the transfusion
			• Rule out hemolysis
			• Order acetaminophen for comfort
			• Consider leukocyte-reduced products for future transfusion

Allergic transfusion reaction	• Mediated by IgE antibodies binding to allergens, ultimately resulting in the release of histamine • Typically occurs during transfusion or within 4 h after transfusion	• Hives and/or pruritis • Angioedema • Respiratory wheezing/stridor • Hypotension • Shock and cardiovascular collapse • Anaphylactic or anaphylactoid reactions	• Treat based on reaction severity • Antihistamines • Glucocorticoids • Bronchodilators • Epinephrine for anaphylaxis • Consider washed products for future transfusion
Transfusion-related acute lung injury (TRALI)	• Noncardiogenic pulmonary edema typically within 6 h of transfusion of donor antibodies, resulting in neutrophil activation, endothelial injury, capillary leakage with exudative fluid extravasation, and ultimately acute lung injury • Leading cause of transfusion-associated mortality	• Dyspnea • Tachypnea • Tachycardia • Hypoxemia • Fever, chills • Blood pressure changes • Chest x-ray with bilateral pulmonary interstitial infiltrates	• Supportive care, oxygen and ventilation strategies same as with ARDS
Hemolytic transfusion reaction (HTR) Acute: Occurring within 24 h	• Immune: Antibody-mediated destruction of RBCs due to (ABO) incompatible RBCs or plasma • Most often due to human error: type/ crossmatch collection, blood bank processing, patient identification at time of transfusion	• Immediate hemolytic intravascular response • Fever, chills • Gross hemoglobinuria • Pain • Acute kidney injury • Jaundice • Shock • DIC • Death	Supportive care
Delayed (DHTR) occurring after 24 h	• Alloantibodies from prior transfusion or pregnancy trigger immune response when transfused blood has same antigen (anamnestic response) • Occurs 3–10 days after transfusion	• Extravascular hemolytic response • Vague symptoms, including: • Back pain • Decreased Hb from hemolysis of donated RBCs • Positive direct antiglobulin test • Occasional elevated bilirubin and acute kidney injury	Supportive care
Transfusion-associated graft-versus-host disease (TAGVHD)	• Viable donor lymphocytes survive, engraft, and target recipient • Occurs within 5 to 10 days of transfusion, with complete marrow aplasia within 21 days • Rare but almost universally fatal	• Rash • Fever • Nausea, vomiting, diarrhea • Pancytopenia	Supportive care only

TABLE 9.5: Transfusion Reactions *(continued)*

REACTION	ETIOLOGY	FEATURES	INTERVENTIONS
NON-IMMUNE MEDIATED			
Transfusion-associated circulatory overload (TACO)	Volume overload from transfusion causes cardiogenic pulmonary edema	• New-onset or worsening dyspnea • Tachypnea • Tachycardia • Hypoxemia • Fever, chills • Hypertension • Bilateral pulmonary interstitial infiltrates on chest x-ray • JVD • Peripheral edema • Elevated BNP	• Supportive care: oxygen, respiratory support if needed • Diuresis • Dialysis if indicated • Consider reduced volume or increased infusion time with future transfusions
Septic reaction	• Bacterial growth in a blood product • Platelets with highest rates due to room temperature storage	Symptoms typically occur within 24 h of transfusion • Fever, chills • Hypotension • Leukocytosis • Elevated lactate	• Culture patient and blood product; should have the same microorganism • Sepsis protocol • Rapidly initiate broad spectrum empiric antimicrobial therapy
Massive transfusion-associated reactions	• Consequence of patient factors (liver transplant, traumatic injury, hemorrhagic shock) and factors associated with large volume blood transfusion: sodium citrate, supernatant potassium, refrigerated blood • Ability to breakdown citrate depleted • Results in decreased ionized calcium, hyperkalemia, citrate toxicity, hypothermia	• Tingling, paraesthesias (hypocalcemia) • Cardiac depolarization abnormalities (hyperkalemia) • Blunted left ventricular response (citrate toxicity) • Coagulation abnormalities (hypothermia)	• Monitor electrolytes, supplement as needed • Treat hyperkalemia • Monitor coagulation factors and TEG • Transfuse blood and fluids with inline fluid warmer

For all actual or suspected transfusion reactions:
• Notify the blood bank of all potential and actual transfusion reactions.
• Return the unit and administration set to the blood bank.
• Collect red and lavender top samples and send to the blood bank.

Source: Adapted from A compendium of transfusion practice guidelines (4th ed). https://www.redcrossblood.org/content/dam/redcrossblood/hospital-page-documents/334401_compendium_v04jan2021_bookmarkedworking_rwv01.pdf; Bunn, H. F., & Kaufman, R. (2017). Blood transfusion. In J. C. Aster & H. F. Bunn (Eds.), *Pathophysiology of blood disorders* (2nd ed.). McGraw-Hill. https://accessmedicine.mhmedical.com/content.aspx?bookid=1900&sectionid=137395856; Delaney, M., Wendel, S., Bercovitz, R. S., Cid, J., Cohn, C., Dunbar, N. M, Apelseth, T. O., Popovsky, M., Stanworth, S. J., Tinmouth, A., Van de Watering, L., Waters, J. H., Yazer, M., & Ziman, J. (2016). Transfusion reactions: Prevention, diagnosis, and treatment. *The Lancet, 388*(10061), 2825–2836. https://doi.org/10.1016/S0140-6736(15)01313-6; DeLoughery, T. G. (2018). Transfusion medicine. *MD Edge Hematology and Oncology, 13*(5), 30–44; Raval, J. S., Griggs, J. R., & Fleg, A. (2020). Blood product transfusion in adults: Indications, adverse reactions, and modifications. *American Family Physician, 102*(1), 30–38

Kaufman, 2017). The major transfusion reactions are reviewed in Table 9.5.

In all cases of suspected or actual transfusion reactions, the AGACNP should stop the transfusion, start normal saline through a dedicated line, and assess the patient's cardiac, respiratory, and renal function; treatment is focused on supportive care (Delaney et al., 2016). The AGACNP collaborates with the blood bank team to identify the etiology of the reaction by sending the transfused blood to the blood bank for additional testing. A sample is checked for hemoglobin—if positive, then hemolysis is more likely. Repeat blood typing may help determine if there were patient identification and blood match errors. Direct antiglobulin testing (Coombs test) will be positive if there is hemolysis. A CBC for he-

moglobin and liver function tests for bilirubin are followed for changes to suggest hemolysis (American Red Cross, 2021; Delaney et al., 2016). Supportive care may include respiratory support, as with supplemental oxygen or positive pressure ventilation; cardiac monitoring and blood pressure support; and kidney function monitoring and renal replacement therapy if indicated (Delaney et al., 2016).

PATIENT BLOOD MANAGEMENT

The AGACNP must be knowledgeable about transfusion science for several reasons. First, the blood supply in the United States is not unlimited; it is highly dependent on volunteer blood donors, nonprofit blood centers, and hospital centers, and is very vulnerable to changes in supply and demand, highlighted by shortages during the recent COVID-19 pandemic (U.S. Department of Health and Human Services, 2020). Therefore, the AGACNP must consider transfusion practices in the setting of a limited supply. Second, patients in acute and critical care are at risk for developing iatrogenic anemia due to procedures and phlebotomy losses with laboratory testing. It is estimated that adult ICU patients can lose up to 660 mL of blood per week from diagnostic testing, and over 70% of adult ICU patients are anemic by hospital day 2, with half of those patients needing transfusion (Whitehead et al., 2019). Finally, the medical community is now recognizing that historical transfusion practices have not been evidence based and there is need for better development and dissemination of clinical indications for transfusion (American Red Cross, 2021). While the blood supply may be safer from transmission of infectious diseases, research has shown more positive outcomes from restricting transfusion and the negative outcomes with transfusion, including morbidity, increased length of stay, and increased costs (Association for the Advancement of Blood & Biotherapies [AABB], 2015).

AGACNPs can contribute to the goals of an adequate blood supply that is safe for patients by using patient blood management (PBM) strategies. PBM is an evidence-based, multidisciplinary approach to the transfusion process, starting with recipient identification and evaluation through the decision to transfuse or not, with the ultimate goal of reducing the need for transfusion (AABB, 2015). PBM strategies include the optimization of RBC volume, the application of appropriate guidelines and transfusion indications, and minimizing blood loss (AABB, 2015). AGACNPs can support these efforts by (a) assessing for necessity one's own practice of ordering daily or serial laboratory work; (b) promoting the use of blood return devices on lines in the practice setting; (c) utilizing guidelines for transfusion indications (AABB, 2015; Whitehead et al., 2019); and following Choosing Wisely® recommendations for best practices (Box 9.1).

9.4: COMMON HEMATOLOGIC CANCERS

ACUTE AND CHRONIC LEUKEMIA

Leukemia is an over proliferation of malignant blood cells having their genesis in the bone marrow. The most common leukemias are those that involve white blood cells (WBCs); for example, acute and chronic myelogenous leukemia and acute and chronic lymphoblastic leukemia (Blum & Bloomfield, 2018; Hoelzer, 2018; Kantarjian & Cortes, 2018; Leukemia and Lymphoma Society [LLS], 2021; Woyach & Byrd, 2018). The leukemic cells are called myeloid blasts and lymphoblasts that effectively diminish normal hematopoiesis (e.g., WBC, red blood cell (RBC), and platelet formation).

EPIDEMIOLOGY

Leukemia is a less common diagnosis compared to solid tumor cancers. A leukemia diagnosis in the 20th century changed from one imbuing a near certain death to one with a potential for cure since the advent of successful allogeneic stem cell transplantation in the 1970s. The National Cancer Institute Surveillance, Epidemiology, and End Results Program (NCI SEER, 2021g) reported that based on 2016–2018 data, 1.6% of people will develop leukemia during their lifetime. In addition, they estimated new cases for 2021 at 4.3 per 100,000 people based on 2014–2018 data; thus leukemia will represent 3.2% of all new cancer diagnoses. The NCI SEER (2021g) also included that the 5-year relative survival rate for leukemia is 65% based on data from 2011–2017 and the death rate is 3.9% using 2015–2019 mortality data. These data indicate that leukemia is comparatively rare, people with leukemia are living longer than historically observed, and overall mortality remains high.

PRESENTING SIGNS AND SYMPTOMS

Regardless of the type of leukemia, patient presentation can be similar. Patients often report nonspecific symptoms like fever, weight loss, fatigue, malaise, paleness, headache, dyspnea, bone pain, and skin changes (Schiffer & Gurbuxani, 2021; Van Etten, 2020). Others reported localizing symptoms of infection and easy or excess bruising or bleeding that is out of proportion to physical trauma.

BOX 9.1 CHOOSING WISELY® CAMPAIGN RECOMMENDATIONS TO OPTIMIZE BLOOD USE

Don't transfuse more units of red blood or other components than absolutely necessary.
Don't transfuse red blood cells for iron deficiency without hemodynamic instability.
Don't routinely use blood products to reverse warfarin.
Don't perform serial blood counts on clinically stable patients.
Don't transfuse O-negative blood except to O-negative patients and in emergencies for women of child-bearing potential of unknown blood group.

Source: From American Board of Internal Medicine Foundation Choosing Wisely. (2014). *AABB partners with the ABIM Foundation on Choosing Wisely campaign; Issues list of recommendations to optimize blood use.* https://www.choosingwisely.org/aabb-partners-with-the-abim-foundation-on-choosing-wisely-campaign-issues-list-of-recommendations-to-optimize-blood-use/?highlight=blood%20management

HISTORY AND PHYSICAL FINDINGS

Subjective and objective physical exam findings for acute leukemias involve a rapid onset of presenting symptoms, whereas patients with chronic leukemias report a gradual increase in symptoms. Pertinent positive objective exam findings may include fever, weight loss, pallor, bruises, hematoma, bleeding (gingival, rectal, or at sites of trauma), and organomegaly (Advani & Aster, 2020; American Society of Hematology [ASH], 2021). Objective findings may also include those indicative of infection, such as purulent sputum, adventitious breath sounds, changes in the percussive note indicating lung consolidation or effusion, and the presence of abscess or other skin changes having purulence.

DIFFERENTIAL DIAGNOSIS AND DIAGNOSTIC CONSIDERATIONS

Diagnostic Considerations

Myeloid Leukemia

Myeloblast evaluation includes the identification of cell type, degree of cell differentiation or maturity, and chromosomal aberrancies (ACS, 2021a; Blum & Bloomfield, 2018; Hoelzer, 2018). Among these factors, myeloid leukemias involving cells in earlier stages of development with high degrees of cellular undifferentiation and chromosomal abnormalities (e.g., gene deletion) portend poorer prognoses (Arber et al., 2017).

Lymphoblastic Leukemia

Lymphoblasts are within either B- or T-lymphocyte cell lines. A diagnosis of lymphoid leukemia involves the identification of cell type, degree of its maturity, and gene mutations (ASH, 2021a; Kantarjian & Cortes, 2018; Woyach & Byrd, 2018). Like myeloid leukemias, cell immaturity, lesser differentiation, and gene mutations are associated with poorer prognoses.

TREATMENT

Treatments for leukemias continue to evolve. Treatment options vary depending on the clinical presentation, leukemic diagnosis, and staging (National Comprehensive Cancer Network [NCCN], 2021a). These include chemotherapy, radiation, immune therapy, and stem cell transplantation and evidence-based guidelines are available (NCCN, 2021a).

TRANSITION OF CARE

The AGACNP may encounter people with leukemia for emergent reasons such as neutropenic fever, active infection, sepsis, or bleeding complications. Other reasons for hospitalization include chemotherapy or stem cell transplantation. Oftentimes, patients have pancytopenia, are immunosuppressed (e.g., corticosteroids), and are hospitalized for several weeks. When these acute issues resolve and permit discharge, it is prudent to ensure that the patient understands the outpatient triage process, has a plan for seeking care when complications occur (these are common and anticipated), and follow-up appointments have been established.

CLINICAL PEARLS

- Leukemias are life-threatening hematologic malignancies
- Infection is a common complication and is the primary cause of death.
- During a hospitalization, consultation with a hematology team is recommended.
- Postdischarge follow-up plans are essential to safe care.

LYMPHOMA

The lymphomas are hematologic cancers that involve the lymph system and organs within it (e.g., lymph nodes and spleen; American Society of Hematology [ASH], 2021b). The type of lymphoma a person has will fall within one of two distinct classifications—Hodgkin's lymphoma (HL) and non-Hodgkin's lymphoma (NHL). In either case, the malignant lymphocytes eventually crowd out normal lymphocytes and thus, if not treated, markedly increase the risk of life-threatening infection.

EPIDEMIOLOGY

The incidence of HL is far less common than NHL. The NCI SEER (2021f) estimated 8,830 new cases and 960 deaths in 2021 which represents 0.5% of all new cancer cases and 0.2% of all cancer deaths in that year, respectively. Furthermore, the 5-year relative survival rate was 88.3%. In contrast, the incidence and mortality due to NHL was higher and estimated at 81,560 new cases (4.3%) and 20,720 deaths (3.4%; NCI SEER, 2021i).

PRESENTING SIGNS AND SYMPTOMS

Many people with HL and NHL report adenopathy. An important triad of symptoms to assess for is the presence of "B symptoms" that include fever, night sweats, and unintentional weight loss (Freedman et al., 2021). The majority of HL and NHL is diagnosed in the outpatient setting. However, the AGACNP may encounter patients with lymphoma who present with an oncologic emergency like airway, gastrointestinal, or superior vena cava (SVC) obstruction or spinal cord compression because of enlarged lymph nodes. Lymphomas can be aggressive or indolent, and certain types of NHL (e.g., Burkitt's) have a high cellular doubling time and may produce tumor lysis syndrome (TLS) and cause hypercalcemia, hyperviscosity, and renal failure (Jacobson & Longo, 2021a; 2021b).

HISTORY AND PHYSICAL FINDINGS

Patients may report previous chemo- or radiation therapy, having a first-degree relative with lymphoma, exposure to pesticides, or a personal history of Epstein-Barr or HIV (Freedman et al., 2021). These factors have been associated with the development of lymphoma; however, the relationship is not to a predictive or causal level. On physical exam, firm and nontender adenopathy is commonly present and hepato- or splenomegaly may be palpable.

DIFFERENTIAL DIAGNOSIS AND DIAGNOSTIC CONSIDERATIONS

The differential diagnosis for adenopathy is vast. Most people will need a thorough evaluation for infection as the cause of the adenopathy. Referral for a biopsy is warranted when HL and NHL are suspected as histopathologic testing of affected lymphoid tissue is required for diagnosis. Imaging and additional testing (e.g., bone marrow evaluation) is often requested by the interventionist obtaining a biopsy or determined by the cancer team.

TREATMENT

Treatments for HL and NHL continue to evolve. Treatment options vary depending on the clinical presentation, diagnosis, and staging. Treatments include chemotherapy, radiation, and immune therapy (e.g., chimeric antigen receptor T-cell therapy). Evidence-based treatment guidelines for B- and T-cell lymphoma guidelines are available (NCCN, 2021b; 2021f; 2021l).

TRANSITION OF CARE

The AGACNP may encounter patients with lymphoma for emergent reasons such as superior vena cava (SVC) syndrome and fever of unknown origin. Other reasons for hospitalization include chemotherapy administration, TLS, or adoptive T-cell therapy. When these acute issues resolve and permit discharge, it is prudent to ensure that the patient understands the outpatient triage process, has a plan for seeking care when complications occur (these are common and anticipated), and follow-up appointments have been established.

CLINICAL PEARLS

- HL is distinct from NHL and is treated differently.
- NHL is an encompassing designation for different types of lymphoma sharing similar characteristics.
- Resection of a lymph node is insufficient to treat HL and NHL because it is a cancer of the lymphoid system and additional treatment is needed.

9.5: COMMON SOLID TUMORS

Solid tumor cancer is a leading cause of death, as evidenced by 8.2 million cancer-related deaths worldwide in 2012 (Torre et al., 2015) and nearly 600,000 people in the United States annually (CDC, 2021). There are numerous types of solid tumor cancers, each with differences in presentation. Because the symptoms that cause patients to access care are often nonspecific, cancer is commonly a part of the differential diagnosis. Cancer epidemiology is thus an essential component of decision-making regarding differential diagnoses and diagnostics.

Information about lung, colorectal, breast, pancreatic, bladder, and ovarian cancers is included in the following sections. These diagnoses are the most common solid tumor cancers in the United States (NCI SEER, 2021h). People with these cancers are commonly diagnosed and cared for by providers in ambulatory care centers. At times and particularly in advanced cancer cases, patients present to, or require care in, acute care settings. A working knowledge of cancer epidemiology, presenting signs and symptoms, history and physical exam findings, differential diagnosis, diagnostic considerations, cancer staging, and standard treatments for these cancers is essential in either setting.

Cancer staging takes place after diagnosis and before treatment because it has implications for treatment and prognosis. Most solid tumors are staged using the TNM system (National Cancer Institute [NCI], 2021a). The TNM staging system for solid tumors takes into consideration the size of the tumor (T), lymph node involvement (N), and the presence of metastases (M). Each component of the TNM system ranges from I to IV. Stage I represents early cancer, II or III indicates locally advanced disease, and IV signifies advanced metastatic cancer.

Finally, the transition of care carries particular importance for cancer patients' care. Thorough and effective communication regarding a cancer workup status and known results is imperative to the cancer care continuum. In some cases, other aspects may impact the transition of care, and these are included where applicable.

LUNG CANCER

EPIDEMIOLOGY

From 2010 to 2016, lung and bronchus cancers were the leading cause of cancer-related deaths and carried an overall 5-year relative survival rate of 20.5% (NCI SEER, 2021h). This overall 5-year survival rate following a lung and bronchus cancer diagnosis was influenced by the cancer stage at diagnosis, representing the extent of cancer in the body. Metastatic disease (beyond the primary tumor or regional lymphatics) was present in 61% of lung and bronchus cancer diagnoses made within this time frame. The 5-year relative survival rate in these cases was 14.1%.

PRESENTING SIGNS AND SYMPTOMS

The most common presenting symptoms reported by patients who were subsequently diagnosed with lung cancer were cough, hemoptysis, chest pain, dyspnea, and weight loss (Latimer, 2018; Midthun, 2021). The presence of certain risk factors for lung cancer was predictive of its diagnosis. The most predictive risk factors were current or remote smoking history, exposure to asbestos, and chronic exposure to secondhand smoke, radon, or other known cancer-causing agents (American Cancer Society [ACS], 2021g; Bade & Dela Cruz, 2020).

HISTORY AND PHYSICAL FINDINGS

Many patients with early-stage lung cancer are asymptomatic and do not have abnormal findings on physical exam. Symptomatic patients often have late-stage cancer and may or may not have abnormal findings on physical exam. In either case, obtaining a detailed health history and performing a complete physical exam is essential to formulate a differential diagnosis.

In addition to pulmonary symptomatology, pertinent positive subjective findings include a personal history or family history of cancer, current or historical environmental exposure to secondhand smoke and toxins, lower socioeconomic status, decreased functional status, pain, chronic cough, dyspnea, hemoptysis, fevers, chills, and unintentional weight loss (Horn & Lovely, 2018). Pertinent positive objective findings on physical examination include male sex, African descent, decreased weight, fever, adventitious breath sounds upon auscultation, decreased breath sounds to percussion and auscultation due to a mass or pleural effusion, digital clubbing, and palpable neck and axillary adenopathy.

DIFFERENTIAL DIAGNOSIS AND DIAGNOSTIC CONSIDERATIONS

Differential Diagnoses

A differential diagnosis stemming from pertinent positive subjective and objective findings includes respiratory tract infection, foreign body in the airway, heart failure, pulmonary embolus (PE), bleeding disorder, toxin exposure, benign respiratory tract tumor, chronic cough syndrome, pleuritis, bronchiectasis, chronic obstructive lung disease, gastroesophageal reflux disease; malignancy-related SVC syndrome and pneumothorax supports an evaluation of the pulmonary organs with radiographic imaging such as x-rays and computed tomography (CT; Thomas et al., 2022; Midthun, 2021; Kassutto & Weinberg, 2021; Silvestri & Weinberg, 2017). Further evaluation of the mass may include bronchoscopy, lymph node evaluation, and additional imaging (e.g., magnetic resonance imaging [MRI]) to obtain a biopsy of the affected tissue to facilitate a timely diagnosis, determine cancer

staging, and discuss treatment options (Latimer & Mott, 2015). Thus, consultation and collaboration with cancer care and surgical teams are needed.

Diagnostic Considerations

Tumor histopathology confirms a lung cancer diagnosis. Nearly all lung cancer tumors are carcinomas; that is, they originate in the cells that line the lung and bronchus (Zheng, 2016). Lung carcinomas are primarily nonsmall cell lung cancers (NSCLC).

NSCLC has two major types, (a) nonsquamous and (b) squamous cell carcinoma. Nonsquamous carcinomas mainly include adenocarcinoma (LUAC), large cell carcinomas, and rare cell carcinomas (Thomas et al., 2022). Squamous cell carcinoma is also known as epidermoid carcinoma. The remainder of lung cancer cases involves small cell lung cancer (SCLC). The genetic and molecular characteristics of an individual tumor aid in prognostication, particularly epidermal growth factor receptor gene mutations in NSCLS (Kim et al., 2020). Staging is assigned using the TNM system where Stage IV involves metastases. Common sites include the lymphatics, central nervous system, and bone (Popper, 2016).

TREATMENT

Treatment can be tailored to lung cancer type, staging, and suitability to patient values and preferences. Treatment for lung cancer includes local and systemic modalities with a goal of a cure for those with limited and nonmetastatic disease (American Society of Clinical Oncology [ASCO], 2021c; Bezjak et al., 2015; NCI, 2021; NCCN, 2021g, Rudin et al., 2015). Local and systemic treatments can be administered to those with advanced and metastatic disease with the goal of palliation. The use of therapies supported by current and best evidence is a goal of many treatment consortium groups within the cancer care community. The more widely used cancer care and treatment guidelines endorsed by the groups listed previously are briefly summarized here (ASCO, 2021c; Bezjak et al., 2015; NCCN, 2021h; NCI, 2021c; Rudin et al., 2015).

Local Treatment

Local treatment modalities include surgery and radiation. Best evidence includes resection of a tumor to decrease tumor bulk before using a subsequent treatment modality. Tumor resection may also be necessary for symptom relief when the tumor compresses the airway causing dyspnea or pain. Involved field radiation is used to treat nonmetastatic disease definitively or administered with palliative intent to decrease tumor size and slow further tumor growth. Radiation may also be directed toward metastases to control cancer-related symptoms, such as to ease or relieve pain due to bone metastasis.

Systemic Treatment

Systemic treatment modalities may be employed with the same intent, including chemotherapy and immunotherapy. The most common chemotherapy regimens are cyclical and platinum-based (cisplatin or carboplatin), with or without paclitaxel. Also, providers may recommend immune system modulating agents with an affinity to a genetic or molecular tumor characteristic (e.g., pembrolizumab or atezolizumab).

Palliative and Supportive Care

All lung cancer treatments have associated side effects, emotional distress, and survivorship issues. Also, patients may choose to forego primary treatment, favoring an individually tailored treatment approach to maximize comfort. The NCI and NCCN provide resources and guidelines for healthcare providers and patients regarding supportive care (NCCN, 2021g; NCI, 2021c).

TRANSITION OF CARE

Some patients who received a lung cancer diagnosis during hospitalization have reported postdischarge challenges related to pain management, preparation to transition to outpatient cancer care, access to cancer services, health insurance coverage, personal finances, and information flow from the inpatient to outpatient care teams (Stiel et al., 2009). Documentation of the workup to date and the known results will help minimize repetition of or unnecessary testing, contribute to cancer staging efforts, and decrease treatment delays.

Cancer care navigators can enhance comprehensive, culturally sensitive cancer care (Oncology Nursing Society [ONS], 2018). Cancer care navigators are nurses with oncology experience who can assist patients in self-advocacy, address barriers to care, and provide individualized education (Phillips et al., 2019). These nursing interventions can impact treatment adherence, optimize communication among care team members, and facilitate the transition into survivorship.

CLINICAL PEARLS

- Presently, lung and bronchus cancers are the leading cause of cancer-related deaths in the United States.
- Common presenting symptoms are cough, hemoptysis, dyspnea, and pain.
- Most people diagnosed with lung cancer have metastatic disease that limits long-term survival.
- There are evidence-based guidelines tailored to cancer type and extent of disease with a treatment goal of palliation in the majority of cases.
- Routine hand-off procedures and cancer care navigators can enhance timely, comprehensive, and culturally sensitive cancer care to all patients, including lung cancer patients.

COLORECTAL CANCER

EPIDEMIOLOGY

Colorectal cancer has been declining since the early 1990s due to the emphasis on screening (NCI SEER, 2021d). However, it was a leading cause of death in adults globally, having a 9% estimated overall mortality rate in 2020 (International Agency for Research on Cancer [IARC], 2021). Colorectal cancer was the third leading cause of cancer-related death in the United States from 2011 to 2015, carrying a 16.9% mortality for males and 11.9% for females (Ward et al., 2019). Providers must understand the importance of screening for colorectal cancer because the significance of early diagnosis cannot be underestimated.

PRESENTING SIGNS AND SYMPTOMS

Many colorectal cancers are diagnosed in asymptomatic patients following an abnormality discovered using standard screening tests such as fecal occult blood testing or colonoscopy (ACS, 2021e). However, the compliance rate for screening tests has been lower than desired (Macrae et al., 2021). Symptomatic patients commonly reported a change in bowel habits, stool characteristics, rectal bleeding, and unintended weight loss. In contrast, highly acute presentations included intestinal obstruction and peritonitis.

HISTORY AND PHYSICAL FINDINGS

Pertinent positive subjective findings include a report of a change in bowel habits (e.g., diarrhea, constipation, narrow stools), abnormal stool characteristics (e.g., thin, dark brown, black, or bloody stool); rectal bleeding (ranging from bright red to black); abdominal pain (generalized to localized), and nonpurposeful weight loss (Horn & Lovely, 2018). Patients with these subjective findings often present to outpatient healthcare providers. During the patient interview, they may describe a high-fat diet, a diagnosis of inflammatory bowel disease, a personal history of colon cancer, or a family history that includes colon cancer, which are all predictive factors for colorectal cancer (Mayer, 2018). Pertinent positive objective findings on physical examination include decreased weight, pain to light or deep abdominal palpation, macroscopic anal bleeding, bright red blood per rectum, hematochezia, melena, a positive occult blood test, and iron deficiency anemia apparent on bloodwork (Macrae et al., 2021).

DIFFERENTIAL DIAGNOSIS AND DIAGNOSTIC CONSIDERATIONS

Differential Diagnoses

A differential diagnosis based on history and physical exam findings includes diagnoses having relevance to the colon and lower abdominal pain, overt or occult lower gastrointestinal bleeding, and iron-deficiency anemia. Some relevant diagnoses include diverticulosis, diverticulitis, infectious colitis, gastrointestinal obstruction and perforation, mesenteric ischemia, inflammatory bowel disease, nonsteroidal anti-inflammatory-related gastrointestinal bleeding, and colorectal and other cancers (Auerbach, 2021a; Penner & Fishman, 2021; Perencevich & Saltzman, 2020; Strate et al., 2012).

Diagnostic Considerations

The majority (96%) of de novo colorectal cancers are adenocarcinomas that develop from adenomatous colon polyps, with a typical colon mucosal cell origin (Ponz de Leon & Gregorio, 2001). Today, many biomarkers have been identified and used to aid in diagnosis, support accuracy in staging and prognostication, and permit individualized and targeted treatments (Alves Martins et al., 2019). The cancer stage is assigned using the TNM system and classified into early- and late-stage categories for treatment-related decisions.

Although less common, there are some inherited syndromes involving colorectal cancer. These include familial adenomatous polyposis coli, Lynch syndrome (also known as hereditary non-polyposis colorectal cancer, or HNPCC), and MUTYH-associated polyposis (Aoki & Taketo, 2007). Of these, Lynch syndrome is the most common hereditary colon cancer (CDC, 2021). Obtaining a family history for patients with this type of presentation is essential to comprehensive care.

TREATMENT

Treatment guidelines for colorectal cancers fall within two groups. The groups are early- and late-stage disease. The following descriptions represent the current consortium- and evidence-based treatment guidelines (ASCO, 2021a; Chiorean et al., 2020; Costas-Chavarri et al., 2019, NCCN, 2021e).

Early-Stage Colorectal Cancer

Surgical resection is recommended for early-stage disease by either laparoscopic or open approaches. Higher stage cases may require colonic stenting or diversion and postsurgical (adjuvant) chemotherapy. Adjuvant chemotherapy regimens are platinum-based (e.g., oxaliplatin) with 5-fluorouracil or capecitabine. While less common in the early-stage group, there may be cases where chemotherapy and radiation therapy may be given before surgery (neo-adjuvant) to reduce tumor bulk before resection.

Late-Stage Colorectal Cancer

Radiation and conventional chemotherapy for late-stage colorectal cancer treatment are most common. There are numerous systemic regimens available, permitting an individualized treatment approach. The most common regimens are those administered for early-stage disease, often with the addition of immune therapy

(e.g., monoclonal antibodies bevacizumab and nivolumab). Radiation or a course of chemotherapy may be effective to the extent that surgical resection would be likely to produce a meaningful outcome. Treatment decisions are influenced by patient preference, the extent of the residual primary tumor, and the effect of chemotherapy on sites of metastases.

TRANSITION OF CARE

While most patients present in an ambulatory setting, those experiencing cancer-related pain, bowel obstruction, and perforation may receive a colorectal cancer diagnosis in an acute care setting. To maximize the successful transition to outpatient care, documentation of the acute problem, cancer workup to date, and any known results will help streamline oncology care transition. Effective and complete communication will also minimize the duplication of tests and imaging, contribute to accurate staging, and maximize treatment expedience.

CLINICAL PEARLS

- Presently, colorectal cancer is the third leading cause of cancer-related death in the United States.
- Common presenting signs and symptoms for colorectal cancer include a change in bowel habits, stool characteristics, rectal bleeding, abdominal pain, and unintended weight loss.
- Treatment, prognosis, and survival are highly dependent on the stage of the disease.
- There are evidence-based guidelines tailored to cancer type and extent of disease with a curative treatment goal in many cases.

BREAST CANCER

EPIDEMIOLOGY

Female breast cancer is the most frequently diagnosed cancer both globally and in the United States (NCI SEER, 2021d). Also, it is a leading cause of cancer-related deaths. Most breast cancer cases are diagnosed in asymptomatic females upon workup for an abnormal finding on routine screening (Esserman & Joe, 2021). Based on 2015–2017 data, approximately 13% of females will develop breast cancer at some point in their lives (NCI SEER, 2021d). Of those diagnosed with breast cancer within that timeframe, the 5-year relative survival rate was 90%, and the death rate was approximately 20%. Breast cancer in males is rare, ranging from 0.5% to 6% globally and 0.5% to 1% in the United States, and routine screening is not recommended (Gradishar & Ruddy, 2020).

PRESENTING SIGNS AND SYMPTOMS

Providers discover most breast masses in asymptomatic females and males as an incidental finding on routine physical examination (ACS, 2021c; 2021d). Symptomatic individuals have reported breast swelling, skin dimpling, breast or nipple pain, nipple inversion, nipple or breast skin erythema or thickening, nipple discharge, and axillary lymphadenopathy (Sabel, 2021). AGACNPs may see patients before a breast cancer diagnosis. These circumstances include hospitalization needed to address the effects of large tumors or metastatic disease (e.g., pain, dyspnea, infection).

HISTORY AND PHYSICAL FINDINGS

Although no symptoms are present, pertinent positive subjective findings—including inquiries about a personal or family history of breast cancer or cancer syndromes—can facilitate the workup for a breast mass. Other informative items include any known genetic risk factor for breast cancer or prior radiation therapy to the neck or chest regions to treat other medical problems or cancers. Pertinent positive objective findings on physical examination of both breasts, chest wall, the inferior anterior neck, and axillae would be a palpable mass of any size or density (soft, firm, or hard; Sabel, 2021). The mass may be discrete (well-defined) and may or may not be mobile or tender. At times, breast tissue changes are lesser defined and better described as skin thickening or dimpling. Erythema, nipple discharge, nipple inversion, and palpable adenopathy (cervical, axillar, or epitrochlear) may also be present.

DIFFERENTIAL DIAGNOSIS AND DIAGNOSTIC CONSIDERATIONS

Differential Diagnoses

The differential diagnoses for a breast mass based on pertinent positives from the history and physical exam findings include benign and malignant processes. Benign breast diseases include fibroadenomas, fibrocystic breast disease, simple cysts, galactoceles, fat necrosis following breast trauma, and abscesses (Sabel, 2021). In addition to these benign processes, cancer diagnoses must also be considered. Histopathologic findings indicative of breast cancer are lobular carcinoma in situ and atypical lobular hyperplasia; that is, localized or invasive disease that is categorized as early, locally advanced, or metastatic and staged using the TNM system (Sabel, 2021).

Diagnostic Considerations

A common risk factor for breast cancer is a family history that includes breast cancer. The risk of breast cancer for a female with more than one first-degree relative diagnosed with breast cancer earlier than age 50 is high (CDC, 2021a; 2021b). Also, there are gene mutations that are predictive of breast cancer in females. Of these, there are two well-known variants; that is, *BRCA1* (BReast CAncer gene 1) and *BRCA2* (BReast CAncer gene 2) mutations. The inheritance of these genes markedly increases a female's risk of developing cancer over a lifetime to over 50% in many cases (Antoniou et al., 2003; NIH, 2021).

Other risk factors for breast cancer include social determinants of health. Low socioeconomic and education status, a disadvantaged location of a primary residence, racial segregation and discrimination, lack of social support, and social isolation influence access to healthcare and screening practices (Coughlin, 2019). The authors reported that these factors delayed breast cancer diagnoses, were associated with advanced disease at initial diagnosis, negatively influenced treatment adherence, and interfered with follow-up care, particularly for young females and females with advanced disease.

TREATMENT

There are many treatment modalities for early-stage or locally advanced ductal carcinoma in-situ (DCIS), early-stage invasive breast cancer, non-metastatic invasive breast cancer, and metastatic and recurrent breast cancer.

Early-Stage or Locally Advanced Ductal Carcinoma In-Situ and Early-Stage Invasive Breast Cancer

Modalities for early-stage or locally advanced ductal carcinoma in-situ (DCIS) and early-stage invasive breast cancer include surgical resection, systemic therapy (chemotherapy, targeted immunotherapy, and endocrine therapy), and radiation. The following descriptions include some current evidence-based treatment recommendations from cooperative cancer treatment groups (ASCO, 2021b; Hassett et al., 2020; Korde et al., 2021; NCCN, 2021d).

Early Stage or Locally Advanced Ductal Carcinoma In-Situ

DCIS is treated with surgical resection, ranging from lumpectomy to total mastectomy, lymph node biopsy to resection, and possibly breast reconstruction. Decisions about postsurgical treatments depend on cancer staging and molecular or genetic tumor features (e.g., estrogen receptor status). Treatments can include observation, adjuvant chemotherapy, or postsurgical radiation. Then, 5 years of endocrine therapy is often recommended (e.g., tamoxifen, aromatase inhibitors).

Nonmetastatic Invasive Breast Cancer

Nonmetastatic invasive breast cancer is treated with cycles of systemic therapy. The choice of chemotherapy regimen depends on disease stage, including risk stratification based on molecular and genetic tumor features (e.g., *HER2* status). The most common systemic treatment regimens include a taxane (e.g., paclitaxel), cyclophosphamide, and an anthracycline (e.g., doxorubicin) or platinum agent (e.g., cisplatin, carboplatin). If needed, a regimen may be administered in a neo adjuvant fashion (before surgery) to facilitate breast conservation by decreasing tumor bulk. Treatment with neoadjuvant chemotherapy can include immune therapy for *HER2* positive breast cancer (e.g., trastuzumab). Neoadjuvant therapy may be beneficial when a patient who will undergo a total mastectomy needs time to decide on breast reconstruction. The systemic regimen continues following surgery (adjuvant treatment), and radiation therapy may also be employed. Similar to other breast cancer diagnoses, decisions about endocrine treatment depend on receptor positivity.

Metastatic and Recurrent Breast Cancer

There are several treatment options in metastatic and recurrent breast cancer and treatment decisions involving assessing tumor characteristics, overall health status, and individual treatment preferences. An alternate chemotherapy regimen may be chosen, with or without targeted immunotherapy or radiation. Likewise, alternate endocrine therapy may be added based on tumor characteristics and the person's health status, values, and preferences.

TRANSITION OF CARE

Breast cancer has a familial tendency, and some predictive genes have been identified (NCI SEER, 2021e). In cases where there are one or more first-degree relatives who have breast cancer, providers consider a referral to a hereditary cancer program (CDC, 2021). Commonly, this consultation occurs in the outpatient setting. Questions about an inpatient consult by the heredity cancer team should be directed to and at the oncology team's discretion.

Support is a concept that many females with breast cancer value (Campbell-Enns & Woodgate, 2015). Family, friends, and community members may provide social support. Participation in support groups outside of this inner circle has benefits, including additional emotional support, resources about cancer, education about the effects of treatment, strategies for coping, available clinical trials, and assistance with the transition to survivorship. Most support groups have a virtual presence, both national and local, and many patients can access them at the cancer treatment location, home, or a local library.

CLINICAL PEARLS

- Breast masses are commonly incidentally found during a routine physical examination, and diagnostic mammography is recommended to evaluate the mass further.
- Most breast cancer diagnoses stem from an evaluation for an abnormal finding on a screening (vs. diagnostic) mammogram.
- Breast cancer treatments are varied and include surgical resection, chemotherapy, immunotherapy, radiation, and endocrine therapies, targeted to tumor histopathology and molecular characteristics.
- Social determinants of health such as low socioeconomic and education status, a disadvantaged location of a primary residence, racial segregation and discrimination, and social disconnectedness impact access to screening practices, ultimately impeding early diagnosis and adherence to treatment and follow-up care.

- Providers can help enhance a patient feeling supported, decrease a sense of isolation, and address fears that people with breast cancer may experience by facilitating a connection to a support group for patients amenable to this strategy.

PROSTATE CANCER

Prostate cancer is the most common cancer in males (NCI SEER, 2021k). Approximately 12% of males will be diagnosed during their lives, based on 2015–2017 data. Data analysis demonstrated that the 5-year relative survival rate was 97.8% within this time frame, and the annual death rate was approximately 19%.

PRESENTING SIGNS AND SYMPTOMS

An overwhelming majority of patients are diagnosed with prostate cancer during the workup for abnormal screening findings, making screening recommendations essential (Montminy et al., 2020). In an early stage, prostate cancer does not often cause symptoms. Common, nonspecific symptoms associated with prostate cancer include urinary urgency and hesitancy, macroscopic hematuria, and blood-tinged semen (Talpin & Smith, 2022). However, it is common that males do not experience symptoms until the cancer is advanced. These symptoms include pain or neurologic dysfunction due to metastatic spread to bones and the spinal cord or related structures.

HISTORY AND PHYSICAL FINDINGS

Pertinent positive subjective findings include the symptoms listed earlier. Patients may also report unintentional weight loss, erectile dysfunction, fatigue, and a personal or family history of prostate cancer or Lynch syndrome. Pertinent positive objective findings include African descent, an elevated prostate-specific antigen in the blood, weight loss, prostate enlargement, induration, lobular asymmetry, and an obscured sulcus. Discreet nodules in the posterior and lateral aspects of the gland (portions that are palpable by digital rectal examination) may also be present. Less commonly, non specific laboratory findings of anemia and renal insufficiency may be present.

DIFFERENTIAL DIAGNOSIS AND DIAGNOSTIC CONSIDERATIONS

Differential Diagnoses

The differential for prostate cancer includes urinary tract infection, benign prostate hyperplasia, and prostatitis (Talpin & Smith, 2022).

Diagnostic Considerations

The diagnostic workup often includes CT and MRI imaging, facilitating a biopsy for histopathology, staging, and discussions about treatment. Prostate cancers are histologically adenocarcinomas (Humphrey, 2017). Cancer staging is performed using the TNM system. It is further categorized into very low, low, intermediate, high, and very high strata using histopathology, imaging, germline testing, and other molecular biomarkers to inform treatment decisions and prognosis.

Social determinants of health have implications for prostate cancer outcomes. The risk and incidence of prostate cancer were higher, and survival lower in low socioeconomic status persons (Coughlin, 2020). Furthermore, immigration and education status, lack of social support, and social isolation influences the cancer stage at diagnosis and survival.

TREATMENT

Treatment options for prostate cancer vary depending on the clinical presentation and staging. A summary of treatment options gleaned from treatment-focused groups is as follows (ASCO, 2021d; NCCN, 2021k). When a patient has an elevated PSA level and no other cancer sign, the PSA level is often monitored over time. For others, local therapy includes radical prostatectomy. Radiation therapy, either targeted (brachytherapy with implanted radioactive beads), conformal (shaped to the affected area), and modulated radiation (varied beam intensity), are other local treatment options. The patient's treatment team may recommend systemic therapy with platinum-based (e.g., carboplatin) chemotherapy, immunotherapy (e.g., pembrolizumab), and androgen deprivation therapy (e.g., abiraterone) for advanced prostate cancer. Patients may opt for interventions solely directed to comfort as well.

TRANSITION OF CARE

Patients undergoing prostatectomy or brachytherapy will need a review of presurgical education, including the risk of exposing others to radiation until bead radioactivity is at a safe level. Reinforcement of the follow-up plan and the subsequent follow-up visit is essential.

Patients treated for prostate cancer with resection, radiation, and androgen deprivation therapy commonly experience long-term sexual dysfunction. Over 75% of spouses reported changes in the quality of their sex life following their partner's treatment (Movsas et al., 2016). While approximately 60% of providers initially recommended sexual treatment, 7% of the cancer survivors were receiving treatment, and 4.1% of spouses were referred to a sex therapist.

CLINICAL PEARLS

- Most prostate cancer diagnoses result from a workup of abnormal findings on screening tests.
- A digital rectal exam (DRE) permits palpation of a portion of the prostate gland; additional screening strategies are essential.
- Symptoms often indicate advanced disease, which are associated with social determinants of health,

such as low socioeconomic and immigration status, lesser education, and social disconnectedness.
- Long-term sexual dysfunction is common after prostate cancer treatment; however, recognizing and treating this adverse effect is uncommon.

PANCREATIC CANCER

PRESENTING SIGNS AND SYMPTOMS

Pancreatic cancer at an early stage does not often cause symptoms. When symptoms manifest, the tumor is usually quite large or has metastasized (ACS, 2021i). Common symptoms are jaundice at presentation or the related symptoms of dark urine; light or greasy stools; epigastric pain; and unintentional weight loss. Patients may also report nausea and vomiting, abdominal and back pain, and puritus (due to hyperbilirubinemia). Given the importance of the pancreas to insulin, some patients may present with symptoms of diabetes (polydipsia, polyphagia, and polyuria).

HISTORY AND PHYSICAL FINDINGS

In addition to the symptoms listed, pertinent subjective findings include recent venous thrombosis and pulmonary embolism and a family history of pancreatic cancer or cancers having genetic linkages. Pertinent positive objective findings on physical exam include weight loss, scleral icterus and jaundice, jugular venous distension, a palpable gallbladder (Courvoisier's sign), a palpable abdominal mass, hepatomegaly, splenomegaly, superficial thrombophlebitis (Trousseau's syndrome), and palpable lymphadenopathy (Von Hoff, 2018).

DIFFERENTIAL DIAGNOSIS AND DIAGNOSTIC CONSIDERATIONS

Differential Diagnoses

Pancreatic masses may be discovered incidentally on imaging performed for other reasons or during the workup for the symptoms listed previously. The symptom triad of jaundice, epigastric pain, and unintentional weight loss is suspicious for pancreatic cancer (Fernandez-del Castillo, 2021). The differential for any of these signs, symptoms, and findings is quite broad and includes neoplastic or nonneoplastic processes such as biliary obstruction, hepatocellular injury, liver failure, pancreatic cysts, pancreatitis, malignancies other than pancreatic in origin.

Diagnostic Considerations

The diagnostic workup often includes imaging with ultrasound and CT. A mass discovered on imaging will be biopsied for histopathology. Serologic evaluation for carbohydrate antigen 19-9 (CA 19-9) is a part of the initial workup. Pancreatic cancers fall within three main categories: resectable, partially resectable, and metastatic. Possible treatments are stratified among these categories. The treatment strategy based on some evidence-based cancer care guidelines are described in the following (ASCO, 2021d; NCCN, 2021k).

TREATMENT

Pancreatectomy is the only curative treatment for pancreatic cancer; however, given that symptoms of pancreatic cancer present when the cancer is extensive or metastatic, only 15% to 20% of individuals diagnosed with pancreatic cancer present early enough for pancreatectomy (Fernandez-del Castillo, 2021). It is more common that extensive resection is needed, with or without ductal stenting and staging laparotomy. There are cases where resection is not possible or preferred by an individual.

In addition to surgery, chemotherapy is a common treatment strategy and regimens consist of 5-fluorouracil and taxane-based (e.g., paclitaxel) regimen or an alternative with gemcitabine (NCCN, 2021k). Chemotherapy may be administered in a neoadjuvant fashion to decrease tumor bulk preoperatively or adjuvant to surgery. In cases where surgery is not an option, these same chemotherapy agents could be administered. Post-chemotherapy treatment may include a course of stereotactic radiation therapy.

Given that pancreatic cancers are commonly extensive, the possibility of death and the experience of cancer- and treatment-related effects are significant. Establishing goals of care, symptom management, maximizing comfort, and attending to quality of life are essential aspects of care (NCCN, 2021k). Palliative care teams can assist patients with extensive cancers that are life-limiting and have a high symptom burden, their families, and providers maximize meaningful care outcomes.

CLINICAL PEARLS

- A common symptom triad is jaundice, epigastric pain, and unintentional weight loss at presentation.
- Aggressive treatment involves surgery, followed by chemotherapy, and then radiation therapy.
- Survival outcomes are poor for patients with pancreatic cancer.
- Palliative care teams assist patients in setting care goals and with symptom management.
- Clinical trials will help guide future therapies.

BLADDER CANCER

There were nearly 84,000 new bladder cancer cases and approximately 17,000 bladder cancer-related deaths anticipated annually (ACS, 2021b). This report includes that the incidence rate is higher in Caucasians, those of male sex, and those 55 years of age and older. However, Black persons were at a slightly higher risk of having advanced cancer at the initial diagnosis. Of all people diagnosed with bladder cancer, including those with local spread, 4% of cases involved distant spread or metastases.

PRESENTING SIGNS AND SYMPTOMS

Hematuria is often the first symptom that patients report when bladder cancer is in an early stage (ACS, 2021b). At times, urinary frequency, urgency, dysuria, and nocturia are reported. When bladder cancer is advanced, patients report weight loss, the inability to void, fatigue, and pain.

HISTORY AND PHYSICAL FINDINGS

Common, pertinent positive subjective findings include the symptoms listed previously, a personal and family history of bladder cancer, and history of other cancers. Pertinent positive objective findings on physical examination include weight loss, grimacing with abdominal palpation or percussion, and macroscopic hematuria.

DIFFERENTIAL DIAGNOSIS AND DIAGNOSTIC CONSIDERATIONS

Differential Diagnoses

Differential diagnoses for these presenting symptoms is broad and includes urinary tract infection and nephrolithiasis. In males, prostatitis and benign prostatic hyperplasia are also included in the differential.

Diagnostic Considerations

When the suspicion for bladder cancer is high, patients undergo cystoscopy. This procedure permits the direct visualization of the bladder wall, and a biopsy for histopathology can be obtained. The oncology team may consider molecular and genomic testing also. Pelvic and abdominal imaging often complete the initial workup, and TNM staging is established to guide treatment recommendations. The following is a summary of some cancer care guidelines for bladder cancer (ASCO, 2021d; NCCN, 2021c).

TREATMENT

Treatment for early-stage bladder cancer without muscle wall invasion can range from observation to intravesicular chemotherapy. Early-stage bladder cancer with muscle wall invasion may consist of transurethral resection of the bladder tumor and a dose of intravesicular (inside the bladder) chemotherapy (e.g., gemcitabine) within 24 hours of surgery. Bacillus Calmette-Guerin (BCG) is an immunotherapy approach to bladder cancer treatment where *Mycobacterium bovis* (live bovine tuberculosis bacteria) may be administered intravesicularly to kill cancer cells. BCG treatment can be repeated, and pembrolizumab may be substituted in BCG-resistant cases.

Treatment of bladder cancer of Stage II to III may involve radical cystectomy, systemic chemotherapy with a platinum-based regimen, and adjuvant radiation therapy. Patients with Stage IV bladder cancer may opt for palliative chemotherapy or radiation and other treatment directed toward comfort.

OVARIAN CANCER

The incidence and death rates for ovarian cancer have been slowly declining since 2000 (NCI SEER, 2021j). NCI SEER reported that the age-adjusted rate of new cases was 11.2 per 100,000 females per year, a death rate of 6.7 per 100,000 females per year, based on data from 2013–2017 and 2014–2018, respectively. In 2020, the estimated incidence among all new cancer cases was 1.2%, and the death rate was 2.3%. Based on 2010–2016 data, the 5-year relative survival rate was 48.6% due to ovarian cancer diagnoses in later stages.

PRESENTING SIGNS AND SYMPTOMS

Ovarian cancer can cause symptoms even at an early stage that are often vague and nonspecific, delaying diagnosis and treatment. Symptoms that cause patients to seek care include weight loss; early satiety; bloating; abdominal, pelvic, and low back pain; and a change in menses (irregular or heavy bleeding; ACS, 2021). Patients may also report fatigue, urinary frequency, constipation, and dyspareunia.

HISTORY AND PHYSICAL FINDINGS

There are no standard screening tests for ovarian cancer; however, transvaginal ultrasound for patients with an elevated CA-125 may be beneficial (Shetty, 2019). Pertinent subjective history findings include the symptoms listed earlier and a personal and family history of ovarian cancer or breast/ovarian cancer syndromes. Pertinent objective physical exam findings include weight loss, a palpably enlarged ovary, and a palpable abdominal mass.

DIFFERENTIAL DIAGNOSIS AND DIAGNOSTIC CONSIDERATIONS

Differential Diagnoses

The differential diagnosis for a patient presenting with the nonspecific symptoms and any associated history and physical exam findings is quite broad, but can include benign adnexal mass or pathology of uterine etiology (Chen & Berek, 2022). Workup of significant symptoms and history and physical exam findings is the first step.

Diagnostic Considerations

Abdominal and pelvic ultrasound are imaging techniques used to evaluate ovarian tumors in addition to blood work for cancer antigen 125, or CA-125. Additional imaging, such as CT or MRI, may be indicated, depending on presentation. Histopathology of involved tissue is required for diagnosis. The types of ovarian cancer include (a) carcinomas, such as carcinosarcoma, clear cell, mucinous, endometrial, and serous; and (b) tumors such as borderline epithelial, malignant sex

cord stromal, and malignant germ cell (NCCN, 2021i). Ovarian cancer is staged using the TNM system, imaging, and molecular testing.

TREATMENT

Surgical resection is commonly employed to debulk disease and complete cancer staging. Single or bilateral salpingo-oophorectomy and hysterectomy are common, sometimes after neoadjuvant immune therapy (e.g., bevacizumab) or chemotherapy per evidence-based guidelines (NCCN, 2021i). The guidelines present treatment decisions based on histopathology, tumor staging, and imaging for people with ovarian cancer Stages I to IV who are treated with platinum- and taxane-based adjuvant chemotherapy regimens, regardless of the presence of germline, *BRCA 1/2*, or somatic gene mutation. Recommended testing to determine biologic response to treatment includes CA-125 levels and imaging. Furthermore, the guideline includes postprimary treatment for Stages II to IV disease with maintenance therapy (e.g., hormonal or combinations of immune therapy agents). Recommendations for persistent primary, progressive, and relapsed disease include different combinations of chemotherapy agents and biologic modifiers in cases where the cancer remains responsive to individual agents.

TRANSITION OF CARE

Treatments for ovarian cancer have evolved over the past few decades. However, advanced disease is common at diagnosis. Although 30% of patients with ovarian cancer survive beyond 5 years, those that survived past this point identified a healthy lifestyle, motivation, persistence, life purpose, and support systems as positive factors influencing their survival (Alimujiang et al., 2019). As potentially modifiable factors, healthy lifestyle changes and enhanced social support may positively impact patients' experience with ovarian cancer.

CLINICAL PEARLS

- There are no standard screening tests for ovarian cancer, and this disease is often in an advanced stage when diagnosed.
- Ovarian cancer can be a part of genetically linked cancer syndromes, so inquiring about a patient's personal and family history is essential.
- Encouraging a healthy lifestyle and identifying a support network may improve a survivor's experience with ovarian cancer and its treatment.

9.6: ONCOLOGIC EMERGENCIES

Oncologic emergencies are acute and potentially life-threatening complications that can arise from a cancer or cancer-related treatment, which may occur at the

TABLE 9.6: Classification of Oncologic Emergencies by Systems

SYSTEM	ONCOLOGIC EMERGENCY	COMMONLY SEEN WITH THESE DISORDERS
Metabolic	Hypercalcemia**	Cancers of lung, head/neck, breast; multiple myeloma; lymphomas; any disease with bone metastases
	Hyponatremia/ SIADH**	Cancers of lung (small cell common), head/neck, pancreas, and urology; treatment with some chemotherapeutics
	Tumor lysis syndrome*	Lymphomas, leukemias
	Hypoglycemia	Pancreatic cancers, aggressive lymphomas
Cardiovascular	Superior vena cava (SVC) syndrome*	Nonsmall cell and small cell lung cancers, Hodgkin and non-Hodgkin lymphoma, cancer with metastases to mediastinum or lymph nodes
	Pericardial effusion and cardiac tamponade**	Lung and breast cancers, lymphomas, leukemias, sarcomas, melanoma
	Deep vein thrombosis (DVT) and pulmonary embolus (PE)**	All malignancies, particularly pancreatic, gastric, and lung cancers; acute promyelocytic leukemia
Infectious	Neutropenic fever*	Recipients of cytotoxic therapies, radiation, and marrow suppressive treatments
	Sepsis**	Recipients of treatment inducing neutropenia, any with relative immune suppression
	Line infection or central line associated blood stream infection (CLABSI)**	Malignancies requiring infusions, pheresis, or other treatments with tunneled or percutaneous central lines
Neurologic	Malignant spinal cord compression (MSCC)*	Lung, breast, prostate, and renal cell cancers, multiple myeloma
	Elevated intracranial pressure (ICP) and seizures**	Primary brain tumors; metastatic disease, particularly from lung and breast cancers, melanoma, renal and colon cancers
Hematologic	Hyperviscosity syndrome (HVS)	Waldenstrom macroglobulinemia, multiple myeloma
	Leukostasis	Acute leukemias
	Disseminated intravascular coagulopathy (DIC)*	Acute leukemias and adenocarcinomas
Respiratory	Malignant airway obstruction	Tongue, oropharynx, thyroid, bronchogenic, and lung tumors, lymphomas
	Acute respiratory failure**	Encephalopathy or weakness-related aspiration, lung cancers
Immunologic	Hypersensitivity reactions and anaphylaxis	Recipients of platinum and taxane agents, cyclophosphamide, bleomycin, monoclonal antibodies
	Cytokine release syndrome	CAR-T recipients
	Immune checkpoint inhibitor adverse events	Recipients of immune checkpoint inhibitors for all malignancies
Chemotherapeutic	Chemotherapy extravasation	Recipients of anthracyclines, vinca alkaloids, mitomycin C, platinum compounds, & taxanes
	Chemotherapeutic toxicities	Recipients of bleomycin, bisulfan, carmustine, and paclitaxel, among others

* Covered in this chapter.

** Covered elsewhere in this text.

Source: Adapted from Demshar, R., Vanek, R., & Mazanec, P. (2011). Oncologic emergencies: New decade, new perspective. *AACN Advanced Critical Care, 22*(4), 337–348. https://doi.org/10.1097/NCI.0b013e318230112b; Lewis, M. A., Hendrickson, A. W., & Moynihan, T. J. (2011). Oncologic emergencies: Pathophysiology, presentation, diagnosis, and treatment. *CA: A Cancer Journal for Clinicians, 61*(5), 287–314. https://doi.org/10.3322/caac.20124; Spring, J., & Munshi, L. (2020). Oncologic emergencies: Traditional and contemporary. *Critical Care Clinics, 37*(1), 85–103. https://doi.org/10.1016/j.ccc.2020.08.004

time the patient presents with an unknown malignancy, through treatments, remission, and up to end-stage disease and death (Yeung & Manzullo, 2016). The patient with an oncologic emergency may be seen by nurse practitioners across all care settings, including those within the scope of the AGACNP. These problems require rapid recognition and urgent intervention to ensure best possible outcomes for those patients.

The "classic" oncologic emergencies are hypercalcemia, tumor lysis syndrome (TLS), syndrome of inappropriate anti-diuretic hormone (SIADH), superior vena cava syndrome (SVC) syndrome, and malignant spinal cord compression (MSCC; Demshar et al., 2011). While some oncologic emergencies are commonly associated with specific cancers, it is important to note that these complications can present atypically with other malignancies. In addition, patients with cancer may be immunocompromised, have bone marrow suppression, and have other comorbidities that make them highly susceptible to urgent complications that are worth considering in the category of "oncologic emergencies." Therefore, a useful way to classify oncologic emergencies is by pathophysiology so the AGACNP can consider oncologic emergencies with a systems approach and not by a specific cancer (Table 9.6).

TUMOR LYSIS SYNDROME

TLS results from excessive tumor and cell breakdown from any treatment, including chemotherapy, radiation, and other treatments, although it has been known to occur spontaneously at the time of presentation (Yeung & Manzullo, 2016). When tumor cells rupture, the contents enter the bloodstream and cause hyperuricemia, hyperphosphatemia, hypocalcemia, and hyperkalemia, leading to risk for acute kidney failure, volume overload, and cardiac arrhythmias (Spring & Munshi, 2020). Anticipating which patients are vulnerable to TLS and use of preventive strategies can greatly reduce the risk of TLS and related sequelae (Demshar et al., 2011).

PRESENTING SIGNS AND SYMPTOMS

Patients may present with vague symptoms early in TLS; with worsening labs, the patient may complain of nausea and/or vomiting, diarrhea or constipation, low urine output, weight gain, and weakness (Yeung & Manzullo, 2016).

HISTORY AND PHYSICAL FINDINGS

The patient with TLS typically has had recent treatment for a malignancy with a high tumor burden or rapidly dividing cells, such as Burkitt's lymphoma and acute leukemias, although it may occur in solid tumors such as SCLC or germ cell tumors (e.g., testicular or ovarian cancers; Lewis et al., 2011). Physical exam findings may include those associated with volume overload and kidney failure, such as tachypnea and crackles on lung exam, tachycardia, and edema. In severe cases, other findings may include those associated with the electrolyte derangements of TLS, such as perioral numbness or tetany from hypocalcemia (Spring & Munshi, 2020).

DIFFERENTIAL DIAGNOSIS AND DIAGNOSTIC CONSIDERATIONS

The diagnosis of TLS is made primary by laboratory findings and the Cairo-Bishop classification system. The criteria start with a laboratory component: a 25% increase in uric acid, potassium, or phosphorus and/or a 25% decrease in calcium within 3 days before and 7 days after the start of a cancer treatment (Lewis et al., 2011). Once the lab criteria are met, the diagnosis of TLS is made if the creatinine is 1.5 times the upper limit of normal, or there is a cardiac arrhythmia or sudden death, or the patient has a seizure (Lewis et al., 2011).

The findings of elevated creatinine with hyperkalemia, hyperphosphatemia, and hypokalemia should lead the AGACNP to consider other possible etiologies of acute kidney injury in the patient with cancer; however, when these findings occur in a patient with a cancer with a high tumor burden and a recent history of completing a cancer therapy, the diagnosis of TLS should be strongly considered.

TREATMENT

Identification of at-risk patients permits clinicians to order interventions that can prevent TLS from developing. The oncology providers should ensure that the patient is adequately hydrated and minimize risk for renal injury (such as avoiding NSAIDs or CT contrast). For the patient who has developed TLS, close monitoring is indicated. Electrolytes should be followed with serial labs, with hyperkalemia and hyperphosphatemia treated as they would be with other patients with these derangements. Hyperuricemia should be treated with rasburicase at 0.15 to 0.2 mg/kg/day as allopurinol is only effective for prevention. A consult with the nephrology service is warranted and urgent hemodialysis is indicated when hyperkalemia becomes life-threatening and cannot be medically managed or there is worsening volume overload (Lewis et al., 2011).

The patient at low risk for TLS can receive preventive measures as an oncology outpatient with oral hydration and oral allopurinol. Allopurinol 100 mg/m² every 8 hours is ordered for low- to moderate-risk patients and rasburicase is ordered for higher-risk patients to decrease uric acid production prior to the cancer therapy (Lewis et al., 2011). The moderate- or higher-risk patient would need admission to the oncology unit if IV hydration is needed or rasburicase is indicated for prophylaxis. TLS can be managed on the oncology unit; however, if the patient requires closer monitoring, more frequent laboratory draws, or becomes more medically unstable, transfer to a progressive care or a critical care unit is warranted.

SUPERIOR VENA CAVA SYNDROME

SVC syndrome occurs when there is obstruction of blood flow through the SVC into the right atrium due to internal obstruction, as with a blood clot, an indwelling vascular device, tumor growth into the vein, or external compression with a tumor or an enlarged lymph node (Yeung & Manzullo, 2016). The obstruction in blood flow causes increased pressure in the venous system of the face, head, and neck, resulting in the signs and symptoms characteristic of this disorder. If the SVC occlusion occurs more slowly, collateral vessels develop as compensation to improve venous return; however, SVC occlusion may occur rapidly in patients with cancer, without time for collateral veins to develop, causing more rapid onset of symptoms and increasing the risk of dangerous sequelae, such as airway compromise or cerebral edema (Spring & Munshi, 2020).

PRESENTING SIGNS AND SYMPTOMS

The patient with SVC syndrome may present with facial swelling, cough, headaches, or visual changes (Spring & Munshi, 2020). The patient may experience syncope or pre-syncope due to the impact of poor venous return on cardiac output (Lewis et al., 2011). Dysphonia or shortness of breath are of great concern due to the possibility that there is airway compromise due to tumor or edema from venous impairment (Lewis et al., 2011).

HISTORY AND PHYSICAL FINDINGS

The most common malignancies that cause SVC syndrome are lung cancers, non-Hodgkin's lymphoma, mediastinal germ cell tumors, and solid tumors with metastasis to the mediastinum (Spring & Munshi, 2020), although it is possible that symptoms of SVC syndrome are what leads the patient to care and to a cancer diagnosis. On physical exam, the patient may have facial edema, upper extremity swelling, facial erythema and flushing (known as facial plethora), or distended chest and neck veins (Lewis et al., 2011). The patient may also demonstrate Pemberton's sign, the development of increased neck and facial erythema and edema with elevation of the arms over the head due to blockage of the venous return from the arms into the right atrium (Keshvani et al., 2018).

DIFFERENTIAL DIAGNOSIS AND DIAGNOSTIC CONSIDERATIONS

Differentials to consider depend on the patient's history and symptoms. For example, if the patient has shortness of breath, exacerbation of comorbidities such as COPD or heart failure should be considered, along with acute problems such as pneumonia or pulmonary embolism. If the patient has an implanted vascular device in the internal jugular or the SVC, a line-related thrombus should also be considered. Headaches or visual changes point toward a neurologic cause to consider, which, in a patient with cancer, should include consideration for brain metastases.

The diagnosis of SVC syndrome is made by imaging, so the AGACNP should order a CT scan of the neck and chest, the imaging modality of choice—this will identify

if there is SVC obstruction, the degree of obstruction, the presence of a thrombus, and the status of the underlying malignancy (Spring & Munshi, 2020). An MRI or venography could also be obtained (Spring & Munshi, 2020); however, the CT scan can likely be obtained in the most timely manner and would also provide information about disease progression in the chest.

TREATMENT

When the SVC obstruction is due to thrombus, treatment with anticoagulation or catheter-directed thrombolysis is preferred over systemic thrombolytics, particularly when it is unclear if the patient has brain metastases (Lewis et al., 2011). External compression on the SVC and the presence of stridor, hemodynamic impairment, or evidence of neurologic impairment calls for more urgent intervention. Endovascular stenting can promptly re-establish flow through the SVC, improving symptoms and venous return; however, the ability to tolerate lying supine for the procedure from comfort and neurologic perspectives may complicate the process (Spring & Munshi, 2020). More importantly, a secure airway is a priority and intubation may be difficult if there is edema or tumor impinging on the trachea, or if the patient cannot tolerate sedation due to hypotension (Spring & Munshi, 2020). Specialty consultation and admission to the critical care unit are warranted. When the patient presents with symptoms, is otherwise stable, and has a tissue diagnosis, endovascular stenting can be performed and chemotherapy or radiation may be possible to shrink the tumor and relieve the obstruction (Yeung & Manzillo, 2016).

MALIGNANT SPINAL CORD COMPRESSION

MSCC (also known as neoplastic epidural spinal cord compression) occurs when cancer cells spread to vertebrae, grow into the epidural space, and impinge on the spinal cord or cause the vertebrae to fracture and collapse, causing pressure on the spinal cord. The tumor injures neurologic structures and the compression obstructs blood flow in the spinal cord, causing ischemia and infarction (Gucalp & Dutcher, 2018). Approximately 10% of patients with cancer develop MSCC and patients with lung, breast, prostate, and renal cell cancers are most affected along with multiple myeloma (Gucalp & Dutcher, 2018). MSCC is truly an oncologic emergency as rapid identification and intervention can improve or preserve neurologic function.

PRESENTING SIGNS AND SYMPTOMS

The most common presenting symptom is back pain, which typically precedes loss of neurologic function. This pain is localized but may become radicular, and is made worse with coughing, sneezing, and lying flat (Spring & Munshi, 2020). Patients may also report sensory symptoms and later, motor symptoms, such as weakness, leg heaviness, or gait problems, with urinary retention/incontinence or constipation/fecal incontinence as late symptoms (Spring & Munshi, 2020). Motor function at the time of MSCC diagnosis determines prognosis, and the presence of bowel and bladder dysfunction portends a poorer prognosis (Spring & Munshi, 2020).

The AGACNP who suspects MSCC must perform a thorough neurologic examination, using light touch, sharp/dull, and vibration to detect sensory deficits. Check deep tendon reflexes, looking for hyperreflexia. Safely observe the patient's gait and test for extremity weakness. For complaints of bowel or bladder dysfunction, assess sphincter tone and post-void residual, respectively (Gucalp & Dutcher, 2018).

DIFFERENTIAL DIAGNOSIS AND DIAGNOSTIC CONSIDERATIONS

Evaluation of back pain starts with a very wide differential. Osteoarthritis, spinal stenosis, disc disease, and epidural abscesses are possibilities (Yeung & Manzullo, 2016). Osteoporosis may also result in pathologic fractures that cause pain. MSCC should be considered in any patient with cancer or a history of cancer who presents with back pain, although it is notable that 10% of patients with MSCC are diagnosed with their malignancies at the same time (Gucalp & Dutcher, 2018). Treatment is more likely to be successful if patients are diagnosed when they have preserved motor function, so delays in diagnosis must be avoided (Gucalp & Dutcher, 2018).

An evaluation of back pain may start with x-rays; however, plain films will not detect cord compression. The gold standard test is MRI because it can detect cord compression but it is also effective in ruling out other diagnoses in the back pain differential (Yeung & Manzullo, 2016). For patients in whom MRI is contraindicated, a CT myelogram is a reasonable alternative, although it is not as effective at ruling out other causes.

TREATMENT

Dexamethasone is urgently initiated to reduce cord edema, typically with a loading dose of 10 mg IV followed by 4 mg four times daily (Yeung & Manzullo, 2016). Surgical decompression and stabilization may be performed on patients who have severe compression, spinal instability, and reasonable hope for neurologic recovery, provided predicted survival is greater than 6 months as the recovery from this surgery is prolonged (Gucalp & Dutcher, 2018). Functional recovery may be better when this surgery is followed by radiation (Yeung & Manzullo, 2016). When patients are not surgical candidates, radiation or radiosurgery can reduce tumor size and relieve pain, while vertebroplasty or kyphoplasty may be used to stabilize a pathologic fracture and reduce pain but will not impact tumor size (Gucalp & Dutcher, 2018).

FEBRILE NEUTROPENIA

Neutrophils are the white blood cells that attack pathogens and are highly active as part of the immune response. Patients receiving chemotherapy, radiation, or have a cancer that impairs hematopoiesis are highly prone to neutropenic fever, generally defined as the state in which the absolute neutrophil count (ANC) is less than 1000/mL (with severe neutropenia equaling an ANC less than 500/mL) with an oral temperature of 38.3°C or 38.0°C for more than 1 hour (Taplitz et al., 2018).

PRESENTING SIGNS AND SYMPTOMS

Patients present with a broad range of symptoms; however, neutropenic fever is of particular concern because the fever may be the only presenting feature of an infection (Lewis et al., 2011). Without neutrophils, the patient with cancer has a limited immune response, so purulence, erythema, edema, or an infiltrate may not be evident. Furthermore, the presence of central lines and disruptions to mucosal membranes from treatment create easy portals of entry and exit for pathogens, making the patient with cancer and neutrophils particularly vulnerable to infections, sepsis, and critical illness (Lewis et al., 2011). For these reasons, neutropenic fever is considered an oncologic emergency.

DIFFERENTIAL DIAGNOSIS AND DIAGNOSTIC CONSIDERATIONS

The primary diagnosis in patients being treated for cancer with fever and ANC <1000/mL is neutropenic fever and treatment with empiric antibiotics is warranted (Taplitz et al., 2018). Other diagnostic possibilities for fever are secondary after antibiotics are started, including drug fever, atelectasis, or activity of the underlying disease, particularly with the acute leukemias.

A full culture workup is indicated. The AGACNP should order two sets of blood cultures, along with at least one set from each port of a central line if the patient has one. Urine for urinalysis and culture should be ordered. If the patient has respiratory symptoms, sputum culture and chest x-ray should also be obtained (Lewis et al., 2011). The AGACNP should also consider ordering viral polymerase chain reaction (PCR) for influenza, respiratory syncytial virus (RSV), and COVID-19 and fungal cultures or antigen screens if indicated by the patient's history.

TREATMENT

Management of neutropenic fever does not necessarily require inpatient admission. If the patient is otherwise stable and can be examined and cultured in the clinic or emergency department, then oral antibiotics and ongoing observation at home are acceptable. This includes patients who are younger, hemodynamically stable, are adequately hydrated and can take oral fluids, with no or mild symptoms and no or few comorbidities (Taplitz et al., 2018). However, if the fever does not resolve after 48 hours or the patient develops other symptoms, then the patient should be instructed to return to the hospital for further management. For patients who are not low risk, evaluation and management in an inpatient setting is recommended (Taplitz et al., 2018).

After cultures are collected, the AGACNP promptly orders anti-infectives with an eye toward the most likely sources of infection. In most cases, a regimen should include broad spectrum antibiotics to cover gram-negative and gram-positive bacteria, including resistant and hospital-associated organisms such as *Pseudomonas*, and with consideration for the patient's past infection history and the local antibiogram. The AGACNP should continue the therapy until the neutropenia has resolved or the patient has been afebrile for 72 to 96 hours while monitoring the patient's condition and the cultures, keeping in mind that approximately 70% of patients with neutropenic fever do not have positive cultures (Halfdanarson et al., 2017).

TRANSITION OF CARE FOR ONCOLOGIC EMERGENCIES

An oncologic emergency is often an unexpected event for the patient. For some patients, an oncologic emergency marks the entry into care with a new cancer diagnosis. For these reasons, the AGACNP must ensure there is clear communication across oncology settings and with the patient's primary providers to ensure safe transitions across these settings. Collaboration with cancer care navigators can be instrumental in transitioning the patient from an acute situation back to primary and ambulatory specialty care. For some patients, such as those with SVC syndrome or MSCC, the oncologic emergency

comes with a poor prognosis. Therefore, in addition to urgent medical treatment, the AGACNP should discuss with patients their goals of care and options for palliative care when delivering this acute cancer care.

CLINICAL PEARLS

- Oncologic emergencies are consequences of cancer or cancer treatments that may present in any setting where AGACNPs practice. These problems should be part of the differential diagnosis when treating a patient with cancer.
- A malignancy should be considered when the patient presents with one of these syndromes, including venous thromboembolism, spinal cord compression, hypercalcemia, and SVC syndrome.
- Tumor lysis syndrome, venous thromboembolism, and hypercalcemia of malignancy can be prevented when at-risk patients are identified and prophylactically treated.

A robust set of instructor resources designed to supplement this text is located at http://connect.springerpub.com /content/reference-book/978-0-8261-6079-9. Qualifying instructors may request access by emailing **textbook@springerpub.com**.

REFERENCES

Full list of references can be accessed at http://connect .springerpub.com/content/reference-book/978-0-8261-6079-9

CHAPTER 10

GASTROINTESTINAL DISORDERS

LEARNING OBJECTIVES

- Identify various acute and chronic gastrointestinal disorders affecting adults and older adults.
- Understand the basic pathogenesis of various acute and chronic gastrointestinal disorders affecting adults and older adults.
- Understand the risk factors associated with development of various acute and chronic gastrointestinal disorders affecting adults and older adults.
- Apply optimal treatment for various acute and chronic gastrointestinal disorders affecting adults and older adults.
- Understand the basic pathogenesis and surgical treatment options for various acute and chronic abdominal and anorectal disorders.

INTRODUCTION

Gastrointestinal disorders comprise a multitude of acute and chronic patient conditions, representing complex presentations with an array of potential differential considerations. This chapter covers the most common gastrointestinal diagnoses, including presenting signs and symptoms, history and physical findings, diagnostic criteria, and current evidence-based treatments.

10.1: GASTROESOPHAGEAL REFLUX DISEASE

Cathy Stepter

Gastroesophageal reflux disease (GERD) is a common disease affecting approximately 10% to 20% of adults in Western countries and nearly 5% of adults in Asian countries at least weekly (Young et al., 2020). Prevalence continues to increase and is parallel with increasing obesity rates. GERD involves gastric content reflux into the esophagus, oral cavity or lung and its associated symptoms and complications (Katz et al., 2013). Contributing factors for the development of GERD include hiatal hernia, lower esophageal sphincter relaxation and pressure, obesity, delayed gastric emptying (Young et al., 2020). Gastroesophageal disease may be further classified as erosive or nonerosive.

PRESENTING SIGNS AND SYMPTOMS

Acid reflux symptom presentation typically includes heartburn and regurgitation. Symptom reports may include retrosternal burning, acidic taste in mouth, eructation, hiccups, and dysphagia. Symptoms can worsen in the recumbent position and especially after meals. Accompanying alarm symptoms (Box 10.1) warrant early endoscopy to rule out a GERD complication (Young et al., 2020). Associated problems resulting from GERD may include erosion of dental enamel, sinusitis, chronic laryngitis, pharyngitis, asthma, chronic cough, and idiopathic pulmonary fibrosis (Katz et al., 2013; Young et al., 2020).

GERD is a common problem during pregnancy and can occur at any trimester (Katz et al., 2013). Symptom severity may increase throughout pregnancy, and is associated with increasing gestational age, pre-existing heartburn before pregnancy, and parity (Katz et al., 2013).

HISTORY AND PHYSICAL FINDINGS

Medical History

The most common symptom of GERD is heartburn. Heartburn commonly occurs 30 to 60 minutes after meals or in the recumbent position and is often relieved with antacids. However, some patients do not experience heartburn, but report regurgitation of gastric contents into the mouth. Dysphagia may be the presenting complaint, which may reflect esophageal involvement. An accurate clinical history is valued and a pragmatic approach to diagnosing and treating GERD (Gyawali et al., 2018).

BOX 10.1 GASTROESOPHAGEAL REFLUX DISEASE ALARM SYMPTOMS

The following symptoms warrant early endoscopy to rule out a GERD complication:
- Anemia
- Bleeding
- Dysphagia
- Early satiety
- Odynophagia
- Vomiting
- Weight loss

BOX 10.2 DIFFERENTIAL DIAGNOSES FOR GASTROESOPHAGEAL REFLUX DISEASE

- Angina pectoris
- Barrett's esophagus
- Cytomegalovirus, herpes, or *Candida* infection
- Dyspepsia
- Eosinophilic esophagitis
- Esophageal motility disorder
- Esophageal stricture
- Erosive esophagitis
- Myocardial infarction
- Peptic ulcer disease

Physical Examination

Physical exam findings and laboratory data are generally noncontributory.

DIFFERENTIAL DIAGNOSIS AND DIAGNOSTIC CONSIDERATIONS

It is essential to distinguish presenting symptoms of pain between cardiac and noncardiac origin. First rule out a cardiac condition, such as myocardial infarction, before considering GERD. The differential diagnoses for GERD are summarized in Box 10.2.

DIAGNOSTIC CONSIDERATIONS

The majority of patients with mild, intermittent symptoms will not require diagnostic testing. Lifestyle modifications and pharmacotherapeutics involving histamine-2 receptor antagonists (H2RAs) and antacids may successfully alleviate symptoms. Patients experiencing moderate symptoms should be treated with a proton pump inhibitor (PPI) daily for a period of 8 to 12 weeks. Diagnostic indications may include upper endoscopy and esophageal pH monitoring. Barium swallow testing is indicated for complaints of dysphagia but is not recommended to diagnose GERD.

Upper Endoscopy

Patients presenting with alarming symptoms or who do not respond appropriately to PPI therapy require upper endoscopy evaluation (Young et al., 2020). Patients can have objective evidence of GERD, such as erosive esophagitis or Barrett's esophagus, without having any reflux symptoms. Biopsies of the esophagus help rule out eosinophilic esophagitis; however, routine biopsy of the esophagus to diagnose GERD is not recommended (Katz et al., 2013). Severity of disease in the elderly is worse than in younger patients, although symptom presentation is generally less. For this reason, an early decision for endoscopic evaluation should occur in the elderly (Young et al., 2020). There is controversial evidence for screening patients who use long-term PPI therapy for *Helicobacter pylori* infection. The Los Angeles (LA) classification system describes the endoscopic appearance of erosive esophagitis from A (mild) to D (severe). Patients with LA Grade A or B may need further diagnostic testing to confirm the presence of GERD; an LA grade C or D esophagitis is conclusive evidence for GERD (Gyawali et al., 2018; Katz et al., 2013).

Esophageal pH Manometry

Esophageal pH manometry is not useful for primary diagnosis of GERD. However, pH manometry testing should be used preoperatively for patients who have persistent symptoms despite normal endoscopic findings to rule out achalasia or severe hypomotility for patients who require any reflux surgery (Katz et al., 2013; Young et al., 2020). Manometry testing is performed in an ambulatory setting either with a telemetry capsule or via a transnasal catheter, and may be done either concurrent with PPI therapy, or without (Gyawali et al., 2018).

Barium Swallow

A barium swallow test is not performed to diagnose GERD. It may be used for evaluation of dysphagia or for esophageal complications, such as stricture or ring.

TREATMENT

Lifestyle Modifications

The first treatment option for most patients is lifestyle modifications including weight loss and sleep position. Studies show that weight loss and waist reduction can significantly lessen or completely resolve symptoms (Katz et al., 2013; Park et al., 2017; Young et al., 2020). Additionally, studies have found that sleeping with the head of the bed elevated using foam blocks or wedges, in the left lateral position, and avoiding meals 2 to 3 hours before bedtime reduces nocturnal reflux symptoms (Allampati et al., 2017; Young et al., 2020). Despite lifestyle modifications including elimination of specific foods, caffeine, alcohol, chocolate, or smoking; no study has found definitive evidence of symptom improvements with these approaches (Young et al., 2020).

H2 Receptor Antagonists and Antacids

Mild, infrequent symptoms may be managed effectively with H2RA, such as famotidine, ranitidine, or cimetidine. H2RAs are effective if there is no erosive disease and the patient experiences relief of symptoms. H2RAs decrease gastric acid by reversibly binding to the histamine-2 receptors on gastric parietal cells. It is important to monitor for tachyphylaxis, or diminished response to successive doses, after several weeks of usage. Antacids, such as Maalox or calcium carbonate, neutralize acid and may provide infrequent symptomatic relief.

Proton Pump Inhibitors

First line treatment for GERD is the use of PPIs. PPIs have been found to be superior to H2RAs and prokinetic therapy for heartburn relief (Gyawali et al., 2018; Katz et al., 2013). PPI therapy, such as omeprazole, lansoprazole, and pantoprazole can be used empirically to confirm diagnosis in patients with typical symptoms. PPIs are irreversible inhibitors, suppressing gastric acid secretion by inactivating the hydrogen potassium ATPase molecules of the parietal cell. PPIs should be taken once daily either prior to meals for daytime symptoms, or in the evening for nighttime symptoms for a period of 8 to 12 weeks, and are safe in pregnancy (Katz et al., 2013; Young et al., 2020). A change in medication or a twice-daily trial may be considered for aggressive acid suppression. There have been no major differences in efficacy identified between the different PPIs, which include both over-the-counter and prescription options. Additionally, there are no data to support switching drug therapies more than once for partial or incomplete therapy response. Long-term maintenance therapy in the lowest effective dose is necessary for patients who have continued symptoms after PPI discontinuation, hiatal hernia, erosive esophagitis, Barrett's esophagus complications, or lack of compliance.

Common mild side effects associated with PPIs include headache and dyspepsia (Katz et al., 2013). Long-term adverse effects may include chronic kidney disease, dementia, bone fracture and *Clostridium difficile* infection (Young et al., 2020). Long-term therapy requires a close evaluation of risk, which may include acute gastroenteritis (Hayes et al., 2019).

Surgical Treatment

Surgery options are generally not recommended for patients who do not respond to PPI therapy. Reasons for surgical consideration include desire to discontinue medical therapy, noncompliance, side effects associated with medical therapy, the presence of a large hiatal hernia, esophagitis refractory to medical therapy, or persistent symptoms from refractory GERD. Preoperative ambulatory pH monitoring is needed in patients who show no evidence of erosive esophagitis to rule out achalasia or scleroderma-like esophagus prior to undergoing surgery. Laparoscopic Nissen fundoplication is a surgical intervention used to reduce hiatal hernia and restore the lower esophageal sphincter barrier. Roux-en-Y gastric bypass is preferred for obese patients with GERD.

CLINICAL PEARLS

- A GERD diagnosis is primarily symptom-based by heartburn and acid regurgitation.
- Weight loss can help reduce and eliminate GERD symptoms.
- PPIs are the first line for initial treatment and considered the therapy of choice for erosive esophagitis.
- PPIs should be taken 30 to 60 minutes prior to a meal for optimal pH control.

- Patients who present with alarm symptoms (Box 10.1) or who do not respond to PPI therapy should promptly undergo upper endoscopy.
- Endoscopy and surgical options are considered only if medical therapy fails.

10.2: GASTROINTESTINAL BLEED

Adrienne Markiewicz and Alyssa Profita

Gastrointestinal bleeding (GIB) is a common presentation in hospital emergency departments, inpatient wards, and critical care units. The total incidence of GIB is estimated to be 40 to 150 per 100,000 persons annually and is estimated to cost $2.5 billion. GIB has been classically described by anatomical location of the bleeding diathesis. Upper gastrointestinal bleeds (UGIB) occur proximal to the ligament of Treitz and can involve tissue in the oropharynx, esophagus, stomach, and upper duodenum. Two percent to 11% of UGIB are caused by variceal bleeding (Navuluri et al., 2012). Figure 10.1 displays anatomical landmarks associated with GIB. Despite significant morbidity, total incidence of UGIB has dropped 20% over the last 20 years due to eradication of *Helicobacter pylori*, use of PPIs, and advances in endoscopic therapy. By contrast, lower GIB occurs distal to the ligament of Treitz, encompassing the colon and anorectum (Tielleman et al., 2015). Lower gastrointestinal bleeding (LGIB) hospital incidence is 20.5 in 100,000 persons annually (Navuluri et al., 2012). Early identification, accurate assessment of clinical stability, appropriate resuscitation efforts, and early endoscopic intervention has decreased hospital mortality from GIB of all sources from 3.5% to 10% down to 2.1% (Cai & Saltzman, 2018).

PRESENTING SIGNS AND SYMPTOMS

Symptomology is largely driven by blood loss in the patient with acute GIB and can vary in conjunction with the degree and location of hemorrhage. Melena and hematemesis are most often associated with overt UGIB, while LGIB more commonly presents as hematochezia (Cappell & Friedel, 2008). Patients with a brisk UGIB may present with bright red blood per rectum and orthostasis (Samuel et al., 2018). As acute blood loss continues, loss of effective circulating volume may lead patients to present with dizziness, syncope, and weakness. Loss of hemoglobin oxygen-carrying capacity reduces cerebral perfusion and patients may present with altered mentation.

HISTORY AND PHYSICAL FINDINGS

Medical History

The most common cause of nonvariceal GIBs is peptic ulcer disease (PUD). The second and third most common causes are gastritis and esophagitis (Samuel et al., 2018). The use of nonsteroidal anti-inflammatory drugs (NSAIDs) further increase risk of PUD. Etiologies of GIB

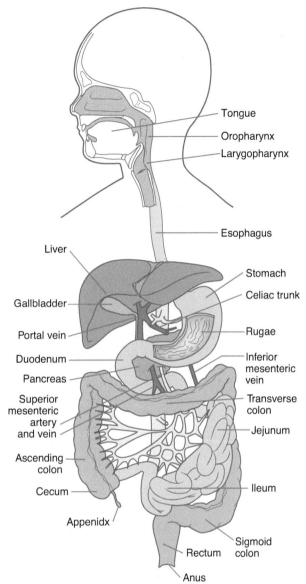

FIGURE 10.1: Anatomical landmarks associated with gastrointestinal bleeding.
Source: Reproduced from Chiocca, E. M. (2019). *Advanced pediatric assessment* (3rd ed.). Springer Publishing Company, Fig. 19.2

TABLE 10.1: Etiologies of Gastrointestinal Bleeding

UPPER GASTROINTESTINAL BLEEDING (NONVARICEAL)	LOWER GASTROINTESTINAL BLEEDING
• Aortoenteric fistula • Cameron lesions • Dieulafoy's lesion • Foreign body ingestion • Gastric antral vascular ectasia (GAVE) • Gastritis • Hematobilia • Ulcer disease • Malignant neoplasm • Mallory-Weiss tear • Portal hypertensive gastropathy • Small bowel arteriovenous malformation	• Angioectasia • Colitis, ischemic or infectious • Colon polyps • Dieulafoy's lesion • Diverticulitis • Hemorrhoids • Malignant neoplasm • Postpolypectomy bleeding

Acute hemorrhage reduces effective circulating volume causing vasoconstriction, end organ hypoperfusion, and eventually hemorrhagic shock as oxygen delivery becomes insufficient to support aerobic metabolism (Cannon, 2018). Evaluation of clinical stability in patients with suspected or confirmed active bleeding cannot rely on measurement of blood pressure alone. As much as 30% of the total circulating blood volume can be lost prior to the onset of hypotension due to the body's significant vasoconstrictive compensatory mechanisms (Cannon, 2018). Instead, assessment of clinical stability hinges on evaluation of vital signs in the context of other subtle clinical findings signaling reduced organ perfusion such as altered mental status, paleness, tachypnea, cool skin temperature, poor capillary refill, and oliguria. Tachycardia in patients not blunted by medications is often the first indicator of developing hemorrhagic shock (Cannon, 2018). The practitioner should attempt to quantify the volume of blood loss, although this is not always possible. Table 10.2 highlights exam findings signaling progressive hemorrhagic shock in the setting of ongoing blood loss.

DIAGNOSTIC CONSIDERATIONS

Localization of acute bleeding is critical. Several modalities are available to both localize and quantify intraluminal bleeding. GI lavage via nasogastric tube can be used to quickly determine potential location and severity of bleeding. Aspiration of bile does not rule out an UGIB—in 18% of the cases of UGIB the aspiration is bile. Gastrointestinal lavage can also be used to improve visualization for endoscopy by clearing contents out of the stomach prior to intervention (Laine & Jensen, 2012).

Endoscopy is both a diagnostic and therapeutic intervention in patients with a GIB. In cases of suspected

are further described in Table 10.1. Comorbid conditions may both increase risk for GIB and alter the compensatory mechanisms of the body to blood loss, predisposing the patient to incur end organ damage more rapidly. Patients with existing coronary artery disease are particularly vulnerable as loss of ventricular preload from bleeding reduces coronary artery perfusion during diastole.

Physical Exam Findings

The bleeding patient presents with physical findings that vary widely in conjunction with the degree of blood loss.

TABLE 10.2: Advanced Trauma Life Support Classification for Hemorrhagic Shock

PARAMETER	CLASS I	CLASS II (MILD)	CLASS III (MODERATE)	CLASS IV (SEVERE)
Approximate blood loss	<15%	15%–30%	31%–40%	>40%
Heart rate	↔	↔/↑	↑	↑/↑↑
Blood pressure	↔	↔	↔/↓	↓
Pulse pressure	↔	↓	↓	↓
Respiratory rate	↔	↔	↔/↑	↑
Urine output	↔	↔	↓	↓↓
Glasgow coma score (GCS)	GCS score ↔	GCS score ↔	GCS score ↓	GCS score ↓↓
Base deficit	0 to −2 mEq/L	−2 to −6 mEq/L	−6 to −10 mEq/L	−10 mEq/L or more
Need for blood products	Monitor	Possible	Yes	Massive transfusion

Source: Data from the American College of Surgeons. (2018). *Advanced trauma life support* (10th ed.). American College of Surgeons, Committee on Trauma.

small bowel bleeding or an obscure source suspected to be originating in the small bowel, push enteroscopy can be a useful diagnostic tool (Hayat et al., 2000). Capsule endoscopy is utilized when the source of an UGIB is unable to be identified by traditional endoscopy and it is not a life-threatening bleed such that embolization or surgical intervention is required. Prior to swallowing the capsule, the patient must undergo bowel prep to clean out the small intestine and the colon. Once the prep is completed, the patient will swallow the capsule and wear a belt with sensors that capture the images.

Alternatively, CT with angiography is used when a GIB is unable to be visualized on endoscopy or attempts have been made to achieve hemostasis with endoscopy and have been unsuccessful. Once the vessel responsible for the GIB has been localized, decisions can be made regarding appropriate intervention (Laine & Jensen, 2012).

TREATMENT

Initial Management

Intravenous Access

The bleeding patient should have large bore peripheral IV access in two locations. Large bore access provides the ability to quickly transfuse blood products in severe bleeding and ensures the blood products being administered will not be damaged. If peripheral IVs cannot be established and bleeding is severe, a central line with capability for massive transfusion should be placed.

Fluid Resuscitation

If blood products are not immediately available, resuscitation should begin with bolus infusion of balanced IV solutions, such as Ringer's lactate. Chloride-rich solutions, such as normal saline, should be avoided in critically ill patients with bleeding as chloride further reduces renal blood flow and accelerates acute kidney injury (Bellomo et al., 2012; Semler et al., 2018). Crystalloid fluid resuscitation should not replace resuscitation with blood products. Packed red blood cells (PRBCs) should be transfused to maintain serum concentrations of hemoglobin >7 g/dL in most patients (Villanueva et al., 2013). Patients with coronary artery disease may benefit from higher transfusion thresholds, though data are mixed (Barkun et al., 2019). In patients with massive bleeding, resuscitation with blood products should be also targeted to improvement in clinical symptoms of hemorrhagic shock rather than lab values alone as the degree of blood loss will quickly invalidate these numbers. Patients anticipated to require more than 4 units PRBCs in a 1-hour period should have clotting factors and platelets repleted using a 1:1:1 transfusion strategy where possible, as this reduces patient mortality (Cotton et al., 2009).

Reversal of Anticoagulation

Inappropriate bleeding is the number one complication of chronic anticoagulation therapy. Reversal of these agents depends on the type of agent used, etiology requiring anticoagulation, severity of bleeding, and extent of coagulopathy. This section discusses warfarin-induced coagulopathy. In patients with a significant GIB on warfarin, fresh frozen plasma (FFP) should be utilized to quickly reverse anticoagulation via repletion of clotting factors, though the clinician should note that reversal is partial and will not be sustained. Check pre- and posttransfusion international normalized ratio (INR) to evaluate coagulation status. Vitamin K can also be given either orally or intravenously to reverse anticoagulation due to warfarin and provides a more sustained response. Vitamin K should not be used alone if bleeding is significant as the onset of action is much slower than FFP. Prothrombin complex concentrate (PCC) should be utilized for complete reversal in patients suffering a massive GIB with warfarin-induced coagulopathy (Yee & Caide, 2019). In recent years, the advent of direct oral anticoagulants (DOAC) and novel oral anticoagulants (NOAC) has posed unique challenges to bleeding management. Currently, idarucizumab is approved for dabigatran reversal and andexanet alpha for apixaban and rivaroxaban reversal in life-threatening hemorrhage. PCC has also been used off-label for DOAC-related bleeding. These agents can be cost prohibitive to healthcare organizations and therefore a case-specific, multidisciplinary approach should be utilized to manage bleeding in these patients (Rawal et al., 2019).

Proton Pump Inhibitors

Initial management of undifferentiated UGIB should assume the possibility of PUD and include PPI therapy. PPIs irreversibly block gastric acid secretion, raising the pH of the stomach and allowing clot formation and stabilization. Therapy is usually comprised of an 80 mg bolus followed by a continuous infusion of 8 mg/h. Duration of therapy will be dependent on endoscopy findings; however, for patients found to have gastric or small bowel ulcers with high-risk stigmata, continuous IV therapy is recommended for 72 hours. More recent studies have suggested that intermittent, high-dose PPI therapy is noninferior to continuous infusion and may be more feasible in patients with difficult vascular access (Cai & Saltzman, 2018).

Elective Airway Management

Patients presenting with brisk UGIB experiencing significant vomiting are at elevated risk for aspiration of bloody contents into the airways and subsequent respiratory arrest. Elective intubation to secure the patient's airway while awaiting definitive treatment via endoscopy or other means should be considered in these cases; however, there is no clear guideline dictating management of these patients (Perisetti et al., 2019). Outcomes, including mortality, for patients requiring prophylactic endotracheal intubation prior to endoscopy are generally much poorer than those not requiring airway management, though the data are mixed (Alshamsi et al., 2017). The AGACNP should carefully weigh the potential benefit of elective intubation with the risks of induction. Sedation for intubation and mechanical ventilation reduces systemic vascular resistance and may lead to peri-intubation arrest in the absence of adequate effective circulating volume. Patients may experience vomiting and aspiration during intubation particularly with the use of neuromuscular blockade. Furthermore, pharmacologic interventions should be chosen carefully as some agents may cause myocardial suppression, worsening end organ dysfunction and shock.

Interventions

Endoscopy

Timing of endoscopy is classified as low versus high risk and depends on the acuity of the patient. The Rockall or Blatchford bleeding score should be utilized to risk stratify patients who present with an UGIB into a high or low risk category and help determine timing of endoscopy (Laine & Jensen, 2012). Endoscopy may utilize epinephrine injections, thermal therapy, and clip placement to achieve hemostasis. Clips may be used for both hemostasis and localization of the bleed if the patient is at elevated risk for rebleeding. A repeat endoscopy within 24 hours of hemostasis is not recommended. If the patient suffers rebleeding, repeat endoscopy could be warranted.

Patients may require intervention by embolization or surgical intervention for bleeding refractory to endoscopy. Embolization is a minimally invasive procedure where an interventional radiologist cannulates the celiac artery and uses contrast to visualize the vasculature and selectively embolize the bleeding vessel(s). Correction of coagulopathy, consultation with the gastroenterology team, and CT angiography as needed for localization should be completed prior to embolization. Surgical intervention for GIBs is less common given advances in endoscopic and angiographic interventions. Patients who have a GIB where hemostasis is not achieved via endoscopic intervention or embolization, or have a bleed in a location where either of those interventions is not amenable, may require surgical intervention. When surgical intervention is required, laparoscopic interventions are attempted to control bleeding or remove the source of bleeding.

TRANSITION OF CARE

Findings on endoscopy will determine patient disposition. Certain high-risk stigmata such as active hemorrhage, visible clot, or nonbleeding visible vessel requires close monitoring in an intensive care unit setting, as well as at least 3 days of hospitalization. In patients with concern for rebleeding, starting a clear liquid diet is acceptable as endoscopy can be done within 2 hours of their last oral intake. These patients should stay on a clear liquid diet for 48 hours to ensure there is no rebleeding post endoscopy and/or intervention. Patients with a clean ulcer base, flat pigmented spot, or Mallory-Weiss tear are considered low risk and can be started on an oral diet. If the low-risk patients have a stable hemoglobin as well as hemodynamic stability, discharge can be considered (Laine & Jenson, 2012).

CLINICAL PEARLS

- Gastrointestinal bleeding is described as upper or lower, depending on location of the bleeding either proximal or distal to the ligament of Treitz.
- Bright red blood per rectum with hemodynamic instability or features of shock should always be presumed as a brisk upper source of bleeding.
- Most gastrointestinal bleeding requires endoscopic evaluation within 24 to 48 hours.
- Significant blood loss can occur in the absence of overt hypotension.

10.3: HEPATORENAL SYNDROME

Liza Rieke

Hepatorenal syndrome is a rare, but life-threatening condition that has an extremely poor prognosis. It is caused by a critical decompensation of acute or chronic liver disease associated with acute kidney injury. Advanced liver disease such as severe alcoholic hepatitis, cirrhosis, or cancer is often the inciting cause of this syndrome. The resultant portal hypertension causes arterial vasodilation in the splanchnic circulation, thus creating a reduction in renal perfusion that can no longer be compensated by increased cardiac output, and results in an acute kidney injury that leads to hepatorenal syndrome (Best et al., 2019; Wadei et al., 2006).

PRESENTING SIGNS AND SYMPTOMS

Presenting signs and symptoms are characterized for those who have evidence of acute or chronic liver disease with advanced hepatic failure and portal hypertension. Laboratory data reflect a progressive increase in serum creatinine of 0.3 mg/dL or more within 48 hours or an increase from baseline by 50% or more within 7 days. Patients may present with oliguria or anuria, no or minimal proteinuria (<500 mg/day), as well as a low rate of sodium excretion (urine sodium concentration<10 mEq/L). Additionally, ascites that are resistant to diuretics are not uncommon, as well as hypotension that is unresponsive to fluids. Hepatorenal syndrome should be considered in the absence of other apparent causes for acute kidney injury, including shock, nephrotoxic medications, no evidence of obstructive kidney disease, and appropriate treatment of bacterial infections (Best et al., 2019; Wadei et al., 2006).

DIFFERENTIAL DIAGNOSIS AND DIAGNOSTIC CONSIDERATIONS

It is important to remember that hepatorenal syndrome is a diagnosis of exclusion and based solely on clinical findings. All other causes of acute kidney injury need to be excluded, including shock, hypovolemia, nephrotoxic medications, obstruction, or parenchymal kidney disease including prerenal azotemia (acute kidney injury acute kidney injury responds to volume resuscitation), glomerulonephritis, acute tubular necrosis (presence of granular casts in urine sediment and urine osmolality equal to plasma osmolality), postrenal urinary obstruction (evaluated by renal ultrasound), and bacterial peritonitis.

TREATMENT

Critically ill patients should be treated in an intensive care unit. Short-term, temporary treatment with dialysis or continuous veno-venous hemofiltration are for candidates with a reasonable chance for improved liver function or are a candidate for liver transplant and are hemodynamically stable enough to tolerate the intervention. In patients with hepatorenal syndrome, 30% to 50% of those that required renal replacement therapy survived to liver transplantation (Allegretti et al., 2018).

Medical therapy is used to treat the AKI-increase mean arterial pressure by 10 to 15 mmHg to a mean arterial pressure (MAP) greater than 82 mmHg using norepinephrine or vasopressin and IV albumin 1 g/kg/day × minimum of 2 days. In noncritically ill patients, a combination treatment with terlipressin (not available in the United States), midodrine, octreotide, and albumin can be used to increase MAP. As the perfusion pressure increases, the serum creatinine should decrease (Velez & Nieter, 2011). If there has been no improvement in renal function after 2 weeks, it is considered medical failure. If there is improvement, patients often need to remain on midodrine long term (Singh et al., 2012).

Long-term treatment involves treating the underlying cause such as alcohol cessation or completing antiviral therapy for hepatitis or transplant. Resolution of hepatorenal syndrome is defined as serum creatinine less than 1.5 mg/dL and no dialysis requirement. One study found a 76% rate of recovery from hepatorenal syndrome in 62 patients who underwent a liver transplant (Wong et al., 2015).

TRANSITION OF CARE

Patients with hepatorenal syndrome are optimally treated in an intensive care unit where IV norepinephrine, IV albumin, and other supportive treatments can be given in a timely manner under close observation and monitored for effectiveness. If a patient is failing medical management and is not a candidate for liver transplantation, palliative care and hospice should be consulted. Without therapy, most patients with hepatorenal syndrome die within weeks of onset of renal impairment. If a patient does recover from hepatorenal syndrome, they should be followed by hepatology and nephrology for optimal medical management.

CLINICAL PEARLS

- Patients with cirrhosis, ascites, and serum creatinine >1.5 mg/dL that does not improve with volume resuscitation should be evaluated for hepatorenal syndrome.
- Hepatorenal syndrome is a diagnosis of exclusion; there is no specific test for it.
- Medical therapy should be initiated immediately for optimal results.

KEY TAKEAWAYS

The key treatment for hepatorenal syndrome is optimizing blood pressure with vasopressors, albumin, and other supportive measures while treating the underlying cause of liver dysfunction.

10.4: ACUTE HEPATITIS

Liza Rieke

Acute hepatitis involves a recent onset of inflammation of the liver. Acute hepatitis has several subcategories of viruses including acute viral hepatitis A, B, C, D, and E as well as alcoholic hepatitis and autoimmune hepatitis. Each subcategory is unique and some can overlap. The most commonly encountered by healthcare providers are hepatitis B, hepatitis C, and alcoholic hepatitis, which require acute supportive care because they can lead to chronic conditions. Table 10.3 provides a summary of acute hepatitis (Centers for Disease Control and Prevention [CDC], 2020a, 2020b).

10.4A: HEPATITIS A

Hepatitis A is spread among humans via the fecal–oral route and contaminated food. Hepatitis A is often encountered in developing countries with poor water quality. Hepatitis A can be sexually transmitted but has not been found to be transmitted in breast milk (Rac & Sheffield, 2014). Individuals infected with hepatitis A are contagious as soon as they are infected during the incubation period and remain contagious for 1 to 2 weeks after presenting with symptoms (Richardson et al., 2001).

PRESENTING SIGNS AND SYMPTOMS

In general, signs and symptoms occur more in adults and rarely in children. Early symptoms include nausea, vomiting, anorexia, fever, malaise, and abdominal pain.

Late symptoms include dark urine, gray stools, and jaundice. Rarely does hepatitis A cause liver failure. It is possible to have a hepatitis A supra-infection in the setting of an underlying chronic hepatitis. In those situations, the outcomes are less optimal (Eui-Cheol & Sook-Hyang, 2018).

DIAGNOSTIC TESTS

Hepatitis A is diagnosed with serum laboratory levels for hepatitis A immunoglobin M (IgM). One may also see elevations of serum aminotransferases >1,000 IU/dL and elevated serum bilirubin up to 10 mg/dL.

TREATMENT

Most of the time hepatitis A is self-limiting within a couple of weeks without medical intervention; however, some individuals have lasting symptoms for up to a year. Infected individuals should not share a restroom and should practice excellent hand hygiene. Medications and supplements that can contribute to liver injury and alcohol should be avoided during recovery. Once infected, one has life-long immunity.

There is a vaccination available. In the United States, children are given two doses, the first at age 12 to 23 months and the second 6 months after the first dose (CDC, 2020b). High-risk adults who were not vaccinated as children should also obtain the vaccine.

CLINICAL PEARLS

- Patients with acute onset of gastrointestinal symptoms that have not had a hepatitis A vaccination should be checked for hepatitis A immunoglobin M.

TABLE 10.3: Summary of Acute Hepatitis

TYPE OF HEPATITIS	SPREAD	TEST	TREATMENT	VACCINE	CHRONIC
Hepatitis A	Fecal/contaminated food and water	IgM antibodies	Supportive care	Yes	Rarely
Hepatitis B	Infected blood and body fluids	HBsAg; anti-HBc	Acute-supportive care Chronic-antivirals	Yes	Rare in adults (5%) Often in children (95%)
Hepatitis C	Infected blood and body fluids	Hep C antibody; HepC RNA	Antivirals	No	Common (75%–85%), but can be cured
Hepatitis D	Infected blood and body fluids	HDAg; HDV RNA	Interferons	No	Common if also have chronic Hep B
Hepatitis E	Fecal/contaminated food and water	Anti-HEV IgM assay; HEV RNA	Supportive care	No	Sometimes
Alcoholic	Self-contained	None	ETOH cessation and liver transplant	No	Common
Autoimmune	Self-contained	None	Glucocorticoids	No	Common

- Patients with suspected or confirmed hepatitis A should understand they are highly contagious and instructed on how to prevent further contamination.
- Hepatitis A is usually self-limiting and requires supportive care at home.

KEY TAKEAWAYS

Hepatitis A is known worldwide, transmitted via the fecal–oral route, is highly contagious, but usually self-limiting. There is a vaccine available.

10.4B: HEPATITIS B

Acute hepatitis B virus is by definition an infection lasting less than 6 months. Hepatitis B can become a chronic infection, especially in those who contract the virus as an infant or child. Around 90% of infants and 25% to 50% of children age 1 to 5 years will remain chronically infected with hepatitis B (Fattovich et al., 2008). Most adults recover and are not chronically infected. Hepatitis B is spread through contact with blood, semen, or other body fluids of an infected person; sexual contact; sharing needles or syringes; and from mother to baby at birth. There is a vaccine for hepatitis B.

PRESENTING SIGNS AND SYMPTOMS

Some newly infected patients with the hepatitis B virus will remain asymptomatic. Others may present with fatigue, poor appetite, abdominal pain, nausea, and jaundice. Rarely, a patient will present with fulminant hepatitis, in which signs and symptoms of liver failure are present.

DIAGNOSTIC TESTS

Hepatitis B is diagnosed with a serum laboratory test for hepatitis B surface antigen (HBsAg) and IgM antibodies to hepatitis B core antigen (anti-HBc). All pregnant women, immunosuppressed individuals, substantial risk individuals, and donors of blood, plasma, organs, and tissues should be screened for hepatitis B.

TREATMENT

The best treatment for acute hepatitis B is prevention with the hepatitis B vaccine and practicing safe sex. For those who do contract the virus treatment is usually supportive. The majority of the time the virus is self-limiting with symptoms lasting from a few weeks for up to 6 months. If a patient presents with a severe case with persistent symptoms, develops a coagulopathy in which the INR is greater than 1.5, or has continued jaundice with a bilirubin greater than 3 mg/dL for more than 4 weeks, it is recommended to treat with antiretroviral medication, tenofovir or entecavir (Terrault et al., 2018). Treatment should be stopped after confirming the patient has cleared HbsAg with two consecutive tests at least 4 weeks apart.

CLINICAL PEARLS

- Hepatitis B is preventable with vaccination.
- Hepatitis B is usually acute in adults.
- Hepatitis B often becomes chronic if diagnosed in infancy or childhood.
- Hepatitis B is often self-limited with supportive care.

KEY TAKEAWAYS

Hepatitis B is known worldwide; spread through contact with blood, semen, or other body fluids; is usually self-limiting in adults and more often becomes chronic in infants and children. There is a vaccine available.

10.4C: HEPATITIS C

Acute hepatitis C is the most serious of the viral hepatitis diseases because more than half of individuals presenting with acute hepatitis C progress to chronic hepatitis C (U.S. Department of Veterans Affairs, 2020). Like hepatitis B, hepatitis C is spread through contact with blood, semen, or other body fluids of an infected person; sexual contact; sharing needles or syringes; and from mother to baby at birth.

PRESENTING SIGNS AND SYMPTOMS

Most cases of acute hepatitis C typically have no symptoms. Those that do have symptoms can present 2 to 12 weeks after exposure with jaundice, dark urine, white-colored stool, nausea, malaise, and pain in the right upper quadrant of the abdomen.

DIAGNOSTIC TESTS

Hepatitis C is diagnosed with a serum laboratory test for HCV antibody. Patients usually have an elevated serum alanine aminotransferase (ALT) level greater than 200 IU/L.

TREATMENT

Acute cases of hepatitis C are usually asymptomatic and do not require treatment. Early screening should take place in those who are in high-risk situations with a known hepatitis C–positive patient. Patients with suspected or confirmed hepatitis C infections should be educated on preventing further spread via sexual activity or needle sharing. In addition, while there is no vaccination to prevent hepatitis C, recommendations for those diagnosed are to receive the hepatitis A and B vaccinations. Those diagnosed with acute hepatitis C are recommended to start treatment with direct-acting antivirals (DAAs) because of the elevated risk of converting to chronic hepatitis C (U.S. Department of Veterans Affairs, 2020). Once treatment is completed, the virus is undetectable in the blood and the risk of transmitting to others is greatly reduced. Those who completed treatment and confirm undetectable viral loads are considered cured.

CLINICAL PEARLS

- Acute hepatitis C often continues to chronic infection.
- Acute hepatitis C often presents with no or few symptoms.
- After confirming hepatitis C infection, treatment with direct-acting antivirals is recommended.

KEY TAKEAWAYS

Infection with acute hepatitis C often leads to chronic hepatitis C that can result in liver failure and death if left untreated. There is no vaccine, but there is treatment to suppress the virus to prevent further spread and liver damage.

10.4D: HEPATITIS D

Hepatitis D is caused by the hepatitis D virus, which is also known as delta virus or satellite virus. The hepatitis D virus requires the simultaneous presence of the hepatitis B virus for complete virion assembly and secretion. Thus, individuals with hepatitis D are always coinfected with hepatitis B. Acquiring hepatitis D after being diagnosed with hepatitis B is considered a supra-infection. Like hepatitis B, hepatitis D is spread through infected blood and body fluids. Hepatitis D is not common in the United States and usually occurs in those that travel and/or have had sexual contact or shared needles with those from other countries where it is more common (CDC, 2020a).

PRESENTING SIGNS AND SYMPTOMS

Signs and symptoms of hepatitis D are similar to all of the hepatitis viruses: fever, fatigue, loss of appetite, nausea, malaise, abdominal discomfort, dark urine, clay-colored bowel movements, and jaundice. Most patients who are coinfected with both hepatitis B and hepatitis D will have a spontaneous recovery. Those diagnosed with a supra-infection of hepatitis D progress quickly to chronic hepatitis B and D infection and have an increased risk of developing liver cirrhosis and liver failure. Seventy percent to 80% of those with both chronic viruses develop liver failure within 5 to 10 years (CDC, 2020b).

DIAGNOSTIC TESTS

Hepatitis D is diagnosed with a serum laboratory test for antibodies against HDV (HDAg) and HDV RNA. Anyone who has severe viral hepatitis symptoms or diagnosed with hepatitis B (HBsAg) should be tested for hepatitis D.

TREATMENT

While there is no vaccine for hepatitis D, prevention does occur with the hepatitis B vaccine. Treating those with hepatitis D with PEGylated interferon alpha has shown some efficacy, but viral clearance is less than 25% (Farci & Niro, 2018).

CLINICAL PEARLS

- Acute hepatitis D infection occurs in association with hepatitis B infection.
- Coinfections with hepatitis D and hepatitis B have better outcomes that supra-infection of hepatitis D on hepatitis B.
- There is no vaccine for hepatitis D, but the hepatitis B vaccine will prevent a hepatitis D infection.

KEY TAKEAWAYS

Hepatitis D is rare in the United States, is spread through infected blood and body fluids, can only occur in the setting of hepatitis B, and has a good prognosis if coinfected rather than supra-infected.

10.4E: HEPATITIS E

The hepatitis E virus causes hepatitis E. Hepatitis E is spread via the fecal–oral route related to contaminated water and poor sanitation practices and is uncommon in the United States. Hepatitis E can also spread to certain mammals and result in transmission to humans when consuming raw or undercooked meat from an infected animal (Feagins et al., 2007).

PRESENTING SIGNS AND SYMPTOMS

As with all of the previously mentioned hepatitis viruses, symptoms can range from nonexistent to full liver failure. Symptoms of hepatitis remain the same for all of the viruses and include fever, fatigue, loss of appetite, nausea, malaise, abdominal discomfort, dark urine, clay-colored bowel movements, and jaundice. Those who are more prone to symptoms include older adolescents, young adults (age 15 to 44 years old), and pregnant women.

DIAGNOSTIC TESTS

Patients infected with hepatitis E have elevated serum concentrations of bilirubin, ALT, and aspartate aminotransferase as well as anti-HEV IgM assay. When there is a chronic infection, detection of HEV RNA is present in serum or stool for longer than 6 months.

TREATMENT

Management for acute hepatitis E virus is supportive care and prevention of further spread. Virus excretion in stool has been detected from as early as 1 week prior to onset of symptoms to 30 days after. Those few who develop chronic hepatitis E will shed the virus indefinitely. There is no FDA-approved vaccine for hepatitis E at this time.

CLINICAL PEARLS

- Hepatitis E is contracted from contaminated stool, water, and food.
- Care is supportive.
- Rarely does hepatitis E become chronic.
- There is no vaccine for hepatitis E.

KEY TAKEAWAYS

Hepatitis E is rare in the United States, treatment is supportive and rarely does it progress to chronic liver injury.

10.4F: ALCOHOLIC HEPATITIS

Acute alcoholic hepatitis occurs from chronic alcohol abuse. It is most common in adults 40 to 60 years of age who have been drinking heavily, more than 80 grams per day for more than 20 years (European Association for the Study of the Liver, 2018). The CAGE or AUDIT questionnaires can help to determine the likelihood of excessive alcohol use.

PRESENTING SIGNS AND SYMPTOMS

Patients with acute alcoholic hepatitis usually present with jaundice, anorexia, tender hepatomegaly, ascites, and fever. Some may have right upper quadrant and epigastric pain, hepatic encephalopathy, and signs of malnutrition. Patients with more advanced liver disease may also have spider angiomas, palmar erythema, and gynecomastia.

DIAGNOSTIC TESTS

No particular set of laboratory findings or radiographic tests are uniquely specific for acute alcoholic hepatitis. Generally, patients with acute alcoholic hepatitis will have moderate elevations in AST and ALT. The only laboratory variation unique to acute alcoholic hepatitis is a disproportionate elevation of serum AST compared to ALT at a ratio greater than 2 (Sorbi et al., 1999). Patients also have elevated serum bilirubin, INR, and gamma-glutamyl transferase (GGT), anemia, thrombocytopenia, and electrolyte abnormalities. Other forms of hepatitis and liver diseases should be eliminated with laboratory testing and transabdominal ultrasound with Doppler. Similar presenting illnesses include nonalcoholic steatohepatitis, ischemic hepatitis, HELLP (hemolysis, elevated liver enzymes, and low platelets) syndrome, Wilson disease, and drug-induced liver injury caused by acetaminophen, herbal supplements, and illicit drugs. Ultimately, the diagnosis of alcoholic hepatitis is a clinical diagnosis based on jaundice, elevated AST, and a history of heavy alcohol use.

TREATMENT

By calculating a Maddrey's Discriminant Function score using the PT and total bilirubin, one may be able to determine a short-term prognosis. A score greater than 32 indicates the patient may benefit from corticosteroids (Maddrey et al., 1978). However, those patients treated with corticosteroids had nearly twice as high rate of infection and no statistically significant improvement in 28-day mortality (Thursz et al., 2015). Another model, the Lille Model has helped providers to limit the duration of steroid therapy in nonresponders based on the bilirubin level on day 4 of treatment and thus help reduce the risk of infection (Louvet et al., 2007). Calculating a MELD score can also be helpful in predicting the 30- and 90-day morality rate in patients with alcoholic hepatitis. A score of 21 or greater has a high mortality risk (Dunn et al., 2005).

Treatment for acute alcoholic hepatitis requires abstinence from alcohol and supportive care for failing organ systems. An inflamed liver can impair bleeding as production of coagulation factors, and blood products are often necessary to correct coagulopathy. Other supportive care includes supplementing B-complex vitamins for Wernicke's encephalopathy, using lactulose and rifaximin to treat hepatic encephalopathy, and salt restriction to treat ascites (European Association for the Study of the Liver, 2018). Optimization of nutrition is also an essential component of recovery. A target of 35 to 40 kcal/kg of body weight and daily protein intake of 1.2 to 1.5 g/kg of body weight is recommended (European Association for the Study of the Liver, 2018). In some cases, patients can benefit from a liver transplant with survival rate of 94% at 1 year and 84% at 3 years (Lee et al., 2018).

CLINICAL PEARLS

- Acute alcoholic hepatitis usually results from more than 20 years of alcohol abuse.
- There is no specific test for alcoholic hepatitis; it is a diagnosis of exclusion.
- Determining treatment can be complex with several tools and models available to calculate risk.

KEY TAKEAWAYS

Alcoholic hepatitis is a complex disease that requires specialty care, cessation of alcohol abuse, and often a liver transplant for survival.

10.4G: AUTOIMMUNE HEPATITIS

Autoimmune hepatitis is rare and occurs when one's own antibodies cause inflammation of the liver. The exact cause is unknown and it more often occurs in women than men.

PRESENTING SIGNS AND SYMPTOMS

As with all forms of acute hepatitis, symptoms are similar and include fatigue, abdominal discomfort, and joint pain.

DIAGNOSTIC TESTS

Autoimmune hepatitis is a diagnosis of exclusion. While there is no specific test for autoimmune hepatitis, it is expected to find an elevated ALT and AST at least two times the upper limit. Often an elevation in gamma globulins is seen, especially immunoglobulin G (IgG). Antibodies, particularly antinuclear antibody (ANA), anti-smooth muscle antibody (ASMA), anti-liver-kidney microsomal-1 antibody (anti-LKM-1) and anti-mitochondrial antibody (AMA) are also commonly found in those with autoimmune hepatitis.

TREATMENT

Autoimmune hepatitis can be treated, but not cured. Initial treatment for acute autoimmune hepatitis is low dose prednisone. For those with a more severe case, a combination of prednisone and azathioprine is the typical course of treatment.

CLINICAL PEARLS

- Autoimmune means the immune system is attacking the liver.
- Autoimmune hepatitis is a diagnosis of exclusion.
- Treatment with steroids helps symptoms, but there is no cure.

KEY TAKEAWAYS

Autoimmune hepatitis is a rare and chronic condition more common among women, in which the immune system causes inflammation in the liver.

10.5: INFLAMMATORY BOWEL DISEASE

Kendra J. Kamp, Jeffrey D. Jacobs, and Kindra Clark-Snustad

Inflammatory bowel disease (IBD) includes Crohn's disease (CD), and ulcerative colitis (UC). Although the majority of care is outpatient, hospitalization is indicated for severe disease flares that cannot be managed in the outpatient setting and for disease-related complications. Up to 50% of IBD patients will require hospitalization over the course of their disease (Huh et al., 2019). Inpatient management is complex and requires a multidisciplinary approach. In the following we present the management of the hospitalized patient with UC or CD.

10.5A: ULCERATIVE COLITIS

UC is a chronic inflammatory autoimmune disease, characterized by mucosal inflammation that begins in the rectum and extends proximally throughout the colon. Untreated UC results in relapsing remitting mucosal inflammation that causes symptoms including diarrhea, hematochezia, tenesmus (sensation of needing to pass stool even when the rectum is empty), and urgency. While UC may range from mild to severe, around 25% of patients will require hospitalization for acute severe UC (ASUC; Dinesen et al., 2010). Of those hospitalized, approximately 20% will undergo colectomy during their first admission for ASUC (Dinesen et al., 2010).

PRESENTING SIGNS AND SYMPTOMS

ASUC is characterized by ≥6 bloody stools daily plus at least one of the following: fever (≥37.8°C), tachycardia (≥90 beats/min), anemia (hemoglobin <10.5 g/dL), and/or an elevated inflammatory marker (Truelove & Witts, 1955). Fulminant colitis describes patients presenting with the aforementioned symptoms, who also have ≥10 bloody stools daily with fecal urgency, and often accompanied by abdominal pain and distention (Rubin et al., 2019). Toxic megacolon is a potentially lethal complication with total or segmental nonobstructive dilation of the colon in the setting of systemic toxicity (Table 10.4). Colonic perforation may present as acute chest or abdominal pain, with or without fever. Patients may be hemodynamically unstable and may have altered mental status. Patients may also present with extraintestinal manifestations (EIM) of IBD which can involve the joints (e.g., peripheral arthritis), eye (e.g., uveitis, iritis), skin (e.g., erythema nodosum, pyoderma gangrenosum), liver (e.g., primary sclerosing cholangitis), and lungs. UC flare is a hypercoagulable

TABLE 10.4: Characteristics of Acute Severe Ulcerative Colitis, Fulminant Colitis, and Toxic Megacolon

ACUTE SEVERE ULCERATIVE COLITIS	FULMINANT COLITIS	TOXIC MEGACOLON
≥6 bloody stools daily AND at least one of the following: • Fever (≥37.8°C) • Tachycardia (≥90 beats/min) • Anemia (hemoglobin <10.5 g/dL) • Elevated inflammatory marker	The features of acute severe ulcerative colitis PLUS: ≥10 bloody stools daily with fecal urgency, often accompanied by abdominal pain and distention	Radiographic evidence of colonic distention AND ≥3 of the following: • Fever (≥37.8°C) • Tachycardia (>120 beats/min) • Neutrophilic leukocytosis >10,500/mcL • Anemia AND ≥1 of the following • Electrolyte disturbances • Hypotension • Dehydration • Altered sensorium

state and patients should be monitored for venous and arterial thromboembolism. Anemia may result from hematochezia or because of systemic inflammation.

HISTORY AND PHYSICAL FINDINGS

For the hospitalized patient with UC, providers should obtain a comprehensive UC history including disease location, extent and duration, symptoms, IBD medication history and response to therapy, surgical history, EIM, and prior disease complications. Providers should assess for signs of systemic inflammatory response such as fever, tachycardia, and hypotension and conduct an abdominal exam assessing bowel sounds, distention, and tenderness with guarding or rebound. Patient symptoms should be tracked, including the number of loose stools daily, urgency, tenesmus, and presence of hematochezia.

DIFFERENTIAL DIAGNOSIS AND DIAGNOSTIC CONSIDERATIONS

For patients presenting with suspected UC flare, evaluation should include laboratory studies (complete blood count [CBC] to assess for leukocytosis, anemia, or thrombocytosis and comprehensive metabolic panel [CMP] to assess electrolyte status, liver and kidney status, and inflammatory markers (C-reactive protein [CRP], erythrocyte sedimentation rate and/or fecal calprotectin). Blood cultures should be ordered for patients with leukocytosis and fever. Stool studies should be ordered to rule out enteric pathogens (e.g., *Clostridioides difficile, Salmonella, Shigella, Campylobacter, Yersinia, Giardia,* and parasitic infection for at- risk patients). Flexible sigmoidoscopy assesses the severity of flare and biopsies can rule out infections such as cytomegalovirus. Colonoscopy should be avoided if there is concern for colonic dilation or perforation (Makkar & Bo, 2013). Imaging with plain abdominal radiography should be completed to assess colonic diameter. Colonic diameter of ≥5.5 cm is suggestive of colonic dilation and a diameter of ≥6 cm with signs of systemic toxicity is consistent with toxic megacolon. Further imaging with computed tomography (CT) or magnetic resonance imaging (MRI) can evaluate for disease complications such as peritonitis from colonic perforation. Attention should be given to any signs of CD (e.g., ileal or upper gastrointestinal involvement, patchy colitis, perianal disease, fibrostenotic complications) as the evaluation and treatment of CD and related complications differs (Table 10.5).

TREATMENT

The short-term goals of the treatment of UC flare include hemodynamic stability and symptom improvement; long-term goals include steroid-free clinical and endoscopic remission.

General Care

Providers should monitor patient vital signs, conduct focused gastrointestinal physical examinations, and assess

TABLE 10.5: Endoscopic Scoring for Ulcerative Colitis

SEVERITY	ENDOSCOPIC FINDINGS
Remission	No evidence of inflammation
Mild	Erythema, decreased vascular pattern, and mild friability
Moderate	Marked erythema, lack of vascular pattern, friability, and erosions
Severe	Spontaneous bleeding and ulceration

Source: Data from Schroeder, K. W., Tremaine, W. J., & Ilstrup, D. M. (1987). Coated oral 5-aminosalicylic acid therapy for mildly to moderately active ulcerative colitis. A randomized study. *The New England Journal of Medicine, 317*(26), 1625–1629. https://doi.org/10.1056/NEJM198712243172603

laboratory results and symptoms for response to treatment throughout the hospitalization. Patients may require IV fluid and electrolyte repletion. Parenteral nutrition (PN) may be indicated if inability to tolerate adequate caloric intake results in malnutrition. Individuals with IBD are at higher risk for venous thromboembolism (VTE) and should receive VTE prophylaxis (Grainge et al., 2010). Treatment of anemia via iron infusions or blood transfusions may be indicated. Oral iron should be avoided as gastrointestinal symptoms can be worsened and systemic inflammation limits absorption (Niepel et al., 2018). Patients should receive adequate pain management with pharmacologic and nonpharmacologic methods. Opioids should be used cautiously as they increase the risk of dilation and perforation and may not effectively manage pain (Berry et al., 2020).

Surgical Consultation

For patients admitted with ASUC, obtain surgical consultation with a colorectal surgeon early during hospitalization. This builds a therapeutic relationship between the patient and both medical and surgical teams and reduces surgical delays if colectomy is indicated. While medical therapy is effective in many patients, indications for colectomy include non response to medical therapy, toxic megacolon, colonic perforation, uncontrolled severe hematochezia, or multiorgan dysfunction (Gallo et al., 2018). In this setting, surgery generally includes a restorative proctocolectomy with ileal pouch–anal anastomosis (IPAA), which is completed in a two-step or three-step procedure. Importantly, providers should thoroughly evaluate for any signs of CD prior to recommending surgical treatment, as colectomy is not curative and IPAA is not recommended as surgical management of CD.

Medical Therapy

First-Line Medical Therapy

IV glucocorticoids, including methylprednisolone and hydrocortisone, are the first-line medical therapy for ASUC. Dosing is typically hydrocortisone 100 mg every 8 hours or methylprednisolone 40 to 60 mg every 24 hours. Higher doses of corticosteroids are not more effective or recommended (Feuerstein et al., 2020). Clinical response is evaluated daily including assessment of symptoms (e.g., hematochezia and stool frequency) and laboratory results (e.g., C-reactive protein [CRP], anemia, leukocytosis). Patients are considered nonresponders if no significant improvement is observed after 3 to 5 days of steroid therapy. Response rates to IV glucocorticoids range from 40% to 60% (Verdon et al., 2019).

Escalation of Medical Therapy

Escalation of medical therapy to infliximab or cyclosporine is recommended for nonresponders to IV corticosteroids (Feuerstein et al., 2020). One meta-analysis indicated a higher colectomy-free survival for infliximab compared to cyclosporine for the first 3 years; but no significant difference in colectomy-free survival beyond 3 years (Szemes et al., 2020). Guidelines do not currently recommend one therapy option over the other. Therapy choice should be based on patient factors, on provider comfort/experience, and available resources (Sternthal et al., 2008).

Infliximab is an IgG1 monoclonal antibody that binds tumor necrosis factor-alpha (TNFα). Theoretically, patients with ASUC may have increased metabolism and fecal wasting of biologic therapy due to high inflammatory burden, and potentially lower drug levels due to malnutrition given that infliximab is an albumin-bound drug. However, given lack of high quality evidence comparing infliximab dosing in hospitalized UC patients, current guidelines make no recommendation for use of standard versus intensified infliximab dosing as initial treatment for hospitalized UC patients (Feuerstein et al., 2020). Typically, a standard induction regimen of 5 mg/kg IV at week 0, 2, and 6 is given. One approach in the patient with nonresponse to the initial infusion after 3 to 5 days is to administer a second dose of infliximab 10 mg/kg. If nonresponse to the second infusion after 5 days, then consideration should be given to colectomy.

Prior to starting infliximab, patients should be screened for tuberculosis and hepatitis B. Contraindications to infliximab include latent tuberculosis, congestive heart failure, demyelinating disease, active infection, malignancy, and prior exposure to infliximab. Given high rates of immunogenicity to biologic therapy, especially in the setting of breaks in therapy, outpatient follow-up and continuation of infliximab induction and maintenance infusions are essential. This can be challenging as insurance authorization for outpatient infliximab must be obtained and infusions coordinated with the patient's primary gastroenterology provider.

Cyclosporine is a calcineurin inhibitor dosed intravenously at 2 mg/kg/day in two divided doses initially and can be increased by 0.5 mg/kg per day as tolerated, up to 4 mg/kg/day. The suggested goal trough level is 300 mg/mL (Cohen et al., 1999). Cyclosporine drug levels should be checked every 1 to 2 days initially, after each dose change, then every 2 to 3 days when on stable dosing. Rounding doses to the nearest 25 mg will assist in conversion to oral dosing. Response is assessed after 3 days of therapy. If response is achieved, the patient may be converted to oral modified cyclosporine by doubling the IV dose and administering oral cyclosporine in divided doses every 12 hours. Cyclosporine drug levels are checked prior to the fourth oral dose, with a goal level of 200 to 300 ng/mL. Outpatient follow-up should be arranged to continue drug monitoring and to transition the patient to a maintenance regimen (e.g., biologic or small molecule) as cyclosporine is not effective as maintenance therapy.

Contraindications to cyclosporine treatment include hypertension, renal disease, history of seizure disorder, and low serum total cholesterol (<120 mg/dL), low magnesium, or low albumin (<2.3 g/dL). Prophylaxis against *Pneumocystis* pneumonia is recommended during cyclosporine therapy. Drug interactions are common and may be serious. Patients are monitored for infection, nephrotoxicity, neurotoxicity, hypertension, and electrolyte abnormalities.

While guidelines do not currently recommend rescue therapy with small molecules such as tofacitinib, small case studies have suggested that there may be a role for small molecule therapy for treatment of ASUC given the rapid onset of action and reliable pharmacokinetics of tofacitinib (Verdon et al., 2019).

Surgery

If the patient has nonresponse to either infliximab or cyclosporine, or if the patient develops a UC complication at any point, then the patient should be evaluated for colectomy by a colorectal surgeon.

TRANSITION OF CARE

Discharge considerations can be made upon clinical improvement including normal vital signs, improvement in bowel symptoms and abdominal pain, and ability to tolerate an oral diet. Patients on IV steroids should be transitioned to an oral prednisone taper with a plan to transition to steroid-free maintenance therapy as an outpatient. If infliximab has been used, ensure continuation of therapy as outpatient as breaks in therapy increase risk of immunogenicity. Patients on IV cyclosporine are typically transitioned to oral cyclosporine. To promote transition of care, ensure outpatient follow-up with an IBD specialist to achieve and maintain steroid-free clinical and endoscopic remission.

10.5B: CROHN'S DISEASE

CD is a chronic, transmural, inflammatory condition that involves the alimentary tract anywhere from the oral cavity to the anus. The terminal ileum and colon are the most commonly affected areas, and about a quarter of those affected will develop perianal disease (Peyrin-Biroulet et al., 2010). Because the inflammation in CD is transmural, (meaning it can involve the full thickness of the bowel) a variety of complications not seen in UC can occur. These complications include diarrhea and malnutrition, intestinal strictures and subsequent obstruction, fistulas, or intraabdominal or perianal abscesses.

PRESENTING SIGNS AND SYMPTOMS

Patients with CD will have various presenting symptoms depending on the severity and location of inflammation. Extensive small bowel or colonic inflammation, or fistulas that bypass large segments of the bowel, will lead to diarrhea and nutrient malabsorption. As a result, patients with CD may present with weight loss, decreased oral intake, malnutrition, and fatigue. The rectum is spared of inflammation in CD in 40% to 50% of cases, so urgency and tenesmus is less common when compared to UC (Peyrin-Biroulet et al., 2010; Waye, 1977). Rectal bleeding is also less common in CD than UC but may still occur with extensive or left-sided colonic inflammation.

Transmural inflammation may lead to intestinal strictures and stenosis, which can be fibrotic, inflammatory, or more commonly, a mix of fibrosis and inflammation (Bettenworth et al., 2019). If severe enough, strictures can lead to bowel obstruction, often in the terminal ileum. Gastric or duodenal CD can progress to gastric outlet obstruction or colonic strictures, and a possible large bowel obstruction (LBO). However, gastric outlet obstruction and LBO are inherently less common as the stomach and duodenum are not as frequently involved in CD and the larger diameter of the colon means that a colonic stricture is less likely to lead to an obstruction (Laube et al., 2018). Presenting symptoms of an obstructing stricture include abdominal pain, bloating, nausea, vomiting, and obstipation. In CD especially, intestinal inflammation may be minimally symptomatic or asymptomatic until severe enough to cause a partial or complete bowel obstruction. Anal strictures may also arise from anal and rectal inflammation and can often be asymptomatic and only detected on digital rectal exam or colonoscopy.

Transmural inflammation can also cause fistulas to form, which are abnormal connections between two epithelial-lined organs. The presenting symptoms of a fistula vary depending on the involved organs. Fistulas from bowel to the skin or perianal area may lead to pain and drainage, whereas fistulas to the vagina or bladder can cause recurrent urinary tract infections, pneumaturia, or passage of stool from the vagina. Fistulas between two bowel segments—whether enteroenteric, enterocolonic, or colocolonic—may be asymptomatic unless large segments of bowel are bypassed, in which case diarrhea and malabsorption will result. If the penetrating bowel inflammation does not lead to a fistula, an abscess or phlegmon (soft tissue infection and inflammation not confined to a discrete fluid collection) can develop, either within the abdomen or in the perianal area. Presenting symptoms of an abscess may include pain and fever.

Lastly, patients with CD are at increased risk for a number of EIM. EIM in CD include inflammatory arthritis, ocular manifestations including uveitis and episcleritis, pyoderma gangrenosum of the skin, osteoporosis, kidney stones, and gallstones.

HISTORY AND PHYSICAL FINDINGS

The physical exam findings in patients with CD can be variable and may be normal in some patients. A partial or complete bowel obstruction will present with abdominal distention and abdominal tenderness. Intraabdominal abscess may present with fever and abdominal tenderness, and potentially with a palpable mass in the right lower quadrant, as the terminal ileum is the most commonly affected location. Perianal disease can be evident as skin tags or small fistula openings. Perianal abscesses are often erythematous, quite tender, and indurated or fluctuant.

DIFFERENTIAL DIAGNOSIS AND DIAGNOSTIC CONSIDERATIONS

The initial evaluation of a patient with CD should include a thorough history to obtain information on the duration of disease; known involved bowel segments; history of prior complications including stricture, fistula, or abscess; current and prior IBD medications; and any prior operations.

Laboratory evaluation should include complete blood count; chemistry panel including renal function, electrolytes, and liver function tests; and C-reactive protein (CRP). The plasma half-life of CRP is about 19 hours and can be assessed daily to monitor therapy response in hospitalized patients (Pepys & Hirschfield, 2003). Especially high CRP values in patients with CD warrants evaluation for perforation or an abscess with cross-sectional imaging. Micronutrient deficiencies are common in CD. Iron studies, vitamin B_{12}, and zinc levels are also often measured. Enteric infections, particularly *Clostridioides difficile*, should be ruled out in IBD patients presenting to the emergency department or those hospitalized.

Imaging is typically warranted in patients with abdominal pain, fever, or an abdominal mass on exam to evaluate for bowel obstruction or an intraabdominal abscess. Options include ultrasound, CT, or MRI. However, it is important to keep in mind that patients with CD are at increased risk for harmful amounts of ionizing radiation exposure from repeated imaging studies, especially for patients diagnosed under the age of 17 years (Desmond et al., 2008; Kroeker et al., 2011). In stable patients, enterography is the preferred imaging technique in which oral contrast allows for optimal evaluation of the small bowel and can be done with CT or MRI. Because the sensitivity for the detection of small bowel disease and abscesses is similar for computed tomography enterography (CTE) and magnetic resonance enterography (MRE), MRE is often preferred for young patients to avoid the radiation that comes with CT imaging (Seastedt et al., 2014; Siddiki et al., 2009). However, due to cost and availability, MRE may not be an option everywhere, and enterography is not typically adequate for the assessment of perianal disease.

In patients with known or suspected perianal disease, pelvic imaging is critical to characterize the anatomy of the perianal fistula or fistulas and to evaluate for a perianal abscess. MRI of the pelvis, exam under anesthesia (EUA), and endoscopic ultrasound (EUS) are all modalities that can be used in this setting. These three modalities have similar diagnostic accuracy, with the best results coming when two of the three are combined (Schwartz et al., 2001).

TREATMENT

The management of CD-related complications depends on the complications, and there is frequent overlap in the presenting complications and treatment.

Diarrhea and Malnutrition

Once an infection has been ruled out or treated, corticosteroids can be used to treat an acute flare of luminal inflammation to help with symptoms. IV methylprednisolone at a dose of 40 to 60 mg per day can be used and transitioned to oral prednisone at discharge. Due to the multitude of side effects of corticosteroids and their lack of efficacy for maintenance of clinical remission, corticosteroids are a bridge to effective maintenance therapy, typically with an immunomodulator or biologic therapy as an outpatient. It is important to be aware that while corticosteroids can often decrease inflammation and help with symptoms, rates of mucosal healing are low (Yang & Lichtenstein, 2002).

Malnutrition, defined as the loss of more than 5% body weight in 1 month or 10% in 6 months, will sometimes require parenteral nutrition (PN) (White et al., 2012). However, due to associated thrombosis and infection risks, the decision to use PN is delicate, and should made in conjunction with a registered dietitian. While there are no universally accepted indications for PN in CD, patients with severe stenosis, especially proximal, or a high output enterocutaneous fistula may need PN. In patients who will be undergoing surgery, malnutrition is associated with an increased risk of complications. For this reason, malnourished patients who are unable to receive enteral nutrition are often started on PN preoperatively (Alastair et al., 2011; Semrad, 2012). Malnourished patients started on PN will also be at risk for refeeding syndrome, in which severe electrolyte abnormalities can occur, most importantly potassium, magnesium, and phosphorus. These electrolytes need to be monitored closely and repleted aggressively, and the rate of nutritional support may need to be slowed or stopped temporarily.

Intraabdominal Abscess

If an intraabdominal abscess is suspected or has been diagnosed with cross-sectional imaging, antibiotics should be started. Intraabdominal abscesses and fistulas often form near the site of intestinal stenosis and will often ultimately require bowel resection, but drainage prior to an operation is beneficial (Yamaguchi et al., 2004). Intraabdominal abscesses larger than 3 cm will need to be drained, whereas abscesses smaller than 3 cm may be managed with antibiotics alone. If feasible, percutaneous drainage (PD) is the preferred approach, but surgical drainage is also an option if PD is not possible. Reimaging in 3 to 5 days after the initiation of antibiotics with or without PD is recommended to confirm improvement (Feagins et al., 2011). Once the infection is controlled, surgery can often be delayed. Delaying surgery will allow for resolution of intraabdominal sepsis, increase the chances of avoiding a diverting ostomy, and may decrease the risk of operative complications (Clancy et al., 2016; Zerbib et al., 2010). A subset of patients with CD with an intraabdominal abscess may not require surgery, particularly those without an associated stricture, but antibiotics, drainage, and subsequent medical therapy are still needed (Clancy et al., 2016; Lichtenstein et al., 2018). Corticosteroids do not have a role in the treatment of penetrating CD unless there is significant bowel inflammation or a bowel obstruction, and corticosteroids may in fact increase the risk of developing an abscess (Agrawal et al., 2005).

Fibrostenosing Complications

Initial management of a complete bowel obstruction requires decompression with placement of a nasogastric tube along with optimization of volume status and correction of electrolyte abnormalities. Cross-sectional imaging is necessary to confirm the diagnosis and location of the obstruction, generally with CT, but if the obstruction is partial then CT or MRI with enterography is ideal. Because imaging is not typically helpful at distinguishing between a fibrotic or inflammatory stricture, IV corticosteroids may be used initially in attempt to reduce any inflammatory component contributing to the bowel narrowing and obstruction (Rimola & Capozzi, 2020). Once the obstruction has resolved, patients can be transitioned to oral prednisone with a plan to transition to biologic therapy as an outpatient. Additionally, once a bowel obstruction has occurred, some patients will ultimately need surgery to resect the stenosed segment, although endoscopic balloon dilation is also an option for strictures without associated fistulas. Endoscopic balloon dilation has high rates of immediate technical success, defined as the ability to traverse the stricture with the colonoscope, but about 40% will still require an operation within 3 years (Bettenworth et al., 2017; Winder et al., 2019). However, initiating a bowel prep for a colonoscopy in a patient who is obstructed or recently obstructed may be high risk and not possible. A nonresolving bowel obstruction will therefore require surgery.

Perianal Abscess

Once a perianal abscess has been diagnosed by examination and imaging, drainage is required with the exception that small abscesses (<5 mm) may be managed without drainage (Lichtenstein et al., 2018). Antibiotics are often used in conjunction with surgical drainage of a perianal abscess and may decrease output and symptoms in patients with perianal fistulas. Antibiotics will not typically lead to fistula healing except for some simple fistulas (such as a single fistula tract that is superficial and distal to the dentate line). However, patients with perianal fistulas will ultimately need advanced biologic therapy, of which infliximab is the best studied, and potentially surgical intervention depending on the fistula anatomy (Sands et al., 2004). The inpatient management of perianal CD is typically limited to surgical drainage of perianal abscesses followed by outpatient medical therapy. As with intraabdominal abscesses, corticosteroids may help with signs and symptoms of luminal inflammation (i.e., diarrhea) but will not otherwise be helpful for the management of perianal fistulas.

CLINICAL PEARLS

Ulcerative colitis
- UC is a chronic inflammatory autoimmune disease. Symptoms include diarrhea, hematochezia, tenesmus, and urgency.
- The initial evaluation of patients with ASUC includes history and physical exam, blood and stool tests, imaging to assess for colonic dilation and/or complications, and flexible sigmoidoscopy.
- Providers should assess for complications including fulminant colitis, toxic megacolon, and colonic perforation.
- Initial treatment is with IV corticosteroids with short-term goals of hemodynamic stability and symptom improvement, and long-term goals of steroid-free clinical and endoscopic remission. If nonresponse to corticosteroids, then treatment is escalated to infliximab or cyclosporine.
- If nonresponse to escalated therapy or if the patient develops toxic megacolon, colonic perforation, uncontrolled severe hematochezia, or multiorgan dysfunction, then colectomy is indicated.

Crohn's disease:
- CD is characterized by transmural inflammation, with potential complications that include diarrhea, malnutrition, bowel obstruction, fistulas, and intraabdominal and perianal abscesses.
- Glucocorticoids are useful for patients with moderate-to-severe disease for symptom relief, but due to a multitude of side effects, they are not used long term, are not helpful, and may in fact be harmful for the treatment of fistulas.
- Other complications such as abscess, obstruction, and fistula require a multidisciplinary approach with gastroenterologists, surgeons, nurse practitioners, nutritionists, and radiologists to achieve the best outcome.
- Intraabdominal abscesses should be treated with antibiotics and potentially percutaneous or surgical drainage, with a goal of delaying surgery.
- Obstruction should be treated initially with decompression followed by corticosteroids to decrease any inflammatory component of the intestinal stricture. Even if the obstruction resolves, patients will be at high risk for needing surgery although a large subset will be able to avoid an operation.

10.6: ESOPHAGITIS

Bimbola Akintade

Esophagitis is characterized by the inflammation of the esophageal lining. Esophagitis is most commonly caused by gastroesophageal reflux disease (GERD) (Dellon et al., 2013; Katz et al., 2013; Lee et al., 2016). GERD occurs when the stomach acid moves into the throat, causing inflammation and damage to the esophagus. Other documented causes of esophagitis include compromised immune systems, medications, infections, and hernias (Groetch et al., 2017).

PRESENTING SIGNS AND SYMPTOMS

Though there are many different causes of esophagitis, the most common presenting symptom is dyspepsia, which is characterized as a burning sensation in the midchest caused by the retrograde contact of stomach acid within the esophageal mucosa (Groetch et al., 2017). Other common symptoms include epigastric and abdominal pain or discomfort, nausea, bloating, and fullness. Less common symptoms include dysphagia, retrosternal pain, odynophagia, drooling, hematemesis, and respiratory distress with wheezing, hoarseness, cough, stridor, fever, sepsis, and anorexia with weight loss. Symptoms tend to worsen after ingestion of a large meal or liquids (Dellon et al., 2013; Groetch et al., 2017; Katz et al., 2013).

Patients often present with chest pain indistinguishable from coronary artery disease. The chest pain is often described as midsternal, with radiation to the neck or arm, and may or may not be associated with shortness of breath and diaphoresis. This requires providers to rule out cardiac etiologies during patient workup (Dellon & Liacouras, 2014; Lee et al., 2016).

HISTORY AND PHYSICAL FINDINGS

The history and physical findings vary based on the type of esophagitis. In uncomplicated esophagitis, unfortunately, physical examination may not be helpful in confirming the diagnosis. However, the history and physical examination may help rule in or out other potential sources of chest or epigastric/abdominal pain (Groetch et al., 2017; Katz et al., 2013).

DIFFERENTIAL DIAGNOSIS AND DIAGNOSTIC CONSIDERATIONS

Due to the varying causes of esophagitis and the cross-systemic nature of symptoms experienced by patients, it is important that providers workup patients for each individual system implicated to rule out life-threatening conditions (Dellon et al., 2013; Katz et al., 2013). Differential diagnoses for esophagitis include coronary artery disease, pericarditis, aortic aneurysm, achalasia, non-ulcer reflux disease, functional dyspepsia, esophageal stricture, and other providers must also consider systemic conditions including systemic lupus erythematosus, acquired immunodeficiency syndrome, scleroderma, and so on, but most importantly, cardiac origins must be ruled out first (Dellon & Liacouras, 2014; Dellon et al., 2013).

In esophagitis, laboratory tests may not be helpful except if complications such as gastrointestinal hemorrhage are present. A complete blood cell (CBC) count is performed to evaluate for a decrease in hemoglobin and hematocrit in bleeding patients and to identify the presence of an infection by trending white blood cell (WBC) counts (Dellon & Liacouras, 2014; Lee et al., 2016). Electrocardiography and cardiac markers (creatine kinase [CK] and troponins) are indicated when patients present with cardiac symptoms. For patients with risk factors for HIV, CD4 count and HIV tests are performed. For patients suspicious of connective tissue diseases, a collagen disorder workup may be conducted. Unless complications including perforation, obstruction, bleeding, and so on are suspected, routine radiographic tests are not indicated (Lee et al., 2016).

For patients presenting with dysphagia or to investigate structural complications such as strictures, a double-contrast esophageal barium study is recommended as the initial imaging study (O'Rourke, 2015). However, an esophagogastroduodenoscopy (EGD) is considered the gold standard for evaluating upper endoscopic conditions as it provides more diagnostic information including mucosal visualization, inflammatory characteristics, shallow ulcers, extrinsic compression of the esophagus, procurement of mucosal biopsies for pathologic examination, and viral and bacterial cultures. For the diagnosis of infectious esophagitis, an EGD with biopsy and cultures is required (Dellon et al., 2013; O'Rourke, 2015).

TREATMENT

Treatment of esophagitis begins with proper diagnosis and management of cardiac-related conditions if present, followed by addressing pain. Since chest pain cannot be accurately distinguished from pain associated with esophageal origin, protocols for chest pain should be followed until ruled out. Subsequent care is directed toward complications of esophagitis that require volume resuscitation, hemodynamic stabilization, and surgical intervention (Dellon et al., 2013; Groetch et al., 2017; Katz et al., 2013).

Therapy after initial management of symptoms depends on the underlying cause of esophagitis and the presence of complications. For patients with esophagitis secondary to chronic GERD refractory to medical treatment, fundoplication—a surgical procedure where the fundus of the stomach is wrapped around the esophagus and sutured into place—may be indicated (Moole et al., 2017). In patients with odynophagia or those unable to consume food orally for extended periods of time, gastric or parenteral feeding may be indicated, otherwise no dietary restrictions are necessary (Moole et al., 2017).

According to the American College of Gastroenterology guidelines, patients who present with symptoms of regurgitation and dyspepsia, separately or in conjunction, should be evaluated and treated for GERD (Dellon et al., 2013). Other forms of esophagitis should be treated based on symptomology, which may range from observation, a trial of proton pump inhibitors (PPIs), oral or aerosolized steroids, prophylactic antibiotics, or esophageal dilation. Infectious esophagitis should be treated with appropriate antibiotics based on results from biopsy and culture samples (O'Rourke, 2015).

CLINICAL PEARLS

- In esophagitis patients with chest pain, potential cardiac sources should be ruled out first.
- Patients who present with symptoms of regurgitation and dyspepsia, separately or in conjunction, should be evaluated and treated for GERD.
- In patients with symptomatic esophageal eosinophilia, the use of proton pump inhibition is suggested over no treatment.

10.7: ACUTE PANCREATITIS

Adrienne Markiewicz and Alyssa Profita

The pancreas is located behind the stomach and under the liver and has several exocrine and endocrine functions. Acute pancreatitis (AP) is an acute inflammatory process of the pancreas. AP has several etiologies; however, gallstones and chronic alcohol abuse account for two thirds of cases (Tenner et al., 2013). AP is classified by timing and severity using the revised Atlanta Classification. Early pancreatitis is defined as symptom onset within 1 week of presentation, whereas late pancreatitis is defined as symptom onset that was greater than 1 week. Late pancreatitis is associated with complications including peripancreatic fluid collection, necrotizing pancreatitis, pseudocyst, or walled off cyst (Tenner et al., 2013). Box 10.3 lists etiologies of AP. Table 10.6 further describes the revised Atlanta Classification of AP.

PRESENTING SIGNS AND SYMPTOMS

The presentation of AP is driven by the extent of pancreatic inflammation. Patients may present with acute or sudden epigastric pain that radiates to the back, nausea, and vomiting with intolerance of oral intake. These presenting symptoms may be difficult to distinguish from an acute cardiovascular event or other acute abdominal etiologies.

HISTORY AND PHYSICAL EXAM FINDINGS

Medical History

Consideration of medical history is important with AP as it is most often triggered by a comorbid condition. AP has been increasing in the United States due to the rising incidence of obesity. Hyperlipidemia and alcohol use also are common etiologies of AP.

Patients with AP will have manifestations of a systemic inflammatory process on physical exam: fevers, tachycardia, and tachypnea. Abdominal pain, guarding, and significant nausea and vomiting are often present. Patients presenting with severe pancreatitis may have more tenderness over the epigastric region versus a patient with mild pancreatitis. Abdominal distention as well as hypoactive to absent bowel sounds may also be a common finding secondary to ileus from pancreatic inflammation. Patients with gallstone pancreatitis with obstruction may present with jaundice. Patients who have alcohol-related pancreatitis may have hepatomegaly or sequelae of chronic liver disease on exam (Tenner et al., 2013). Other possible exam findings include periumbilical (Cullen's sign) and lateral abdominal wall ecchymoses (Grey Turner's sign). Though these have been much described, the true incidence of one or both in AP approximates 1% to 3%. In addition, the average onset of both Cullen and Grey Turner sign in AP is 3 days and both are nonspecific findings which can be seen in any process causing intraabdominal hemorrhage. Therefore, the AGACNP should never use the absence of these findings to exclude the diagnosis of pancreatitis and should consider alternative diagnoses based on the patient history and clinical context even if one or both are present (Bosmann et al., 2009).

DIFFERENTIAL DIAGNOSIS AND DIAGNOSTIC CONSIDERATION

In patients presenting with acute abdominal pain, life-threatening cardiac and gastrointestinal conditions must be excluded. These include aortic aneurysm rupture or dissection, myocardial infarction, gastrointestinal bleed, and peptic ulcer disease (PUD) with perforation. The history and review of systems is pivotal, identifying the most likely etiology of pain. If the clinical history and exam suggest AP, several diagnostic tests can be used to confirm the diagnosis. The AGACNP should obtain serum amylase or lipase levels, which will be elevated at least three times the upper limit of normal. Abdominal CT imaging with contrast may show evidence of pancreatic inflammation, edema, and may show necrosis or local complications depending on the timing of the patient's presentation (Tenner et al., 2013). The AGACNP should proceed cautiously in attempting to use imaging to quantify severity of disease early in the patient's illness course, as imaging findings correlate poorly with clinical severity, and imaging sensitivity for necrotizing pancreatitis is decreased in the first few days of symptomatology.

BOX 10.3 ETIOLOGIES OF ACUTE PANCREATITIS

- Alcohol
- Direct-bile duct injury (penetrating trauma)
- Drug-induced
- Gallstones
- Genetic mutations
- Hypertriglyceridemia
- Postendoscopic retrograde cholangiopancreatography

TABLE 10.6: Classification of Acute Pancreatitis

MILD ACUTE PANCREATITIS	MODERATELY SEVERE ACUTE PANCREATITIS	SEVERE ACUTE PANCREATITIS
Abdominal pain Serum amylase or lipase 3 times the normal value Imaging with pancreatitis No organ failure No local complications	Criteria from mild AP AND Local complications AND/OR (peripancreatic fluid collection, necrotizing pancreatitis, pseudocyst or walled off cyst) Transient organ failure resolving within 48 hours	Criteria from mild/moderate AP AND Organ failure of two or more systems as defined by the Marshall scoring system

Local complications often occur later in the disease course; thus if there is suspicion of complications, repeat imaging may be warranted (Shah et al., 2018).

Once the diagnosis of AP is confirmed, the next step is to determine etiology. In most cases, the history makes this clear. Based on the clinical context, the AGACNP could obtain a medication, recent procedures and substance use history, serum triglyceride levels, and a right upper quadrant ultrasound to assess for the presence of gallstones. Magnetic resonance cholangiopancreatography (MRCP) may identify or exclude gallstones, a disconnect in the pancreatic ducts, pancreatic or parenchymal fluid collections, hemorrhage, or pseudocyst (Shah et al., 2018).

TREATMENT
Volume Resuscitation

Most patients with mild AP recover with aggressive fluid resuscitation, bowel rest and supportive treatment of nausea and vomiting. Patients with moderate to severe pancreatitis often require intensive care unit-level care due to complex management of concomitant organ failure. Frequent assessment of the patient's intravascular volume status and aggressive volume resuscitation to clinical euvolemia is imperative as patients with AP have gastrointestinal losses from vomiting, poor oral intake, and high insensate losses with distributive physiology. Lactated Ringer's is the preferred crystalloid for large volume resuscitation to avoid hyperchloremic acidosis associated with normal saline. The American College of Gastroenterology Guidelines recommends maintenance fluids in appropriate patients of 250/500 mL/h of crystalloid solution for the initial 12 to 24 hours (Tenner et al., 2013).

Endoscopic Retrograde Cholangiopancreatography

Most patients with AP caused by choledocholithiasis pass the stone without intervention; however, some may require endoscopic retrograde cholangiopancreatograpy (ERCP) for stone removal. Persistent choledocholithiasis resulting in pancreatic duct occlusion and biliary tree obstruction requires ERCP to reduce the risk of downstream complications such as cholangitis. This decision should be made cautiously as ERCP can worsen AP. In these patients, cholecystectomy is recommended to prevent recurrence of pancreatitis.

Pancreatitis causes a hypercatabolic state where fat and protein are rapidly metabolized. Providing early nutrition can reduce the catabolic effects. Additionally, nutrition can maintain gut motility as well as the gut barrier reducing the risk of bacterial gut translocation. Bacterial gut translocation can result from breakdown of the gut barrier from immobility, bacterial overgrowth, and increased intestinal permeability (Tenner et al., 2013).

Timing of introducing nutrition depends on the severity of the pancreatitis. Patients with mild pancreatitis who are demonstrating signs of improvement (improvement in pain, nausea, vomiting) can be started on a soft/bland diet immediately. Patients with severe pancreatitis should be started on enteral nutrition within 48 hours of presentation (Tenner et al., 2013). PN is not recommended if there is an option to use enteral nutrition.

COMPLICATIONS
Infection

Pancreatitis is an inflammatory process but not always infectious. The infectious risk rises with associated cholangitis and necrotizing pancreatitis. When there is concern an infectious workup and antimicrobial therapy should be considered.

Necrosis

Necrotizing pancreatitis is a complication with pancreatitis that increases patient morbidity and mortality, thus early identification and appropriate management is important. Necrotizing pancreatitis is identified on imaging such as a CT scan with contrast. Utilization of antibiotics to prevent sterile necrotizing pancreatitis from becoming infected is not recommended (Tenner et al., 2013).

Patients with peripancreatic necrosis who show signs of clinical deterioration 7 to 10 days into their course may have infected necrotizing pancreatitis. Treatment for these patients includes antimicrobials as well as a CT-guided needle aspiration to obtain a culture. Carbapenems, quinolones, and metronidazole are the antimicrobials of choice (Tenner et al., 2013). In patients who are showing signs of clinical stability or improvement, surgical or endoscopic intervention is not recommended for at least 4 weeks to allow the necrosis to demarcate. Patients who are showing signs of ongoing deterioration or instability should undergo surgical debridement.

CLINICAL PEARLS

- AP is commonly caused by gallstones, alcohol, or hyperlipidemia.
- AP is diagnosed using amylase or lipase three times the normal level, abdominal pain, and imaging.
- Pancreatitis is classified by the severity using the Atlanta criteria.
- Nutrition should be started as soon as symptoms improve in patients with pancreatitis.

10.8: PEPTIC ULCER DISEASE

Cathy Stepter

Peptic ulcer disease (PUD) is a disease manifested by a break or defect in the gastric or duodenal wall mucosa where erosion and ulceration forms. These ulcerations are created by acid that denudes the mucosa extending into the deeper wall layers. Two major causes include the presence of *Helicobacter pylori* infection or nonsteroidal anti-inflammatory drug (NSAID) ingestion (Fashner et al., 2015; Kavitt et al., 2019). Prevalence has decreased since the availability of H2RAs, proton pump inhibitors (PPIs), and *H. pylori* eradication treatment (Tonolini et al., 2017). However, PUD is still estimated to affect about 10% of people in the United States, with a higher incidence noted among males, smokers, those with chronic medical conditions, and increasing age (Kavitt et al., 2019; Narayanan et al., 2018). Stress ulcerations due to hospitalization have also been identified as a risk factor, particularly for patients in the intensive care unit (Cook & Guyatt, 2018). The spectrum of disease may include a range from asymptomatic to life-threatening presentations, including dyspepsia, gastrointestinal bleeding (GIB), gastric outlet obstruction and perforation (Gururatsakul et al., 2010; Kavitt et al., 2019).

H. pylori is a gram-negative bacterium that causes inflammation and epithelial cell degeneration and injury and is present in the majority of patients with gastric and duodenal ulcers (Narayanan et al., 2018). Bacteria invasion is usually acquired in childhood, colonizes in the gastric mucosa, and can progress to gastritis, PUD, and gastric cancer (Chey et al., 2017). A large segment of the world's population has *H. pylori* colonization, but only a small percent will develop clinical symptoms (Kavitt et al., 2019; Narayanan et al., 2018). The use of NSAIDs including aspirin (acetylsalicylic acid) is another common risk factor, with many cases associated with *H. pylori* colonization and NSAID use (Fashner et al., 2015; Kavitt et al., 2019; Narayanan et al., 2018).

Other risk factors for ulcer formation and bleeding include coadministration of corticosteroids and bisphosphonates with NSAIDs, selective serotonin reuptake inhibitors (SSRIs), 5-fluorouracil, anticoagulants, aldosterone antagonists, sirolimus, as well as neoplasms or idiopathic causes (Kavitt et al., 2019; Narayanan et al., 2018).

PRESENTING SIGNS AND SYMPTOMS

The most common presenting symptom with PUD is dyspepsia, often characterized as "gnawing" epigastric pain, that may be accompanied by bloating, abdominal fullness, nausea, vomiting, bleeding, weight loss, postprandial fullness, or early satiety (Kavitt et al., 2019; Narayanan et al., 2018). Many patients are asymptomatic, however, and a range of GIB presentations from occult to hemorrhage may be the first indication of ulceration (Gururatsakul et al., 2010). The most common complica-

tion associated with PUD is acute upper gastrointestinal hemorrhage, with worse outcomes seen in advanced age, shock presentation, and associated comorbid disease (Kavitt et al., 2019).

HISTORY AND PHYSICAL FINDINGS

Medical History

PUD includes both gastric and duodenal ulcers, and a detailed history of symptoms can help distinguish location. Gastric ulcers are more common between the ages of 55 and 65 years, while duodenal ulcers are more common between the ages of 30 and 55 years. Upper abdominal pain is the most common symptom, which may be worse in the right or left upper quadrants and may radiate to the back.

Classic gastric ulcer presentation is described as worsening pain with eating, often with subsequent epigastric fullness, early satiety, nausea, vomiting, and weight loss. Classic presentation for duodenal ulcers is worsening abdominal pain on an empty stomach, with relief of pain after eating (Gururatsakul et al., 2010; Narayanan et al., 2018; Tonolini et al., 2017). These complaints, combined with a history of NSAID use or a history of *H. pylori* infection, confirms suspicion for PUD.

The most common complication of PUD is GIB, which has significant associated morbidity (Kavitt et al., 2019). It is important to ascertain any history of GIB which includes hematemesis, melena, and hematochezia. Hematemesis, which may be either bright red or coffee ground, and melena, a black or tarry stool, may result from a peptic ulcer formation. Hematochezia, which is red or maroon blood in the stool, may be from ulceration and indicates a massive gastrointestinal bleed, which can lead to orthostatic hypotension (de Melo et al., 2013). Complaints of dyspepsia along with family history of gastrointestinal malignancy, age >60 years, weight loss, early satiety, GIB, iron deficiency anemia, and vomiting are considered alarm symptoms, warranting endoscopic evaluation (Kavitt et al., 2019).

Physical Examination

Physical examination may be unremarkable with the exception of mild epigastric tenderness or worsening abdominal pain in the right or left upper quadrants. Clinical presentation may be related to bleeding which includes melena, hematemesis or coffee-ground emesis, or symptoms of gastric outlet obstruction including nausea, vomiting, and abdominal distention. There is high clinical suspicion for perforation in patients who present with sudden development of severe, diffuse abdominal pain accompanied by abdominal rigidity.

DIFFERENTIAL DIAGNOSIS AND DIAGNOSTIC CONSIDERATIONS

Upper endoscopy testing in the presence of suspected or actual GIB is the most accurate initial test for PUD because of its diagnostic and therapeutic benefit (Kavitt et al., 2019).

Patients who are actively bleeding should generally be hospitalized and undergo timely evaluation depending on severity of bleed, hemodynamic stability, and risk, but generally within 24 hours of hospital admission (Laine & Jensen, 2012). Direct visualization of the ulcer via upper endoscopy allows for definitive diagnosis of PUD. Upper endoscopy is considered the mainstay of diagnostic testing for PUD, but ulcerations can also be detected via CT imaging (Tonolini et al., 2017). Routine repeat endoscopy is not recommended and should only be performed when there is evidence of continued bleeding (Laine & Jensen, 2012).

H. pylori infection is an important cause of PUD and its detection is paramount in treating the disease (Chey et al., 2017). A rapid urease test and direct histological testing is performed on biopsy specimens to detect *H. pylori* (Crowe, 2019; Fashner et al., 2015). All patients with active or past history of untreated PUD, a low-grade gastric mucosa-associated lymphoid tissue (MALT), or history of endoscopic resection of gastric cancer should be tested for *H. pylori* infection (Chey et al., 2017). Routine *H. pylori* screening is not recommended, but other risk factors, such as unexplained iron deficiency anemia, idiopathic thrombocytopenia purpura, or those taking long-term low-dose aspirin, may warrant testing (Chey et al., 2017).

The American College of Gastroenterology recommends testing for *H. pylori*, using a test-and-treat strategy for patients with dyspepsia and no alarm symptoms (Chey et al., 2017; Fashner et al., 2015). Several noninvasive mechanisms are available which include urea breath testing, stool monoclonal antigen tests, and serologic tests. Urea breath testing can be used for initial diagnosis of *H. pylori*, as well as for cure. This noninvasive test involves ingestion of urea labeled with nonradioactive isotopes and yields extremely high sensitivity (97%) and specificity (100%). To reduce false-negative results, PPI therapy must be discontinued for at least 2 weeks before re-testing for cure (Fashner et al., 2015).

Stool antigen testing is a more cost-effective monoclonal test that detects active *H. pylori* infection and requires less equipment than urea breath tests. This test can also be used as a test of cure. To reduce false-negative results, PPI therapy must be discontinued at least 2 weeks before testing (Fashner et al., 2015). Rapid urease testing is an invasive rapid test to detect cure, which is comparatively inexpensive, yielding 95% sensitivity and 100% specificity. Serologic antibody testing can be used to detect *H. pylori*-specific immunoglobulin G levels for patients who are unable to stop taking PPIs. However, this test cannot distinguish between active and past infection (Fashner et al., 2015).

Box 10.4 summarizes key differentials and diagnostic alarm symptoms.

TREATMENT

Proton Pump Inhibitors

PPI therapy promotes ulcer healing through acid suppression and is effective to heal >90% of peptic ulcers

---

BOX 10.4 PEPTIC ULCER DISEASE DIFFERENTIALS AND ALARM SYMPTOMS

PEPTIC ULCER DISEASE DIFFERENTIALS

Gastrointestinal infections	Gastritis
Crohn's disease	Esophagitis
Ischemia	Gastroesophageal reflux disease (GERD)
Gastrointestinal malignancy	Celiac disease
Biliary fistula	Esophageal perforation
Pancreatic fistula	

PEPTIC ULCER DISEASE ALARM SYMPTOMS*

Unexplained weight loss	Family history of gastrointestinal cancer
Progressive dysphagia	Overt gastrointestinal bleeding
Odynophagia	Abdominal mass
Recurrent vomiting	Iron deficiency anemia
	Jaundice

*Fashner, J., & Gitu, A. C. (2015). Diagnosis and treatment of peptic ulcer disease and H. pylori infection. American Family Physician, 91(4), 236–242. https://www.aafp.org/afp/2015/0215/p236.html

---

when NSAIDs are discontinued. Treatment duration is based upon etiology and ulcer complications, such as bleeding, perforation, penetration, or gastric outlet obstruction. Patients with complicated peptic ulcers, including bleeding, perforation, penetration, or gastric outlet obstruction should initially receive IV PPI therapy prior to endoscopic evaluation and while hospitalized (Kavitt et al., 2019; Laine & Jensen, 2012). They can then switch to oral high dose therapy twice daily, then daily after 4 weeks. Duration of PPI therapy depends on location and cause of the ulcer. Generally, a duodenal ulcer requires PPI therapy for 4 to 8 weeks, and a gastric ulcer requires therapy for 8 to 12 weeks (Wolfe & Sachs, 2000).

PPI therapy, such as omeprazole 20 to 40 mg, provides faster control of PUD symptoms and higher ulcer healing rates compared with H2RAs, and heals NSAID-related ulcers more effectively (Kavitt et al., 2019). Discontinuation of NSAIDs, including aspirin, is strongly recommended for NSAID-related ulcerations. Patients who must remain on NSAIDs or ASA should continue daily PPI maintenance therapy to reduce risk of complications or recurrence (Kavitt et al., 2019; Laine & Jensen, 2012). Ulcers not caused by *H. pylori* or NSAID use may be more difficult to heal, have a higher rate of recurrence, and require long-term PPI therapy.

Acid suppression prophylaxis and the prevention of stress-induced ulcers for hospitalized patients has been a long-time practice, and extensively reviewed. A recent review and recommendations warn of widespread acid suppression prophylaxis as common practice. PPI prophylaxis may be reasonable for patients at elevated risk for developing a gastrointestinal bleed (GIB), such as those receiving concurrent NSAID or anticoagulant

TABLE 10.7: Recommended Therapies for *H. pylori* Eradication

Standard Triple Preferred First-Line Therapy Option 1	Standard Triple Therapy Option 2
• PPI • Amoxicillin 1 g • Clarithromycin 500 mg • Twice daily for 7–10 days	• PPI • Clarithromycin 500 mg • Metronidazole 500 mg • Twice daily for 10–14 days
Quadruple Therapy (May Also Be Used if First-Line Therapy Fails) • Bismuth subsalicylate 525 mg or subcitrate 300 mg • Metronidazole 250 mg • Tetracycline 500 mg • Four times daily for 10–14 days • Additionally, take PPI twice daily	

therapy (Cook & Guyatt, 2018). However, the risk for development of hospital-acquired pneumonia or *Clostridioides difficile* (*C. difficile*) infection must also be considered. Routine use of PPI therapy for low-risk hospitalized patients may actually cause harm (Cook & Guyatt, 2018).

Helicobacter pylori *Eradication*

The American College of Gastroenterology recommends eradication of *H. pylori* for all patients with PUD (Fashner et al., 2015). For an uncomplicated ulcer, standard first line triple therapy regimen of a PPI, amoxicillin 1 g, and clarithromycin 500 mg twice daily for 7 to 10 days is effective to eradicate *H. pylori*. Antibiotic resistance to clarithromycin may necessitate substitution of metronidazole for amoxicillin. Additionally, probiotic usage with lactobacillus has shown success with increasing eradication. Failed first-line therapy may warrant use of a quadruple therapy regimen with the addition of bismuth and tetracycline for 10 to 14 days (Table 10.7; Fashner et al., 2015).

The American College of Gastroenterology recommends confirmation of *H. pylori* infection eradication after completion of initial therapy (Chey et al., 2017). To reduce false-negative results, PPIs must be held 1 to 2 weeks prior to testing. An ulcer that persists >5 mm after 8 to 12 weeks of PPI therapy is refractory to treatment. Smoking, prior ulcer history, and some comorbid conditions may affect the overall healing process, requiring prolonged acid suppression therapy.

CLINICAL PEARLS

- Most peptic ulcers are caused by *H. pylori* infection and/or NSAID use.
- Upper endoscopy is the mainstay of PUD diagnosis. Routine repeat endoscopies are not recommended.
- PPIs suppress acid formation and are first line therapy for PUD.
- *H. pylori* must be eradicated and requires triple therapy with antibiotics and PPIs. If first line therapy fails, quadruple therapy may be effective. Noninvasive testing is available.
- Long-term PPI therapy may be required for those requiring continued NSAIDs.
- Providers must consider risk prior to prophylaxis PPI therapy to prevent stress-induced ulcers.

10.9: GASTRITIS

Cathy Stepter

Gastritis is a condition where there is inflammation in the epithelial tissue of the stomach and can be erosive or nonerosive. The condition occurs most commonly in those taking NSAIDs, alcoholics, chronically ill and critically ill patients. Gastritis is prominent worldwide and is strongly associated with the presence of *Helicobacter pylori* (*H. pylori*) infection, with serious implications if undetected and untreated. There has been a decline in prevalence, which is parallel with the decline in *H. pylori* infection (Sipponen & Maaroos, 2015).

Chronic gastritis is a progressive and often lifelong inflammation that can cause a loss of mucosal glands, resulting in atrophic gastritis in the antrum, fundus, or both. These further result in metaplasia of displaced immature intestinal or small bowel cells. Chronic mucosal atrophy leads to decreased production of hydrochloric acid and intrinsic factor, which causes malabsorption of vitamin B_{12}, iron, calcium, magnesium, zinc, and some medications (Sipponen & Maaroos, 2015). The pathogenesis of gastritis and chronic *H. pylori* infection is strongly linked to the development of peptic ulcers and gastric cancers. Because of hypochlorhydria, colonization of microbes that produce carcinogens like acetaldehyde and nitrosamines can occur, which can lead to peptic ulcer formation and gastric cancer (Sipponen & Maaroos, 2015).

Gastritis may be acute or chronic, with acute inflammation histology showing neutrophilic infiltration, and chronic inflammation histology showing mixed mononuclear lymphocytes, plasma cells, and macrophages (Dixon et al., 1997). Certain histological distinctions further classify gastritis, including an autoimmune chronic gastritis. Autoimmune metaplastic gastritis (AMAG) is distinguished by the disruption of gastric acid secretion not associated with ongoing *H. pylori* infection (Sipponen & Maaroos, 2015). This atrophic gastritis results from autoimmune destruction of the parietal cells and intrinsic factor and is commonly associated with vitamin B_{12} deficiency and pernicious anemia. Destruction of the gastric fundus mucosa and resultant achlorhydria leads to hypergastrinemia, which can lead to cancerous cell growth (Minalyan et al., 2017; Park et al., 2013). It is not known if *H. pylori* infection causes an autoimmune reaction in some patients that triggers chronic inflammation, or if there is a pure autoimmune etiology (Sipponen & Maaroos, 2015).

A rare and life-threatening form of necrotizing gastritis can occur from rapidly, progressive acute bacterial Streptococci, Staphylococci, *Proteus, Clostridium,* or *Escherichia coli* infections, particularly in immunocompromised patients. Prompt diagnosis and management with antimicrobial therapy are required, and may require emergency gastrectomy (Iqbal et al., 2018). Cytomegalovirus viral infections or *Candida* fungal infections may also cause gastritis in immunocompromised or diabetic patients.

Stress-induced gastritis is also an important clinical management issue among critically ill patients due to the risk for bleeding. Bleeding can be in the esophagus, stomach, or duodenum (Ye et al., 2020). Risk factors for stress-induced gastritis among critically ill patients include mechanical ventilation for at least 48 hours; coagulopathy defined as a platelet count <50,000, an INR >1.5, or a >2× partial-thromboplastin time; males; age >50; and trauma, burns, shock, sepsis, hepatic, and kidney injury (Bardou et al., 2015).

PRESENTING SIGNS AND SYMPTOMS

Gastritis presentation can range from asymptomatic to mild diffuse inflammation, peptic or gastric ulcer formation, or gastric cancer. Associated signs and symptoms may include recurrent epigastric pain or dyspepsia, anorexia, nausea, vomiting, and abdominal pain. In the critically ill patient, relevant clinical manifestations may include occult bleeding found in stool or nasogastric aspirate, or overt bleeding manifested by frank bright red blood, coffee-ground hematemesis, or melena (Bardou et al., 2015). The associated mortality can be high considering underlying illness and associated comorbidities.

HISTORY AND PHYSICAL FINDINGS

Medical History

A thorough history and review of systems, with review of medications, specifically NSAIDs and aspirin therapy, along with diet and excessive alcohol consumption are important. A past medical history of ulcers, GIB, renal or hepatic disease, coagulation disorders, or a family history of gastric cancers should also be assessed.

Physical Examination

Physical examination may be noncontributory.

DIFFERENTIAL DIAGNOSIS AND DIAGNOSTIC CONSIDERATIONS

Evaluation of complete blood count (CBC) is important to establish presence of anemia, and its severity. Patients with alarm symptoms including severe abdominal pain, GIB, vomiting, or significant weight loss should undergo

> ### BOX 10.5 DIFFERENTIAL DIAGNOSES FOR GASTRITIS
>
> - Biliary tract disease
> - Esophageal varices
> - Food poisoning
> - Gastric cancer
> - Gastrointestinal ischemia
> - Mallory-Weiss tear
> - Perforating ulcer
> - Peptic ulcer disease
> - Viral gastroenteritis

upper-endoscopy diagnostic testing. Noninvasive testing for *H. pylori* with fecal antigen immunoassay and urea breath test, and invasive endoscopy testing when indicated, is covered in the peptic ulcer disease section of this chapter. Differential diagnoses are summarized in Box 10.5.

TREATMENT

Treatment for gastritis includes PPIs therapy for a period of 2 to 4 weeks and discontinue use of NSAIDs when possible. Mild cases may respond and benefit from short-term H2RAs, antacids, or mucosal coating agents such as sucralfate. If unable to discontinue NSAIDs and symptoms do not improve with PPI therapy, consider need for upper endoscopy diagnostic evaluation. Treatment for *H. pylori* infection is covered in the peptic ulcer disease section of this chapter.

Stress Ulcer Prophylaxis in Critically Ill Patients

Prophylactic treatment with use of PPIs or H2RAs to reduce stress ulcer incidence among critically ill patients has been a focus for many years. Available evidence continues to shape clinical guideline recommendations. Current guidelines recommend that critically ill patients with a 4% or higher risk of GIB be placed on prophylactic acid suppression therapy with PPIs or H2RAs (Ye et al., 2020). High risk includes mechanical ventilation without enteral nutrition, chronic liver disease, concerning coagulopathy, and those with two or more of the following risk factors: shock, sepsis, acute kidney injury, and mechanical ventilation with enteral nutrition. Low risk includes critically ill patients without any risk factor, acute hepatic failure, use of steroids or immunosuppression, use of anticoagulants, cancer, and male gender (Ye et al., 2020).

The concerns for PPI and H2RA therapy use among critically ill patients include outcomes risks for pneumonia, *C. difficile* infection, impact on intensive care length of stay and mortality. Current studies indicate that PPIs reduce bleeding risk more than H2RAs, but there is no other significant difference in outcomes of care. Sucralfate is not recommended in critically ill patients (Ye et al., 2020).

CLINICAL PEARLS

- Gastritis is an inflammatory condition of the gastric mucosa and may be caused by *H. pylori* infection, autoimmune disease, infection, or be stress-induced.
- Development of GIB is a serious concern.
- Untreated erosive gastritis pathogenesis causes metaplasia, which can lead to gastric cancer.
- PPI or H2RA therapy is usually effective to treat gastritis. *H. pylori* infection must be eradicated. Prophylactic therapy with PPIs or H2RAs is warranted among high-risk critically ill patients.

10.10: END-STAGE LIVER DISEASE

Amy Stoddard

Patients who have liver diseases that have progressed to failure are considered end-stage liver disease (ESLD). For patients who have reached ESLD, a referral to a transplant center is needed to determine if the patient is a liver transplant candidate. ESLD has several complications that require identification and treatment. The complications discussed in this section include cirrhosis, hepatic encephalopathy, ascites, and variceal bleeding.

10.10A: CIRRHOSIS

Cirrhosis is a complication due to the inflammation and hepatic fibrosis from chronic liver disease (Smith et al., 2019). Eventually, structures within the liver will collapse, nodules within the liver will develop, the vasculature within the liver becomes distorted, and the hepatic parenchyma distorts, leading to a decrease in liver function (Smith et al., 2019). Pathophysiologic changes in the liver lead to decreased function, which causes increased bilirubin, coagulopathy due to diminished production of clotting factors and thrombopoietin, and splenic platelet sequestration (Smith et al., 2019). In addition, portal pressure increases causing portal hypertension, which leads to the development of ascites and variceal bleeding (Smith et al., 2019). Cirrhosis is the 12th leading cause of death in the United States and is reversible if caught before the irreversible fibrotic changes develop (Smith et al., 2019).

PRESENTING SIGNS AND SYMPTOMS

Presenting signs and symptoms of cirrhosis are summarized in Table 10.8.

TABLE 10.8: Presenting Signs and Symptoms of Cirrhosis

Compensated Cirrhosis	Decompensated Cirrhosis
• Fatigue	• Ascites
• Loss of appetite	• Hepatic encephalopathy
• Right upper quadrant (RUQ) pain	• Jaundice
• Unexplained weight loss	• Peripheral edema
• Weakness	• Portal hypertension (HTN)

HISTORY AND PHYSICAL FINDINGS

If the patient has compensated cirrhosis, they are typically asymptomatic but may present with the symptoms listed in Table 10.8 (Smith et al., 2019). Decompensated patients present with many different signs and symptoms, as noted in Table 10.8 (Smith et al., 2019). Physical exam findings for both types of cirrhosis include: general muscle wasting asterixis, drowsiness, confusion, fetor hepaticus, jaundice, parotid enlargement, scleral icterus, gynecomastia, spider nevi, ascites, caput medusae, enlarged liver, splenomegaly, nail clubbing, Dupuytren contracture of the fingers/hands, palmar erythema, terry nails, testicular atrophy in men, and distal erythema, edema, and petechiae in the lower extremities (Smith et al., 2019)

DIFFERENTIAL DIAGNOSIS AND DIAGNOSTIC CONSIDERATIONS

Possible differentials that need to be ruled out are malignancy, heart failure, pericarditis, Budd-Chiari syndrome, portal vein thrombosis, splenic vein thrombosis, and infection (Bethea & Chopra, 2018). Laboratory tests that should be considered are AST (aspartate transaminase)/ALT to check hepatocellular injury, alkaline phosphatase, serum bilirubin, GGT, and 5'-nucleotidase to monitor cholestasis, serum albumin to assess synthetic liver function, and PT/INR to determine coagulation status (Bethea & Chopra, 2018). Diagnostic tests include viral hepatitis panel, iron studies to check for Wilson's disease, alpha-1 antitrypsin (A1AT) level, and protease inhibitor type to check for A1AT deficiency, tissue transglutaminase to check for celiac disease, serum immunoglobulins, and autoantibodies to check for autoimmune causes (Box 10.6; Bethea & Chopra, 2018). Abdominal ultrasound is the most helpful imaging study because it can detect ascites and bile duct dilation, and duplex Doppler studies can be obtained to check for vascular patency (Bethea & Chopra, 2018). Liver biopsy is the gold standard for diagnosing cirrhosis currently (Bethea & Chopra, 2018).

TREATMENT

Prevention of further complications, decompensation, and death is key when a patient presents with cirrhosis (Smith et al., 2019). If the patient has portal hypertension, the risk of varices increases, these patients should

BOX 10.6 IMPORTANT DIAGNOSTIC TESTS FOR CIRRHOSIS

- **Labs:** AST/ALT, alkaline phosphatase, serum bilirubin, GGT, 5'- nucleotidase, albumin, PT/INR
- **Imaging:** Abdominal ultrasound with Doppler
- **Liver Biopsy:** Gold standard for diagnosis

be screened for esophageal varices via endoscopy routinely (Smith et al., 2019). Monitoring and treating ascites are vital as it increases mortality, decreases quality of life, and increases the risk of further complications such as infection, hernias, and respiratory compromise (Smith et al., 2019). Any development of hepatic encephalopathy, ascites, or variceal bleed warrants referral to a hepatologist (Smith et al., 2019).

CLINICAL PEARLS

- Decompensated cirrhosis leads to further complications and death if left untreated.
- Labs are monitored closely, and prognostic score updated (such as the Model for End-Stage Liver Disease [MELD] Score, Child-Pugh Score and others).
- The gold standard for diagnosis is a liver biopsy.
- Treatment is the prevention of further complications such as hepatic encephalopathy, ascites, and variceal bleed; if these complications occur, referral to hepatologist/transplant center is warranted.

10.10B: HEPATIC ENCEPHALOPATHY

One of the common complications of liver disease is hepatic encephalopathy (HE). HE is defined as a metabolic disorder that leads to neuropsychiatric disturbances that are reversible (Jaffe et al., 2020). HE occurs most commonly in chronic liver failure; however, it may occur in the acute liver failure setting (Allampati & Mullen, 2018). HE can be due to hepatocellular failure or portosystemic shunting (PSS; Jaffe et al., 2020). The HE patient may present along a broad spectrum of symptoms varying from mild cognitive impairment to a comatose state (Jaffe et al., 2020). There is a high morbidity rate associated with HE in acute and chronic liver failure patients; in decompensated cirrhosis patients, HE represents the most common reason for hospital admission (Jaffe et al., 2020).

PRESENTING SIGNS AND SYMPTOMS

Patients with HE may present with varying neuropsychiatric symptoms that range from mild deficits, altered sleep patterns, short-term memory loss, anxiety, depression, and euphoria to a comatose state (Dellatore et al., 2020).

HISTORY AND PHYSICAL FINDINGS

Patients who present with HE have a history of liver disease (hepatocellular failure) or PSS (Dellatore et al., 2020). Due to the spectrum of possible presenting symptoms, HE is mostly a diagnosis of exclusion (Shawcross, 2018). When obtaining the history, it is crucial to determine if precipitating factors are present (Box 10.7). The precipitating factors of HE are infection, gastrointestinal bleeding (GIB), recent transjugular intrahepatic portosystemic shunt (TIPS) procedure, vomiting and diarrhea, large-volume paracentesis, electrolyte imbalance due to

BOX 10.7 HISTORY AND PHYSICAL FINDINGS

- Check for precipitating factors such as infection, gastrointestinal bleed, metabolic derangements/electrolyte disturbances, recent transjugular intrahepatic portosystemic shunt (TIPS) procedure, vomiting, diarrhea, or hypovolemia.
- In patients with known cirrhosis, suspect hepatic encephalopathy but always rule out differentials.
- Findings may be subtle and present as insomnia, hypersomnia, euphoria, anxiety, depression, lack of awareness, loss of attention span, or inability to do basic math.

possible recent dosing of diuretics, constipation, and any ingestion of any sedating medications or alcohol (Shawcross, 2018).

When examining the patient, a thorough neurologic exam is crucial. While the patient may be alert and oriented to person, place, time, and situation, subtle neurologic changes such as anxiety, bizarre behavior, euphoria, lack of awareness, or short attention span may be noticeable (Dellatore et al., 2020). The patient may also present on the opposite end of the spectrum and may be confused, disoriented, somnolent, or comatose (Dellatore et al., 2020). Further examination may reveal ataxia, asterixis, bradykinesia, hyperactive deep tendon reflexes, nystagmus, and slurring of speech (Dellatore et al., 2020). The physical findings of liver disease that one might find are jaundice, ascites, palmar erythema, and spider telangiectasias (Dellatore et al., 2020).

DIFFERENTIAL DIAGNOSIS AND DIAGNOSTIC CONSIDERATIONS

In any patient with known liver disease who presents with neurologic dysfunction, one should suspect hepatic encephalopathy (Allampati & Mullen, 2018). However, the differentials that need to be ruled out are intracranial abnormalities such as ischemic or hemorrhagic stroke, other metabolic derangements/electrolyte disturbances, ingestion of toxic substances, a possible overdose of medications, and sepsis (Shawcross, 2018).

Diagnostic tests are obtained that not only assist in proving but also excluding HE. A full set of laboratory tests that include a complete blood count (CBC), comprehensive metabolic panel (CMP), serum ammonia, urinalysis, and blood cultures are obtained upon presentation; also, a paracentesis should be performed if the patient has ascites to rule out spontaneous bacterial peritonitis (SBP; Shawcross, 2018). This may also determine if a precipitating factor such as GIB or infection is present. If this is an acute presentation, obtain a head CT to rule out intracranial abnormalities (Shawcross, 2018). In the awake patient, the neuropsychometric tests needed to classify overt and covert HE should be obtained (Table 10.9). The Psychometric Hepatic Encephalopathy Score (PHES) test evalu-

TABLE 10.9: West Haven Criteria for Classification of Hepatic Encephalopathy

GRADE	DESCRIPTION	RECOMMENDED TESTS
0	No abnormality detected	–
Minimal (covert)	Normal mental status and neurologic examination Abnormal psychometric tests	>2 SD on two or more tests in PHES ICT: >5 lures CFF: Cutoff frequency 39 Hz
I	Trivial lack of awareness Euphoria or anxiety Shortened attention span Impairment of addition or subtraction	Naming ≤7 animals in 120 sec Orientation in time and space
II	Lethargy or apathy Disorientation for time Obvious personality change Inappropriate behavior	Disorientation in time (≥3 items incorrect): Day of the week Day of the month The month The year Orientation to place
III	Somnolence to semistupor Responsiveness to stimuli Confusion Gross disorientation Bizarre behavior	Disorientation to place (≥2 items incorrect): State/country Region/county City Place Floor/ward Disorientation to time (as above) Reduction of Glasgow coma score (8–14)
IV	Coma, inability to test mental state	Unresponsiveness to pain stimuli (Glasgow coma score <8)

CFF, Critical Flicker/Fusion Frequency; HE, hepatic encephalopathy; ICT, inhibitory control test; PHES, Psychometric Hepatic Encephalopathy Score; SD, standard deviation.

Source: From Allampati, S., & Mullen, K. (2018). Hepatic encephalopathy. In P. Martin & L. S. Friedman (Eds.), *Handbook of liver disease* (4th ed., pp. 207–216). Elsevier. https://doi.org/10.1016/B978-0-323-47874-8.00015-8

ates the cognitive function and psychomotor processing speed and visuomotor coordination using five written exams (Shawcross, 2018). The Inhibitory Control Test (ICT) is a test taken on the computer that tests response inhibition and working memory (Shawcross, 2018). The naming seven animals test can also be used at the bedside in addition to asking baseline exam questions to determine the neurocognitive function (Shawcross, 2018).

TREATMENT

Most patients who present with HE have a precipitating factor initiated at the onset of the episode; correction of any precipitating factors is key to treatment (Allampati & Mullen, 2018). Empiric treatment includes a low to zero protein diet, gut cleansing with an enema or gastric lavage, and lactulose administration (Box 10.8; Allampati & Mullen, 2018). Second-line treatment is summarized in Table 10.10.

Long-Term Management

Long-term management for HE (Box 10.9) requires patient adherence, which includes following a prescribed regime of lactulose and rifaximin and a vegetable based-low protein diet at home. (Allampati & Mullen, 2018).

For recurrent HE, the patient should be referred for a liver transplant evaluation (Allampati & Mullen, 2018). If the patient has a portosystemic shunt or transjugular

BOX 10.8 EMPIRIC TREATMENT OF HEPATIC ENCEPHALOPATHY

- Empiric treatment consists of a low to zero protein diet, gut cleansing with enemas or gastric lavage, and lactulose administration.
- Lactulose should be given 15 mL every 2 hours until liquid bowel movements are noted, then change to 30 mL every 4 hours to maintain 2 to 3 bowel movements per day.

TABLE 10.10: Second-Line Treatment for Hepatic Encephalopathy

MEDICATION	ADMINISTRATION INSTRUCTIONS
Rifaximin	550 mg BID
Metronidazole	250 mg PO QID (short-term use)
Neomycin	500 mg PO QID (use higher doses with caution)
Vancomycin	250 mg PO QID
Sodium benzoate	Not approved for use in the United States
Other cathartic agents and branched-chain amino acids are beneficial	Not approved for this use by the U.S. Food and Drug Administration

BOX 10.9 LONG-TERM MANAGEMENT OF HEPATIC ENCEPHALOPATHY

- The patient should be discharged with lactulose to take orally; the frequency should be enough to have 2 to 3 BMs per day.
- The patient should also be discharged on rifaximin, which is given in addition to lactulose to decrease HE episode frequency.
- The patient should eat a vegetable-based protein diet at home.
- If the patient has recurrent episodes of HE, a referral for a liver transplant should be made. If the patient has a portosystemic shunt, the patient should be referred back to the surgeon to determine if it can be closed or the diameter reduced.

intrahepatic portosystemic shunt (TIPS), referral back to a hepatobiliary surgeon may be necessary as this may be amenable to closure or reduction in diameter (Allampati & Mullen, 2018).

CLINICAL PEARLS

- HE is a complication of liver disease that is reversible.
- Physical exam findings will vary with each patient, depending on the severity of the HE.
- Obtaining a history from the patient or family member to determine if there is a precipitating factor is critical for treatment.
- Treatment of precipitating factors and empiric therapy should begin immediately.
- Second-line therapy may be needed to obtain control of the HE.
- Long-term therapy will include lactulose and rifaximin in addition to diet changes.
- Referral of refractory HE to a liver transplant center is necessary, or referral to a surgeon or gastroenterologist for portosystem shunt options.

10.10C: ASCITES

Ascites is an accumulation of fluid in the peritoneal cavity that occurs due to the increase in portal hypertension (Patidar & Sanyal, 2018). Ascites is the most common complication of cirrhosis; approximately 85% of patients with ascites have cirrhosis (Patidar & Sanyal, 2018). When a patient with cirrhosis develops ascites, this is considered the transition from compensated to decompensated cirrhosis (Patidar & Sanyal, 2018). Ascites will typically develop in about 50% of patients with cirrhosis within the first 10 years of diagnosis. Once ascites is present, the risk of spontaneous bacterial peritonitis (SBP) and renal complications increases (Figure 10.2; Patidar & Sanyal, 2018).

PRESENTING SIGNS AND SYMPTOMS

Patients may present with abdominal distention, lower extremity edema, possible difficulty breathing, and caput medusae on the abdomen (Patidar & Sanyal, 2018).

HISTORY AND PHYSICAL FINDINGS

Physical examination reveals a full and enlarged abdomen with flank dullness on percussion and a positive fluid wave. Shifting dullness may represent greater than 1500 mL of fluid in the abdomen (Patidar & Sanyal, 2018). If the fluid collection is extensive, the patient may have difficulty breathing as well. The patient will also have the typical exam of a patient with cirrhosis, as mentioned previously.

DIFFERENTIAL DIAGNOSIS AND DIAGNOSTIC CONSIDERATIONS

It is always important to rule out possible differentials such as underlying malignancy, congestive heart failure, infection such as tuberculosis, or renal disease (Patidar & Sanyal, 2018). The confirmation diagnostic exam is the abdominal ultrasound because it can detect as little as 100 mL of fluid in the abdomen (Patidar & Sanyal, 2018).

TREATMENT

Treatment of ascites in the cirrhosis patient is to induce and maintain a negative sodium balance of at least 78 mmol per day, which is accomplished by a strict sodium-restricted diet and the use of spironolactone (an aldosterone antagonist/distal convoluted tubule-acting diuretic; Patidar & Sanyal, 2018). Lasix may be combined with spironolactone but not used alone, because lasix does not adequately allow for sodium removal (Patidar & Sanyal, 2018).

Refractory ascites is divided into two categories: diuretic resistant and diuretic intractable; these are treated with large-volume paracentesis and are considered for a TIPS procedure (Box 10.10; Patidar & Sanyal, 2018). There is a 10% annual risk of a SBP infection, which requires prompt administration of broad-spectrum antibiotics (Patidar & Sanyal, 2018).

CLINICAL PEARLS

- Ascites is the most common complication of cirrhosis, and 50% of cirrhosis patients will develop ascites within 10 years, the risk of ascites being infectious is 10% each year.
- Classic physical findings are a large full abdomen, lower extremity edema, and dullness on percussion.
- Abdominal ultrasound is the preferred diagnostic exam due to the ability to pick up small amounts of fluid.
- Treatment begins with a sodium-restricted diet and spironolactone; Lasix (furosemide) may be added.
- Refractory ascites requires large volume paracentesis or consideration of TIPS (transjugular intrahepatic portosystemic shunt)

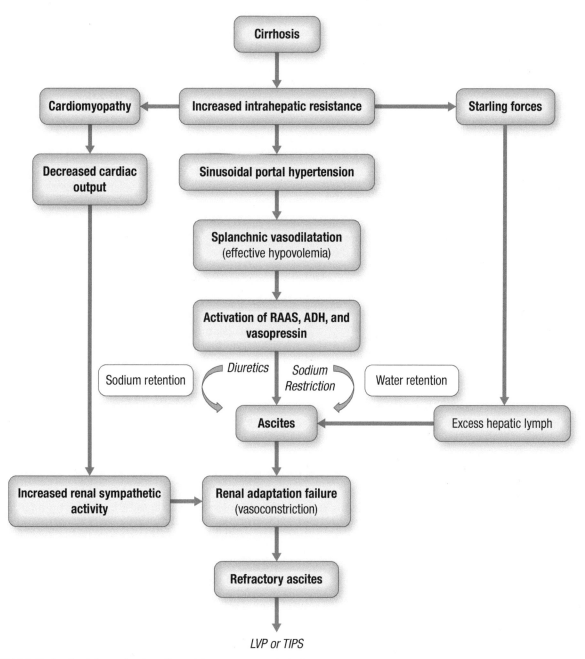

FIGURE 10.2: Pathophysiology of ascites. Potential treatments are in italics.
ADH, Antidiuretic hormone; LVP, large-volume paracentesis; RAAS, renin-angiotensin-aldosterone system; TIPS, transjugular intrahepatic portosystemic shunt.
Source: From Patidar, K. R., & Sanyal, A. J. (2018). Hepatic encephalopathy. In P. Martin & L. S. Friedman (Eds.), *Handbook of liver disease* (4th ed., pp. 182–196). Elsevier.

10.10D: VARICEAL BLEEDING

Patients with decompensated cirrhosis may have portal hypertension, which is defined as a hepatic venous portal gradient (HVPG) greater than 10 mmHg (Grace et al., 2018). Blood vessels in the esophagus become enlarged over time, despite the development of collaterals; the portal hypertension increases causing rupture and bleeding (Grace et al., 2018). In those patients with alcoholic cirrhosis, approximately 50% will develop esophageal varices within 2 years; other liver diseases have less risk of developing varices (Grace et al., 2018). Esophageal variceal

BOX 10.10 DEFINITION AND DIAGNOSTIC CRITERIA OF REFRACTORY ASCITES

Diuretic-resistant ascites: **Inability to mobilize ascites or prevent the early recurrence of ascites after a large- volume paracentesis because of the lack of response to dietary sodium restriction and intensive diuretic therapy (maximum doses of spironolactone and furosemide).**

Diuretic-intractable ascites: **Inability to mobilize ascites or prevent the early recurrence of ascites after a large-volume paracentesis due to the development of diuretic-induced complications that preclude the use of an effective diuretic dose.**

Diagnostic Criteria

- *Treatment duration:* **Patients must be on intensive diuretic therapy for at least 1 week and on a salt-restricted diet of <88 mmol/day.**
- *Lack of response:* **Mean weight loss of <0.8 kg over 4 days and urinary sodium output less than the sodium intake (i.e., urine sodium-to-potassium ratio <1).**
- *Early ascites recurrence:* **Recurrence of grade 2 or 3 ascites within 1 month of initial mobilization.**
- *Diuretic-induced complications:* **Hepatic encephalopathy, renal impairment, and diuretic-induced hyponatremia (<125 mEq/L).**

Source: From Patidar, K. R., & Sanyal, A. J. (2018). Hepatic encephalopathy. In P. Martin & L. S. Friedman (Eds.), *Handbook of liver disease* (4th ed., pp. 182–196). Elsevier.

TABLE 10.11: Pharmacological Treatment of the Acute Variceal Bleed

DRUG	ROUTE	DOSE
Terlipressin	IV	Initially 1–2 mg every 4 hours until control of bleeding; then 1 mg every 4 hours maintenance
Somatostatin	IV	Initial bolus of 250 mcg followed by continuous infusion of 250–500 mcg/h
Octreotide	IV	Initial bolus of 50 mcg followed by continuous infusion of 50 mcg/hr

Treatment should be continued for 5 days IV.
Source: Data from Grace, N. D., Stoffel, E. M., & Puleo, J. (2018). Hepatic encephalopathy. In P. Martin & L. S. Friedman (Eds.), *Handbook of liver disease* (4th ed., pp. 172–181). Elsevier.

hemorrhage has a mortality rate of 15% to 20% with each bleeding episode (Grace et al., 2018).

HISTORY AND PHYSICAL FINDINGS

Cirrhosis patients who present with hematemesis may have esophageal or gastric varices due to portal hypertension (Grace et al., 2018). Physical examination findings will be the same as those with decompensated cirrhosis (Grace et al., 2018).

DIFFERENTIAL DIAGNOSIS AND DIAGNOSTIC CONSIDERATIONS

Possible differentials could be aortic-esophageal fistula—particularly if the patient has had aortic surgery—an upper gastrointestinal bleeding ulcer, or underlying malignancy. Once the patient is stable, the patient should undergo diagnostic and therapeutic endoscopy (Grace et al., 2018).

TREATMENT

Acute variceal bleeds should be treated as life-threatening; an airway should be established in those who are unable to protect their airway, large-bore IV access should be obtained, and preparation for possible blood product or factor administration are part of the initial resuscitation (Grace et al., 2018). The only measure of establishing source control is endoscopy with direct banding or Cyanoacrylate glue as well as incorporating local and systemic vasoactive agents. (Grace et al., 2018). Cyanoacrylate glue does carry the risks of bacteremia and glue embolization (Grace et al., 2018). The vasoactive pharmacological agents listed in Table 10.11 are used to treat acute bleed (Grace et al., 2018). The TIPS procedure is the treatment of choice for gastric variceal bleeds that fail pharmacological therapy, and balloon tamponade may be used if emergent endoscopy is unavailable (Grace et al., 2018).

Prevention of recurrent variceal bleed is crucial, and the risk of rebleed is highest in the first 6 months from the first bleed (Table 10.12; Grace et al., 2018). Endoscopic variceal ligation (EVL) is the preferred therapy to prevent recurrent bleeding (Grace et al., 2018). Beta-blockers are also used for the prevention of variceal bleeds in addition to frequent EVLs (Grace et al., 2018).

CLINICAL PEARLS

- Portal hypertension (HVPG >10 mmHg) will cause varices to form and bleed.
- Mortality with esophageal variceal hemorrhage is high.
- Acute bleeds need to be treated as life-threatening, and resuscitation measures should be taken.
- Source control of an acute esophageal bleed is only accomplished by endoscopy; vasoactive agents will sometimes be used locally and systemically to treat the acute bleed.
- TIPS is the treatment of choice for variceal bleeds that fail endoscopic and pharmacologic therapy.
- Prevention of rebleeding is crucial and is accomplished with beta-blockers.

TABLE 10.12: Pharmacological Prevention of Variceal Bleeding

DRUG	INITIAL DOSE	THERAPEUTIC DOSE RANGE
Propranolol	40 mg twice/day	40-320 mg/day
Nadolol	40 mg/day	40-160 mg/day
Timolol	10 mg/day	5-40 mg/day
Carvedilol	6.25 mg/day	6.25-12.5 mg/day
Isosorbide 5-mononitrate	20 mg twice/day	20 mg 3-4 times/day

Source: Data from Grace, N. D., Stoffel, E. M., & Puleo, J. (2018). Hepatic encephalopathy. In P. Martin & L. S. Friedman (Eds.), *Handbook of liver disease* (4th ed., pp. 172–181). Elsevier.

10.11: SURGICAL ABDOMEN/ACUTE ABDOMINAL PAIN

Bimbola Akintade

Surgical abdomen, sometimes referred to as acute abdomen, is an intraabdominal condition of abrupt onset and severe pain requiring emergency surgical intervention due to infection, obstruction, perforation, vascular occlusion, inflammation, infarction, or rupture of abdominal organs and vessels (Di Saverio et al., 2020; Snyder et al., 2018).

Due to the large number of possible causes of a surgical abdomen, the approach to evaluating such patients includes a thorough history and physical exam. Symptoms such as the location of pain to the presence of free air on radiographic examination may help clinicians narrow down differential diagnoses (Dumas et al., 2018; Elhardello & MacFie, 2018). Causes of a surgical abdomen include but are not limited to the following: appendicitis, acute cholecystitis, cholangitis, peritonitis, intussusception, bowel infarction, obstruction, perforation, and diverticulitis (Di Saverio et al., 2020; Elhardello & MacFie, 2018; Snyder et al., 2018).

Surgical abdomen may be caused by acute peritonitis and can result from a complication of IBD or malignancy or rupture of a hollow viscus organ. Mesenteric ischemia and ruptured abdominal aortic aneurysm are examples of vascular events causing a surgical abdomen. Other uncommon causes of surgical abdomen include urologic conditions (ureteral colic and pyelonephritis) and obstetric and gynecologic causes (ruptured ectopic pregnancy and ovarian torsion; Di Saverio et al., 2020; Elhardello & MacFie, 2018).

10.11A: APPENDICITIS

Appendicitis is defined as an inflammation of the inner lining of the appendix leading to increased mucus production and bacterial overgrowth, leading to wall tension and potentially necrosis and perforation (Di Saverio et al., 2020; Dumas et al., 2018; Snyder et al., 2018). It also

accounts for approximately 10% of all emergency department visits and the most common diagnosis made in young patients admitted to the hospital with an acute abdomen. In the United States, more than 300,000 appendectomies are performed annually (Huang et al., 2017).

A major complication of appendicitis is perforation. Perforation rates for individuals with appendicitis varies with a higher frequency occurring in the younger population and the elderly. Compared to nonperforating appendicitis, perforating appendicitis is associated with increased morbidity and mortality (Dumas et al., 2018).

PRESENTING SIGNS AND SYMPTOMS

In patients suffering from appendicitis, the clinical presentation is very inconsistent (Di Saverio et al., 2020). Though most patients present with right lower quadrant abdominal pain, periumbilical pain, nausea and vomiting, anorexia, progressive fever, abdominal bloating, constipation and diarrhea, flatulence, the classic presentation of periumbilical pain, anorexia, nausea and vomiting only occurs in approximately 50% of patients. Other symptoms include abdominal distention and severe abdominal cramps (Di Saverio et al., 2020; Elhardello & MacFie, 2018; Snyder et al., 2018).

HISTORY AND PHYSICAL FINDINGS

Appendicitis when accurately and efficiently diagnosed can prevent perforation and other complications thereby reducing morbidity and mortality (Elhardello & MacFie, 2018). A comprehensive history and physical examination are more helpful at ruling in the diagnosis. Table 10.13 summarizes physical findings of appendicitis (Di Saverio et al., 2020; Elhardello & MacFie, 2018; Snyder et al., 2018).

DIFFERENTIAL DIAGNOSIS AND DIAGNOSTIC CONSIDERATIONS

Appendicitis can mimic several abdominal conditions making the diagnosis of the condition a challenge (Di Saverio et al., 2020; Elhardello & MacFie, 2018). Many other acute and surgical abdominal processes present with symptoms similar to appendicitis. Some of the

TABLE 10.13: Physical Findings of Appendicitis

FINDING	COMMENTS AND DESCRIPTION
Rebound tenderness and right lower quadrant tenderness	Most specific finding
Rovsing's sign	Peritoneal irritation demonstrated by pain in the right lower quadrant with palpation of the left lower quadrant
Psoas sign	An inflamed appendix located along the course of the right psoas muscle, demonstrated by right lower quadrant pain with the extension of the right hip or with flexion of the right hip against resistance
Obturator sign	An inflamed appendix located deep in the right hemipelvis demonstrated by right lower quadrant pain with internal and external rotation of the flexed right hip
Dunphy sign	Localized peritonitis demonstrated by sharp pain in the right lower quadrant while coughing

symptoms include pelvic inflammatory disease, diverticulitis, Crohn's disease, cholecystitis, endometriosis, biliary or renal colic, urinary tract infections, enterocolitis, pancreatitis, perforated duodenal ulcer, colonic carcinoma, ovarian cyst, and torsion (Dumas et al., 2018; Snyder et al., 2018).

Due to the wide range of differential diagnoses, laboratory tests are not specific. However, when combined with signs and symptoms or in combination with imaging studies as part of a structured evaluation, laboratory tests are helpful (Dumas et al., 2018; Huang et al., 2017). Laboratory tests include a complete blood cell (CBC) count (to evaluate the presence of infection), C-reactive protein (CRP; to determine inflammation), liver and pancreatic function tests (to rule out liver and pancreatic etiologies), urinalysis (to rule out a urinary tract infection), and urinary beta-hCG (to rule out pregnancy or confirm the presence of an ectopic pregnancy; Dumas et al., 2018; Huang et al., 2017).

Though the use of specific imaging modalities is widely debated, this represents an important part of the diagnostic process. For the evaluation of patients with suspected acute appendicitis ultrasonography, CT, and MRI are viable options (Kearl et al., 2016). Several factors including cost, duration since symptoms began, diagnostic accuracy, availability of experienced sonographers, and potential radiation exposure, should be evaluated when ordering imaging studies for this patient population. Due to its availability and limited risk, ultrasonography should be the first imaging study ordered to evaluate for appendicitis (Elhardello & MacFie, 2018; Kearl et al., 2016). In patients with appendicitis, an ultrasound will demonstrate a noncompressible tubular structure. When the ultrasound is negative or inconclusive (which may occur in obese patients), a CT scan is indicated. In pregnant patients, a MRI may be indicated (Di Saverio et al., 2020; Kearl et al., 2016).

TREATMENT

Appendectomy, via laparoscopy or via open laparotomy through a right lower quadrant incision remains the gold standard treatment for appendicitis (Dumas et al., 2018; Huang et al., 2017). Laparoscopic appendectomies resulted in a lower incidence of wound infection, shorter length of stay, and fewer postoperative complications, but a longer operation time compared to open laparotomies (Dumas et al., 2018; Huang et al., 2017). Based on the results of a standard health-status measure for nonsurgical patients with appendicitis, and according to the Comparison of the Outcomes of Antibiotic therapy in Appendectomy (CODA) Collaborative, antibiotics were noninferior to appendectomy, and should be considered (Flum et al., 2020).

CLINICAL PEARLS

- The classic presentation of periumbilical pain, anorexia, nausea and vomiting only occurs in approximately 50% of patients.
- Due to the wide range of differential diagnoses, laboratory tests are not specific.
- Appendectomy, via laparoscopy or via open laparotomy through a right lower quadrant incision, remains the only curative treatment of appendicitis.

10.11B: ACUTE CHOLECYSTITIS

Acute cholecystitis can be defined as the chemical or bacterial inflammation of the gallbladder usually caused by a gallstone leading to an obstruction of the cystic duct (Burmeister & Schafmayer, 2018; Giles et al., 2020). Calculous cholecystitis (presence of gallstones) accounts for approximately 95% of this population, while the rest are considered acalculous (lack of gallstones) and can be classified as acute or chronic (Pisano et al., 2019). Gangrenous cholecystitis occurs when untreated acute cholecystitis leads to necrosis of the gallbladder. Twenty percent of individuals admitted for biliary tract disease are diagnosed with acute cholecystitis. Acute calculous cholecystitis is three times more common in women than in men up to age 50, and thereafter, approximately one and one-half times more common (Giles et al., 2020; Okamoto et al., 2018).

Due to its vague presentation, other conditions such as acute and chronic pancreatitis, peptic ulcer disease (PUD), irritable bowel disease, and cardiac disease could be confused with acute cholecystitis. Though more common in women, acute cholecystitis is seen in some populations more than others (Okamoto et al., 2018). Acute illness, dramatic weight loss, obesity, pregnancy, contraceptives, estrogen replacement therapy, and women in their 40s present an increased risk of acute cholecystitis. In addition, patients with sickle cell disease are at increased risk for acute calculous cholecystitis due to the breakdown of blood cells (Giles et al., 2020; Pisano et al., 2019).

PRESENTING SIGNS AND SYMPTOMS

The presence of gallstones or inflammation causes patients with acute cholecystitis to present with constant epigastric right upper quadrant pain that lasts for greater than 6 hours. Other presenting symptoms include anorexia, nausea, vomiting, low-grade fever, abdominal bloating, chills, and clay-colored stool (Burmeister & Schafmayer, 2018; Giles et al., 2020; Pisano et al., 2019).

HISTORY AND PHYSICAL FINDINGS

It is important to perform a comprehensive history, physical examination, and a rectal examination in all patients presenting with abdominal pain including pelvic examinations in women (Okamoto et al., 2018). Patients with acute cholecystitis typically present with progressing right upper quadrant abdominal pain with bloating; sometimes pain may also be present in the midback or shoulder (this is often mistaken for cardiac issues and a myocardial infarction must be ruled out), greasy and spicy food intolerances, jaundice, increased gas, nausea, and vomiting (Giles et al., 2020; Okamoto et al., 2018).

Upon assessment, patients with cholecystitis are usually ill appearing and may present with fever, tachycardia, and or hypotension suggesting early stages of shock. Patients with chronic cholecystitis may appear jaundiced. Physical exam reveals a positive Murphy sign in approximately 93% of patients (demonstrated by an inspiratory pause on palpation of the right quadrant) and palpable fullness in the right upper abdominal quadrant. The presence of peritoneal signs suggests complicated acute cholecystitis and may be a surgical emergency (Burmeister & Schafmayer, 2018; Giles et al., 2020; Pisano et al., 2019).

DIFFERENTIAL DIAGNOSIS AND DIAGNOSTIC CONSIDERATIONS

A comprehensive history and physical examination remain the hallmark of properly diagnosing patients with acute cholecystitis. Differential diagnoses for acute cholecystitis include biliary colic, cholelithiasis and renal calculi, pregnancy, urinary tract infections, small bowel obstruction (SBO), hepatitis, gastroenteritis, abdominal aneurysm, myocardial infarction, pancreatitis, mesenteric ischemia, diverticulitis, and irritable bowel obstruction (Burmeister & Schafmayer, 2018; Giles et al., 2020).

In uncomplicated cholecystitis, biliary obstruction is limited to the gallbladder; therefore, elevation in certain serum markers may be absent. Laboratory tests including a complete blood cell (CBC) count (to evaluate the presence of infection); AST, ALT, bilirubin, and alkaline phosphatase (ALP) may be elevated in cholecystitis (Giles et al., 2020). It is important to note that they are not sensitive to excluding cholecystitis; therefore, normal values do not rule out the condition. Serum amylase and lipase levels should be evaluated to rule out pancreatitis. A urinary beta-hCG should be evaluated to rule out pregnancy, and cardiac enzymes and an electrocardiography should be conducted to rule out myocardial infarction (Giles et al., 2020; Okamoto et al., 2018).

For the diagnosis of cholecystitis, nuclear medicine studies and ultrasonography are considered the most effective, with ultrasonography being recommended as the initial test. Though the hepatic 2,6-dimethyliminodiacetic acid (HIDA) scan has a high sensitivity and specificity for acute cholecystitis (94% and 85%, respectively), it is not practical in the emergency department setting and may not be available in other settings (Okamoto et al., 2018). CT scan is often recommended only for the evaluation of abdominal pain if the diagnosis is uncertain and is not considered an ideal routine test for cholecystitis. For patients with acute calculous cholecystitis, an endoscopic retrograde cholangiopancreatography (ERCP) may be appropriate as it provides both diagnostic endoscopic and radiographic visualization of the biliary tract, and therapeutic removal of common bile duct stones. An ERCP should be considered in cholecystitis patients with an elevated clinical suspicion of biliary stones (Burmeister & Schafmayer, 2018; Giles et al., 2020; Pisano et al., 2019).

TREATMENT

The curative treatment for cholecystitis is a cholecystectomy and the most appropriate surgical approach is the laparoscopic approach. Laparoscopic cholecystectomies have demonstrated lower morbidity and mortality rates with quick recovery compared to open cholecystectomies. For patients who are not candidates for the laparoscopic procedure, an open cholecystectomy will be performed (Burmeister & Schafmayer, 2018; Pisano et al., 2019). Perforation, empyema, or emphysematous cholecystitis are indications for urgent surgical intervention. Patients who are poor candidates for laparoscopic or open cholecystectomy may benefit from temporizing percutaneous gallbladder drainage and placement of a cholecystostomy tube (Giles et al., 2020).

CLINICAL PEARLS

- ■ Through cholecystitis can occur in young and older adults, the highest incidence is in the fourth decade.
- ■ The risk of cholecystitis increases in individuals who fit in the "fat, forty, fertile, and flatulent" categories.
- ■ Proper diagnosis can be made with a complete history and physical examination with food intolerances being the initiating factor for an acute attack.
- ■ The preferred recommended treatment is a laparoscopic cholecystectomy.

10.11C: CHOLANGITIS

Acute cholangitis is a life-threatening condition that is a bacterial infection of the biliary tract (Lan Cheong Wah et al., 2017). With infection-causing stones in the common bile duct leading to partial or complete obstruction of the biliary system, choledocholithiasis is the most common reported cause of cholangitis (Lindor et al., 2015; Miura et al., 2018). Though acute cholangitis is a treatable condition when properly and effectively managed, if left untreated it can cause significant morbidity and mortality. Different types of cholangitis include primary sclerosing cholangitis, primary biliary cholangitis, IgG4-related autoimmune cholangitis, and acute bacterial cholangitis, which is the most common (Miura et al., 2018; Ramchandani et al., 2017).

In the United States, there are approximately 200,000 cases of acute cholangitis annually affecting individuals in their fifth and sixth decades of life. Of patients with gallstone disease, approximately 6% to 9% are diagnosed with acute cholangitis. The condition occurs mostly in adults and is diagnosed more among Native American and Hispanic patients. African American patients with sickle cell disease are also at risk. Complications of cholangitis include acute renal failure, pyogenic liver abscess, portal hypertension, and liver failure (Lan Cheong Wah et al., 2017; Ramchandani et al., 2017).

PRESENTING SIGNS AND SYMPTOMS

Patients with cholangitis may be admitted with a wide clinical range of presentations from mild illness to overwhelming fulminant sepsis. Symptoms may include generalized abdominal pain, but often include fever with chills, malaise, rigors, right upper quadrant pain, jaundice, pruritus, and pale stools (Lindor et al., 2015; Ramchandani et al., 2017).

HISTORY AND PHYSICAL FINDINGS

Medical or recent history of cholelithiasis, recent biliary tract manipulation or cholecystectomy, endoscopic retrograde cholangiopancreatography (ERCP) procedure or prior history of cholangitis, increase the clinical suspicion of cholangitis (Miura et al., 2018). Patients with cholangitis tend to appear quite ill with over 80% presenting

with fever, right upper quadrant pain, and jaundice. It is also common for patients to present in severe sepsis or septic shock. Other characteristic presentations of cholangitis include abdominal distention, altered mental status, or hemodynamic instability (Lan Cheong Wah et al., 2017; Lindor et al., 2015).

Due to the wide range of presentations and levels of acuity, clinical criteria such as Charcot triad (intermittent fever with chills, right upper quadrant pain, and jaundice), Reynold's Pentad (fever, right upper quadrant pain, jaundice, confusion, and hypotension), and the Tokyo guidelines have been adopted in clinical practice (Miura et al., 2018; Ramchandani et al., 2017). The following five predictors have improved the ability of clinicians to properly diagnose cholangitis and determine its level of severity: age 75 or older, the presence of systemic inflammatory response syndrome upon presentation, serum albumin level below 3.0 g/dL, platelet count below 120,000/mcL, and blood urea nitrogen (BUN) level above 20 mg/dL (Lindor et al., 2015; Miura et al., 2018; Ramchandani et al., 2017).

DIFFERENTIAL DIAGNOSIS AND DIAGNOSTIC CONSIDERATIONS

A comprehensive history, physical examination, and proper workup remain the hallmark of properly diagnosing patients with acute cholangitis as it is based on a combination of typical clinical features, laboratory data, and imaging findings (Lindor et al., 2015). Understanding of the Charcot triad as a typical clinical presentation of acute cholangitis remains important. Differential diagnoses for cholangitis include acute cholecystitis, acute pancreatitis (AP), mesenteric ischemia, diverticulitis, septic shock, hepatitis, liver cirrhosis and failure, perforated peptic ulcer disease (PUD), and pyelonephritis (Lan Cheong Wah et al., 2017; Miura et al., 2018; Ramchandani et al., 2017).

Further confirmation of the diagnosis of cholangitis can then be made via abnormal laboratory results and imaging studies implying infection and biliary obstruction. Laboratory tests for acute cholangitis include complete blood count (to evaluate the presence of infection), complete metabolic profile (to evaluate electrolyte imbalances and kidney involvement), liver function tests (to evaluate or rule out hepatic failure), C-reactive protein (to evaluate inflammation), and serum amylase and/or lipase levels (to rule out pancreatitis; Lindor et al., 2015; Ramchandani et al., 2017). Common findings in cholangitis include leukocytosis with neutrophil predominance, leukopenia in septic or immunocompromised patients, and liver function test results consistent with cholestasis (hyperbilirubinemia and increased alkaline phosphatase). Other findings include elevation of transaminases and serum amylase levels due to possible concurrent pancreatitis from stone impaction (Lan Cheong Wah et al., 2017; Miura et al., 2018).

The first-line imaging study of choice for cholangitis is abdominal ultrasonography. It has shown both significant sensitivity and specificity in examining the gallbladder and investigating for biliary duct dilatation (Lan Cheong Wah et al., 2017; Lindor et al., 2015). Additional imaging studies that may serve as an adjunct used to investigate coexisting conditions such as hepatic/pancreatic disease, metastasis, or hepatic abscess diagnose is the CT scan as it better examines the intrahepatic and extrahepatic ducts, as well as inflammation of the biliary tree. CT scans may also help rule out diagnoses including AP, mesenteric ischemia, and diverticulitis (Lan Cheong Wah et al., 2017; Lindor et al., 2015).

Magnetic resonance cholangiopancreatography (MRCP) is the most sensitive diagnostic and therapeutic modality for detecting common bile duct stones. It is noninvasive and involves no exposure to radiation (Lindor et al., 2015; Miura et al., 2018).

TREATMENT

Managing both biliary infection and obstruction are the goals of treating acute cholangitis. Percutaneous or endoscopic biliary drainage and decompression have replaced surgery as the initial treatment of acute cholangitis (Miura et al., 2018). Biliary drainage or decompression can be achieved by endoscopic retrograde cholangiopancreatography (ERCP), percutaneous transhepatic cholangiography (PTC), or endoscopic ultrasound-guided drainage or surgical drainage. Effective in approximately 96% of cases, ERCP remains the gold standard and treatment of choice for biliary decompression. Surgical procedures are reserved for patients with cholangitis who decompensate despite optimal medical management and endoscopic/percutaneous biliary drainage due to high rates of complications (Lan Cheong Wah et al., 2017; Miura et al., 2018; Ramchandani et al., 2017).

CLINICAL PEARLS

- Acute cholangitis if untreated leads to significant mortality and morbidity.
- Though important in the diagnostic process, cholangitis rarely presents with the classic Charcot triad of fever, jaundice, and right upper quadrant abdominal pain.
- MRCP is the most sensitive diagnostic and therapeutic modality for detecting common bile duct stones.
- Managing both biliary infection and obstruction are the goals of treating acute cholangitis.

10.11D: PERITONITIS

Peritonitis is defined as an inflammation of the serous membrane lining the abdominal cavity and organs within the abdominal cavity (Brahmbhatt & Tapper, 2017; Li et al., 2016; Lobo et al., 2016). With a uniform inflammatory response, the peritoneum that is otherwise sterile becomes infected through organ perforation or from irritants such as a lacerated liver or bile from a perforated gallbladder, foreign bodies, or a perforated ulcer. An infected fallopian tube, ectopic pregnancy, or a ruptured ovarian cyst may also cause a localized peritonitis in women (Ross et al., 2018; Tolonen et al., 2019).

Peritonitis can be classified as primary (usually seen in immunocompromised patients), secondary (usually seen in pathologic processes in visceral organs due to trauma, etc.) and tertiary (usually seen in patients resistant to adequate initial therapy (Li et al., 2016; Ross et al., 2018).

The abdomen is the second most common source of sepsis and secondary peritonitis. Spontaneous bacterial peritonitis (SBP), a form of secondary peritonitis, is most often seen in patients with chronic liver disease. Often, in the absence of the original visceral organ pathology or misdiagnosis, tertiary peritonitis develops (Li et al., 2016).

PRESENTING SIGNS AND SYMPTOMS

Patients with peritonitis may be admitted with a wide clinical range of presentations from mild illness to septic shock (Brahmbhatt & Tapper, 2017; Tolonen et al., 2019). Symptoms often include fever with chills, unexplained or worsening encephalopathy, generalized abdominal pain, nausea, vomiting, and diarrhea, paralytic ileus, renal failure, and ascites (Brahmbhatt & Tapper, 2017; Ross et al., 2018). Patients in shock may present with intravascular hypovolemia from anorexia, tachycardia due to the release of inflammatory mediators, vomiting and fever, and third-space losses into the peritoneal cavity. Patients with severe peritonitis or in septic shock may present with hypothermia, hypotension, oliguria, or anuria (Li et al., 2016; Lobo et al., 2016; Ross et al., 2018; Tolonen et al., 2019).

HISTORY AND PHYSICAL FINDINGS

A comprehensive history and physical examination are key factors in making a timely and accurate diagnosis of peritonitis (Lobo et al., 2016). During the comprehensive history, previous episodes of peritonitis, abdominal surgery, travel history, and use of immunosuppressive agents should be investigated. This includes conditions such as peptic ulcer disease (PUD), diverticulitis, and inflammatory bowel disease (IBD) as they may predispose patients to intraabdominal infections (Brahmbhatt & Tapper, 2017; Ross et al., 2018).

Patients with peritonitis generally appear unwell and in acute distress on physical examination. Like other surgical abdominal conditions, a broad range of signs and symptoms are seen in patients suffering from peritonitis. While caring for critically ill patients with worsening ascites, a high index of suspicion for peritonitis must be maintained because up to 30% of patients are completely asymptomatic (Li et al., 2016; Ross et al., 2018; Tolonen et al., 2019).

The most common chief complaint of patients with peritonitis is abdominal pain. The pain, which may be acute or insidious, can initially present as dull and poorly localized demonstrating visceral peritoneal involvement. Other confirmatory peritoneal signs may include psoas sign, obturator sign, Rovsing's sign, or Dunphy's sign (Li et al., 2016). If untreated, it may progress to steady, severe, and more localized pain demonstrating parietal peritoneal involvement. In patients with peritonitis, coughing, hip flexion, and local pressure may exacerbate the abdominal pain (Brahmbhatt & Tapper, 2017; Li et al., 2016).

Signs of dysfunction of other organs and abdominal distention may be noted in patients with peritonitis. In critically ill, hospitalized patients, patients on corticosteroids, elderly patients, and patients with advanced neuropathy secondary to diabetes, symptoms may be subtle or underrepresented. Decreased friction between the visceral and parietal peritoneal surfaces may reduce the symptoms of abdominal pain in the presence of ascites (Brahmbhatt & Tapper, 2017; Lobo et al., 2016; Tolonen et al., 2019).

DIFFERENTIAL DIAGNOSIS AND DIAGNOSTIC CONSIDERATIONS

The diagnosis of peritonitis is largely based on a comprehensive history and clinical presentation. Differential diagnoses for patients suffering from peritonitis include empyema, pyelonephritis, cystitis, acute urinary retention, rectus hematoma, chemical irritants introduced into the peritoneal space including bile, blood, gastric juice, barium, enema, chronic peritoneal dialysis, fungal infection, gynecologic disorders, opportunistic organisms from HIV, perforated viscus, mesenteric ischemia/embolus, vasculitis, appendicitis, and urinary tract infection (Li et al., 2016; Ross et al., 2018; Tolonen et al., 2019).

Further diagnostic confirmation can be made via abnormal laboratory results, fluid cultures, and imaging studies. Laboratory tests that may be helpful in diagnosing peritonitis include: complete blood count (CBC; to evaluate the presence of infection), complete metabolic profile (CMP; to evaluate electrolyte imbalances and kidney involvement), liver function tests (to evaluate or rule out hepatic failure) along with prothrombin time (PT), partial thromboplastin time (PTT), and INR, procalcitonin levels (which may be an indicator of severity and mortality in patients with peritonitis). A urinalysis may be helpful in ruling out urinary tract disease. Common findings in peritonitis include leukocytosis with a left shift suggesting severe infection (Brahmbhatt & Tapper, 2017; Li et al., 2016; Ross et al., 2018).

In patients with inconclusive signs on physical examination, or who cannot provide an adequate history, diagnostic peritoneal lavage may be helpful. Patients with a clinical suspicion of SBP without indwelling peritoneal catheters are candidates for a paracentesis. Ascitic fluid neutrophil count along with bacterial cultures are typically used in guiding therapy (Brahmbhatt & Tapper, 2017; Ross et al., 2018).

Imaging provides definitive data in conjunction with physical examination and laboratory results in the diagnosis of peritonitis. The first imaging studies obtained in patients presenting with peritonitis are plain films of the abdomen, and though their value is limited, it may provide information suggestive of free air. To identify free air under the diaphragm in patients with a perforated viscus, upright films are indicated. It is important to note that plain films are not the most sensitive or specific radiographic tests as small amounts of free air are often missed (Brahmbhatt & Tapper, 2017; Li et al., 2016; Lobo et al., 2016).

Ultrasonography use in the diagnosis of peritonitis is advantageous due to low cost, portability, and availability. It may be helpful in the evaluation of solid organ pathology and detection of fluid in the peritoneal space. Unfortunately, its use is sometimes limited due to patient habitus, discomfort, abdominal distention, and bowel gas interference. Its ability to detect low quantities of fluid is also limited (Brahmbhatt & Tapper, 2017; Ross et al., 2018). In cases where the diagnosis cannot be established on clinical grounds and the findings on abdominal plain films and ultrasonography are inconclusive, a CT scan (if possible, with IV contrast) is indicated. For peritoneal abscess and related visceral pathology, CT scans of the abdomen and pelvis remain the diagnostic study of choice as it detects areas of inflammation, small quantities of fluid, and other gastrointestinal tract pathology (Brahmbhatt & Tapper, 2017; Ross et al., 2018). For patients with intraabdominal abscesses, an MRI may be indicated. High cost, limited availability, patient's ability to tolerate, and MRI-compatible support equipment limit its usefulness in this patient population (Li et al., 2016).

TREATMENT

Identifying and resolving the underlying process with operative management directed at controlling the infectious source, administration of systemic antibiotics, and supportive therapy to prevent organ system failure are the treatment goals of peritonitis (Li et al., 2016; Ross et al., 2018; Tolonen et al., 2019). As such, adequate source control with resolution of sepsis and clearance of all residual intraabdominal infection defines treatment success. Since peritonitis is caused by an array of intraabdominal processes or conditions, the type and extent of surgery indicated depends on the underlying disease process and the severity of intraabdominal infection (Tolonen et al., 2019). Abdominal surgery utilizing a laparoscopic approach for early and definitive source control in addition to eliminating bacteria and toxins remains the cornerstone of peritonitis treatment. Though a second or a third procedure may be required, this can typically be achieved during a single operation in certain situations (Li et al., 2016; Ross et al., 2018).

CLINICAL PEARLS

- Peritonitis is caused by an array of intraabdominal processes or conditions.
- Surgery utilizing a laparoscopic approach remains a cornerstone of peritonitis treatment.
- Surgical procedures for the treatment of peritonitis should focus on early and definitive source control in addition to eliminating bacteria and toxins.

10.11E: INTUSSUSCEPTION

Intussusception in the adult population is defined as the telescoping of one segment of the bowel into an immediately adjacent segment causing an obstruction and eventually intestinal ischemia (Figure 10.3; Marsicovetere et al., 2017). If untreated, intussusception may lead to multiple complications including bowel ischemia, bowel obstruction, bowel necrosis, and sepsis. Intussusception is uncommon in adults accounting for less than 5% of bowel obstructions, but when present is likely acute and may lead to significant morbidity and mortality (Aydin et al., 2016; Marsicovetere et al., 2017).

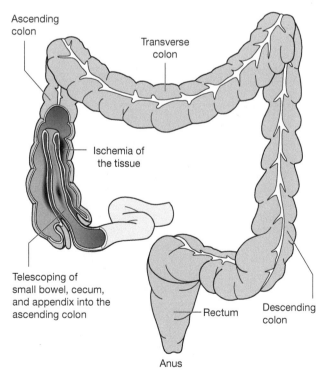

FIGURE 10.3: Intussusception.
Source: From Small, A. (2019). Advanced health assessment of the abdomen, rectum, and anus. In K. M. Myrick & L. M. Karosas (Eds.), *Advanced health assessment and differential diagnosis: Essentials for clinical practice* (pp. 240–280). Springer Publishing Company. Fig. 8.39.

In the adult population, intussusception is divided into four categories based on anatomical location. The four common types are enteric, ileocolic, ileocecal, and colonic. The enteric and colonic types only appear in the small and large intestine, respectively. Ileocolic intussusceptions occur when a segment of the ileum protrudes into the colon through the ileocecal valve demonstrated by the ileocecal valve as the lead point (Marsicovetere et al., 2017).

Intussusception is also challenging in adults due to the vagueness of its presenting symptoms and can cause severe complications and poor patient outcomes if not properly diagnosed (Gange et al., 2020; Marsicovetere et al., 2017).

PRESENTING SIGNS AND SYMPTOMS

In the adult population, the clinical presentation of intussusception can be vague and rarely presents with the classic triad of abdominal pain, palpable mass, and bloody stool; instead, variable but generally marked abdominal pain and signs of bowel obstruction are common (Aydin et al., 2016; Gange et al., 2020). Other symptoms consistent with bowel obstruction include abdominal cramping, nausea, vomiting, obstipation, gastrointestinal bleeding (GIB), change in bowel habits, and bloating (Aydin et al., 2016).

Patients typically present appearing ill with acute symptoms that have been present for days to weeks. Symptoms consistent with acute presentations secondary to necrosis, sepsis, peritonitis, or bowel perforation, and include hypothermia or hyperthermia, hypotension, and tachycardia (Aydin et al., 2016).

HISTORY AND PHYSICAL FINDINGS

A comprehensive history and physical examination are important in patients with intussusception. Adult patients with intussusception typically complain of abdominal pain, and abdominal pain remains one of the most common complaints treated in the acute care settings (Marsicovetere et al., 2017).

The physical exam can show diffuse or localized abdominal pain, bloating, and decreased bowel sounds. A distended abdomen with tenderness ranging from mild (parietal irritation) to severe (consistent peritoneal irritation), an abdominal mass or guaiac-positive stool may be revealed on a physical exam (Aydin et al., 2016; Gange et al., 2020). Patients may also present with pain out of proportion to physical exam findings suggestive of peritonitis or bowel ischemia (Gange et al., 2020).

DIFFERENTIAL DIAGNOSIS AND DIAGNOSTIC CONSIDERATIONS

The rarity of intussusception in adults, along with the nonspecific nature of its presentation, results in a broad list of differential diagnoses. These include volvulus, gastritis, small or large bowel obstruction, ileus, fibroids, pelvic inflammatory disease, pyelonephritis, ovarian torsion, pancreatitis, diverticulosis, diverticulitis, abdominal aortic aneurysm, irritable bowel disease, inflammatory bowel syndrome, peptic ulcer disease, cholecystitis, cholelithiasis, mesentery ischemia, constipation, and gastroparesis (Aydin et al., 2016; Gange et al., 2020; Marsicovetere et al., 2017).

Physical assessment and management of abdominal pain are dependent on the severity of signs and symptoms in patients who present with intussusception. Laboratory evaluation may not be helpful without imaging studies (Aydin et al., 2016; Gange et al., 2020). Laboratory tests that may be useful in the diagnostic workup include a complete blood count, complete metabolic profile, liver function tests, C-reactive protein, and serum amylase and/or lipase levels. Laboratory values typically reveal elevated inflammatory markers including leukocytosis, elevated CRP, and electrolyte imbalances (Aydin et al., 2016; Gange et al., 2020).

Ultrasonography has a documented sensitivity and specificity of over 97%, when detecting ileocolic intussusception. Plain abdominal supine and upright radiographs are important as they are diagnostic in approximately 60% of cases. Though they may be normal in early cases, as intussusception progresses, abdominal radiographs demonstrate an absence of air in the right lower and upper quadrants suggesting the diagnosis. CT scan (though considered unreliable in some cases with risks associated with IV contrast administration, radiation exposure, and sedation) has been proposed as a useful tool to diagnose intussusception if abdominal radiographs and ultrasonography are inconclusive (Aydin et al., 2016; Gange et al., 2020; Marsicovetere et al., 2017). Intussusception on CT scan may present as a target sign (also known as the donut sign or bull's eye sign). Due to the invagination of the bowel, the target sign is caused by alternating echogenic and hypoechoic concentric bands (Figure 10.4; Carroll et al., 2017).

TREATMENT

Surgical management is indicated in patients with persistent small bowel intussusception nonresponsive to enema reduction, close observation, or the presence of perforation. Due to the high incidence of malignancy, adult patients with ileocolic, ileocecal, and colonic intussusception necessitates surgical resection using appropriate oncologic techniques (Aydin et al., 2016; Gange et al., 2020).

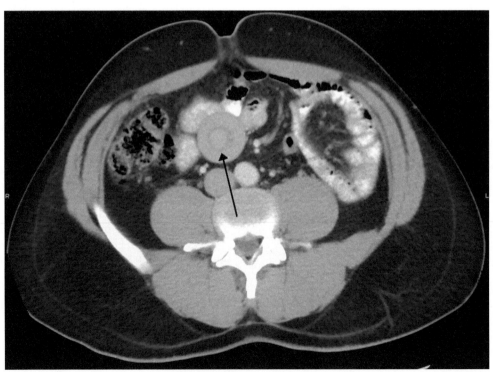

FIGURE 10.4: "Donut" or "target" sign seen with intussusception on CT.
Source: Courtesy of James Heilman, MD.

CLINICAL PEARLS

- Intussusception is an uncommon diagnosis with vague presentations requiring a strong clinical suspicion for the condition.
- Early diagnosis and treatment are essential to decreasing mortality and morbidity.
- Surgical intervention is the definitive treatment as most resolve spontaneously; surgical options are only required if nonoperative treatment fails.

10.11F: BOWEL INFARCTION

Bowel infarction, also known as mesenteric ischemia, may be defined as a sudden interruption of the blood supply to a segment of the small intestine or colon, leading to ischemia, irreversible cellular damage, intestinal necrosis, and, if untreated, death (Ananthan et al., 2017; Bala et al., 2019). Although bowel infarction is relatively rare, it is a life-threatening condition. In addition to obstruction of venous outflow, bowel infarction can be caused by occlusive or nonocclusive obstruction of the arteries (Bala et al., 2019).

The four major etiologies of bowel infarction include (a) mesenteric arterial embolism which accounts for approximately 50% of cases and occurs when emboli lodge in the superior mesenteric artery (SMA), which supplies the small intestine; (b) mesenteric arterial thrombosis, which accounts for 15% to 25% of cases and occurs due to atherosclerosis either secondary to gradual build up until there is critical stenosis or acute plaque rupture; (c) mesenteric venous thrombosis, which accounts for approximately 5% of cases and occurs due to pathologies such as inflammatory bowel disease that cause increases in the resistance of mesenteric venous blood flow; and (d) nonocclusive mesenteric ischemia, which accounts for approximately 20% of cases, and typically involves SMA spasms leading to hypoperfusion to the small intestine and colon.

Elderly patients, especially those with cardiovascular disease, are at higher risk for bowel ischemia, compared to venous thrombosis, which is the cause of bowel ischemia in younger patients without cardiovascular disease (Ananthan et al., 2017; Bala et al., 2019; Lim et al., 2019).

PRESENTING SIGNS AND SYMPTOMS

All patients with bowel infarction typically present with similar symptoms; however, based on the etiology, there are some differences in clinical appearance for each type (Ananthan et al., 2017; Bala et al., 2019). Pain, which is described as sometimes colicky, moderate to severe, diffuse, nonlocalized, and constant that is disproportionate to physical examination findings is the most common finding (Ananthan et al., 2017; Bala et al., 2019). Other presenting symptoms of bowel infarction include nausea, vomiting, anorexia, diarrhea, obstipation, abdominal distention, and GIB. Signs of sepsis, including tachycardia, tachypnea, hypotension, fever, and altered mental status, develop as the bowel becomes gangrenous (Ehlert, 2018; Lim et al., 2019).

Bowel infarction should be considered in any patient (especially over the age of 60) with abdominal pain disproportionate to physical findings. Otherwise, if not properly diagnosed and managed, morbidity and mortality are typically significantly elevated. Untreated acute mesenteric infarction has a catastrophic outcome (Ehlert, 2018).

HISTORY AND PHYSICAL FINDINGS

Obtaining a comprehensive personal and family history is important along with physical examination especially in patients with a personal or family history of bowel infarction (Bala et al., 2019). Approximately 30% of patients who present with bowel infarction have a prior history of an embolic event. In addition, approximately 50% of patients with acute mesenteric venous thrombosis have a personal or family history of deep vein thromboses or pulmonary emboli (Ananthan et al., 2017; Bala et al., 2019; Ehlert, 2018).

The most common presenting symptom in all types of bowel infarction is abdominal pain. Though peritoneal signs are only present when transmural bowel infarction and necrosis develop, patients may have mild abdominal distention on admission (Ehlert, 2018; Lim et al., 2019). Sudden, severe, periumbilical pain associated with nausea and vomiting is characteristic of an arterial embolism. Pain that is worse after eating (also known as "food fear") is usually associated with thrombotic mesenteric arterial occlusion. Patients that present with slow-onset, intermittent abdominal pain are typically diagnosed with mesenteric venous thrombosis (Bala et al., 2019; Lim et al., 2019).

DIFFERENTIAL DIAGNOSIS AND DIAGNOSTIC CONSIDERATIONS

Bowel ischemia is a condition with an unclear initial presentation requiring a high clinical index of suspicion especially in patients over age 60, otherwise substantial morbidity and mortality are imminent (Ananthan et al., 2017; Bala et al., 2019; Ehlert, 2018). Differential diagnoses in patients with bowel infarction include perforated bowel, bowel obstruction, ruptured abdominal aortic aneurysm, acute surgical abdomen, abdominal abscess, ovarian torsion, Crohn's disease, ulcerative colitis, hepatic disease, acute cholecystitis, acute pancreatitis (AP), acute pyelonephritis, aortic dissection, appendicitis, cholangitis, cholecystitis, diverticulitis, cholelithiasis, postoperative ileus, multiple organ dysfunction syndrome, myocardial infarction, septic shock, small bowel obstruction, and testicular torsion (Ananthan et al., 2017; Bala et al., 2019; Ehlert, 2018).

Laboratory studies including white blood cell count, d-Dimer, and lactate may be evaluated to aid in the diagnosis of bowel infarction, but they will not establish the diagnosis. The gold standard for the diagnosis of bowel infarction is mesenteric angiography. However, due to access and availability without delay, other effective imaging studies include CTA or MRA (Ananthan et al., 2017; Ehlert, 2018).

TREATMENT

Prevention of tissue damage and bowel necrosis is the goal for treatment. Patients diagnosed with bowel infarction typically need immediate surgical intervention (Lim et al., 2019). Early surgical laparotomy with embolectomy is the treatment of choice for mesenteric arterial occlusion from an embolism. Typically, surgical revascularization or stenting is indicated in patients with mesenteric arterial thrombosis. Depending on the severity, mesenteric venous thrombosis may be managed with systemic anticoagulation. Eliminating the underlying cause of ischemia is the treatment goal for nonocclusive mesenteric ischemia (Bala et al., 2019; Ehlert, 2018; Lim et al., 2019). Patients with bowel infarction are usually treated with systemic anticoagulation after surgical intervention in the absence of contraindications (Ehlert, 2018).

CLINICAL PEARLS

- Mesenteric arterial embolism, typically from a cardiac source, is the most common cause of bowel infarction.
- A comprehensive personal and family medical history is important as patients or family may have experienced bowel infarction or embolism.
- Surgical intervention for bowel infarction depends on the type and most patients are anticoagulated after surgery.

10.11G: BOWEL OBSTRUCTION

Bowel obstruction is defined as a mechanical or functional obstruction of the small or large intestines preventing forward flow of intestinal content (Baiu & Hawn, 2018; Jackson & Vigiola, 2018; Ten Broek et al., 2018). It is an emergency condition requiring early identification and intervention to reduce mortality and morbidity. Small bowel obstructions (SBOs) are more common with intraabdominal adhesions accounting for more than 70% of cases. Large bowel obstructions (LBOs), which may result from dilation of the colon in the absence of an anatomic lesion or mechanical interruption of the flow of intestinal contents, is usually age dependent. Bowel obstructions are classified as complete (true obstruction), partial (pseudo-obstruction), or closed loop (an obstruction in which two points along the course of a bowel are obstructed at a single location thus forming a closed loop; Jackson & Vigiola, 2018; Ten Broek et al., 2018).

Etiologies of small SBOs and LBOs can be classified as extrinsic, intrinsic, or intraluminal. In SBOs, extrinsic causes include postsurgical adhesions, cancer, and inguinal and umbilical hernias. The most common cause of intrinsic SBO is Crohn's disease. Foreign body ingestion is the main cause of intraluminal SBOs, which are far less common. Approximately 15% of all intestinal obstructions are attributed to LBOs with the most common causes being adenocarcinoma, diverticulitis, and volvulus. The sigmoid colon is the most common location for colonic obstruction (Baiu & Hawn, 2018; Jackson & Vigiola, 2018; Ten Broek et al., 2018).

PRESENTING SIGNS AND SYMPTOMS

Due to the different types and varying degrees of bowel obstruction, patients typically present with a myriad of symptoms (Ten Broek et al., 2018). Initials goals include attempting to distinguish complete from partial obstruction, which may be associated with passage of some stool or flatus. Signs and symptoms of SBO include nausea, vomiting, abdominal discomfort/distention, absence of passage of flatus and/or feces. Signs and symptoms in LBO include abdominal distention, nausea, vomiting, and crampy abdominal pain. Additional symptoms may include anorexia, feculent vomiting, dehydration, and electrolyte disturbances. Late findings include tachycardia, tachypnea, hypotension, fever, and altered mental status (Baiu & Hawn, 2018; Jackson & Vigiola, 2018).

HISTORY AND PHYSICAL FINDINGS

Risk factors include prior abdominal surgery, chronic intestinal inflammatory disease, colon or metastatic cancer, and foreign body ingestion (Baiu & Hawn, 2018; Ten Broek et al., 2018). SBOs and LBOs have many overlapping symptoms making the diagnosis challenging; however, quality, timing, and presentation differ. More focal tenderness on palpation is seen in patients with SBO as compared to diffuse tenderness on palpation experienced by patients with LBO. Abdominal pain in SBO is described as intermittent and colicky but improves with frequent and bilious vomiting; patients who suffer from LBO remain in continuous pain associated with intermittent vomiting of fecal matter. Patients with LBO may also demonstrate peritoneal signs including rebound tenderness, rigid abdomen, guarding, and pain out of proportion to the examination (Baiu & Hawn, 2018; Jackson & Vigiola, 2018; Ten Broek et al., 2018).

Due to colonic involvement, abdominal distention is more marked in LBOs compared to SBOs. In cases with ileocecal valve incompetence, LBOs may mimic SBOs due to insufflation of air from the large bowel into the small bowel, which may present with symptoms of SBO (Baiu & Hawn, 2018).

DIFFERENTIAL DIAGNOSIS AND DIAGNOSTIC CONSIDERATIONS

Differential diagnoses in patients with bowel obstruction include: infarction, abdominal hernias, ruptured abdominal aortic aneurysm, acute surgical abdomen, Crohn's disease, ulcerative colitis, acute cholecystitis, acute pancreatitis (AP), acute pyelonephritis, aortic dissection, appendicitis, cholangitis, cholecystitis, diverticulitis, cholelithiasis, postoperative ileus, multiple organ dysfunction syndrome, myocardial infarction, septic shock, chronic or toxic megacolon, endometriosis, intussusception, and diabetic ketoacidosis (Jackson & Vigiola, 2018; Ten Broek et al., 2018).

Laboratory tests that may be helpful in diagnosing peritonitis include complete blood count, complete metabolic profile, and serum lactate. Common findings in bowel obstruction include leukocytosis, hypochloremic metabolic alkalosis, elevated hemoglobin, hematocrit and blood-urea-nitrogen levels that suggest dehydration, and elevated lactic acid which may suggest bowel ischemia (Baiu & Hawn, 2018; Jackson & Vigiola, 2018).

Although bowel obstruction alone can be suspected with a comprehensive patient history and presentation with an emphasis on risk factors, the current standard of care for the diagnosis and management of SBOs and LBOs is an abdominal CT with oral contrast. An abdominal radiography is an appropriate initial examination in patients with suspected intestinal obstruction. While supine views show dilation of multiple loops of small bowel, with a paucity of gas in the large bowel, upright or lateral decubitus views may show air–fluid levels in a stepladder fashion. In 60% of cases, radiographic findings, in conjunction with lack of gas and stool in the distal colon and rectum, are highly suggestive of mechanical intestinal obstruction. In the diagnosis of partial SBO in clinically stable patients, contrast fluoroscopy studies can be helpful, particularly in those with intermittent or low-grade obstruction (Baiu & Hawn, 2018; Jackson & Vigiola, 2018; Ten Broek et al., 2018).

Ultrasound evaluation of the abdomen historically had diagnostic sensitivity of over 80%; however, even at baseline, operator expertise is necessary to obtain and interpret high-grade intestinal obstruction in adults with intraluminal gas and typical patient body habitus which significantly obscures images. MRI, though superior to other imaging modalities in the evaluation of intestinal obstruction, remains adjunctive in the diagnosis of bowel obstruction due to its increased cost, lack of easy accessibility, and the technical expertise required (Baiu & Hawn, 2018; Jackson & Vigiola, 2018; Ten Broek et al., 2018).

TREATMENT

The key to reducing mortality in patients with SBOs and LBOs is early diagnosis and operative intervention. Surgical intervention depends on the etiology and sever-ity of the obstruction (Baiu & Hawn, 2018). However, in stable patients with partial or low-grade obstruction, nonsurgical management approaches are recommended including nasogastric tube decompression and supportive measures. In patients who clinically deteriorate at any point during hospitalization due to signs of peritonitis, clinical instability, worsening leukocytosis, leukopenia, acidosis and are concerning for abdominal sepsis, ischemia, or perforation, immediate surgical exploration is indicated (Baiu & Hawn, 2018; Ten Broek et al., 2018). In patients with an irreducible or strangulated hernia, immediate surgery is required. After reduction of a hernia, patients with resolution of SBO should be scheduled for an elective hernia repair. As the risk of ischemia increases, complete or high-grade obstructions often require urgent or emergent surgical intervention (Ten Broek et al., 2018).

In most patients with uncomplicated intestinal obstruction, advancements in minimally invasive surgical techniques have made laparoscopy an accepted approach for initial exploration. When appropriate patients are selected for surgery to treat abdominal obstructions, laparoscopic approaches have shown lower rates of complications, shorter hospitalizations, and lower healthcare costs (Baiu & Hawn, 2018; Jackson & Vigiola, 2018).

CLINICAL PEARLS

- The key to preventing the high morbidity and mortality following a bowel obstruction is early diagnosis, resuscitation, and operative intervention.
- The most important step in the initial management of bowel obstruction is identifying the type, severity, and cause.
- Most bowel obstructions will require hospital admission and surgical consultation.

10.11H: BOWEL PERFORATION

Bowel perforation (commonly referred to as intestinal perforation) is a condition associated with considerable morbidity and mortality (Borofsky et al., 2015; Pouli et al., 2020). Defined as a loss of continuity of the bowel wall, bowel perforation is a potentially devastating condition caused by several different etiologies (Borofsky et al., 2015; Kothari et al., 2017; Pouli et al., 2020). It can be categorized as free (when bowel contents spill into the abdominal cavity causing diffuse peritonitis) or contained (when contiguous organs prevent spillage). In adults, there are numerous causes of bowel perforation and these causes are categorized into four sections: (a) ischemia caused by bowel obstruction and necrosis, (b) infectious processes including appendicitis and diverticulitis, (c) malignancy, and (d) physical disruption, which involves trauma or other iatrogenic causes.

Perforations from duodenal ulcers are two to three times more common than gastric ulcer perforations with gastric carcinoma accounting for approximately 30% of gastric perforations. Free air perforation may be seen in up to 15% of patients with acute diverticulitis, and patients occasionally present with signs of generalized peritonitis even though perforated diverticula are confined to the pelvis (Borofsky et al., 2015; Kothari et al., 2017; Pouli et al., 2020).

PRESENTING SIGNS AND SYMPTOMS

Though the most common presenting symptom of bowel perforation is abdominal pain, depending on the mechanism of perforation, associated symptoms are important in determining an early and accurate diagnosis (Kothari et al., 2017). Other presenting symptoms of a bowel perforation include sharp, severe, sudden-onset epigastric pain that awakens the patient from sleep (suggestive of perforated peptic ulcer), abdominal cramping, shoulder pain (suggestive of diaphragmatic involvement), nausea and vomiting, fever, chills (suggestive of peritonitis), abdominal distension, tachycardia and hypotension (suggestive of sepsis; Borofsky et al., 2015; Kothari et al., 2017). Late findings associated with acute peritonitis include tachycardia, tachypnea, hypotension, fever, and altered mental status (Pouli et al., 2020).

HISTORY AND PHYSICAL FINDINGS

The importance of a comprehensive history and physical examination cannot be overstated and is usually sufficient to accurately diagnose bowel perforation (Borofsky et al., 2015). Obtaining pertinent information related to location and duration of pain, prior episodes, recent procedures, exacerbating, and relieving factors can be helpful in determining the cause of the perforation. A comprehensive history should serve to rule out etiologies such as penetrating injuries or blunt trauma, aspirin or NSAIDs or steroid overdose, perforation of a peptic ulcer, history of recent travel or lower endoscopic procedures such as colonoscopies, or history of chronic inflammatory disease (Kothari et al., 2017; Pouli et al., 2020).

On physical examination, it is important to ensure the patient is hemodynamically stable as any deterioration in condition may indicate the need for emergent surgical intervention. The patient's abdomen should be examined for signs of abrasion, injury or ecchymosis, surgical scars, visible hernias, and distention (Pouli et al., 2020). Perforation, peritonitis, or localized abscess usually elicits discomfort and may yield peritoneal signs when palpating the abdomen. Intraabdominal hemorrhage may present as abdominal fullness. In assessing conditions such as acute appendicitis, perforated acute diverticulitis and ruptured tubo-ovarian abscess, bimanual pelvic examinations and rectal examinations may be conducted (Borofsky et al., 2015; Pouli et al., 2020).

DIFFERENTIAL DIAGNOSIS AND DIAGNOSTIC CONSIDERATIONS

Differential diagnoses for bowel perforation include bowel obstruction, ruptured abdominal aortic aneurysm, tubo-ovarian abscess, ovarian torsion, endometriosis, Crohn's disease, ulcerative colitis, acute cholecystitis, acute pancreatitis, acute pyelonephritis, appendicitis, cholangitis, cholecystitis, diverticulitis, cholelithiasis, acute gastritis, multiple organ dysfunction syndrome, and septic shock (Borofsky et al., 2015; Pouli et al., 2020).

Laboratory tests that may be helpful in diagnosing bowel perforation include complete blood count, complete metabolic profile, and serum lactate. Aerobic and anaerobic blood cultures are indicated in bowel perforation. Common findings in bowel perforation include leukocytosis (which may be absent in the elderly), and lactic acid may suggest sepsis from acute peritonitis (Borofsky et al., 2015; Kothari et al., 2017; Pouli et al., 2020).

Abdominal and upright radiographs are recognized as the most appropriate first-line investigation when investigating perforated bowel. Typically, free air in the subdiaphragmatic locations and a visible falciform ligament are suggestive of bowel perforation. Ultrasonography may also be useful to evaluate the liver, spleen, pancreas, kidneys, adrenals, ovaries, and uterus and may be able to detect the site of perforation and free intraperitoneal air.

To diagnose bowel perforation effectively and accurately, CT of the abdomen and pelvis remains the most sensitive and specific imaging test. CT scan can readily identify disease processes such as diverticulitis, appendicitis, and bowel obstructions, in addition to complications of bowel perforation. To visualize potential areas of ischemia, the use of IV contrast is recommended. Complications from a perforation such as an abscess and secondary bowel obstruction can also be identified and guide management (Borofsky et al., 2015; Kothari et al., 2017).

TREATMENT

The mainstay of treatment for bowel perforation is surgical intervention. Prior to surgery, contraindications such as severe heart failure, respiratory failure, or multiorgan failure should be assessed (Borofsky et al., 2015). Cases unaccompanied by sepsis and peritonitis may be managed by noninvasive modalities while patients in septic shock secondary to peritonitis are likely to require surgery. In patients undergoing surgery for bowel perforation, a laparoscopic approach is considered acceptable and associated with lower rates of complications, shorter hospitalizations, and lower healthcare costs (Borofsky et al., 2015; Kothari et al., 2017; Pouli et al., 2020).

CLINICAL PEARLS

- The key to reducing the high morbidity and mortality associated with bowel perforation is early diagnosis, resuscitation, and surgical intervention.
- The most important step in the initial management of bowel perforation is identifying the etiology of the condition.
- Patients with peritonitis and sepsis secondary to bowel perforation will likely require surgery.

10.11I: DIVERTICULITIS

Diverticula are sacular outpouchings of the colonic wall, diverticulitis occurs when these become inflamed or infected. (Hall et al., 2020; Huston et al., 2018; Schultz et al., 2020). Diverticulosis occurs most commonly in the left colon where the outpouching in the inner layers of the colon push through weaknesses in the outer muscular layers. An overgrowth of bacteria due to obstruction of the diverticular base by feces with micro-perforations is the presumed mechanism of diverticulitis (Hall et al., 2020; Schultz et al., 2020).

The prevalence of diverticulitis increases with age and is present in approximately 50% of individuals over the age of 60, with the incidence rising to 70% after 80 years of age. Only approximately 4% of individuals will develop diverticulitis in their lifetime despite the significant prevalence of diverticulosis (Hall et al., 2020).

PRESENTING SIGNS AND SYMPTOMS

The most common presenting symptom of diverticulitis is pain in the left lower quadrant of the abdomen. The severity of the inflammatory process, location of the affected diverticulum, and the presence of complications determine the clinical presentation of diverticulitis. Other symptoms may include nausea, vomiting, constipation, obstipation, fever, bloating, and diarrhea. Findings associated with acute diverticular rupture with peritonitis and septic/hypovolemic shock include tachycardia, tachypnea, hypotension, fever, and altered mental status (Hall et al., 2020; Schultz et al., 2020).

HISTORY AND PHYSICAL FINDINGS

The importance of a comprehensive history and physical examination in patients with diverticulitis is important as this may be sufficient to arrive at a diagnosis in most cases (Schultz et al., 2020). The presence of diverticula is commonly identified incidentally during colonoscopy or radiologic studies as most patients with diverticulosis are asymptomatic. On physical examination, patients with diverticulitis typically demonstrate localized abdominal tenderness, abdominal distention, tympanic abdomen to percussion, and findings suggestive of fistula formation (colovesicular or colovaginal fistula; Hall et al., 2020; Huston et al., 2018).

DIFFERENTIAL DIAGNOSIS AND DIAGNOSTIC CONSIDERATIONS

Differential diagnoses for diverticulosis include ovarian cysts, acute cholecystitis, acute pancreatitis, acute pyelonephritis, appendicitis, cholangitis, cholecystitis, cholelithiasis, mesenteric ischemia, constipation, irritable bowel disease, pelvic inflammatory disease, and ectopic pregnancy (Hall et al., 2020; Huston et al., 2018; Schultz et al., 2020)

Laboratory tests that may be helpful in diagnosing diverticulitis include complete blood count, complete metabolic profile, liver function tests, urinalysis/urine culture, and aerobic/anerobic blood cultures (bowel perforation). Common findings in diverticulitis include leukocytosis and metabolic alkalosis in patients with significant vomiting (Hall et al., 2020; Huston et al., 2018; Schultz et al., 2020).

In addition to laboratory tests, imaging modalities should be useful to confirm the diagnosis of diverticulitis. Different imaging modalities, including plain abdominal films, ultrasonography, and barium enema, may be used to diagnose diverticular disease. However, the gold standard imaging study for the diagnosis of diverticulitis is a CT scan of the abdomen and pelvis with IV and oral contrast which has a sensitivity and specificity of approximately 97%. The CT scan can detect colonic diverticula, bowel wall thickening, soft tissue inflammatory masses, abscesses, and phlegmon. It is important to assess renal function prior to administering IV contrast (Huston et al., 2018; Schultz et al., 2020).

TREATMENT

The standard of care of acute noncomplicated diverticulitis remains medical management with pain control, hydration, and antibiotics (Huston et al., 2018). Selection criteria for elective surgery should be individualized according to the number, severity, and frequency of diverticulitis episodes, persistent symptomatology after an episode of diverticulitis, and the immunologic status of the patient.

When performing an open, laparoscopic, or robotic elective sigmoid colectomy for diverticulitis, curative treatment requires removing the entire sigmoid colon. Emergent surgical intervention is indicated in patients presenting with signs of peritonitis or sepsis (Huston et al., 2018). A Hartmann procedure, which includes resection of the sigmoid colon, preservation of the rectum in the form of a rectal pouch, and creation of an end colostomy is the traditional surgical method when intraoperative findings confirm perforated diverticulitis (Hall et al., 2020; Schultz et al., 2020). In 3 to 6 months, patients are candidates for colostomy reversal. Unfortunately, approximately 30% of patients undergoing a Hartmann procedure never undergo a colostomy reversal due to complications, associated comorbidities, or frailty (Hall et al., 2020; Schultz et al., 2020).

CLINICAL PEARLS

- The prevalence of diverticulosis increases with age and is present in approximately 50% of individuals over the age of 60.
- The most common presenting symptom of diverticulitis is pain in the left lower quadrant of the abdomen.
- The gold standard imaging study for the diagnosis of diverticulitis is a CT scan of the abdomen and pelvis with IV and oral contrast.
- When performing an open, laparoscopic, or robotic elective sigmoid colectomy for diverticulitis, curative treatment requires removing the entire sigmoid colon.

10.12: ANORECTAL DISORDERS

Bimbola Akintade

Anorectal disorders such as rectal abscess, anal fissure, and hemorrhoids occur at the junction of the anal canal and the rectum, and include structural, neuromuscular, and functional conditions (Lohsiriwat, 2016; Wald et al., 2014). They are common, often distressing, and in some cases debilitating, and significantly add to the healthcare burden. Diagnostic and management dilemmas are encountered when working up patients with anorectal disorders as symptoms frequently overlap obscuring the underlying pathology. As such, a thorough history and physical examination including a digital rectal examination may provide an appropriate roadmap to diagnosis and treatment (Rao & Tetangco, 2020).

10.12A: RECTAL ABSCESS

A rectal abscess usually originates from an infected anal gland in the anal mucosa forming an abscess in the anorectal region with its opening at the level of the dentate line (Beck et al., 2019; Rao & Tetangco, 2020). Abscesses may form in several different areas including the perianal region, deep postanal space, ischiorectal fossa or, rarely, the supralevator space. Anal fistulas characterized as epithelialized tunnels that connect an infected gland inside the anal canal to the skin are a complication of rectal abscesses and occur in up to 40% of patients. Risk factors for rectal abscesses include pregnancy, diabetes mellitus, foreign objects placed in the rectum, immunosuppression, Crohn's disease, and sexually transmitted diseases (Beck et al., 2019; Lohsiriwat, 2016; Wald et al., 2014).

PRESENTING SIGNS AND SYMPTOMS

The most commonly reported symptom of a rectal abscess is acute and throbbing perianal pain, which may be aggravated by coughing, sitting, or defecation. Other presenting symptoms may include fatigue, fever, constipation, and perirectal drainage that may be mucoid, purulent, or bloody (Beck et al., 2019; Wald et al., 2014).

HISTORY AND PHYSICAL FINDINGS

Physical exam and a rectal examination may reveal a tender lump, tissue hardening, or inflammation of the affected area. External findings may include erythema, induration, or fluctuance (Beck et al., 2019; Lohsiriwat, 2016; Wald et al., 2014).

DIFFERENTIAL DIAGNOSIS AND DIAGNOSTIC CONSIDERATIONS

Differential diagnoses of rectal abscesses include rectal prolapse, inflammatory bowel disease, hemorrhoids, anal fissures and fistulas, abdominal pain, and acute prostatitis (Rao & Tetangco, 2020). The clinical workup of patients that present with rectal abscesses rely heavily on a comprehensive history and physical examination as there are no specific laboratory studies indicated in diagnosing the condition.

Though imaging studies are typically not indicated in patients with a rectal abscess, three-dimensional endoanal ultrasonography or CT scan and MRI (gold standard) of the pelvis may provide some additional information on the location and extension of the abscess or confirm the clinical suspicion of an intersphincteric or supralevator abscess.

TREATMENT

The presence of a rectal abscess requires aggressive treatment including incision and drainage. To shorten the length of potential subsequent fistula tract that may form as a complication, the drainage should be performed close to the anal verge. Patients with extensive infection or on immunosuppressive medications should receive IV antibiotics in addition to surgical incision & drainage (I&D). Following I&D, warm sitz baths, adequate pain control, and the prevention of constipation are recommended (Beck et al., 2019; Rao & Tetangco, 2020).

CLINICAL PEARLS

- A rectal abscess usually originates from an infected anal gland in the anal mucosa.
- A comprehensive history and clinical examination with a digital rectal exam (if the patient is able to tolerate) may positively diagnose the disease.
- The presence of a rectal abscess is an indication for incision and drainage.
- Delaying surgical intervention for a rectal abscess may lead to significant complications.

10.12B: ANAL FISSURE

An anal fissure is a painful linear or irregularly shaped tear in the distal anal canal that typically involves only the epithelium, and if left untreated, may involve the full thickness of the anal mucosa (Altomare et al., 2011; Jahnny & Ashurst, 2020). Forceful passage of a hard stool and trauma are the most common causes. An acute fissure gives the appearance of a simple tear. Fissures can be extremely painful during defecation. Rectal pain and spasm may predispose patients to chronic anal fissures (Altomare et al., 2011; Rao & Tetangco, 2020).

PRESENTING SIGNS AND SYMPTOMS

Patients suffering from anal fissures report specific symptoms, and the diagnosis of the condition may be attained with only a comprehensive history and physical examination (Rao & Tetangco, 2020). Patients typically report painful defecation lasting several minutes to hours accompanied by the passage of blood. Patients with anal fissures experience recurring painful defecation which may discourage them from having bowel movement resulting in a cycle of worsening constipation, harder stools, and more anal pain and spasm (Altomare et al., 2011; Jahnny & Ashurst, 2020; Rao & Tetangco, 2020).

HISTORY AND PHYSICAL FINDINGS

In patients reporting a recent history of painful defecation, a small shallow tear in the anal mucosa is evident without the need of digital rectal examination (DRE) and is diagnostic of the condition (Beck et al., 2019; Rao & Tetangco, 2020). Fissures lasting for more than 8-12 weeks are considered chronic and will often have swelling and scar tissue present. Chronic fissues may appear wide and/or raised with the presence of skin tags and hypertrophied anal papilla. (Altomare et al., 2011; Jahnny & Ashurst, 2020; Rao & Wald, 2014).

DIFFERENTIAL DIAGNOSIS AND DIAGNOSTIC CONSIDERATIONS

Differential diagnoses for anal fissures include perianal ulcers, anal abscesses, anal carcinoma, Crohn's disease, and AIDS (Altomare et al., 2011; Lohsiriwat, 2016; Wald et al., 2014). A comprehensive history, in conjunction with a gentle perianal examination with inspection of the anal mucosa typically helps providers make the diagnosis. For anal fissures located in the anterior or posterior anal mucosa, laboratory tests are not indicated. Anal fissures located laterally should raise concerns of other anorectal disorders including Crohn's disease and squamous cell cancer (Beck et al., 2019; Wald et al., 2014). In this situation, additional laboratory tests including stool and viral cultures, erythrocyte sedimentation rate, complete blood cell count and HIV testing should be conducted. In patients with anal fissures that are not easily visualized, an anoscopy with topical lidocaine is indicated (Beck et al. 2019; Wald et al., 2014).

TREATMENT

Treatment goals of anal fissures include symptom relief, ease of defecation, healing, and prevention (Beck et al., 2019; Rao & Tetangco, 2020). Management approaches usually fall into three different categories: conservative, interim, and surgical. In patients with acute anal fissures, healing occurs within a few weeks in the conservative approach. This approach includes adequate pain control with topical nitroglycerin or topical 2% diltiazem, high-fiber diet, stool softeners, laxatives, antiinflammatory and analgesic creams and/or suppositories, warm sitz baths, and local anesthetic injections. Patient education is also essential to prevent or minimize disease recurrence (Altomare et al., 2011; Hang et al., 2017; Lohsiriwat, 2016; Wald et al., 2014).

Chronic anal fissures can reduce the quality of life of patients. In patients with persistent anal fissures symptoms despite 8 weeks or more of conservative treatment, the interim approach involving endoscopy is indicated to rule out irritable bowel disease. Treatment for chronic fissures may include botulinum A toxin injections into the internal anal sphincter or surgery. Botulism A toxin helps relieve spasm by relaxing the anal sphincter and allowing the fissure to heal (Rao & Tetangco, 2020).

In patients with anal fissures unresponsive to conservative or interim management approaches, surgical intervention is indicated. In these patients, a lateral internal sphincterotomy is indicated. Patients who do not qualify for a sphincterotomy may benefit from a fissurectomy with botulinum A toxin injections (Jahnny & Ashurst, 2020; Lohsiriwat, 2016).

CLINICAL PEARLS

- An anal fissure is a clinical diagnosis made essentially by physical exam alone, which must be done to rule out other possible causes of rectal pain.
- Treatment goals of anal fissures include symptom relief, ease of defecation, healing, and prevention.
- Most anal fissures heal spontaneously. Frequent sitz baths, analgesics, stool softeners, and a high-fiber diet are also recommended.

10.12C: HEMORRHOIDS

Hemorrhoids, described as abnormally enlarged, bleeding, or protruding vascular structures in the lower rectum, are among the most common anorectal conditions (Muldoon, 2020; Rao & Tetangco, 2020). Though common, the prevalence of hemorrhoids remains unclear, as many patients are too embarrassed to report them. Risk factors for hemorrhoids include pregnancy, portal hypertension with anorectal varices, rectal surgery, episiotomies, anal intercourse, and colonic malignancy (Lohsiriwat, 2016; Rao & Tetangco, 2020; Wald et al., 2014).

The two types of hemorrhoids are internal and external hemorrhoids. Internal hemorrhoids occur in the lower rectum, while external hemorrhoids develop under the skin around the anus. Due to the overlying skin becoming irritated causing erosion, external hemorrhoids are the most uncomfortable (Beck et al., 2019; Muldoon, 2020; Wald et al., 2014).

PRESENTING SIGNS AND SYMPTOMS

The most common presenting symptom of hemorrhoids is rectal bleeding. The quantity of blood expelled may range from streaks on toilet paper to bright red blood that may drip into the toilet bowl. Clinical suspicion of a more proximal cause of bleeding should be considered with the presence of melena. Symptoms of hemorrhoids include painful defecation, pain and irritation around the anus, pruritus, and fecal leakage (Muldoon, 2020; Rao & Tetangco, 2020).

HISTORY AND PHYSICAL FINDINGS

Prior to the diagnosis of hemorrhoids, a comprehensive history and physical examination should be conducted to rule out other anorectal conditions including anal fissures, abscesses, viral or bacterial skin infection, condylomata, and so on (Beck et al. 2019; Muldoon, 2020; Wald et al., 2014). The disease-specific history should focus on the onset, duration, and degree of the symptoms and risk factors. Due to concerns for increased bleeding, the patient's coagulation history and immune status should be evaluated in addition to characterizing change in bowel habits, bleeding, pain, or protrusion (Beck et al., 2019; Muldoon, 2020).

To guide the therapeutic approach, classification of the grade of internal hemorrhoids is useful. There are four classifications of internal hemorrhoids: first-degree often bleeds without prolapsing, second-degree may protrude with spontaneously reducing prolapse when straining ceases, third-degree produces spontaneously and prolapse requires manual reduction, and fourth-degree if prolapse is irreducible. Though internal hemorrhoids are typically painless, if completely prolapsed, they can be painful (Rao & Tetangco, 2020; Wald et al., 2014).

DIFFERENTIAL DIAGNOSIS AND DIAGNOSTIC CONSIDERATIONS

Painless bleeding with defecation and reducible protrusion are cardinal signs of hemorrhoids and they are typically not associated with other medical conditions. Other anorectal conditions including, Crohn's disease and ulcerative colitis must be ruled out prior to management of hemorrhoids. Differential diagnoses for hemorrhoids include rectal prolapse, anal fissures, anal fistulae, acute prostatitis, proctitis, condyloma acuminatum, pendulated polyps, perianal abscesses, pruritus ani, colorectal tumors, and anal cancer.

In patients who present with hemorrhoids, a complete blood cell count is indicated to evaluate for potential infection or anemia. If the physical examination suggests coagulopathy, coagulation studies are also indicated. To evaluate bright-red rectal bleeding, a flexible sigmoidoscopy or anoscopy should be conducted. For patients with negative anorectal examinations or strong risk factors for colonic malignancy, a colonoscopy should be considered.

TREATMENT

Though the treatment goals in patients with hemorrhoids are to correct constipation and treat complications, clinicians should avoid treatment of asymptomatic hemorrhoids despite how inflamed they look. After hemorrhoids are characterized, treatment is based on symptoms and internal grade (Muldoon, 2020; Rao & Tetangco, 2020). First-line therapy for uncomplicated hemorrhoids includes increasing fluid and fiber intake, stool softeners, warm sitz baths, and counseling regarding defecation habits and dietary modification (AGA, 2004). If grade 1 to 3 internal hemorrhoids are unresolved with the aforementioned management strategies, various minimally invasive procedures, including sclerotherapy, infrared coagulation, ligation, and banding, should be considered. Patients with large grade 3 or grade 4 internal hemorrhoids refractory to conservative management should be referred for a surgical consultation. Management of external hemorrhoids depends solely on symptom management. For patients with acute thrombosis, excision is indicated, and operative resections are indicated in hemorrhoids with problematic skin tags (AGA, 2004; Muldoon, 2020; Rao & Tetangco, 2020; Wald et al., 2014).

CLINICAL PEARLS

- Hemorrhoids can be diagnosed with a comprehensive history and physical examination.
- Treatment goals in patients with hemorrhoids are to correct constipation and treat complications.
- Internal hemorrhoids grades 1 to 3 can be managed conservatively, while large grade 3 or grade 4 conditions may require surgical intervention.

KEY TAKEAWAYS

- Most anorectal disorders can be diagnosed with a comprehensive history and physical examination.
- Laboratory tests including a complete blood cell count is indicated to determine the presence of infection and to evaluate for blood loss. If the physical examination suggests coagulopathy, coagulation studies are also indicated.
- Required imaging studies in anorectal disorder vary based on symptoms, severity, and potential complications.
- Prior to making the specific anorectal diagnosis, other potentially life-threatening diseases and conditions must be ruled out.

A robust set of instructor resources designed to supplement this text is located at **http://connect.springerpub.com/ content/reference-book/978-0-8261-6079-9.** Qualifying instructors may request access by emailing **textbook@springerpub.com.**

REFERENCES

Full list of references can be accessed at http://connect .springerpub.com/content/reference-book/978-0-8261-6079-9

CHAPTER 11

NUTRITIONAL CONSIDERATIONS IN ACUTE CARE

Paula S. McCauley

LEARNING OBJECTIVES

- Learn to perform a thorough nutritional assessment.
- Determine basic nutritional needs for a highly stressed individual.
- Differentiate indications for enteral versus parenteral nutrition (PN).
- Identify common complications of enteral and PN.

INTRODUCTION

As the provider and prescriber, the AGACNP must have a basic understanding of the nutritional needs of acutely ill patients, including a fundamental ability to conduct a comprehensive nutritional assessment and establish standard nutritional needs for supplemental feeding. Basic knowledge of enteral versus parental nutrition and the complications encountered with both is necessary. Dietary consults and resources are readily available to the AGACNP to assist with nutritional needs but may be limited based on settings or off-shift routines in acute care. A comprehensive nutritional assessment will require a thorough history and physical as well as laboratory data. It is necessary to incorporate the patient's medical and surgical history, associated comorbidities, dietary and bowel habits, level of stress, and current medications when initiating nutritional therapies (Baron, 2019).

NUTRITIONAL ASSESSMENT

A comprehensive nutritional assessment incorporates clinical observations along with weight gain or loss, nitrogen balance, muscle mass and function, as well as supportive laboratory data.

The benefits of adequate nutrition include wound healing, enhanced immune system function and maintenance of gastrointestinal structure and function, all of which are linked to improved clinical outcomes, decreased length of stay, and decreased mortality. Providing adequate nutrition is not without risks or complications and strategies to maximize the benefits and minimize the risks are considered when selecting the appropriate means of support (Heyland et al., 2014).

ESTIMATING CALORIC NEEDS

The gold standard for estimating needs is indirect calorimetry (IC), which measures oxygen consumption and carbon dioxide production to calculate energy expenditure. Due to cost (i.e., the expense of the machinery and training of personnel to perform IC), it is not often used and predictive equations have been incorporated. The Academy of Nutrition and Dietetics and the American Society for Parenteral and Enteral Nutrition (ASPEN) have developed standardized diagnostic criteria for defining and documenting adult malnutrition in the clinical setting and include energy intake, fluctuations in weight, body fat, muscle mass, fluid accumulation, and grip strength. Examples of predictive equations include the Penn-State equation or the Ireton Jones equation. These equations incorporate body mass index (BMI) along with temperature, minute ventilation, age, ventilator support, and presence or absence of trauma or burns (Aldeguer et al., 2017).

For a generalized assessment, body weight and Basal Metabolic Index are largely utilized as markers of nutritional assessments. These can be incorporated in an initial calculation by the AGACNP followed by a dietary/nutrition consultation for a more comprehensive evaluation. Utilization of the actual versus ideal body weight (IBW) is important when calculating caloric needs as BMI in acute and critically ill patients may be altered by associated issues such as fluid shifts or volume status. IBW utilizes standard formulas that calculate using height and weight (Bedi & Robinson, 2017). IBW calculations are shown in Box 11.1.

Basic requirements include total daily calories with specifics for various aspects including protein, carbohydrates, and fat. Nutritional requirements are commonly expressed as recommended dietary allowances (RDAs); in healthcare dietary reference intakes (DRIs) go beyond

BOX 11.1 IDEAL BODY WEIGHT CALCULATIONS AND STANDARD REFERENCES

- **Female:** 100 pounds for the first 5 feet of height, an additional 5 pounds for each additional inch
- **Males:** 106 pounds for the first 5 feet of height, additional 6 pounds for each additional inch
- **Standard references:**
    - Underweight is a BMI less than 18 kg/m²
    - Overweight is a BMI greater than 25 kg/m²
    - Obese is a BMI greater than 30 kg/m²

BMI, body mass index.

Source: Data from Aldeguer, Y., & Wilson, S., & Kohli-Seth, R. (2017). Nutrition support. In J. M. Oropello, S. M. Pastores, & V. Kvetan (Eds.), *Critical care*. McGraw Hill. https://accessmedicine-mhmedical-com.ezproxy.lib.uconn.edu/content.aspx?bookid=1944&sectionid=143517561

the RDAs to address long-term health and reduction of chronic risk stratified by age and gender-specific groups (Saunders & Igel, 2022b). The level of energy required to maintain basic physiologic functions is considered when calculating caloric needs. In healthy individuals the level of basal energy expenditure (BEE) and physical activity are included. These may both be altered or reduced in the acute and critically ill individual, thus impacting their minimum requirements. On the other hand, these patients may have a high metabolic demand secondary to a catabolic state seen in illnesses and syndromes such as sepsis or diabetic ketoacidosis.

PROTEIN

Protein provides 4 kcal/g and is needed for tissue growth and maintenance and should account for approximately 20% of daily kilocalories. Protein required per day ranges from 0.8 to 2 g/kg of body weight. Highly stressed patients (e.g., trauma, burns, sepsis) require 1.5 to 2 g or more per kilogram of body weight. Excessive protein intake increases the amount of nitrogenous waste (urea) that must be excreted through the urine. Patients with acute kidney injury or chronic kidney disease will require restriction of protein to prevent exacerbation of kidney injury (Saunders & Igel, 2022b).

CARBOHYDRATE

Carbohydrates consist of 4 kcal/g. They account for the largest proportion of kilocalories in most diets and should provide approximately 50% to 60% of daily need. More oxygen—and release of more carbon dioxide—is required to metabolize carbohydrates than protein or fat, thus patients with compromised respiratory function would benefit from less than average carbohydrate content (Saunders & Igel, 2022b).

FAT

Fat or lipid needs and should account for 20% of daily need. Fats consist of 9 kcal/g. Fat has the lowest respiratory quotient or uses the least amount of oxygen and produces the least amount of carbon dioxide as a byproduct of metabolism. Substituting fat for carbohydrates can reduce stress on the respiratory system, particularly if the patient has minimal lung capacity (Saunders & Igel, 2022b).

BASIC LABORATORY MEASUREMENTS

Basic laboratory measurements for nutritional assessment are one part of your assessment but must be used in combination with physical findings. There is no reliable laboratory marker for diagnosis of malnutrition or response to feeding. For example, serum albumin or prealbumin are good markers of the patient's nutritional status but are impacted by volume status, inflammation, acute illness, liver failure, renal failure, and medications, all of which can alter their sensitivity and specificity. An important factor is the trend in these indicators (Jensen, 2018).

Basic metabolic parameters will also need to be monitored and trended especially if receiving parenteral nutrition (PN). Careful monitoring of triglycerides with propofol is necessary; with inclusion of the lipid calories it provides, you may need to restrict fat intake if maintained for any length of time (Baron, 2019; Druyan et al., 2012).

A comprehensive review and trend of the following values may be considered but used with caution.

SERUM ALBUMIN

Albumin lacks sensitivity or specificity for malnutrition. Less than 3.5 g/dL indicates protein malnutrition.

Albumin's half-life is 20 days and synthesis requires adequate amino acids and hepatic function. Due to its osmotic function you can expect edema if values are less than 2.7 g/dL. Values may be skewed if there is concomitant liver or renal disease, heart failure, or inflammation. Albumin is a principal drug carrier and dosage adjustments may be necessary when reduced. It is a positive predictor for increased morbidity and mortality if significantly reduced.

PREALBUMIN

Normal reference values are 20 to 50 mg/dL, moderate depletion is 10 to 15 g/dL, and less than 10 g/dL indicates severe depletion. Its half-life is approximately 2 days and thus it reflects changes in nutritional status more quickly than albumin. Prealbumin is affected by renal dysfunction, hepatic dysfunction, hydration status, and inflammation. Trends are important and usually done once or twice weekly.

TRANSFERRIN

Transferrin or total iron binding capacity (TIBC) is a common marker used for nutritional evaluation. Normal concentration is 170 to 250 mg/dL; 151 to 200 mg/dL indicates mild depletion; 100 to 150 mg/dL moderate depletion and less than 100 mg/dL severe depletion. Its half-life is 8 to 10 days; it also reflects changes more quickly than albumin. Transferrin is synthesized in the liver and values can be skewed in liver disease, renal disease, congestive heart failure or inflammation. Its concentration is also influenced by iron status. Trends are important and transferrin is often checked with pre-albumin once or twice weekly.

C-REACTIVE PROTEIN

C-reactive protein is a positive acute phase reactant. Elevation is indicative of an active inflammatory process and nutrition assessment may indicate a negative nitrogen balance (Bedi & Robinson, 2017; Jensen, 2018).

PRESENTING SIGNS AND SYMPTOMS

Presenting signs and symptoms may include rapid or gradual weight loss, edema, anorexia, altered or limited nutritional intake, and specific physical findings discussed in the following.

HISTORY AND PHYSICAL FINDINGS

Rapid cellular turnover is noted in many body systems and nutritional deficiencies in these areas quickly become obvious. Emphasis is on history and physical findings specific and sensitive to the chief complaint, including pertinent positive/negative findings. IBW calculations are based on height and weight with adjustments for skeleton size.

Focused assessment of the following will help identify many vitamin, mineral, or fatty acid deficiencies. Common assessments are included in Box 11.2.

Common physical findings seen with malnutrition are included in Box 11.3 and specific physical exam findings are included in Box 11.4.

SPECIAL CONSIDERATIONS IN THE ELDERLY

Nutritional needs may change with aging. Obesity and/or malnutrition become more prevalent with aging. Lean body mass and muscle mass declines by middle age. Dietary recommendations for the elderly are similar to middle-aged adults with recommendations for higher calcium and vitamin D intake. B$_{12}$ and D deficiencies are also common. The Mini Nutritional Assessment (MNA®) is a standardized screening tool for geriatric patients. It includes changes in food intake, weight loss, mobility,

neuropsychological problems such as dementia, and BMI to assess overall nutritional status (Sheffrin & Yukawa, 2021).

Weight loss that is unintentional has been shown to be a reliable measure of malnutrition. A loss of more than 5% in 1 month or 7.5% over 3 months is considered clinically significant (Bedi & Robinson, 2017).

BOX 11.2 SYSTEMATIC NUTRITIONAL ASSESSMENTS

- **Skin:** Should be smooth and free of color irregularities.
- **Mucous membranes:** Should be smooth, pink, and moist.
- **Hair:** When healthy, hair is shiny, not easily plucked or brittle.
- **Skin tone:** When well-nourished, skin is muscular, some fat should be present.
- **Skeleton:** Evaluate for erect posture versus kyphosis or scoliosis; evaluate for joint irregularities.
- **Nails:** Should be regularly shaped and free of ridges.

Source: Data from Baron, R. B. (2019). Nutritional disorders. In M. A. Papadakis, S. J. McPhee, M. W. Rabow, & T. Berger (Eds.), *Current medical diagnosis & treatment 2019*. Lange Medical Books; Jensen, G. L. (2018). Malnutrition and nutritional assessment. In J. Jameson, A. S. Fauci, D. L. Kasper, S. L. Hauser, D. L. Longo, & J. Loscalzo (Eds.), *Harrison's principles of internal medicine* (20th ed.). McGraw Hill. https://accessmedicine-mhmedical-com.ezproxy.lib.uconn.edu/content.aspx?bookid=2129&sectionid=192283158

BOX 11.3 INDICATIONS OF MALNUTRITION

- Loss of muscle mass leading to temporal muscle wasting or clavicular prominence
- Loss of subcutaneous fat in the cheeks or orbital area, between the thumb and forefinger
- Localized or generalized fluid accumulation
- Diminished functional status assessed by handgrip strength

Source: Data from Bedi, N. M., & Robinson, M. K. (2017). Nutrition and metabolic support. In S. C. McKean, J. J. Ross, & D. D. Dressler, & D. B. Scheurer (Eds.), *Principles and practice of hospital medicine* (2nd ed.). McGraw Hill. https://accessmedicine-mhmedical-com.ezproxy.lib.uconn.edu/content.aspx?bookid=1872&sectionid=138891217

BOX 11.4 PHYSICAL EXAM FINDINGS THAT SUPPORT NUTRITIONAL DEFICIENCIES

- Dry brittle hair, hair loss (protein, vitamin A, vitamin E, biotin deficiencies)
- Dry cracking skin (niacin deficiency)
- Petechiae, ecchymosis (vitamin A, vitamin C, vitamin K)
- Visual disturbances (vitamin A)
- Stomatitis, glossitis, and cheilosis
- Paresthesia, memory disturbance, hyporeflexia (thiamine, B_{12} deficiencies)
- Dermatitis, wounds and pressure injuries, poor dentition, tooth loss, ataxia, loss of muscle mass and strength and balance are associated with multiple deficiencies and compromised nutritional status

Source: Data from Sheffrin, M., & Yukawa, M. (2021). Defining adequate nutrition. In L. C. Walter, A. Chang, P. Chen, G. Harper, J. Rivera, R. Conant, D. Lo, & M. Yukawa (Eds.), *Current diagnosis & treatment geriatrics* (3th ed.). McGraw Hill. https://accessmedicine-mhmedical-com.ezproxy.lib.uconn.edu/content.aspx?bookid=2984&sectionid=250006969

DIFFERENTIAL DIAGNOSIS AND DIAGNOSTIC CONSIDERATIONS

Differentials for malnutrition or weight loss should include:

- **Medical factors:** Malignancy, gastrointestinal (GI) disorders (e.g., motility disorders, dysphagia, peptic ulcers), dementia, heart failure, and end-stage renal disease.
- **Psychosocial factors:** Isolation, depression, paranoia, alcoholism.
- **Medications:** Numerous medications may impact nutrition and intake with side effects such as anorexia, nausea/vomiting (e.g., opiates, digoxin, selective serotonin reuptake inhibitors [SSRIs], antibiotics), dry mouth (e.g., anticholinergics, loop diuretics, antihistamines), or altered taste and smell (e.g., angiotensin-converting enzyme [ACE] inhibitors, calcium channel blockers, spironolactone, iron, antiparkinsonian medications, opiates; Sheffrin & Yukawa, 2021).

TREATMENT

Initiation of nutritional support should be considered early on in admission to the acute care setting. The most appropriate route with lowest risk and lowest cost possible should be considered with oral intake being the best route. Modified diets such as clear or full liquids are considered in special situations but should be advanced as quickly as possible to meet the patient's full nutritional needs. Oral supplements may also be considered to meet adequate nutritional needs. If oral intake is not possible, decisions regarding types of nutritional support rely on the guidelines that enteral feeding is safer and less expensive; if the GI track is nonfunctional, parenteral (intravascular) feeding is appropriate (Saunders & Igel, 2022b).

Supplemental nutritional support is indicated for at least four groups of adult patients:

- Inadequate bowel syndromes: short gut syndrome, malabsorption, irritable bowel disease
- Severe prolonged hypercatabolic states seen with extensive burns, trauma, mechanical ventilation
- Patients requiring prolonged therapeutic bowel rest: post surgery, pancreatitis

Severe protein–calorie malnutrition with a treatable disease who have sustained a loss of 10% body weight at 6 months or 20% body weight at 1 year (Saunders & Igel, 2022c)

Before initiation of feedings in the acute care population a thorough assessment should include evaluation of weight loss and previous nutrient intake before admission, level of disease severity, comorbid conditions, and function of the GI tract (Saunders & Igel, 2022a).

The patient's level of stress will contribute to the number of calories the AGACNP will provide. Stressed patients first receive full nutritional support in the later stage of the stress response. In the early stage of stress and treatment the focus is on correcting fluid and electrolyte imbalances, generally in the first 24 to 48 hours.

Utilizing kilocalories per kilogram (kcal/kg) of body weight when determining nutritional needs is a general rule of thumb and 25 to 30 kcal/kg is necessary for maintenance of weight. The average adult requirement is 30 kcal/kg or 13 kcal/lb of body weight per 24 hours. Stressed individuals require 25 to 35 kcal/kg and include those with hypercatabolic states such as trauma, burns, sepsis, or neurologic diagnoses. For weight gain, 35 or more kcal/kg is necessary (Saunders & Igel, 2022a).

Special considerations in your calculations will be necessary for patients with elevated body temperature and renal and liver disorders. There is an approximate 10% increase in kilocalories per 24 hours required for each degree above 98.6°F. With renal and liver dysfunction the amount of protein, amino acids, and electrolytes will need to be adjusted and monitored closely (Saunders & Igel, 2022b).

ENTERAL NUTRITION

Enteral nutrition (EN) should be used if the GI tract is functional. EN is any feeding that uses the GI tract and is the preferred form of feeding. There are significant physiologic advantages to EN including preservation of gut integrity and prevention of transmigration of GI bacteria through the intestinal wall to the bloodstream with resulting sepsis (Druyan et al., 2012).

Forms of enteral feeding include nasogastric, nasoduodenal, or nasojejunal tubes. Surgically created openings include surgical gastrostomy or percutaneous endoscopic gastrostomy (PEG) or percutaneous endoscopic jejunostomy (PEJ). The choice of route is influenced by the expected length of time of enteral feeds. If the patient is expected to require support for more than 4 to 6 weeks, enterostomal tubes are preferred as prolonged nasogastric and nasoenteric tubes increase the potential risk for sinus infections and oral complications.

Tube feeds can be administered by bolus, intermittent, or continuous modalities. Formulas have been developed that are standard but also rich in calories with low volume, as well as specialized for disease-specific conditions such as low in carbohydrates for hyperglycemia and chronic lung disease, and low protein for renal dysfunction. Routes that enter into the duodenal or jejunum are utilized to reduce incidence of aspiration and require elemental or hydrolyzed formulas as the stomach and its digestive enzymes are bypassed (Aldeguer et al., 2017).

DETERMINE GOAL RATE OF FEEDING

- Estimate caloric needs
- Choose a formula (this will depend on the formulary that your facility utilizes)
- Divide goal calories by kcal/mL to determine daily volume of formula
- Divide daily volume by number of hours feeding will infuse to determine goal rate

Example: For a 60 kg individual requiring 25 kcal/kg, the desired kg is 1,500 and the AGACNP wishes to utilize a 24-hour continuous infusion. If using a semi elemental formula that provides 1.2 kcal/mL for a caloric estimate of 1500 kcal (Aldeguer et al., 2017):

1,500 kcal/1.2 mL = 1250 mL
1,250 mL per 24 hour = 52 mL/hour

COMPLICATIONS OF ENTERAL FEEDING

Enteral feeds are typically started at a low rate and gradually advanced to infusion goal within 24 to 48 hours. Patients are evaluated for symptoms that may indicate intolerance or complications. Complications of enteral feeding include GI effects such as diarrhea or constipation. Gastric retention may contribute to potential aspiration. Alterations in osmolarity and volume status may also occur with derangements in electrolytes including sodium, potassium, and glucose.

Frequent comprehensive metabolic panels are required to monitor electrolytes and the need for supplemental free water, vitamins, and minerals. Alterations in formulas with fiber rich or reduced fiber may aid in complications such as diarrhea or constipation (Aldeguer et al., 2017).

ASPEN recommends monitoring gastric residual volumes; if residual volume is greater than 250 mL for two residual checks, consider adding a motility agent such as metoclopramide. Hold feedings for residuals greater than 500 mL and evaluate for abdominal distention, ileus, or impact of motility agents. If intolerance persists, consideration of PN may be necessary (Bedi & Robinson, 2017).

PARENTERAL NUTRITION

PN should be provided under very specific conditions. Evidence has shown that PN therapy provided for a duration of less than 5 to 7 days does not impact outcomes and may result in increased risk to the patient. In the standard population consider the use of PN only after the first 7 days of hospitalization when EN is not available unless there is evidence of protein-calorie malnutrition on admission and EN is not feasible, or if the patient is expected to undergo major upper GI surgery. PN may be considered if unable to meet energy requirements (100% of target goal calories) after 7 to 10 days by the enteral route alone. Exceptions include the patient who is malnourished and requires a surgical intervention. PN should be initiated 5 to 7 days preoperatively and continued into the postoperative period (Aldeguer et al., 2017; Druyan et al., 2012).

PN can be delivered through a peripheral vein which limits the percent of dextrose to a maximum of 10% due to a high incidence of phlebitis and infiltration. Higher concentrations of dextrose require a central line. Formulations include dextrose, amino acids, electrolytes, and minerals. Supplemental lipid solutions must be included 3 to 7 times per week depending on the patient's needs. If the patient is receiving propofol this must be included in the lipid calculations (Aldeguer et al., 2017; Bedi & Robinson, 2017).

CALCULATING NEEDS FOR PARENTERAL NUTRITION

Differing from EN, PN calculations require specific calculations for each subset and are divided into protein needs and nonprotein calories which includes carbohydrate and fat/lipid needs. Fluid and electrolyte replacements are adjusted daily based on comprehensive metabolic panels. Micronutrients may be added for wound healing and to avoid complications from deficiencies. Box 11.5 provides a basic example of PN calculations.

COMPLICATIONS OF PARENTERAL NUTRITION

Complications of parenteral nutritional support are many and include mechanical, infectious, and metabolic complications.

Mechanical complications include catheter occlusion and thrombosis. Infectious complications include catheter-related infection. PN places the patient at higher risk for infection due to its high glycemic content. Metabolic complications include hyperglycemia, hypoglycemia, and hypercapnia. There is also increased risk of pancreatitis and hypertriglyceridemia with lipid infusion. Cholestasis and gallbladder sludge or stones

BOX 11.5 CALCULATING PARENTERAL NUTRITION NEEDS

Example (using 60 kg body weight): Total calories: 1,500 kcal

1. Protein (AA): 60 kg × providing 1.5 g/kg = 90 g
   90 g × 4 kcal/g (AA concentration) = 360 kcal
2. Carbohydrate (dextrose): 1,500 kcal × .5 = 750 kcal
   750 kcal/3.4 kcal/g (standard dextrose concentration) = 220 g
3. Fat (lipid): 1,500 kcal − 750 kcal (from carbohydrate) − 360 kcal (from protein) = 390 kcal 390 kcal/10 kcal/g = 39 g (can be rounded to 40 g)

AA, amino acids.

Source: Data from Aldeguer, Y., Wilson, S., & Kohli-Seth, R. (2017). Nutrition support. In J. M. Oropello, S. M. Pastores, & V. Kvetan (Eds.), *Critical care*. McGraw Hill. https://accessmedicine-mhmedical-com.ezproxy.lib.uconn.edu/content.aspx?bookid=1944&sectionid=143517561

are associated with PN. Decreased enteral stimulation may also result from PN and supplemental trickle enteral feeding is often employed to combat complications while receiving PN (Aldeguer et al., 2017).

Box 11.6 includes routine monitoring and considerations when PN is utilized that will help identify and address complications.

SPECIAL CONSIDERATIONS IN THE ELDERLY

Social or cognitive issues that may impact overall nutrition in the older adult include underlying medical conditions and medications. Older adults often eat better

BOX 11.6 CONSIDERATIONS WHEN ADMINISTERING PARENTERAL SUPPORT

- Monitor blood glucose every 6 hours
- Monitor electrolytes, CBC, Ca, Phos, Mg, LFTs, as well as triglyceride levels daily
- Infuse fat emulsions slowly over 12 to 24 hours
- Involve pharmacist, dietitian, and physician in planning parenteral support
- Trend nutritional laboratory results a minimum of weekly and adjust additives accordingly

Source: Data from Druyan, M. E., Compher, C., Boullata, J. I., Braunschweig, C. L., George, D. E., Simpser, E., & American Society for Parenteral and Enteral Nutrition Board of Directors. (2012). Clinical guidelines for the use of parenteral and enteral nutrition in adult and pediatric patients: applying the GRADE system to development of ASPEN Clinical Guidelines. *Journal of Parenteral and Enteral Nutrition*, *36*(1), 77–80. https://doi.org/10.1177/0148607111420157

and more when fed by family members or when eating with others. Always consider the use of oral supplements and appetite stimulants before initiating artificial feeding (Sheffrin & Yukawa, 2021).

Goals of care should be discussed prior to initiating artificial feeding. Consider a therapeutic or predetermined limit of time to trial with plans to discontinue if the overall goals of care are not achieved or the patient is able to resume adequate nutrition without supplementation (Sheffrin & Yukawa, 2021).

TRANSITION OF CARE

Patients should be monitored for adequacy of treatment and to prevent or detect complications. Because estimates of nutritional requirements are imprecise, frequent reassessment is necessary. Daily intakes should be recorded and compared with estimated requirements. Body weight, hydration status, and overall clinical status should be followed. Patients who do not appear to be responding as anticipated can be evaluated for nitrogen balance (Saunders & Igel, 2022a).

Patients with positive nitrogen balances can be continued on their current regimens; patients with negative balances should receive moderate increases in calorie and protein intake and then reassessed. Monitoring for metabolic complications includes daily measurements of laboratory tests including serum glucose, sodium, chloride, potassium, phosphorus, magnesium, calcium, creatinine, and blood urea nitrogen (BUN). Once the patient is stabilized, these laboratory tests should be obtained at least twice weekly. Folate, zinc, and copper should be checked at least once per month (Saunders & Igel, 2022a).

When transitioning from unit or facility goals of care, baseline weight, electrolytes, minerals and trended evaluations of prealbumin and transferrin should be included in the transfer data. Documentation of complications and effective treatment should also be provided.

CLINICAL PEARLS

- Nutritional assessment is done upon admission to acute and critical care.
- Initiation of nutrition should take place within 24 to 48 hours of admission.
- If the gut works, use it!
- EN helps prevents transmigration of bacteria through the intestinal wall to the bloodstream.
- Complications of PN are many.
- When utilizing PN, monitor blood glucose every 6 hours and electrolytes, liver functions, and triglycerides daily.
- Trend nutritional laboratory results weekly.

KEY TAKEAWAYS

- A comprehensive nutritional assessment will identify most deficiencies; laboratory values will validate those findings.
- EN is the preferred route of feeding unless the GI track is nonfunctional.
- PN for less than 7 days may not impact outcomes and may result in risk.
- Consider PN only after 5 to 7 days when EN is not available, when a patient is undergoing upper major GI surgery, or as supplemental when EN is inadequate.
- Utilize an interprofessional team approach including pharmacist and dietitian for best practice.

EVIDENCE-BASED RESOURCES

ASPEN:

Clinical Guidelines for the Use of Parenteral and Enteral Nutrition in Adult and Pediatric Patients

Applying the GRADE System to Development of A.S.P.E.N. Clinical Guidelines https://aspenjournals .onlinelibrary.wiley.com/doi/full/10.1177/ 0148607111420157

Guidelines for the provision of nutrition support therapy in the adult critically ill patient: The American Society for Parenteral and Enteral Nutrition. (2022). *Journal of Parenteral and Enteral Nutrition, 46,* 12–41. https://doi .org/10.1002/jpen.2267.

Mini Nutritional Assessment: https://www.mna-elderly .com/sites/default/files/2021-10/mna-mini-english.pdf

Simplified Nutrition Assessment: https://www.msdmanuals .com/professional/multimedia/figure/nut_simplified_ nutritional_assessment

Seniors in the Community: Risk Evaluation for Eating and nutrition. https://www.phsd.ca/resources/research -statistics/research-evaluation/reports-knowledge -products/seniors-community-risk-evaluation-eating -nutrition/

A robust set of instructor resources designed to supplement this text is located at **http://connect.springerpub.com/ content/reference-book/978-0-8261-6079-9.** Qualifying instructors may request access by emailing **textbook@springerpub.com.**

REFERENCES

Full list of references can be accessed at http://connect .springerpub.com/content/reference-book/978-0-8261-6079-9

KIDNEY DISORDERS

INTRODUCTION

Injury to the kidney can develop acutely or chronically, ranging from acute kidney injury (AKI) to chronic or end-stage kidney disease (ESKD). The mechanisms contributing to kidney dysfunction can be acquired such as hypertension, iatrogenic occurring after contrast administration, or as a consequence of another pathology such as volume depletion, renal artery stenosis (RAS), or rheumatologic disorder. Consequences associated with kidney injury and failure can be life-threatening and require complex management considerations.

12.1: ACUTE KIDNEY INJURY

Jacqueline Ferdowsali

PRESENTING SIGNS AND SYMPTOMS

The signs and symptoms of acute kidney injury (AKI) may be attributed to the underlying pathology causing the AKI or due to the loss of renal filtration and elimination. Box 12.1 provides a summary of common signs and symptoms. For some patients there may be no complaints of symptoms initially.

HISTORY AND PHYSICAL FINDINGS

The most common causes of AKI include sepsis and hypovolemia followed by nephrotoxic drugs (Hoste et al., 2015). The history should include pertinent findings of signs or symptoms of infection such as fever, nausea, vomiting, or cough. Additionally, attention should be given to oral intake status and physical findings suggestive of dehydration such as skin tenting, low jugular venous pressure, or orthostatic hypotension. Other etiologies leading to hypovolemia should also be explored such as bleeding. A review of medications should be undertaken to determine any potential nephrotoxic agents that may be contributing to the AKI. Other potential etiologies to explore include evidence to support vasculitis such as butterfly rash or purpuras or jaundice to support a liver pathology.

> **BOX 12.1 PRESENTING SIGNS AND SYMPTOMS OF ACUTE KIDNEY INJURY**
>
> - Decrease in urine production
> - Lower extremity edema or periorbital edema
> - Fatigue
> - Dyspnea
> - Confusion
> - Chest pain

BOX 12.2 DEFINITION OF ACUTE KIDNEY INJURY

- Increase in SCr by greater than or equal to 0.3 mg/dL (greater than or equal to 26.5 mol/L) within 48 hours
- Increase in SCr to ≥1.5 times baseline, which is known or presumed to have occurred within the prior 7 days
- Urine volume <0.5 mL/kg/h for 6 hours
- SCR, serum creatinine

Source: Data from Kidney Disease Improving Global Outcomes, 2012a, p. 8.

BOX 12.3 DIAGNOSTIC TESTING CONSIDERATIONS IN ACUTE KIDNEY INJURY

- Serum creatinine and blood urea nitrogen
- Serum electrolytes
- Complete blood count
- Fractional excretion of sodium or urea
- Urine sodium
- Urine protein
- Urine osmolality
- Urine albumin to creatinine ratios
- Serum and urine protein electrophoresis (rule out monoclonal gammopathy and multiple myeloma)
- Renal ultrasound
- Computed tomography (CT) noncontrast scan
- Urine sediment examination
- Kidney biopsy

Note: Not all tests are indicated for every patient. The history and physical exam should guide test selection.

DIFFERENTIAL DIAGNOSIS AND DIAGNOSTIC CONSIDERATIONS

The diagnosis of AKI is based on either serum creatinine or urine output. AKI is defined as any of the following criteria listed in Box 12.2. In addition to diagnosing AKI, a staging system can also be applied (Table 12.1). The staging of AKI is helpful in guiding treatment interventions. It is important to also recognize those individuals at risk for developing AKI prior to any changes in urine output or creatinine levels.

TABLE 12.1: Staging System for Kidney Disease

STAGE	SERUM CREATININE	URINE OUTPUT
1	Any one of the following: • 1.5–1.9 times baseline • ≥0.3 mg/dL (≥26.5 mmol/L) increase	<0.5 mL/kg/h for 6-12 hours
2	2.0–2.9 times baseline	<0.5 mL/kg/h ≥ 12 hours
3	Any one of the following: • 3 times baseline • Increase in serum creatinine to ≥4.0 mg/dL (≥353.6 mmol/L) • Initiation of renal replacement therapy • In patients <18 years, decrease in eGFR to <35 mL/min per 1.73 m²	<0.3 mL/kg/h for ≥24 hours or anuria for ≥12 hours

Source: Data from Kidney Disease Improving Global Outcomes, 2012a, p. 8.

Differential Diagnosis

One approach to the differential diagnosis of AKI is to determine if the etiology is prerenal, intrarenal, or postrenal in origin (Esquivel, 2019; Table 12.2). It is possible that the injury started as a prerenal cause such as sepsis and progressed to intrarenal tubular injury. Several diagnostic tests may be helpful in determining the etiology of the AKI. Urinary indexes such as fractional excretion of sodium (FeNa) and urea may provide a clue to a prerenal etiology. Evaluating the urine sodium can also be helpful. A FeNa ($\% = 100 \times (S_{Cr} \times U_{Na})/(S_{Na} \times U_{Cr})$) less than 1% and a urine sodium less than 20 suggests a prerenal etiology. Caution should be used in interpreting a FeNa or urine sodium in the presence of diuretic use, chronic kidney disease (CKD), urinary obstruction, or acute glomerular disease. Routine renal ultrasounds should only be performed if obstructive etiology is a concern. Urine sediment suggests acute tubular necrosis if muddy brown casts are observed. Box 12.3 provides a summary of diagnostic testing to consider.

TREATMENT

A clear goal of AKI management is to prevent further injury and allow renal function to improve, and is largely supportive care. Initially, a fluid challenge may be administered to determine the patient's fluid responsiveness and observe for improvement in renal function prior to a definitive diagnosis of the AKI. Volume resuscitation is a cornerstone of AKI management (Ostermann et al., 2020). Specific fluid selection should be based on the underlying etiology. For patients with sepsis, fluid resuscitation should follow current guideline recommendations. If hemorrhagic shock is present, then volume resusci-

TABLE 12.2: Differential Diagnosis Framework for Acute Kidney Injury

PRERENAL	INTRARENAL	POSTRENAL
Intravascular volume depletion • Gastrointestinal loss • Renal loss • Skin and mucous membrane loss • Hemorrhage • Third spacing	Tubular injury • Ischemia • toxin	Mechanical • Stones • Tumors • Hematoma • Benign prostatic hyperplasia • Strictures Neurogenic bladder
Decreased effective circulation volume • Heart failure • Cirrhosis • Pulmonary hypertension, pulmonary embolism	Interstitial • Acute interstitial nephritis (medications, infection or systemic diseases) • Pyelonephritis	
Systemic or renal vasodilation • Sepsis • Cirrhosis • Anaphylaxis • Anesthesia or medication induced	Glomerular • Nephritic • Nephrotic syndromes	
Impaired renal autoregulation • Medication induced • Abdominal aortic aneurysm • Hepatorenal syndrome • Renal artery thrombosis or embolism	Vascular (either large or small vessels) • Renal artery thrombosis • Renal vein thrombosis • Atheroembolism • Thrombotic microangiopathies • Malignant hypertension • Vasculitis	

Source: Data from Esquivel, E. (2019). Acute kidney injury. In S. D. C. Stern, A. D. Cifu, & D. Altkorn (Eds.), *Symptom to diagnosis: An evidence-based guide* (4th ed.). McGraw-Hill Education.

tation with blood products would be most beneficial. Assessment of fluid responsiveness should be used to guide volume resuscitation. All nephrotoxic drugs should be discontinued. Box 12.4 provides a summary of important nephrotoxic drugs for which to evaluate. Also, medication dosages may need to be adjusted based on changing glomerular filtration rates (GFR). It is important to consider the unreliability of the GFR in changing creatinine levels as seen in AKI (Moore et al., 2018).

Glycemic control is important in AKI although exact targets are still debated (Moore et al., 2018). It is important to consider that hyperglycemia is associated with worse morbidity and mortality in AKI but the patient with AKI is also more at risk for developing hypoglycemia. The main complications associated with AKI include hyperkalemia, metabolic acidosis, volume overload, and symptoms of uremia.

The Kidney Disease Improving Global Outcomes (KDIGO) guidelines (2012a) recommend the use of diuretics in those patients who are volume overloaded only. Treatment of hyperkalemia should follow established medical therapy interventions.

Renal replacement therapy may be indicated for some patients with AKI. The indications for renal replacement therapy are summarized in Box 12.5. The selection of either continuous renal replacement therapy (CRRT) or intermittent hemodialysis is dependent on many factors such as patient hemodynamics and resources available.

BOX 12.4 COMMON DRUGS ASSOCIATED WITH ACUTE KIDNEY INJURY DEVELOPMENT

- Aminoglycosides
- Nonsteroidal anti-inflammatory drugs
- Angiotensin-converting enzyme inhibitor or angiotensin receptor blocker
- Amphotericin
- Foscarnet
- Iodine contrast
- Pentamide
- Tenofovir
- Zolendronic acid

Source: Data from Moore, P., Hsu, R., & Liu, K. (2018). Management of acute kidney injury: Core curriculum 2018. *American Journal of Kidney Disease, 72*(1), 136–148. https://doi.org/10.1053/j.ajkd.2017.11.021

TRANSITION OF CARE

AKI may resolve quickly or, in the case of acute tubular necrosis, take weeks or months. Kidney function may

BOX 12.5 INDICATIONS FOR RENAL REPLACEMENT THERAPY

- Acidosis
- Electrolyte abnormalities (hyperkalemia)
- Intoxicants
- Fluid overload
- Uremia symptoms (nausea, seizure, pericarditis, bleeding)

also not return to baseline and CKD may develop. Recommendations include the measurement of serum creatinine 3 months after AKI to evaluate for resolution or new or worsened CKD.

12.2: CHRONIC KIDNEY DISEASE

R. Brandon Frady

According to the National Vital Statistics Reports (2019), chronic kidney disease (CKD) is the ninth-leading cause of death in the United States ("Deaths: Final Data for 2017," 2019). In the United States, 14% of adults have some stage of CKD. Adults over the age of 70 make up more than half of patients with Stage 3 to 5 CKD ("Deaths: Final Data for 2017," 2019). CKD is a progressive disease that may lead to a total loss of all kidney function. Medicare patients with CKD not on dialysis have triple to quadruple the hospitaliza-

tion rate (Tuttle et al., 2018). Also, patients with CKD are more likely to have readmission to the hospital, eventually culminating in worsening kidney function (Tuttle et al., 2018). The fatal readmission rate between 2012 and 2014 Medicare patients was 2.5-fold for Stage 5 CKD patients (Tuttle et al., 2018). In a 9-year study of veterans, the decline in kidney function rate led to higher hospitalizations, readmissions, and prolonged lengths of stay (Xie et al., 2015).

The definition of CKD includes abnormal kidney structure and or function for greater than 3 months. With structure and function abnormalities being albuminuria, urine sediment abnormalities, abnormalities associated with tubular dysfunction, histological abnormalities, structural abnormalities, history of kidney transplantation, and/or an estimated glomerular filtration rate (eGFR) less than 60 mL/min/1.73 m^2 (Kidney Disease Improving Global Outcomes [KDIGO], 2013). CKD should be classified based on the cause, GFR, and albuminuria. The staging of CKD is essential for the evaluation and management of patients. Staging is depicted in Figure 12.1. The albumin-creatinine ratio (ACR) is the optimal quantification of albuminuria (Brown et al., 2017; Smith, 2016). Albuminuria is categorized as follows: A1 is an ACR less than or equal to 30 mg/g, A2 is 30 to 300 mg/g, and A3 is greater than 300 mg/g. Figure 12.1 defines the relationship between GFR and albuminuria when attempting to predict worsening kidney function. A rising GFR and albuminuria are associated with the progression of kidney disease (KDIGO, 2013).

Prognsosis of CKD by GFR and Albuminuria Categories: KDIGO 2012				Persistent albuminuria categories Description and range		
				A1	**A2**	**A3**
				Normal to mildly increased	Moderately increased	Severely increased
				<30 mg/g <3 mg/mmol	30-300 mg/g 3-30 mg/mmol	>300 mg/g >30 mg/mmol
GFR categories (ml/min/ 1.73 m²) Description and range	G1	Normal or high	≥90			
	G2	Mildly decreased	60-89			
	G3a	Mildly to moderately decreased	45-59			
	G3b	Moderately to severely decreased	30-44			
	G4	Severely decreased	15-29			
	G5	Kidney failure	<15			

White: low risk (if no other markers of kidney disease, no CKD); Light gray: moderately increased risk; Gray: high risk; Dark gray: very high risk

FIGURE 12.1: Prognosis of CKD by GFR and albuminuria categories.
Source: Reproduced from Kidney Disease Improving Global Outcomes. (2013). KDIGO 2012 Clinical Practice Guideline for the Evaluation and Management of Chronic Kidney Disease. *Kidney International Supplements, 3*(1). https://doi.org/10.1038/kisup2012.73

Loss of kidney function is mostly asymptomatic. Proper evaluation, diagnosis, and management are essential for the care of the patient with CKD. Ideal management of CKD includes cardiovascular risk reduction, monitoring and treatment of albuminuria, avoiding nephrotoxic agents, and managing pharmacologic dosing of medication.

PRESENTING SIGNS AND SYMPTOMS

CKD patients may initially be asymptomatic until they reach Stage 3 CKD or greater. CKD is often an incidental finding during routine healthcare visits. The discovery of CKD typically consists of serum electrolytes abnormalities, urine studies, and clinical presentation. The early detection or prediction of CKD is difficult given the lack of correlation between symptoms and stage of CKD (Brown et al., 2017). CKD patients' complaints are frequently associated with weakness, decreased appetite, anorexia, nausea, nocturia, polyuria, urinary frequency, hematuria, edema, flank pain, hypertension, and pallor (Chen et al., 2019). As kidney disease progresses, the primary driver of CKD symptoms is uremia. Table 12.3 outlines signs and symptoms based on the organ system. In addition to uremic-driven signs and symptoms, patients with advanced CKD disease stages may present with drug toxicities as an initial finding (Papadakis et al., 2021).

HISTORY AND PHYSICAL FINDINGS

The vague signs and symptoms of CKD make a comprehensive history and physical essential to detection and diagnosis. Chief complaints in patients with CKD are often nonspecific, ambiguous, or frequently a silent condition alone. The initial history and physical should focus on differentiation between acute kidney injuries (AKI), CKD, and other causes of the patient's symptoms.

History of Present Illness

The knowledge that CKD symptoms are vague and often difficult to ascertain makes a detailed history of present illness crucial to CKD evaluation and may provide data supporting CKD. Assessment of the chronicity of signs and symptoms is essential to the diagnosis of CKD. Clinicians should inquire about the timing of symptoms, any aggravating events, any attempts to alleviate symptoms, and successful treatments for symptoms.

Review of Systems

The review of systems for a patient with CKD is essential to the patient's overall diagnosis and management. While the initial presentation may be vague, a closer look at a review of systems may reveal the following:

- **General:** Fatigue, signs of volume overload, decreased mental acuity, intractable hiccups
- **Skin:** Uremic frost, pruritic excoriations, ashen appearance
- **Pulmonary:** Dyspnea, pleural effusions, pulmonary edema, and uremic lung
- **Cardiovascular system:** Pericardial friction rub, congestive heart failure, pitting edema
- **Gastrointestinal:** Anorexia, nausea, vomiting, weight loss, stomatitis
- **Neuromuscular:** Muscular twitching, peripheral sensory and motor neuropathies, muscle cramps, restless legs, sleep disorders, hyperreflexia, seizure encephalopathy, coma
- **Endocrine:** Amenorrhea, impotence, decreased libido
- **Hematologic:** Anemia and bleeding

TABLE 12.3: Signs and Symptoms of Uremia and Chronic Kidney Disease

BODY SYSTEM	SYMPTOMS	SIGN
General	Fatigue, malaise	Pale, chronic ill appearance
HEENT*	Metallic taste in mouth, epistaxis	Pale conjunctiva
Pulmonary	Shortness of breath,	Pleural effusion, rales
Cardiovascular	Dyspnea on exertion, retrosternal chest pain	Hypertension, cardiomegaly, friction rub
Gastrointestinal	Anorexia, nausea, vomiting, hiccups	
Genitourinary	Nocturia, erectile dysfunction, decreased libido	
Musculoskeletal	Restless legs, numbness, and cramps in legs	
Integumentary	Pruritus, bruising easy	Pallor, ecchymoses, edema, xerosis
Neurologic	Irritability, inability to concentrate	Stupor, asterixis, peripheral neuropathy, myoclonus

HEENT, head, eyes, ears, nose, and throat.

Physical Examination

A comprehensive physical exam looking for findings consistent with CKD aids in the diagnosis and management of patients. Physical exams should be systematic and focus on the cardiovascular, pulmonary, integumentary, and neurologic systems. Special attention to the volume status of the patient is also crucial in the examination of CKD patients. Patients with volume overload from CKD are likely to experience weight gain, peripheral or sacral edema, and crackles.

Hypertension is a common finding in patients with CKD. Patients with arteriovenous nicking or retinopathy suggest long-standing hypertension and or diabetes that may elevate suspicion of CKD. Assessment for cardiovascular bruits may raise suspicion of renovascular disease. Pulmonary findings are significant for crackles, diminished breath sounds, or dullness with the lung bases' percussion associated with pleural effusions. Integumentary findings are rashes, palpable purpura, petechiae, telangiectasias, or sclerosis. Neurologic findings are neuropathies, altered mental status, inattention, weakness, or poor ability to concentrate. Musculoskeletal findings are neuromuscular irritability, tetany, and possible seizures secondary to hypocalcemia due to reduced vitamin D production. CKD patients with advanced CKD may exhibit pallor, skin excoriations, muscle wasting, asterixis, myoclonus, altered mental status, and pericardial friction rub (Chen et al., 2019).

A thorough review of all prescribed and over-the-counter medications is essential in patients suspected of having CKD. Special attention to medications and supplements that are metabolized and or excreted by the kidneys is key to evaluating and managing CKD patients. Additionally, a thorough review of the family history, paying particular attention to familial or hereditary kidney disorders, is important.

DIFFERENTIAL DIAGNOSIS AND DIAGNOSTIC CONSIDERATIONS

The differential diagnosis for patients with suspected or confirmed CKD focuses on determining an underlying cause contributing to the CKD. The CKD presentation is also a presentation that may be similar to heart failure, nephrotic syndrome, obstructive uropathy, AKI, nephrolithiasis, pyelonephritis, or polycystic kidney disease (Chen et al., 2019). Additionally, vasculitis, amyloidosis, systemic lupus erythematosus (SLE), and scleroderma are on the differential list.

Laboratory/Diagnostic Findings

CKD patients are at risk for severe electrolyte imbalances and or worsening metabolic acidosis that may be life-threatening. Patients with CKD should have electrolytes evaluated including sodium, potassium, chloride, carbon dioxide, blood urea nitrogen (BUN), creatinine, calcium, magnesium, and phosphorus. In addition to electrolyte monitoring, acid-base balance monitoring is essential to the management of CKD patients. Although there is controversy over the definition, patients with metabolic acidosis may be considered chronic if more than 5 days. While the exact mechanism is unknown, the resulting chronic metabolic acidosis may contribute to negative protein balance and worsen CKD (Patschan et al., 2020). Additionally, Banerjee et al. found that elevated serum anion gap levels increased CKD risk (Banerjee et al., 2019).

Additionally, eGFR and albuminuria are essential in patients with CKD. Albuminuria is a crucial laboratory finding in the diagnosis and management of CKD. The best albuminuria study is the urine-albumin serum creatinine ratio. There are additional urine studies that substitute for urine albumin creatinine ratio, including urine protein/serum creatinine ratio and automated urinalysis with reagent strip for total protein; the last and least reliable study to assess albuminuria is the manual reading of urinalysis via a reagent strip. As renal function worsens, patients will need more frequent monitoring to follow the progression of CKD and monitor for electrolyte and acid-base disturbances.

Diagnostic imagining that may be useful in diagnosing and managing CKD is chest radiography to evaluate pulmonary edema. Renal ultrasound and renal vascular imaging may also provide additional data on the kidney's structure and blood supply.

TREATMENT

Treatment for CKD focuses on early detection and prompt treatment of further decline in kidney function. In addition to treating kidney dysfunction, evaluating, and treating cardiovascular risk, blood pressure, anemia, diabetes, lipids, nephrotoxic medications, dietary management, mineral-bone disorders, and hepatitis C are part of a comprehensive care plan for a patient with CKD.

Cardiovascular Risk Reduction

Patients with CKD are at a greater risk of developing cardiovascular disease resulting in worsening CKD (Chen et al., 2019). Patients with a GFR G3a to G4 have a two to three time higher rate of cardiovascular disease mortality (Sarnak et al., 2019). Consistent with other risk reduction guidelines, management of hypertension and lifestyle modifications will improve long-term cardiovascular outcomes. CKD patients should maintain a healthy weight, eat a low sodium diet (less than 2 grams per day), limit alcohol intake to no more than two standard drinks per day (KDIGO, 2012c), and exercise a minimum of five times per week for at least 30 minutes. Exercise recommendations are based on the overall health, including cardiovascular ability. Smoking cessation is recommended for all CKD patients.

Hypertension Management

Patients with CKD should have individualized targeted blood pressures according to age, comorbidities, risk of CKD progression, and presence of diabetes (KDIGO, 2012c). All CKD patients should have blood pressure control targeted at systolic blood pressures less than 140 mmHg and diastolic blood pressures less than 90 mmHg (KDIGO, 2012c). Patients with albuminuria greater than 30 mg in 24 hours (with or without diabetes) should have a target blood pressure of systolic less than 130 mmHg and diastolic less than 80 mmHg. Initial treatment should use angiotensin-converting enzyme inhibitor (ACE-I) or angiotensin receptor blocker (ARB) to treat the blood pressure (KDIGO, 2012c). ACE-I or ARB therapy should be titrated to maximum dosing as tolerated to achieve the blood pressure goal. Evaluation of potassium and serum creatinine levels are used to adjust ACE-I/ARB therapy. In patients that develop hyperkalemia secondary to ACE-I/ARB therapy initial attempts should be made to reduce the potassium level and continue ACE-I/ARB therapy (de Boer et al., 2020).

Anemia

Patients with CKD should have hemoglobin concentrations measured when clinically relevant (KDIGO, 2012b): at a minimum of annually with CKD Stage 3, biannually with CKD Stage 4–5, and every 3 months with CKD Stage 5 on hemodialysis and or peritoneal dialysis (PD; KDIGO, 2012b). Evaluation of anemia should include complete blood count, absolute reticulocyte count, ferritin level, serum transferrin saturation (TSAT), vitamin B12 levels, and folate levels (KDIGO, 2012b). Treatment of anemia is iron replacement, erythropoietin- (EPO) stimulating agents (ESA), and/or red blood cell transfusions (KDIGO, 2012b).

Iron Supplementation

CKD patients with iron deficiency should have iron supplementation risk-benefit evaluated before prescribing IV or oral supplementation. The use of iron has the benefit of minimizing and possibly avoiding the use of blood transfusion or the use of ESAs (KDIGO, 2012b). This risk of iron transfusion is possible anaphylaxis or other adverse events. Patients should receive an IV iron trial; if the patient cannot tolerate this, then a 1- to 3-month trial of oral iron for patients that are not on hemodialysis is acceptable. The goal with iron replacement is to increase the hemoglobin concentration without using ESA treatment. A TSAT <30% and ferritin less than 500 ng/mL is the goal (KDIGO, 2012b). For patients taking an ESA, IV iron replacement to reduce the ESA dosing is recommended. Patients on an ESA should have TSAT and ferritin studies monitored at least every 3 months and with ESA dose increases (KDIGO, 2012b).

Erythropoietin-Stimulating Agents

Before initiating ESA agents, all correctable causes of anemia should be evaluated (KDIGO, 2012b). ESAs in patients with CKD and hemoglobin less than 10 g/dL is reasonable. This evaluation includes the rate of hemoglobin decline and another risk (active malignancy, history of stroke, and malignancy history). For a patient in CKD Stage 5 and on dialysis, ESA is to avoid a hemoglobin level less than 9 g/dL (KDIGO, 2012b).

Red Blood Cell Transfusion

Avoid the use of red blood transfusions when possible to minimize the risk associated with blood product transfusions. Overall the decision to transfuse patients outside of symptomatic acute blood loss anemia, acute hemorrhage, and unstable coronary artery disease (CAD) should not be based on hemoglobin level alone but rather symptoms of anemia (KDIGO, 2012b).

Diabetes Management

Ideal management of patients with CKD and diabetes includes a comprehensive approach including a multidisciplinary team focused on kidney management, cardiovascular disease management and risk reduction, and control of diabetes. The cardiovascular risk reduction and patient management were outlined previously in the cardiovascular risk section.

Blood Glucose Monitoring

Monitoring of people with diabetes includes hemoglobin A1C (HgbA1C) and self-monitoring practices. Once a CKD patient reaches stage G4 to G5, especially in dialysis, the HgbA1C has low reliability, and redundant, blood glucose monitoring via continuous methods or self-monitoring methods is more accurate and is essential for hypoglycemia detection and to improve compliance with overall glycemic control. For patients who cannot monitor their blood sugar, renally adjusted antihyperglycemic medications that pose the lowest hypoglycemia risk are preferred. HgbA1C goals for CKD and diabetes range from less than 6.5% to less than 8%. HgbA1C differences are related to eGFR and overall risks. The severity of CKD, macrovascular complications, comorbidities, life expectancy, hypoglycemia awareness, hypoglycemia management, and treatment causing hypoglycemia are all considered when establishing HgbA1C goals (de Boer et al., 2020).

Glycemic Treatment

A comprehensive antihyperglycemic management approach includes exercise, nutritional awareness, smoking cessation, blood pressure control, lipid management, administration of insulin or oral antihyperglycemics. For people with type 1 diabetes, supplemental exogenous insulin is the mainstay of therapy. Patients with CKD and an eGFR greater than 30 mL/min/1.73 m², metformin and sodium-glucose cotransporter-2 inhibitor (SGLT2) inhibitors are the treatment of choice (de Boer et al., 2020). Metformin formulation is immediate or sustained release. Initially, for immediate release, 500 mg or 850 mg daily with titration up by 500 mg or 850 mg weekly to a maximum dosing of 2000 mg daily should be prescribed (de Boer et al., 2020). Extended release appears to have fewer gastrointestinal side effects. Once the eGFR is less than 45 mL/min/m², metformin dosing is adjusted, and for some patients, dosing adjustment for eGFR between 45 and 59 mL/min/m² is necessary. For patients that require dose adjustments, metformin initiation is half the dose (250 mg) with up-titration weekly to half the maximum dose (1000 mg; de Boer et al., 2020). If patients are on metformin for longer than 4 years, vitamin B12 level monitoring is essential (de Boer et al., 2020; Navaneethan et al., 2020). For type 2 diabetes and CKD, patients with eGFR less than 30 mL/min/1.73 m² should not receive metformin but keep should receive SGLT2 inhibitors. The selection of SGLT2 inhibitors should account for the renal and cardiovascular benefits. Concomitant diuretics and SGLT2 inhibitor use increase the risk for hypovolemia, and patients need to monitor for signs and symptoms of dehydration. If type 2 diabetes remains uncontrolled, then the addition of a third-line agent is considered. The patient's preferences, comorbidities, eGFR, and cost acceptance must contribute to medication selection. Long-acting glucagon-like peptide-1 receptor agonists are commonly preferred (de Boer et al., 2020).

Lipid Management

In patients with a new diagnosis or current diagnosis of CKD, lipid profile evaluation is recommended. CKD patients over the age of 50 and eGFR less than 60 mL/min/1.73 m² not on chronic dialysis or post kidney transplant are treated with statin or statin/ezetimibe therapy (Wanner et al., 2014). For patients over 50 and eGFR greater than 60 mL/min/1.73 m², the recommended treatment is with statin therapy alone (Wanner et al., 2014). In patients aged 18 to 49 years with nondialysis CKD and one or more of the following: known CAD, diabetes mellitus, prior ischemic stroke, and or greater than 10% risk of fatal myocardial infarction or coronary death within the next 10 years statin therapy is recommended. (Wanner et al., 2014). For dialysis-dependent CKD patients do not use statin or stain/ezetimibe, unless that patient is already on a lipid lowering agent, continuing current therapy is reasonable (Wanner et al., 2014). For patients with kidney transplantation, statin therapy is recommended. In addition to pharmacologic therapy, patients with hypertriglyceridemia are counseled on lifestyle changes.

Nephrotoxic Agents and Medication Dosing

As the eGFR declines, a frequent review of medications is necessary for dose adjustments. When the eGFR reaches <60 mL/min/1.73 m², medications excreted by the kidney require dose adjustment. Patients with CKD should avoid herbal supplements and review all over-the-counter medicines with a clinician before taking them. Avoid the routine use of nonsteroidal anti inflammatories (NSAIDs). Standard medication classes requiring dose adjustments are antibiotics, direct oral anticoagulants, oral hypoglycemic agents, chemotherapy, and opiates. Finally, patients with CKD should avoid phosphate-based bowel preparations.

CKD patients should avoid NSAIDs except aspirin. Acetaminophen is a safe pain reliever for CKD patients noting that they should consume based on safe dosing. Initially, this may be difficult as patients with CKD have vague symptoms or are even a symptomatic until their kidney disease is severe. Plantinga et al. found that 10.2% of patients with CKD had a current prescription for NSAIDs, and up to 66% had used NSAIDs for a year or more (Plantinga et al., 2011). Even patients with disease awareness did not have reduced use of NSAIDs.

Dietary Management

Patients with CKD should have a low protein diet (0.8 g/kg/day) with reduced GFR and 1.3 g/kg/day for at-risk patients. CKD patients are to avoid excessive protein consumption as it leads to excessive phosphorus production in the body. Additionally, the patient should avoid excessive consumption of dietary acids and follow a low sodium diet. Patients with CKD may benefit from accredited nutritional consultation to make appropriate food choices.

Mineral Bone Disorders

Patients with CKD have serum calcium, phosphorus, parathyroid, alkaline phosphate, and calcitriol [25(OH)D] levels monitored beginning with CKD level G3a. The frequency of monitoring these levels is based on the progression of CKD. Patients found to have vitamin D deficiency are to have vitamin D replacement included in the treatment plan. Patients with CKD risk factors, suspected of having osteoporosis, or evidence of CKD-MBD should have bone mineral density testing. Parathyroid hormone (PTH) and alkaline phosphate are monitored to evaluate bone disease. Patients with suspected vascular calcification should have lateral abdominal radiographs to assess vascular calcification and an echocardiogram to look for valvular calcifications.

Patients with elevated phosphorus levels are to have phosphorus levels targeted to a normal level. Treatment with phosphate-lowering agents is based on progressively or persistently elevated phosphate levels. Long-term use of aluminum-based phosphate binders should be avoided in patients with CKD G5D. Limiting dietary phosphate intake is a crucial component of phosphorus management in CKD patients. While the exact level of PTH in CKD is unknown, if rising or persistently high PTH levels are found, patients should have modifiable factors of hyperphosphatemia, hypocalcemia, increased phosphate intake, and vitamin D deficiency evaluated and treated as necessary. The goal for intact PTH level should be maintained between 2 and 9 times the upper limit of normal. The suggested treatment for lowering iPTH is calcimimetics, calcitriol, vitamin D analogs, or calcimimetics plus calcitriol or vitamin D analogs.

Patients with CKD and osteoporosis or have a high risk of fracture are treated consistently with the current osteoporosis guidelines.

COVID-19 and CKD

Severe Acute Respiratory Syndrome Coronavirus 2 (SARS-CoV-2) is a viral pandemic changing the healthcare landscape. Data are limited on the direct effects of SARS-CoV-2 on the kidney. A recent study evaluated 4264 hospitalized intensive care unit patients across 68 ICUs in the United States and found that patients with CKD regardless of dialysis dependence had higher 28-day mortality rates than non-CKD patients. Additionally, CKD patients with SARS-CoV-2 are more likely to develop AKI and a decline in overall renal function leading to worsening CKD stages and including end-stage renal disease requiring hemodialysis (Coca et al., 2020; Flythe et al., 2021).

Hepatitis C and Chronic Kidney Disease

Chronic kidney disease patients should be screened for hepatitis C infection. A patient that has progressive CKD to the point of needed hemodialysis requires hepatitis C screening before admittance into a dialysis center, initiation of PD, or starting home dialysis regime (KDIGO, 2018). Follow-up hepatitis screening should occur at a 6-month interval. For patients that are positive for hepatitis C, liver function monitoring for liver fibrosis is essential (KDIGO, 2018). A patient that needs to undergo hepatitis C treatment and has a coexisting CKD is treated with consideration given the eGFR. Patients with eGFR greater than or equal to 30 mL/min/1.73 m² are treated with usual antiviral therapies. Patients with eGFR less than 30 mL/min/1.73 m² are to be treated with ribavirin-free antiviral regimens (KDIGO, 2018).

Nephrology Referral

Patients with progressive kidney disease (eGFR < 30 mL/min/1.73 m², albuminuria >300 mg/24 hours), a swift decline in eGFR, CKD with hypertension on four or more antihypertensives, persistent electrolyte abnormalities, or CKD progressing needing renal replacement therapy should have a prompt referral to a nephrologist (KDIGO, 2013).

12.3: END-STAGE KIDNEY DISEASE

Molly Lillis Cahill, Jennifer Branch, and Suzanne James

End-stage kidney disease (ESKD), formerly known as end-stage renal disease (ESRD; Kidney Disease Improving Global Outcomes [KDIGO], 2018), is the final stage (Stage 5) of chronic kidney disease (CKD), when kidney function has declined to the point that the kidneys no longer function on their own. According to the National Center for Chronic Disease Prevention and Health Promotion ([CDC], 2021) 30 million people, or 15% of adults in the United States are estimated to have CKD. Some risk factors for developing CKD include uncontrolled diabetes, high blood pressure, heart disease, drug abuse, chronic NSAID use, obstructive or reflux diseases of the urinary tract, family history of CKD, inflammation, and various genetic disorders. Without good control of these comorbid conditions, CKD can progress more quickly to ESKD and ultimately require dialysis or kidney transplantation as life-sustaining treatment. Conservative management is also an option for patients who do not wish to start dialysis or pursue transplant.

The prevalence of CKD in U.S. adults in 2016 was 47 million (14%–15% of the adult U.S. population). This accounts for 20% of all Medicare costs ($52 billion/year in 2014). The prevalence of ESKD in the United States in 2002 was 435,000; in 2016 it was 660,000.

CKD is a progressive disease that will worsen over time (Figure 12.1). Factors that will lead to a quicker progression to ESKD include uncontrolled diabetes, uncontrolled systemic hypertension, hyperlipidemia, smoking, proteinuria, hyperphosphatemia with calcium phosphate deposition, decreased perfusion (severe dehydration, sepsis, or shock) and nephrotoxic medications (nonsteroidal antiinflammatory drugs [NSAIDs], IV contrast media). Many patients in the early stages of CKD do not experience any symptoms or have many electrolyte or acid base disturbances but as CKD progresses these become more common.

PRESENTING SIGNS AND SYMPTOMS

Electrolyte and metabolic disorders most often manifest with CKD Stages 4–5 (GFR <30 mL/min/1.73 m²). Patients with tubulointerstitial disease, cystic diseases, nephrotic syndrome, and other conditions associated with polyuria, hematuria, and edema are more likely to develop signs of disease at earlier stages.

Hyperkalemia

Hyperkalemia is a common electrolyte abnormality seen in ESKD patients. Potassium is the most important electrolyte to monitor in CKD patients due to the risk of cardiac arrest. Hyperkalemia usually does not develop until the GFR falls below 20–25 mL/min/1.73 m², at which point the kidneys have decreased capacity to excrete potassium. Hyperkalemia may be seen sooner in patients with a high potassium diet or low serum aldosterone levels. Common causes of low aldosterone levels are diabetes mellitus, use of angiotensin-converting enzyme inhibitors and angiotensin II receptor blockers (ARBs), NSAIDs, and beta-blockers.

Metabolic Acidosis

Metabolic acidosis in Stage 5 may manifest as protein-energy malnutrition, loss of lean body mass, and muscle weakness. Altered salt and water regulation by the kidney in CKD can cause peripheral edema, hypertension, and potentially pulmonary edema.

Uremic Manifestations

Uremic manifestations in patients with CKD Stage 5 are usually secondary to an accumulation of multiple toxins; as these waste products build up, uremic symptoms increase. Patients may have a metallic taste in their mouth and their breath may smell of ammonia. Uremia causes alteration in taste and halitosis. In ESKD patients it is common to stop eating certain meats due to poor taste and they begin to lose weight with poor intake. Progressive uremia can cause nausea and vomiting.

Skin Rash/Itching

As kidney function decreases, waste products accumulate systemically which can cause severe itching.

Heart Failure

The incidence of heart failure is directly correlated to an increased risk of worsening CKD. Changes to the myocardium with overload from chronic uncontrolled hypertension, volume overload adds to ventricular dysfunction and heart failure (see also Chapter 3 for further information on heart failure). Diastolic dysfunction can occur early in CKD prior to the development of left ventricular hypertrophy (LVH). Individuals with heart failure experience significant fatigue, activity intolerance, and fluid retention. Fluid volume overload, peripheral edema associated with heart failure, or pulmonary edema can be critical if under dialyzed. Shortness of breath is often multifactorial with fluid build-up and anemia. Nitrates (oral, topical, or IV) can be temporarily effective for patients with fluid overload.

Cardiac Dysfunction

Cardiac dysfunction and chest pain in ESKD occurs frequently during dialysis. For patients presenting with chest pain, a cardiac origin should be considered due to the high prevalence of coronary disease in ESKD patients. Cardiac arrest in a patient with ESKD may be due to hyperkalemia. The AGACNP should consider treatment with IV calcium and IV bicarbonate while awaiting laboratory confirmation. Nebulized albuterol may also be used for temporary lowering of serum potassium levels, when appropriate. In the setting of pulseless electrical activity (PEA), the AGACNP should consider pericardial tamponade. If tamponade is suspected, pericardiocentesis may be required. If bedside ultrasound is available, this can confirm the diagnosis and guide pericardiocentesis.

Hypotension

Hypotension in ESKD patients on dialysis may be due to bleeding, cardiac dysfunction, or sepsis. Treatment requires careful consideration of their kidney function due to risk for fluid overload. If IV fluid is required, small bolus doses of normal saline (200-250 mL) should be used. Lactated Ringers solution should be avoided given it's potassium content. Ringer's should not be used due to potassium content.

Anemia

Anemia, which in CKD develops primarily because of decreased renal synthesis of EPO, manifests as fatigue, reduced exercise capacity, impaired cognitive and immune function, and reduced quality of life. Anemia is also associated with the development of cardiovascular disease, the new onset of heart failure, worsening heart failure, and increased cardiovascular mortality.

Bleeding

Bleeding may be due to uremic coagulopathy or from anticoagulation during hemodialysis. In the latter case, the heparin effect may be reversed with protamine. Desmopressin (DDAVP) by nasal, subcutaneous, or IV routes and cryoprecipitate are effective in correction of uremic coagulopathy. Applying firm but nonocclusive pressure for 10 to 15 minutes best treats bleeding from a vascular access site.

PRESENTING SIGNS AND SYMPTOMS

The typical presenting complaints of ESKD in the acute care setting include abdominal pain, chest pain, uremic pericarditis (cardiac tamponade risk), myocardial ischemia, dyspnea, congestive heart failure exacerbations, electrolyte abnormalities (e.g., hyperkalemia), fever (bloodstream infections from infected dialysis access), hypotension or syncope (commonly due to rapid fluid removal during dialysis treatment).

The generalized symptoms related to inadequate dialysis include volume overload, peripheral edema, pulmonary edema, hypertension or hypotension, fatigue, reduced exercise capacity associated with anemia in CKD, impaired cognitive and immune function, reduced quality of life, development of cardiovascular disease, new onset of heart failure, worsening heart failure, and increased cardiovascular mortality (Arora, 2022; KDIGO, 2012).

HISTORY AND PHYSICAL FINDINGS

For dialysis dependent patients it is important to gather outpatient dialysis orders and history including the first date of dialysis, dialysate prescription, baseline vital signs, estimated dry weight, in-center medications, and missed dialysis treatments. Some patients have uni- or bilateral kidneys removed for cancer, blood pressure control, or other disease-related causes. It is important to know/note if post nephrectomy. Residual renal function, including urine output, is imperative to note and can aid in fluid removal goal setting.

Past Medical History

The cause (biopsy proven or not) and baseline stage of kidney disease should be stated. When gathering the patient history, it is important to note the onset and duration of specific disease states: diabetes mellitus, presence of microalbuminuria, prehypertension, albuminuria, retinopathy, and hypertension, which if present for over 5 to 10 years may have resulted in irreversible end-organ damage.

Pertinent family history includes autosomal dominant polycystic kidney disease (affects men and women in every generation), autosomal recessive polycystic kidney disease, Alport syndrome (x-linked recessive, affects men in every generation), and Fabry disease.

Physical Exam

A comprehensive physical exam is important for all patients in the acute care setting but for those with ESKD there are additional assessments that are important not to miss (Table 12.4).

Labs

ESKD patients in the acute care setting will need specific labs checked at admission and will also need a daily metabolic panel if on dialysis (Table 12.5). Additionally, residual kidney function should be assessed using one of the methods in Table 12.6.

If the patient is admitted in CKD Stage 5 with little or no known history of CKD, additional tests may be ordered as part of the evaluation to determine etiology of disease. Serum and urine protein electrophoresis (SPEP, UPEP) and free light chains are ordered to screen for a monoclonal protein possibly representing multiple myeloma. Antinuclear antibodies (ANA) and double-stranded DNA antibody levels are used to screen for systemic lupus erythematosus (SLE). Serum complement levels are also commonly ordered and may be depressed with some glomerular diseases. Cytoplasmic and perinuclear pattern antineutrophil cytoplasmic antibody (C-ANCA and P-ANCA) levels can aid in the diagnosis of granulomatosis with polyangiitis (Wegener granulomatosis). The P-ANCA is also helpful in the diagnosis of microscopic polyangiitis. Antiglomerular basement membrane (anti-GBM) antibodies are suggestive of Goodpasture syndrome. hepatitis B and C, HIV, and Venereal Disease Research Laboratory (VDRL) serology may be related to some glomerular diseases (Benjamin & Lappin, 2021).

Considerations for hypercoagulable workup include antithrombin, protein C, protein S, Factor V Leiden, and antiphospholipid antibodies. Table 12.7 lists imagining studies that may be used in the diagnosis of CKD (KDIGO, 2012).

TABLE 12.4: Physical Exam Findings in End-Stage Kidney Disease

PHYSICAL EXAM	POSSIBLE EXAM FINDINGS IN ESKD
General	Subtle changes in LOC could be attributed to uremia
HEENT	Hearing loss could be indicative of ototoxicity or some kidney specific diseases (e.g., Alports)
Neck	Assess if the patient has had parathyroidectomy. Note presence of IJ line or CVC or any signs of infection
Respiratory	Rales/crackles, peripheral edema, or diffuse anasarca
Cardiac	Uremic pericarditis (tamponade), pericardial friction rub
Abdomen	Tenderness or pain (peritonitis), ascites (common in dialysis patients and may be due to congestive heart failure or liver disease), hematochezia, constipation (PD patients with constipation may have drainage problems), bowel sounds (slow gastric emptying is common in dialysis patients); presence of or tenderness over allograft
Genitourinary	Some patients with ESKD do not make urine or may be anephric. Presence of nephrostomy tube or Foley catheter. Assess output and insertion site
Extremity	Access sites (AVF/AVG), assess for audible bruit or palpable thrill; if absent this may suggest access thrombosis. AVF/AVG site assess for infection; inflammation, redness, warmth, drainage
Skin	Any diabetic ulcers or wounds present, uremic frost, discolorations related to vascular access infection of blood flow (dialysis patients with vascular access issues may present with discolored or gangrenous fingers/toes)
Neuro	Restless legs syndrome history, decreased or altered LOC (may be related to uremia); lethargy, mental fogginess, ataxia, confusion, and ophthalmoplegia, focal neurologic deficits. Hypocalcemia presents with tetany like symptoms.

AVF, arteriovenous fistula ; AVG, arteriovenous graft; CN, cranial nerves; CVC, central venous catheter; LOC, level of consciousness; PD, peritoneal dialysis; RRR, regular rate and rhythm.

TABLE 12.5: Specific Laboratory Considerations in End-Stage Kidney Disease

LAB TEST	FREQUENCY	WHAT TO WATCH	NOTE AT DISCHARGE
Comprehensive metabolic panel (CMP), basic metabolic panel (BMP), or renal panel	On admission and as needed daily, directs dialysis prescription/timing	K+, CO_2 for dialysis prescription; BUN indicator of uremia; Cr indicator of kidney function; address diet and medications for elevated phosphorus, K+	Communicate to outpatient unit which K+, Ca dialysis bath used
Complete blood count	On admission, may need daily if severe anemia, neutropenia, leukopenia, infection	White blood cells for infection, Hgb/Hct for anemia, ESA, transfusion; uremic platelet dysfunction	Transfusions, ESA dose
Urinalysis	On admission and as needed	Infection, proteinuria, hematuria	Infection/Rx, new onset or increased proteinuria, hematuria; change in urine output may alter dialysis prescription
International normalized ratio/prothrombin tim	On admission and as needed	Levels with anticoagulants, procedures; over-heparinization	Starting, stopping, or any change in dose of any anticoagulant
Lipid panel	As needed	Aid in diagnosis renal artery stenosis, cardiac baseline, risk factors, genetic risk	Starting, stopping, or any change in lipid-lowering medications
Serum calcium, intact calcium	On admission and as needed (especially hypocalcemia)	Hypocalcemia can be life-threatening, prompt treatment; neurologic signs/ symptoms; hypercalcemia is a cardiovascular risk factor	Starting, stopping, or any change in medications
Parathyroid hormone (PTH)	As needed	Coordinate with medication doses	Continue outpatient regimen for BMD, communicate any changes to outpatient dialysis
Albumin, pre-albumin	On admission, as needed; frequent with hypocalcemia until corrected	Nutritional status, if nutritionally depleted use corrected calcium: 0.8× (normal albumin - patient albumin) + serum Ca)	Communicate any hypocalcemia, TPN, supplements started
Iron studies	On admission, as needed	T-sat <20 to dose IV iron; ferritin >800 can indicate acute phase reactant, infection	Do not give iron supplementation in presence of infection

BMD, bone mineral density; BUN, blood-urea-nitrogen; ESA, erythropoiesis-stimulating agents; s/s, signs and symptoms;TPN, total parenteral nutrition.

DIFFERENTIAL DIAGNOSIS AND DIAGNOSTIC CONSIDERATIONS

Table 12.8 lists the differential diagnosis considerations for ESKD.

TREATMENT

Kidney Replacement Therapy Options

Hemodialysis

Extracorporeal circuit removes water and solutes across a semipermeable dialyzer membrane.

- **Typical treatment time:** 3 to 4 hours
- **Frequency:** 3 days per week

Adequate dialysis, indicated by Kt/V >1.2 per session, is calculated by K = dialyzer clearance, t = dialysis duration/v = urea volume of distribution. Hemodialysis (HD) can be done in-center, at home, or nocturnally (6–9 hours 3 times weekly). Advantages of HD include rapid toxin removal, lower cost, reduced exposure to anticoagulation, and treatments can be individualized. Disadvantages of HD include hypotension with rapid fluid removal, dialysis disequilibrium syndrome, and it requires specialized training and staff.

Indications for HD include ESKD, AKI with uremic complications (encephalopathy, pericarditis, uncontrolled bleeding, BUN >100 to 150, persistent nausea and vomiting), anuria/oliguria, or ingestion of unknown substances. Toxins and overdose substances that can be cleared by HD can be remembered by the mnemonic "I STUMBLED": (Isopropanol, Salicylates, Theophylline, Tenormin (Atenolol), Uremia, Methanol, Barbiturates (e.g., phenobarbital), Lithium, Ethylene Glycol.

TABLE 12.6: Methods to Estimate Residual Kidney Function

FORMULA	CALCULATION	RELIABILITY
Chronic Kidney Disease Epidemiology Collaboration Equation or CKD-EPI (preferred standard	eGFR = 141 × min (SCr/κ, 1)α × max (SCr/κ, 1) −1.209 × 0.993 age × 1.018 [if female] × 1.159 [if Black]	Newest equation; more accurate for wider population versus MDRD
MDRD	eGFR = 175 × (SCr) −1.154 × (age) − 0.203 × 0.742 [if female] × 1.212 [if Black]	Validity tested in African Americans, diabetic kidney disease, kidney transplant recipients
Cockcroft-Gault	CrCl (mL/min) = (140 − age) × (body weight in kg) (72) × (serum Cr in mg/dL)	Oldest equation, not accurate if GFR >60 mL/min, tends to overestimate GFR

GFR, glomerular filtration rate; MDRD, modification of diet in renal disease.

TABLE 12.7: Imaging Studies Used in the Diagnosis of Chronic Kidney Disease

STUDY	INTERPRETATION OF FINDINGS
Renal ultrasonography	Useful to screen for hydronephrosis, which may not be observed in early obstruction or in dehydrated patients; or for involvement of the retroperitoneum with fibrosis, tumor, or diffuse adenopathy; small, echogenic kidneys are observed in advanced kidney failure
Retrograde pyelography	Useful in cases with high suspicion for obstruction despite negative renal ultrasound, as well as for diagnosing renal stones
CT scanning	Useful to better define renal masses and cysts usually noted on ultrasound; also the most sensitive test for identifying renal stones
MRI	Useful in patients who require a CT scan but who cannot receive IV contrast; reliable in the diagnosis of renal vein thrombosis
Renal radionuclide scanning	Useful to screen for renal artery stenosis when performed with captopril administration; also quantifies the kidney contribution to the glomerular filtration rate (GFR)
Kidney biopsy	Percutaneous or ultrasound-guided kidney biopsy is indicated when kidney impairment and/or proteinuria approaching the nephrotic range are present and the diagnosis is unclear after appropriate workup. Indications include hematuria and low creatinine clearance or proteinuria, nephrotic range proteinuria, chronic kidney failure with normal or large kidneys, acute kidney injury unknown cause. Contraindications include kidney length <9 cm, severe hypertension, multiple large cysts, bleeding tendency, hydronephrosis, or acute infection
Echocardiogram	Remains the gold standard for diagnosis of LVH and heart failure. LVH can be related to anemia in people with early CKD (Kidney Disease Improving Global Outcomes, 2017)

Continuous Renal Replacement Therapy

Continuous renal replacement therapy (CRRT) is an established modality for treatment of kidney failure in the ICU setting. It allows solute and fluid removal in critically ill, hemodynamically unstable patients with shock who may also have high fluid intake requirements due to nutritional needs and various IV medications. Because of the gentle solute removal and ultrafiltration (UF), it is the preferred treatment for brain injury patients at risk for cerebral edema and ischemia. Most often the treatment is performed by specially trained ICU staff. Different terms for CRRT are continuous veno-venous hemofiltration (CVVH); continuous venovenous hemodialysis (CVVHD); continuous veno-venous hemodiafiltration (CVVHDF); slow continuous ultrafiltration (SCUF); and sustained low efficiency dialysis (SLED). Disadvantages of CRRT include prolonged exposure to anticoagulation, immobilization, hypothermia, and increased cost.

Peritoneal Dialysis

Fluid and solute removal can be achieved by using the peritoneal membrane which is a semipermeable membrane. Fluid removal in peritoneal dialysis (PD) occurs at the capillary level by osmotic and oncotic pressures

TABLE 12.8: Differential Diagnosis Considerations for End-Stage Kidney Disease

DIALYSIS DEPENDENT	NONDIALYSIS DEPENDENT

• Missed dialysis treatment
• Fluid overload
   Hyperkalemia
• Chest pain
• Vascular revision
• Other nondialysis related admissions
   ○ Gastrointestinal bleed
   ○ Surgery
	• Acute kidney injury (AKI)
	   ○ Dehydration
	   ○ Sepsis
	   ○ Congestive heart failure exacerbation
	   ○ Postcardiac procedure
	• New end-stage kidney disease
	   ○ Diabetes mellitus
	   ○ Hypertension
	   ○ HIV, hepititis pC
	   ○ Glomerular disease
	   ○ Genetic disorder
	   ○ Urologic

generated via hypertonic peritoneal fluid (dialysate). Concentration of the dextrose in dialysate solution and the dwell time determine the amount of solute and fluid removed. Hydraulic pressure minimally contributes to fluid removal.

There is increasing use of PD (urgent/rapid start PD) in ESKD patients first starting dialysis in the hospital. There is increased focus by the Centers for Medicare and Medicaid Services (CMS) to increase utilization of home dialysis therapies in the United States. Understanding the concepts of PD is important to recognizing the complications. Urgent-start PD is for patients who need to start kidney replacement therapy (KRT) within 2 weeks. It allows earlier PD treatments without the need for HD and without waiting 4 to 6 weeks for the catheter to heal. The frequency of leaks or other position complications continue to be evaluated in the data (Xu et al., 2017).

PD patients are taught strict infection control and most often will participate in their PD care even while hospitalized. If the effluent (drained fluid) is cloudy, they are taught to take the bag with them to the hospital or emergency department for culture evaluation of infection. It is recommended to drain the abdomen of dialysate prior to any procedures.

Vascular Access Types and Recommendations

- **Fistulas (autogenous subcutaneous access):** Preferred long-term, most common HD permanent access in the United States, lower risk of infection, lower risk of thrombosis than with other graft or CVC. Radiocephalic, brachiocephalic are most common, requiring months to mature for use.
- **Arteriovenous grafts (AVG):** Indicated when a patient needing long-term HD access does not have native vessels needed for AVF placement, typically made of Dacron and polytetrafluoroethylene. Can be used quickly, some within 24 to 48 hours.
- **Central venous catheters (CVC):** Can be temporary or tunneled; can be used after discharge. Temporary vascular access can be double-lumen HD catheter

or CVC inserted in various sites-internal jugular vein, femoral vein or subclavian vein. CVCs move large blood flow volumes. Infection risk with CVCs is high and placement of these catheters should be done using strict aseptic technique. CVCs are primed with heparin to prevent clotting at the start of treatment.

- **Venipuncture:** Avoid venipuncture in the access arm. Avoid blood draws from the CVC line or fistula (unless an emergency without other access). Avoid taking blood pressure in the access arm.

Vascular Access and Complications

Maintaining vascular access in CKD is costly for hospitalizations and outpatient procedures, costing more than $1 billion/year in the United States (and increasing) (Padberg, et al., 2008). Arteriovenous fistula (AVF), AVG, and CVC complications that potentially require admission to acute care include bleeding, thrombosis (or stenosis from intimal hyperplasia), and steal syndrome (limb ischemia; Table 12.9).

Complications in Hemodialysis

- **Hypotension:** Most often related to excessive UF volume or rate of UF, investigate other causes to exclude bleeding, electrolyte disturbances, infection
- **Hypersensitivity reaction:** Includes anaphylaxis, possibly related to the HD membrane, phthalate (in PVC tubing), ethylene oxide used when disinfecting the HD machine, polyacrylonitrile (in HD membrane)
- **Hemolysis:** Associated with dialysate components
- **Air embolism:** Rare in United States with current technology
- **Electrolyte abnormalities:** Sodium, potassium, calcium, magnesium, osmolality
- **Bloodstream infections:** Associated with hemodialysis
- **Graft stenosis or thrombosis:** Common; flow may be assessed via ultrasound. It is important to attempt to repair and declot to preserve vascular access. Methods that may be utilized include graft thrombectomy,

TABLE 12.9: Vascular Access Complications

ACCESS COMPLICATIONS	SIGNS/SYMPTOMS	TREATMENT	NOTE AT DISCHARGE
Infiltration of fistula or graft	Swelling, pain, ecchymosis	Rest of access arm, ice, mild pain relievers	ANY change in vascular access should be communicated to the outpatient dialysis team, missed treatments, date of infiltration
Thrombosis of graft	Absence of bruit or thrill	Discuss with nephrologist, vascular surgeon, interventional radiology asap; timing of revascularization depends on patient status; a CVC may be needed	ANY change in vascular access should be communicated to the outpatient dialysis team
Thrombosis of CVC	Lack of or sluggish blood return from line, difficult flush	Thrombolytics may be instilled; exchange of CVC	ANY change in CVC should be communicated to the outpatient dialysis team; provide CXR for placement confirmation
Infection	Systemic fever, fatigue, hypoxia, dyspnea; localized warmth, redness, pain, swelling	Systemic antibiotics; CVC removal, replacement	ANY infection should be communicated to the outpatient dialysis team including antibiotic, dosing; change of access
Steal syndrome	Pain, numbness, tingling, pale, weakness distal to access	Coil embolization of collateral veins, access ligation and banding	
Hemorrhage		Direct pressure to cannulation sites posttreatment; protamine 0.01 mg/IU heparin; gelatin sponges; tourniquet if severe	

*When dialysis access is needed, CVC placement is typically recommended with internal jugular (IJ) vein or femoral vein to preserve subclavian vessels and protect upper extremities for future permanent vascular access.

CVC, central venous catheter; CXR, chest x-ray.

catheter-directed thrombolysis, embolectomy balloon, and urokinase

- **Calciphylaxis:** Vascular calcification secondary to severe abnormal metabolism of calcium and phosphorus; this can be from undiagnosed or undertreated hyperparathyroidism

Complications of Peritoneal Dialysis

- **Access:** The PD catheter and catheter exit site are at risk for infection after placement and great care is taken to train the patient to prevent infection using sterile technique with all PD care. Exit site infection may present with purulent discharge (with or without erythema) at the catheter epidermal interface. A tunnel infection may present with inflammation and/or pain along the tunneled track or ultrasound evidence of a collection along the catheter tunnel.
- **Peritonitis:** Treat empirically with coverage for *Staphylococcus aureus* using a penicillinase-resistant penicillin or first-generation cephalosporin. If the patient has a history of methicillin-resistant *S. aureus* (MRSA), use clindamycin or a glycopeptide. Peritonitis treatment

should follow general guidelines. Modify the empiric therapy as soon as PD effluent culture results are available using the International Society for Peritoneal Dialysis (ISPD) guidelines. Recommendations are available at https://ispd.org/ispd-guidelines.

- **Constipation:** Can obstruct the catheter or cause problems with inflow/outflow. Severe constipation can contribute to catheter migration or peritonitis. Prevention of constipation requires daily stool softeners or laxatives. Abdominal x-rays can help diagnose constipation and check for catheter tip dislodgement.
- **Inflow or outflow problems:** Noted difficulty with filling or draining PD fluid from the peritoneum could be emergent as it prevents dialysis. Troubleshooting would include looking for physical obstruction, clamps, kinks, or constipation. Repositioning the patient might move the fluid or the catheter into a different position that allows for increased flow. Plain films of the abdomen can be used to assess the PD catheter and position.
- **Dialysate leak:** Can be external or internal. External leaks can be seen after initiation of PD, and near the

catheter exit site. Occasionally, leaks can occur after abdominal surgeries at surgical incision sites. To determine the presence of a leak, a glucometer or a urine dipstick can be used to test for dialysate containing glucose. Internal leaks can be subcutaneous and appear like edema in the scrotum, labia, or into the thorax (Leblanc et al., 2008). An internal dialysate leak can be diagnosed with CT or MRI using contrast in the peritoneal fluid.

- **Hernias:** PD increases intraabdominal pressure, increasing risk for hernias. Most hernias are identified and corrected before initiation of PD. New hernias can develop after starting therapy—most often umbilical, inguinal, and incisional (Shah et al., 2006). Evaluate hernias frequently and refer for surgical correction if enlarging. Surgical correction requires holding PD and using HD temporarily. Rarely patients can continue PD with lower fill volumes while healing from hernia surgery.

- **Encapsulating peritoneal sclerosis (EPS):** Progressive fibrosis of the peritoneal membrane seen with changes in solute and UF transport and ultimate UF failure. Fibrosis encapsulating the bowel may cause intermittent obstruction and ileus. EPS is likely caused by inflammation of the peritoneal membrane and subsequent fibrin deposition. Ongoing fibrin deposition can form a dense capsule that surrounds, and at times traps, the bowel (Burkart, 2017). Risk is increased in patients on PD for more than 5 years (Burkart, 2017).

- **Anemia:** Treat anemia of CKD/ESKD when the hemoglobin level is below 10 g/dL, with ESAs, which include epoetin alfa and darbepoetin alfa after iron saturation and ferritin levels are at acceptable levels. While anemia of CKD is common, always evaluate for other causes of bleeding and treat accordingly. Baseline hemoglobin is typically poor due to decreased EPO (ESAs not always appropriate or contraindicated in acute care), hemolysis, and bleeding diathesis. Transfusion should be reserved as a life-saving measure (hematocrit <18%). All patients should be considered potential kidney transplant recipients and exposure to anything foreign, including blood products, increases antibody levels and immune sensitization.

- **Disorders of mineral bone metabolism and hyperphosphatemia:** CKD-mineral and bone disorder (CKD-MBD) is a complex group of disorders that involves bone, minerals, and hormones as well as significant abnormalities in the cardiovascular system and coronary arteries caused by a process of calcification (KDIGO, 2017). CKD-MBD increases the patient's risk of mortality due to the damages caused to the cardiovascular system. Treat with dietary phosphate binders and dietary phosphate restriction, use oral vitamin D analogs and/or calcimimetics (e.g., cinacalcet), which are part of the dialysis prescription.

If unable to control secondary hyperparathyroidism (SHPT) medically, consider referral for surgical partial parathyroidectomy. Monitor serum calcium levels frequently post parathyroidectomy. Treat hypocalcemia aggressively using calcium supplements with or without calcitriol.

- **Hyperkalemia:** Caused by increased potassium intake or decreased potassium excretion. Seen in AKI, CKD Stages 4 and 5, constipation, hemorrhage, blood transfusions, and some medications: ACE inhibitor/ARB, potassium-sparing diuretics, NSAIDs, and cyclosporine. Treatment is based on the cause of hyperkalemia or changes to or discontinuation of medications. Discontinue any potassium supplements or any medications that increase the potassium level. Kayexalate (sodium polystyrene sulfonate) is a resin-exchanger that removes serum potassium via the gut; reserved use is due to potential bowel necrosis. Veltassa (patiromer) and Lokelma (sodium zirconium cyclosilicate) bind potassium in the GI tract and is excreted in stool. Use with caution with GI abnormalities including ostomy. For ESKD patients, potassium (K) dialysate is ordered based on laboratory values. Zero K dialysate is not recommended except in severe hyperkalemia as it can cause rapid decline in serum potassium and increased risk for cardiac arrhythmias/cardiac arrest. A dialysate bath of K-2 or K-3 (2 mEq/L or 3 mEq/L) is the most commonly used concentration. Potassium K-4 (4 mEq/L) is used in cases of hypokalemia.

- **Volume overload:** Treat with loop diuretics or increased UF with dialysis.

- **Metabolic acidosis:** The kidneys play an essential role in acid-base homeostasis by controlling serum bicarbonate (HCO_3^-) concentration through excretion or reabsorption of filtered HCO_3^-, excretion of metabolic acids, and synthesis of new HCO_3^- (Morrow & Malesker, 2019). Metabolic acidosis is common in advanced CKD and can lead to poor health outcomes. Measured in arterial blood gas or venous carbon dioxide. As nephron mass decreases, the kidney's ability to excrete acid diminishes which typically occurs when GFR is less than 20 to 25 mL. Treat with oral or IV alkali supplementation.

- **Uremic manifestations:** Treat with long-term KRT (hemodialysis, PD, or renal transplantation). Acute indications for initiation of KRT include: severe metabolic acidosis, hyperkalemia, pericarditis, encephalopathy, intractable volume overload, failure to thrive and malnutrition, peripheral neuropathy, intractable gastrointestinal symptoms. For asymptomatic patients, a GFR of 5 to 9 mL/min/1.73 m², irrespective of the cause of the CKD or the presence/absence of other comorbidities, is also an indication.

- **ESKD specific CHF management/pulmonary edema management:** Consider emergent HD if weight >5 pounds over baseline weight (dry weight), missed dialysis, severe electrolyte derangements, or respiratory distress. Administer diuretics if appropriate, nitroglycerin, oxygen, Bi-PAP if indicated.

■ **Air embolism (rare):** Exam presentation with chest pain, dyspnea, hypotension (or cardiac arrest), access lines should be clamped, position patient in Trendelenburg and supine or left lateral decubitus position, oxygen.

Medications and Special Consideration in ESKD Population

■ **Avoid use in CKD or ESKD**: Metformin in setting of metabolic acidosis, bisphosphonates if GFR <30, NSAIDs, bowel preparation (use polyethylene glycol [PEG] instead of magnesium or phosphorus preparations), use caution with contrast dye, caution with dosing of medications for GFR <30. Avoid NSAIDs. Recommend cautious use of antibiotics, check recommendations for dosages based on eGFR.

■ **Anemia—ESAs (espogen, aranesp, procrit, mircera):** Indicated for hemoglobin <9 mg/dl. Use caution with ESA use with Hgb >12 mg/dL due to increased risk of cerebrovascular accident. Iron supplementation: Parenteral replacement is preferred due to decreased oral absorption. Non-dextran IV iron is preferred due to less anaphylaxis (e.g., ferumoxytol [feraheme], iron sucrose [venofer], or sodium ferric gluconate [Ferrlecit], ferric pyrophosphate [triferic]). Hypoxia inducible factor medication stimulates endogenous EPO. Do not use iron supplements in the setting of sepsis/infection.

■ **Depression:** Management with antidepressants either short term or long term; chronic use of SSRIs may cause hyponatremia/SIADH.

■ **Nausea and vomiting:** Minimize uremia with adequate dialysis frequency, ondansetron 4 mg orally every 8 hours, metoclopramide (Reglan) 5 mg twice daily. May need GI referral.

■ **Pruritus:** Minimize uremia with adequate dialysis frequency; be sure, if related to phosphorus, the patient is on phosphate binders, standard dry skin therapy (e.g., barrier creams). Some medications include hydroxyzine (Atarax or Vistaril), 25 mg orally every 6 hours, naltrexone (Revia) 50 mg orally daily, and phototherapy (UV-B Light).

■ **Insomnia:** Treat restless legs syndrome, treat obstructive sleep apnea, Zolpidem 5 mg orally at bedtime, temazepam (Restoril) 15 mg orally at bedtime.

Advance Directives and Hospice

Advance care planning is crucial when establishing ESKD treatment plans. Conservative management when a patient chooses not to initiate dialysis includes symptom management and referral to palliative care or hospice. Patients on dialysis can be referred to hospice or palliative care and continue to receive dialysis as long as the primary indication for hospice is not ESKD related.

TRANSITION OF CARE

ESKD patients have unique transitions and challenges. Standardizing the communication process between inpatient and outpatient dialysis units when patients are discharged from the hospital has shown the potential to reduce adverse events related to poor communication and improve patient care during this transition (Erickson, et al., 2015). Interprofessional collaboration has the potential to create solutions to this complex problem and foster a culture of multidisciplinary care, recognizing the complex interactions among multiple providers and patients and the importance of communication.

Key information to communicate to the outpatient facility at discharge:

■ Assess/adjust target weight at first treatment back from the hospital
■ Review new medications or modifications, or discontinued medications
■ Note any change to heparinization (ICHD/HHD)
■ Note any change to IV/IP antibiotics
■ Any new/protocol labs required upon readmission
■ Record any follow-up from hospital
■ Notify the facility and provider/specialist of appointments or follow-up
■ Confirm advance directives
■ Update any patient/caregiver education
■ Review changes in treatment plan with IDT
■ Notify the facility of any durable medical equipment or home health referrals that could impact their treatment schedule

Inpatient to Outpatient Dialysis

Communication is crucial to ongoing care especially medication changes, changes to the dry weight. Many dialysis providers and hospital systems have put in place a tool to communicate the hand off inpatient to outpatient ESKD.

12.4: SECONDARY HYPERPARATHYROIDISM

R. Brandon Frady

Secondary hyperparathyroidism (SHPT) is associated primarily with chronic kidney disease (CKD). Also, SHPT is associated with mineral and bone disease, malnutrition, or failure of one or more of the calcium (Ca) homeostasis mechanisms. The mainstay of SPHT therapy is hyperphosphatemia management, vitamin D replacement, calcium, and parathyroid hormone (PTH) monitoring (Mizobuchi et al., 2019). Estimates are that 30% to 50% of Stage 5 CKD patients have significantly elevated iPHT levels. Over time, as kidney failure worsens, patients develop chronic kidney disease-metabolic bone disorder (CKD-MBD; Gasparri et al., 2015).

CKD-MBD is a combination of Ca, P, PTH, and vitamin D metabolism abnormalities, abnormalities in bone turnover, mineralization, volume, and growth, and vascular and soft tissue calcifications. The recognition and management of SHPT include evaluating biochemical mineral profiles and adjustments in the medications with the goal of normal biochemical profiles.

Parathyroid Function and Regulation

Multiple mechanisms control the production, synthesis, and secretion of PTH. PTH releases from chief cells in response to decreased circulating ionized Ca levels. Ca-sensing receptors (CaSR) located on the parathyroid gland are responsible for detecting the extracellular free ionized Ca. Small fluctuations in ionized Ca^{++} levels result in significant PTH changes (Portillo & Rodríguez-Ortiz, 2017). Figure 12.2 outlines the role of PTH in the regulation of Ca and its effects on other mineral stability. In addition to Ca^{++} homeostasis, phosphorus (P) is another factor that regulates PTH. Elevated P levels stimulate PTH production. The exact mechanism of how elevated P exerts its effect on PTH is unknown. PTH is negatively regulated by calcitriol ($1,25D_3$) through direct inhibition of PTH synthesis and secretion (Gasparri et al., 2015).

Additionally, the increased Ca level secondary to $1,25D_3$ suppresses PTH secretion. Fibroblast Growth Factor 23 (FGF23) is a hormone synthesized by osteoblast and osteocytes secondary to elevated serum P levels and elevated $1,25D_3$ levels (Mizobuchi et al., 2019). FGF23 is a significant regulator of P. FGF23 binds to the FGF23-Klothor receptor in the parathyroid gland inhibiting parathyroid function. FGF23 increases the expression of CaSR and vitamin D receptors, making the parathyroid gland more sensitive to Ca and 1,25D3 level inhibitory actions. Figure 12.3 summarizes critical mechanisms of mineral homeostasis. Hyperphosphatemia or decreased kidney production of 1,25-dihydrooxycolecalciferol (1,25[OH]2D3) in patients with CKD can lead to hypocalcemia resulting in parathyroid gland hyperplasia.

PRESENTING SIGNS AND SYMPTOMS

Given that diagnosing SHPT is based primarily on biochemical profiles of Ca, P, vitamin D, and PTH, signs and symptoms are associated with alterations in the serum levels. The initial presenting symptom for SHPT may be related to hypocalcemia. Hypocalcemia features are expressed as neuro excitability, muscle twitching and spasms, numbness and tingling, and carpopedal spasms. Numbness and tingling are typically present as peri-oral and digital (Hassan-Smith & Gittoes, 2017). These neurologic and muscle symptoms may progress to tetany and seizures. Neuromuscular excitability is associated with the rate of development and degree of hypocalcemia (Hassan-Smith & Gittoes, 2017). Chronic hypocalcemia may lead to neuropsychiatric symptoms.

HISTORY AND PHYSICAL FINDINGS

The diagnosis of SHPT is primarily based on biochemical profiles of Ca, P, vitamin D, PTH levels. The history and physical exam include the initial and ongoing evaluation of patients at risk for or progressing through CKD stages (Fraser, 2009). Hyperphosphatemia has little to no symptoms. The history and physical exam should have a focus on the development of CKD mineral bone disorders. The assessment of bone pain and fracture history is essential in the history and physical.

DIFFERENTIAL DIAGNOSIS AND DIAGNOSTIC CONSIDERATIONS

Differential Diagnoses

The differential diagnoses of SHPT includes gastrointestinal causes, vitamin D causes, kidney disorders, cellular mediated, genetic, hungry bone syndrome, bisphosphonate therapy, lactation, and metastatic prostate cancer (Chandran & Wong, 2019).

Diagnostic Considerations

SHPT identification and management are based on measuring biochemical levels of calcium (Ca), phosphorus (P), vitamin D, and PTH levels. Additional to serum mineral levels, the assessment of bone density, the risk for bone fractures, and the development of vascular calcifications should be factored in. A key to diagnostic considerations relates to the development and progression of CKD (Ketteler et al., 2017).

Biochemical Profiles

The measurement of Ca, P, $1,25D_3$, and PTH levels are essential in the care of SHPT. With CKD stage 3, serum Ca and P levels are monitored every 6 to 12 months. As CKD stages advance to Stage 4 through 5 with dialysis, monitoring frequency should increase to every 3 months, even monthly. PTH level monitoring begins with CKD Stage 4 every 6 to 12 months and increases to every 2 to 3months with CKD Stage 5 with or without hemodialysis (Ketteler et al., 2017).

Bone Diagnostics

SHPT in combination with serum mineral abnormalities contributes to bone disease in CKD patients. PTH and alkaline phosphatase levels are associated with increased bone turnover. Bone disease may be evident by bone fractures, bone pain, bone deformities, and growth abnormalities. In addition to the biochemical profiles outlined previously, dual-energy X-ray absorptiometry (DXA) can predict bone fractures for patients with CKD Stages 3 to 5. Mineral testing, alkaline phosphatase measurement, and DXA cannot determine low, normal, or high bone turn over and therefore, in certain patients, a bone biopsy may be necessary (Portillo & Rodríguez-Ortiz, 2017).

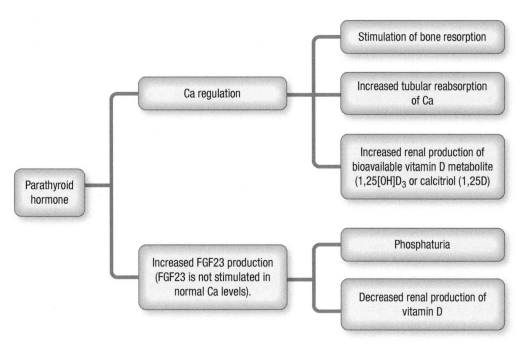

FIGURE 12.2: Parathyroid hormone and calcium regulation.

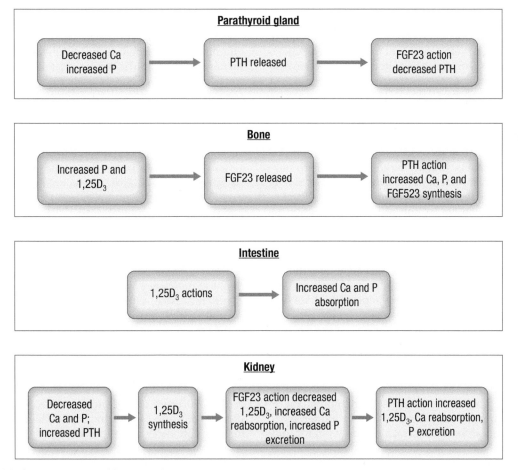

FIGURE 12.3: Mechanisms in mineral homeostasis.

Vascular Calcification

SHPT patients are at risk for the development of vascular calcification secondary to extraosseous calcification deposits in the vascular bed. As CKD progresses, the development of vascular calcification increases. Abnormal mineral metabolism contributes to the development of vascular calcification (Mizobuchi et al., 2019). Patients with CKD have vascular calcification assessed by lateral kidney-ureter-bladder (KUB) x-ray, echocardiogram (ECHO), or computed tomography (CT) calcium score. The lateral x-ray and ECHO may provide enough information to assess vascular calcification.

TREATMENT

The treatment of SHPT consists of prevention and intervention. The treatment of SHPT is focused on the measurement and management of Ca, P, PTH, and vitamin D levels with the possibility of surgical intervention if conservative medical management does not adequately control SHPT. A large multicenter study COSMOS set thresholds for Ca, P, and PTH levels. P levels are targeted to 3.6 mg/dL to 5.2 mg/dL. Ca levels goals are 7.9 mg/dL to 9.5 mg/dL. PTH levels targeted to 168 to 174 pg/mL (Gasparri et al., 2015). Acceptable PTH levels between CKD 3 and 4 are currently unknown. For CKD 5 with dialysis, a target PTH level of two to nine times the upper limit of normal is the target. Treatment goals are based on the development and progression of CKD. Starting with CKD Stage 3, monitoring of biochemical minerals is essential to the treatment of SHPT. As CKD advances, the measurement of PTH level monitoring is started at CKD Stage 4.

Prevention

Prevention of SHPT is focused on the measurement of Ca, P, and PTH levels. Initially targeting P levels to normal is a crucial component in the management of SHPT. Prevention and reduction of P include reducing P intake, decreasing intestinal absorption of P, and promotion of renal clearance of P. An additional prevention strategy is the replacement of vitamin D (Portillo & Rodríguez-Ortiz, 2017). Vitamin D replacement in nutritional intake is the primary source. Active replacement of vitamin D is done cautiously due to the increased risk for the development of hypercalcemia and hyperphosphatemia.

Phosphate Binders

Treatment of phosphorus is initiated when the level is above the normal range. The primary action of phosphate binders is related to the binder's ability to bind phosphorus in the gastrointestinal tract preventing P absorption. There are multiple preparations on P binders. Aluminum-based binders are no longer used secondary to toxic bone, central nervous system, and bone marrow effects. Ca++-based binders replaced aluminum binders Ca++ acetate and carbonate. While the elemental Ca++ varies among binders, the overall

undesirable side effect is the accumulation of Ca++. There are several nonaluminum and non-Ca++-based binders. A widely studied and used binder, sevelamer hydrochloride, has demonstrated reductions in mortality over time in multiple studies. Sevelamer is a synthetic polymer that is a nonabsorbable phosphate binder (Qunibi et al., 2008). In addition, to lower all-cause cardiovascular mortality, sevelamer is associated with a lower rate of progression of extraosseous calcification (Qunibi et al., 2008). Sevelamer is more costly compared to other formulations of P binders. Lanthanum carbonate is another nonaluminum non-Ca binder. Lanthanum is effective at binding phosphate without hypercalcemia (Portillo & Rodríguez-Ortiz, 2017). Finally, there are two new iron-based P binders available for patients: ferric citrate and sucroferric oxyhydroxide. These are iron based. Ferric citrate releases iron as a part of the binding process. This release of iron is desirable in CKD Stage 3 to 5 patients by improving iron-related parameters. Sucroferric oxyhydroxide is another iron-based binder with minimal iron absorption (Portillo & Rodríguez-Ortiz, 2017). Table 12.10 provides the dosing and side effects of selected P binders.

Vitamin D Replacement

Calcitriol levels fall in patients with CKD. Over time, the deficiency in $1,25D_3$ contributes to SHPT. For this reason, vitamin D replacement is an essential component in the management of SHPT. Active vitamin D should not be routinely used for CKD patients below Stage 4. It is reasonable that patients with CKD Stages 4 to 5 with or without dialysis need to use active vitamin D for replacement (Friedl & Zitt, 2017; Portillo & Rodríguez-Ortiz, 2017). Patients having active vitamin D replacement should have close monitoring of Ca++ and P levels. The initiation of active vitamin D replacement is done in conjunction with monitoring Ca, P, and PTH level altogether. The use of $1,23D_3$ (the active form of vitamin D) is associated with a higher risk of hypercalcemia. Paricalcitol is a vitamin D analog that is associated with less hyperphosphatemia and hypercalcemia. Paricalcitol is effective in predialysis and dialysis patients (Portillo & Rodríguez-Ortiz, 2017).

CKD patients are also deficient in $25D_3$. Generally, vitamin D deficiency is defined as serum levels less than 20 ng/mL. Also, vitamin D levels between 20 ng/mL and 30 ng/mL are insufficient and need to have vitamin D supplementation started. Correction of vitamin D insufficiency and deficient patients are based on recommendations for the general population. The recommended daily allowance (RDA) for vitamin D is 600 IU/day for patients 19 to 70 years of age, with patients greater than 70 years of age increased RDA to 800 IU/day (Portillo & Rodríguez-Ortiz, 2017). The max daily doing for any patient 19 and older is 400 IU/day. Nutritional vitamin D replacement may be achieved with vitamin D_2 (ergocalciferol) or vitamin D_3 (cholecalciferol; Portillo & Rodríguez-Ortiz, 2017). Although studies using

TABLE 12.10: Phosphate Binders

BINDER NAME	RECOMMENDED DOSING	SIDE EFFECTS
Calcium acetate	1.5 g–3 g	Hypercalcemia GI upset
Calcium carbonate	2 g–3 g	Hypercalcemia Extraskeletal calcification PTH suppression GI upset
Magnesium carbonate/calcium acetate	3–9 tablets	Hypermagnesemia GI upset
Sevelamer-HCl	1.2 g–2.4 g	Decreased bicarbonate level GI upset
Sevelamer carbonate	2.4 g	GI upset
Lanthanum carbonate	1.5 g–3 g	GI upset
Ferric citrate	6 g	GI upset
Sucroferric oxyhydroxide	1.5 g–2 g	GI upset

GI, gastrointestinal; PTH, parathyroid hormone

nutritional vitamin D replacement have variable results, normalizing 25D$_3$ levels in CKD patients may contribute to risk reduction in CKD patients.

PTH Management

The use of calcimimetics is an essential strategy for the management of SHPT. Calcimimetics act on the CaSR receptor. Calcimimetics increase sensitivity of PTH to Ca++ levels, resulting in a lower Ca++ level producing the desired effect on the PTH. Calcimimetics also reduce Ca, P, and FGF23 levels. Cinacalcet and etelcalcetide are the currently approved calcimimetics for use in end-stage renal disease. The significant side effects of cinacalcet are nausea, vomiting, and the potential for hypocalcemia (Jeong et al., 2016; Portillo & Rodríguez-Ortiz, 2017). Studies on calcimimetics have demonstrated some impact on bone, vascular calcification, and reduction in the need for parathyroidectomy. However, calcimimetics use should not be based on the advantage of patient survival (Jeong et al., 2016).

Parathyroidectomy

A parathyroidectomy is an option for patients with SHPT. Patients with nodular hyperplasia are excellent candidates for parathyroidectomy (Portillo & Rodríguez-Ortiz, 2017). Additionally, patients resistant to medical therapy and who have significant ongoing SHPT should be evaluated for parathyroidectomy. Several surgical complications are associated with parathyroidectomy, including persistent hyperparathyroidism, transient or recurrent laryngeal nerve paralysis, and hungry bone syndrome.

12.5: RENAL ARTERY STENOSIS

Mary S. Haras

Renal artery stenosis (RAS) is the progressive narrowing of one or both of the arteries that carry blood from the aorta to the kidneys, most often caused by the plaque buildup of atherosclerosis and contributes to approximately 5% of all causes of secondary hypertension. Atherosclerotic RAS (ARAS) accounts for 90% of all RAS cases and is seen more commonly in older populations. A less common cause of RAS is the nonatherosclerotic, noninflammatory abnormal growth or development of cells on the renal artery walls, known as fibromuscular dysplasia (FMD), contributing to approximately 10% of renovascular hypertension cases. FMD is seen primarily in women (90%) and in younger populations; recent data suggest the average age at diagnosis is 54 years. Other rarer causes of RAS include traumatic thrombosis or avulsion, hypercoagulable states resulting in nontraumatic thrombosis, renal or aortic dissection, renal artery aneurysm, congenital, William syndrome, or Takayasu arteritis (Colyer et al., 2011). Blood flow obstruction from inadvertent partial or complete coverage of the renal artery after endovascular aortic repair (EVAR) can also cause nonatherosclerotic RAS (Brinster & Sternbergh, 2021). The prolonged reduced blood supply to the kidneys can result in chronic kidney disease (CKD) progressing to end-stage kidney disease, and persons with RAS are at a greater risk for coronary artery disease, stroke, and peripheral vascular disease. Early detection and prompt treatment can result in improved blood pressure and kidney function.

PRESENTING SIGNS AND SYMPTOMS

Most often, no symptoms are present until the RAS is more advanced. Often, RAS is detected as a secondary finding in diagnostic imaging for other vascular conditions or in preparation for living kidney donor transplant. The majority of cases of RAS are due to ARAS, and patients present with the same atherosclerotic risk factors of family history, smoking, diabetes, hypertension, and hyperlipidemia (Simon, 2021). Smoking has also been implicated in FMD, along with vessel wall ischemia, hormonal imbalance, and genetic factors. The patient may present with new onset or difficult to treat or worsening hypertension, or decreased kidney function, or a combination of both.

Hypertension

In persons under 30 years of age, new onset hypertension may be noted. In persons greater than 50 years of age with a history of controlled hypertension, sudden worsening of their hypertension may be noted, despite maximum dosing of at least three different medications, including a diuretic.

Chronic Kidney Disease

If there is evidence of decreased kidney function, the patient may present with the typical signs and symptoms of CKD, including increased or decreased urination, lower extremity edema, fatigue, dry skin, pruritus, nausea/vomiting, sleep disturbances, difficulty concentrating, appetite and weight loss, or muscle cramps. See section on CKD for more information.

HISTORY AND PHYSICAL FINDINGS

History

A thorough cardiac history should be taken to determine the cause of hypertension, including age of onset and medication history to treat the hypertension. RAS is refractory to antihypertensive medications, so it is important to determine the inability to treat the hypertension with at least three or more different medications including a diuretic, or intolerance to maximum dosing of three anti-hypertensive medications. Evaluate history of atherosclerosis, coronary artery disease including history of myocardial infarction, coronary artery bypass graft (CABG) or prior cardiac stenting, peripheral artery disease, stroke, and hypertension. Assess family history for hypertension as well. Smoking history is important to determine in both ARAS and FMD.

Determine if there is a family history for kidney disease/disorders or a personal history for kidney disease. Determine if there has been a decrease in kidney function, particularly after starting an angiotensin converting enzyme inhibitor (ACEI). RAS is associated with at least a 30% increase in serum creatinine after starting an ACEI. Determine if there has been an increase or decrease in urinary output, presence of lower extremity edema, fatigue, pruritus, nausea/vomiting/decreased appetite, muscle cramps, difficulty sleeping, or difficulty concentrating.

Determine the presence/absence of less common causes of RAS including FMD, most often diagnosed in younger individuals.

Physical Findings

Hypertension will be the main presenting problem; determine whether it is accelerated, malignant, or resistant. Auscultate the abdomen for presence of abdominal bruit, assess for pulmonary edema and peripheral arterial disease. Determine if body mass index (BMI) is greater than 25. In younger males, assess for gynecomastia.

- **Review diagnostic findings for kidney asymmetry by ≥1.5 cm:** This size difference is diagnostic and occurs in over two thirds of patients with renovascular hypertension.
- **Kidney Doppler ultrasound:** Considered the first-line screening method for RAS. Reduced kidney blood flow via kidney Doppler ultrasound revealing peak systolic velocity (PSV) >250 cm/sec, peak diastolic velocity (PDV) >150 cm/sec, renal to aortic ratio (RAR) >3.5, acceleration time >100 msec are indicative of RAS.
- **Review diagnostic imaging to determine the presence of stenosis of 60% to 99%:** There are two types of FMD, the more common being medial multifocal (68% to 91%) and more prevalent in females, and the less common unifocal intimal, more prevalent in men. Angiography in persons with FMD reveals a classic "string of beads'"imaging in multifocal RAS, and typically involves the distal main renal and intrarenal branches. The decreased perfusion to the kidneys in multifocal FMD does not allow for the degree of RAS to be determined from imaging (Gottsater & Lindblad, 2014).
- **Angiography:** In persons with ARAS angiography most often reveals stenosis in the ostium and proximal third of the main renal artery, and the degree of stenosis is able to be determined from imaging.
- **Kidney function:** Before undertaking any noninvasive or invasive diagnostic imaging, it is important to assess the patient's current kidney function as there is a greater risk of developing AKI, defined as a minimum increase in SCr of 1.5 times baseline over 7 days, or an increase of ≥0.3 mg/dL in 48 hours, from IV contrast agents or systemic sclerosis. Pretreatment with hydration and n-acetylcysteine may be warranted if these tests are needed to determine the severity of the RAS.
- **Magnetic resonance angiography (MRA):** MRA has a sensitivity of 90% to 100% and a specificity of 76% to 94%. It is superior to Doppler ultrasound, and equivalent to CT angiography.
- **Computed tomography angiography (CT angiography):** CT angiography has a sensitivity of 59% to 96% and a specificity of 82% to 99%. It is superior to Doppler ultrasound, and equivalent to MRA.

■ **Nuclear renography:** Nuclear renography is a non-invasive test used to document differences in kidney function. If there is <20% differential, it is unlikely to contribute to worsening kidney function. Nuclear renography is used to determine if revascularization or removal of the kidney is necessary. Renography without an ACEI is necessary to establish baseline nucleide uptake. ACEIs should be discontinued 2 to 7 days before the test (Blaufox et al., 2018). Follow-up renography after ACEI administration will restrict uptake of the nuclear agent Tc-diethylenetriamine-pentaacetic acid (DTPA) and can then be compared to the baseline exam (Sarkodieh et al., 2013). Imaging will show uptake in both kidneys without the captopril, and in only one kidney after the captopril of RAS is present. Unlike other diagnostic imaging, captopril renograms will directly determine renovascular hypertension (Blaufox et al., 2018) and provide information about the function, rather than the structure of the kidney (Greco & Umanath, 2019). Because the interventional treatment for RAS is restricted to specific high-risk populations, the use of captopril renography is declining. Additionally, long-term ACEI use will diminish the effectiveness of the study (Blaufox et al., 2018). Instead, the ACEI is prescribed in the medical management of the condition.

■ **Direct digital subtraction angiography:** Digital subtraction angiography (DSA) is recommended after a positive noninvasive test. DSA is considered the gold standard for diagnosing RAS; however, there are risks associated since it is an invasive procedure. Patients should be monitored closely for access site bleeding, contrast-induced nephropathy, and aortic dissection (Rickey & Geary, 2019; Simon, 2021). It has a sensitivity of 88% and a specificity of 90%. For patients with reduced kidney function, prehydration is warranted to reduce the risk of contrast-induced nephropathy.

Laboratory Findings

■ Review basic metabolic panel (BMP) to assess sodium, potassium, blood-urea-nitrogen (BUN) and serum creatinine for elevations. Assess for acute kidney injury (AKI) after initiating an ACEI or ARB.

■ Serum cholesterol levels to determine presence of hypercholesterolemia.

■ Urinalysis to determine presence of blood or protein.

■ Renal vein renin sampling and plasma renin activity are no longer recommended as useful screening tools (Level of Evidence: B; Anderson et al., 2013).

■ Labs to rule out other causes of secondary hypertension:
  ● Dexamethasone suppression test (Cushing's syndrome)
  ● 24-hour urinary fractionated metanephrines and normetanephrine (pheochromocytoma)
  ● Plasma renin-aldosterone ratio (hyperaldosteronism)

DIFFERENTIAL DIAGNOSIS AND DIAGNOSTIC CONSIDERATIONS

Differential Diagnoses

■ Essential hypertension
■ Other causes of secondary hypertension:
  ● Renal parenchymal disease
  ● Endocrine abnormalities (Cushing's syndrome, hyperaldosteronism)
  ● Adverse effects of a drug(s)
  ● Coarctation of the aorta
■ Arterial dissection
■ Vasculitis
■ Neurofibromatosis
■ Extrinsic compression of renal arteries

Diagnostic Considerations

ARAS

Screening for ARAS is indicated for persons with known risk factors of RAS: hypertension <30 or >55 years of age, presence of accelerated, malignant or resistant hypertension, unexplained kidney dysfunction, azotemia with initiation of ACEI or ARB, variation in kidney size by >1.5 cm, and flash pulmonary edema, and may be reasonable in persons with unexplained kidney failure, multivessel CAD, unexplained congestive heart failure or refractory angina (Anderson et al., 2013). The 2016 American College of Cardiology/American Heart Association (ACC/AHA) guideline on the management of patients with lower extremity peripheral artery disease recognizes that persons with peripheral artery disease (PAD) are at higher risk of atherosclerotic disease in other locations, and does not recommend screening asymptomatic individuals with PAD unless revascularization will improve the clinical outcome. Therefore, for persons with asymptomatic PAD, invasive and noninvasive angiography should not be performed to assess other anatomic disease (Gerhard-Herman et al., 2017).

The Renal Artery Stenosis Prediction Rule developed by Krijnen and colleagues in 1998 and revalidated in 2005 identified clinical characteristics of age, sex, vascular disease, recent onset of hypertension, smoking, BMI, abdominal bruit, serum creatinine and hypercholesterolemia as predictors of RAS. The rule can be found on EBMcalc Complete for clinical use on iOS (cost associated with app). Use of the prediction rule in calculating risk of RAS may reduce unnecessary invasive procedures.

Cohen and colleagues (2005) developed a simple prediction rule for significant RAS in patients undergoing cardiac catheterization. They identified independent predictors of significant RAS to be older age, elevated creatinine levels, peripheral vascular disease, the number of cardiovascular drugs the patient is taking, hypertension, female, and three-vessel coronary artery disease (CAD) or previous coronary artery bypass graft surgery (CABG).

Any invasive procedure has associated risks for complications. In digital subtraction angiography (DSA), access site complications include hematoma, thrombosis, bleeding, and pseudoaneurysm. Catheter-associated complications include vessel wall damage, causing dissection or perforation of the vessel, and embolization. Systemic complications are associated with contrast, radiation, and anticoagulation (Desai & Hodgson, 2019).

TREATMENT

Treatment of RAS is aimed at controlling blood pressure, treating heart failure and/or pulmonary edema, and preventing kidney disease. No treatment is necessary for persons with asymptomatic RAS.

Pharmacologic Therapy

First-line treatment for RAS should be medical therapy. The 2013 ACC/AHA (Anderson et al., 2013) and the 2017 European Society of Cardiology (ESC; Aboyans et al., 2018) recommend that patients be treated with antihypertensive medications that block the renin-angiotensin-aldosterone system (RAAS), including ACEIs or ARBs, and calcium channel blockers for unilateral RAS. ACEI therapy is contraindicated in bilateral RAS and in RAS in a person with a single kidney. Monitoring of kidney function is essential to avoid AKI in patients on ACEI or ARB therapy.

For hypertension related to ARAS, the ACC/AHA also recommends beta-blockers. The ESC recommends antiplatelet and statin medications as best practice to prevent MI and stroke in persons with atherosclerotic disease. For persons with heart failure or pulmonary edema, a diuretic should be considered. In persons with RAS due to FMD, blood pressure should be controlled with an ACEI or ARB.

Nonpharmacologic Therapy

Atherosclerotic Renal Artery Stenosis

Revascularization with stent placement should be reserved to persons with hemodynamically significant RAS, defined as ≥70% narrowing, or moderate RAS defined as 50% to 69% narrowing by visual estimation and confirmation of hemodynamic severity of the stenosis with a resting mean pressure gradient >10 mmHg or systolic hyperemic pressure gradient >20 mmHg or renal fractional flow reserve (FFR) ≤0.8 (Bailey et al., 2019; Spinowitz, 2020). According to the ACC/AHA guidelines and consistent with the ACC/AHA 2005 Guidelines for the Management of Patients with Peripheral Artery Disease (Bailey et al., 2019), percutaneous revascularization should occur in patients with:

- Poorly controlled hypertension who are on maximally tolerated doses of three blood pressure medications that include a diuretic
- Uncontrolled hypertension who cannot tolerate maximum dosing of three antihypertensive medications

The following clinical criteria must be met:
- Accelerated, resistant, or malignant hypertension
- Hypertension with asymmetrical kidney
- Hypertension with intolerance to maximum medication therapy
- Progressive CKD with RAS
- Recurrent, unexplained heart failure
- Sudden, unexplained pulmonary edema or recurrent unstable angina

Fibromuscular Dysplasia

Revascularization with balloon angioplasty is generally sufficient to cure RAS due to FMD. A systematic review and meta-analysis conducted by Trinquart and colleagues (2005) revealed that only moderate benefit was seen after revascularization, and that patient age had a strong influence on blood pressure outcomes. Stenting is not appropriate in persons with FMD. Renal artery bypass may be warranted in persons with recurrent FMD or in persons who have not had an improvement in blood pressure after angioplasty.

12.6: CONTRAST ASSOCIATED AND CONTRAST INDUCED ACUTE KIDNEY INJURY

David S. Goede and Kelly K. Nye

Imaging studies are a vital component in diagnosing, treating, and monitoring many of today's medical conditions. Clear and accurate images are required so the radiologist can properly diagnose and ultimately guide the provider in developing an effective treatment plan. Iodinated contrast media (ICM) is used for many medical imaging studies such as x-ray, CT, angiography, myelograms, arthrograms, venography, and occasionally ultrasound. ICM can be administered via catheter, IV, intraarterial, orally, rectally, and via intrathecally. ICM are renally cleared; the use of ICM has been long associated with the development of acute kidney injury (AKI; Nelson et al., 2017).

DIFFERENTIAL DIAGNOSIS AND DIAGNOSTIC CONSIDERATIONS

The criteria for diagnosing contrast-induced nephropathy (CIN) have been the focus of many studies and at the center of great debate for years. According to the American College of Radiology (ACR) and the National Kidney Foundation consensus statement "Use of Iodinated Contrast Media in Patients with Kidney Disease," there is a difference between contrast *associated* acute kidney injury (CA-AKI) and contrast *induced* acute kidney injury (CI-AKI). CA-AKI is described as any deterioration in renal function occurring within 48 hours following intravascular administration of contrast medium. CA-AKI is said to occur from contrast media event that is coincidental, but not necessarily caused by the exposure. CA-AKI is also referred to as postcontrast AKI (PC-AKI). CI-AKI is a subset of CA-AKI and implies a causative deterioration in renal function which is directly associated with the administration of contrast medium (ACR, 2021; Davenport et al., 2020). The National Kidney Foundation Kidney Disease Outcomes Quality Initiative (NKF-KDOQI) 2012 guideline defined AKI as an abrupt decrease in kidney function over 7 days or less (Kellum et al., 2012). The Acute Kidney Injury Network (AKIN) defines AKI in three stages based on a rise in the serum creatinine 48 hours post insult (Table 12.11). Although there are no standard criteria, an absolute increase of 0.5 mg/dL over a baseline serum creatinine is also commonly used (ACR, 2021; Mehta et al., 2007). Studies on CA-AKI and CI-AKI use serum creatinine as a measurement of renal injury. Serum creatinine levels are indirect, nonspecific, and take time to accumulate after an exposure to a nephrotoxic event. Serum creatinine is also affected by age, diet, muscle mass, and has daily variations making it somewhat unreliable. estimated glomerular filtration rate (eGFR) has been found to be a better predicator of risk than using serum creatinine even through the calculation of eGFR uses the serum creatinine. The risk of development of CA-AKI is 5% in patients with eGFR ≥60 mL/min/1.73 m², 10% for eGFR of between 45 and 59 mL/min/1.73 m², 15% for eGFR of between 30 and 44 mL/min/1.73 m², and 30% if eGFR is <30 mL/min/1.73 m². The risk of development of CI-AKI is significantly lower due to the limitations of observational studies. The risk for CI-AKI in patients is 0% in patients with an eGFR ≥45 mL/min/1.73 m², 0% to 2% for eGFR of 30 to 44 mL/min/1.73 m², and 0% to 17% if eGFR is <30 mL/min/1.73 m² (Davenport et al., 2020; Faucon et al., 2019; Rudnick et al., 2020). There has also been concern about increased risk of CIN when multiple doses of ICM are given within a short amount of time. Most low osmolar contrast medium (LOCM) have a half-life of 2 hours. If renal function is normal, it would take approximately 20 hours for the patient to eliminate the contrast. It is suggested to avoid dosing intervals shorter than 24 hours apart unless the situation is emergent and the benefits outweigh the risks (ACR, 2021). There are additional patient-related risk factors proposed for the development of CA-AKI that require provider consideration. Box 12.6 summarizes predisposing patient risk factors. Providers should be aware

> ### BOX 12.6 PATIENT RISK FACTORS FOR DEVELOPMENT OF CONTRAST ASSOCIATED ACUTE KIDNEY INJURY
>
> - Age 60 or older
> - History of renal disease, including:
>   - Dialysis
>   - Kidney transplant
>   - Single kidney
>   - Renal cancer
>   - Renal surgery
> - Proteinuria
> - Gout
> - History of hypertension requiring medical therapy
> - History of diabetes mellitus
> - Aboriginal or Torres Strait Islander ethnicity (GCM)
> - History of vascular disease—previous acute MI or stroke (GCM)
> - History of smoking (GCM)
> - BMI >30 (GCM)

that patients taking metformin or metformin-containing drug combinations who develop AKI are at increased risk of developing lactic acidosis. The decision as to whether to hold metformin or metformin-containing drug combinations should be based on the patient's eGFR. According to the ACR Committee on Drugs and Contrast Media, if no evidence of AKI exists and the eGFR is ≥30 mL/min/1.73 m², metformin may be continued and not held prior to or after the administration of ICM. If the patient has AKI or severe CKD (Stage 4, Stage 5, eGFR <30 mL/min/1.73 m²), or is having an arterial catheter study, metformin should be held at the time of or prior to the procedure. Metformin may be restarted 48 hours post procedure after the renal function has been reevaluated and is deemed to be normal. Metformin does not need to be held for GCM administration assuming the dose does not exceed the radiology recommended dose range (ACR, 2021). It is critical to understand each patient's risk prior to ordering any test that can cause an adverse reaction.

Pathophysiology

Contrast media (CM) negatively impacts renal function through renal/glomerular hemodynamic alterations. ICM induces vasoconstriction of the vascular bed in the renal medullary region. This results in release of vasoactive agents like adenosine, endothelin, and cytotoxic agents. The CM also inhibits the production of nitric oxide, a potent vasodilator, within the renal bed. This leads to acute tubular necrosis (ATN) and ischemia of outer regions of the renal medulla (Azzalini et al., 2016). In addition to the direct effect of the CM on the renal tubulars, the properties of the CM, specifically the osmolarity and viscosity, can also impact renal function. Osmolarity is the ratio of solutes to solution. Our serum osmolarity range

TABLE 12.11: Acute Kidney Injury Stages per the Acute Kidney Injury Network

Stage 1	Serum creatinine increases by ≥ 0.3 mg/dL or rises to 1.5- to 2-fold from baseline
Stage 2	Serum creatinine increases to 2- to 3-fold above baseline
Stage 3	Serum creatinine increases ≥4 mg/dL or rises greater than 3-fold above the baseline

is between 285 and 295 mmol/kg. The early iodine-based contrast media was high-osmolar contrast medium (HOCM). The osmolarity was 1,500 to over 2,000 mOsm/kg, thus HOCM had direct negative effects on renal function. HOCM was replaced with low-osmolar contrast medium (LOCM), 400 to 800 mOsm/kg and iso-osmolar CM (IOCM) (290 mOsm/kg). The LOCM and IOCM have a higher viscosity then plasma. This increase in viscosity leads to hypoperfusion of the renal medullary. To avoid the negative effects of the CM viscosity, the CM is administered as a warm solution and the patient is hydrated at the time of administration (Azzalini et al., 2016; Faucon et al., 2019).

Studies evaluating the relationship between CM and CA-AKI have dominantly focused on patients who were exposed during cardiac angiography. During cardiac angiography, the contrast injection is delivered from a catheter located within the arterial system and supra-renally. This differs from the IV route used for other contrast enhanced studies. Consequently, the dose of contrast medium via intraarterial injection reaches the kidneys in a more abrupt and concentrated manner. Studies have in fact shown a higher incidence of CA-AKI post cardiac angiography; however, the results may be exaggerated as dislodged atheroemboli from the injection catheter placement, hemodynamic instability during the procedure, and intraarterial versus IV administration may contribute to the higher incidence of AKI. Unfortunately, these findings are not generalizable to standard IV contrast injections which leads to an overestimated risk for CA-AKI (Davenport et al., 2014).

If a patient is scheduled for a routine intravascular study but does not have any of the aforementioned risk factors, they do not require a renal function assessment prior to ICM administration. Patients with AKI or severe CKD (Stage 4 and Stage 5) are at increased risk of CIN. The use of ICM should be avoided if possible unless the benefits outweigh the risks. Anuric patients with end-stage renal disease have nonfunctioning kidneys so they may receive ICM without risk of CIN or further damage to the kidneys (ACR, 2021).

TREATMENT

Preventing CA-AKI through identification of the best test to achieve the intended outcome is the best strategy. This requires interdisciplinary discussion between the providers and radiologist regarding desired outcome of the test. There are two primary strategies to minimize risk of developing CA-AKI and CI-AKI, volume expansion and pharmacologic therapy. The major preventive strategy is volume expansion. The AGACNP should consider the role of IV hydration prior to ICM exposure in patients who are deemed to be high risk, eGFR <30 mL/min/1.73 m², and presence of individual risk factors (Box 12.6). Volume expansion with normal saline is the preferred method. Volume expansion is thought to reduce the renin activation and the release of cytotoxic agents through dilution of the CM. Typically, most protocols

begin IV hydration 1 hour prior to CM exposure and continues IV hydration for up to 12 hours post CM exposure. The rate of infusion ranges between 1 and 3 mL/kg/h or may consist of a single infusion of 500 mL of normal saline. The POSEIDON trial was the first randomized control study to compare different rates of normal saline infusion in the prevention of CA-AKI (Brar et al., 2014). The rate of normal saline infusion was based on the patient's left ventricular end diastolic pressure (LVEDP), a hemodynamic measure of the patient's volume status. If the LVEDP was lower than 13 mmHg, then the rate of infusion of the normal saline was 5 mL/kg/h. If the LVEDP was 13 to 18 mmHg, the rate was 3 mL/kg/h and if the LVEDP was higher than 18 mmHg, the rate of infusion was 1.5 mL/kg/h. The infusion of the normal saline began at the beginning of the procedure prior to CM exposure and continued for 4 hours post procedure. The findings of the POSEIDEN study demonstrated a 68% relative reduction (6.4% absolute reduction) of CA-AKI as compared to the control group (Brar et al., 2014). Oral hydration has not been well studied in high-risk patient groups. The two most common pharmacologic therapies used to reduce the risk of CA-AKI include the use of IV hydration with sodium bicarbonate solution or the use of either the IV or oral form of N-acetylcysteine (NAC). Free oxygen radicals produce an acidic environment. The administration of sodium bicarbonate causes an alkalization, thus reducing the effect of the free oxygen radicals through reduction in their production as well as acting as a scavenger. This results in a decrease in vasoconstriction and cytotoxic affects. N-acetylcysteine is thought to be renally protective through its indirect role as an antioxidant and reducing vasoconstriction through stabilizing nitric oxide production (Xie et al., 2021). The use of either IV or oral form of NAC in prevention of CA-AKI continues to have mixed reviews in the literature as evidence demonstrates that NAC reduces serum creatinine without improving eGFR. Both sodium bicarbonate and NAC administration should not be considered a substitute for appropriate volume expansion (Faucon et al., 2019; Mamoulakis et al., 2017). Other pharmacologic agents under review include ascorbic acid, statins, and phosphodiesterase 5 inhibitors. There are insufficient data in the literature to support their role in CIN protocols at this point.

CLINICAL PEARLS

- Acute tubular injury is a severe form of AKI rather than a separate pathology.
- Most patients with kidney disease have vague symptoms and may even be asymptomatic.
- A decline in GFR over time is consistent with CKD.
- Patients with kidney disease are at high risk for cardiovascular disease.
- Initiate a nephrology referral when there is a need for renal replacement therapy and or GFR <30 mL/min/1.73 m².

- Acute presentations of ESKD patients
  - Fluid overload
  - Hyperkalemia
  - Pericarditis
  - Fever/sepsis
    - Access related? Check fistula, CVC, or PD catheter
- New ESKD needing dialysis
  - Check hepatitis B series; if positive will need to run in ISO
  - Start off with shorter run times, minimal UF to avoid dialysis disequilibrium syndrome.
- Additional fluid removal can be achieved by ordering dry ultrafiltration (DUF) which is typically a 2- to 3-hour treatment that removes only fluid and does not provide solute clearance.
- Do not give ESAs in patients with malignancies.
- For treatment of anemia, assess for and treat iron deficiency.
- Avoid removing UF too much or too quickly to prevent myocardial stunning.
- Avoid contrast with gadolinium to avoid renal fibrosis.
- In CKD Stage 5, closely monitor blood glucose and insulin doses as it is not metabolized at normal rates. Avoid hypoglycemia.
- During hospitalizations, the AGACNP should educate regarding limb restrictions on that arm to ensure venipunctures and blood pressure readings are not taken on that arm.
- If ESKD patient is on diuretic, ensure they still make urine. If anuric this can be discontinued. Review the Centers for Disease Control and Prevention guidelines for additional recommendations on vaccinating patients on dialysis; the guidelines can be found at https://www.cdc.gov/dialysis/PDFs/Vaccinating _Dialysis_Patients_and_Patients_dec2012.pdf
- Measurement of serum calcium, phosphorus, vitamin D, and PTH levels are essential to the diagnosis of SHPT.
- Patients with CKD especially starting at Stage 3, should be evaluated for SHPT.
- As CKD progresses, monitoring for SHPT is essential.
- Management of SHPT includes vitamin D replacement, phosphate binders, and calcimimetics.
- RAS is most often an incidental finding with no presenting symptoms.
- Patients with atherosclerotic risk factors should be considered for ARAS.
- Patients presenting with hypertension and an abdominal bruit should be evaluated for RAS.
- DSA is the gold standard for diagnosing RAS, however persons with asymptomatic PAD should not undergo invasive or noninvasive angiography.
- Consider RAS in persons who develop AKI or azotemia after initiation of an ACEI or ARB.
- ARAS is most commonly seen in older adults, and FMD is most commonly seen in women in their 30s and 40s with normal kidney function.

KEY TAKEAWAYS

- CKD is progressive and required close monitoring, especially during periods of acute illness.
- Co-management of cardiovascular disease, diabetes, and peripheral vascular disease is essential in managing CKD.
- An acute decline in GFR and or a clinical presentation consistent with dialysis needs are reasons for nephrology consultation.
- The number one cause of ESKD in the United States is diabetic nephropathy, followed by hypertension. Other etiologies can include glomerulonephritis, cystic kidney disease, recurrent kidney infection, chronic obstruction.
- ESKD is a glomerular filtration rate of less than 15 mL/min and requires either kidney replacement therapy or conservative care with palliative care.
- Monitor GFR and proteinuria in diabetics and nondiabetics for managing disease and preventing progression in patients with CKD.
- Understanding early referral to specialists for timely dialysis or kidney transplant planning.
- Specialized AGACNPs play a vital role in educating the patient about lifestyle modifications necessary to prevent the progression of CKD.
- In patients with advanced CKD, it is crucial to protect an arm for future fistula placement.
- During hospitalizations, the AGACNP should educate regarding limb restrictions on that arm to ensure venipunctures and blood pressure readings are not taken on that arm.
- Once a patient is diagnosed with ESKD, a significant number will require dialysis, or kidney transplant.
- End-stage kidney failure significantly increases morbidity and mortality.
- ESKD is a significant cost to the healthcare system. With early referral and management of disease control can improve outcomes for these patients.
- PD patients rely on residual kidney function to maintain dialysis adequacy, reservation of residual kidney function is very important to maintain patients on PD therapy. When hospitalized it is important to flag their chart regarding procedures and therapies that may increase risk of loss of residual kidney function from contrast dye.
- Measurement of serum calcium, phosphorus, vitamin D, and PTH levels are essential to the diagnosis of SHPT.
- Patients with CKD especially starting at Stage 3 should be evaluated for SHPT.
- Management of SHPT includes vitamin D replacement, phosphate binders, and calcimimetics.

- Management of RAS is aimed at controlling hypertension, preventing cardiac mortality, and restoring kidney function.
- Radiologic intervention should be restricted to patients with severe disease with the goal of restoring kidney function.
- Systematic reviews and meta-analyses comparing revascularization to medical therapy generally do not show significant differences in clinical outcomes or blood pressure control except in patients with rapidly declining kidney function or pulmonary edema (Balk et al., 2016).

EVIDENCE-BASED RESOURCES

American Nephrology Nurses Association. (2017). *Nephrology nursing scope and standards of practice* (3rd ed.).

Bodin, S. (Ed.). (2017). *Contemporary nephrology nursing* (3rd ed.).

Counts, C. (2020). *Core curriculum for nephrology nursing* (7th ed.). Lulu Press.

Daugirdas, J., Blake, P., & Ing, T. (Eds.). (2015). *Handbook of dialysis* (5th ed.). Wolters Kluwer.

Gilbert, S., Weiner, D., Bomback, A., Parazella, M., & Tonelli, M. (2018). *Primer on kidney diseases* (7th ed.). Elsevier.

Kidney Disease Improving Global Outcomes. https://kdigo.org

Lerma, E., & Weir, M. (Eds.). (2017). *Henrich's principles and practice of dialysis* (5th ed.). Wolters Kluwer.

Management of patients with peripheral artery disease (Compilation of 2005 and 2011 ACCF/AHA guideline recommendations)

Nephrology Nursing Journal: The Official Journal of the American Nephrology Nurses Association

2016 AHA/ACC Guideline on Management of Patients With Lower Extremity Peripheral Artery Disease: Executive Summary

2017 ESC guidelines on the diagnosis and treatment of peripheral arterial diseases, in collaboration with the European Society for Vascular Surgery (ESVS)

ACC/AHA/SCAI/SIR/SVM 2018 Appropriate Use Criteria for peripheral artery intervention: A report of the American College of Cardiology Appropriate Use Criteria Task force, American Heart Association, Society for Cardiovascular Angiography and Interventions, Society of Interventional Radiology, and Society for Vascular Medicine.

A clinical prediction rule for renal artery stenosis. *Annals of Internal Medicine, 129*(9), 705–711. https://doi.org/10.7326/0003-4819-129-9-199811010-00005

A robust set of instructor resources designed to supplement this text is located at **http://connect.springerpub.com/content/reference-book/978-0-8261-6079-9.** Qualifying instructors may request access by emailing **textbook@springerpub.com.**

REFERENCES

Full list of references can be accessed at http://connect.springerpub.com/content/reference-book/978-0-8261-6079-9

CHAPTER 13

GENITOURINARY AND GYNECOLOGIC DISORDERS

Margaret J. Carman, Whitney Haley, Jeanne Martin, Beth McLear, and Diane Fuller Switzer

LEARNING OBJECTIVES

- Describe patient risk factors, subjective, and objective data to differentiate complicated and uncomplicated urinary tract infections (UTI).
- Identify risk factors and subjective and objective data to differentiate cystitis, asymptomatic bacteriuria (ASB) and catheter associated UTIs.
- Design an evidence-based treatment plan according to the type of UTI for a patient presenting in the inpatient or outpatient setting.
- Utilizing the classification system PALM-COEIN, differentiate (identify) the causes of abnormal uterine bleeding (AUB) in nonpregnant patients.
- Describe the new terminologies of AUB.
- Compare/contrast the medical management of emergent from nonemergent acute AUB.

13.1: URINARY TRACT INFECTION

Urinary tract infections (UTIs) are frequently encountered in healthcare (Tandogdu & Wagenlehner, 2016). In adults, UTIs occur far more commonly in females than in males until 50 years of age. Obstruction of the prostate from prostatic hypertrophy becomes common in males after 50 years of age, and the occurrence of UTI increases and approaches that of females (Gupta & Trautner, 2018). A UTI may be asymptomatic (subclinical infection) or symptomatic (disease). The term *urinary tract infection* encompasses a spectrum of clinical entities, including asymptomatic bacteriuria (ASB), cystitis, prostatitis, and pyelonephritis. These distinctions are significant as the treatments are based on the location of infection and the presence of symptomatic UTI versus ASB. They are further categorized as uncomplicated or complicated. The term "complicated" suggests there is a predisposing reason for the infection, including the presence of abnormal voiding (e.g., neurogenic bladder, stricture, benign prostatic hypertrophy) or a foreign body (e.g., stone, stent, catheter)

immunosuppression or pregnancy (Gupta, n.d.). Recent studies also reveal that many uropathogens in complicated UTI exhibit multidrug resistance (Bader, 2017). These distinctions, along with knowledge of common causative pathogens and local susceptibility patterns, are crucial as they provide a guide for the choice and duration of antimicrobial therapy (Coyle & Prince, 2017).

CYSTITIS

Acute cystitis is an infection of the bladder, most often caused by *Escherichia coli*. In most guidelines and recommendations, cystitis is categorized as uncomplicated if it is present in any patient that is a premenopausal, nonpregnant woman with no known urological abnormalities or comorbidities (Gupta et al., 2011). All others are considered complicated. Risk factors for uncomplicated cystitis include sexual intercourse, use of spermicides, previous UTI, a new sex partner (within the past year), and a history of UTI in a first-degree female relative. In older females, risk factors include estrogen deficiency, functional or mental impairment, and a UTI history before menopause (Sobel & Kaye, 2014).

PRESENTING SIGNS AND SYMPTOMS

Cystitis commonly presents with dysuria, frequency, urgency, and suprapubic discomfort. Hematuria may occasionally occur in females. Symptoms often appear following sexual intercourse. The patient's history has a high predictive value in uncomplicated cystitis. A meta-analysis evaluating the probability of acute UTI based on history and physical findings concluded that, in females presenting with at least one symptom of UTI (dysuria, frequency, hematuria, or back pain) and without complicating factors, the probability of acute cystitis or pyelonephritis is 50%. The likelihood is even higher for those with a history of recurrent UTI. If vaginal discharge and complicating factors are absent and risk factors for UTI are present, then the probability of UTI is close to 90%, and no laboratory evaluation is needed (Gupta & Trautner, 2018).

HISTORY AND PHYSICAL FINDINGS

A history of dysuria, frequency, urgency, and suprapubic discomfort are often elucidated with cystitis. Hematuria may also be reported. Symptoms may be reported to occur after sexual intercourse in females. Suprapubic tenderness may be elicited on palpation, although the physical exam is often unremarkable.

DIFFERENTIAL DIAGNOSIS AND DIAGNOSTIC CONSIDERATIONS

Differential Diagnoses

Vulvovaginitis and pelvic inflammatory disease (PID) should be considered in females with cystitis-like symptoms. In males, uncomplicated cystitis is rare and other causes such as infected stones, prostatitis, and urethritis should be considered.

Noninfectious causes of cystitislike symptoms should also be considered, including pelvic irradiation, chemotherapy, carcinoma of the bladder, interstitial cystitis, voiding function disorders, and psychosomatic disorders.

Diagnostic Testing

Urinalysis will show pyuria and bacteriuria, and varying degrees of hematuria. A urine culture will be positive for the causative organism; however, colony counts <105 colony-forming units [CFU]/mL are not diagnostic of UTI, a urine culture is not routinely recommended for uncomplicated cystitis. However, culture should be done on all cases of pyelonephritis and complicated UTI as well as males with UTI. Assessment for pyuria and bacteriuria is often performed with the use of dipsticks that also test for leukocyte esterase and for nitrites. Understanding the dipstick test is essential in interpreting results. Members of the family Enterobacteriaceae are the only organisms that convert nitrate to nitrite, and a certain amount of nitrite must accumulate in the urine to reach the threshold of detection. Increasing fluids and voiding frequently makes the dipstick test for nitrite less likely to be positive, even when *E. coli* is present. The leukocyte esterase test detects this enzyme in polymorphonuclear leukocytes in the host's urine, in intact or lysed cells. The diagnostic accuracy of dipstick testing has been the subject of many reviews. An important point to remember for clinicians is that in a patient with a reasonably high pretest probability of UTI, a urine dipstick test can confirm the diagnosis of uncomplicated cystitis in a patient—either nitrite or leukocyte esterase positivity can be interpreted as a positive result. Blood in the urine also may suggest a diagnosis of UTI. A dipstick test negative for both nitrite and leukocyte esterase should trigger consideration of other explanations for the patient's symptoms and collection of urine for culture. In pregnant patients, for whom it is important to detect all episodes of bacteriuria, a negative dipstick test is not sensitive enough to rule out bacteriuria (Gupta & Trautner, 2018).

In the case of complicated cystitis, a urine culture is indicated, and computed tomography (CT) or ultrasound (US) is often indicated to determine the underlying cause. Bacteriuria may be present in the absence of urinary symptoms. ASB is defined as the presence of one or more species of bacteria growing in the urine at specified quantitative counts (≥105 CFU/mL or ≥108 CFU/L), with or without the presence of pyuria, without signs or symptoms attributable to UTI (Nicolle et al., 2019).

TREATMENT

Uncomplicated

After confirming the diagnosis of uncomplicated UTI, empiric therapy with narrow spectrum antibiotics is indicated. Most (95%) of uncomplicated UTIs are monobacterial. The most common bacteria for uncomplicated UTIs is *E. coli* (75%–95%). It is important to consider local antimicrobial susceptibility patterns of *E.coli* when considering therapy. *Klebsiella pneumoniae, Staphylococcus saprophyticus, Enterococcus faecalis*, group B *streptococcus*, and *Proteus mirabilis* are other bacteria most frequently seen in uncomplicated UTI (Sobel & Kaye, 2014). Other gram-negative and gram-positive species are rarely isolated in uncomplicated UTIs.

Uncomplicated UTIs are most often treated in the outpatient setting. However, in patients who present with fever or systemic symptoms of infection (e.g., systemic inflammatory response with a suspected urinary source), hospitalization and treatment with parenteral antibiotics should be considered.

The first-line empiric therapies for acute uncomplicated bacterial cystitis in otherwise healthy adult nonpregnant females is a 5-day course of nitrofurantion or a 3-g single dose of fosfomycin. Second-line options include fluoroquinolones and beta-lactams, such as amoxicillin-clavulanate (Table 13.1). The utilization of fluoroquinolones for empiric treatment of UTIs should be restricted due to increased rates of resistance (Bader, 2017). If pyelonephritis, is suspected, a urine culture and susceptibility test should always be performed, and initial empirical therapy should be tailored appropriately on the basis of the infecting uropathogen (Gupta et al., 2011).

Because cystitis can cause significant bladder discomfort, urinary analgesics can be considered. Phenazopyridine is commonly used but can cause significant nausea. Combination analgesics containing urinary antiseptics (methenamine, methylene blue), a urine-acidifying agent (sodium phosphate), and an antispasmodic agent (hyoscyamine) also are available (Gupta & Trautner, 2018).

TABLE 13.1: Antibiotic Therapy Recommendations for Uncomplicated Urinary Tract Infections

FIRST LINE		
Medication	Dose and Frequency	Comments
Nitrofurantoin monohydrate/macrocrystal	100 mg PO BID 5 days	
Trimethoprim/sulfamethoxazole 160/800 mg	PO BID 3 days	Increasing resistance rates, use if susceptible
Trimethoprim 100 mg	PO BID 3 days	Increasing resistance rates, use if susceptible
Fosfomycin	3 g PO once	
ALTERNATIVE AGENTS		
Amoxicillin/clavulanate	500/125 mg PO Q8hr 5–7 days	
Cefpodoxime proxetil	100 mg PO BID 5–7 days	
Cephalexin	500 mg PO BID 5–7 days	Commonly used; limited data
Ciprofloxacin	250 mg PO BID 3 days	Use empirically if *E. coli* resistance to fluoroquinolones is <10%
Levofloxacin	250–500 mg PO daily 3 days	Use empirically if *E. coli* resistance to fluoroquinolones is <10%

Source: Data from Bader, M. S., Loeb, M., & Brooks, A. A. (2017). An update on the management of urinary tract infections in the era of antimicrobial resistance. *Postgraduate Medicine, 129*(2), 242–258. https://doi.org/10.1080/00325481.2017.1246055; Gupta, K., Hooton, T. M., Naber, K. G., Wullt, B., Colgan, R., Miller, L. G., Moran, G. J., Nicolle, L. E., Raz, R., Schaeffer, A. J., Soper, D. E., Infectious Diseases Society of America, & European Society for Microbiology and Infectious Diseases. (2011, March 1). International clinical practice guidelines for the treatment of acute uncomplicated cystitis and pyelonephritis in women: A 2010 update by the Infectious Diseases Society of America and the European Society for Microbiology and Infectious Diseases. *Clinical Infectious Diseases, 52*(5), e103–e120. https://doi.org/10.1093/cid/ciq257; Gupta, K., & Trautner, B. W. (2018). Urinary tract infections, pyelonephritis, and prostatitis. In J. Jameson, A. S. Fauci, D. L. Kasper, S. L. Hauser, D. L. Longo, & J. Loscalzo (Eds.), *Harrison's principles of internal medicine* (20th ed.). McGraw-Hill. https://accessmedicine.mhmedical.com/content.aspx?bookid=2129&sectionid=186949849

Complicated

Treatment of complicated cystitis should be guided by host factors and susceptibility patterns. The range of species of uropathogens and their susceptibility to antimicrobial agents are varied. Therefore, therapy for any complicated urinary tract infection (UTI) must be individualized and guided by urine culture results. Frequently, a patient with complicated UTI may have prior urine culture results that can be used to guide empirical therapy while current culture results are pending.

CLINICAL PEARLS

- Uncomplicated cystitis is uncommon in men.
- Prostatitis should be considered in a male with symptoms consistent with cystitis.
- Although antibiotics are indicated in UTI, overuse and misuse have contributed to the growing problem of resistance among uropathogenic bacteria; therefore, selecting the antibiotic most focused on the genitourinary tract for the shortest duration is important for antibiotic stewardship.

KEY TAKEAWAYS

- Diagnose uncomplicated cystitis in females who have no other risk factors for complicated UTIs based on:
  o A focused history of lower urinary tract symptoms (LUTS) (dysuria, frequency and urgency);
  o The absence of vaginal discharge or irritation.
- Treat uncomplicated cystitis empirically.
- Urine culture is indicated if suspect pyelonephritis or complicated UTI.

13.2: PYELONEPHRITIS

PRESENTING SIGNS AND SYMPTOMS

Acute pyelonephritis is an infection of the urinary tract that involves the kidney including renal tissue and renal pelvis (Colgan et al., 2011). Patients presenting with acute pyelonephritis may exhibit symptoms of nausea, vomiting, high fevers, malaise, flank pain, dysuria, frequency, urinary hesitancy, or suprapubic tenderness. Presentation can vary in degrees of severity from flank tenderness to septic shock (Johnson & Russo, 2018). Elderly or immunocompromised patients may not present with classic symptoms or may be asymptomatic early in disease trajectory. Elderly patients with unexplained altered mental status, falls, or other nonspecific symptoms may be a less common presentation of pyelonephritis.

HISTORY AND PHYSICAL FINDINGS

Pyelonephritis may be uncomplicated or complicated. Uncomplicated pyelonephritis typically occurs in young patients without known abnormalities of the urinary tract or known preexisting medical comorbidities (Colgan et al., 2011). Pyelonephritis is considered complicated if there is a known functional or structural abnormality of the urinary tract, immunocompromise, history of resistant organisms, or associated relevant medical condition such as polycystic kidney disease, renal transplant, or renal malignancy (Kalra & Raizada, 2009). Antimicrobial therapy considerations may differ depending upon whether the infection is classified as complicated or uncomplicated.

Physical examination should consist of assessment for costovertebral angle (CVA), abdominal, or suprapubic tenderness. CVA tenderness aids in differentiating pyelonephritis from nephrolithiasis because CVA tenderness is typically not present with nephrolithiasis. In sexually active females, a pelvic examination may be warranted to assess for cervical motion tenderness. Additionally, males may warrant rectal examination to assess for edema of the prostate or tenderness that may suggest prostatitis. Patients that have progressed to develop sepsis may develop tachycardia, flushed appearance, fever, or tachypnea due to a hypermetabolic state.

DIFFERENTIAL DIAGNOSIS AND DIAGNOSTIC CONSIDERATIONS

First line in diagnostic testing for acute pyelonephritis is urinalysis (UA) and urine culture. In patients with a supporting physical examination, positive UA results confirm a diagnosis of pyelonephritis (Johnson & Russo, 2018). Nearly all urinary infections have pyuria and leukocyte esterase identified on the UA. Additionally, the UA may have presence of bacteria and nitrites. White blood cell casts are diagnostic for a renal etiology of pyuria; however, it is infrequently identified on UA (Colgan et al., 2011). Presence of blood in a UA may prompt the clinician to consider nephrolithiasis as a differential diagnosis. *Escherichia coli* is the most common causative organism. *Klebsiella, Enterococci, Proteus*, and *Pseudomonas* species are also commonly identified urinary pathogens (Colgan et al., 2011). A complete blood count is beneficial as leukocytosis is frequently associated with this illness. A basic metabolic panel should be obtained to evaluate renal function (Colgan et al., 2011). A clinician should obtain blood cultures to ensure that bacteremia has not developed as a result of this significant infection in patients requiring hospitalization.

Patients presenting with symptoms suggestive of acute pyelonephritis must have consideration to additional differential diagnoses including PID and prostatitis.

Diagnostic imaging is typically reserved for atypical presentations, patients that do not respond to conventional treatment, or immunocompromised individuals. It should be done immediately on presentation if the patient is septic or there is clinical suspicion for urolithiasis or obstruction and should be repeated if there is no clinical improvement after 24 to 48 hours of treatment (Johnson & Russo, 2018). Suspect urinary obstruction if there is a noted decrease in renal function despite appropriate medical therapy (Colgan et al., 2011). Urinary obstruction and preexisting diabetes mellitus are risk factors for development of complications. CT scan can reveal information regarding possible formation of abscess or emphysematous pyelonephritis as well, which

is characterized by gas formation (Johnson & Russo, 2018). Emphysematous pyelonephritis is a necrotizing infection of the perinephric tissue and parenchyma. Most commonly this occurs in diabetics, however this remains a rare complication of pyelonephritis. Identification of one of the previously mentioned obstructions requires prompt consultation with a urology specialist for appropriate, often surgical, interventions.

TREATMENT

Empiric antibiotics should be initiated promptly according to disease severity and risk of drug-resistant organisms. AGACNPs should familiarize themselves with their local antibiogram when making antibiotic selections. Appropriate therapies for uncomplicated pyelonephritis are shown in Box 13.1.

Patients who present with evidence of volume depletion or septic shock should receive IV fluid resuscitation guided by the most updated sepsis guidelines (Hooton et al., 2019).

BOX 13.1 THERAPIES FOR UNCOMPLICATED PYELONEPHRITIS

Outpatient treatment:
- Ciprofloxacin 500 mg twice daily for 7 days +/− initial 400 mg IV dose.
- Bactrim DS 160–800 mg twice daily for 3 days.
- Beta-lactam agents in 3- to 7-day regimens may be used when the previously recommended agents cannot be used. If these are used, they should receive an initial dose of ceftriaxone 1 g or a consolidated 24-hour dose of an aminoglycoside (e.g., gentamycin).

Hospitalization:
- Patients should receive parenteral antibiotics therapy. Current recommendations suggest one of the following:
  o Fluoroquinolone
  o Aminoglycoside
  o Extended spectrum cephalosporin or penicillin
  o Carbapenem

Source: Data from Gupta, K., Hooton, T. M., Naber, K. G., Wullt, B., Colgan, R., Miller, L. G., Moran, G. J., Nicolle, L. E., Raz, R., Schaeffer, A. J., Soper, D. E., Infectious Diseases Society of America, & European Society for Microbiology and Infectious Diseases. (2011, March 1). International clinical practice guidelines for the treatment of acute uncomplicated cystitis and pyelonephritis in women: A 2010 update by the Infectious Diseases Society of America and the European Society for Microbiology and Infectious Diseases. *Clinical Infectious Diseases, 52*(5), e103–e120. https://doi.org/10.1093/cid/ciq257

TRANSITION OF CARE

Mildly ill patients with the ability to take an appropriate oral antibiotic, stable comorbidities, and stable hemodynamics may be appropriate for discharge home to continue treatment. Intractable nausea or vomiting should prompt hospitalization to ensure adequate hydration and antimicrobial therapy. Patients exhibiting signs of sepsis associated with pyelonephritis or urinary obstruction should be admitted to the hospital for IV antibiotics and fluid resuscitation (Colgan et al., 2011).

CLINICAL PEARLS

- CVA tenderness with flank pain is a hallmark sign of pyelonephritis.
- Urinalysis is the most important diagnostic test to be performed in a patient suspected to have pyelonephritis.

13.3: UROSEPSIS

PRESENTING SIGNS AND SYMPTOMS

Urosepsis is a systemic inflammatory response or dysregulated immune response that arises from an infection involving the urogenital tract (Bonkat et al., 2018). Patients presenting with urosepsis may have similar complaints to those with a UTI or pyelonephritis. Urinary frequency, urgency, hematuria, flank pain, fever, myalgias, malaise, and fever often accompany a diagnosis of urosepsis. Gastrointestinal symptoms such as abdominal pain, nausea, and vomiting commonly develop and require a thorough evaluation to rule out additional differential diagnoses. Immunocompromised or elderly patients often do not develop classic symptoms or may not demonstrate symptoms at all until later in the trajectory of urosepsis. Elderly patients often present with nonspecific changes in mental status and confusion without specific urinary symptoms.

HISTORY AND PHYSICAL FINDINGS

Recent treatment of a urinary infection or a history of frequent UTI should prompt a differential diagnosis of urosepsis. Urinary infections occasionally are complications of recent urologic procedures, including catheter placement, and should guide workup as a potential source of sepsis. Immunocompromised status precludes an appropriate response to infection and is an important aspect of a provided history when considering presenting signs or symptoms and physical examination, which may not be specific to urosepsis. Patients with urosepsis often present with a hyperdynamic state including tachycardia, fever, and flushed appearance (Kalra & Raizada, 2009). If this is not promptly addressed, septic shock can develop quickly. Cyanosis, decreased pulse, poor circulation of the extremities, and signs of organ dysfunction may be present in a patient presenting in septic shock and is associated with higher risk of mortality. Suprapubic and abdominal tenderness may be present on palpation, and costovertebral angle (CVA) tenderness often accompanies underlying pyelonephritis.

DIFFERENTIAL DIAGNOSIS AND DIAGNOSTIC CONSIDERATIONS

Urinalysis and urine culture are the first tests to be performed if a diagnosis of urosepsis is suspected. Presence of bacteria, nitrites, leukocyte esterase, and white blood cells in a UA often suggests infection of the urinary tract. Commonly, an obstructive process of the upper urinary tract, most often nephrolithiasis, induces urosepsis. Red blood cells present on UA may suggest presence of nephrolithiasis. Obstructive processes commonly encountered in clinical practice also include stricture of the urethra or ureters, tumors, and prostatic hypertrophy. Plain abdominal x-ray (KUB) can be helpful in identifying calculi and monitoring movement of renal calculi; however, in patients with sepsis, CT scan and MRI are more beneficial in making a diagnosis and determining if complications exist within the urinary tract (Kalra & Raizada, 2009). Once appropriate antibiotic therapy has been initiated, patients should begin to improve within 48 to 72 hours. Failure to improve during this time period should prompt further evaluation for complication such as obstruction or abscess formation.

Determining if an infection of the urinary tract has progressed to sepsis is based on a set of criteria listed in Table 13.2. Urosepsis is often associated with signs of organ dysfunction such as renal failure, encephalopathy, thrombocytopenia, coagulopathy, and hypoxemia. Table 13.2 also lists examples of organ dysfunction commonly identified with a sepsis syndrome. Once tissue hypoperfusion persists despite appropriate fluid resuscitation the patient is considered to be in septic shock. Hypotension or lactic acidosis suggests hypoperfusion and confirms ongoing septic shock. Once sepsis or septic shock has been identified blood cultures should be obtained prior to initiation of antimicrobials. Empiric antibiotics should be broad to cover potential organisms and should be deescalated once a specific organism is isolated.

Urine culture is the most accurate diagnostic method in confirming if a patient has an infection of the urinary system. The most common organisms associated with urosepsis are gram-negative bacilli. Common organisms encountered are *Escherichia coli*, *Pseudomonas*, *Serratia*, and *Enterobacter* species. Recent urological instrumentation increases the risk of pseudomonas species (Kalra & Raizada, 2009).

TABLE 13.2: Severe Sepsis and Septic Shock Criteria

SEVERE SEPSIS	SEPTIC SHOCK

All three must be met within 6 hours:
1. Documentation of a **suspected source** of infection
2. Two or more manifestations of **SIRS** criteria:
  a. Temperature >38.3°C/101°F or <36°C/96.8°F
  b. Heart rate >90
  c. Respiratory rate >2-0
  d. WBC >12 or <4 or >10% bands
3. **Organ dysfunction,** evidenced by any one of the following:
  a. SBP <90 or MAP <654, or a SBP decrease of more than 40 pts
  b. Cr >2.0 or urine output <0.5 cc/kg/h for 2 hours
  c. Bilirubin >2 mg/dL (32.4 mol/L)
  d. Platelet count <100
  e. INR <1.5 or PTT >60
  f. Lactate >2 mmol/L
4. Or if a provider documents severe sepsis, rule out sepsis, possible sepsis, or septic shock
	1. There must be documentation of septic shock present and
	2. **Tissue hypoperfusion** persisting in the hour after crystalloid fluid administration, evidenced by:
	  a. **systolic blood pressure** <90
	  b. Mean arterial pressure <65
	  c. Decrease in SBP by >40 points from the patient's baseline
	  d. Lactate ≥4
	3. Or, if the criteria are not met, but there is provider documentation of septic shock or suspected septic shock

Source: Data from Weiss, S. L., Peters, M. J., Alhazzani, W., Agus, M., Flori, H. R., Inwald, D. P., Nadel, S., Schlapbach, L. J., Tasker, R. C., Argent, A. C., Brierley, J., Carcillo, J., Carrol, E. D., Carroll, C. L., Cheifetz, I. M., Choong, K., Cies, J. J., Cruz, A. T., De Luca, D., … Tissieres, P. (2020). Surviving sepsis campaign international guidelines for the management of septic shock and sepsis-associated organ dysfunction in children. *Intensive Care Medicine, 46*(Suppl. 1), 10–67. https://doi.org/10.1007/s00134-019-05878-6

TREATMENT

If left untreated, urosepsis may progress to septic shock. The Surviving Sepsis Campaign frequently updates treatment recommendations including guidance of fluid administration, IV steroid use, and vasopressor choices (https://www.sccm.org/SurvivingSepsisCampaign/Home). Current guidelines support obtaining blood cultures prior to the initiation of antibiotics. After obtaining cultures empiric broad-spectrum antibiotics should be initiated within 1 hour of identified sepsis, and timely antibiotic administration is associated with improved outcomes in urosepsis (Weiss et al., 2020). Appropriate first-line antibiotic choices for urosepsis include a third-generation cephalosporin, piperacillin plus beta lactamase inhibitor, or fluoroquinolone (Kalra & Raizada, 2009). Antibiotic choices should be reevaluated once finalized urine culture results are available and a minimum of 7 to 10 days of therapy should be completed, although 14 to 21 days are required at times (Bonkat et al., 2018). Clinicians should always reference a local antibiogram and avoid antimicrobials with high resistance patterns. If obstruction or complication such as abscess is identified, obtaining control of the source within 6 hours is recommended (Weiss et al., 2020). Depending on the severity of illness, this may occur in a stepwise approach such as drain or stent placement prior to total removal of the offending agent.

Fluid resuscitation with crystalloid or colloid solutions should be initiated in patients identified to have signs of tissue hypoperfusion or volume depletion. Current guidelines support 30 mL/kg of rapid fluid administration on initial identification of sepsis or septic shock. In scenarios where hypotension persists despite adequate fluid resuscitation, vasopressor therapy should be initiated to titrate for a mean arterial pressure (MAP) greater than 65 mmHg (Weiss et al., 2020). If hemodynamic stability cannot be achieved with fluid resuscitation and vasopressor therapy, the Surviving Sepsis Campaign guidelines currently support the addition of hydrocortisone 200 mg/d IV (Weiss et al., 2020).

TRANSITION OF CARE

Treatment of urosepsis should be performed in a hospital with IV antibiotics. Mildly ill patients may be treated in a regular medical room; however, significantly ill patients and those in septic shock should be transferred to an intensive care unit for close monitoring and stabilization of hemodynamics. Vasopressors should be administered in the ICU with frequent blood pressure monitoring. Once sepsis has resolved, an organism has been identified, and the patient can reliably maintain hydration and nutrition, they should be transitioned to an appropriate oral antibiotic.

CLINICAL PEARLS

- Elderly or immunocompromised patients may have atypical presentation.
- Urinalysis is the most important diagnostic tests in identifying urosepsis.
- Early treatment of urosepsis is associated with improved mortality.
- Empiric antibiotics should be initiated within 1 hour of identified urosepsis.

- Blood cultures should be obtained prior to initiation of antibiotics unless this will delay care.
- Patients that do not respond to appropriate therapy within 48 to 72 hours should be evaluated for potential complications.

13.4: PROSTATITIS

The prostate is a walnut-shaped secretory sex gland in males that sits at the base of the bladder. Its purpose is to develop fluid which enhances sperm mobility, containing proteolytic enzymes necessary for the liquefaction of semen (Bajpayee et al., 2012). The prostate gland is comprised of both glandular and stromal epithelium. The glandular epithelial cells make up the tubular structures that provide the drainage of prostatic fluid into the ejaculatory ducts that reside in the prostatic urethra. The stromal epithelial cells aid in the rapid discharge of prostatic fluid during ejaculation. The term "prostatitis" is a broad, nonspecific phrase that has been commonly used to describe male genital and/or pelvic discomfort (Quallich, 2020). It is the third most common urinary tract disease in males after prostate cancer and benign prostatic hyperplasia (BPH).

Epidemiology

In 1995, the National Institutes for Health (NIH) first developed and then later refined a classification system for prostatitis that has gained international acceptance and use (Krieger et al., 1999). The NIH classification categorizes prostatitis into four separate groups: Category I, acute bacterial prostatitis (ABP); Category II, chronic bacterial prostatitis (CBP); Category III, chronic prostatitis/chronic pelvic pain syndrome (CP/CPPS) which is further broken down into subcategory IIIa/inflammatory and IIIb/noninflammatory; and Category IV, asymptomatic inflammatory prostatitis (Nickel, 2003). Worldwide, prostatitis accounts for approximately 25% of office visits for urogenital symptoms (Khan et al., 2017). The prevalence of ABP comprises roughly 5% to 10% of all prostatitis diagnoses (Ha et al., 2021; Krieger et al., 2008). The incidence of CBP has been reported as 1.26 cases per 1000 males in population-based studies. Approximately 10% of males with ABP will go on to develop CBP and roughly 10% of those males will develop CP/CPPS (Wagenlehner et al., 2013).

Pathophysiology

Bacterial prostatitis generally occurs in a bimodal distribution affecting males ages 20 to 40 years with a second peak of males >60 years old (Davis & Silberman, 2022; Pontari, 2020). It is typically caused by an ascending colonization of a urinary tract pathogen that ultimately results in infection of the prostate (Hua & Schaeffer, 2004). Risk factors include unprotected vaginal/anal intercourse,

phimosis, and conditions that can cause urine stasis such as BPH and urethral stricture. Transrectal prostate biopsy and instrumentation of the urinary tract are also causes and tend to occur in older males. In rare cases, it can be caused by hematogenous spread of bacteria such as tuberculosis in the setting of bacterial sepsis (Pontari, 2020). Typical causative pathogens are gram-negative bacteria, most commonly *Escherichia coli* (Kim et al., 2014; Wagenlehner et al., 2014; Yoon et al., 2012) along with Klebsiella, Serratia, Enterobacter, Pseudomonas, and Proteus species (Paulis, 2018; Yoon et al., 2012). Neisseria gonorrhea, Chlamydia trachomatis, Ureaplasma urealyticum, and Trichomonas vaginalis should be considered in sexually active males while Cryptococcus, Salmonella, and Candida species should be considered for those who have human immunodeficiency disease (Khan et al., 2017; Paulis, 2018).

PRESENTING SIGNS AND SYMPTOMS

Acute bacterial prostatitis (ABP; NIH Category I) presents with a sudden onset of fever, malaise and occasionally myalgias along with dysuria, urinary frequency, and hesitancy with associated perineal/pelvic pain (Davis & Silberman, 2022; Hua & Schaeffer, 2004; Krieger & Thumbikat, 2016). Chronic bacterial prostatitis (CBP; NIH Category II) presents more gradually as dysuria, urinary frequency and urgency, and recurrent UTI (typically with the same organism) without the acute prostatitis symptoms of fever, malaise, and myalgia. Dysuria and pain typically respond to antimicrobial treatment and the patients remain asymptomatic between episodes (Pontari, 2020). Chronic prostatitis/chronic pelvic pain syndrome (CP/CPPS; NIH Category IIIa/b) is a diagnosis of exclusion with the main complaints being perineal pain and prostatic tenderness lasting 3 months or longer without evidence of a UTI. This is the most common form of prostatitis. It is further distinguished between inflammatory (IIIa) and noninflammatory (IIIb) determined by the presence or absence of leukocytes in semen, expressed prostatic secretions or urine obtained after prostatic massage (Schaeffer, 2002). These patients should be referred to a urologist for a thorough workup of symptoms (Pontari, 2020). NIH Category IV, asymptomatic inflammatory prostatitis, does not present with any symptoms and is found on histological sampling of the prostate.

HISTORY AND PHYSICAL EXAMINATION

For patients suspected of ABP, it is important to document a chronology of the onset of symptoms along with obtaining a thorough sexual and procedural history to help confirm the diagnosis. History should also include any complicating past medical history factors such as diabetes, HIV, neurologic diseases, and recent antibiotic usage (Pontari, 2020). An abdominal exam should be performed to assess for bladder distention and/or suprapubic discomfort. A gentle rectal exam should also be performed to assess for prostatic swelling, tenderness, warmth, and induration (Kim et al., 2014). For those with CBP, the physical exam should include an abdominal exam to evaluate for suprapubic fullness and/or pain which may indicate urinary retention and bladder outlet obstruction. Postvoid residuals >180 mL have been associated with increased risk of UTIs (Truzzi et al., 2008). A scrotal exam should be performed to assess for possible infection or inflammation of the epididymis and testes, as well as a digital rectal exam to evaluate the prostate for tenderness, enlargement, or nodules suggestive of prostate cancer. Patients who meet the definition of Category IIIa/b (CP/CPPS) should be referred to a urologist for evaluation as the history and physical examination is quite detailed and multifactorial, requiring a comprehensive pain assessment, voiding and sexual history, and extensive review of systems including neurologic, gastroenterological, rheumatological, and psychological symptoms. Physical exam is the same as in Category II (CP) with addition of assessment of the pelvic floor during digital rectal exam by palpation of the muscles lateral to the prostate and extending to the coccyx. These maneuvers can help identify myofascial trigger points that can be targeted for therapy (Berger et al., 2007). Category IV (asymptomatic prostatitis) does not have any specific workup as it is detected only on prostate biopsy or by the presence of leukocytes in expressed prostatic secretions or semen during evaluation for infertility.

DIFFERENTIAL DIAGNOSIS AND DIAGNOSTIC CONSIDERATIONS

Pertinent laboratory testing for ABP should include a complete blood count (CBC), serum chemistries, midstream clean-catch UA, and urine culture. If the UA is suggestive of contamination, a catheterized sample should be obtained. If fever and hypotension are present, blood cultures should also be obtained (Dielubanza et al., 2014). If urethral discharge is present, a urine sample should be sent for nucleic acid amplification testing for gonorrhea and chlamydia (Pontari, 2020). Prostatic massage to obtain prostatic fluid for culture is contraindicated in the setting of ABP for fear of hematogenous seeding of bacteria. PSA testing is also not recommended due to the elevated levels circulating during the acute phase of inflammation (Game et al., 2003). An assessment of postvoid residuals should be established, preferably through noninvasive methods such as transabdominal US or bedside bladder scanning rather than catheterization. Other imaging studies such as CT, MR imaging, or transrectal USs are not necessary unless there is suspicion of a prostatic abscess, which is rare (Lee et al., 2016). However, abscess should be suspected in males with high fever or history of immunosuppressive disease states such as HIV and diabetes or who do not respond to initial therapy after 48 hours of initiation (Ha et al., 2021). For CBP, the diagnosis is made from premassage and postmassage prostatic urine samples that are obtained and sent for culture (Nickel et al., 2006). Hematuria should be assessed via urinalysis (UA) along with urine culture. Hematuria present in the setting of infection should be reevaluated in 4 to 6 weeks after the resolution of infection. If hematuria persists, a full hematuria workup is warranted to rule out other entities such as malignancy and urolithiasis. For patients with CP/CPPS, this diagnosis should only be made after other causes for pelvic pain have been eliminated (irritable bowel syndrome, fibromyalgia, chronic fatigue syndrome). Other potential causes outside of the pelvis such as psychological issues and neurologic problems should also be explored and ruled out (Pontari, 2020).

TREATMENT

Treatment of ABP depends upon initial clinical presentation. If no signs of systemic illness (fever, hypotension) are present, urinary retention is absent, and if oral fluids and medications can be tolerated, then treatment can take place on an outpatient basis with oral antibiotic therapy. The antimicrobial selection of choice is a either a fluoroquinolone or trimethoprim-sulfamethoxazole for 2 to 4 weeks (Yoon et al., 2012). Urologic follow-up is required to determine if treatment is complete with a repeat urine culture obtained after 1 week of treatment. It is critical to completely treat acute prostatitis to prevent progression to CBP (10.2%) or CP/CPPS (9.6%; Yoon et al., 2012). For those who are ill-appearing upon presentation or have fever and urinary symptoms after prostate biopsy, admission to hospital is recommended for parenteral administration of antibiotics, IV fluids, and monitoring of laboratory values (Pontari, 2020). Due to the high rates of resistance to fluoroquinolones and incidence of expanded spectrum beta-lactam (ESBL) bacteria reported in this population, broad spectrum antibiotics such as carbapenems, second- or third-generation cephalosporin, or amikacin should be administered after collection of blood and urine cultures. After initial symptoms have improved and fever has subsided, transition to oral antimicrobial therapy can be initiated and continued on an outpatient basis. Ciprofloxacin 500 mg twice daily or levaquin 500 mg once daily are appropriate choices (Brede & Shoskes, 2011; Yoon et al., 2012). However, selection must be targeted to the susceptibilities of urine and blood cultures. Again, repeat urine cultures after 1 week of therapy should be obtained to check for clearance of infection (Dielubanza et al., 2014). Adjunctive therapies to alleviate pain and inflammation include NSAIDs if able to tolerate. For males with lower urinary tract symptoms (LUTS; frequency, urgency, hesitancy), alpha blockers can be utilized.

For the rare case of prostatic abscess found on imaging studies, treatment is dictated by the size of the abscess. For lesions <2 cm, conservative treatment with broad spectrum antibiotics is appropriate (Ackerman et al., 2018); for larger lesions, or if no improvement after 2 weeks of therapy, percutaneous drainage versus transurethral resection to unroof the abscess should be considered depending on the location and size of abscess (Abdelmoteleb et al., 2017; Ackerman et al., 2018).

Treatment for CBP is targeted at antibiotics that have a high penetrance into prostatic tissue. Fluroquinolones have excellent prostatic penetrance (Pontari, 2020). Additional antimicrobial selections include tetracyclines, macrolides, and trimethoprim (Charalabopoulos et al., 2003), as well as fosfomycin (Karlowsky et al., 2014). Duration of therapy is based on expert opinion although guidelines published in 2015 by the Prostatic Expert Reference Group from the United Kingdom recommends at least 4 to 6 weeks (Rees et al., 2015). Based on a Cochrane review in 2013 examining treatment of chronic prostatitis, no definitive conclusion could be drawn regarding optimal antimicrobial therapy duration with treatment ranging from 4 to 12 weeks (Perletti et al., 2013). Alpha-blockers are considered first line therapy for treatment of pelvic discomfort and other urinary symptoms (Rees et al., 2015).

Patients with CP/CPPS should be managed by urology providers and may require multimodal therapy. Validated instruments including the NIH Chronic Prostatitis Symptom Index (NIH-CPSI) questionnaire, the American Urological Association's (AUA) International Prostate Symptom Score (I-PSS), and the UPOINT (urinary, psychosocial, organ-specific, infection, neurogenic/systemic, tenderness of skeletal muscles) classification systems can be used to quantify symptoms and target therapy (Pontari, 2020; Quallich, 2020). Treatment modalities include medications such as long-term suppressive antibiotics, alpha blockers and 5-alpha reductase inhibitors (5ARIs) to reduce LUTS, NSAIDs for inflammation and pain control, pelvic floor physical therapy, trigger point injections, Sitz's baths, phytotherapy and mental health counselling (Nickel et al., 2013; Shoskes & Nickel, 2013).

TRANSITION OF CARE

All patients diagnosed with either acute or chronic prostatitis of any kind should follow up with a urologist for further monitoring and potential workup.

CLINICAL PEARLS

- Acute bacterial prostatitis must be considered in any male with a febrile UTI.
- Aggressive palpation of the prostate on initial physical exam should be avoided in suspected cases of ABP.
- Always obtain urine cultures before starting antimicrobial therapy.

KEY TAKEAWAYS

- Refer patients who are diagnosed with ABP to a urologist for follow-up.
- Incomplete treatment of ABP can lead to CBP and/or CPPS.
- CP/CPPS is treated in a multimodal fashion.

EVIDENCE-BASED RESOURCES

National Institutes of Health Chronic Prostatitis Symptom Index (NIH-CPSI)
http://www.proqolid.org/instruments/national_institute_of_health_chronic_prostatitis_symptom_index_nih_cpsi?private=yes&fromSearch
American Urological Association International Prostatism Symptom Score
https://www.uptodate.com/contents/calculator-international-prostatism-symptom-score-ipss
UPOINT clinical phenotyping system for CP/CPPS to guide multimodal treatment
http://www.upointmd.com/index.php

13.5: BENIGN PROSTATIC HYPERPLASIA

Benign prostatic hyperplasia (BPH) is a common urologic condition among males with increasing frequency in aging men. BPH is defined as the nonmalignant proliferation of smooth muscle and glandular epithelial cells within the transition zone of the prostate (Parsons et al., 2020). Clinical BPH is a histologic diagnosis representing a progressive enlargement of the prostate gland, or benign prostatic enlargement (BPE) caused by increased production of fibroblasts and glandular cells near the urethra (Egan, 2016). Rate of proliferation is inevitable and varies among individuals (Vuichoud & Loughlin, 2015). BPH alone is not a pathologic diagnosis. It causes symptomatology when BPH progresses to BPE and causes bothersome lower urinary tract symptoms (LUTS) such as urinary frequency, urgency, hesitancy, nocturia, incomplete bladder emptying, and urinary retention. BPH symptoms can have a profound negative impact on quality of life leading to anxiety, depression, lack of sleep, decreased mobility, increased risk of falls, impairment of activities of daily living, and decreased leisure and sexual activities (Gacci et al., 2014; Raheem & Parsons, 2014). Untreated clinical BPH can also lead to serious complications such as urinary retention, renal insufficiency, and possible renal failure (Lee et al., 2017).

Epidemiology

BPH increases with age starting at approximately 40 years, increasing to roughly 60% in males 60 years of age and 80% in males 80 years of age (Lerner et al., 2021a). BPH can lead to BPE which can cause increasing bothersome LUTS, leading males to seek consultation and treatment. The incidence of new cases of BPH worldwide in 2019 were reported as 11.26 million (Xu et al., 2021). Prevalence data vary from region to region due to a lack of a globally accepted definition of BPH (Roehrborn & Strand, 2020). In the United States, it has been reported to range from 29% to 36%, with higher rates up to 45% in African American male-only studies (Yeboah, 2016). Incidence rates in the United States as of 2014 were reported as 38.1 million males (age >30), with 12.9 million males seeking consultation from a healthcare provider and 12.2 million males who are actively managed for BPH with LUTS (Vuichoud & Loughlin, 2015). The approximate annual cost in U.S. healthcare dollars to treat BPH is $4 billion. This accounts for direct costs (office visits, medications, office procedures, surgery), indirect costs (decreased productivity due to time off work), and intangible costs of pain and suffering (Taub & Wei, 2006).

Pathophysiology

The prostate is a walnut-shaped gland in males and is responsible for developing fluid necessary for sperm mobility and liquefaction of semen (Bajpayee et al., 2012). The prostate consists of two types of epithelial cells: Glandular cells make up the structures that provide drainage of prostatic fluid into the ejaculatory ducts in the prostatic urethra; stomal cells aid in the rapid discharge of prostatic fluid during ejaculation. The prostate is comprised of three distinct zones: the central zone, peripheral zone, and the transitional zone, which contains the prostatic urethra. The exact mechanism of action is unknown but is thought that hyperplasia results from remodeling of normal prostatic tissue in the transitional zone driven by a series of hormonal processes resulting in an imbalance between cell proliferation and cell death (Lerner et al., 2021a; Roehrborn & Strand, 2020). BPH requires the presence of male androgens which are present during prostatic development, puberty, and aging (Roehrborn, 2008). The two main androgens are testosterone and dihydrotestosterone (DHT) which is a byproduct of testosterone after it is converted by steroid enzymes called 5-alpha reductase enzymes with DHT being the more potent androgen. The majority (90%) of testosterone is produced by the testes with the adrenal gland contributing to 10% of production. Testosterone diffuses directly into the epithelial and stromal prostatic cells where it is converted to DHT through enzymatic conversion. Local growth factors regulate cell homeostasis within the prostate. Interactions between growth factors and steroid hormones can change the balance of cell proliferation versus cell death. An imbalance of DHT occurs when there is an alteration between growth factors and steroids leading to decreased cell death and increased cell proliferation, causing hyperplasia of the prostate gland (Roehrborn, 2008).

PRESENTING SIGNS AND SYMPTOMS

Men can present with LUTS to both primary care providers and urologists. They typically present with a wide variety of complaints ranging from irritative urinary tract symptoms such as urinary frequency, urgency, urge incontinence, nocturia to obstructive urinary tract symptoms including weakening of urinary stream, feelings of incomplete bladder emptying, intermittent stream/hesitancy, straining to void, overflow incontinency and urinary retention. The correlation between degree of bothersome symptoms and the actual size of the prostate is very little and symptoms can vary greatly among individual patients (Powley & Briolat, 2020).

HISTORY AND PHYSICAL EXAMINATION

A thorough intake of medical and sexual history as well as medications and lifestyle habits should be obtained. A meta-analysis by Raheem & Parsons in 2014 demonstrated that certain modifiable risk factors such as obesity, decreased physical activity, and diet can substantially increase the risk of developing BPH and LUTS (Raheem & Parsons, 2014). The American Urological Society's guidelines on BPH initial workup recommend using a validated questionnaire such as the AUA's I-PSS to quantify LUTS. This is a self-administered, seven-item questionnaire that also includes one quality of life question and is considered the gold standard tool to use as it is universally accepted and utilized worldwide (Roehrborn & Strand, 2020). Physical examination should include a digital rectal exam, external genitalia exam, and a focal neurologic exam. Digital rectal exam should focus on size and symmetry of the prostate along with assessment of rectal tone. Increased tone may be indicative of pelvic floor dysfunction while decrease tone may denote a neurologic condition. Examination of external genitalia can rule out abnormalities such as meatal stenosis, phimosis, or palpable urethral masses which may impede urinary outflow.

DIFFERENTIAL DIAGNOSIS AND DIAGNOSTIC CONSIDERATIONS

Differential diagnoses include cauda equina syndrome which can present as acute urinary retention. Other neurologic conditions such as Parkinson's disease and multiple sclerosis can also present with urinary retention. Bladder cancer and prostate cancer are also to be considered as they can present with both irritative and obstructive urinary tract symptoms. Additional diagnoses include bladder stones and urethral strictures which can cause obstruction of the urinary stream. Urinary tract infections (UTIs), sexually transmitted infections (STI), and prostatitis can present with irritative symptoms similar to BPH.

According to the latest AUA Guidelines on BPH, laboratory testing should include a urinanalysis and an assessment of urine flow rate and postvoid residuals. Evidence of postvoid residuals can help determine baseline ability of the bladder to empty. Severe retention may not be amenable to therapies other than surgical intervention (Lerner et al., 2021a). PSA testing was removed from the updated AUA guidelines in 2018 due to its unreliability to correctly evaluate prostate size (Doolin et al., 2021). A basic metabolic panel to check for renal function is also not a guideline recommendation in the workup of BPH.

TREATMENT

The two main goals of treatment are to reduce bothersome symptoms and to decrease/delay the long-term physiological effects of BPH. These include possible development of bladder diverticula, hydronephrosis, bladder calculi, and renal insufficiency due to prolonged bladder outlet obstruction from BPH (Powley & Briolat, 2020). Treatment for BPH is often multimodal and includes strategies such as behavior modification, medications, and surgical interventions.

First-line therapy should be aimed at behavior and lifestyle modifications such as diet, physical activity, and weight management, as well as reducing fluid intake and eliminating substances that have a diuretic effect such as caffeine, alcohol, and certain medications if possible (Dornbier et al., 2020). Increased physical activity has been observed to have a protective effect on BPH outcomes in several studies (Wolin et al., 2015). Increased adiposity and waist circumference have both been associated with increase prostate volume as determined by ultrasound (US) and magnetic resonance imaging (MRI) studies (Raheem & Parsons, 2014). If modification of lifestyle factors does not provide any significant symptom improvement, then counseling on either medical therapy and/or referral to a urologist for surgical intervention are the next steps (Lerner et al., 2021a).

The mainstays of medical therapy have traditionally included alpha blockers and 5-alpha-reductase inhibitors (5-ARIs) either as monotherapy or in combination. However, in recent years, additional medications such as antimuscarinics, beta-3 agonists, and phosphodiesterase type 5 inhibitors (PDE5Is) have also been utilized in medical treatment of BPH (Serati et al., 2019).

Alpha blockers target alpha receptors located in the prostatic urethra and bladder neck thereby relaxing smooth muscle tone thus allowing for improved urinary flow. The 5-ARIs block the conversion of testosterone to dihydrotestosterone, causing apoptosis or cell death of prostatic epithelial cells which can lead to a reduction of prostatic tissue over a 3- to 6-month interval. AUA guidelines recommend starting with alpha blockers which include terazosin, doxazosin, tamsulosin, alfuzosin, and silodosin. Terazosin and doxazosin are nonselective alpha-1 receptor blockers that were originally approved for hypertension and therefore have a higher potential for orthostatic hypotension and syncope. Tamsulosin and silodosin are selective alpha 1-a receptor blockers and alfuzosin is a selective alpha 1-b receptor blocker. Although the more selective alpha blockers impact blood pressure significantly less, they also have been found to cause ejaculatory dysfunction and are more common in the alpha 1-a class (Lerner et al., 2021a). In a study by Hellstrom & Sikka in 2006, alfuzosin demonstrated less ejaculatory dysfunction as compared to tamsulosin (Hellstrom & Sikka, 2006). Therefore, selection of which alpha blocker to use should take into consideration patient's age and existing comorbidities. Additional consideration must be given to patients who may need cataract surgery as use of alpha blockers have a higher risk of developing intraoperative floppy iris syndrome (IFIS; Lerner et al., 2021a). These

patients should be advised to discuss this risk with their ophthalmologist before therapy can be initiated.

Use of 5-ARI medications finasteride and dutasteride is considered in instances of significant prostatic enlargement and concern of possible urinary retention due to BPH. Finasteride selectively inhibits the 5-alpha reductase type II isoenzyme and dutasteride inhibits both types I and II. Serum DHT levels are reduced by 70% by finasteride and 95% with dutasteride; however, the type II isoenzyme is more prevalent in prostatic tissue. Only one head-to-head comparison study to date has been performed comparing both medications and showed no differences in prostate volumes, symptom score, and urinary flow rates (Nickel et al., 2011). Patients should be counseled on side effects including gynecomastia, decreased libido, erectile dysfunction, ejaculatory disorder, and depression (Lee & Cho, 2018). Both alpha blockers and 5-ARIs can be used alone or in combination as a treatment option to reduce LUTS and decrease the risk of urinary retention and need for surgical intervention (Lerner et al., 2021a).

Antimuscarinic agents such as oxybutynin, hyoscyamine, darifenacin, solifenacin, and trospium have been used to treat irritative urinary symptoms such as frequency, urgency, urge incontinence, and nocturia. Their mechanism of action is through antagonism at muscarinic M3 receptors located at the neuromuscular junctions in the bladder detrusor muscle allowing for increased bladder storage capacity. Side effects of these drugs include dry mouth, constipation, fatigue, blurry vision, and cognitive impairment, particularly in the elderly (Huang et al., 2020). Beta-3 agonists are a newer class of drugs that have been used to treat irritative voiding symptoms. They work by acting on the beta-3 adrenergic receptors located in the detrusor smooth muscle of the bladder. Their side effect profile includes hypertension, nasopharyngitis, and UTIs (Huang et al., 2020). According to AUA guidelines, both antimuscarinic agents and beta-3 agonists can be used alone or in combination with an alpha blocker for those patients with irritative voiding symptoms (Lerner et al., 2021a). Choice of which agent to use should be based on patient profile.

Use of PDE5Is has been studied to assess their impact on BPH/LUTS with the majority of trials using tadalafil 5 mg. Although results demonstrated no statistical difference in symptoms score (IPSS) as compared to placebo, a relative effect was noted suggesting that tadalafil could provide subjective symptom improvement. Therefore, AUA guidelines recommend tadalafil as an option in selected patients or those who have concomitant erectile dysfunction (Lerner et al., 2021a).

Of note, medical therapy is required long term to maintain effectiveness. Patients whose symptoms do not improve with behavior modification and/or medical therapy or do not wish to remain on medication indefinitely should be referred to a urologist for consideration of surgical intervention (Lerner et al., 2021b).

Current surgical interventions to treat BPH are divided into three categories: transurethral surgery (TURP); simple prostatectomy; and minimally invasive surgical therapies (Lerner et al., 2021b). Each category has its risks and benefits. The choice of the optimal approach should be decided by the urologist and patient taking into consideration prostatic size, patient characteristics, and procedural risks (Lerner et al., 2021b).

TRANSITION OF CARE

BPH with mild to moderate LUTS can be managed by both primary care providers and urologists. For those patients managed by primary care providers, they should be referred to a urologist once their symptoms become progressively bothersome to prevent long-term sequelae of BPH with LUTS.

CLINICAL PEARLS

- Treatment plans should be individualized to each patient.
- Incidence of BPH increases with age and treatment is dependent on severity of LUTS.
- Medical therapy for BPH is life-long to maintain symptom relief.

KEY TAKEAWAYS

- Goals of treatment include reduction of bothersome LUTS and decrease/delay the long-term physiological effects of BPH.
- Use of validated tool (IPSS) to quantify LUTS is key in determining treatment options.
- Refer to a urologist for patients with moderate to severe LUTS or who do not wish to take life-long medications.

EVIDENCE-BASED RESOURCES

American Urological Association International Prostatism Symptom Score https://www.uptodate.com/contents/calculator-international-prostatism-symptom-score-ipss

Lerner, L. B., McVary, K. T., Barry, M. J., Bixler, B. R., Dahm, P., Das, A. K., Gandhi, M. C., Kaplan, S. A., Kohler, T. S., Martin, L., Parsons, J. K., Roehrborn, C. G., Stoffel, J. T., Welliver, C., & Wilt, T. J. (2021). Management of lower urinary tract symptoms attributed to benign prostatic hyperplasia: AUA guideline part I-initial work-up and medical management. *Journal of Urology*, *206*(4), 806–817. https://doi.org/10.1097/JU.0000000000002183

Lerner, L. B., McVary, K. T., Barry, M. J., Bixler, B. R., Dahm, P., Das, A. K., Gandhi, M. C., Kaplan, S. A., Kohler, T. S., Martin, L., Parsons, J. K., Roehrborn, C. G., Stoffel, J. T., Welliver, C., & Wilt, T. J. (2021). Management of lower urinary tract symptoms attributed to benign prostatic hyperplasia: AUA guideline part II—Surgical evaluation and treatment. *Journal of Urology*, *206*(4), 818–826. https://doi.org/10.1097/JU.0000000000002184

13.6: NEPHROLITHIASIS

Nephrolithiasis, commonly referred to as kidney stones, represents an obstructive process in which crystals migrate through the ureter toward the bladder (Khan et al., 2016). During this process, bradykinin and other proinflammatory cytokines, as well as mechanical irritation, typically result in severe pain with microscopic or even gross hematuria on presentation. The prevalence of nephrolithiasis increases with age and has become more common in the general population over time (Scales et al., 2012; Ziemba & Matlaga, 2017).

PRESENTING SIGNS AND SYMPTOMS

Stones can form in the renal calyces and pelvis or develop within the urinary tract due to supersaturation of mineral solutes. The majority of kidney stones will pass through the ureteropelvic junction (UPJ) on exiting the kidney and enter the bladder at the ureterovesicular junction (UVJ; Figure 13.1), at which time pain should resolve with cessation of the inflammatory process.

Complications requiring immediate intervention include hydronephrosis, which is the backflow of urine into the kidney and can lead to postobstructive nephropathy. Infection can occur in the presence of urinary stasis due to a stone, which can become a urological emergency requiring surgical intervention. Ultimately, goals of care include preservation of baseline renal function, prevention and early treatment of infection, and effective analgesic therapy.

HISTORY AND PHYSICAL FINDINGS

History taking should include questions about recent fluid intake and the possibility of dehydration or heat-related illness (Johnson et al., 2019). Other risk factors include hypercalciuria, hyperuricosuria, or low urine pH (Spivacow et al., 2016). Obesity, cardiovascular disease, diabetes, hypertension, and metabolic syndrome increase the risk for stone formation and recurrence (Khan et al., 2016); the AGACNP should ask the patient about these conditions, as well as a personal or familial history of nephrolithiasis. Certain medications, including thiazide diuretics, allopurinol, or some antiviral agents can promote supersaturation and crystal formation (Fontenelle & Sarti, 2019; Palsson et al., 2019).

Patients may report a progressive onset of symptoms, but most often can describe rapid onset of cramping pain radiating from the flank toward the ipsilateral lower abdomen. Pain in patients with acute nephrolithiasis is usually constant but worsening in episodic waves. This may be accompanied by urinary frequency or urgency, referred pain to the groin, testicle, or labia, or nausea and vomiting (Manthey & Nicks, 2020).

Differential diagnoses to consider include abdominal aortic dissection, renal artery infarction, pyelonephritis, appendicitis, or other acute abdominal inflammation

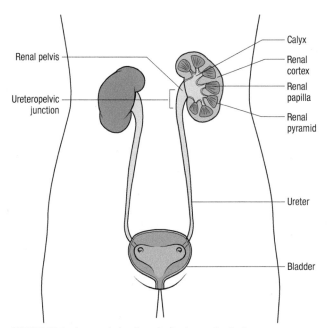

FIGURE 13.1: Anatomic landmarks in the urological system.

Labels: Renal pelvis, Ureteropelvic junction, Calyx, Renal cortex, Renal papilla, Renal pyramid, Ureter, Bladder

or infection. Clinical diagnoses such as musculoskeletal back pain may be viable differentials but should be supported by findings on the clinical exam, especially for initial presentations. Special populations at risk for nephrolithiasis, as well as the complications, include pregnant patients (Semins & Matlaga, 2013), obese patients (Kelly et al., 2019), and those with previous chronic kidney disease (AUA, n.d.).

Physical assessment in the patient with nephrolithiasis is helpful in identifying complications, such as infection or associated dehydration. There are no specific clinical signs or findings in the literature to support a definitive diagnosis of nephrolithiasis.

Vital signs may reflect pain; the AGACNP should be alerted to the presence of fever, tachycardia, and hypotension as these may represent impending sepsis or hypovolemia. The presence of an abdominal bruit should be correlated with the patient history and investigated for potential abdominal aortic aneurysm (AAA) or renal artery occlusion. The presence of these findings should prompt consideration of alternative diagnoses involving abdominal or pelvic pathology, as well as pyelonephritis. Pain that is exacerbated by movement and characterized by reproducible tenderness to a muscular distribution may represent strain or sprain; this should be a diagnosis of exclusion if accompanied by a history supportive of kidney stones.

DIFFERENTIAL DIAGNOSIS AND DIAGNOSTIC CONSIDERATIONS

Laboratory Analysis

The diagnostic evaluation of patients with suspected nephrolithiasis should include testing for pregnancy in all females of childbearing age; especially if imaging will be needed. Urinalysis should be performed to investigate for hematuria, which occurs in 84% of cases (Minotti et al., 2020). A complete blood count (CBC) may be useful if the patient is febrile or at risk for infection. Renal function should be assessed. During an obstructive process, the unaffected kidney will normally double its filtration rate (Manthey & Nicks, 2020), resulting in little if any increase in serum creatinine. A significant elevation in creatinine above baseline may indicate that the patient has only one kidney or that there is underlying renal disease.

Patients should be instructed to use a urine filter to catch the stone for analysis once it is passed. Analysis can tell a story, aiding in targeted treatment and prevention. Struvite stones are directly associated with urinary tract infections (UTIs) and due to their irregular, spiky contours are more likely to become lodged in the urinary tract. Calcium oxalate or phosphate are the most common type of stone formed (Khan et al., 2016; Schwaderer & Wolfe, 2017), and may be better controlled with improved hydration and dietary adherence. Uric acid stones may be connected to systemic gout and also controlled with nutritional counseling. Increasing attention has been given to the role of genetic counseling for patients with recurrent nephrolithiasis, and this should be a consideration for follow-up upon discharge (Palsson et al., 2019).

Diagnostic Imaging

Diagnostic imaging may not be required in patients with a history of recurrent nephrolithiasis and no indication of acute complications if symptoms are typical. In the acute care setting, there is often a question of whether an alternative diagnosis is likely or whether hydronephrosis is present. For patients experiencing their initial episode, the clinician should determine which imaging modality will be least harmful and cost-effective, while providing the information needed to facilitate diagnosis and management decisions. This should be weighed against potential harm such as radiation dose, resource depletion, and cost (AUA, n.d.).

Renal ultrasound (US) has arisen as a rapid, simple, and cost-effective strategy for identifying nephrolithiasis without the risks of ionizing radiation (American Urologic Association [AUA], n.d.; Semins & Matlaga, 2013). US can confirm the presence of obstruction indicated by hydronephrosis in the acute care setting (Vijayakumar et al., 2018). Doppler US provides additional information on urine flow, or ureteral jet, which is useful in determining whether there is obstruction (Brisbane et al., 2016). The reliability of US has been questioned with sensitivities as low as 24% to 69% (Vijayakumar et al., 2018), although it is highly dependent on operator skills and aided by the use of both Doppler and different US modalities (Vijayakumar et al., 2018). Sensitivity and specificity are also affected by stone size which translates directly to visibility.

US should be considered in patients at low risk for other acute processes or as a step in rapid narrowing of the differentials while waiting for other studies to be completed. Overall, while renal US has become a very popular diagnostic tool in the diagnosis of nephrolithiasis, current recommendations continue to support the use of low-dose CT as first-line imaging for suspected nephrolithiasis (Brisbane et al., 2016; Kocher et al., 2011; *The Journal of Urology*® home study course 2013 volume 189/190, 2013; Türk et al., 2016).

Kidney, ureter, and bladder (KUB) radiographs are a relatively low cost, low risk (effective radiation exposure of 0.7 mSv) option for imaging of patients with suspected nephrolithiasis (AUA, n.d.). Traditional KUB technology exhibits low sensitivity and specificities of 57% and 76%, respectively (AUA, n.d.; *The Journal of Urology*® home study course 2013 volume 189/190, 2013), making this a less utilized diagnostic resource. Digital tomosynthesis, an emerging technology, provides additional views similar to CT scanning and may have an increased role for diagnosis in the future.

Low-dose noncontrasted renal CT scanning remains the preferred imaging modality for evaluation of patients presenting with an initial presentation for suspected nephrolithiasis or for those with suspected complications (Fulgham et al., 2013; Türk et al., 2016). Use of CT allows for rapid identification of the stone, which may appear on scout films, as well as the presence of hydronephrosis, stranding (indicative of infection or severe inflammation), or other intraabdominal or pelvic processes. The test is reliable, with 95% sensitivity and up to 98% specificity (Brisbane et al., 2016). While the amount of fluid collection itself does not correlate with surgical interventions, there is a relationship between CT findings and performance of shock wave lithotripsy or ureteroscopic retrieval (Fulgham et al., 2013).

TREATMENT

Nonsteroidal antiinflammatory drugs are a staple in the symptomatic management of nephrolithiasis pain, particularly because of their ability to block the production of prostaglandins which have a vascular effect on the irritated smooth muscle lining of the affected ureter. In addition, reducing prostaglandin may have an effect on stone development (Buck et al., 1983). Consideration should be given to the baseline renal function of the patient. Ketorolac, 30 mg IV, has demonstrated effectiveness in pain management for nephrolithiasis (Prina et al., 2002), although effectiveness is related to stone size. Parenteral administration of NSAIDs has demonstrated a higher level of comfort achieved, and although less commonly available, IV Ibuprofen may have a more rapid effect than Ketorolac (Forouzanfar et al., 2019).

IV lidocaine exhibits great potential for the management of pain associated with nephrolithiasis and should be considered as a safe alternative to opioids ("IV Lidocaine Safe Alternative to Opioids for Kidney Stone Pain," n.d.). The American College of Emergency Physicians (ACEP) recommends dosing 1.5 mg/kg delivered by IV infusion over a period of 10 minutes via pump, to a maximum of 200 mg. Patients should receive cardiac monitoring during infusion (ACEP, n.d.).

Low dose, subdissociative ketamine is another option for effective analgesia in patients with the pain of renal colic and can be dosed at 0.3 mg/kg IV (Grill et al., 2019).

Nausea frequently accompanies the pain of stone passage through the ureter, and patients may exhibit vagal symptoms including vomiting and diaphoresis. Those requiring opioid analgesics may have additive effects of the medications, increasing the need for antiemetics as part of their treatment. Recommendations for therapy are lacking on agents specific to the management of nephrolithiasis.

The use of tamsulosin (Flomax™), an alpha-adrenergic inhibitor, has long been debated to reduce smooth muscle spasm along the ureter, expediting the passage of ureteral stones. Although many providers continue to prescribe tamsulosin as medically expulsive therapy, the 2018 STONE Trial (Meltzer et al., 2018) demonstrated no significant effect in patients with stones of less than 9 mm in diameter at 28 days. The drug does appear to have a therapeutic effect on individuals with stones 10 mm or greater, with a minimal risk of adverse effects (Wang et al., 2017).

Although commonly prescribed in practice, the use of opioid analgesics for nephrolithiasis is not a first line recommendation. It should be noted that individuals with a history of kidney stones are at increased risk for long-term opiate use. Shared decision-making, cautious prescribing practices, and the use of clinical judgment are essential in cases where alternative therapies are not successful.

Urology should be consulted for patients with obstruction or complicated nephrolithiasis; 5 mm in diameter is a generally accepted cutoff for concern that the stone may not pass spontaneously (Prina et al., 2002). Crystals with irregular conformity such as staghorn calculi are also at increased risk for obstruction. The presence of fever, infection requiring IV therapy, or acute renal insufficiency are indications for consultation and admission (Schwaderer & Wolfe, 2017). Patients who are found to be acutely hypercalcemic may also require hospital admission.

Infected kidney stones, or those associated with UTI due to urostasis should be treated with appropriate antimicrobial coverage with consideration of local antibiograms and resistance patterns. (See Section 13.1, UTIs.)

The approach to interventional decompression of urologic stones has become less invasive over time. Ureteroscopy with or without ureteral stent placement to facilitate passage, or percutaneous nephrolithotomy are first-line options to facilitate stone expulsion, while shock-wave lithotripsy is used less commonly due to increased risk of recurrence and overall costs of therapy (Geraghty et al., 2018; Kartal et al., 2020).

TRANSITION OF CARE

For patients requiring treatment of acute nephrolithiasis, prevention of recurrence is an important factor in the plan of care. Patients should promote urinary flow by drinking adequate amounts of water and recognizing the need to increase water intake during exposure to hot environments (e.g., hot weather, saunas), or increased physical exertion. Awareness of dietary sources rich in purines (uric acid stones) or oxalate such as chocolate, sweet potatoes, or peanuts, can promote formation of calcium deposits. The timing of ingestion can also reduce the risk of recurrence, as taking in calcium with oxalate promotes binding in the upper GI tract (National Kidney Foundation, n.d.).

Patients should be instructed to complete their full course of antibiotics in the case of infection, and arrangements made for follow up with urology if this was a recurrence or if intervention was required.

Urology can provide recommendations if the patient is expected to remove a ureteral stent at home, and guidance on returning for fever, flank, or abdominal pain, inability to urinate, hematuria, or uncontrolled pain, nausea, or vomiting should be conveyed.

13.7: EPIDIDYMITIS

Jeanne Martin

Epididymitis is a clinical syndrome consisting of pain, swelling, and inflammation of the epididymis, a long tubular structure located on the superior/posterior side of each testis. This structure connects the vas deferens to the testis and its main purpose is to confer sperm to maturity after leaving the testis (James et al., 2020). Epididymitis can be caused by both infectious and noninfectious etiologies (Taylor, 2015). It can affect males of all ages; however, the most common age group affected is 20 to 39 years old, mostly associated with sexually transmitted infections (STIs; Rupp & Leslie, 2022). Epididymitis can be classified as acute epididymitis and chronic epididymitis depending on duration of symptoms of < or > than 6 weeks (Taylor, 2015; Workowski et al., 2021).

Epidemiology

It is estimated that the prevalence of acute epididymitis is approximately 600,000 cases annually in the United States (Ching, 2020; Rupp & Leslie, 2022). Incidence rates are 1 in 1,000 males per year (Ching, 2020). Chronic epididymitis is estimated to account for up to 80% of patients presenting to a urology clinic for scrotal pain (Tracy et al., 2008).

Pathophysiology

Although the true etiology of acute epididymitis is unclear, it is postulated that it is caused by retrograde flow of infected urine into the ejaculatory duct (Tracy et al., 2008). Acute epididymitis can be caused by an infectious or noninfectious process (Taylor, 2015; Tracy et al., 2008). The most common cause in males 14 to 35 years of age is an STI, typically *Chlamydia trachomatis* and *Neisseria gonorrhea* (Louette et al., 2018; Rupp & Leslie, 2022). In prepubertal boys and males >35 years, it is often caused by nonsexually transmitted urinary tract pathogens (Pilatz et al., 2015; Trojian et al., 2009). For males who have practice insertive anal intercourse, coliform bacteria such as *Escherichia coli* are often the pathogens to be considered (Smith & Angarone, 2015). Mumps is also a known infectious cause of acute epididymitis (Rupp & Leslie, 2022). Non infectious causes of acute epididymitis include prostate biopsy, urinary instrumentation, disease states such as sarcoidosis and Bechet's disease, and medications such as amiodarone (Taylor, 2015; Tracy et al., 2008). Chronic epididymitis can be categorized as inflammatory (infective, granulomatous caused by tuberculosis, and drug induced), obstructive (congenital, acquired, or iatrogenic obstruction of the vas deferens or epididymis), and idiopathic (Nickel et al., 2002).

PRESENTING SIGNS AND SYMPTOMS

Acute epididymitis presents over several days with increased scrotal pain and swelling localized to the posterior testis (Rupp & Leslie, 2022; Trojian et al., 2009). Pain may spread to the contralateral testis though typically rare (4% of cases; Michel et al., 2015). It is often associated with fever and chills (75%) and, in 30% of cases, irritative voiding symptoms such as dysuria, frequency, and urgency (Michel et al., 2015). Urethral discharge may or may not be present (Chirwa et al., 2021). Additional signs may include hematospermia, lower abdominal pain, groin pain, and pain with intercourse or ejaculation (Montgomery & Bloom, 2011).

HISTORY AND PHYSICAL EXAM

History intake should outline the circumstances of the onset of symptoms. A thorough history should include the possibility of injury from repetitive activities such as sports (running, jumping, biking) or a traumatic injury to the scrotum. A detailed sexual history should be obtained including any history of prior STI exposure along with any past medical history of genitourinary tract problems or procedures (Pontari, 2020; Rupp & Leslie, 2022). Physical exam will reveal a tender, edematous and often indurated epididymis that is painful to palpation. Swelling typically begins at the tail of the epididymis located in the lower pole of the testis and spreads in a cephalad fashion toward the head of the epididymis located in the upper pole (Trojian et al., 2009). The spermatic cord usually becomes edematous and tender to palpation and the testis is in its normal position (Pontari, 2020). The cremasteric reflex remains intact (contraction of the cremaster muscle causing elevation of testis upon stroking the upper medial thigh) and Prehn sign will be positive which is elicited when elevation of the affected testis relieves pain (Trojian et al., 2009).

DIFFERENTIAL DIAGNOSIS AND DIAGNOSTIC CONSIDERATIONS

Diagnosis is made mainly by history and physical exam. If the patient is unclear about onset of pain (hours vs. days) or has physical findings consistent with testicular torsion, a scrotal ultrasound (US) should be obtained as this is a true surgical emergency and requires urological consultation (Rupp & Leslie, 2022). Other differential diagnoses include torsion of the appendix testis, isolated orchitis associated with mumps, hydrocele, spermatocele, testicular mass, epididymal congestion following vasectomy, and urinary tract infections (UTIs; Pontari, 2020; Rupp & Leslie, 2022). The Centers for Disease Control and Prevention (CDC) recommends one of the following tests be performed: Gram stain of urethral secretions; urinalysis to test for presence of leukocyte esterase; or microanalysis of urine to evaluate ≥10 WBCs/HPF (Workowski et al., 2021). In sexually active men, urine should be obtained for nucleic acid amplification testing to check for *Chlamydia trachomatis* and *Neisseria gonorrhoeae* A urine culture should be obtained for prepubertal boys, males who practice insertive anal intercourse, and males who have recently undergone vasectomy, prostate biopsy, or genitourinary instrumentation. The CDC also recommends screening all sexually active males for STIs including syphilis and HIV (Workowski et al., 2021).

TREATMENT

Treatment goals of acute epididymitis include symptom relief, reduction of STI transmission if present, cure of microbiological infection if present, and reduce risks of potential complications including infertility, abscess, recurrent epididymitis, chronic testicular pain (Workowski et al., 2021). For treatment of acute epididymitis likely due to *Chlamydia* or *Gonorrhea*, administer ceftriaxone 500 mg IM × 1 plus doxycycline 100 mg orally twice daily for 10 days. For acute epididymitis most likely caused by *Chlamydia*, *Gonorrhea*, or an enteric organism, administer ceftriaxone 500 mg IM × 1 plus levofloxacin 500 mg orally once daily for 10 days. If acute epididymitis is most likely caused by enteric organisms only and gonorrhea has been ruled out by Gram stain (prostate biopsy, vasectomy, urinary tract instrumentation), administer levofloxacin 500 mg orally once daily for 10 days (Workowski et al., 2021). Nonsteroidal antiinflammatory drugs (NSAIDs) can be administered to aid with fever, pain, and swelling. Other adjuvant therapies include bed rest, ice, and scrotal elevation (Rupp & Leslie, 2022; Workowski et al., 2021).

TRANSITION OF CARE

Advise males with suspected or confirmed *N. gonorrhea* or *C. trachomatis* to refer all sexual partners within 60 days before onset of symptoms and diagnosis for evaluation, testing, and treatment. If the last sexual encounter was >60 days, only the last partner needs to be referred. Abstinence from sexual activity until all partners have been treated and are symptom free is of paramount importance (Workowski et al., 2021). In prepubertal boys and older males, perform follow-up urine cultures. Although symptoms generally resolve within 72 hours, it may take several weeks after completion of antimicrobial therapy for complete symptom resolution. If no symptom improvement is noted in 3 days, follow-up is recommended for reevaluation (Pontari, 2020). For pain that lasts longer than 6 weeks (chronic epididymitis), refer to a urologist.

CLINICAL PEARLS

- Ages 14 to 35 typically due to STI (*N. gonorrhea, C. trachomatis*).
- Prepubertal boys and males >35 years old, typically due to UTI.
- Males who practice insertive anal intercourse typically due to coliform/enteric organisms.
- Pain is gradual (days) as opposed to acute (hours), differentiating from testicular torsion.

KEY TAKEAWAYS

- If history and/or physical exam are unclear, obtain scrotal US to rule out testicular torsion (surgical emergency).
- Counsel all males suspected of STI to refer sexual partner(s) for evaluation, testing, and treatment.
- Symptom improvement usually within 72 hours; complete symptom resolution may take up to several weeks.
- If no symptom relief is noted within 3 days, follow up with provider for reevaluation.
- Refer to a urologist if symptoms persist longer than 6 weeks

13.8: TESTICULAR TORSION

Testicular torsion is a mechanical twisting of the spermatic cord, resulting in neurovascular compromise to the organ. The presence of testicular torsion is considered a surgical emergency and if suspected, should prompt early urological consultation. Torsion typically affects young males with a bimodal distribution during the neonatal and prepubescent periods (Sharp et al., 2013), but undetected structural defects may lead to intermittent torsion or a delay in diagnosis. The mean incidence of torsion occurs in males aged 1 to 25 years, making this an important consideration on the differential for any patient presenting with testicular pain (Lee et al., 2014; Schick & Sternard, 2020).

Pathophysiology

While common sense would lead the AGACNP to assume that arterial occlusion may be the result of torsion, ischemia is first the result of venous congestion. Continued edema, as well as the production of pro-inflammatory cytokines, will increase the risk of arterial occlusion and subsequent necrosis and orchiectomy (Lysiak, 2004; Schuppe et al., 2017). Even with timely intervention, this process can lead to permanent atrophy and oligospermia or complete lack or sperm production (Schick & Sternard, 2020).

HISTORY AND PHYSICAL FINDINGS

Evaluation for testicular torsion should be done in a timely manner for efficient consultation and definitive treatment. The Testicular Workup for Ischemia and Suspected Torsion (TWIST) score (Table 13.3) is a validated tool for assessment by urologists as well as nonurological providers (Sheth et al., 2016) and appears to be reliable for use in the adult population (Barbosa et al., 2021). Patients with a score of 2 or lower may be suitable for further evaluation with testicular ultrasound (US), while those with a score of 5 or more would likely benefit from immediate urology consultation.

Patients with torsion typically report a sudden or abrupt onset of unilateral pain in the affected teste, often associated with nausea and vomiting (Sharp et al., 2013). Shortening of the spermatic cord due to twisting may result in elevation or a "high riding" testicle.

Congenital defects or adhesions of the tunica vaginalis to the teste may promote acute or intermittent torsion with the presence of a bell clapper deformity (Figure 13.2) on exam (Al-Kandari et al., 2017); this increases the risk of twisting of the spermatic cord, which may be intermittent. It is helpful to ask the patient whether they have had transient episodes of pain or injury to the area. Increasing mass of the testicles occurs in puberty and may also contribute to torsion (Bandarkar & Blask, 2018).

TABLE 13.3: The Testicular Workup for Ischemia and Suspected Torsion Scoring System

	POINTS	
Testicular swelling	2	
Hard testicle	2	
Absence of cremasteric reflex	1	
Nausea/vomiting	1	
High riding testis	1	
Total (7 Points total)		

A positive Prehn sign, or relief of pain with scrotal elevation, is nonspecific for the diagnosis of torsion (What is the role of the cremasteric reflex and Prehn sign in the evaluation of testicular torsion?, n.d.) but is worthy of noting in the exam. Lack of a cremasteric reflex on the affected side, although not diagnostic, is a significant finding and increases concern for the presence of torsion (Mellick et al., n.d.).

The presence of a "blue dot sign" or a pinpoint area of blue discoloration along the superior aspect of the epididymis, may represent torsion of the testicular appendix (Figure 13.3), and is accompanied by a similar abrupt onset of pain.

DIFFERENTIAL DIAGNOSIS AND DIAGNOSTIC CONSIDERATIONS

Obtaining an expedited testicular US and rapid urological consultation are the priorities in caring for the patient with suspected testicular torsion. As with any ischemic injury, definitive treatment is needed to restore perfusion to the compromised tissue. Notation of a whirlpool

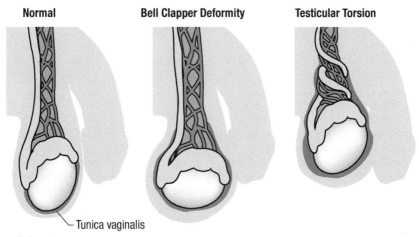

Normal   **Bell Clapper Deformity**   **Testicular Torsion**

Tunica vaginalis

FIGURE 13.2: Bell Clapper deformity.

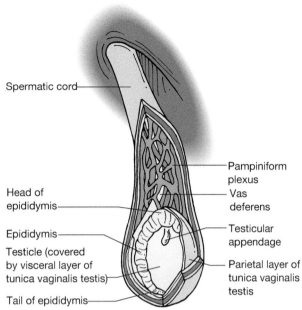

FIGURE 13.3: Scrotal anatomy showing testicular appendage.
Source: Yedinak, C., Hurtado, C. R., Leung, A. M., Annon, M., Harbison, H. S., Spatz, D. L., Polidori, G. P., & Fischer, V. (2021). Endocrine system. In N. C. Tkacs, L. L. Herrmann, & R. L. Johnson (Eds.), *Advanced physiology and pathophysiology: Essentials for clinical practice*. Springer Publishing Company. Fig 17.37.

sign on US is considered diagnostic for testicular torsion (DaJusta et al., 2013; McDowell, 2018).

Patients should remain NPO if there is suspicion for torsion. While manual reversal is possible, surgical exploration should never be delayed as infarction and permanent infertility may result within as little as 4 to 6 hours (Sharp et al., 2013). Manual detorsion may be attempted in cases when surgical intervention is delayed or unavailable at the clinical site; providing adequate analgesia and sedation allows for relaxation of fibers in the cremasteric muscle, with the provider applying gentle rotation from medial to lateral sides, in a fashion similar to opening a book (Davis, 2020; Gordhan & Sadeghi-Nejad, 2015).

Timely surgical detorsion with orchiopexy may restore perfusion to the teste; frank necrosis would likely require orchiectomy with removal (Taskinen et al., 2008). Postoperatively, the patient undergoing orchiectomy may be referred for placement of a testicular prosthesis approximately 6 months after surgery. Recent attention has focused on preservation of germ cell function by limiting the effects of reperfusion injury on the affected organ. Nonsteroidal antiinflammatory agents (NSAIDs) may be prescribed for pain as well as their antagonizing effects on the cyclo-oxygenase pathway. Phosphodiesterase inhibitors such as sildenafil and supplements including lycopene have also been studied in animal models but are not included in authoritative guidelines at this time.

In summary, testicular torsion represents an acute ischemic emergency which, if not identified rapidly, can result in testicular necrosis and male infertility. Although there is no definition for the time at which ischemia progresses to irreversible necrosis; it is the clinician's duty to recognize indications on the history and exam, and to initiate rapid urologic consultation in suspicious cases, and obtaining expedited testicular US for timely intervention.

13.9: SEXUALLY TRANSMITTED INFECTIONS

Sexually transmitted infections (STIs) include any infection transmitted through sexual contact and can involve not only the lower genitourinary tract but oral and anal ports of entry and can result in serious complications including pelvic inflammatory disease (PID), tubo-ovarian abscess, infertility, disseminated infection, and sepsis. Public awareness and prevention education are therefore a key role for the nurse practitioner.

The Centers for Disease Control and Prevention (CDC) reports that in 2018, nearly 68 million people in the United States had a STI on any given day, resulting in a cost of $13.7 million to the U.S. healthcare system (CDC, n.d.-a). To limit the spread of STI, treatment strategies include screening individuals at risk for STIs, empiric antimicrobial therapy, single-dose therapy when possible, and reporting to local health departments for notification and treatment of all sexual partners (Workowski et al., 2015). Prevention includes patient education and is a core competency of the AGACNP role.

STIs continue to trend upward across the United States, although the incidence of infection by various organisms has shifted. Chlamydial infections have outpaced *Neisseria gonorrhoeae* with over 1.7 million cases in 2018, although both continue to rise in occurrence. Cases of syphilis have also increased, prompting the CDC to issue a warning on the risk of newborn deaths from congenital disease (CDC, n.d.-b).

PRESENTING SIGNS AND SYMPTOMS

The CDC categorizes STIs as notifiable or nonnotifiable based on the risk to public health. Notifiable conditions include chancroid, *C. trachomatis*, *N. gonorrhoeae*, or various forms of syphilis, infection caused by the spirochete *Treponema pallidum* (congenital, primary, secondary, early nonprimary nonsecondary, unknown duration or late, or syphilitic stillbirth, or complicated/tertiary). Nonnotifiable STIs include genital herpes and genital warts, granuloma inguinale, lymphogranuloma venereumm, mucopurulent cervicitis, nongonococcal urethritis, or PID (CDC, n.d.-a; Horner & Martin, 2017). Trichomoniasis is a parasitic infection which is highly curable and seen more commonly in females aged 14 to 59 years (CDC, n.d.-c). The wide variety of STIs and their potential to cause long-term morbidity reinforces the need to collect samples for both surveillance and screening. These infections can manifest as asymptomatic or mild conditions such as epididymitis or urethritis, which may not be tracked if treated empirically. Conversely, the

AGACNP should not presume that a patient with genitourinary complaints is experiencing an STI, when in fact the cause may be related to neoplasm, obstruction, allergic or autoimmune response, or some other infectious etiology.

HISTORY AND PHYSICAL FINDINGS

The AGACNP should collect a detailed history of present illness to assess the risk for STI, alternative diagnoses, and clues regarding acute versus chronic illness, disseminated infection, or other complications. The presence of rash or skin lesions, vaginal or urethral discharge, associated burning, pain, or pruritis can aid in identifying the causative agent.

A thorough sexual history should be obtained using the 5 Ps: partners, practices, protection from STIs and pregnancy, and past history of STIs. It is important to establish rapport and a relationship which conveys a sense of safety in disclosing sensitive information. Assure patients that the discussion is confidential, that the purpose of questions is to promote their health and that questions are asked routinely of patients with similar presenting complaints (CDC, 2020). Patients should be asked for their current pronouns as well as sexual identity or any other information that would facilitate sharing.

The AGACNP should inquire about partners they have had over a lifetime as well as whether they have multiple partners simultaneously, and the length of current relationships. A thorough history can help identify multiple ports of entry for infection; the AGACNP should inquire about oral, anal, and genital contact as well as the use of barrier protection and contraceptive protection.

The AGACNP should recognize the risk of STI in vulnerable populations, including transgender individuals (Van Gerwen et al., 2020), sex workers, men who have sex with men, people who inject drugs, prison inmates, mobile populations and adolescents (World Health Organization [WHO], 2019) and take this into account when making decisions regarding single-dose therapy, probability that the patient may not have access to follow-up, and cost of medications prescribed.

The review of systems for an individual at risk for STIs should be broad and include constitutional questions about fever, unintentional weight loss, fatigue, and night sweats. Neurologic symptoms may represent complications of HIV or syphilis infection (New York City Department of Health, n.d.). In the acute care setting, altered mental status may also represent disseminated disease. Review pertinent positives or negatives related to the eye/nose/throat (pharynx), gastrointestinal, and certainly the genitourinary system should be included.

Physical Assessment

The physical assessment on individuals with STIs can range from an unremarkable exam, to one of septic shock, depending on the causative agent. It has been reported that up to 95% of cases of gonorrhea and chlamydia may be asymptomatic, again supporting the need for screening, as the physical assessment may not yield significant findings (Farley et al., 2003).

A thorough inspection should be done, observing for chancres, ulcerations, or other lesions to the skin or mucosa. This includes the oropharynx, which may reveal posterior exudate as seen with N. gonorrhoeae or tender ulcerations with HSV-2. Encephalopathy is concerning and will prompt a comprehensive workup.

The abdominal exam can help to identify the need for imaging, particularly in females, as the risk for progression to peritonitis or rupture of tubo-ovarian abscess can become rapidly life-threatening.

The genitourinary exam may reveal signs more supportive of urinary tract infection (UTI), with costovertebral tenderness (CVAT) and a lack of purulent penile or vaginal discharge. It should be noted that there is a significant rate of coinfection and that the presence of one should not rule out the other (Armed Forces Health Surveillance Center, 2014; Mead & Grüneberg, 1978). Trichomonas in particular can produce severe dysuria, and the presence of CVAT may be associated with upper UTI (Kissinger, 2015).

DIFFERENTIAL DIAGNOSIS AND DIAGNOSTIC CONSIDERATIONS

Testing Mechanisms for Sexually Transmitted Infections

Nucleic acids amplification tests (NAATs) use fluorescence to detect the presence of antigenic DNA, typically by polymerase chain reaction (PCR) testing (Meyer, 2016). This has become the gold standard over traditional culture due to its high sensitivity and reduction in time to diagnosis (Budkaew et al., 2017). Self-collection has become a topic of interest in recent years, as this increases the likelihood of patients to test, reducing embarrassment and fear of the discomfort of a female pelvic exam. Self-swabbing for chlamydia and gonorrhea has demonstrated accuracy and better detection in some trials (Korownyk et al., 2018).

Improved testing methods have also begun to dispel the need for a first-void or "dirty" urine collection; midstream urine samples can also provide reliable results (Mangin et al., 2012), although in females vaginal collection remains more common as the pelvic examination is important to diagnosis of complicated STIs. Vaginal herpetic ulcerations should be swabbed separately for confirmation of HSV-2 infection, also by PCR (Sauerbrei, 2016).

Trichomonas vaginalis may be observed on the urinalysis or with wet mount microscopy; once again, NAAT is found to be more sensitive, with a three-fold increase in detection of the organism (CDC, n.d.-d; Kissinger, 2015).

Serologic testing for HIV and syphilis should be offered to patients with suspected STI, as these can be asymptomatic for prolonged periods, leading to severe long-term consequences. Rapid syphilis testing (RST), while less reliable than rapid plasma regain testing (RPR), may be more desirable for use in patients who can become easily lost to follow-up. The RPR has become the gold standard serology testing for *T. pallidum* (New York City Department of Health, n.d.; Trinh et al., 2017). (Recommendations for HIV testing and prophylaxis are found in Chapter 19, Infectious Diseases.)

TREATMENT

Due to increasing antimicrobial resistance patterns in the United States, the CDC released updated recommendations for empiric treatment of gonorrheal infections in December 2020 (St Cyr et al., 2020). Patients should now receive a one-time dose of 500 mg of a third-generation cephalosporin, typically ceftriaxone. Cefixime may be substituted, but it should be noted that this is less effective if there is pharyngeal involvement (n.d., 2021). For patients with cephalosporin allergy, the recommendation is a combination dosage of gentamicin, 240 mg IM plus azithromycin 2 g PO given as a single dose (St Cyr et al., 2020).

Empiric treatment for *C. trachomatis* includes azithromycin, 1-g PO as a single dose regimen.

There is growing support for the use of doxycycline, 100 mg PO BID in lieu of azithromycin, given increases in macrolide resistance (Tien et al., 2020; Workowski et al., 2015). The AGACNP should, as with all antimicrobial practice, remain conscious of local antibiogram data and weigh these with the risk of noncompliance due to dosing regimens or low tolerance for gastrointestinal side effects.

Primary or secondary syphilis can be treated with a one-time dose of benzathine penicillin, 2.4 million units IM, with the alternative of doxycycline 100 mg PO twice daily or tetracycline 500 mg PO QID in individuals who are penicillin allergic. Given emerging patterns of macrolide resistance, azithromycin is not a first-line alternative to treatment (Workowski et al., 2015).

Genital warts and human papilloma virus (HPV) are also included in the category of STI but have not been discussed at length here due to the long-term nature of complications. Health promotion and disease prevention, patient education and counseling are a core aspect of APRN practice and should be included in the management of patients with all suspected STIs or high-risk behaviors.

STIs are the primary cause of both urethritis and epididymitis in younger males. Replication and invasion in local tissues can cause an inflammatory response resulting in pain, swelling, and vascular congestion. In males, infertility may be the result of thrombosis and infarction of the testes and fibrosis with scarring of the vas deferens and epididymis (Schuppe et al., 2017).

13.10: ABNORMAL UTERINE BLEEDING

Abnormal uterine bleeding (AUB) is a common condition of females of reproductive age with a prevalence of 10% to 30% impacting quality of life, emotional well-being, health, and personal finances. AUB in the postmenopausal female (postmenopausal bleeding [PMB]) is

cancer until proven otherwise; however, in the premenopausal female it may also be a symptom of endometrial cancer which demands prompt evaluation and diagnosis (Link, 2016). AUB has replaced the term dysfunctional uterine bleeding (DUB) which more clearly describes the type of bleeding patterns and etiologies.

In 2011, a classification system, PALM-COEIN (polyp, adenomyosis, leiomyoma, malignancy and hyperplasia, coagulopathy, ovulatory dysfunction, endometrial, iatrogenic, not yet classified) was developed by the International Federation of Gynecology and Obstetrics (FIGO) Menstrual Disorders Working Group to better describe abnormalities in patterns of uterine bleeding referring to structural or nonstructural etiologies for AUB in nonpregnant females of reproductive age (Munro et al., 2011). This classification system has been adopted and approved by the FIGO Executive Board and accepted worldwide (Table 13.4).

To understand the causes and treatments of AUB, a clear understanding of the normal menstrual cycle is necessary.

Normal Menstrual Cycle

Menstrual cycles occur every 24 to 38 days and are under the influence of fluctuating hormone levels secreted by the hypothalamus, ovaries, and pituitary gland. Day 1 of the menstrual cycle is when menstrual flow begins and lasts for an average of 4.5 to 8 days with a volume loss of 5 to 80 mL (Fraser et al., 2011). This is the preovulatory phase where low estrogen and progesterone blood levels stimulate the secretion of gonadotropin-releasing hormone (GnRH) by the hypothalamus. This hormone in turn stimulates the secretion of the follicle-stimulating hormone (FSH) and luteinizing hormone (LH) by the anterior pituitary gland. As the FSH levels rise, so do the LH levels. Day 6 is the beginning of the proliferative or follicular phase which lasts until day 14 during which

TABLE 13.4: PALM-COEIN Classification System for Abnormal Uterine Bleeding

PALM - Structural		
P	Polyps	(AUB-P)
A	Adenomyosis	(AUB-A)
L	Leiomyoma	(AUB-L)
M	Malignancy and hyperplasia	(AUB-M)
COEIN - Nonstructural		
C	Coagulopathy	(AUB-C)
O	Ovulatory dysfunction	(AUB-O)
E	Endometrial	(AUB-E)
I	Iatrogenic	(AUB-I)
N	Not yet classified	(AUB-N)

Source: Reproduced from Munro, M. G., Critchley, H. O. D., Broder, M. S., & Fraser, I. S. (2011). FIGO classification system (PALM-COEIN) for causes of abnormal uterine bleeding in nongravid women of reproductive age. *International Journal of Gynecology & Obstetrics, 113*(1), 3–13. https://doi.org/10.1016/j.ijgo.2010.11.011

time the FSH and LH hormones stimulate the ovarian follicle to secrete estrogen, causing the thickening of the endometrium. Estrogen levels peak at midcycle with a decrease in FSH secretion and an increase in LH secretion, then estrogen levels fall, the follicle matures, and ovulation occurs.

The luteal or secretory phase begins on day 15 and lasts until day 28 which is characterized by declining FSH and LH levels as well as estrogen and progesterone levels as the corpus luteum begins functioning producing progesterone. The progesterone stimulates the endometrium to become thick and secretory in preparation for implantation. If implantation does not occur, the corpus luteum dies, estrogen and progesterone levels drop sharply around 10 to 12 days after ovulation, and the lining is shed as menses, beginning a new cycle (Figure 13.4).

New Terminologies/Definitions

AUB has replaced DUB as the overarching term to describe the symptom of disturbed menstrual bleeding as evidenced by changes in frequency, duration, volume, and regularity that occur outside of a normal pattern of menstruation (Fraser et al., 2011; Munro et al., 2011; Wouk & Helton, 2019). The term "heavy menstrual bleeding" (HMB) has been proposed to replace "menorrhagia," and terminologies such as "heavy and prolonged menstrual bleeding (HPMB), intermenstrual bleeding (IMB), and PMB are gaining popularity to describe menstrual symptoms (Fraser et al., 2011). Chronic AUB has replaced "menometrorrhagia" and "menorrhagia" which is characterized by an increase in volume, regularity, and timing for 6 months. Although chronic AUB does

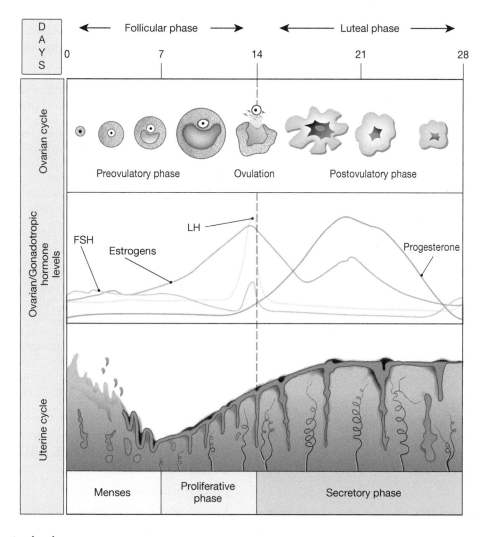

FIGURE 13.4: Menstrual cycle.
Source: Bumpus, S., & Carriveau, A. (2021). Evidence-based assessment of the female genitourinary system. In K. Gawlik, B. Melnyk, & A. Teall (Eds.), *Evidence-based physical examination: Best practices for health and well-being assessment*. Springer Publishing Company. Fig. 20.7.

TABLE 13.5: New Terminologies and Definitions

TERM	DEFINITION
AUB (abnormal uterine bleeding)	Any deviation in menstrual bleeding from the normal menstrual cycle
HMB (heavy menstrual bleeding)	Most common, excessive blood loss, interferes with quality of life
HPMB (heavy and prolonged menstrual bleeding)	Menstruation exceeding 8 days in duration on a regular basis
IMB (intermenstrual bleeding)	Random or unpredictable bleeding between regular menstrual cycles
PMB (postmenopausal bleeding)	Common, occurring >1 year after menopause
Chronic AUB	Increase in volume, regularity, and timing for 6 months
Acute AUB	Single episode of heavy bleeding in a nonpregnant female of reproductive age

not require immediate intervention, it is the first sign of endometrial cancer and requires further evaluation. Acute AUB is defined as a single episode characterized by heavy bleeding requiring prompt intervention to stop severe and possibly life-threatening blood loss. Acute AUB can occur with chronic AUB or alone. IMB has replaced "metrorrhagia" to describe random or unpredictable bleeding between regular menstrual cycles (Deneris, 2016; Fraser et al., 2011; Table 13.5).

The differential diagnosis of AUB in the nonpregnant female is broad, and in addition to utilizing new terminologies to describe bleeding patterns, (e.g., light, intermenstrual, heavy, heavy and prolonged, and PMB) with the PALM-COEIN classification system, approaching AUB by age helps to narrow the diagnosis even further (Table 13.6).

In addition to the PALM-COEIN classification system, two additional causes for AUB must be considered. Pregnancy (abortion, abruption or subchorionic hemorrhage) must be ruled out first in every female of childbearing age, as well as infection (acute or chronic endometritis and pelvic inflammatory disease [PID]; Wouk & Helton, 2019).

Another way to simplify the confusing and complicated approach to evaluating AUB is by separating the causes into three major categories: "The woman has caught something, is growing something, or is experiencing anovulatory bleeding" (Halloran, 2011).

HISTORY AND PHYSICAL FINDINGS

History

- The initial evaluation of AUB for females in all age groups begins with gathering a detailed history regarding the bleeding patterns (frequency, duration regularity, and volume), and determining hemodynamic stability/instability due to blood loss.
- Determining the volume of blood loss is difficult, so gathering a history regarding blood clot passage or the number of pads/tampons changed per hour may be helpful in determining if the menstrual bleeding is heavy (Wouk & Helton, 2019).
- As coagulopathies exist in patients with AUB, asking detailed questions about a family and/or personal

history of HMB and symptoms of bleeding (e.g., epistaxis, frequent bruising, postpartum hemorrhage) may indicate an undiagnosed coagulopathy that requires further evaluation.
- Pregnancy testing (premenopausal) and risk for endometrial carcinoma must be assessed based on bleeding patterns and age.
- Reproductive history: the first day of last menstrual cycle, age of menarche, use of birth control, sexual activity (number of partners, history of sexually transmitted diseases), pelvic pain, vaginal discharge, pregnancies, age of menopause, cycle length and predictability, number of days of each menstrual cycle and pads/tampons/day. A history of current symptoms and association with the menstrual cycle.
- Past medical history of thyroid disease, polycystic ovarian syndrome (PCOS), anemia, recent illnesses, and medication history.

Physical Exam

A comprehensive physical exam must be performed, including vital signs to assess for hemodynamic instability as evidenced by hypotension, tachycardia, tachypnea, pallor, oxygen saturation, temperature, and prolonged capillary refill time. Frequent assessment for signs of altered mentation may indicate worsening hemodynamic instability. A pelvic exam must be performed to evaluate for pain/tenderness, infection, uterine consistency, size, and shape, and confirming the cervix is the source of bleeding rather than nongynecological sites (e.g., bladder, anus, perineum).

DIFFERENTIAL DIAGNOSIS AND DIAGNOSTIC CONSIDERATIONS

Laboratory Studies

The following tests should be ordered:
- A urine or serum human chorionic gonadotropin pregnancy test must be performed on all females of childbearing age, even if the patient denies any possibility of pregnancy.

TABLE 13.6: Signs and Symptoms According to the PALM-COEIN Classification System

	POLYPS	ADENOMYOSIS	LEIOMYOMA	MALIGNANCY/HYPERPLASIA
AGE	Older than adolescents Increase with age	Older than adolescents Increase with age	Older than adolescents Increase with age	Postmenopausal Increase with age
INCIDENCE	8%–35% and increases with age	5%–70%	80%	Occurs in one fourth of new diagnoses in females <55 years old
BLEEDING PATTERN	Asymptomatic or intermenstrual bleeding	Asymptomatic or painful, heavy, or prolonged menstrual bleeding	Asymptomatic or heavy/prolonged menses with larger leiomyomas	Highly variable. AUB most common symptom
MALIGNANCY RISK	Low in premenopausal/95% of symptomatic are benign		Benign tumors	Due to long-term unopposed estrogen exposure

	COAGULOPATHY	OVULATORY DYSFUNCTION	ENDOMETRIAL	IATROGENIC	NOT OTHERWISE CLASSIFIED
AGE	Adolescents	Adolescents, perimenopausal	Older than adolescents		
INCIDENCE /CAUSE	20% with heavy bleeding have underlying bleeding disorder (von Willebrand disease/platelet disorder) higher in adolescents	Endocrine dysfunction	Vasoconstriction disorders, inflammation, infection (Diagnosis of exclusion)	Medical treatments, hormonal contraception, medications that interfere with sex steroid hormone function or synthesis	Poorly understood conditions
BLEEDING PATTERN	Heavy menstrual bleeding/irregular menstrual bleeding	Irregular, heavy, or prolonged		Breakthrough bleeding	
MALIGNANCY RISK					

Source: Wouk, N., & Helton, M., (2019). Abnormal uterine bleeding in premenopausal women. *American Family Physician*, *99* (7), 435–443.

- Hemoglobin and hematocrit in females who present with excessive bleeding and/or hemodynamic instability.
- Complete blood count (CBC) to evaluate for anemia, thrombocytopenia, and infection.
- Coagulation studies to rule out coagulopathies.
- If a pelvic infection is suspected, test for *Chlamydia trachomatis*, *Neisseria gonorrhoeae*, and *Trichomoniasis vaginalis*.
- Thyroid stimulating hormone to rule out hypothyroidism as a cause for AUB.

Imaging

Premenopausal

Perform transvaginal ultrasonography to evaluate for pregnancy (intrauterine or ectopic), adnexal masses, leiomyomas, endometrial thickening, or a focal mass and if performed within 10 days following the menses can measure endometrial thickness. An endometrial biopsy is indicated for a measurement greater than 7 mm (Deneris, 2016).

Postmenopausal

Transvaginal ultrasonography can be measured at any time; if >4 mm an endometrial biopsy is indicated as a thickened endometrium (>4 mm) may indicate an underlying lesion or excess estrogen.

TREATMENT

Emergent Management

For hemodynamic instability:
- Treat the same as for hemorrhagic shock with blood products.
- For rapid and temporary control of blood loss, create a uterine tamponade with a Foley catheter or gauze packing.
- Administer IV conjugated equine estrogen (CEE) 25 mg IV every 4 to 6 hours for 24 hours or until the bleeding stops.
- Progesterone alone or a combination oral contraceptive (COC) can follow for 10 to 14 days.

- Obtain urgent surgical and gynecological consultations for emergency interventions such as dilation and curettage, uterine artery embolization, or hysterectomy (Wouk & Helton, 2019).

Nonemergent Acute Management

A wide variety of medical and surgical options are available for the treatment of nonemergent acute uterine bleeding. Choice is dependent on several factors including contraindications, type of bleeding, PALM-COEIN classification system, fertility desires, and side effects.

Some available options for nonemergent acute AUB are listed in the following (Bradley & Gueye, 2016; Cheang & Umland, 2020; Poor & Tibbles, 2018; Wouk & Helton, 2019):

- Estrogen-progestin oral contraceptives: 35 mcg of ethinyl estradiol three times daily for 7 days, then daily dosing for 3 weeks. COC work by cycle regulation and counteract unopposed estrogen effects on the endometrium.
- Oral progestins: Medroxyprogesterone acetate (MPA) 20 mg three times daily for 7 days (for patients with contraindications to COC).
- Oral tranexamic acid (TXA): 1.3 g PO every 8 hours for 5 days (indicated in ovulatory patients with excessive menstrual bleeding). As this is a prothrombotic agent, contraindications include any current or past thromboembolic disease, acquired impaired color vision, and cannot be used with combined oral contraceptives (COC).
- Nonsteroidal antiinflammatory drugs (NSAIDs): Naproxen 500 mg orally twice daily while bleeding. Avoid in patients with coagulopathies.

TRANSITION OF CARE

Patients who are hemodynamically stable, can be discharged home safely with oral contraceptives or oral TXA with follow-up with gynecology within 1 week.

CLINICAL PEARLS

DIFFERENTIAL DIAGNOSES BY AGE
Adolescents:
- Undiagnosed coagulopathy
- Pelvic infection
- Hypothalamic-pituitary-ovarian axis dysregulation due to physiologic immaturity or PCOS
- Pregnancy

Older than adolescents:
- Structural lesions (polyps, leiomyomas)
- Endometrial hyperplasia
- Anovulation secondary to PCOS or preceding conditions
- Pregnancy

Older than 40 years but not yet postmenopausal:
- Pregnancy
- Anovulatory bleeding due to perimenopause
- Endometrial carcinoma
- Hyperplasia
- Leiomyoma

Postmenopausal:
- Endometrial carcinoma

KEY TAKEAWAYS

- AUB has replaced DUB
- HMB has replaced "menorrhagia"
- HPMB, IMB, and PMB are used to describe menstrual symptoms.
- IMB has replaced "metorrhagia."
- Chronic AUB has replaced "menometrorrhagia" and "menorrhagia."
- The PALM-COEIN classification system should be utilized to characterize AUB in nonpregnant females of reproductive age.
- In patients with acute AUB and hemodynamic instability, treat as hemorrhagic shock with blood products and seek urgent gynecological and surgical consults.
- Coagulopathies are common and evaluate for the presence in adolescents that are perimenopausal.
- A pregnancy test must be performed in all females of childbearing age to rule out intrauterine, ectopic pregnancy, or miscarriage.
- AUB may be a sign of endometrial cancer in pre- and post-menopausal females
- Contraindications must be reviewed prior to initiating pharmacologic therapies for AUB.

A robust set of instructor resources designed to supplement this text is located at http://connect.springerpub.com/content/reference-book/978-0-8261-6079-9. Qualifying instructors may request access by emailing **textbook@springerpub.com**.

REFERENCES

Full list of references can be accessed at http://connect.springerpub.com/content/reference-book/978-0-8261-6079-9

CHAPTER 14

INTEGUMENTARY DISORDERS

LEARNING OBJECTIVES

- Identify, differentiate, and treat common skin and soft tissue infections (SSTI).
- Recognize signs and symptoms of extravasation/infiltration injury and identify appropriate assessment scales and pharmacologic and nonpharmacologic management interventions.
- Describe the etiology of pressure injuries and demonstrate accurate differentiation and evaluation/staging of pressure injuries according to the National Pressure Injury Advisory Panel (NPIAP).
- Outline treatment options, including dressing types, for pressure injuries based on injury staging.
- Identify necrotizing soft tissue infections (NSTIs), based on clinical history and physical exam; determine appropriate treatment and management.
- Compare and contrast pressure ulcer and diabetic foot ulcer (DFU); discuss risk factors and treatment options for DFUs and DFU infections.
- Identify a herpes zoster infection based on clinical history and physical exam; determine appropriate treatment and management.
- Correctly identify type and extent of burn, calculate resuscitation requirements, anticipate potential complications, describe treatment options, and discuss necessary consultation.
- Analyze data influencing the selection of laboratory and diagnostic tests for the patient with a rash; develop an appropriate management plan for the adult patient with a rash.
- Describe the identification of and treatment for superficial and deep frostbite injuries.

INTRODUCTION

The skin is widely recognized as the largest organ in the human body and as such is involved in a wide variety of functions including temperature regulation, protection, and sensation. It is also in constant contact with the environment. This interaction with the environment exposes the skin to almost constant assault and both major and minor injuries. The skin has the capacity to heal itself in most instances. The following discusses both the process by which the skin heals and some of the ways the skin can be assisted to heal faster.

The skin is responsible for protection, temperature regulation, moisture regulation, and sensation reception and transmission (Childs & Murthy, 2007). Given its constant exposure to the outside environment, the skin is prone to both minor and major disruptions in integrity.

14.1: ACUTE WOUNDS

Steven J. Gort

PRESENTING SIGNS AND SYMPTOMS

Skin wounds are often classified by the mechanism of injury. There are two primary categories in the classification of skin injuries. The first category is trauma which is usually subcategorized into blunt trauma and penetrating trauma. The second category is environmental exposure which is subdivided into chemical exposure, extreme temperature exposure (both very high and very low temperatures), prolonged or excessing pressure, and radiation (Lee & Hansen, 2009).

HISTORY AND PHYSICAL FINDINGS

Acute wound management begins with a complete history and physical examination including obtaining information regarding the mechanism of injury. This can be difficult in the setting of many acute wounds due to their traumatic nature and the sometimes-chaotic emergency department (ED) backdrop. Nevertheless, the initial evaluation (after airway and circulation stabilization) should be focused on identification of all wounds and ruling out the presence of occult wounds (Gurney & Westergard, 2014; Ramasastry, 2005).

One important factor to be elucidated in the initial history and physical is a determination of the age of the injury. An acute wound is considered chronic when healing does not fall within the expected normal healing arc (Whitney, 2005). While there are similarities in the treatment of both chronic and acute wounds, there are also critical differences. The treatment plan will depend heavily on the length of time the wound has been present (Whitney, 2005).

DIFFERENTIAL DIAGNOSIS AND DIAGNOSTIC CONSIDERATIONS

The extent of trauma in blunt force injuries can be difficult to determine since the injury is often below the surface and can extend beyond what is easily seen. These injuries require careful examination including imaging studies and potentially surgical exploration to determine the extent of the injury (Gurney & Westergard, 2014; Lee & Hansen, 2009).

The extent of injury in penetrating trauma wounds can be difficult to determine initially; the injury is usually limited to the area around the zone of penetration, but can, however, extend into the underlying tendons, nerves, and blood vessels (Lee & Hansen, 2009). As with blunt injury, imaging and surgical exploration,should be considered to determine the extent of the injury (Gurney & Westergard, 2014).

This initial evaluation may include invasive and noninvasive imaging and assessment techniques including computed tomography, radiographs, magnetic resonance imaging, angiography, ultrasound, bronchoscopy, endoscopy, exploratory surgery, and others (Gurney & Westergard, 2014). It is important to remember that damage from both blunt force and penetrating trauma can extend beyond what is easily seen. It should never be assumed that injuries are limited to what can be visually observed (Gurney & Westergard, 2014; Lee & Hansen, 2009).

TREATMENT

Wound Healing

Wound healing generally occurs in four stages.

- **Stage one—Hemostasis:** The initial insult causes a disruption of the skin and/or vascular endothelium. This results in extravasation of blood and blood components and initiation of the clotting cascade. Platelet aggregation, in addition to clotting, also involves the activation of growth factors involved with the creation of an extracellular matrix upon which epithelization will take place (Childs & Murthy, 2017; Janis & Harrison, 2016; Ramasastry, 2005).
- **Stage two—Inflammation:** Within 1 to 2 days the platelet aggregation is followed by infiltration of inflammatory cells. Polymorphonuclear leukocytes, neutrophils, monocytes, fibroblasts, and endothelial cells are all deposited on the extracellular matrix formed after the hemostasis step. The monocytes are rapidly activated into macrophages. Macrophages play a critical role in wound healing. They are responsible for tissue debridement and for secretion of additional growth factors that promote wound healing (Childs & Murthy, 2017; Gonzalez et al., 2016; Janis & Harrison, 2016; Ramasastry, 2005).
- **Stage three—Proliferation:** This stage is marked by epithelialization, angiogenesis, formation of granulation tissue, and deposition of collagen. This stage involves increased metabolic requirements and is highly dependent on an increased oxygen supply. The formation of new blood vessels through angiogenesis helps to improve oxygen supply which is important for reepithelialization.
- **Stage four—Maturation and Remodeling:** This involves reorganization of the new collagen into a structured, mechanically sound network. During this stage, the wound strength increases to a level approaching that of intact skin (Childs & Murthy, 2017; Gonzalez et al., 2016; Janis & Harrison, 2016; Sorg et al., 2017; Whitney, 2005).

Wound Treatment

Discoveries related to germ theory led to the development of the first antiseptic dressing by Joseph Lister in 1867. This first antiseptic dressing was simply gauze soaked in carbolic acid (phenol; Broughton et al., 2006). Dressing and wound research has progressed significantly since that time. For example, more current research has shown occlusive dressings help to retain moisture which improves wound healing. The wound's natural moisture contains proteins and cell signaling agents that facilitate debridement, angiogenesis, and the formation of granulation tissue. Occlusive dressings also help to create a hypoxic environment which stimulates angiogenesis and a restoration of the body's natural oxygen supply (Broussard & Powers, 2013).

The choice of dressing is based on several factors including the initial cause of the tissue damage, tissue and wound bed perfusion, and the presence of bacterial contamination. The ideal wound dressing has the general characteristics of being easy to apply, cost-effective, easy to store, and nonallergenic. The dressing should facilitate healing by maintaining a moist environment, absorbing excess moisture to avoid additional trauma and maceration to the wound edges, retaining body warmth, and facilitating gas exchange. Finally, the dressing should minimize the risk of infection by debriding necrotic tissue, absorbing excess moisture, and minimizing environmental contamination (Broussard & Powers, 2013; Korting et al., 2011).

Moisture-Retaining Dressings

Alginate

Alginate dressings are made from polysaccharides obtained from kelp. The alginate gel is highly absorbent, and these dressings are useful for wounds with large amounts of exudate. This type of dressing has been reported to absorb as much as 15 to 20 times their weight in fluid. Due to their high absorbency, they may dry and adhere to the wound bed. Dressing changes can, consequently, be very painful (Broussard & Powers, 2013; Korting et al., 2011).

Film

Film dressings are clear sheets of polyurethane with a self-adherent base. Films are permeable to gas and water vapor but provide a barrier against fluid and bacteria.

This type of dressing is flexible and elastic. They can fit to wounds of a wide variety of shapes and sizes. Films are nonabsorbent. Excess exudate produced by wounds can lead to maceration and destruction of wound edges (Broussard & Powers, 2013; Korting et al., 2011).

Foam

Foam dressings have a polyurethane or silicone surface with an outer backing. The backing has varying degrees of permeability to gas and fluid depending on the manufacturer. The backing layer does provide protection against entry of bacteria from the environment. The dressings are absorbent, but only on a limited basis. Foam dressings should be changed when they become soaked with exudate (Broussard & Powers, 2013; Korting et al., 2011).

Hydrocolloid

Hydrocolloid dressings have a cross-linked backbone impregnated with adhesives and biopolymers such as starch, cellulose, gelatin, pectin, and guar. The material readily absorbs exudate. When a backing is present the material can also provide a cushion. The dressing is opaque which can make observing the underlying wound problematic (Broussard & Powers, 2013; Korting et al., 2011).

Hydrofiber

Hydrofiber dressings are made of sheets of sodium carboxymethylcellulose. They are highly absorbent. In the presence of exudate, they transform into gels. These dressings help provide a moist environment and a level of autolytic debridement (Broussard & Powers, 2013; Korting et al., 2011).

Hydrogel

Hydrogels are crosslinked starch polymers and contain up to 96% water. They are ideal for dry wounds as they can help to rehydrate the wound bed and can help to maintain a moist environment optimal for wound healing (Broussard & Powers, 2013; Korting et al., 2011).

Antimicrobial Dressings

All the dressings mentioned previously can be impregnated with antimicrobial substances such as iodine, silver, or a host of other antimicrobial compounds. This type of impregnated dressing can be useful for superficially infected wounds and can help to improve the rate of wound healing (Broussard & Powers, 2013; Korting et al., 2011).

14.2: BITES

Kristopher J. Jackson

Bite injuries and bite wounds are common complaints among patients seeking acute care services in the United States. Taken together, the bite wounds from cats, dogs, insects, spiders, and other humans result in millions of emergency department visits in the United States each year (Bula-Rudas & Olcott, 2018; Hareza et al., 2020). In light of these statistics, it is very likely that the AGACNP will encounter a variety of bite wounds in the course of their work. As such, it is imperative that any clinician caring for a patient with a bite injury recognizes the risks and relevant diagnostic considerations. The management of bite wounds varies significantly based upon several key factors, including the organism that created the wound, the location of the wound, and the characteristics and/or severity of the resultant injury.

PRESENTING SIGNS AND SYMPTOMS

While many bite wounds result in urgent or emergent evaluation by a clinician, other patients with bite wounds may initially defer evaluation because the wound was initially perceived as "minor." Late patient presentations are typically prompted by signs of localized infection (e.g., pain, erythema, swelling) that worsen in the hours or days following the initial injury (Bula-Rudas & Olcott, 2018). Most insect bites typically present as mild, localized allergic reactions at the site of the bite wound (Lee et al., 2016). According to Juckett (2013), there are only two poisonous spider species in the United States: the black widow (*Latrodectus mactans*) and the brown recluse (*Loxosceles reclusa*). Envenomation with neurotoxin following a black widow spider bite results in severe pain, nausea/vomiting, muscle spasticity, and even localized paralysis (Ibister & Fan, 2011). *Loxosceles* spiders, such as the brown recluse, can cause intense pain and even necrotic ulceration (Ibister & Fan, 2011). Poisonous spiders aside, most spider bites in the United States require nothing more than diligent wound care with soap and water and symptomatic management with cool compresses and/or antihistamines (Mayo Clinic, 2018).

HISTORY AND PHYSICAL FINDINGS

When taking an initial history from a patient with a bite wound, emphasis should be placed on gathering as much information as possible about the patient's past medical history as well as any pertinent information about the organism responsible for the wound. AGACNPs should be sure to inquire about any conditions, medications, or surgical history that would cause the patient to be immunocompromised. Clinicians should also obtain and thoroughly document the patient's immunization history, being sure to note the patient's hepatitis B, tetanus, and rabies vaccine status (Bula-Rudas & Olcott, 2018).

In the case of human bite wounds, AGACNPs should try to elicit information about the health status of the individual responsible for creating said wound. Particularly pertinent information is any history of bloodborne illnesses including HIV, hepatitis B, or hepatitis C (Bula-Rudas & Olcott, 2018). The social circumstances surrounding human bite wounds, not infrequently referred to as "fight bites," may preclude such history taking. Thus, obtaining baseline serologic testing for HIV, hepatitis B, and hepatitis C is prudent. For all bite wounds; cat, dog, or human, it is essential that clinicians obtain a detailed history about when and how the bite injury occurred. Delayed treatment and delayed wound care significantly increase a patient's risk of developing an infection (Jaindl et al., 2015). In the case of bite wounds perpetrated by cats or dogs, the treating clinician should gather as much information as possible about the health of the offending organism, being sure to document any known information pertaining to the animal's most recent rabies vaccine administration (Bula-Rudas & Olcott, 2018).

History taking for patients with suspected insect bites should focus on recent environmental exposures, such as any recent travel or proximity to stagnant water, grassy areas, or woodlands that would make exposure to a particular species of insect more likely. For all suspected insect or arachnid bites, patients should be asked if they were able to identify the offending organism. AGACNPs should also inquire if the patient happened to save the offending insect or arachnid; species identification and/ or testing of the organism may prove useful in guiding patient management.

Evaluation of a bite wound should include careful evaluation of the severity and location of the wound or wounds, paying particular attention to any wound occurring over a joint. Bite wounds can be very deceptive; a small puncture wound from a tooth at the skin's surface may not look severe, but tiny puncture wound may be a harbinger of infection (Raval et al., 2014). AGACNPs should carefully inspect the skin around the bite wound, being sure to note any erythema. The wound bed must be carefully assessed for any foreign debris, necrotic tissue, or purulent discharge (Bula-Rudas & Olcott, 2018). Older canines and felines tend to have poor dentition and thus bite wounds perpetrated by cats or dogs should be carefully inspected for any retained foreign bodies or tooth fragments (Ellis & Ellis, 2014).

Deep wounds should be assessed for possible tendon rupture or injury. A patient with tendon rupture may present with weakness, immobility, and/or impaired range of motion in the affected extremity (Ellis & Ellis, 2014). Wounds occurring over joints are considered high risk for bacterial infections such as septic arthritis, osteomyelitis, tenosynovitis, and/or tendonitis (Bula-Rudas & Olcott, 2018). Thus, AGACNPs who encounter wounds situated over joints or who encounter patients with a suspected tendon injury as a result of a bite wound should seek out prompt surgical consultation.

DIFFERENTIAL DIAGNOSIS AND DIAGNOSTIC CONSIDERATIONS

Human and animal bite wounds are generally diagnosed based upon the patient's history and the evaluating clinician's visual inspection of the presenting wound. Radiographs of the affected site are indicated if there is concern for infection or osteomyelitis, particularly if the bite wound is located over a joint. Radiographs may also be useful in identifying any retained foreign bodies or tooth fragments not noticed during physical inspection of the wound.

Unlike most mammalian bite wounds, insect or arachnid bites oftentimes mimic other soft tissue inflammatory or infectious conditions. Most insect or arachnid bites trigger a mild localized allergic reaction manifested by localized swelling, erythema, and/or pruritis (Lee et al., 2016). Spider bites commonly mimic soft tissue infections or cellulitis. Therefore, AGACNPs should keep infection high on their list of differential diagnoses for the patient who presents with a chief complaint of an alleged "spider bite" perpetrated by an unwitnessed spider (Juckett, 2013).

Insects are common vectors of disease. Therefore, history taking is crucial to ensure patients receive the appropriate screening and education. Mosquitos carry a variety of diseases, such as chikungunya virus, dengue fever, malaria, West Nile virus, and yellow fever (Lee et al., 2016). Ticks are also common vectors of disease; common tick-borne illnesses include babesiosis, borrelia Lyme disease, anaplasmosis, ehrlichiosis, and Rocky Mountain spotted fever (Lee et al., 2016). Patients who have traveled to or inhabit regions of the world where these conditions are endemic should be carefully evaluated for signs or symptoms of these conditions at the time of initial presentation. Prior to being discharged from care, patients should be instructed to monitor for the signs and symptoms of any relevant conditions for which they are at increased risk based on the history gathered by the assessing clinician.

TREATMENT

Wound Management: Cat, Dog, and Human Bites

Meticulous wound care is perhaps the most important aspect of treatment for patients presenting with any bite wound. Following an initial evaluation of a patient's bite wound, the wound bed should be vigorously irrigated to remove debris, retained foreign bodies, and nonviable tissue to reduce the risk of infectious complications (Thibault & Rosseau, 2018). A 20 to 30 mL (or larger) syringe should be used to irrigate the wound bed using a *minimum* of 250 cc of either sterile water, saline, or a dilute povidone-iodine solution (Bula-Rudas & Olcott, 2018; Ellis & Ellis, 2014). Should a 20 mL syringe be unavailable, a 20 gauge catheter should be connected to a smaller syringe in order to generate sufficient pressure for high-quality wound irrigation (Ellis & Ellis, 2014).

Once the bite wound has been assessed and generously irrigated, the location of the bite wound should be used to guide wound closure strategy. In general, cat, dog, and human bite wounds should be left open and allowed to heal by secondary intention (Thibault & Rosseau, 2018). If a bite wound is particularly large or the evaluating provider feels the wound borders *must* be secured in some fashion, any such closure must be one that is both temporary and easily removed to reassess for potential infection (e.g., steri-strips, several nylon sutures). Exceptions to delayed closure include bite wounds inflicted upon the patient's face, neck, or genital region. In general, wounds in these areas should be closed by primary intention (Thibault & Rosseau, 2018). Further consideration should be given to closed-fist injuries or bite wounds that occur over a joint. Again, these wounds warrant consultation with a hand surgeon given the increased risk of osteomyelitis, tenosynovitis, and/or tendinitis (Bula-Rudas & Olcott, 2018; Harper et al., 2020).

Wound Management: Insect Bites and Stings

According to Callahan (2018), hymenoptra—the order of insects to which ants, bees, and wasps belong—account for the vast majority of human sting injuries. Envenomation injuries from these stinging insects can cause a host of reactions, ranging from mild localized erythema and discomfort to life-threatening anaphylaxis (Sukmawati, 2018). Some hymenoptra, such as honeybees, have a barbed stinger that is left behind in the wake of their attack (Callahan, 2018). Other hymenoptra, such as wasps and hornets, do not. To remove a retained stinger, the National Library of Medicine (NLM, 2019) recommends using a blunt object with a straight edge (e.g., a credit card or the back of a knife) to scrape over the site of the retained stinger. There is conflicting evidence over whether using tweezers to remove a retained stinger will release more venom into the wound (see, e.g., Callahan, 2018; NLM, 2019). After thoroughly washing the affected area with soap and water, residual inflammation and discomfort are generally managed with a combination of oral nonsteroidal antiinflammatory medications (NSAIDs), topical antihistamines, and/or cold compresses (Callahan, 2018; NLM, 2019).

Other insect bite injuries, such as those caused by flies and mosquitos, generally cause only local inflammation and discomfort. In these instances, the affected area should thoroughly cleansed with soap and water. After cleansing a 0.5% or 1% hydrocortisone cream, calamine lotion, or a baking soda paste should be applied several times per day to help reduce pruritic symptoms (Mayo Clinic, 2021). In cases of severe discomfort, oral antihistamines may also help in ameliorating pruritic symptoms.

While most tick bites are asymptomatic, cases of "tick paralysis," a form of ascending, flaccid paralysis caused by tick saliva, have been reported in the literature (Centers for Disease Control and Prevention [CDC], 2019). More common, however, are tick-borne illnesses such as Lyme disease. To remove a tick embedded in a patient's subcutaneous tissue, the treating clinician or family member should use a pair of tweezers to grip the tick at the surface of the patient's skin before pulling back firmly. Ticks' mouths are equipped with many barbed hooks that afford the tick a firm grasp within the subcutaneous tissue of its victim (Richter et al., 2013). Avoid twisting or rocking the tick to loosen its grip to facilitate removal (CDC, 2019). Any twisting or rocking motion during removal of the tick may cause the tick's mouth to separate from the rest of its body. Should the tick's mouth separate from its body during attempts to remove the tick, use tweezers to extract any visible tick remnants from the bite wound. Once the tick and any mouth parts have been removed, the bite wound should be thoroughly cleansed with alcohol and/or soapy water. Patients should be counseled on the importance of monitoring for concerning signs of infection following a tick bite. Fever, chills, muscle, or joint aches and/or the development of a slowly expanding, bullseye rash, are symptoms concerning for Lyme disease (CDC, 2021). This bullseye rash is also commonly referred to as erythema migrans (EM) or erythema chronicum migrans.

Wound Management: Arachnid Bites

Poisonous spiders notwithstanding, the care of a patient following a spider bite is similar to that of other insect bites. Treatment for these wounds involves wound care, symptom management, and patient education in terms of monitoring for signs of any resultant, evolving infectious process (Mayo Clinic, 2018). Care following an attack from a poisonous spider such as the black widow spider (*Latrodectus mactans*) is largely supportive in the form of pain medication and antispasmodics. Antivenom is commercially available but in short supply; antivenom should be administered in concert with a toxicologist (Barish & Arnold, 2020). Brown recluse (*Loxosceles reclusa*) spider bites become intensely more painful in the 30 to 60 minutes after the initial attack; these wounds can become necrotic and may require surgical debridement. The constellation of systemic systems that result from a brown recluse spider bite is known as loxoscelism. Loxoscelism can vary widely in terms of severity and can include mild symptoms such as nausea, vomiting, and fever, but can also result in much more severe symptoms including renal failure and disseminated intravascular anticoagulation (DIC).

Antimicrobial Considerations

Recommendations for prophylactic antibiotic coverage following a bite wound vary depending on wound location, offending organism, wound severity, and health history of the patient (Kwak et al., 2017). For patients presenting with dog or cat bites, the Infectious Disease Society of America recommendation is for 3 to 5 days of empiric antimicrobial therapy for any patient who is immunocompromised, asplenic, has advanced liver disease, has a bite wound on the hand or face, or a bite wound involving the joint capsule or periosteum (Stevens et al., 2014).

In general, human bites carry a greater risk of infection than cat or dog bites (Kwak et al., 2017). Thus, the threshold for empiric antimicrobials should be lower for patients presenting with a human bite wound or "fight bite." When offering empiric coverage or treating a bite wound for suspected infection, coverage against both aerobic and anaerobic bacteria is critical. The antibiotic of choice for most bite wounds is typically amoxicillin/clavulanate 875/125 mg orally dosed twice daily (Bula-Rudas & Olcott, 2018; Ellis & Ellis, 2014; Kwak et al., 2017). In the event of allergy or intolerance, trimethoprim/sulfamethoxazole 160/800 mg twice daily or levofloxacin 750 mg daily **plus** anaerobic coverage with metronidazole 500 mg three times daily or clindamycin 300 mg three times daily are suitable alternative regimens (Bula-Rudas & Olcott, 2018; Ellis & Ellis, 2014; Kwak et al., 2017). Macrolides should be avoided because they offer no coverage against *Pasteurella* spp., the most common organism found in bite wounds perpetrated by dog or cat bites (Kwak et al., 2017).

Vaccine Considerations

Tetanus toxoid is recommended for patients presenting with a bite wound and who have not had a tetanus vaccine during the preceding 10 years (Stevens et al., 2014). Patients without a prior history of vaccination against rabies who are bitten by a wild animal, or any domesticated animal not known to them should receive rabies postexposure prophylaxis (Kwak et al., 2017). A patient presenting for care following a human bite wound who has not completed or received vaccination against hepatitis B should be offered such vaccination (Porter-Jones, 2016).

TRANSITION OF CARE

Most insect bites require little, if any, follow-up. Patients who have suffered animal or human bites, on the other hand, must have a coordinated follow-up plan no more than 48 hours after the initial wound assessment to re-evaluate the wound for signs of evolving infection (Bula-Rudas & Olcott, 2018; Thibault & Rousseau, 2018).

CLINICAL PEARLS

- Meticulous, high-quality wound irrigation with sterile water, saline, or a dilute povidone-iodine solution is crucial to minimizing a patient's risk of infectious complications.
- Wounds occurring over joints are considered high risk for bacterial infections such as septic arthritis, osteomyelitis, tenosynovitis, and/or tendonitis and warrant surgical consultation.
- Most bite wounds should be left to close by secondary intention; premature wound closure may lead to serious infectious complications and abscess formation.
- Bite wounds deemed high risk for infectious complications should receive empiric coverage with amoxicillin/clavulante 825/125 mg tablets for 3 to 5 days.

- AGACNPs should keep cellulitis or soft tissue infection on the list of differentials for any patient that presents for the evaluation of an alleged spider bite by an unwitnessed spider.

KEY TAKEAWAYS

- Millions of Americans seek out care for the evaluation and treatment of bite wounds every year; bite wounds are a very common complaint in the acute care setting.
- The management of bite wounds varies significantly based upon several key factors, including the organism that created the wound, the location of the wound, and the characteristics and/or severity of the resultant injury.
- When managing the patient with a bite wound, thorough history taking is critical to ensuring that patients get the appropriate care both in the acute setting and in terms of continued follow-up.
- A wound should not be dismissed as "low risk" merely because it appears small; even a small puncture wound can be a serious harbinger of infection.
- Most insect and arachnid bites, while unpleasant, warrant nothing more than diligent wound care.

EVIDENCE-BASED RESOURCES

Bula-Rudas, F. J., & Olcott, J. L. (2018). Human and animal bites. *Pediatrics in Review, 39*(10), 490–500. https://doi.org/10.1542/pir.2017-0212

Callahan, M. V. (2018). Bites, stings, and envenoming injuries. In J. S. Keystone, D. O. Freedman, P. E. Kozarsky, B. A. Connor, & H. D. Nothdurft (Eds.), *Travel medicine* (pp. 437–447). Elsevier, Health Sciences Division.

Ellis, R., & Ellis, C. (2014). Dog and cat bites. *American Family Physician, 90*(4), 239–243.

Kwak, Y. G., Choi, S. H., Kim, T., Park, S. Y., Seo, S. H., Kim, M. B., & Choi, S. H. (2017). Clinical guidelines for the antibiotic treatment for community-acquired skin and soft tissue infection. *Infection and Chemotherapy, 49*(4), 301–325. https://doi.org/10.3947/ic.2017.49.4.301

Stevens, D. L., Bisno, A. L., Chambers, H. F., Dellinger, E. P., Goldstein, E. J., Gorbach, S. L., Hirschmann, J. V., Kaplan, S. L., Montoya, J. G., Wade, J. C., & Infectious Diseases Society of America. (2014). Practice guidelines for the diagnosis and management of skin and soft tissue infections: 2014 update by the Infectious Diseases Society of America. *Clinical Infectious Diseases, 59*(2), e10–e52. https://doi.org/10.1093/cid/ciu444

14.3: BURNS

Roxanne Buterakos

Burn injuries are one of the most common and most devastating skin injuries across the United States and globally, with more than 700,000 emergency department

(ED) visits annually in the United States alone (Roth & Hughes, 2016). Approximately 40,000 admissions to hospital critical care units are burn related with a 96.7% survival rate and with burns ranging from fire/flame (43%), scalding (34%), contact (9%), electrical (4%), chemical (3%), or other (7%) (American Burn Association, 2015). To determine the appropriate plan of care, the clinician caring for patients presenting with burns must be able to identify the type of burn, the extent of the burn, and the total body surface area (TBSA) affected. While burns (<10%TBSA) may be diagnosed as minor and not large by burn standards, 10% is a significant size and most are admitted for at least a short period of time for assessment, initial wound management, teaching, and arrangement for follow-up. The threshold for most clinicians to send the patient to the burn unit is often very low. Patients with moderate to severe burns (>10%–20% TBSA) will need hospital admission and/or admission to a burn unit for extensive pain management, fluid resuscitation, and surgical intervention. Burns have inherent risks for complications and are fraught with the need for close assessment and monitoring and will need early consultations to physical therapy, occupational therapy, nutrition, and mental health practitioners for optimal functional outcomes.

PRESENTING SIGNS AND SYMPTOMS, DIFFERENTIATION OF BURNS, AND DIAGNOSTICS

The initial assessment of burns is to determine the type and extent of the the burn and classify the type of burn.

Type of Burn Injury

Burn injuries to the skin or mucous membranes have unique etiologies which can be due to excessive heat or cold (thermal or radiation), chemicals, or electric current (Sheikh et al., 2020). This chapter focuses on thermal burns, but each type of burn warrants special consideration (Table 14.1).

Extent of Burn

Burns are classified by the damage to the layers of tissues affected. Superficial burns (SB) are limited to the epidermis. Partial-thickness burns (PTB) can be either superficial (SPTB) which involve the more superficial dermis or deep (DPTB) which would include the deeper dermis. Full-thickness burns (FTB) extend through the dermis and into the underlying subcutaneous fat. Subdermal burns (SDB) extend to deeper structures such as fascia, muscle, and bone. It is important to keep in mind that burn wounds can continue to mature and damage skin for several hours after initial insult secondary to edema and coagulation of small vessels when burned, therefore the depth of a burn may not be clear for several days. Each depth is associated with different signs and symptoms and predicted times to heal. The clinician

should recognize that burns are often irregular and/or mixed with areas of varying depth (Table 14.2).

HISTORY AND PHYSICAL FINDINGS

Evaluation of the Burn Patient via Primary Survey

Burn patients are trauma victims. Given the extreme seriousness of the injury, a primary survey with priority given to stopping the burning process, ensuring that airway and ventilation are adequate, and managing circulation by establishing IV access are required (American College of Surgeons [ACS], 2018). To stop the burning process, remove all clothing unless adhered to the burn and avoid any contact with chemical contaminants. Dry chemicals should be brushed from the skin and the area thoroughly rinsed with copious amounts of warm water or saline.

Patients who are at increased risk for airway obstruction secondary to the burn and inflammatory response include those with increasing burn size and depth, burns to the face and head, inhalation injury, any associated trauma, and/or burns to the mouth. Clinicians must be alert to signs of inhalation injury which would warrant consideration for bronchoscopy and early intubation as airway injuries can remain subtle and not appear for 24 hours. Signs of inhalation injury are burns and/or edema to the mouth, face, or neck; singed eyebrow or nasal hairs; carbon deposits in the mouth, nose, or sputum; any acute inflammatory changes in the oropharynx; difficulty swallowing; hoarseness; signs of respiratory compromise; change in mentation and trouble maintaining airway; history of confinement in a burning structure; explosion with injuries to head and torso; and a carboxyhemoglobin level >10% (ACS, 2018).

Circulation will be addressed primarily through resuscitation to ensure there is no signs of bleeding and that the patient has a blood pressure compatible with organ perfusion. Disability would be the evaluative process in which gross deformities, penetrating injuries, and neurological examination would be noted (Roth & Hughes, 2016). To expose any further areas of injury or burns, the patient will need to be completely disrobed and examined head to toe, including the perineum and rectum. To monitor urine output (UOP) and for abdominal compartment syndrome, a temperature sensing Foley catheter with pressure transducer should be inserted. To ensure gastric decompression, a nasogastric tube (NGT) should also be placed.

History and Secondary Survey

Simultaneous examination with history and physical intake must utilize a systematic methodological approach (Jeschke et al., 2020). This should be accomplished while keeping the environment as warm as possible to avoid hypothermia (ideally between 28° and 32°C) as an unintentional drop of temperature increases mortality in trauma patients, especially those with burns (Podsiadło et al.,

TABLE 14.1: Types of Burns

TYPE OF BURN	RESULTS FROM	CONCERNS	IMMEDIATE ACTION REQUIRED	CARE
Chemical	Exposure to acids, alkalis, cement, calcium oxide (lime) and petroleum products Either ingested or by contact	Alkalis are more serious than acids as they penetrate deeper by liquefaction necrosis of tissue	Rapid removal of the chemical and immediate wound care Obtain Material Safety Sheet to address systemic toxicity	Remove dry powders from wound and then flush with copious amounts of warm water for at least 20 minutes
Electrical	Power source makes contact with a patient and a current is either transmitted through the body or as an electrical flash Can be low voltage (v) of <1000 v or high >1000 v	Body serves as a conductor of the current, suffering thermal injury to deep tissues with muscle necrosis; currents travel inside vessels and nerves causing thrombosis and nerve injury Flash injuries can be very damaging as well Can be low voltage <1000 volts or high voltage >1000 volts	Burn damage is more serious than appears Severe injuries usually result in contractures of the affected extremity A clenched hand is indicative of a deep soft tissue injury that is much more extensive than it appears Causes forced contraction of muscles, thus, there are risks of skeletal fractures of the spine	Ensure adequate airway, obtain EKG and continuous telemetry as will be at risk for serious cardiac arrhythmias Prone to rhabdomyolysis, immediate evaluation of urine is warranted and if pigmented, start prompt fluid resuscitation with 4 mL/kg/h titrating to clear urine with urine output of 0.5 mL/kg/h
Tar burns	Hot tar or asphalt to skin	Molten tar temperature can be 450°F or greater	Tar adheres to skin, melting through clothing with continued transmission of heat	Rapid cooling of the tar; avoid further injury while removing from skin Remove with mineral oil
Patterns suggestive of abuse	Intentional burns occur in both adults and children (especially very young and old)	Look for circular burns, burns with clear edges and with unique patterns	Soles of the feet are consistent with immersion scald burns Be suspicious of old burn injuries in the setting of a new trauma	X-ray for fractures (old and new) All mechanism and pattern of injury should match history of injury

Source: Data from American College of Surgeons. (2018). *Advanced trauma life support* (10th ed.).; Schweizer, R., Pedrazzi, N., Klein, H. J., Gentzsch, T., Kim, B. S., Giovanoli, P., & Plock, J. A. (2021). Risk factors for mortality and prolonged hospitalization in electric burn injuries. *Journal of Burn Care and Research, 42*(3), 505–512. https://doi.org/10.1093/jbcr/iraa192; Shih, J. G., Shahrokhi, S., & Jeschke, M. G. (2017). Review of adult electrical burn injury outcomes worldwide: An analysis of low-voltage versus high-voltage electrical injury. *Journal of Burn Care and Research, 38*(1), e293–e298. https://doi.org/10.1097/BCR.0000000000000373

2019; Roth & Hughes, 2016). When taking the injury history, note any activities that may have caused associated internal or fracture injuries sustained while trying to escape the fire, the time of injury, if the patient was in a closed space, any risk for inhalation, anoxic injuries, and/or loss of consciousness. Notations of comorbidities and medications, tetanus immunization status, allergies and drug sensitivities, social history, and advance directives are important. Look for any possibility of suicide or abuse such as inconsistencies between burn pattern and history of the injury (ACS, 2018; Roth & Hughes, 2016; Sheridan, 2012).

Burn-Specific Physical Exam

A complete physical exam must be done to uncover any injuries and abnormalities and determine baseline normal findings such as respiratory or neurologic status. Table 14.3 summarizes burn-specific points of the physical exam and basic workup.

Total Body Surface Area

When noting the extent of bodily injury from a burn, the area must be described with notation of the depth of the burn, whether the burn crosses joints, or if it is circumferential (Roth & Hughes, 2016). To determine resuscitative therapy, the clinician will need to evaluate the patient for the extent of burn in terms of the TBSA. The Wallace Rule of Nines—wherein parts of the body are assigned 9% proportions of body surface area (BSA)—is a useful method of estimation for the adult patient. All surfaces added together equal 100% and are calculated as shown in Table 14.4.

To best describe the burn, a Lund and Browder chart (Figure 14.1) incorporates the Rule of Nines and guides the clinician in outlining the burn on the diagram with different patterns that differentiate thickness. The palmar rule is applied for very small areas: Any area that is the size of the patient's palm, including the fingers (together not spread apart) would grossly approximate 1% of the TBSA (Cheah et al., 2018).

TABLE 14.2: Classification of Burns

CLASSIFICATION OF BURN	DESCRIPTION OF BURN INJURY	SIGNS AND SYMPTOMS	EXPECTED HEALING
Superficial burns (SB)	Epidermis only	Burns are red, blanch with light pressure, are painful and tender. No vesicles or bullae	Resolve without scarring within 3–5 days
Superficial partial-thickness burns (SPTB)	Papillary dermis	Burns blanch with pressure, are painful and tender. Vesicles and bullae develop within 24 hours. The bases of the vesicles and bullae are pink and develop fibrinous exudate	Usually nonfatal, are the most common. Usually cures after epithelialization in 1–3 weeks and leave no hypertrophic scar. Have been known to progress to deep or full thickness burns which can confound diagnosis, treatment selection, and outcome
Deep partial-thickness burns (DPTB)	Reticular dermis Involves hair follicles and sweat glands	Burns may be white, red, or mottled white and red. No blanching with pressure and less painful and tender than the more superficial burns. Will have difficulty discerning pinprick–will be described as pressure instead of sharp. Vesicles or bullae may develop; these burns are usually dry	Requires 3–4 weeks until cure by epithelization, healing in approximately 10 weeks and likely to leave scar tissue and contractures over joint lines
Full-thickness burns (FTB)	Below the dermal layers of the skin into adipose	Burns may be white or pliable, black or charred, brown or leathery, or bright red secondary to fixed hemoglobin in the subdermal region. Pale FTB may appear to be normal skin except that the skin does not blanch to pressure. Can be anesthetic or hypoesthetic. Hairs can be pulled easily from follicles. Vesicles and bullae do not usually develop	Slow to heal, require surgical intervention, lead to hypertrophic scarring with increased risk of infection, shock, and death. Because epithelization progresses only from the margin of the injury, 1–3 months or longer are needed for cure, and hypertrophic scar or contractures occur without skin grafting
Subdermal burns (SDB)	Extend through the skin and subcutaneous tissue into the fascia, muscle, or bone	The burn goes through both layers of skin and underlying adipose, muscle, and/or bone is involved. Hypoesthesia exists in the area since the nerve endings are destroyed.	

Source: Data from Jeschke, M., van Baar, M., Choudhry, M., Chung, K., Gibran, N., & Logsetty, S. (2020). Burn injury. *Nature Reviews Disease Primers, 6*, 11. https://doi.org/10.1038/s41572-020-0145-5; Johnson, C. (2018). Management of burns. *Surgery, 36*(8), 435–440. https://doi.org/10.1016/j.mpsur.2018.05.004; Lateef, Z., Stuart, G., Jones, N., Mercer, A., Fleming, S., & Wise, L. (2019). The cutaneous inflammatory response to thermal burn injury in a murine model. *International Journal of Molecular Sciences, 20*(3), 538. https://doi.org/10.3390/ijms20030538; Yin, S. (2017). Chemical and common burns in children. *Clinical Pediatrics, 56*(Suppl. 5), 8S–12S. https://doi.org/10.1177/0009922817706975; Yoshino, Y., Ohtsuka, M., Kawaguchi, M., Sakai, K., Hashimoto, A., Hayashi, M., Madokoro, N., Asano, Y., Abe, M., Ishii, T., Isei, T., Ito, T., Inoue, Y., Imafuku, S., Irisawa, R., Ohtsuka, M., Ogawa, F., Kadono, T., Kawakami, T., … Wound/Burn Guidelines Committee. (2016). The wound/burn guidelines–6: Guidelines for the management of burns. *Journal of Dermatology, 43*(9), 989–1010. https://doi.org/10.1111/1346-8138.13288

TREATMENT

Fluid Resuscitation

Due to the inflammatory response to burns, increased capillary permeability contributes to fluid shifts, hypovolemia, and hypoperfusion. Fluid resuscitation is initiated to counteract the volume shifts into the interstitial space and provide volume for circulation and perfusion of vital organs. As circulation is compromised, immediate IV access—peripheral with large bore access or central venous access—is imperative. Sites and lengths of angiocatheters should be chosen with the knowledge that the peripheral IV may become dislodged with anticipated soft tissue edema in response to the inflammatory changes and the fluid resuscitation that is needed for any DPTB and FTB larger than 20% TBSA (ACS, 2018).

To avoid hypothermia, all IV fluids should be warmed. The recommended fluid of choice is lactated Ringer's solution to avoid hyperchloremic acidosis. According to the ACS (2018), the rate of resuscitation is suggested to be the lower range set by the Parkland formula which is 2 mL per the patient's body weight in kilograms times the percent TBSA for DPTB and FTB injuries, but many clinicians adhere to the 2 to 4 mL per kg × the TBSA range with UOP targeted for resuscitation goals. Pediatric burns (for children <14 years and those <30 kg) should be resuscitated at 3 mL/kg times percent TBSA (DPTB and FTB); please note that children <30 kg will need maintenance fluid requirement added to the resuscitation fluid which would be half normal saline with 5% dextrose (D5.45NS) or lactated Ringer's solution with 5% dextrose (D5LR) utilizing the 4:2:1 method for maintenance rate (Roth & Hughes, 2016; Sheridan, 2012). One half of the

TABLE 14.3: Burn Specific Exam and Basic Workup

HEENT	• Examine corneas for abrasions or epithelial losses with fluorescein if possible • Evaluate and record visual acuity in each eye using a pocket Snellen chart • Clouded appearance of the cornea may indicate burns to the globe • Avoid pressure to burned ear or occiput • Evaluate oral cavity for signs of perioral and intraoral burns, carbonaceous materials, or progressive hoarseness • If facial scald injury hot liquid can be aspirated and result in airway compromise warranting intubation emergently • Ensure that the endotracheal tube (ETT) is secured with ties or harness, not tape
Neck	• X-ray as per mechanism of injury • If extremely deep, circumferential wounds may need escharotomy to facilitate venous drainage of the head
Cardiac	• Patient should be placed on telemetry monitoring, especially if electrical injury, at least 24–72 hours
Pulmonary	• If chest wall compliance and ventilation are impaired by compartmentalization, chest escharotomy is indicated
Vascular	• Perfusion of burned extremity should have serial hourly evaluations for any indication of compartment syndrome. Indications for escharotomy includes temperature signs, slow capillary refill and diminished doppler flow in the distal vessels • Fasciotomy is indicated after electrical or deep thermal burns when distal flow is compromised
Abdomen	• NGT should be placed to decompress the stomach and avoid vomiting and possible aspiration • If deep circumferential abdominal wall burns exist, there is a potential risk for compartmentalization and need for torso escharotomies to facilitate ventilation • Immediate ulcer prophylaxis with histamine receptor blockers and antacids is indicated for all patient with severe burns to prevent Curling's ulceration
Genitourinary	• Bladder catheterization is required to facilitate urine output as a resuscitative endpoint in fluid resuscitation; it is prudent to utilize a catheter with a temperature probe and pressure transducer so that core temperature and intraabdominal pressures can be measured
Neurologic	• Early neurologic exam is important for baseline information; if sensorium is altered, then CT of the head may be warranted to rule out any incidental injury • Pain and sedation medications should be given with care for safety and airway protection
Extremities	• Extremities are at risk for ischemia especially if circumferential or electrical, and will need dressings that allow serial exams • Tense extremities should be decompressed promptly by escharotomy and/or fasciotomy if exam reveals decreased temperature, slow capillary refill, and diminished doppler flow in the distal vessels
Wound	• Examine and determine type of burn, extent of burn, and TBSA
Laboratory and other studies	• Complete blood count, type and screen, comprehensive metabolic profile, magnesium and phosphorus, arterial blood gas, carboxyhemoglobin (if warranted), PT/INR/PTT, urinalysis, creatine kinase, urine myoglobin, pregnancy test if appropriate, initial (and then weekly) prealbumin • Any radiologic exams warranted by injuries discovered including noncontrast head CT scans for patients with altered mental status • Chest x-ray • EKG
Lines	• Two large bore peripheral IVs and/or central line access, arterial line, NGT for decompression and early nutrition (until postpyloric access placed)
Chemoprophylaxis	• DVT prophylaxis • GI prophylaxis (histamine-2 [H2]-receptor blockers) • Tetanus (Tdap, IgG)

INR, international normalized ratio; NGT, nasogastric tube; PT, prothrombin time; PTT, partial thromboplastin time.

Source: Data from Roth, J., & Hughes, W. (2016). *The essential burn unit handbook* (2nd ed.). CRC Press Press, Taylor & Francis Group; Sheridan, R. (2012). *Burns: A practical approach to immediate treatment and long-term care*. Thieme Medical Publishers

total volume will be given within the first 8 hours (from time of burn, not time of arrival at the medical facility with the caveat that all fluids given from time of the burn is credited toward this total resuscitation) of resuscitation and the second half will be given over the final 16 hours (from time of burn) of resuscitation. When transitioning between the first and second half of the initial resuscitation (first 24 hours), remember that when the rate is decreased for the next 16 hours, these calculations are but a guide for resuscitation and to monitor for signs of decreased circulatory perfusion secondary to decreasing the dose too quickly as it risks hypotension and/or decreased urine output (ACS, 2018; Roth & Hughes, 2016). A Foley catheter should be in place to monitor

TABLE 14.4: Rule of Nines for Adults and Adolescents

BODY PART	% FOR ADULTS	% FOR 10–14 YEARS
Head (entire)	9	13
Right arm	9	9.5
Left arm	9	9.5
Anterior thorax	9	32 (includes the entire trunk and perineum anterior and posterior)
Posterior thorax	9	
Anterior abdomen	9	
Posterior abdomen	9	
Right anterior leg	9	18
Right posterior leg	9	
Left anterior leg	9	18
Left posterior leg	9	
Perineum	1	Included in trunk
Total %	100%	100%

Source: Data from Roth, J., & Hughes, W. (2016). *The essential burn unit handbook* (2nd ed.). CRC Press Press, Taylor & Francis Group; Sheridan, R. (2012). *Burns: A practical approach to immediate treatment and long-term care*. Thieme Medical Publishers

accurate UOP. To help prevent overresuscitation, hourly evaluation of the urine output, which is the best indicator of the circulating blood volume and perfusion, can be utilized for titration of these fluids. The target hourly urine output is 0.5 mL/kg/h for adults (at least 30–50 mL/hour). Different types of injuries necessitate increased fluid requirements such as electrical injuries in which the fluids would be titrated for UOP of 1 to 1.5 mL/kg/h until urine clears and is no longer dark and pigmented (ACS , 2018).

Use of colloids for severe burns >30% TBSA, is controversial as studies projected that this would enable infusion of lower total volume of crystalloid in the first 24 hours, where colloids can increase oncotic pressure which would decrease fluid leakage. This administration may reduce complications associated with fluid overload such as adult respiratory distress syndrome (ARDS), acute kidney injury (AKI), and abdominal compartment syndrome (Clark et al., 2017; Jeschke et al., 2020; Legrand et al., 2020). It is important to explore the facility of practice for its protocols on this matter.

Targets for resuscitation includes several objective signs such as improved sensorium; systolic blood pressure adequate for perfusion 90 to 120 mmHg for adolescents and adults; easily palpable distal pulses and warm extremities; urinary output of 0.5 mL/kg/h; and a base deficit of <2 (Sheridan, 2017).

During resuscitation, monitor soft tissues closely for signs of compartment syndrome where there might be areas of circumferential burns such as chest, abdominal wall, and/or extremities (Sheridan, 2012). It is especially important during resuscitation to monitor electrolytes closely and correct in a timely manner. After the initial 24 hours, the fluids are changed to maintenance fluids which can be calculated using the 4:2:1 method adapted from the early works of Holliday and Segar where they recommended that 24-hour maintenance fluids for the first 10 kg should be 100 mL/kg; then the second 10 kg should be 50 mL/kg; and every remaining kilogram above 20 kg would be 20 mL/kg (Holliday & Segar, 1957). Clinicians have noted that if the 24 hours maintenance dose was divided by 24 hours, to get a quick approximated maintenance dose, the 4:2:1 (100/24; 50/24; 20/24) method can be used so that the first 10 kg times 4 equals 40 mL/h; the second 10 kg times 2 equals 20 mL/h; and every kg above 20 kg times 1 equals that number per hour and adding each line gives maintenance mL/h. An example of the calculation for a 70 kg patient would be as demonstrated in Table 14.5.

Wound Care

Covering the wound is the first step to care and pain relief. Prophylactic systemic antibiotics are not recommended, but often topical antibacterial preparations such as Silvadene or bacitracin are utilized. The goal of wound care is to wash off the debris and superficial dead skin, apply an antibacterial cream or ointment of choice, and cover with a nonadherent dressing. Early removal of devitalized tissue (excision) is vital for attenuation of the hypermetabolic state and to eliminate the biological nidus for infection and decreasing the risk for sepsis (Jeschke et al., 2020).

1. Rule of Palm (1%) 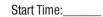   Start Time:_____

Total burn % estimation: _____   End Time: _____

2. Rule of Nines   Start Time:_____

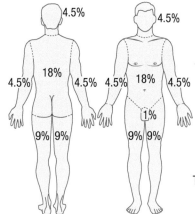

Total burn % estimation: _____   End Time: _____

3. Lund and Browder Chart   Start Time:_____

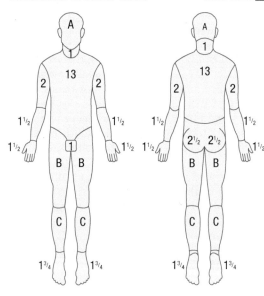

Region	Partial thickness (%) [NB1]	Full thickness (%)
Head		
Neck		
Anterior trunk		
Posterior trunk		
Right arm		
Left arm		
Buttocks		
Genitalia		
Right leg		
Left leg		
Total burn		
NB1: Do not include erythema		

Area	Adult
A = Half of head	3½
B = Half one thigh	4½
C = Half of one lower leg	3½

End Time: _____

4. 3D Burn Resuscitation Application Start Time:_____

Total burn % estimation: _____ End Time: _____

Thank You

FIGURE 14.1: Estimating total body surface area of burn wounds.
Source: Courtesy of Cheah, A. K. W., Kangkorn, T., Tan, E. H., Loo, M. L., & Chong, S. J. (2018). The validation study on a three-dimensional burn estimation smart-phone application: Accurate, free and fast? *Burns and Trauma, 6,* 7. https://doi.org/10.1186/s41038-018-0109-0

TABLE 14.5: Utilizing the 4:2:1 Method for Maintenance Fluids

70 KG PATIENT	24 HOUR 100:50:20 METHOD	HOURLY 4:2:1 METHOD
First 10 kg	Times 100 mL/24h = 1000 mL/24h	Times 4 mL = 40 mL/h
Second 10 kg	Times 50 mlL24h = 500 mL/24h	Times 2 mL = 20 mL/h
Every kg above 20 kg (50)	Times 20 mL/24h = 1000 mL/24h	Times 1 mL = 50 mL/h
Total maintenance fluid	2500 mL/24h = 104 mL/h	110 mL/hour

For DPTB and FTB, surgical intervention with early excision and coverage of the wound depends upon the extent of the burn and the stability of the patient, but usually takes place within 24 to 72 hours (Johnson, 2018). This early intervention is key to decreased infection, morbidity, mortality, and hospital length of stay.

Photo documentation of the initial wound and progression of healing is essential for clinicians to gauge wound healing. Photos remove the subjectivity of documentation and enable better interrater reliability when evaluating wounds for evidence of healing or infection (Koetsier et al., 2019).

Pain Management and Sedation

Unavoidable acute pain is challenging to control with multiple debridement, therapies, interventions, and dressing changes. The AGACNP needs to be innovative in their approach to pain control, ensuring that the patient is premedicated prior to any intervention such as dressing changes, physical therapy, debridement, split thickness grafting, and others. Ketamine may be utilized to make these procedures more tolerable and less traumatic. Analgesics should be scheduled and not "as needed" in the acute period of the burn injury. Pain should be managed per patient report because vital signs are not reliable indicators of pain (Lundy et al., 2016). A bowel regimen should be in place to avoid constipation or ileus secondary to the narcotics. Sedation for agitation or anxiety can induce amnesia or suppress neurologic function and metabolic demand making painful interventions much more tolerable (Lundy et al., 2016). These interventions are important for the care of the severely burned patient, especially in the acute phase when there is increased pain and inflammation, multiple procedures, debridement, and dressing changes.

Nutrition

Severely burned patients are challenged by hypermetabolism, which increases oxygen consumption and is associated with substantial increases in resting energy expenditure (REE; Wise et al., 2019). Clinicians need to anticipate the dynamic phases of the burn and plan nutritional support accordingly. Although indirect calorimetry (IC) is considered the gold standard to determine energy requirements of a patient, its use is often inconsistent (Wise et al., 2019). Studies focus on nutritional targets based on IC measurements of severely burned patients. During the initial acute resuscitative period of the burn, duodenal feeding tube placement, trophic feeds, and protein are recommended; for the postacute period (days to weeks after initial burn), tube feeds may be advanced as tolerated to initial targets in the 25 to 30 kcal/kg/day range with 1 to 2 g/kg protein supplementation for wound healing (Wise et al., 2019). Increases in tube feeding are outlined by Roth and Hughes (2016) when the trophic feeds have been tolerated and ready to advance to goal, then ½ strength at 25 mL/h × 4 hours, then ¾ strength at 25 mL/h × 4 hours, then full strength at 25 mL/h × 4 hours, then increase to 15 mL Q4h to goal. As with all tube feeds, glycemic control is necessary. Total parenteral nutrition is rarely warranted.

Ancillary Consultation

Mental Health

There is a high association between preexisting mental health conditions and burn injuries (Cleary et al., 2018) and these patients are likely to experience worse outcomes, increased hospital lengths of stay, more complications with increased morbidity and mortality (Mahendraraj et al., 2016). Studies have noted that up to 25% of people who sustain burn injuries are likely to develop a mental health condition such as posttraumatic stress disorder, sleep disturbance, altered body image, anxiety, and depression (Lawrence et al., 2016; Mahendraraj et al., 2016). Mental health consultation and treatment presents an opportunity to mediate these issues during hospitalization. Patients with known mental health history may require evaluation and medication adjustments to better tolerate increased mental stressors. For those patients without a mental health history, this consultation may nonetheless be an opportunity to meet and discuss, diagnose, and treat any mental health issues that may have arisen during hospitalization. Early consultation can help set the foundation for healthy coping skills, medication, and therapy during hospitalization, rehabilitation, and transfer to home.

Physical and Occupational Therapy

When planning for functional outcomes, the physical and occupational therapy teams should be consulted early in the hospitalization of the burn patient. Physical and occupational therapy initiated at admission can help minimize scarring and contractures. Active and passive range of motion can begin almost immediately, thereby facilitating the patient's adaptation to activities of daily living by providing assistive devices and training patients and families how to use them (Aghajanzade et al., 2019) This team can fit compression garments for the patient as well. Compression garments are designed to help control hypertrophic scarring, burn contracture, and keloids that result from severe burns and skin grafting by exerting uniform pressure across the affected tissue (Coghlan et al., 2019).

TRANSITION OF CARE

Surviving burn patients will transition from the critical care unit to either a step-down unit, rehabilitation, or home. The care initiated in the unit will continue at a different level depending upon the discharge disposition. Physical and occupational therapy will continue in all these settings either as inpatient or outpatient. The goal remains to obtain optimal functional outcomes. The transition of care will be mediated by case management and social work in conjunction with the healthcare team and family input. The patient should continue to be seen in a burn clinic until completely healed.

End-of-Life Issues and Support

Despite extensive critical and resuscitative efforts, patients with severe thermal injuries may not survive. Often APACHE, frailty, and/or injury severity scores alert the care team that the patient may not survive care. The care team and family together take into consideration the extensive care required, the low likelihood of returning to prior quality of life, or even survival, to transition from the goal of sustaining life to comfort measures (Lundy et al., 2016). It is important to refer to the patient's advance directive if available. Comfort care usually foregoes invasive treatment, concentrating instead on quality family time with the patient and providing end-of-life care that is peaceful, considerate, dignified, and comforting for both the patient and the family.

CLINICAL PEARLS

- Always look for signs that allude to burn depth such as the presence of large blisters (bullae) which would be consistent with a partial thickness burn; and painless burns with decreased sensation, with a dry eschar and the ability to easily remove or pull hairs would be suggestive of full thickness burns.
- Burns with >10% TBSA will need fluid resuscitation with actated Ringer's guided by the lower Parkland formula during the first 24 hours after the burn occurs. Fluids are usually initiated by EMS prior to arrival to the hospital and would be counted in the total volume to be infused. Clinical response (such as urine output) would be the key indicator for ade-

quate resuscitation and should lead the clinician in fluid adjustments accordingly.
- Any circumferential burn is of concern for constriction. Be prepared for emergent escharotomy if constriction is suspected or if there are signs of compartment syndrome with a compartmental pressure >30 mmHg.
- Adequate pain control is essential for the care of the burn patient. All dressing changes should be premedicated and done in a warm heated room to prevent hypothermia.
- Nutrition should be initiated early on any burns that are >20%TBSA; total parenteral nutrition is rarely necessary.
- Transfer to a burn center if the partial thickness (or deeper) burns involve hands, feet, joints, or perineum; if the partial thickness (or deeper) burns are >5% TBSA; are >1% TBSA and are full thickness; if the patient is >60 or <2 years in age or cannot adhere to home care measures.
- Early surgical intervention if eschar is present and/or if the burns are full or deep partial thickness.
- Topical antimicrobial nonadherent dressings are recommended for prevention of infection. Burns should be thoroughly inspected daily for early signs of infection or other complications with systemic antibiotics when needed for infected wounds.
- Early physical and occupational therapy is key to minimize scarring and risk of contractures.
- Early psychological consults are key to addressing the mental stress and psychological scarring from the burn experience.
- If the patient has a history of full vaccination and has not had a booster within the past 5 years when presenting with greater than a minor burn, a tetanus toxoid booster is recommended.

KEY TAKEAWAYS

- There are four major types of burns: thermal, radiation, chemical, and electrical.
- Burns are classified by how deep the damage is (superficial, deep partial thickness, and full thickness) and by the TBSA of tissue injured.
- Burn patients are at risk for complications such as hypovolemic shock, inhalation injury, infection, sepsis, ATN, AKI, rhabdomyolysis, fluid overload, heart failure, compartment syndrome, scarring, contractures, and mental duress/depression.
- Remember the ABCDEs when assessing the burn patient: Airway, Breathing, Circulation, Debility and Exposure.
- Any time a burn patient presents with respiratory symptoms (such as a cough or dyspnea), carbonaceous sputum, perioral burns, singed nasal hairs or were inside when exposed to the fire (inside the house or car), suspect inhalation

injury and be prepared to assess the airway (with a bronchoscope if possible) and intubate if needed.

- It is important to monitor for electrolyte imbalance and to replace the electrolytes in a timely manner.
- The deeper and larger the burn, the higher the mortality rate.
- If the burn is >20% TBSA, the patient will require fluid resuscitation utilizing an algorithm such as the Parkland formula.
- Treatment will include topical antibacterial nonadherent dressings, regular assessment and cleaning of the wounds, elevation, warm environments, and (most times) skin grafting.
- Consultation with physical therapy, occupational therapy and mental health professionals is important as the patient will need intensive rehabilitation, splinting, compression garments, and therapy.

14.4: DIABETIC FOOT ULCERS AND INFECTIONS

Steven J. Gort

Diabetes affects over 22 million people in the United States and over 422 million people worldwide. Up to 15% to 20% of those are at risk for diabetic foot ulcers (DFUs; Bandyk, 2018; Monterio-Soares et al., 2020). The cost of treating a DFU is two times that of any other chronic ulcer and the added cost to the healthcare system is estimated to be between $9 and $13 billion annually (Hurlow et al., 2018; Rice et al., 2014). DFUs are a result of common complications of diabetes, specifically neuropathy and peripheral arterial insufficiency.

PRESENTING SIGNS AND SYMPTOMS

DFUs typically develop as a result of one or more of the three following pathologies: (a) diabetic neuropathy, (b) reduced perfusion related to peripheral artery disease (PAD), or (c) skin infection due to breakdown from repetitive trauma (Bandyk, 2018).

Neuropathy

Up to 85% of DFUs can be attributed, at least in part, to peripheral neuropathy (Boulton, 1996). Diabetic neuropathy can result in a loss of both motor and sensory function (Bandyk, 2018). Persistently elevated blood glucose levels sometimes seen in diabetes can result in oxidative damage to nerve cells due to the production of cytokines and advanced glycation end products. The damaged neurons can also lead to changes in gait and weight bearing which can accelerate tissue damage resulting in ulcer formation (Lim et al., 2017).

Peripheral Artery Disease

Diabetic changes in glucose metabolism including hyperglycemia lead to endothelial damage and, over time, atherosclerosis. This atherosclerosis leads to poor perfusion of the foot. It becomes impossible to perfuse the foot at a level that would maintain tissue integrity and can lead to an ischemic ulcer (Lim et al., 2017).

Repetitive Trauma and Infection

Peripheral neuropathy leads to muscle atrophy which can lead to changes in the functional anatomy of the foot. This may result in the development of zones of uneven or increased pressure on the plantar surface of the foot. Repetitive motion from walking coupled with decreased sensation resulting from diabetic neuropathy leads to skin injury and ulceration and often to the development of a soft tissue infection (Bandyk, 2018). The risk of ulceration is significantly higher in the presence of diabetic neuropathy, foot deformity, and prior digit amputation (Bandyk, 2018).

HISTORY AND PHYSICAL FINDINGS

Some have argued the presence of any ulcer (including pressure ulcers) on the foot of a person with diabetes should be classified as a DFU (Vowden & Vowden, 2015). The primary reason behind this recommendation is the misdiagnosis of DFUs often leads to an ulcer of increased severity, delayed wound healing, and other complications including infection (Chadwick, 2021).

A DFU can be classified based on the severity of the wound and the presence of infection. The severity of the wound ranges from a superficial ulcer to a deeper wound with exposed bone, joint, or tendon, and involvement of the heel. The infection is typically graded based on the severity of the infection and ranges from a localized infection that may or may not include purulent drainage to an infection that has spread and includes systemic signs and symptoms including sepsis and septic shock (Monteiro-Soares et al., 2020). Several DFU classification systems have been published in the literature. However, there is no consensus regarding the best classification system. The selection of a single system will be controversial since the utility of the system will vary depending on the population served and the resource availability of the clinicians making the assessment (Monteiro-Soares et al., 2020).

DIFFERENTIAL DIAGNOSIS AND DIAGNOSTIC CONSIDERATIONS

One important diagnosis in the differential is cutaneous squamous cell carcinoma. Cutaneous squamous cell carcinoma usually presents as a scaly, red, or bleeding lesion and can be mistaken for a DFU. While it usually presents on sun-exposed areas of the skin, it may present on the feet. Diagnosis is confirmed through an abnormal cytology study from a skin biopsy (Waldman & Schmults, 2019).

The presence of diabetic neuropathy and ischemia can help to point toward the diagnosis of a DFU. The Ipswich Touch Test and the monofilament test can help to identify the loss of sensation often present in the diabetic foot. An abnormal ankle brachial index can identify the presence of arterial disease of the lower extremities. If sensation and circulation are both abnormal in the presence of a foot ulcer, the diagnosis of a DFU is confirmed (Chadwick, 2021).

A DFU infection usually occurs in an open DFU. The open wounds are often colonized by microorganisms; however, colonization alone cannot be used to define an infection. A DFU infection is defined clinically as the presence of an inflammatory process below the level of the malleoli in a person with diabetes (Lipsky et al., 2020).

TREATMENT

Prevention

A key intervention for DFUs is prevention. It has been shown that promotion of podiatry services within a community leads to a reduction in both hospital admissions and the number of preventable amputations (Gibson et al., 2014). Risk stratification of the likelihood of DFU can help to target individuals most at risk and, therefore, those who could most benefit from preventive care and screening.

Patient education can also be an effective measure for prevention of DFUs. Education should include information on foot care and self-screening, appropriate footwear, and wound care (Lim et al., 2017).

Treatment

Intensive glycemic control has been shown to delay the onset and progression of diabetic neuropathy in patients with insulin-dependent diabetes (Diabetes Control and Complications Trial Research Group, 1993; Pop-Busui et al., 2013). Of course, intensive glycemic control must be complemented with increased monitoring since tighter glycemic control can lead to severe hypoglycemia.

Foot deformities, limited joint mobility, and neuropathy contribute to high pressure and/or uneven pressure distribution on the diabetic foot. These pressure abnormalities are associated with the development of DFUs. A mainstay for prevention and treatment of DFUs is offloading the area of high pressure to reduce the risk for ulcer development or to prevent further damage once an ulcer has formed. Offloading devices include crutches, walkers, wheelchairs, custom shoes, depth shoes, shoe modifications, custom inserts, custom relief orthotic walkers, diabetic boots, forefoot and heel relief shoes, and total contact casts (Lavery et al., 2016).

If an ulcer has formed, prevention of infection and wound healing become the priority. Necrotic or devitalized tissue becomes a site for bacterial proliferation. Debridement of this tissue by surgical, enzymatic, mechanical,

biological, or autolytic methods is recommended to reduce the bacterial bioburden (Lavery et al., 2016).

While routine cultures of DFUs are not recommended, if an infection is suspected or if there is no improvement after 2 weeks despite proper debridement and offloading therapy, anaerobic and aerobic cultures from tissue biopsy or validated swab techniques should be obtained (Lavery et al., 2016). Antibiotic therapy is recommended for all patients with a DFU infection. The choice of empiric antibiotics should be made based on the clinician's best guess regarding the causative organism, local patterns of antibiotic resistance, and other factors such as patient drug allergies, recent hospitalization, and comorbidities (e.g., kidney disease) (Lipsky et al., 2020).

DFU infections are often polymicrobial. Treatment should be directed against the more virulent pathogens identified (e.g., *Staphylococcus aureus* or beta-hemolytic streptococci). Nonpathogenic isolates (e.g., corynebacterial or coagulase-negative staphylococci) are usually contaminants and can be ignored. Antibiotic therapy should be tailored to work against the virulent pathogens. The contaminants do not need to be targeted (Lipsky et al., 2020).

Antibiotic therapy should last 1 to 2 weeks. Extending treatment to 3 to 4 weeks should be considered if the infection is not improving or if the initial infection was severe (Lipsky et al., 2020).

Surgical consultation is recommended in the case of extensive infection involving gangrene, necrotizing infection, deep abscess, compartment syndrome, severe lower extremity ischemia, or osteomyelitis (Lipsky et al., 2020). In the case of osteomyelitis, bone biopsy is recommended, and antibiotics should be tailored based on the culture results. If the infected bone can be removed, antibiotic therapy only needs to be continued for a few days after removal of the infected bone. If unable to remove the bone, antibiotic therapy should last up to 6 weeks (Lipsky et al., 2020).

14.5: EPIDERMAL NECROLYSIS–STEVENS-JOHNSON SYNDROME AND TOXIC EPIDERMAL NECROLYSIS

Valerie J. Fuller

Stevens-Johnson syndrome (SJS) and toxic epidermal necrolysis (TEN) are two rare, life-threatening disorders that affect the skin and mucous membranes. The two conditions are considered variants of the same disease and differ only in the extent of body surface involvement (Wolff et al., 2017). Patients are classified by the amount of body surface area (BSA) affected by epidermal detachment: SJS <10% of BSA, SJS/TEN overlap 10% to 30% of BSA, and TEN >30% of BSA (Micheletti et al., 2018). The mortality ranges from <10% for SJS to as high as 30% for TEN (Creamer et al., 2016). Scoring systems have been developed to assess mortality risk including the SCORTEN (severity-of-illness score of TEN) system but diagnostic criteria have not yet been established (Maverakis et al., 2017).

The syndrome is predominantly drug-induced but it has been suggested that more than 20% of cases are idiopathic or caused by infection (Mockenhaupt & Roujeau, 2019). The exact pathophysiology of SJS/TEN is not completely understood. Risk factors include advanced age, HIV infection, autoimmune illness (like systemic lupus erythematosus [SLE]), and in persons with certain genetic HLA allotypes.

PRESENTING SIGNS AND SYMPTOMS

Prodromal symptoms of fever, malaise, headache, arthralgias, and upper respiratory infections (URI) symptoms typically precede the onset of skin lesions by 1 to 3 days (Creamer et al., 2016).

HISTORY AND PHYSICAL FINDINGS

In gathering the history, the AGACNP should inquire about prodromal symptoms and any new or recently added medications. The time from drug exposure to the onset of symptoms can be 1 to 3 weeks in duration (Wolff et al., 2017).

The skin changes begin as diffuse erythema or as a maculopapular rash and progresses to necrotic, target-like lesions, bullae, and sheetlike loss of the epidermis (Wolff et al., 2017). Mucous membrane lesions may precede the cutaneous rash (Figure 14.2).

Fever and tachycardia are often present, and patients will report severe pain and burning of the skin and mucous membranes. If the disease is systemic, sepsis, metabolic derangements, pulmonary complications, and multisystem organ failure may be seen.

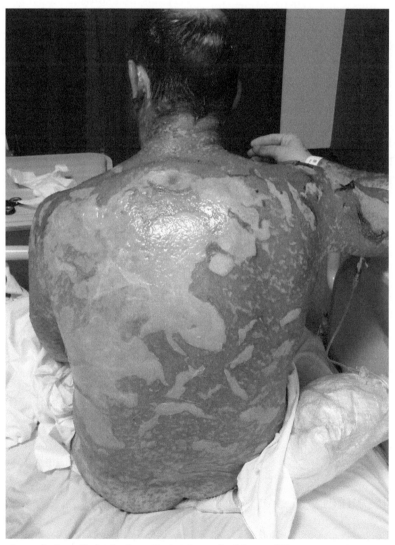

FIGURE 14.2: Toxic epidermal necrolysis on the back of a patient at the peak of the condition.
Source: Courtesy of Jay2Base.

DIFFERENTIAL DIAGNOSIS AND DIAGNOSTIC CONSIDERATIONS

Differential diagnoses include exanthematous drug eruptions, scarlet fever, toxic shock syndrome, acute graft-versus-host disease, thermal burns, and staphylococcal scalded-skin syndrome (Wolff et al., 2017).

Separation of the skin when lateral traction is applied (Nikolsky sign) is a positive and important diagnostic clue in SJS/TEN (Basko-Plluska et al., 2014).

Diagnosis is often suggested by the physical signs and symptoms, but histopathology should be confirmed with skin biopsy (Creamer et al., 2016).

TREATMENT

Treatment is largely supportive and there is currently no consensus on the most effective treatment for SJS/TEN (Micheletti et al., 2018). The UK Guidelines for the management of SJS/TEN in adults is an excellent resource for AGACNPs caring for individuals with this syndrome.

TRANSITION OF CARE

Like burns, the epidermal detachment seen in SJS/TEN can cause significant fluid losses, electrolyte abnormalities and hemodynamic instability (Creamer et al., 2016). Patients who are suspected to have SJS/TEN should be admitted to the hospital and may require ICU level of care if skin involvement is extensive (>10% BSA). Dermatology and wound care teams should be involved early.

CLINICAL PEARLS

- Mucosal involvement is common; be sure to examine the eyes, lips, buccal mucosa, and genital and anal skin.
- Fever is often present. A fever associated with mucous lesions and/or a new rash should alert the AGACNP to the possibility of SJS/TEN.
- Assess for Nikolsky sign.
- Look for any new or recently added medications. Prompt removal of the offending drug is essential.

KEY TAKEAWAYS

- A rare mucocutaneous reaction characterized by epidermal detachment.
- Most often drug-induced and numerous medications have been implicated.
- Systemic involvement can occur and portends a poor prognosis.

EVIDENCE-BASED RESOURCES

https://www.nhs.uk/conditions/stevens-johnson
-syndrome/
https://dermnetnz.org/topics/stevens-johnson-syndrome
-toxic-epidermal-necrolysis

14.6: FROSTBITE

Lori Hull-Grommesh

Frostbite is a cold injury that occurs when a body part is exposed to cold. It is estimated that frostbite begins to occur when skin is exposed to temperatures below the freezing point of tissue at −0.55°C(Carceller et al., 2019). The most common body parts affected are hands, feet, fingers, toes, ears, and nose. Affected skin will begin to frostbite within 30 minutes in subzero temperatures and can occur in as little as 15 minutes in extreme conditions (i.e., extreme wind, rain, or snow). Frostbite injuries are classified as superficial or deep, where first- and second-degree injuries are classified as superficial and third- and fourth-degree injuries are classified as deep (Zonnoor & Elston, 2020). Initial vasodilation occurs in response to the cold, followed by vasoconstriction, the formation of ice crystals, and subsequent damage to tissue and bone below the skin (Handford et al., 2014). The goal of treatment is to preserve tissue and prevent deep tissue injury.

Frostbite most often occurs in young healthy individuals and can significantly impact quality of life and activities of daily living if a deep injury is sustained. Patients at risk for frostbite are those who enjoy outdoor activities such as skiing and hiking (Carceller et al., 2019). Occupational exposure is an additional risk factor for those working in cold environments, such as ski patrol, cold chain, and construction.

PRESENTING SIGNS AND SYMPTOMS

Superficial Frostbite Injury (First- and Second-Degree)

The patient with first- or second-degree injury will present with whiteness to the affected part which may be discolored, swollen, and numb (Basit et al., 2021). In second-degree injury, large clear or milky-white blisters will usually appear. The blisters will develop within 23 hours of prolonged exposure and will enlarge. The blisters may need to be drained if presenting with significant pain or if infection is suspected. The blisters will begin to heal and form eschar, which will be replaced by new tissue over 6 months, depending on the amount of surface area. Superficial injuries only damage the skin and not tissue (Basit et al., 2021).

Deep Frostbite Injury (Third- and Fourth-Degree)

Patients with a third-degree frostbite injury will have blisters that may be smaller but are hemorrhagic (Handford et al., 2017). The patient will have edema, discoloration, and numbness as with a superficial injury.

The hemorrhagic blisters then extend through the dermis with necrosis of skin, muscle, and bone, which results in a fourth-degree injury (Handford et al., 2017). The tissue will die within 10 days. The affected body part will appear black and necrotic. Cyanosis is a clue that a necrotic process may be taken place and is seen with deep injury.

HISTORY AND PHYSICAL FINDINGS

Obtaining an accurate history and physical examination in patients presenting with frostbite is key. The patient with suspected deep frostbite injury should be examined quickly to ensure that they are hemodynamically stable and not in a shock state or in hypothermia. The AGACNP must assess for any trauma and thoroughly examine all body parts for frostbite. Questioning the patient as to their past medical history, past surgical history, medications, allergies, and immunization history is vital and any co-morbidities (e.g., diabetes, hypertension, heart failure). As frostbite worsens, vasoconstriction occurs and a patient with known Raynaud's syndrome would be at risk for complications. Patients will complain of being cold and anxious, often due to the amount of time it may have taken to seek treatment, as often patients are on mountains, working, or hiking in the cold. The AGACNP should assess the patient's affected body parts for degree of injury: Is there discoloration (white, red, blue, or purple)? Does the patient complain of pain? Does the patient have numbness anywhere? Has the patient lost the sensation of pain in the affected body part? Additional critical questions to ask include: Did you pass out? Were there others affected? Was there any environmental exposure to chemicals? Accurately obtaining a complete history and physical and determining the suspected level of frostbite injury can help to quickly guide therapy, especially with deep injury where in an equipped hospital the patient may receive angiography with thrombolytics.

DIFFERENTIAL DIAGNOSIS AND DIAGNOSTIC CONSIDERATIONS

Frostbite diagnosis is made by the patient's signs and symptoms, obtaining an accurate history, and physical examination. It is imperative that the patient be questioned as to their activities and location, along with an estimated time that the frostbite began. The timing of frostbite initiation is often difficult to assess as the patient may have been alone in the cold and often patients may not suspect frostbite until they feel pain or discoloration of the affected area is noted (i.e., whitish color, erythema, or a bluish-purple color). The AGACNP must thoroughly examine the skin for appearance, any breakage of the skin, and exposure of any vessels or underlying tissue. Identification of frostbite that occurs in a patient who is experiencing homelessness or living in a home without heat alerts the AGACNP to ensure that social support and resources are provided. The goal is to prevent tissue damage and amputation. The patient presenting with a deep injury will have a body part that is black/blue/purple, numb, and the patient at this point may feel no pain. Deep injury occurs within 24 to 48 hours of prolonged exposure to cold. Differential diagnosis of frostbite includes identification of the degree of injury, superficial or deep. The body part may look necrotic; thus, a strong history and physical exam is required to determine the cause. Frostnip, exposure to nonfreezing cold may result in blanching of the skin with numbness and paresthesia that does not persist. Trench foot should also be on the differential as this is where the body part is exposed to damp, wet, nonfreezing cold and can result in pain, pallor, numbness, and even lack of pulses. The AGACNP must always be aware as hypothermia (body temperature <35°C) is often occurring concurrently and that a superficial injury can become a deep injury depending on timing and success of treatment. Frostbite rarely results in mortality, but rather, with deep injuries and loss of body parts (Basit et al., 2021). Other co-morbidities seen with frostbite are alcohol and drug use with high-risk behavior. X-rays are warranted for patients presenting with frostbite if trauma is suspected. Bone scanning and angiography, when available, are used for deep injuries. SPECT scanning, as well as MRI, may be used to assess the viability of tissue.

TREATMENT

Superficial injuries do not often result in a hospital stay, whereas deep injuries often do. With cold injuries, the patient should be warmed and treated for any other life-threatening conditions (Zonnoor & Elston, 2020). All wet clothes should be removed. Rewarming, wound care, and advanced treatment can prevent amputation and preserve quality of the body part. Rewarming should take place with warm water at 37°C to 39°C. Ideally the warm water should be circulating, such as the use of a whirlpool. The affected frostbitten area should not be rewarmed if there is a possibility of refreezing, as this will create substantially more tissue damage. The rewarming can take up to 30 minutes and the AGACNP must be aware that this is a painful process and to treat the patient with ibuprofen; for more severe pain the patient may need opioids. Antibiotics may be given depending on the presentation and other co-morbidities; however, they are not routinely given for frostbite. Superficial injuries should be managed with a nonadherent dressing and the wound should be dry. The blisters may be drained, depending on pain and if there is limited mobility. Topical aloe may be applied with the dressing changes. Deep frostbite injury may be treated with angiography and intraarterial tissue plasminogen activator (TPA), as the tissue inflammation and vasoconstriction contribute to microvascular changes and thrombus formation. Pandey et al. (2018) found altitude to be a significant risk factor for frostbite and for amputation in severe frostbite. These authors noted improved treatment outcomes with IV or TPA and the vasodilator iloprost if the patient receives treatment within 48 hours of the frostbite and is most effective within 24 hours of injury. TPA is often used with arteriography as TPA is a fibrinolytic agent that is found in endothelial cells and can dissolve the thrombus and emboli that form with frostbite. Iloprost is a prostacyclin analogue, a potent vasodilator that inhibits platelet aggregation. In a study by Pandey et al. (2018), the IV iloprost dose was titrated up to 2 mg/kg/min for 6 hours daily x 5 days. A meta-analysis by Lee et al. (2020) examined the use of TPA in 209 severe frostbite patients with 1109 digits at risk for amputation and found that in 926 patients that received TPA there was a 76% salvage rate. Prior to the use of TPA and iloprost, the prevention of infection, trauma, and amputation with reconstructive surgery were the only treatments used. Treatment of frostbite is dependent on the degree. Early recognition of the severity is key and with suspicion for deep injury, the appropriate surgical and plastic surgery consult should be made. The patients with deep injury will have a long course of treatment that may include amputation. The patient should be up to date on their tetanus.

TRANSITION OF CARE

Patients with superficial wounds may not need treatment, but should be given instructions to monitor for any further discoloration, and so forth . Patients with deep injury require hospitalization and close collaboration with all providers. The AGACNP can ensure follow-up with the appropriate specialists, home healthcare at discharge, and ensure communication of instructions.

CLINICAL PEARLS

- Always determine the degree of frostbite injury and assess for co-occurring conditions.
- Be aware that superficial frostbite can become deep frostbite.
- Do not rewarm if there is a chance that body part will be exposed to cold again.
- Timeliness of treatment is key and early diagnosis prevents loss of tissue.
- Be aware that patients at higher risk for frostbite are those with alcohol/drug and or high-risk behavior disorders/problems.
- Treatment for deep injury may include the use of angiography and TPA.

KEY TAKEAWAY

- Frostbite is a disorder of morbidity versus mortality. The AGACNP should quickly identify the degree of injury and rewarm the affected areas. Prevention of deep injury is the goal, as deep tissue injury can result in amputation and or a significant impact on the patient's quality of life. Advanced treatment with angiography and TPA can be used when available, outside the use of traditional treatments.

EVIDENCE-BASED RESOURCES

Basit, H., Wallen, T. J., & Dudley, C. (2021, January 24). Frostbite. In *StatPearls*. StatPearls Publishing. https://www.ncbi.nlm.nih.gov/books/NBK536914/
Zonnoor, B., & Elston, D. M. (2020, October 13). Frostbite. *Medscape*. https://emedicine.medscape.com/article/926249-overview

14.7: HERPES ZOSTER

Bradley Goettl

Herpes zoster (shingles) is a common viral infection that usually leads to a painful dermatomal rash. Herpes zoster is caused by the reactivation of a dormant varicella-zoster virus (chickenpox). Herpes zoster infections are typically divided into three phases: the preeruptive or prodromal phase, the acute or eruptive phase, and the chronic or healing phase (Dworkin et al., 2007).

PRESENTING SIGNS AND SYMPTOMS

Presenting signs and symptoms can differ for each phase of the herpes zoster infection. The painful preeruptive phase can last up to 10 days, without obvious skin changes. Patients presenting during the preeruptive phase will often complain of a persistent burning or stinging pain in the affected area. Patients presenting during the eruptive phase will have continued pain and a new rash or skin lesions. Rash can present as patchy erythema, induration, and/or vesicles. Once the vesicles rupture, the patient might complain of a clear drainage, crusting, or exhibits signs of secondary infection/cellulitis. The eruption phase usually lasts 1 to 2 weeks. In some cases, it can take longer for the lesions to heal completely. Once the lesions heal, some patients will experience persistent pain known as postherpetic neuralgia (PHN; Dworkin et al., 2007). Pain and skin changes are typically unilateral, do not cross the midline, and are found along a skin dermatome. Herpes zoster affecting the upper dermatomes can cause additional signs and symptoms such as eye pain, conjunctival/scleral injection, tearing, hearing changes/loss, facial weakness/paralysis, and dizziness (Niederer et al., 2021; Shin et al., 2016). Occasionally, patients will have systemic symptoms that are like other viral illnesses (e.g., fatigue, fever, headache).

HISTORY AND PHYSICAL FINDINGS

Uncomplicated Herpes Zoster

Herpes zoster can usually be diagnosed from the clinical history and physical examination alone. A clear understanding of the timeline and progression of symptoms is helpful in making a diagnosis. During the prodromal or pre-eruption phase, patients will have subjective pain complaints often without obvious physical exam findings. During the eruption phase, the classic exam findings include a painful erythematous/vesicular rash that aligns with a skin dermatome. These skin changes are typically unilateral and do not cross the body's midline (Dworkin et al., 2007). Any dermatome can be affected; however, infections along the thoracic, trigeminal, and cervical dermatomes are most common (Cohen, 2013). Localized lymphadenopathy may be present. Exam findings can vary, based on the location of the infection.

Herpes Zoster Ophthalmicus

Herpes zoster ophthalmicus (HZO) occurs when the ophthalmic branch of the trigeminal nerve is affected. On physical exam, patients with HZO will have a unilateral erythematous/vesicular rash on the scalp, forehead, eyelid, and/or nose. Approximately 50% of patients with HZO will have eye involvement (Niederer et al., 2021). Patients that have lesions at the tip of the nose are more likely to have ocular involvement (Hutchinson's sign). Conjunctivitis is common with HZO; on exam the conjunctiva can appear injected or inflamed. Inflammation can occur throughout the eye causing uveitis, scleritis, and in severe cases optic neuritis or retinal necrosis (Niederer et al., 2021). A slit lamp or Wood's lamp examination, using fluorescein dye, can be performed to evaluate for corneal defects or pseudodendrites. If HZO is suspected, an urgent comprehensive eye exam should be performed by an ophthalmologist. Delays in recognition and treatment can lead to severe ocular complications including vision loss (Niederer et al., 2021).

Herpes Zoster Oticus

Herpes zoster oticus (Ramsey-Hunt syndrome) can occur with facial nerve involvement. Classic physical exam findings include painful vesicles in the ear canal or on the tympanic membrane. Patients can also have dizziness, facial nerve paralysis, and auditory disturbances (Shin et al., 2016).

Disseminated Herpes Zoster

When additional vesicles appear outside the primary and adjacent dermatomes, it can be described as disseminated herpes zoster. This type of infection is rare in healthy individuals and more common with immunocompromised patients. Patients with disseminated herpes zoster should be monitored closely for visceral organ involvement. Brain or lung involvement, causing encephalopathy or pneumonitis, can be life-threatening. Severe cases can cause alterations in vital signs and physical exam findings consistent with systemic infection (Stratman, 2002).

DIFFERENTIAL DIAGNOSIS AND DIAGNOSTIC CONSIDERATIONS

Differential diagnoses and diagnostic consideration can vary based on the clinical presentation, location of the infection, and the phase of the infection.

A herpes zoster diagnosis can be more difficult during the pre-eruption phase. Based on the location of the pain, additional causes for the patient's complaints might be considered. Herpes zoster affecting the thoracic dermatomes can lead to chest pain that can mimic cardiac or pulmonary diagnoses. Herpes zoster affecting the upper dermatomes can cause headache, dizziness, facial paralysis, and eye complaints that can mimic neurologic diagnoses, Bell's palsy, inner ear pathology, or ocular diagnoses.

A painless rash is less likely to be herpes zoster and the clinician should consider other conditions such as contact dermatitis, viral exanthems, herpes simplex, eczema, cellulitis, impetigo, or systemic causes for skin changes.

TREATMENT

Uncomplicated herpes zoster is usually self-limiting, will resolve with time, and can be treated as an outpatient. Fewer patients will have severe or systemic symptoms or complications that require inpatient management and/or specialty consultation.

Antiviral Medications

Antiviral medications, like acyclovir, famciclovir, and valacyclovir, can prevent the replication of the varicella-zoster virus (Dworkin et al., 2007). Early administration of antivirals can shorten the duration of the infection and reduce pain. Antivirals are most effective if administered within 72 hours from the onset of symptoms. Antivirals administered past the 72-hour mark can still help with PHN. Oral antivirals should be prescribed for 7 to 10 days (Conceicao, 2018). Immunocompromised patients or patients with severe/disseminated herpes zoster will require prolonged or IV antiviral treatment (Stratman, 2002). For these complicated or disseminated zoster cases, an infectious disease specialist should be consulted.

Corticosteroids

The use of corticosteroids is controversial. If there are no medical contraindications, corticosteroids can be used in conjunction with antiviral therapy. Steroids should be reserved for patients with facial paralysis or other neurologic symptoms and for patients with moderate to severe pain. Prednisone 40 to 60 mg can be prescribed for 1 week followed by a short taper. Like antiviral therapy, steroids are most effective and started early in the disease process (Dworkin et al., 2007).

Pain Control

Pain is the most common complication of a herpes zoster infection. In the acute phase over-the-counter nonsteroidal antiinflammatory drugs (NSAIDs) and acetaminophen can be recommended. Some patients will experience more severe pain and require a short course of opioids. Gabapentin has been proven to help with acute zoster-associated pain and PHN (Dworkin et al., 2007).

Prevention

The Centers for Disease Control and Prevention (CDC) recommends that immunocompetent patients over 50 years old receive the recombinant zoster vaccine series (Shingrix). Shingrix is effective at preventing herpes zoster and PHN (Syed, 2018). Isolation can help prevent spreading of the varicella-zoster virus to people who have never had the chickenpox or are unvaccinated. Postexposure prophylaxis, with varicella-zoster immune globulin, can be considered for certain high-risk patients (Lachiewicz & Srinivas, 2019).

TRANSITION OF CARE

Most herpes zoster infections will resolve with time and will require little follow-up. Ophthalmology should be consulted if HZO is suspected. Patients with complicated or disseminated herpes zoster should be evaluated by an infectious disease specialist. A pain management specialist can be consulted for pain that is refractory to standard treatments.

CLINICAL PEARLS

- There are three phases to the herpes zoster infection.
- The typical herpes zoster presentation includes a painful, unilateral, dermatomal, erythematous/vesicular rash.
- Early antiviral therapy can shorten the duration of the herpes zoster infection and reduce pain.
- Gabapentin can be prescribed for both acute zoster-associated pain and PHN.

KEY TAKEAWAYS

- To prevent herpes zoster, the CDC recommends the recombinant zoster vaccine series (Shingrix) for all immunocompetent patients over 50 years old.
- Immunocompromised patients are at an increased risk for herpes zoster and complications.
- Herpes zoster involving the face should trigger urgent ophthalmology consultation to evaluate for HZO.

EVIDENCE-BASED RESOURCE

https://www.cdc.gov/shingles/index.html

14.8: INFECTIONS OF THE SKIN AND SOFT TISSUE

Steven J. Gort

Skin and soft tissue infections (SSTIs) are commonly encountered in the healthcare system. Patients with SSTI account for 14.2 million healthcare interactions (physician office, outpatient hospital, emergency department visits) each year with a total estimated direct healthcare cost of around $15 billion (Tun et al., 2018). Many of these infections are treated on an outpatient basis with empiric treatment against gram-positive cocci (Golan, 2019). More serious infections may require treatment for sepsis and surgical intervention for certain types of necrotizing infections in addition to treatment with broad spectrum antibiotics (Chahine & Sucher, 2015; Stevens et al., 2014).

PRESENTING SIGNS AND SYMPTOMS

Outpatient Skin and Soft Tissue Infections

Impetigo

Impetigo usually occurs in children. Multiple erythematous, vesicular, and pruritic lesions appear on the face and extremities (Chahine & Sucher, 2015). The condition typically takes one of two forms: bullous or nonbullous. Bullous presents as vesicles that progress into bullae filled with yellow fluid. These bullae usually rupture leaving behind a brown crust (Chahine & Sucher, 2015). Nonbullous presents as small fluid filled pustules. These pustules often rupture leaving behind yellow crusts (Chahine & Sucher, 2015). Bullous impetigo is usually caused by *Staphylococcus aureus* and nonbullous is usually caused by beta-hemolytic streptococci or by *S. aureus* either separately or together (Stevens et al., 2014).

Cutaneous Abscess, Furuncle, Folliculitis, and Carbuncle

Folliculitis, furuncles, and carbuncles are infections of hair follicles. They may affect any area of the body except the palms of the hands and the soles of the feet (where there is no hair; Chahine & Sucher, 2015). Folliculitis is a superficial infection of a hair follicle, and any pus is limited to the epidermis. Furuncles are deeper infections of the hair follicle. In this case the infection spreads through the dermis into the subcutaneous tissue ending with the formation of a small abscess (Stevens et al., 2014). Both initially present as a red dot that progresses to a white purulent tip. A furuncle appears as a painful swollen boil on the skin (Chahine & Sucher, 2015). A carbuncle is an infection of several adjacent hair follicles. It may have an opening that drains pus and could be associated with fever, swollen lymph nodes, and fatigue (Chahine & Sucher, 2015).

A cutaneous abscess is a collection of pus within the dermis and may spread into the deeper tissues of the skin. Like a carbuncle, a cutaneous abscess may have an opening that drains pus or fluid and may be associated with systemic symptoms including fever, swollen lymph nodes, and fatigue (Chahine & Sucher, 2015; Stevens et al., 2014)

Inpatient Skin and Soft Tissue Infections

Cellulitis

Cellulitis is an infection of the skin including the dermis and epidermis. It may also extend into the superficial facia. The infection is characterized by inflammation of the superficial structures of the skin causing a bright red lesion. The lesion is not raised and usually has a poorly defined margin. The inflamed area is usually associated with a burning pain (Chahine & Sucher, 2015; Stevens et al., 2014).

Surgical Site Infections

Surgical site infections are typically placed into three categories: superficial, deep, and organ or space. Surgical site infections usually present with pain, swelling, and tenderness around the site in addition to purulent discharge (Chahine & Sucher, 2015).

HISTORY AND PHYSICAL FINDINGS

General Findings

SSTIs are diagnosed based on clinical indications including warmth, erythema, and pain around the site of the infection. Depending on the severity of the infection, systemic signs may be present including fever, leukocytosis, and elevated inflammatory markers such as C-reactive protein. In patients with severe disease or those with significant comorbidities, liver and kidney function should be tested due to the possibility of progressive organ dysfunction (Ramakrishnan et al., 2015). Blood cultures are not typically recommended for cellulitis. In cases of systemic disease or if sepsis is suspected, blood cultures would be indicated (Stevens et al., 2015)

Impetigo

Cultures of purulence or exudate may be useful in determining whether *Streptococcus pyogenes* or *S. aureus* is the causative agent, but empiric treatment is reasonable in uncomplicated cases (Stevens et al., 2015).

Cutaneous Abscess, Furuncles, Folliculitis, and Carbuncles

Gram stain and cultures of pus from carbuncles and abscesses are recommended but not required for treatment in nonsevere disease (Chahine & Sucher, 2015)

Cellulitis

Blood, aspirate, or swab cultures are not typically recommended unless the patient is immunocompromised. Similarly, biopsies are not routinely recommended unless there is some other clinical indication for the biopsy (Chahine & Sucher, 2015).

Surgical Site Infections

Surgical site infections usually do not develop until at least 4 days postoperatively. A surgical site infection may present with erythema 5 cm or more from the surgical site, temperature over 38.5°C, tachycardia, and leukocytosis (Chahine & Sucher, 2015).

DIFFERENTIAL DIAGNOSIS AND DIAGNOSTIC CONSIDERATIONS

Cellulitis, Pyoderma Gangrenosum, Gas Gangrene, Necrotizing Fasciitis, and Deep Vein Thrombosis

Cellulitis generally presents with erythema, edema, and warmth. Systemic symptoms such as fever and leukocytosis may be present but patients with cellulitis are generally hemodynamically stable. While cellulitis is generally associated with burning pain, it is usually not severe. Elevated creatine kinase may suggest involvement of the muscle or fascia which would be more consistent with necrotizing fasciitis (Chahine & Sucher, 2015).

Pyoderma gangrenosum is difficult to distinguish from necrotizing fasciitis. This is problematic since the main treatment for necrotizing fasciitis (surgical debridement) can worsen pyoderma gangrenosum and steroids, a mainstay for treatment of pyoderma gangrenosum, can worsen necrotizing fasciitis. Pyoderma gangrenosum does not resemble cellulitis; it has a slow progression and blood cultures are almost always negative. Pyoderma gangrenosum typically presents as a painful lesion on the lower extremities and is often associated with inflammatory bowel disease. The lesion usually progresses to a necrotic ulcer (George et al., 2019).

Gas Gangrene

Both gas gangrene and necrotizing fasciitis may show gas in the soft tissue radiographically. Necrotizing fasciitis will have the characteristic firmness of the underlying subcutaneous tissues. The most important differentiating factor is the appearance of the fascial planes during surgical debridement. Additionally, the Gram stain of cultures from gas gangrene will be very different than necrotizing fasciitis. Gram stain in gas gangrene will usually show only gram-positive rods (*Clostridium* species are typically the causative agent). Gas-producing necrotizing fasciitis is usually polymicrobial and may show gram-positive rods and cocci as well as gram-negative rods and cocci (Chahine & Sucher, 2015).

Deep vein thrombosis is also characterized by extremity pain, swelling, and warmth. However, the pain is less severe than necrotizing fasciitis. An ultrasound of the lower extremities can identify clots and can be used to diagnose deep vein thrombosis (Thachil, 2014).

- A number of infectious and noninfectious conditions should also be included in the differential diagnosis:
  - Herpes zoster presents as a unilateral rash covering one or two adjacent dermatomes and does not cross the body's midline. The erythematous, macropapular rash eventually converts to pustules that rupture, crust over, and heal within 2 to 4 weeks (Chahine & Sucher, 2015).
  - Contact dermatitis is usually a pruritic lesion with erythema, edema, vesicles, bullae, and oozing fluid.

The site is limited to the site of contact with the irritant. The patient may complain of burning or stinging pain at the site (Usatine & Riojas, 2010).

- Acute gout is associated with severe pain, warmth, erythema, and swelling over a single joint. Diagnosis can be confirmed by analysis of synovial fluid. The fluid will contain urate crystals in the case of gout and calcium pyrophosphate crystals in the case of pseudogout (Dalbeth et al., 2019).
- Vasculitis may present as macular or papular lesions in an area of nonblanchable erythematous skin. The definitive diagnosis for vasculitis is a skin biopsy (Watts & Robson, 2018).

TREATMENT

Impetigo

Treatment for impetigo may be either oral or topical antibiotics. Topical mupirocin or retapamulin is given twice daily for 5 days. Oral antibiotics should be considered if the lesions are widespread or if the case is part of an outbreak. An agent effective against methicillin-susceptible *S. aureus* (MSSA; dicloxacillin or cephalexin) should be used unless culture results are positive for streptococci only (penicillin) or if cultures identify methicillin-resistant *S. aureus* (MRSA). In a case where MRSA has been cultured or is strongly suspected, doxycycline, clindamycin, or sulfamethoxazole-trimethoprim is recommended (Stevens et al., 2015).

Cutaneous Abscess, Folliculitis, Furuncles, and Carbuncles

Incision and drainage (I&D) is recommended for treatment of abscesses, carbuncles, and large furuncles. Gram stain and culture of the pus is recommended but treatment may be appropriate without these results. Systemic antibiotics do not improve abscess cure rates but are appropriate in systemic disease. Antibiotics to treat *S. aureus* in addition to I&D should be considered in the presence of systemic inflammatory response syndrome (SIRS). An antibiotic effective against MRSA should be considered for patients who are immunocompromised or have risk factors. (Chahine & Sucher, 2015).

Cellulitis

Current guidelines recommend against routine cultures of blood, aspirates, or swabs although cultures should be considered in immunocompromised patients or if cellulitis is thought to be a result of an animal bite. Mild cellulitis should be treated with an antibiotic with activity against streptococci. For systemic disease, many clinicians use an antimicrobial with coverage against MSSA although the evidence for this is weak. If the cellulitis is associated with blunt trauma, confirmed MRSA infection at another source, nasal colonization with MRSA, injection drug use, or SIRS, an antimicrobial with activity against MRSA (e.g., vancomycin) should be used.

In immunocompromised patients it is appropriate to start with broad empiric coverage including vancomycin and piperacillin-tazobactam or imipenem/meropenem (Stevens et al., 2015). Systemic corticosteroids are not recommended for most patients but should be considered in adult nondiabetic patients with cellulitis (Stevens et al., 2015).

Recurrent cellulitis is often associated with a predisposing condition such as edema, obesity, eczema, venous insufficiency, and toe web abnormalities. Whenever possible these pre-existing conditions should be treated to help prevent cellulitis as a complication of the primary disease process (Stevens et al., 2015).

Surgical Site Infections

Removal of sutures along with I&D is recommended for surgical site infections. In the absence of systemic symptoms, antibiotic therapy is not always indicated. If antibiotic therapy is required, a penicillin with activity against MSSA or a first-generation cephalosporin is adequate. For surgical site infections following surgery on the axilla, gastrointestinal tract, perineum, or the female genital tract, a cephalosporin or fluroquinolone along with metronidazole should provide adequate coverage (Stevens et al., 2014).

TRANSITION OF CARE

Antibiotic coverage should always be adjusted (escalated or deescalated) depending on culture results (Golan, 2019).

14.9: INTRAVENOUS INFILTRATION AND EXTRAVASATION

Kathryn E. Smith, Michelle Wang, and Alice X. Wang

Extravasations and infiltrations are iatrogenic injuries associated with IV administration of medications or solutions and can contribute significantly to patient morbidity. Risk factors may be related to the infusion site, patient characteristics, healthcare received, and physiochemical properties of the infusate. Early recognition of signs and symptoms is key to limiting the extent of injury. A suspected extravasation/infiltration is best assessed and managed using a systematic and collaborative approach that involves the patient, administering nurse, treating provider, and pharmacist. While evidence-based guidance is sparse, a treatment strategy involving nonpharmacologic methods and pharmacologic antidotes, when appropriate, should be employed.

Extravasation and infiltration are known complications of IV administration of medications and solutions that place the patient at significant risk of iatrogenic morbidity. The terms "extravasation "and "infiltration" are often used interchangeably. Extravasation is defined as an inadvertent infiltration of a vesicant, a medication or solution that has potential for severe tissue or cellular damage into surrounding tissue (Gorski et al., 2021). Infiltration is defined as the inadvertent extraneous administration of any nonvesicant or irritant solution into surrounding tissue (Gorski et al., 2021).

The true incidence of extravasation/infiltration is unknown due to inconsistent documentation and lack of reporting. The incidence of peripheral vein extravasation in adult patients is reported to be 0.1% to 6% (Kreidieh et al., 2016; Reynolds et al., 2014). The most commonly affected sites are the dorsum of the hand, forearm, or antecubital fossa (Firat, 2013). Extravasation injury with central venous access devices occurs less frequently, with a reported incidence of 0.3% to 4.7% (Kreidieh et al., 2016).

Extravasation/infiltration may occur as a result of dislodgement of the device, venous irritation, or poor practitioner technique during insertion (Dougherty, 2010). Infiltration of a medication into the subcutaneous space places pressure on surrounding structures and can affect local blood supply, impede lymphatic drainage, alter sensation, and compromise tissue viability (Amjad et al., 2011). The larger the amount of fluid infiltrated, the greater the potential damage. The mechanical pressure on the subdermal plexus can obstruct and deform blood vessels, which may result in ischemic injuries. The physiochemical properties of the extravasated medication or solution can also impact the degree of damage. The mechanism of injury based on physiochemical property is discussed in the treatment section that follows.

PRESENTING SIGNS AND SYMPTOMS

Early recognition of signs and symptoms of extravasation/infiltration is key to limiting the extent of injury (Gorski et al., 2021). Immediate manifestations seen during drug administration include pain, absence of blood return, a change in the quality of infusion, or pressure or resistance at the syringe barrel during injection (Dougherty, 2010). Leakage around the needle or cannula site and blanching of skin may also be noted. Pain may manifest as severe stinging or burning and may continue beyond 24 hours after extravasation/infiltration and intensify over time. Delayed manifestations of extravasation/infiltration injury, occurring 24 hours after the insult, include redness, swelling, and local tingling or other sensory deficits. Ulceration, blistering, and necrosis can occur within 48 to 96 hours but may take weeks to develop. Patients should be evaluated every day for 1 week, then weekly until resolution of symptoms (Pérez Fidalgo et al., 2012).

A standardized tool for assessment of extravasation/infiltration is recommended for documentation and monitoring of injuries (Gorski et al., 2021). Multiple grading scales exist to classify the severity of extravasation/infiltration (Amjad et al., 2011). The most widely accepted scale for infiltration injury is the Infusion Nurses Society Infiltration Scale of Intravenous Infiltrations (Table 14.6; Gorski et al., 2021). The Common Terminology Criteria for Adverse Events (CTCAE V5) is often used to grade extravasation injury in oncology clinical trials (U.S. Department of Health and Human Services, & National Institutes of Health—National Cancer Institute, 2017).

The burden of disease associated with extravasation/infiltration injuries can be significant. The infiltration of a noncytotoxic medication still has the possibility of causing local tissue inflammation or discomfort to the patient. If left untreated, severe pain, discomfort, or compartment syndrome may occur. Long-term consequences may include chronic pain, limitations in mobility, decreased function, permanent nerve damage, soft tissue sloughing, tendon damage, loss of limb function, and

TABLE 14.6: Comparison of Grading Tools for Infusion Site Extravasation/Infiltration Injuries

	INS CLINICAL CRITERIA	CTACE ADVERSE EVENT (V5.0)
INS Grade 0 / CTACE Grade 1	No symptoms	Painless edema
INS Grade 1 / CTACE Grade 2	Skin blanched, edema <1 inch in any direction, cool to touch, with or without pain	Erythema with associated symptoms (e.g., edema, pain, induration, phlebitis)
INS Grade 2 / CTACE Grade 3	Skin blanched, edema 1–6 inches in any direction, cool to touch, with or without pain	Ulceration or necrosis; severe tissue damage; operative intervention indicated
INS Grade 3 / CTACE Grade 4	Skin blanched, translucent, gross edema >6 inches in any direction, cool to touch, mild to moderate pain, possible numbness	Life-threatening consequences; urgent intervention indicated
INS Grade 4 / CTACE Grade 5	Skin blanched, translucent; skin tight, leaking; skin discolored, bruised, swollen; gross edema >6 inches in any direction; deep pitting tissue edema; circulatory impairment; moderate to severe pain; infiltration of any amount of blood product, irritant, or vesicant	Death

CTACE, Common terminology criteria for adverse events; INS, Infusion Nurses Society.

Source: Data from Infusion Nurses Society. (2006). Infusion nursing standards of practice. *Journal of Infusion Nursing, 29*(Suppl. 1), S1–S92. http://doi.org/10.1097/00129804-200601001-00001; United States Department of Health and Human Services, & National Institutes of Health–National Cancer Institute. (2017, November 27). *Common terminology criteria for adverse events (CTCAE)* (5.0 version). https://ctep.cancer.gov/protocoldevelopment/electronic_applications/docs/CTACE_v5_Quick_Reference_8.5x11.pdf

even mortality. Up to 25% of extravasation/infiltration injuries may cause a burden of disease that is more severe than the admitting diagnosis (Reynolds et al., 2014).

HISTORY AND PHYSICAL FINDINGS

Identification of risk factors and appropriate monitoring is imperative to the prevention of extravasation/infiltration injuries. Vascular access devices should be assessed regularly by the bedside nurse prior to intermittent and continuous IV infusions for appropriateness and patency (Gorski et al., 2021). Infusion-specific, patient-specific, and healthcare-specific risk factors for extravasation/infiltration should be evaluated and addressed (Gorski et al., 2021). Major infusion-specific risk factors include duration of infusion, infusion rate, catheter location at a point of flexion, and infiltration volume (Reynolds et al., 2014). Patient-specific risk factors include extremes of age and altered mental status that impede the patients' ability to report pain and discomfort, disease states that reduce peripheral circulation (e.g., hypotension, Raynaud's disease, peripheral vascular disease), and alterations to sensory perception (e.g., peripheral neuropathy). Healthcare-specific risk factors include lack of knowledge, distraction, or lack of monitoring for infiltration during high-risk drug administration, or infiltration during overnight shift. Finally, the physiochemical properties (pH, osmolarity, vasoconstrictive, cytotoxic) properties of medications or solutions administered should be considered. Increased frequency of monitoring should be employed, and alternative vascular access options should be considered if risk factors are present (Gorski et al., 2021).

DIFFERENTIAL DIAGNOSIS AND DIAGNOSTIC CONSIDERATIONS

Distinguishing extravasation/infiltration from other local reactions can be challenging due to the variability in manifesting signs and symptoms. The differential diagnoses include chemical phlebitis, and, with chemotherapy agents, flare reaction and venous shock. Chemical phlebitis is venous inflammation which may be followed by thrombosis or sclerosis of the vein. Symptoms associated with phlebitis include a burning sensation at the cannula site and cramping along the vein proximal to the cannula site (Pérez Fidalgo et al., 2012). The most notable difference from extravasation/infiltration injury is the presence of a palpable hard venous cord (Gil et al., 2017). Flare reaction is a transient streaking erythema along the cannula site and vein associated with anthracycline administration (Kreidieh et al., 2016; Pérez Fidalgo et al., 2012). It is often associated with itching, burning sensation, and pain that typically resolves within 1 to 2 hours. It can be differentiated from extravasation/infiltration as no swelling or change in blood return occurs. Venous shock is associated with the administration of very cold agents, resulting in venous muscle spasm and loss of

blood flow return. This can be managed with warm dry compresses to help relax the vein (Kreidieh et al., 2016).

TREATMENT
Principles of Management

The primary goal of extravasation/infiltration management is to attenuate potential complications. Early recognition and prompt treatment is essential. The European Society of Medical Oncology/European Oncology Nursing Society (ESMO-EONS) has published clinical practice guidelines on the management of chemotherapy extravasation (Pérez Fidalgo et al., 2012). However, there are currently no evidence-based consensus guidelines available for nononcologic extravasation/infiltration injuries. For both chemotherapy and nononcologic extravasation/infiltrations, there is a lack of clinical trials, thus recommendations are based on literature reviews, expert opinion, and case reports.

The principles of approach to extravasation/infiltration injuries include nonpharmacologic management, pharmacologic antidotes, and surgical intervention (Reynolds et al., 2014). The physiochemical properties of pharmacologic agents determine the mechanism of tissue injury and treatment strategies. Pharmacologic agents and solutions associated with extravasation/infiltration injury can be broken down into four categories: acidic/alkaline, hyperosmolar, vasoconstrictive, and cytotoxic and are examined in detail in the following. The antidotes utilized for extravasation/infiltration injury, along with their indications, mechanisms of action, and dosing are presented in Table 14.7. Figure 14.3A and B summarize the nonpharmacologic and pharmacologic management of oncologic and nononcologic extravasation/infiltration injuries.

Nonpharmacologic Management Overview

Regardless of the causative agent, nonpharmacologic interventions should always be applied first as soon as extravasation/infiltration is suspected (Doellman et al., 2009; Reynolds et al., 2014). The IV push or infusion should be discontinued immediately and disconnected from the IV tubing to prevent further extravasation/infiltration. The catheter/needle should be maintained in place to attempt to aspirate fluid (3–5 mL) from the extravasated area and potentially reduce the size of injury. The catheter/needle should then be removed, and the extent of extravasation/infiltration should be marked for monitoring. Elevation of the affected limb for 24 to 48 hours after extravasation/infiltration can minimize swelling and encourage lymphatic resorption of the drug by decreasing capillary hydrostatic pressure (Doellman et al., 2009). Thermal treatments (warm dry or cold compress) should be applied to the affected site after extravasation/infiltration occurs. Cold compresses decrease extravasation/infiltration site reaction and absorption of infiltrate via vasoconstriction. Warm dry compresses cause vasodilation and enhance dispersion

TABLE 14.7: Targeted Treatments for Extravasation/Infiltration

ANTIDOTE	MECHANISM	INDICATION	DOSING AND ADMINISTRATION
Hyaluronidase	Modifies connective tissue permeability through hyaluronic acid hydrolysis to increase distribution and absorption	Acidic Alkaline Hyperosmolar	15 units as five 0.2 mL SC injections around the site
		Vinca alkaloids Taxanes Etoposide	150 units as five 0.2 mL SC injections around the site
Phentolamine	Alpha-1 antagonist to promote vasodilation	Vasoconstrictive	5 mg as five 1 mg/2 mL SC injections around the site within 12 hours of injury. May repeat if symptoms persist
Topical nitroglycerin 2% ointment	Increase vasodilation of capillaries	Vasoconstrictive (alternative)	1-inch strip on the affected site. May repeat after 8 hours if needed. Monitor for hypotension
Terbutaline	Beta-2 agonist to increase smooth muscle relaxation	Vasoconstrictive (alternative)	Large extravasation site: 1 mg diluted in 10 mL 0.9% normal saline injected locally across symptomatic sites Small/distal extravasation site: 1 mg diluted in 2 mL 0.9% normal saline injected locally across symptomatic sites
Sodium thiosulfate 25%	Free-radical scavenger	Calcium salts	12.5–25 g IV three times weekly
		Mechlorethamine	2 mL of 1/6 molar solution per 1 mg mechlorethamine SC around site
DMSO	Free-radical scavenger	Mitomycin C	4 drops per 10 cm^2 for twice the affected area topically every 8 hours for 7 days. Do not cover with dressing. May cause mild local burning sensation
Dexrazoxane (Totect)	Iron chelation, free-radical scavenger, inhibition of topoisomerase II	Anthracyclines	Days 1–2: 1,000 mg/m^2 (max. 2,000 mg) Day 3: 500 mg/m^2 (max. 1000 mg) Administer IV over 1–2 hours using unaffected arm and separate from cooling procedures by at least 15 minutes. Avoid in combination with DMSO and hepatic impairment. Dose reduce by 50% if CrCl <40 mL/min

CrCl, creatinine clearance; DMSO, dimethyl sulfoxide.

Source: Data from Clinigen Group PLC. (2020). *Totect®*. Package insert.; Kreidieh, F. Y., Moukadem, H. A., & El Saghir, N. S. (2016). Overview, prevention and management of chemotherapy extravasation. *World Journal of Clinical Oncology, 7*(1), 87–97. http://doi.org/10.5306/wjco.v7.i1.87; Le, A., & Patel, S. (2014). Extravasation of noncytotoxic drugs: A review of the literature. *Annals of Pharmacotherapy, 48*(7), 870–886. http://doi.org/10.1177/1060028014527820; Pérez Fidalgo, J. A., García Fabregat, L., Cervantes, A., Margulies, A., Vidall, C., Roila, F., & ESMO Guidelines Working Group. (2012). Management of chemotherapy extravasation: ESMO-EONS Clinical Practice Guidelines. *Annals of Oncology, 23*(Suppl. 7), vii167–vii173. http://doi.org/10.1093/annonc/mds294; Reynolds, P. M., MacLaren, R., Mueller, S. W., Fish, D. N., & Kiser, T. H. (2014). Management of extravasation injuries: A focused evaluation of noncytotoxic medications. *Pharmacotherapy, 34*(6), 617–632. http://doi.org/10.1002/phar.1396

of infiltrated vesicant, decreasing drug accumulation in local tissues. The appropriateness of thermal treatments for each physiochemical category is assessed in the following.

The extravasation/infiltration event and pertinent details should be documented in the patient's chart. A wound care consult should be considered as one third of injuries will ulcerate and may require specific dressings. Surgical management may be required in up to one third of cases. Surgical debridement and excision of necrotic tissue can be considered if pain continues for more than 1 to 2 weeks (Froiland, 2007; Reynolds et al., 2014).

Acidic/Alkaline Medications

Extravasation/infiltration of nonphysiologic pH agents can lead to severe tissue injury. Alkaline solutions (pH >7.45) have a propensity for severe tissue injury due to the formation of dissociated hydroxide ions that can penetrate tissues deeply and cause cellular apoptosis. Acidic solutions (pH <7.35) can cause cellular desiccation, coagulation necrosis, and eschar formation (Reynolds et al., 2014). Central line administration has been recommended for agents with pH < 5 or > 9 (Coyle et al., 2014).

General management of acidic or alkaline agent extravasation/infiltration remains largely nonpharmacologic. Warm dry compresses and hyaluronidase, in refractory cases, can be used to promote absorption of extravasated drugs. If intraarterial extravasation occurs, systemic heparin and stellate ganglion blocks may be indicated (Reynolds et al., 2014).

Hyperosmolar Medications or Solutions

Hyperosmolar agents (osmolarity >375 mOsm/L) cause direct fluid shifts from the intracellular space to the extracellular space, resulting in osmotic stress and ulti-

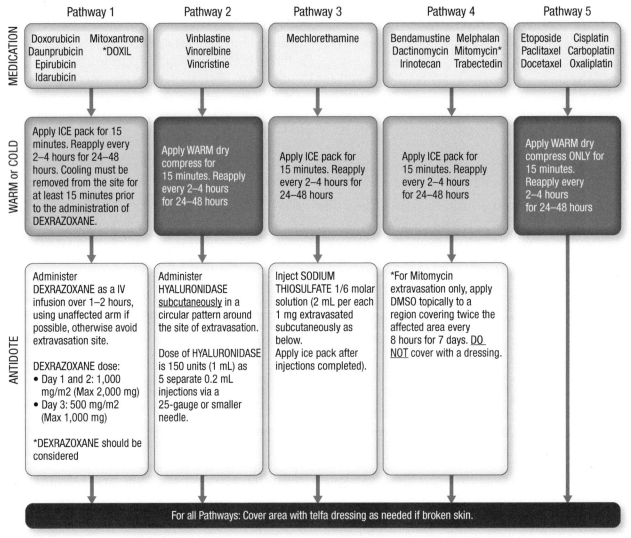

If extravasation is suspected:
1. Immediately **STOP** the infusion and disconnect the IV tubing from the IV device. Do NOT flush.
2. Leaving the needle in place, **aspirate/withdraw** as much of the drug as possible, using a small (1-3 mL) syringe.
3. **Remove** the peripheral IV device or port needle and **assess** the site of the suspected extravasation. **Mark** the affected area.
4. **Initiate** appropriate management measures in accordance with Appendix A.
5. **Notify** provider and pharmacist to determine if further treatment is necessary.
6. **Document** site assessment in electronic medical record. **Submit** safety report.

	Pathway 1	Pathway 2	Pathway 3	Pathway 4	Pathway 5
MEDICATION	Doxorubicin Mitoxantrone Daunprubicin *DOXIL Epirubicin Idarubicin	Vinblastine Vinorelbine Vincristine	Mechlorethamine	Bendamustine Melphalan Dactinomycin Mitomycin* Irinotecan Trabectedin	Etoposide Cisplatin Paclitaxel Carboplatin Docetaxel Oxaliplatin
WARM or COLD	Apply ICE pack for 15 minutes. Reapply every 2–4 hours for 24–48 hours. Cooling must be removed from the site for at least 15 minutes prior to the administration of DEXRAZOXANE.	Apply WARM dry compress for 15 minutes. Reapply every 2–4 hours for 24–48 hours	Apply ICE pack for 15 minutes. Reapply every 2–4 hours for 24–48 hours	Apply ICE pack for 15 minutes. Reapply every 2–4 hours for 24–48 hours	Apply WARM dry compress ONLY for 15 minutes. Reapply every 2–4 hours for 24–48 hours
ANTIDOTE	Administer DEXRAZOXANE as a IV infusion over 1–2 hours, using unaffected arm if possible, otherwise avoid extravasation site. DEXRAZOXANE dose: • Day 1 and 2: 1,000 mg/m2 (Max 2,000 mg) • Day 3: 500 mg/m2 (Max 1,000 mg) *DEXRAZOXANE should be considered	Administer HYALURONIDASE subcutaneously in a circular pattern around the site of extravasation. Dose of HYALURONIDASE is 150 units (1 mL) as 5 separate 0.2 mL injections via a 25-gauge or smaller needle.	Inject SODIUM THIOSULFATE 1/6 molar solution (2 mL per each 1 mg extravasated subcutaneously as below. Apply ice pack after injections completed).	*For Mitomycin extravasation only, apply DMSO topically to a region covering twice the affected area every 8 hours for 7 days. DO NOT cover with a dressing.	

For all Pathways: Cover area with telfa dressing as needed if broken skin.

(A)

FIGURE 14.3: Example Extravasation Management Algorithms for Oncology and Nononcology Vesicants/Irritants. (a) and (b) provide an overview of nonpharmacologic and pharmacologic interventions for oncologic and nononcologic extravasations/infiltrations. The physiochemical properties of different medications determine the type of thermal compress and pharmacologic antidote indicated.
Source: Adapted from Kreidieh, F. Y., Moukadem, H. A., & El Saghir, N. S. (2016). Overview, prevention and management of chemotherapy extravasation. *World Journal of Clinical Oncology, 7*(1), 87–97. http://doi.org/10.5306/wjco.v7.i1.87; Le, A., & Patel, S. (2014). Extravasation of noncytotoxic drugs: A review of the literature. *Annals of Pharmacotherapy, 48*(7), 870–886. http://doi.org/10.1177/1060028014527820; Pérez Fidalgo, J. A., García Fabregat, L., Cervantes, A., Margulies, A., Vidall, C., Roila, F., & ESMO Guidelines Working Group. (2012). Management of chemotherapy extravasation: ESMO-EONS Clinical Practice Guidelines. *Annals of Oncology, 23*(Suppl. 7), vii167–vii173. http://doi.org/10.1093/annonc/mds294; Reynolds, P. M., MacLaren, R., Mueller, S. W., Fish, D. N., & Kiser, T. H. (2014). Management of extravasation injuries: A focused evaluation of noncytotoxic medications. *Pharmacotherapy, 34*(6), 617–632. http://doi.org/10.1002/phar.1396

If extravasation is suspected:
1. Immediately **STOP** the infusion and disconnect the IV tubing from the IV device. Do NOT flush.
2. Leaving the needle in place, **aspirate/withdraw** as much of the drug as possible, using a small (1–3 mL) syringe.
3. **Remove** the peripheral IV device or port needle and **assess** the site of the suspected extravasation. **Mark** the affected area.
4. **Initiate** appropriate management measures in accordance with Appendix B.
5. **Notify** provider and pharmacist to determine if further treatment is necessary.
6. **Document** site assessment in electronic medical record. **Submit** safety report.

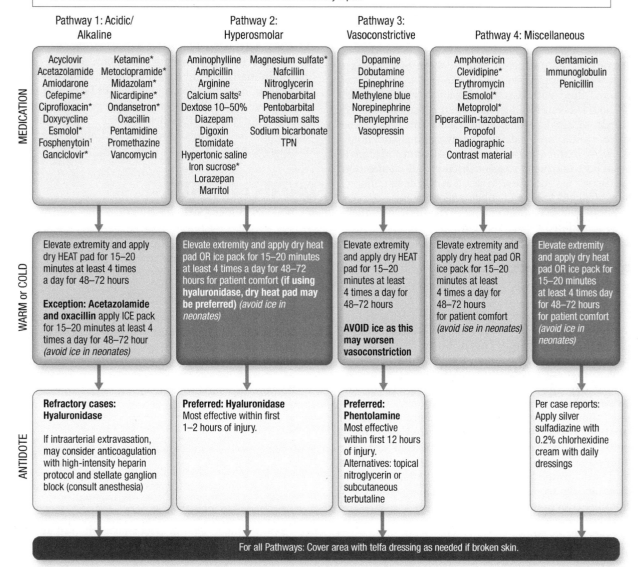

Pathway 1: Acidic/Alkaline

MEDICATION

Acyclovir	Ketamine*
Acetazolamide	Metoclopramide*
Amiodarone	Midazolam*
Cefepime*	Nicardipine*
Ciprofloxacin*	Ondansetron*
Doxycycline	Oxacillin
Esmolol*	Pentamidine
Fosphenytoin[1]	Promethazine
Ganciclovir*	Vancomycin

WARM or COLD

Elevate extremity and apply dry HEAT pad for 15–20 minutes at least 4 times a day for 48–72 hours

Exception: Acetazolamide and oxacillin apply ICE pack for 15–20 minutes at least 4 times a day for 48–72 hour *(avoid ice in neonates)*

ANTIDOTE

Refractory cases: Hyaluronidase

If intraarterial extravasation, may consider anticoagulation with high-intensity heparin protocol and stellate ganglion block (consult anesthesia)

Pathway 2: Hyperosmolar

Aminophylline	Magnesium sulfate*
Ampicillin	Nafcillin
Arginine	Nitroglycerin
Calcium salts[2]	Phenobarbital
Dextose 10–50%	Pentobarbital
Diazepam	Potassium salts
Digoxin	Sodium bicarbonate
Etomidate	TPN
Hypertonic saline	
Iron sucrose*	
Lorazepan	
Marritol	

Elevate extremity and apply dry heat pad OR ice pack for 15–20 minutes at least 4 times a day for 48–72 hours for patient comfort **(if using hyaluronidase, dry heat pad may be preferred)** *(avoid ice in neonates)*

Preferred: Hyaluronidase
Most effective within first 1–2 hours of injury.

Pathway 3: Vasoconstrictive

Dopamine
Dobutamine
Epinephrine
Methylene blue
Norepinephrine
Phenylephrine
Vasopressin

Elevate extremity and apply dry HEAT pad for 15–20 minutes at least 4 times a day for 48–72 hours

AVOID ice as this may worsen vasoconstriction

Preferred: Phentolamine
Most effective within first 12 hours of injury.
Alternatives: topical nitroglycerin or subcutaneous terbutaline

Pathway 4: Miscellaneous

Amphotericin	Gentamicin
Clevidipine*	Immunoglobulin
Erythromycin	Penicillin
Esmolol*	
Metoprolol*	
Piperacillin-tazobactam	
Propofol	
Radiographic	
Contrast material	

Elevate extremity and apply dry heat pad OR ice pack for 15–20 minutes at least 4 times a day for 48–72 hours for patient comfort *(avoid ise in neonates)*

Elevate extremity and apply dry heat pad OR ice pack for 15–20 minutes at least 4 times day for 48–72 hours for patient comfort *(avoid ice in neonates)*

Per case reports: Apply silver sulfadiazine with 0.2% chlorhexidine cream with daily dressings

For all Pathways: Cover area with telfa dressing as needed if broken skin.

†: For infiltration of non-vesicant drugs and IV fluids, follow supportive nonpharmacologic measures as outlined above.
*: No current case reports or data, treat according to chemical properties
1: Monitor for signs of purple glove syndrome (e.g., painful purple-blue discoloration and edema around IV site, cullae formation, absence of arterial flow, skin necrosis, compartment sundrome)
2: Consider surgical resection and sodium thiosulfate for severe cases of delayed tissue injury (calcinosis cutis)

Disclaimer: most data is derived from case reports and clinical judgement supersedes the recommendations in this guideline. Practice changes from institution to institution.

(B)

FIGURE 14.3: *(Continued)*

mately cellular apoptosis. Central line administration has been recommended for solutions with osmolarity >600 mOsm/L (Coyle et al., 2014). The extravasation site should be closely monitored for the "six Ps" of compartment syndrome (pain, pallor, paresthesia, pulselessness, poikilothermia, paralysis) which may require emergent surgical decompression (Coyle et al., 2014; Reynolds et al., 2014).

Warm dry compresses may be applied to promote fluid removal into the capillaries. The preferred antidote is hyaluronidase administered within 1 hour of extravasation. It works rapidly, within 10 minutes, to diffuse extravasated fluid with tissue permeability restored in 24 to 48 hours. Hyaluronidase has been successfully used for dextrose, total parenteral nutrition, calcium, potassium, mannitol, and nafcillin extravasations (Reynolds et al., 2014). Extravasation of calcium salts can additionally cause necrosis due to vasoconstriction and calcification of the tissues. Severe cases can result in calcinosis cutis, erythematous and hardened subcutaneous masses or papules that may take weeks to manifest. Sodium thiosulfate may be considered if calcinosis cutis is debilitating, unresolving, or life-threatening (Reynolds et al., 2014).

Vasoconstrictive Medications

Vasoconstrictive agents cause increased hydrostatic pressure in the circulation and ischemia as a result of direct alpha-adrenergic-mediated vasospasm. Central line administration is recommended for prolonged (>12–24 hour) infusions (Loubani & Green, 2015).

Prompt nonpharmacologic intervention is paramount to prevent morbidity from vasopressor necrosis. Warm dry compresses should be applied to the site of extravasation to promote vasodilation. Cool compresses should be avoided due to the possibility of exacerbating vasoconstriction. The preferred antidote is phentolamine, which is most effective within 12 hours of injury. Phentolamine promotes vasodilation and has been demonstrated to reduce skin loss. Alternative antidotes include topical nitroglycerin or subcutaneous terbutaline (Reynolds et al., 2014).

Cytotoxic Medications

Antineoplastic agents cause direct cellular toxicity. The severity of the injury is often worse with DNA-binding agents (e.g., anthracyclines) compared to non-DNA-binding agents (e.g., vinca alkaloids; Sauerland et al., 2006). The general principles and management of chemotherapy extravasation are similar to that of nononcologic extravasations. Notable differences include use of drug-specific pharmacologic antidotes and indications for thermal compresses. Vinca alkaloids, taxanes, and oxalipatin should be managed with warm dry compresses to increase reabsorption of the extravasated agent, while cold compresses are recommended for other chemotherapy agents (Pérez Fidalgo et al., 2012). Conflicting recommendations

exist for other platinum agents (Pérez Fidalgo et al., 2012; Rubach, 2018).

TRANSITION OF CARE

Nursing and staff education is key to extravasation prevention. Healthcare facilities should establish policies and procedures for the prevention, prompt recognition, and treatment of extravasation infiltration injuries (Gorski et al., 2021; Pérez Fidalgo et al., 2012). Creation of order sets that incorporate clinical decision support can be helpful in managing injuries quickly and effectively. An extravasation/infiltration injury should be considered a sentinel event and documented appropriately in a risk management system (Doellman et al., 2009). Patients should also be informed and educated about treatment and management of the condition (Dougherty, 2010).

CLINICAL PEARLS

- Prevention is key. Assess patient-specific, infusion-specific, healthcare-specific, and pharmacologic-specific risk factors.
- Recognition of signs and symptoms and rapid treatment are essential to minimizing severity of injury.
- Warm dry compresses should be used with extravasation/infiltration of vasopressors, vinca alkaloids, taxanes, and platinum-based agents. Cold compresses may worsen injury in these cases.
- The most commonly utilized antidotes for extravasation/infiltration are phentolamine for vasoconstrictives and hyaluronidase for hyperosmolar agents.

KEY TAKEAWAYS

- Oncologic or nononcologic medication extravasations/infiltrations occur at a low frequency but can be associated with significant morbidity.
- Employ strategies to prevent the occurrence of extravasation/infiltration, recognize when an event occurs, and document the severity of the injury.
- Nonpharmacologic measures may be used to provide comfort, reduce swelling, and minimize risk of deep tissue injury.
- Pharmacologic antidotes are dependent on the physiochemical properties of the extravasated/infiltrated medication and should be utilized rapidly if indicated.

EVIDENCE-BASED RESOURCES

Gorski, L. A., Hadaway, L., Hagle, M. E., Broadhurst, D., Clare, S., Kleidon, T., Meyer, B. M., Nickel, B., Rowley, S., Sharpe, E., & Alexander, M. (2021). Infusion therapy standards of practice, 8th edition. *Journal of Infusion Nursing, 44*(Suppl. 1), S1–S224. http://doi.org/10.1097/NAN.0000000000000396

Kreidieh, F. Y., Moukadem, H. A., & El Saghir, N. S. (2016). Overview, prevention and management of chemotherapy extravasation. *World Journal of Clinical Oncology, 7*(1), 87–97. http://doi.org/10.5306/wjco.v7.i1.87

Pérez Fidalgo, J. A., García Fabregat, L., Cervantes, A., Margulies, A., Vidall, C., Roila, F., & ESMO Guidelines Working Group. (2012). Management of chemotherapy extravasation: ESMO-EONS Clinical Practice Guidelines. *Annals of Oncology, 23*(Suppl. 7), vii167–vii173. http://doi.org/10.1093/annonc/mds294

Reynolds, P. M., MacLaren, R., Mueller, S. W., Fish, D. N., & Kiser, T. H. (2014). Management of extravasation injuries: A focused evaluation of noncytotoxic medications. *Pharmacotherapy, 34*(6), 617–632. http://doi.org/10.1002/phar.1396

14.10: NECROTIZING SOFT TISSUE INFECTION

Bradley Goettl

Necrotizing soft tissue infections (NSTIs) are relatively rare but are potentially life-threatening. This aggressive soft tissue infection spreads rapidly though the subcutaneous tissues and along the fascial planes causing tissue necrosis. NSTIs can trigger a systemic inflammatory response, septic shock, and death (Chen et al., 2020). Morbidity and mortality are high (Wong et al., 2003). Early recognition, surgical debridement, and broad-spectrum antibiotics are key to reducing morbidity and mortality. Patients with NSTI often need serial debridement, prolonged antibiotic therapy, and intensive care management by a multidisciplinary team (Stevens & Bryant, 2017).

PRESENTING SIGNS AND SYMPTOMS

Patients with NSTIs can present with a wide range of signs and symptoms. Symptoms will vary based on the location and severity of the infection (Goh et al., 2014). Although a portal of entry is not required, patients will often describe an injury or initial break in the skin near the infection site. Patients who seek care early may have minor symptoms that can mimic a more superficial soft tissue infection (Goh et al., 2014). Initially, the patient may have mild discomfort and/or subtle skin changes. As the infection advances, patients will often describe an intense pain. Some patients will have more obvious skin changes including erythema, edema, discoloration, necrosis, blistering, crepitus, and/or drainage from a wound (Chen et al., 2020; Goh et al., 2014). Systemic symptoms can include fever, chills, malaise, fatigue, and nausea. In severe cases, patients can experience shock-like symptoms including altered mentation.

HISTORY AND PHYSICAL FINDINGS
Clinical History

A thorough clinical history will describe the onset and progression of symptoms and help identify high-risk patients. NSTIs should be considered with any rapidly spreading soft tissue infection. In general, immunocompromised patients are at an increased risk for severe infections. NSTIs are more common in patients with uncontrolled diabetes and multiple comorbidities (Goh et al., 2014). An open wound (lacerations/abrasions, foreign body, new surgical sites, diabetic wounds) or a recent cutaneous infection (cellulitis or abscess) are common precursors to an NSTI (Goh et al., 2014). Intravenous drug users are at a significant risk. Suspicion should be heightened for soft tissue infections following saltwater exposures or marine activity. Patients who seek evaluation multiple times or have soft tissue infections not responsive to antibiotic therapy should be evaluated for possible NSTI.

Physical Exam

It is important to perform a detailed physical exam as NSTI can occur anywhere in the body. The extremities and perineum/genital area are common locations. Fournier's gangrene is an NSTI that occurs in the perineum/genital region (Broner, 2020). The physical exam findings of NSTIs can vary based on the location and severity of the infection. Early in the infection, the patient may not have obvious exam findings, or they might only have subtle skin changes that mimic a wound or simple infection (Goh et al., 2014). Pain that is out of proportion to exam findings should heighten suspicion. The more classic skin findings include erythema, edema, discoloration, necrosis, blistering, bullae, and/or crepitus (Chen et al., 2020; Goh et al., 2014). Edema can expand beyond the erythematous area. As edema increases, the skin can feel tense. Marking the skin can show the expansion of edema and erythema. Crepitus, or subcutaneous emphysema, may be palpated when subcutaneous gas is present. A gloved finger may be able to be inserted directly into a necrotizing wound, without difficulty, dissecting through the soft tissues (finger test). Wound drainage can be foul-smelling and gray-colored and is often described as "dirty dishwater" (Goh et al., 2014; Stevens & Bryant, 2017). Serial physical exams should be performed to evaluate for disease progression. As the infection worsens, the patient may have exam findings consistent with severe sepsis or shock.

DIFFERENTIAL DIAGNOSIS AND DIAGNOSTIC CONSIDERATIONS

Diagnostic accuracy depends on the severity of the infection at the time of presentation. Early NSTIs can mimic simple soft tissue infections or injuries, leading to misdiagnosis (Goh et al., 2014). Late presentations are more likely to have classic exam and diagnostic findings.

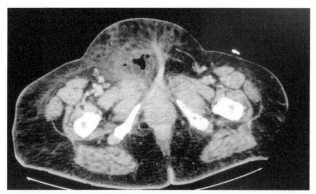

FIGURE 14.4: CT imaging of Fournier's gangrene. CT abdomen/pelvis demonstrating subcutaneous gas and infectious findings consistent with a necrotizing soft tissue infection in the genital region.

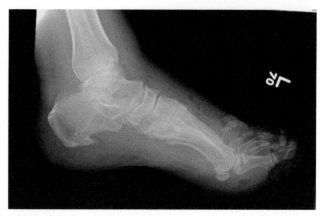

FIGURE 14.5: Plain radiograph of a lower extremity with a necrotizing soft tissue infection. Plain radiograph of the left foot demonstrating subcutaneous gas in a patient with a necrotizing soft tissue infection.

Deep vein thrombosis should be considered for patients with extremity pain, erythema, and/or edema. Venous thrombosis can both mimic a soft tissue infection and be a complication of NSTI.

It is important to note that there is no exam finding or diagnostic test that can fully rule out NSTI. Laboratory studies and diagnostic imaging can be used as decision-making adjuncts. Clinicians should maintain a high index of suspicion for at-risk patients and concerning clinical presentations. Ultimately, if there is a concern for NSTI, the patient should have a surgical evaluation (Stevens & Bryant, 2017).

Laboratory Studies

Uncomplicated cellulitis rarely requires laboratory studies. However, if NSTI is considered, laboratory studies should be obtained. The Laboratory Risk Indicator for Necrotizing Fasciitis (LRINEC) score) can be used to help determine the risk for an NSTI (Wong et al., 2004) A complete blood count (CBC), metabolic panel, and C-reactive protein will provide the data points needed to calculate the LRINEC score. A LRINEC score of 6 or higher indicates an increased risk for NSTI (Table 14.8). Classic laboratory derangement may not occur early in the infectious process. Scoring tools should not replace clinical judgment. If there is a high index of suspicion, initiate immediate surgical evaluation. If there is evidence of systemic infection or sepsis, include blood cultures and a lactate in the workup. An elevated lactate can indicate an advanced infectious process. Gram stain and cultures will help provide a definitive diagnosis and target antibiotic therapy; however, they provide little value during initial management (Stevens & Bryant, 2017).

Radiographic Imaging

Radiographic imaging can be useful, when evaluating for NSTI. The most sensitive form of imaging for NSTI is an MRI with contrast (Malghem et al., 2013). Unfortunately, MRI is not always available and can delay surgical intervention. CT imaging is widely available and can be performed rapidly (Chen et al., 2020). CT is more sensitive than plain films and can reveal inflammatory/infectious changes, abscess, or subcutaneous gas (Figure 14.4). Plain radiographic imaging should not be used to rule out NSTI as gas formation is less likely to be seen (Malghem et al., 2013). If subcutaneous gas is seen on a plain film, it is highly specific for NSTI (Figure 14.5). The absence of subcutaneous gas does not rule out NSTI. Venous dopplers can be obtained to evaluate for deep vein thrombosis. Surgical consultation should not be delayed for advanced imaging (Stevens & Bryant, 2017).

TREATMENT

Early surgical intervention is associated with improved outcomes. Patients with NSTI require immediate and aggressive surgical debridement of all infected tissues. Tissue specimens can be obtained for gram stain and culture (Stevens & Bryant, 2017). Following debridement, patients should be monitored closely for recurrent or expanding tissue infection and may need ICU level of care. It is common for a patient to return to the operating room several times for additional debridement (Chen et al., 2020). Extensive postoperative wound care is required, and patients may benefit from vacuum-assisted closure. Soft tissue reconstruction can be considered in the recovery phase.

The majority of NSTIs are polymicrobial. Common organisms include group A beta-hemolytic *Streptococcus, Staphylococcus aureus, Enterococcus,* Enterobacteriaceae, *Bacteroides,* and Clostridia (Stevens & Bryant, 2017). *Vibrio vulnificus,* a gram-negative rod, is associated with saltwater exposures or marine activities (Wong et al., 2003). Broad spectrum parental antibiotics should be administered early and include coverage for aerobic gram-positive, gram-negative, and anaerobic organisims (examples include piperacillin-tazobactam or carbapenem plus vancomycin

TABLE 14.8: Laboratory Risk Indicator for Necrotizing Fasciitis (LRINEC Score)

VARIABLE	VALUE	SCORE
C-reactive protein	<15 mg/dL (150 mg/L)	0
	≥15 mg/dL (150 mg/L)	4
White blood cell count (×10,000/mcL)	<15	0
	15–25	1
	>25	2
Hemoglobin (g/dL)	>13.5	0
	11–13.5	1
	<11	2
Sodium (mEq/L)	≥135	0
	<135	2
Creatinine	≤1.6 mg/dL (141 mcmol/L)	0
	>1.6 mg/dL (141 mcmol/L)	2
Glucose	≤180 mg/dL (10 mmol/L)	0
	>180 mg/dL (10 mmol/L)	1

NOTE: Scoring tools should not replace clinical judgment. If there is a high index of suspicion, facilitate immediate surgical evaluation.

A LRINEC score of <6: Lower risk for necrotizing soft tissue infection

A LRINEC score of ≥6: Intermediate risk for necrotizing soft tissue infection

A LRINEC score of ≥8: High risk for necrotizing soft tissue infection

Source: Adapted from Wong, C. H., Khin, L. W., Heng, K. S., Tan, K. C., & Low, C. O. (2004). The LRINEC (Laboratory Risk Indicator for Necrotizing fasciitis) score: A tool for distinguishing necrotizing fasciitis from other soft tissue infections. *Critical Care Medicine, 32*(7), 1535–1541. https://doi.org/10.1097/01.ccm.0000129486.35458.7d

or linezolid for methicillin-resistant *Staphylococcus aureus* [MRSA] coverage). Antibiotic monotherapy is not indicated for NSTIs (Dennis et al., 2014; Stevens & Bryant, 2017). Clindamycin has been shown to inhibit toxin production and can be added as a third agent (Dennis et al., 2014).

TRANSITION OF CARE

Surgical consultation should occur early. Depending on the location and severity of the infection, surgical subspecialties may need to be consulted (e.g., Fournier's gangrene will require urology consultation). Facilities that lack surgical services should transfer patients to a hospital with surgical and intensive care capabilities. The appropriate medicine teams should be consulted to manage any acute and chronic medical problems. An infectious disease specialist and clinical pharmacist should be involved to guide antibiotic therapy. A multidisciplinary team of clinicians, wound care specialists, physical/occupational therapists, dieticians, and social services should be engaged early. After discharge, the patient will need follow-up with the surgical and medical teams. Home healthcare should be considered for patients requiring prolonged outpatient management and services.

CLINICAL PEARLS

- NSTIs are severe life-threating infections.
- Surgical debridement is required for NSTIs.
- NSTI is often polymicrobial and requires broad spectrum antibiotics.

KEY TAKEAWAYS

- NSTIs is a surgical emergency.
- Maintain a high index of suspicion for at risk patients and concerning clinical presentations.
- There is no exam finding or diagnostic test that can fully rule out NSTI.

EVIDENCE-BASED RESOURCES

Wong, C. H., Khin, L. W., Heng, K. S., Tan, K. C., & Low, C. O. (2004). The LRINEC (Laboratory Risk Indicator for Necrotizing fasciitis) score: A tool for distinguishing necrotizing fasciitis from other soft tissue infections. *Critical Care Medicine, 32*(7), 1535–1541. https://doi.org/10.1097/01.ccm.0000129486.35458.7d

14.11: PRESSURE INJURIES

Brooke Carpenter

In 2016, the National Pressure Injury Advisory Panel (NPIAP)—formerly the National Pressure Ulcer Advisory Panel (NPUAP)—replaced the name "pressure ulcer" with the term "pressure injury" to more accurately describe and incorporate skin and soft tissue injuries which can present as intact skin or open ulcerations. The NPIAP defines a pressure injury as "localized damage to the skin and underlying soft tissue usually over a bony prominence or related to a medical or other device" (Edsberg et al., 2016, p. 586). Pressure injuries may or may not be painful and develop after prolonged exposure to pressure or pressure in combination with shear.

Pressure injuries are prevalent worldwide in acute and long-term care facilities, posing a major burden on individuals and the healthcare system as a whole. Although precise data are limited, an estimated 1 to 3 million adults are affected annually in the United States. Pressure injuries can result in severe medical complications including pain, cellulitis, osteomyelitis, necrotizing fasciitis, gangrene, and bacteremia. In general, pressure injuries with or without sequelae, are associated with high morbidity and significantly impact an individual's overall quality of life (Mervis & Phillips, 2019).

The pathogenesis of pressure-induced injuries is complex and multifactorial. Ischemia, edema, and ultimately injury will occur when pressure is applied to soft tissues at a higher level than within the blood vessels, generally over a bony prominence (Figure 14.6). Other contributing factors that may impair skin integrity include friction, shearing, and moisture (Ricci et al., 2017).

Numerous individual risk factors increase susceptibility and affect wound healing, including immobilization, malnutrition, frailty, sensory loss (spinal cord injury or neuropathy), neurologic impairment, advanced age, and prolonged hospitalization (Berlowitz, 2021). Furthermore, patients' characteristics, overall health status, and exposure to risk factors, coupled with unrelieved mechanical pressure, are all contributing elements to the inherent variability of pressure injury development (Coleman et al., 2014).

PRESENTING SIGNS AND SYMPTOMS

Pressure injuries are not uniform and can be difficult to identify on physical exam due to varying skin colors, texture, and wound staging. It is important to thoroughly examine the patient from head to toe, focusing on bony prominences (Figure 14.7). When first assessing an ulcer or wound, confirm pressure and/or shearing as the causative agent prior to diagnosing or staging it as a pressure injury. Nonpressure-related wounds can present similarly, such as diabetic foot ulcers (DFUs), skin tears, or venous stasis ulcers, each with their own unique staging/classification system for wound-specific management (Edsberg et al., 2016). The most universally accepted pressure injury staging system was developed by the NPIAP (Table 14.9).

HISTORY AND PHYSICAL FINDINGS

Risk Factors

Completing a comprehensive history and physical is key in determining any reversible predisposing factors and identifying individuals with higher susceptibility to pressure injuries. Risk factors can vary depending on the

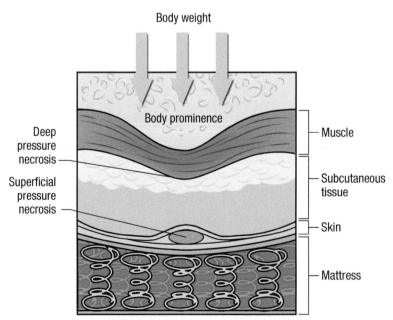

FIGURE 14.6: Pathophysiological development of a pressure injury.

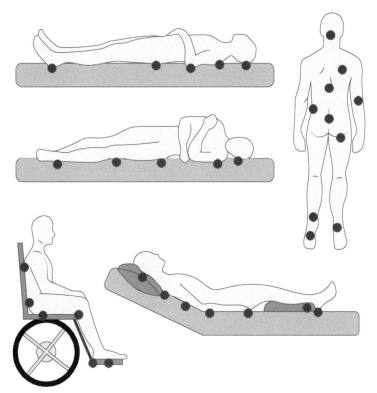

FIGURE 14.7: Common sites associated with pressure-induced injury.
Source: https://www.cdss.ca.gov/agedblinddisabled/res/VPTC2/8%20Paramedical%20Services/Preventing_Pressure_Ulcers_Patient_Guide.pdf

healthcare setting (outpatient, acute care, and long-term facilities); however, immobility, malnutrition, reduced skin perfusion, and sensory loss are the most consistently recognized among all populations (Berlowitz, 2021).

Physical Exam

After a comprehensive health history, a thorough assessment and evaluation of the present wound is indicated to determine staging and treatment. Prior to staging, cleaning of the wound bed is necessary to optimize evaluation and allow for thorough visualization of tissue layers and anatomy. The NPIAP staging system is the most commonly used which consists of four main stages (Table 14.3). This staging system is not intended to suggest that all pressure injuries will progress through all stages nor will wound healing follow a regression pattern from Stages 4 to 1 (Mervis & Phillips, 2019).

DIFFERENTIAL DIAGNOSIS AND DIAGNOSTIC CONSIDERATIONS

Pressure injuries can often present similarly to other wounds such as diabetic neuropathic ulcers, arterial or venous insufficiency ulcers, and cellulitis. Given there are no confirmatory diagnostic or laboratory studies, the diagnosis of a pressure injury is one of exclusion and based on history and clinical examination.

Laboratory Studies

There are several useful but nonspecific laboratory studies which can be utilized for a comprehensive workup. A complete blood count (CBC) with differential may demonstrate an elevated white blood cell (WBC) count suggesting inflammation and/or infection. To evaluate nutritional status for adequate wound healing, albumin, prealbumin, transferrin, and serum protein can be obtained. If there is concern for bacteremia or sepsis, peripheral blood cultures should be obtained (Kirman, 2020).

TREATMENT

The general components for treatment of skin and soft tissue pressure injuries include the following (Bluestein & Javaheri, 2008):

- Relieve pressure/eliminate contributing factors
- Adequate pain control
- Providing local wound care: cleansing, debridement (if necrotic tissue present), manage infection/bacterial colonization
- Optimize nutritional state
- Preventive measures: Repositioning (the gold standard of prevention and treatment), encourage mobile patients to shift weight every 10 minutes and immobile patients require repositioning every 2 hours (even with specialty surface bed), and thorough skin care/hygiene

TABLE 14.9 : National Pressure Injury Advisory Panel Staging System

PRESSURE INJURY STAGE	DESCRIPTION	ADDITIONAL NOTES
Stage 1	Nonblanchable erythema of intact skin	Presence of blanchable erythema or changes in sensation, temperature, or firmness may precede visual changes. Color changes do not include purple or maroon discoloration; these may indicate deep tissue pressure injury
Stage 2	Partial-thickness skin loss with exposed dermis	The wound bed is viable, pink or red, moist, and may also present as an intact or ruptured serum-filled blister. Adipose (fat) is not visible and deeper tissues are not visible. Granulation tissue, slough, and eschar are not present
Stage 3	Full-thickness skin loss with adipose (fat) visible in the ulcer and granulation tissue and epibole (rolled wound edges) often present	Slough and/or eschar may be visible. The depth of tissue damage varies by anatomical location; areas of significant adiposity can develop deep wounds. Undermining and tunneling may occur. Fascia, muscle, tendon, ligament, cartilage and/or bone are not exposed. If slough or eschar obscures the extent of tissue loss this is an unstageable pressure injury
Stage 4	Full-thickness skin and tissue loss with exposed or directly palpable fascia, muscle, tendon, ligament, cartilage, or bone in the ulcer	Slough and/or eschar may be visible. Epibole (rolled wound edges), undermining and/or tunneling often occur. Depth varies by anatomical location. If slough or eschar obscures the extent of tissue loss this is an unstageable pressure injury
Unstageable pressure injury	Obscured full-thickness skin and tissue loss in which the extent of tissue damage within the ulcer cannot be confirmed because it is obscured by slough or eschar	A Stage 3 or 4 pressure injury may be revealed if slough or eschar is removed. Stable eschar on the heel or ischemic limb should not be softened or removed
Deep tissue pressure injury	Persistent nonblanchable deep red, maroon or purple discoloration or epidermal separation revealing a dark wound bed or blood-filled blister	If necrotic tissue, subcutaneous tissue, granulation tissue, fascia, muscle, or other underlying structures are visible, this indicates a full thickness pressure injury (unstageable, Stage 3, or Stage 4). Do not use deep tissue pressure injury to describe vascular, traumatic, neuropathic, or dermatologic conditions

Source: Reproduced with permission from National Pressure Injury Advisory Panel. (2017). *NPIAP pressure injury stages.* https://cdn.ymaws.com/npiap.com/resource/resmgr/online_store/npiap_pressure_injury_stages.pdf

Wound care and appropriate dressings are determined by the stage of skin injury based on the NPIAP staging system (Bluestein & Javaheri, 2008):

- Stage 1: Cover with transparent film, evaluate risk factors for more serious pressure injuries, implement preventive measures.
- Stage 2: Maintain moist wound bed, little to no debridement (avoid wet-to-dry dressings), use a transparent film or occlusive dressing.
- Stage 3 and 4: If necrotic tissue is present, debridement is necessary then cleanse the wound and apply a moist to absorbent dressing (e.g., hydrogel, alginate, foam), consider a surgical consultation.

CLINICAL PEARLS

- Pressure injuries are a result of prolonged pressure with or without friction, shearing, or moisture to bony prominences.
- Variability in chronicity, size, and depth of wounds.
- The NPIAP staging system is utilized to guide treatment/management.
- Consult a wound care specialist for appropriate staging and treatment recommendations.

KEY TAKEAWAYS

- Comprehensive history and physical is pertinent to identifying at-risk individuals.

14.12: RASHES COMMON IN ACUTE CARE

Ameera Chakravarthy and Barbara Miller

Rashes can manifest with multiple morphologies and clinical manifestations. Patients in acute care are at risk for developing skin problems as a result of critical illness as well as from therapeutic interventions aimed at managing the acute insult. Acutely ill patients may be at risk for developing line-related infections, allergic contact dermatitis to adhesives and EKG leads, pressure necrosis from prolonged bedrest, drug-induced reactions from exposure to multiple drugs, secondary infections from indwelling lines and endotracheal tubes, and more. Additional factors to consider and address in the management plan include fluid resuscitation increasing peripheral edema, chronic or acute malnutrition complicating wound healing, secondary skin colonization, and superinfection by commensal organisms or normal skin flora.

PRESENTING SIGNS AND SYMPTOMS

Contact Dermatitis

Contact dermatitis can be either irritant or allergic. Irritant is the more common form. Contact dermatitis that is caused by irritants is characterized by a nonimmune modulated irritation of the skin by a substance while the allergic form is a result of a delayed type IV, T-cell–mediated, hypersensitivity reaction (e.g., poison oak or ivy dermatitis). In both forms, the reaction is characterized by erythema and pruritus (Usatine & Riojas, 2010). Acute allergic dermatitis affects people of all ages, ethnicities, and skin types, with an estimated 25 to 40 million cases requiring treatment yearly (Baer, 1990; Epstein, 1994). The clinical presentation of contact dermatitis is based on the allergen or irritant, the area affected, as well as the duration of time the affected area of skin was in contact with the irritating substance. Contact dermatitis caused by irritants typically affects the hands, causing erythema, burning, pruritus, and pain with a dry and fissured skin appearance and less distinct lesion borders. Contact dermatitis caused by an allergen typically affects the hands with pruritus along with vesicles, bullae, and lesions that have distinct angles, lines, and borders or crusting and oozing (Usatine & Riojas, 2010). The rash that occurs from contact dermatitis can develop minutes or hours from exposure and last for 2 to 4 weeks.

Poison Oak or Ivy Dermatitis

Toxicodendron toxicity causes a form of allergic contact dermatitis by exposure to plants within the Anacardiaceae family. These include poison ivy, poison oak, and poison sumac and is the most common cause of allergic dermatitis in North America (Lofgran & Mahabal, 2021). The plants can vary in appearance and are found throughout continental North America (Lofgran & Mahabal, 2021). This form of allergic contact dermatitis is caused by direct or indirect (e.g., contaminated clothing) contact with the leaves, roots, or branches of poison oak or ivy plants. An allergic reaction occurs when skin comes into contact with the oily coating, urushiol, that is contained in all parts of the plant but especially in the leaves and fruit. Once there is contact, urushiol is absorbed rapidly by the Langerhans cells in the epidermis. Repeated exposure to poison ivy may cause one to become sensitized to the urushiol; there is no intervention to reverse the sensitivity once it occurs. While domestic or wild animals are not affected by poison ivy, urushiol can be transferred through physical contact of animals with humans. The rash or the associated fluid-filled blisters caused by poison oak or ivy are not contagious and can appear within a few hours to 10 days after exposure. The severity of the dermatitis depends on an individual's sensitivity to urushiol as well as degree of exposure.

Drug-Induced Rashes

Drug-induced rashes are very common in the acute care environment and are usually mild and self-limiting. Some forms, however, are serious and can significantly increase morbidity and mortality, including SJS, TEN, drug reaction with eosinophilia and systemic symptoms (DRESS) syndrome, multiple drug hypersensitivity (MDH) syndrome, acute generalized exanthematous pustulosis (AGEP), and drug-induced bullous pemphigoid (DIBP; Frey et al., 2017). SJS and TEN symptoms typically present within 1 to 3 weeks of drug introduction with epidermal detachment along with bullae and erosions, and mucous membrane involvement.

Fungal Infections

Fungal diseases accounted for over 75,000 hospitalizations and nearly 9 million outpatient visits in the United States in 2017 and much of this is underestimated due to underdiagnosis and undercoding (CDC, 2020). *Candida*, followed by *Aspergillus*, are the most common causes of nosocomial fungal infections. The degree of immunosuppression in a patient effects the frequency by which fungi cause infections. *Candida* requires a minimal level of immunosuppression to predispose a patient to a fungal infection whereas *Aspergillosis* tends to occur in patients with an intermediate to severe degree of immunosuppression. Mucorales, fusarium, and other molds (e.g., scedosporium) are relatively less common, and are seen in the most severely immunocompromised hosts or in those who have been immunocompromised for a long period of time (Wilson et al., 2002). Dermatophytes or fungal organisms that cause skin infections prefer environments that are moist and warm (e.g., between toes, genital area, underneath the breasts). Fungal skin infections or tinea are more likely to develop in people living in tropical climates or in those who wear tight, nonbreathable clothing. Additionally, obese and diabetic individuals are also at risk for developing fungal infections due to increased sweating, moisture trapping in larger, thicker skin folds, bacterial overgrowth, and microvascular dysfunction (Hirt et al., 2019). Adolescents and adults are more likely to develop tinea cruris, tinea pedis, and tinea unguium (onychomycosis). Hospital-acquired fungal infections include respiratory infections which are most commonly seen with stem cell or solid organ transplant recipients and patients receiving immunosuppressant medications (e.g., invasive *Aspergillus* infection).

HISTORY AND PHYSICAL FINDINGS

Contact Dermatitis

A thorough history is key to obtaining information about the causative substance and thus, effectively treat the dermatitis and prevent further damage. Certain occupations put adults at risk for contact dermatitis due to the exposure of irritants and allergens including healthcare and dental workers, metal workers, gardeners, or agricultural workers. Exposure to common irritants related to these professions (e.g., solvents and cutting fluids in machining, detergents, pesticides, allergens, medicines, and substances used in dental procedures) may be revealed through adequate patient history. Urushiol is the most common allergen causing the allergic form of contact dermatitis. Allergic contact dermatitis can affect people of all ages, though it is most prevalent in adults. History and physical findings may include complaints of itching and discomfort, acute cases with erythema, vesicles, and bullae. Chronic cases may involve lichen with cracks and fissures.

Poison Oak or Ivy Dermatitis

A detailed history reviewing occupational and environmental exposures within the past few weeks is important, along with the presence of symptoms including intense pruritus, popular, or vesicular rash in a linear pattern. The pattern may also be scattered and there may be black spots (oxidized urushiol) on affected skin or clothing which should be carefully avoided to prevent secondary exposure. Poison ivy and oak dermatitis can be mild, moderate, or severe depending on localization of and severity of symptoms. Mild forms present mainly with localized or linear erythema and/or edema with minimal symptoms. Moderate to severe cases will have more diffuse involvement associated with severe pain, burning, and or pruritus.

Drug-Induced Rashes

A drug-induced reaction should be considered in any patient who is taking medications and who suddenly develops a symmetric cutaneous eruption. A morbilliform (measleslike) drug eruption is a form of allergic reaction, mediated by cytotoxic T-cells and classified as a Type IV immune reaction. The target of attack may be a drug, a metabolite of the drug, or a protein bonded to the drug. The rash often starts on the face and trunk and spreads to the extremities; the distribution is bilateral and symmetrical, urticarial, papulosquamous, pustular, and bullous. If mucosal lesions are present, they can be seen in the mouth, conjunctiva, and in the genital area. On the first occasion, the morbilliform rash usually appears 1 to 2 weeks after starting the drug, but it may occur up to 1 week after stopping it. On re-exposure to the causative (or related) drug, skin lesions appear within 1 to 3 days. It is very rare for a drug that has been taken for months or years to cause a morbilliform drug eruption. Drug-induced rashes in Stevens-Johnson syndrome (SJS)/toxic epidermal necrolysis (TEN) are commonly caused by antibiotics including trimethoprim-sulfamethoxazole, cephalosporins, penicillins, carbapenems, and vancomycin, antiepileptic drugs, NSAIDs, and allopurinol. With regard to antiepileptics, carbamazepine can induce SJS/TEN reactions in Thai, Han, Chinese, Malay, and Indian populations requiring screening for HLA-B* 15:02

prior to starting treatment (Aggarwal et al., 2014; Chang et al., 2011; Godhwani & Bahna, 2016; Hsiao et al., 2014; Khor et al., 2014; Tassaneeyakul et al., 2010). Additionally, oxicams (e.g., meloxicam) and sulfonamides have been associate with TEN in Europeans with HLA-B*12 and allopurinol has induced these reactions in Thai and Chinese patients with HLA-B*58:01 (Hung et al., 2005; Roujeau et al., 1987; Saksit et al., 2017). To differentiate between a blistering and a nonblistering drug eruption or skin condition (e.g., phemphigus group of disorders), a test for Nikolsky sign can be performed by applying lateral or tangential pressure to the mucosa or skin in the perilesional area. If this results in a shearing away of the epidermis in the normal areas, the test is positive and confirms a blistering skin condition (Maity et al., 2020).

Fungal Infections

Common risk factors for fungal infections in acute care include the presence of diabetes, obesity, microbial colonization, broad-spectrum antibiotics, indwelling central catheter, total parenteral nutrition, immunosuppression, burns, and increased severity of illness (Tufano, 2002). Rashes from a fungal skin infection are typically more erythematous with scaling at the border and/or have defined lesions (pustules) at the edge of the rash. Pruritus or burning may be present and the rash can appear anywhere on the body—including the nails—though it is most commonly found in skin folds and on the groin, buttocks, or thighs.

DIFFERENTIAL DIAGNOSIS AND DIAGNOSTIC CONSIDERATIONS

Contact Dermatitis

The history and physical examination findings help to strengthen the diagnosis of contact dermatitis and rule out other differential diagnoses including atopic dermatitis, dyshidrotic eczema, inverse psoriasis, latex allergy, palmoplantar psoriasis, scabies, and tinea pedis. The presence of a bacterial or fungal superinfection should be considered when there is exudate, weeping, and crusting. This can be identified with a bacterial culture or a fungal culture. If scabies or mites are suspected, dermoscopy and microscopy can be used to confirm these diagnoses via direct visualization of the mite with a skin scraping. If a known or suspected allergen or irritant substance is removed and symptoms resolve, the diagnosis of contact dermatitis is established. Consultation with a dermatologist for patch testing (gold standard) for allergic contact dermatitis may be indicated if removing the offending substance and empiric treatment do not resolve the dermatitis and symptoms of a chronic, pruritic, eczematous, or lichenified dermatitis persist (Fonacier et al., 2015).

Poison Ivy or Oak Dermatitis

The diagnosis of poison ivy or oak dermatitis is made by a confirmatory history and physical exam. If allergy patch testing is available, it can be used to identify patients with severe urushiol sensitivity; however, exercise caution to avoid inadvertently sensitizing an unsensitized patient. Confirmation of the diagnosis can be made via dermoscopy to evaluate for black spot dermatitis evidenced by the presence of jagged red-rimmed dark brown lesions (Rader et al., 2012). Other conditions that can be confused with poison oak or ivy dermatitis include herpes zoster as phytophotodermatitis, irritant contact dermatitis, bed bugs (*Cimex lectularius*), or scabies (*Sarcoptes scabiei*). The last two conditions are pruritic; though the rash is not vesicular, there is burrowing pattern and the bites from bed bugs cause immediate skin findings (Lofgran & Mahabal, 2021).

Drug-Induced Rash

A sound history and physical exam is often sufficient to substantiate the diagnosis of a drug-induced rash. There are no routine tests to confirm the diagnosis or identify the offending drug. Differential diagnoses for a drug-induced rash are vast and include acute or chronic urticaria, erythema multiform, irritant contact dermatitis, pityriasis rosea measles, rubella, nonspecific toxic erythema associated with infection, Kawasaki disease, connective tissue disease, and acute graft-versus-host disease. A biopsy of the rash can be useful in confirming the diagnosis of a drug eruption as it may show eosinophils in morbilliform eruptions. Unfortunately, drug-induced rashes can vary histologically with and without the use of immunomodulating drugs (Blume et al., 2020). Laboratory studies (e.g., complete blood count [CBC] with differential) may show leukopenia, thrombocytopenia, and eosinophilia in patients with serious drug eruptions and a complete metabolic panel may show serious lethal liver involvement in persons with hypersensitivity syndromes. Special attention should be paid to the electrolyte balance, renal, and/or hepatic function indices in patients with severe reactions such as SJS, TEN, or vasculitis. Antibody and/or immunoserology tests may be ordered to confirm drug-induced systemic lupus erythematosus (SLE) or drug-induced subacute cutaneous lupus erythematosus (SCLE) and direct cultures can support a primary infectious etiology or secondary infection.

Fungal Infections

Making a clinical diagnosis of a fungal infection can be challenging as there are many mimics that have identical skin lesions (e.g., tinea corporis can be confused with eczema). The diagnosis can be made by visualization, correlating symptoms, use of potassium hydroxide preparation (KOH), skin biopsy, and fungal culture. Use of a KOH preparation is helpful when the diagnosis is uncertain based on history and visual inspection. Additionally, if symptoms worsen after empiric treatment with a topical steroid, dermatophyte infection should be suspected. Alternatively, the nonfungal lesion will not improve or worsen if it is treated with an antifungal cream. Differential diagnoses to consider for fungal infections are extensive and include atopic dermatitis, fixed drug eruption, SLE, contact dermatitis, and psoriasis (Ely et al., 2014).

TREATMENT

Contact Dermatitis

The first priority in treating patients with contact dermatitis is to identify and remove the causative allergen or irritant. Therapeutic treatment in the acute phase includes the use of cool compresses, calamine lotion, and colloidal oatmeal baths to help dry and soothe lesions. If the lesions are acute, allergic, and localized, the use of moderate- to high-potency topical steroids, such as triamcinolone 0.1% (Kenalog, Aristocort) or clobetasol 0.05% (Temovate) is recommended. Flexural surfaces, eyelids, face, anogenital region areas have thinner skin and therefore lower-potency steroids, such as desonide ointment (Desowen), can be helpful and minimize the risk of skin atrophy. If allergic contact dermatitis involves more than 20% of skin area, treatment with systemic steroid therapy is required and may provide relief to symptoms in 12 to 24 hours. The recommended treatment includes 5 to 7 days of prednisone, 0.5 to 1 mg per kg daily. If there is relief with a reduction of severity and successful avoidance of the irritant or allergen, the dose may be reduced by 50%. In severe dermatitis caused by poison ivy, poison oak, or sumac, oral prednisone should be tapered over 2 to 3 weeks because rapid discontinuation of steroids can cause rebound dermatitis. Randomized control data support a longer course of treatment starting with a 5-day regimen of 40 mg of prednisone followed by a prednisone taper of 30 mg daily for 2 days, 20 mg daily for 2 days, 10 mg daily for 2 days, and 5 mg daily for 4 days over a total of 15 days in patients with severe poison ivy dermatitis (Curtis & Lewis, 2014). Prescribing a steroid dose pack is not recommended as it has insufficient dosing and duration of treatment. While antihistamines are generally not effective for pruritus associated with allergic contact dermatitis, they are commonly used. Sedation from more soporific antihistamines (e.g., diphenhydramine [Benadryl], hydroxyzine [Vistaril]) may offer some degree of relief and moisturizers or barrier creams may be instituted as secondary prevention strategies to help avoid continued exposure. To prevent irritant contact dermatitis of the hands, it is helpful to wear non-latex gloves with a cotton liner when working with irritants to keep skin dry.

Poison Ivy and Poison Oak

Poison ivy and oak dermatitis are usually self-limiting and will resolve within a few weeks with no treatment. The initial treatment includes immediate irrigation of the affected area with a mild soap along with removal and decontamination of clothing and cleaning of fingernails. Other treatments include cool, moist compresses, oatmeal baths, calamine lotion, and topical astringents. Topical and oral antihistamines are commonly used to decrease pruritus and are not effective as the primary pathophysiological problem which is not due to histamine release. Instead, primary management should include use of moderate to high dose topical or systemic corticosteroids early, before the appearance of papules or vesicles. A tapered dose of prednisone for severe cases can begin at 1 mg/kg/day for a max dose of 60 mg/day and tapered weekly over 3 weeks to prevent rebound dermatitis. Alternatives for patients who are not candidates for systemic corticosteroids include the application of moderate-strength topical corticosteroids with an occlusive dressing for 24 hours that is then repeated 48 hours after initial application.

Drug-Induced Rashes

The management of drug-induced rashes primarily consists of a thorough review of medications, supportive care, and immediate withdrawal of the causative medication. IV fluids may be used to maintain euvolemia with a urinary output of 0.5 to 1.0 mL/kg per hour. Insertion of an nasogastric feeding tube may be needed to maintain adequate calorie and protein intake, especially in patients with mucosal involvement (McCullough et al., 2017). These patients should be managed in a burn unit and ophthalmology and/or urology should be consulted if the eyes or genitourinary system are affected to mitigate long-term complications. Treatment of drug-induced rashes may include use of IV corticosteroid therapy with or without intravenous immunoglobulin (IVIG) for 5 days. Additionally, cyclosporine combined with plasmapheresis is associated with decreased mortality. TNF-α inhibitors, such as infliximab and etanercept, have produced promising results. Drug-induced rashes may be complicated by infections, including pneumonia, bacteremia, and urinary tract infections (Lofgran & Mahabal, 2021).

Fungal Infection

Tinea corporis, tinea cruris, and tinea pedis are generally responsive to topical creams such as terbinafine (Lamisil) and butenafine (Lotrimin Ultra). The use of oral antifungal agents may be indicated for extensive disease, failed topical treatment, immunocompromised patients, or those with severe moccasin-type tinea pedis. Patients with chronic or recurrent tinea pedis may benefit from wide shoes, drying between the toes after bathing, and placing lamb's wool between the toes. While Nystatin is effective for cutaneous *Candida* infections, it should not be used to treat tinea infections because dermatophytes are resistant to nystatin. Caution should be used with oral ketoconazole when treating tinea infections due to the risk for hepatic toxicity. Combination products such as betamethasone/clotrimazole should not be used as they can aggravate fungal infections (Ely et al., 2014). If central venous catheters (CVCs) are present, they should be removed as early as possible in the course of candidemia when the source is presumed to be the CVC and the catheter can be removed safely (Peter et al., 2016).

TRANSITION OF CARE

Clear communication is essential between all inpatient providers managing the care of patients with irritant or allergic dermatitis as they may present in the emergency department or within the hospital. Following acute treatment in the hospital, management should continue with the patient's primary clinician or dermatologist as corticosteroids are typically prescribed and related side effects will need to be monitored. Patients should be given specific instructions regarding prevention, decontamination, and when to return if symptoms spread or worsen. For those with systemic or respiratory complications, they should be admitted to the hospital for closer observation and management (Lofgran & Mahabal, 2021).

CLINICAL PEARLS

Contact Dermatitis
- Priority is to identify and remove the irritant or allergen.
- Localized acute allergic contact dermatitis lesions are successfully treated with mid- or high-potency steroids (e.g., triamcinolone 0.1% (Kenalog, Aristocort) or clobetasol 0.05% (Temovate).
- Lower potency steroids (e.g., desonide ointment) are effective on thinner skin surfaces (e.g., eyelids or face) and reduce the risk of skin atrophy.
- If allergic contact dermatitis involves >20% of skin, systemic steroid therapy is often required and offers relief within 12 to 24 hours.

Poison Ivy and Oak Dermatitis
- Management includes immediately washing affected skin with soap and water and early application of topical corticosteroids.
- Hospital admission may be warranted with the presence of respiratory or systemic symptoms.

Drug-Induced Rash
- Drug-induced rashes are common and mostly self-limiting; however, some carry a high risk of morbidity and mortality (e.g., SJS, TEN).
- Management includes immediate discontinuation of the suspected drug(s) and supportive treatment.
- Immunomodulatory and/or immunosuppressant agents may be used with caution.

Fungal Infections
- Candida followed by aspergillus are the most common causes of nosocomial fungal infections.
- The degree of immunosuppression correlates with the severity of fungal infection.
- There may be many mimics and the diagnosis can be made by visualization, correlating symptoms, use of KOH, skin biopsy, and fungal culture.
- CVCs should be removed as early as possible in the course of candidemia when the source is presumed to be the CVC.

KEY TAKEAWAYS

Contact Dermatitis
- Identify and remove the irritant or allergen immediately.
- Treatment is based on the severity of symptoms, duration of exposure, location, and extension of the rash.

Poison Ivy and Oak Dermatitis
- The best prevention is to recognize and avoid Toxicodendron plants, use barriers, *and employ decontamination.*
- The rash is self-limiting and irreversible sensitization can occur.
- Treat with moderate to high dose topical or systemic corticosteroids early before the appearance of papules or vesicles.

Drug-Induced Rash
- Most forms are mild though vigilance is needed to recognize severe forms (e.g., Steven-Johnsons syndrome)
- The rash is symmetric and morbilliform, occurring 1 to 3 weeks after a drug is introduced.
- Treatment of drug-induced rashes include use of IV corticosteroid therapy with or without IVIG for 5 days with consideration for cyclosporine combined with plasmapheresis, TNF-α inhibitors.

Fungal Infection
- Risk factors supporting the development of fungal rashes include the presence of diabetes, obesity, increased sweating, microbial colonization, broad-spectrum antibiotics, indwelling central catheter, total parenteral nutrition, immunosuppression, burns, and increased severity of illness.
- Fungal rashes are more erythematous with scaling at the border and or having defined lesions (pustules) at the edge of the rash with complaints of pruritus or burning.
- Topical antifungal creams are useful for tinea corporis, tinea cruris, and tinea pedis whereas oral treatment may be indicated for extensive disease, failed topical treatment, immunocompromised patients, or those with severe moccasin-type tinea pedis.
- Nystatin is effective for cutaneous *Candida* infections though it should not be used to treat tinea infections because dermatophytes are resistant to nystatin.
- Combination products such as betamethasone/clotrimazole should not be used as they can aggravate fungal infections.

EVIDENCE-BASED RESOURCES

American Contact Dermatitis Society. (2020, June 11). *Mission and values.* https://www.contactderm.org/about-acds/mission-and-values

Fonacier, L., Bernstein, D. I., Pacheco, K., Holness, D. L., Blessing-Moore, J., Khan, D., Lang, D., Nicklas, R., Oppenheimer, J., Portnoy, J., Randolph, C., Schuller, D., Spector, S., Tilles, S., & Wallace, D. (2015). Contact dermatitis: A practice parameter–update 2015. *The Journal of Allergy and Clinical Immunology: In Practice, 3*(3), S1–S39. https://doi.org/10.1016/j.jaip.2015.02.009

Food and Drug Administration. (2020, June 11). *Outsmarting poison ivy and other poisonous plants.* https://www.fda.gov/consumers/consumer-updates/outsmarting-poison-ivy-and-other-poisonous-plants

American Academy of Dermatology Association. (2020, June 11). *Poison ivy, oak, and sumac: How to treat the rash.* https://www.aad.org/public/everyday-care/itchy-skin/poison-ivy/treat-rash

Fowler, T., Bansal, A. S., & Lozsádi, D. (2019). Risks and management of antiepileptic drug induced skin reactions in the adult out-patient setting. *Seizure, 72,* 61–70. https://doi.org/10.1016/j.seizure.2019.07.003

Joint Task Force on Practice Parameters; American Academy of Allergy, Asthma and Immunology; American College of Allergy, Asthma and Immunology; Joint Council of Allergy, Asthma and Immunology. (2010). Drug allergy: An updated practice parameter. *Annals of Allergy, Asthma & Immunology, 105*(4), 259–273. https://doi.org/10.1016/j.anai.2010.08.002

Centers for Disease Control and Prevention. (2020, June 11). *Who gets fungal infections?* https://www.cdc.gov/fungal/infections/index.html

Pappas, P. G., Kauffman, C. A., Andes, D. R., Clancy, C. J., Marr, K. A., Ostrosky-Zeichner, L., Reboli, A. C., Schuster, M. G., Vazquez, J. A., Walsh, T. J., Zaoutis, T. E., & Sobel, J. D. (2016). Executive summary: Clinical practice guideline for the management of Candidiasis: 2016 update by the Infectious Diseases Society of America. *Clinical Infectious Diseases, 62*(4), 409–417. https://doi.org/10.1093/cid/civ1194

A robust set of instructor resources designed to supplement this text is located at http://connect.springerpub.com/content/reference-book/978-0-8261-6079-9. Qualifying instructors may request access by emailing textbook@springerpub.com.

REFERENCES

Full list of references can be accessed at http://connect.springerpub.com/content/reference-book/978-0-8261-6079-9.

CHAPTER 15

MUSCULOSKELETAL DISORDERS

Bimbola Akintade, Lisa Fetters, and Sally M. Villaseñor

LEARNING OBJECTIVES

- Recognize the signs and symptoms of a musculo-skeletal injury or disorder.
- Demonstrate a skillful and effective musculo-skeletal examination based on presenting signs, symptoms, and history.
- Differentiate underlying etiologies of musculo-skeletal injuries and disorders.
- Analyze presenting history, pertinent positive and negative examination findings, and differential diagnoses to facilitate an appropriate treatment plan.
- Recognize the need for extensive workup, emergent interventions, hospital admissions, or specialty referrals as indicated.
- Create an effective care plan and transition of care.

INTRODUCTION

AGACNPs who evaluate and care for adults must be able to recognize signs and symptoms and differentiate among the underlying etiologies of musculoskeletal disorders and injuries. A musculoskeletal disorder may arise suddenly and resolve (as in the case of injuries such as fractures, sprains, and strains) but may also progress to lifelong conditions associated with ongoing pain and disability across the lifespan (World Health Organization [WHO], 2019). Musculoskeletal conditions may create disability due to pain, inflammation, loss of dexterity and mobility, or damage to nerve or tissue. Analyzing presenting history, pertinent positive and negative examination findings, and differential diagnoses to facilitate an appropriate treatment plan and transition of care are imperative and may prevent long-term disabilities (WHO, 2019). Recognizing the need for emergent interventions, hospital admissions, or specialty referrals may also mitigate disability and long-term complications.

15.1: ACUTE KNEE INJURY

PRESENTING SIGNS AND SYMPTOMS

Acute knee injuries are one of the most common complaints for which patients seek evaluation and care. Injuries can occur from a variety of mechanisms including overuse; various types of trauma including blunt, rotational, and shear forces caused during sporting activities; or from slips, trips, and falls. The knee is the largest synovial joint in the human body; it is a complex structure, and plays a critical role in a patient's mobility to stand, walk, or run. The bones in the knee joint include the femur, tibia, fibula, and the sesamoid bone (the patella). Along with the soft tissues of the knee, muscles (quadriceps, hamstring, and popliteus), ligaments (medial and lateral collateral ligaments, anterior and posterior cruciate ligaments), and tendons (hamstring, quadriceps, and patellar) provide support and stability to the joint (Figure 15.1).

Patients presenting with knee complaints should have a detailed history taken including mechanism of injury, associated symptoms, location, characteristics of pain, prior surgeries, or injuries to the affected knee area. Characteristics of pain should include rapid or fast onset, location (anterior, posterior, medial, or lateral location), duration, severity, quality of pain (dull vs. sharp), alleviating and exacerbating factors. Patients should be asked if they have noticed any locking of the joint, feeling or hearing a "pop" or "knee giving out." The physical exam of the knee should include inspection above and below the joint and surrounding area assessing for skin color, swelling, ecchymosis, abrasions/lacerations, and observable deformity. If able, the patient should be observed for ability to weight-bear on the lower extremities. The affected knee area should be palpated for warmth, joint tenderness, localized area of discomfort, crepitus, and neurovascular status. Evaluation of the joint should include range of motion (ROM), strength, and knee instability which can indicate internal derangements including meniscal and ligament tears. It is important for the AGACNP to also assess and evaluate the unaffected knee for comparison.

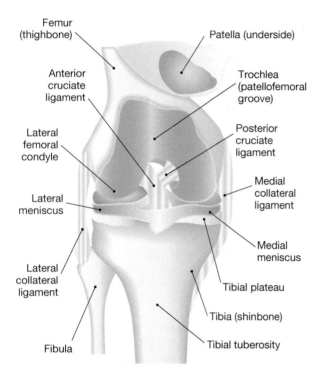

FIGURE 15.1: Anatomical structures of the knee. Frontal view of right knee (with patella reflected).
Source: Stutzman, Z., & Gawlik, K. (2021). Evidence-based assessment of the musculoskeletal system. In K. S. Gawlik, B. M. Melnyk, & A. M. Teall (Eds.), *Evidence-based physical examination: Best practices for health and well-being assessment.* Springer Publishing Company, p. 410, Fig. 15.11.

There are several specialty knee exams which can be utilized to identify specific injuries to the knee (Table 15.1).

HISTORY AND PHYSICAL FINDINGS

Knee Strains

Knee strains occur when there is injury or damage to the muscles and tendons surrounding the knee joint. This can occur from overuse of the joint or increased pressure over the joint area. Signs and symptoms include mild swelling, pain on palpation, and pain with ROM maneuvers.

Knee Sprains (Medial Collateral Ligament, Lateral Collateral Ligament, Anterior Cruciate Ligament, and Posterior Cruciate Ligament)

Knee sprains, on the other hand, occur when there is injury or damage to the ligaments (mMedial collateral ligament [MCL], lateral collateral ligament [LCL], anterior cruciate ligament [ACL[, posterior cruciate ligament [PCL]) of the knee joint and can occur with trauma, slips, trips, falls, or collision with an object.

Medial Collateral Ligament Injury

MCL injuries occur when there is twisting in the leg or by a direct blow causing the knee to move inward into a valgus position stressing the MCL (Brook & Matzkin,

TABLE 15.1: Associated Knee Injuries With Specialty Knee Exam

ASSOCIATED KNEE INJURIES	SPECIALTY KNEE EXAMS
Medial cruciate ligament (MCL) and lateral cruciate ligament (LCL)	• Varus stress test • Valgus stress test
Anterior cruciate ligament (ACL)	• Lachman • Pivot shift • Anterior drawer test
Posterior cruciate ligament (PCL)	• Posterior drawer test • Posterior sag sign
Meniscus injury	• Apley's test • McMurray's test • Thessaly test
Patellar dislocation	• Patella tilt • Patella glide • Apprehension test

2018). Patients often present with point tenderness of the MCL, moderate swelling, and decreased ROM. Patients who experience a full-thickness tear of the MCL will describe severe pain and loss of ROM; they also may develop large effusions (Brook & Matzkin, 2018).

Lateral Collateral Ligament Injury

LCL injuries occur less frequently than MCL injuries. Patient will often present with history of having an injury to the inside of the knee causing varus stress on the LCL. Physical exam demonstrates moderate swelling, point tenderness over LCL and decreased ROM. If the tear in the ligament is full-thickness, the patient can have complete loss of ROM.

Anterior Cruciate Ligament Injury

Patient will report history as a traumatic force during a twisting motion of the knee or sudden change in direction, side stepping, or landing a jump. The patient may describe a "pop" in the knee experienced with extreme pain, immediate swelling, and "knee giving out," and hemarthrosis within 0 to 12 hours after the injury (Logerstedt et al., 2017).

The Lachman test is most sensitive test for ACL tears. It is performed with the patient laying supine or sitting and having the patient bend the knee roughly 20 degrees. The examiner places one hand on the anterior thigh above the patella and the other hand around the tibia and pulls the tibia anteriorly while pushing down on the thigh. A positive Lachman with "soft" end will demonstrate increased anterior tibial translation (Logerstedt et al., 2017).

Posterior Cruciate Ligament Injury

PCL injuries are reported when the knee is in the flexed position and collides with a hard surface. This can be seen when a patient's knee is flexed and strikes the dashboard during a motor vehicle collision. Isolated PCL tears are uncommon and have been estimated at an annual incidence of 2 per 100,000 persons (Sanders et al., 2017)

Patient's typically report severe pain in the posterior knee, the inability to bear weight, instability, decrease in ROM, and hemarthrosis. During the physical exam, the patient can demonstrate a positive sag sign or posterior draw sign. The posterior drawer test is performed with the patient supine; the hip of the affected leg is flexed to approximately 45 degrees, while the knee is flexed 90 degrees, and the foot is left in neutral position. The examiner wraps hands around the patient's proximal tibia with the examiner's thumbs at the tibial tuberosities. Force is applied toward the proximal tibia. Increased posterior displacement greater than the unaffected extremity suggests partial or complete tear of the PCL (Beutler & Alexander, 2021).

Meniscus Injury

Acute MCL injuries typically occur with a twisting motion of the knee while the foot is solidly planted (Babu et al., 2016). Other activities such as cutting, squatting, or testing maneuvers may also cause acute MCL injuries. Patients present with swelling, painful locking of the joint, popping or clicking sensation, as well as feeling like the knee is "giving out." Several specialty knee exams can be completed to help make the diagnosis of a meniscus injury. These exams include Apley's test, McMurray test, and Thessaly test (Babu et al., 2016; Cardone & Jacobs, 2021). The McMurray test involves repeated passive flexion and extension of the knee joint. While performing this test, if the patient reports a painful click while in early to mid-extension, it is suggestive of a meniscal injury (Cardone & Jacobs, 2021).

Knee Dislocation

Knee dislocations can occur as the result of high-energy mechanisms seen in motor vehicle collisions, sport-related activities, all-terrain vehicle accidents, and pedestrians struck by vehicles (Roberson et al., 2016). These injuries can also occur with low-energy injuries such as stepping off a curb in the morbidly obese population (Ockuly et al., 2020). Approximately 50% of knee dislocations can reduce spontaneously before assessment (Gottlieb et al., 2020); providers should remain suspicious of injury based on the mechanism of history and clinical presentation. Symptoms include knee pain, gross swelling, ecchymosis, deformity of knee, hemarthrosis, diffuse ligamentous laxity or instability (Banerjee, 2017; Purcell, Terry, & Allen, 2019). Open injuries have been found in approximately 19% to 35% of cases (Gottlieb et al., 2020); it especially important evaluate the open wound as these injuries require emergency surgical intervention. The most important aspect of the physical exam is to assess for neurovascular status in the distal extremity as 10% to 30% have associated vascular injury which can be limb threatening (Purcell, Terry, & Allen, 2019).

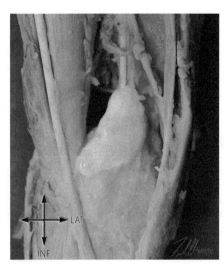

FIGURE 15.2: Baker's Cyst.
Source: Dreviscerator.

Patellar Fracture

Patellar fractures can occur from high or low velocity impacts to the patella. Low velocity fractures can occur after a fall whereas high velocity fractures occur when the knee collides with a dashboard in a motor vehicle collision. Symptoms with this injury are associated with anterior knee pain, swelling, ecchymosis, hemarthrosis, inability for patient to actively extend knee, and gap at the fracture site when palpated (Banerjee, 2017).

Popliteal "Baker's" Cyst

Although a "Baker's" cyst is not associated with an acute knee injury, patients will present for evaluation related to abrupt posterior knee pain and swelling. A Baker's cyst (Figure 15.2) is a fluid-filled pouch located in the popliteal fossa; it is not a true effusion. Often the patient reports pain, swelling, and stiffness with ROM occurring after repetitive flexion and squatting exercises (Carlton & Shmerling, 2021). Physical exam can reveal swelling with a palpable mass located in the popliteal fossa when the knee is extended with the palpable mass disappearing with knee flexion.

Diagnostic Exams: Radiology

When patients present for acute knee pain, a clinical decision rule can help determine the appropriateness of radiology studies. The Ottawa Knee Rule (OKR) provides high diagnostic accuracy for knee fracture (Sims et al., 2020; Stiell, 2021b). Knee studies are required only for patients with knee injuries who meet one of the following requirements:

- Age older than 55 years, OR
- Isolated tenderness of the patella, OR
- Tenderness of the head of the fibula, OR
- Cannot flex knee 90 degrees, OR
- Unable to bear weight immediately and at evaluation for four steps

Plain radiographs, including anterior-posterior, lateral, and sunrise (patella fractures) views of the knee should be obtained to rule out fracture if indicated by the OKR (Stiell, 2021b). Other radiograph films should be considered as an avulsion fracture of the lateral tibia is highly specific for an ACL injury (Banerjee, 2017).

Doppler Ultrasound/Ankle-Brachial Index

In the setting of acute knee injuries when the physical exam is suspicious for neurovascular compromise, especially in the case of knee dislocation, a Doppler ultrasound can be ordered to obtain an ankle-brachial index (ABI) to compare the blood pressure measured at the ankle with the blood pressure measured at the arm. A Doppler ultrasound measures the systolic pressure in the dorsalis pedis or posterior tibial tuberosity by placing a blood pressure cuff around the ankle of the injured knee (Figure 15.3). The ABI value is obtained by dividing the systolic blood pressure in the arm on the same side of the injured limb by the systolic pressure of that limb. Any value above 0.9 suggests normal arterial flow in the extremity. If the value is abnormal then a computed tomography (CT) angiogram should be performed (Hoit et al., 2019).

Magnetic Resonance Imaging

For acute knee injuries, magnetic resonance imaging (MRI) is a useful noninvasive diagnostic exam with high diagnostic accuracy and sensitivity for internal derangements of the knee joint. MRI is considered the gold standard for determining ligamentous and meniscal injuries (Brook & Matzkin, 2018; Hoit et al., 2019; Sharma et al., 2020).

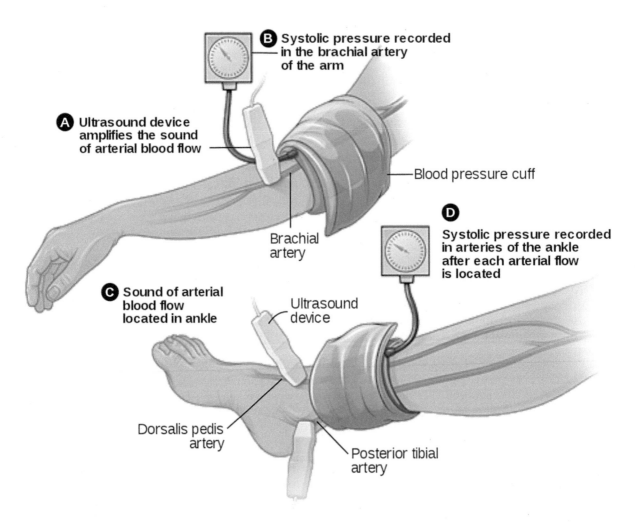

FIGURE 15.3: Ankle brachial index. How to obtain the ABI.
Source: National Heart, Lung, and Blood Institute. (2020). *Peripheral artery disease*. https://www.nhlbi.nih.gov/health-topics/peripheral-artery-disease

DIFFERENTIAL DIAGNOSIS AND DIAGNOSTIC CONSIDERATIONS

Differential diagnoses for knee injury include but are not limited to:

- Sprain/strain
- Fractures—patella, fibula
- Medial and lateral collateral ligament tear
- Anterior or posterior cruciate ligament tear
- Gout
- Patella dislocation
- Meniscus tear
- Osteoarthritis
- Effusion, hemarthrosis
- Septic joint
- Bursitis
- Baker's cyst

TREATMENT

Minor Sprains, Strains, and Contusions

For patients with minor sprains, strains, and contusions after an acute knee injury, nonpharmacologic measures consist of rest, ice, compression, and elevation (RICE) with elevation of the injured knee joint. If applicable, crutches or assistive devices for the patient's mobility may be ordered. In most instances, nonopioid pharmacologicalmanagement can help with minor pain control. Recent research has demonstrated acetaminophen being as effective as NSAIDs in treating pain in adults with minor musculoskeletal injuries (Ridderikhof et al., 2019).

Anterior and Posterior Cruciate Ligament Injuries

Management of patients with acute ACL injuries should include RICE and analgesic medications.

If the knee is unstable, patients should be given crutches and told to avoid bearing weight on the affected limb. The patient should be referred to PT and given a consult to an orthopedic specialist.

Patients should be fitted with a hinged knee brace or knee immobilizer to keep the affected knee extended for 2 weeks. The patient should be given crutches and instructed to have limited weight bearing on the affected limb. Patients can be referred to PT to strengthen muscles around the knee including the quadriceps for optimal recovery (Logerstedt et al., 2017; MacDonald & Rodenberg, 2021).

Medial and Lateral Collateral Ligament Injuries

Management of patients with a moderate sprain or partial tear of the MCL or LCL should include RICE and analgesic medications. If there is instability of the joint, the patient should be fitted with a functional knee brace to prevent valgus stress and given crutches. Patients should be referred to PT to increase proximal muscle strength (Brooke & Matzkin, 2018). Patients with full-thickness tears should be referred for an orthopedic surgical consult.

Meniscus Injury

Management of meniscus injuries consist of RICE and analgesic medications. The patient should be fitted with a patellar-restraining brace, especially if the patient feels the "knee is giving out" often and should be given crutches. The patient should be told to avoid any deep knee flexion movements such as repetitive bending by going up and down stairs, squatting, kneeling, twisting, and pivoting. The patient should be referred to physical therapy (PT) to strengthen the muscles surrounding the knee and referred to orthopedic surgeon for any complaints of knee "locking" (Babu et al., 2016; Cardone & Jacobs, 2021).

Knee Dislocation

Knee dislocations are considered an orthopedic emergency needing prompt diagnosis and treatment to prevent nerve and vascular injuries to the affected extremity. Knee dislocations need prompt reduction by experienced providers. Several items can be completed while waiting for the specialty team to arrive to complete the reduction. Splint the affected knee with a knee immobilizer or rigid splint to provide comfort and protection of soft tissues from additional injuries. The knee immobilizer or rigid splint should extend superior and inferior to the knee joint, the knee slightly flexed 15 degrees to allow normal blood flow. This can be done by placing a rolled towel behind the knee. Obtain prereduction films to identify fractures and perform the ABI. If neurovascular compromise is suspected, consult a vascular surgeon and prep the patient for an arteriogram. Knee dislocations can be extremely painful; provide analgesic medications and prepare the patient for sedation prior to the knee reduction. In cases where there is an open wound associated with a knee dislocation, place an emergent orthopedic surgery consult and prepare the patient for the operating room.

Patellar Fractures

If the patellar fracture is nondisplaced, nonpharmacologic measures consist of RICE with analgesic medication. The patient should be fitted for a knee immobilizer or brace and given crutches. If the patella fracture is displaced or there is loss of extensor function in the affected limb, consult an orthopedic specialist and prepare the patient for the operating room and hospital admission.

Baker's Cyst

Conservative management of a Baker's cyst consists of resting of the extremity and ACE wrap as needed. For pain and discomfort, nonopioid medications including acetaminophen and NSAIDs can be given. If the provider is experienced, the Baker's cyst can be aspirated. Glucocorticoid injections have been found to decrease discomfort and swelling (Helfgott et al., 2021).

CLINICAL PEARLS

- The knee is the largest synovial joint in the human body; it is a complex structure.
- There are several specialty knee exams which can be utilized to identify specific injuries to the knee.
- The OKR provides high diagnostic accuracy for knee fracture.
- Knee dislocations are considered an orthopedic emergency needing prompt diagnosis and treatment.
- The ABI can be used to assess for neurovascular compromise.

EVIDENCE-BASED RESOURCES

The OKR (http://www.theottawarules.ca/knee_rules)
Ottawa Rules App for iPad and iPhone (https://apps.apple
.com/ca/app/the-ottawa-rules/id1104004722)
Ottawa Rules App for Android (https://play.google.com/
store/apps/details?id=ca.ohri.ottawarules&hl=en)

15.2: ACUTE LOW BACK PAIN

PRESENTING SIGNS AND SYMPTOMS

Low back pain (historically called "lumbago") is often chronically related to a combination of overuse, poor posture, gluteal and core muscle deconditioning (National Institutes of Health [NIH], National Institute of Neurological Disorders and Stroke [NINDS], 2020; U.S. Department of Health and Human Resources, Centers for Disease Control and Prevention [CDC], 2020) resulting in symptoms consistent with strain (pain in the muscles and joints of the lower back). The lumbar and sacral spine with associated soft tissues and nerves are the anatomical origins of low back pain (Norris & Lalchandani, 2018a). Axial low back pain, per definition, will involve an isolated area of the back and may include neuropathic radiating pain (NINDS, 2020). Underlying etiology is most commonly nonspecific or mechanical (DePalma, 2020). However, injuries from a variety of traumatic mechanisms such as falls, heavy lifting, motor vehicle accidents, sports-related activities, or work-related activities may be an underlying cause of low back pain resulting in fractures, contusions, or sprains (Norris & Lalchandani, 2018a). Bony/spinal pain-causing etiologies can include osteoarthritis, nerve compression syndromes, and intervertebral disc disruptions (Norris & Lalchandani, 2018a).

The hallmark presenting symptoms of low back pain are self-identified in the areas of the lumbar and/or sacral spine; they involve pain, tightness, spasms which are exacerbated by mechanical movements such as bending, twisting, standing up, sitting down, and walking. The AGACNP may visibly appreciate signs of pain including facial grimacing and crying, bent or stooped posture, slow or guarded gait. The AGACNP may also elicit tender musculature, muscle spasms, decreased or limited range of motion (ROM), loss of function or strength on exam. Sometimes, patients will report symptoms of paresthesia (tingling) in a unilateral lower extremity, and rarely, weakness or hypoesthesia (numbness) in the lower extremity. If new onset or progressively worsening, radicular symptoms should be evaluated promptly and correlated with the physical exam to ascertain if neurologic compromise exists from spinal or nerve root compression (DePalma, 2020).

Risk factors for low back pain can include older age, obesity, poor general health, repetitive physical stress on the spine, pregnancy, and psychological stressors (DePalma, 2020; NINDS, 2020). Anticoagulation, immunocompromise, fever or chills, intravenous drug abuse (IVDA), history of cancer, and history of recent surgery or epidural injection are historical red flags (Table 15.2). Adults older than 50 with a new onset of low back pain are of higher clinical suspicion for compression fractures, cancer/tumors, infection, or intraabdominal processes which could radiate to the low back such as abdominal aortic aneurysm or nephrolithiasis (DePalma, 2020). Individuals that are anticoagulated or take an antiplatelet drug may be at risk for epidural hematoma which could cause spinal cord or nerve root compression. Complaints of fever and chills or findings of elevated temperature can indicate an infectious process; a classic triad of fever, neurologic deficit, and low back pain is present in 10% of patients with an epidural abscess (DePalma, 2020). Immunocompromised individuals and those with history of drug use are at higher risk for infection; epidural abscess from bacteremia could occur in patients that are known intravenous drug abusers. Any combination of weakness or loss of lower extremity function (unilateral or bilateral), perineal numbness ("saddle paresthesia"), loss of bowel or bladder control, decreased or poor rectal tone, reported male sexual impotence indicate a need to rule out cauda equina or conus medullaris nerve root compression.

TABLE 15.2: Red Flag Symptoms and Risk Factors

RED FLAG SYMPTOMS	RED FLAG HISTORICAL RISK FACTORS
• Decreased or poor rectal tone • Fever or chills • Loss of bowel or bladder control • Perineal numbness ("saddle paresthesia") • Reported male sexual impotence • Severe pain • Weakness or loss of lower extremity function (unilateral or bilateral)	• Age over 50 with new onset low back pain • Anticoagulation • History of cancer • History of recent surgery or epidural injection • Immunocompromise • Intravenous drug abusers (IVDAs)

HISTORY AND PHYSICAL FINDINGS

The history and physical examination should identify and evaluate for (a) neurologic deficits such as lumbar or sacral radiculopathies and neurogenic claudication; (b) red flag symptoms of malignancy, fracture, or infections; and (c) psychosocial factors (North American Spine Society, 2020; Pangarkar et al., 2019).

History

Common descriptors from patients may include "my back went out" or "I bent over and couldn't stand up" after describing a simple daily activity or a traumatic episode, such as those listed previously. Parents and grandparents often attribute their low back pain to lifting and carrying their children/grandchildren. There may be a history of similar back issues (chronic or acute on chronic onset) versus new onset (acute onset) of low back pain. Patients with previous episodes might describe, for example, "sciatica flare" or "muscle spasm" or "arthritis acting up." They may also report attempts at self-mitigation such as use of over-the-counter (OTC) analgesics, heating pad, ice packs, or use of old prescription medications for pain or spasm. Patients with new onset may have made the same mitigating efforts but will have no experiential frame of reference for self-treatment.

It is imperative that the AGACNP inquire about location of pain, radiation of pain (buttocks, groin, leg, foot), laterality of pain, intensity of pain, perception of strength loss, and location/laterality of associated symptoms of numbness or tingling (North American Spine Society [NASS], 2020). Presence of bowel and/or bladder incontinence or urinary retention should be queried, along with symptoms of sexual impotence in male patients. Self-treatment attempts should be discussed, focusing on effectiveness versus ineffectiveness. Psychosocial factors such as depression, generalized anxiety, posttraumatic stress disorder, interpersonal stress at home or work, job satisfaction, sleep quality, job-related ergonomics are correlated with chronic low back pain (NASS, 2020). Table 15.2 outlines red flag symptoms and risk factors.

Physical Exam

A focused physical examination of the low back and lower extremities is required of the AGACNP. Physical examination findings may include tender lumbar paraspinal musculature, tender sacroiliac (SI) joints, mild to severe muscle spasms, and decreased ROM with bending or twisting. Less often, midline bony lumbar or sacral spinal tenderness will be found. Numbness or tingling sensations reported by the patient may be distributed along a lumbar or sacral dermatome (Figure 15.4).

First, a visual examination of the low back should occur to check for bruises/ecchymosis, wounds, or pain-inducing rashes (such as varicella zoster). Next, palpation of the lumbar and sacral bony and soft tissues areas will help identify bony and/or muscle tenderness, muscle

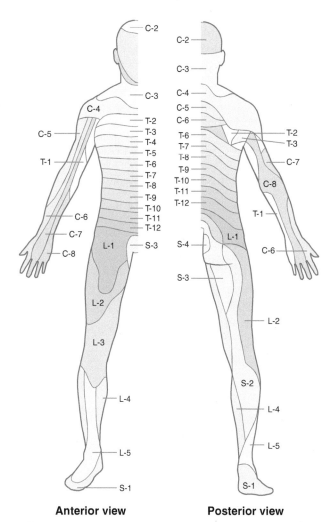

Anterior view   **Posterior view**

FIGURE 15.4: Dermatomes. Anterior and posterior view of dermatomal distribution.
Source: Chiocca, E. M. (2019). Assessment of the neurologic system assessment of the neurologic system of the pediatric patient. In *Advanced pediatric assessment* (3rd ed.). Springer Publishing Company, p. 487, Fig. 22.06.

spasms, and tightness which could be bilateral or unilateral. The AGACNP should then visualize the patient's ability to move through ROM of the lumbar spine (i.e., bending forward, leaning back, side to side tilt, and twisting in both directions) and note any movements that exacerbate or reproduce the pain. To identify decreased ROM, it is best to assist the patient to a standing position.

A focused neurologic examination is necessary to exclude functional abnormalities and strength loss (NASS, 2020; Pangarkar et al., 2019). Testing of functional movements related to lumbar and sacral nerve roots can be done, noting any deficits. Motor and sensory assessments are necessary for complaints of paresthesia or lower extremity weakness. Motor strength should be assessed and compared bilaterally. If paresthesia (tingling) or hypoesthesia (numbness) are reported by the patient, examination of light touch (nylon microfilament or cotton swab) and pin prick should be assessed in the dermatomes to determine the nerve root involved. Bilateral reflex comparisons can assess for hyperreflexia (associated with upper motor neuron lesion) or hyporeflexia (associated with lower motor neuron lesion or compression). A positive Babinski is suggestive of upper motor neuron lesion. A digital rectal exam can be performed if indicated to evaluate anal sphincter sensation and muscle tone (comparing relaxed versus contracted). Table 15.3 outlines various nerve root/dermatome-related evaluations for the focused neurologic examination with low back pain.

Other examination techniques for the low back might involve evaluation of SI joint stability to diagnose SI joint pain or dysfunction. One hypothesis is that SI joint pain is caused by stress from asymmetry within the pelvic ring (anterior or posterior displacement/torsion) creating a positional change within one or both SI joints and stressing the structures attached to the innominates (hip bones of the pelvic girdle). Another theory of SI joint pain is that SI joint hypomobility, with or without concomitant innominate torsional asymmetry, is causative (Levangie, 1999). The five provocative tests for the SI joints are summarized in Table 15.4. Accuracy of detecting SI joint dysfunction is increased when at least three of the five tests are positive (Levangie, 1999). For a test to

TABLE 15.3: Nerve Root/Dermatome-Related Evaluations for the Focused Neurologic Examination of Low Back Pain

LUMBAR AND SACRAL NERVE ROOT	LOCATION OF DERMATOME FOR PIN PRICK/ LIGHT TOUCH ASSESSMENT	MOTOR STRENGTH ASSESSMENT	REFLEX ASSESSMENT
L-1	Back, over trochanter, anterior and inner surfaces of leg	Iliopsoas strength with hip flexion	
L-2	Back, anterior and inner surfaces of thigh	Iliopsoas strength with hip flexion	Patellar
L-3	Back, upper buttock, anterior and inner thigh and knee, medial lower leg	Quadriceps strength with knee extension	Patellar
L-4	Medial buttock, lateral thigh, medial leg, dorsum of foot, medial side of big toe	Anterior lower leg muscles with ankle dorsiflexion	Patellar
L-5	Buttock, posterior and lateral thigh, lateral aspect of leg, dorsum of foot, medial half of sole, and first, second, and third toes	Extensor halucis longus strength with big toe extension/dorsiflexion	
S-1	Buttock, posterior and outer surfaces of thighs, lateral foot, lateral malleolus, and little toe	Gastrocnemius and soleus strength with ankle plantar-flexion	Ankle
S-2	Buttock, posterior and outer surfaces of thighs, lateral heel, perineum	Hamstring strength	Ankle
S-3	Medial thigh to knee, groin, perineum	Not applicable	
S-4	Perineum, genitals, lower sacrum	Not applicable	
S-5	Perineum, skin around rectum	Not applicable	

TABLE 15.4: Tests for Sacroiliac (SI) Joint Dysfunction

TEST	DESCRIPTION
Gaenslen's test	Applies torsional stress on the SI joints with nonaffected side in full flexion
FABER (flexion, abduction, external rotation) test	Applies tensile force on the anterior aspect of the SI joint on the side tested
Femoral shear test	Also known as thigh thrust; applies anteroposterior shear stress on the SI joint
Sacral compression test	Applies compression force across the SI joints with patient lying on one side
Anterior superior iliac spin (ASIS) test	Distraction which applies tensile forces on the anterior aspect of the SI joints with patient supine

Accuracy of detecting SI joint dysfunction is increased when at least 3 of the 5 tests are positive.

be positive, it must reproduce the patient's typical pain in their SI joint region.

DIFFERENTIAL DIAGNOSIS AND DIAGNOSTIC CONSIDERATIONS

Axial low back pain can sometimes be considered a syndrome with both nociceptive and neuropathic pain components (mixed pain). Suboptimal outcomes may result from both missed diagnoses and misdiagnosis (DePalma, 2020; Paganoni, 2018). It is important to consider differential possibilities and ascertain the most likely etiology.

Differential diagnoses for low back pain include but are not limited to:

- Ankylosing spondylitis
- Compression fractures (osteoporosis)
- Infection (IVDA, immunosuppression)
- Intervertebral disc dysfunction (bulging/herniated disc)
- Low back pain (lumbago)
- Low back sprain
- Low back strain
- Osteoarthritis
- SI junction sprain or dysfunction
- Sciatica
- Spinal stenosis
- Spondylolisthesis
- Traumatic injury (fractures)

Routinely obtaining imaging studies or invasive diagnostic tests for patients with acute axial low back pain without red flags (Table 15.2) or clinical suspicion of pathology is not recommended by evidence-based practice guidelines (Jenkins et al., 2018; Pangarkar et al., 2019). However, diagnostic imaging is indicated when red flag symptoms or neurologic deficits are present (Jenkins et al., 2018; Pangarkar et al., 2019). If ankylosing spondylitis, cancer, compression, or traumatic fracture is suspected, a plain film lumbosacral radiographic image (x-ray) could be obtained initially (Pangarkar et al., 2019). In cases with red flag symptoms or physical exam findings pointing to infection, severe spinal stenosis, cauda equina syndrome, or conus medullaris syndrome, an emergent MRI is indicated (Jenkins et al., 2018; Pangarkar et al., 2019). Follow-up MRI can be obtained to further evaluate spinal fractures, intervertebral disc dysfunction, or mild-moderate cases of spinal stenosis.

Any combination of weakness or loss of lower extremity function (unilateral or bilateral), perineal numbness ("saddle paresthesia"), loss of bowel or bladder control, decreased or poor rectal tone, reported male sexual impotence indicate that a thorough evaluation with MRI is needed to exclude cauda equina or conus medullaris nerve root compression and to determine the etiology of said compression (e.g., disc herniation, epidural abscess, or hematoma, tumor). Cauda equina syndrome occurs when the nerve roots of the cauda equina (levels L1–L5) are compressed and disrupt motor and sensory func-

tion to the lower extremities and bladder, potentially leading to permanent paralysis or incontinence. Conus medullaris syndrome results when there is compressive damage to the terminal end of the spinal cord at levels T12–L2. Signs and symptoms of these syndromes are overlapping; patients are often admitted to the hospital as a medical emergency.

TREATMENT

Most cases of acute low back pain remit without complications in 2 to 6 weeks regardless of treatment (DePalma, 2020; Paganoni, 2018; Qaseem et al., 2020). PT, analgesics, and muscle relaxants can help. Very few cases may require surgery (Qaseem et al., 2020). Whenever possible, nonpharmacologic options should be attempted; therapies with the lowest costs and fewest potential harm should be considered (Qaseem et al., 2020). It is within the scope of practice of the AGACNP to educate the patient regarding recommended exercises and stretches, ergonomics, and avoidance of activities that exacerbate pain. Therapeutic measures can also include instructions regarding application of ice packs or heating pad, or advice to seek a therapeutic massage (Qaseem et al., 2020). Chronic cases of low back pain may require referrals for cognitive behavioral therapy if psychosocial etiological association is suspected (Pangarkar et al., 2019). The AGACNP may also educate the patient about methods of mindfulness and stress reduction (Pangarkar et al., 2019).

Acute pain that does not respond to nonpharmacologic measures can be managed with over-the-counter (OTC) analgesics such as acetaminophen, and NSAIDs such as ibuprofen and naproxen (Paganoni, 2018; Pangarkar et al., 2019; Qaseem et al., 2020); dosing and frequency recommendations should be provided for the patient. Acetaminophen is not recommended for chronic low back pain unless it is secondary to osteoarthritis (Pangarkar et al., 2019). Prescription analgesics such as opioids or NSAIDs can be provided if OTC products were reported ineffective by the patient. Muscle relaxants, antidepressants, and benzodiazepines can be adjuvant pain control (Paganoni, 2018; Pangarkar et al., 2019; Qaseem et al., 2017) and are sometimes prescribed alongside an OTC or prescription analgesic. Occasionally corticosteroids are utilized short term if an inflammatory etiology is suspected; however, many guidelines do not support their use (Pangarkar et al., 2019; Qaseem et al., 2020). Neuropathic pain agents (duloxetine, gabapentin, pregabalin) are adjuvant considerations for cases of nerve compression and chronic low back pain (Pangarkar et al., 2019). NSAIDs should be regarded as first line therapy, and opioids and adjuvants as second line (Paganoni, 2018; Pangarkar et al., 2019; Qaseem et al., 2020).

In some settings, it is appropriate to provide rescue measures for moderate to severe pain such as intramuscular injections of opioids (morphine, hydromorphone),

NSAIDs (ketorolac), corticosteroids (solu-medrol, depo-medrol), plus or minus an oral or intramuscular muscle relaxant (diazepam, cyclobenzaprine) (Qaseem et al., 2017). Pain management efforts should always involve joint decision-making with the patient with education regarding safety and potential side effects.

Trigger point injections can be used to treat pain associated with low back pain due to spasm (U.S. Department of Health and Human Resources, Pain Management Best Practices Inter-Agency Task Force [DHHS], 2019). Trigger points are palpable, tense bands of skeletal muscle fibers that, upon compression, can produce both local and referred pain. Using either dry needling or injections of local anesthesia, trigger points can be disrupted, resulting in relaxation and lengthening of the muscle fiber, thereby providing pain relief (DHHS, 2019). Local anesthesia can include lidocaine 1% or 2% or bupivacaine; the anesthetic is sometimes combined with a long-acting corticosteroid like depo-medrol.

PT referrals are often indicated; however, AGACNP ability to independently prescribe PT varies by state.

TRANSITION OF CARE

Typically, the AGACNP will refer the patient back to their PCP for long-term management. At times, it is appropriate for the AGACNP to make a referral for a PT evaluation and treatment of the patient, even if the patient has a PCP. Depending on the history, onset, mechanism of injury, or severity of signs/symptoms, the patient might be referred to physical medicine and rehabilitation (PM&R), pain management services, neurology, orthopedics, sports medicine, or another applicable specialist. Depending on the practice setting of the initial encounter, the patient with red flags or neurologic deficits might be transferred to the emergency department or admitted to the hospital with appropriate specialty consult. Care transitions are best facilitated with thorough documentation of the patient visit and a verbal handoff to ensure understanding of transition rationale.

CLINICAL PEARL

- Nonpharmacologic measures should be recommended with both acute and chronic low back pain.

KEY TAKEAWAYS

- Low back pain is a common complaint treated by NPs in many settings.
- A thorough history and physical examination with ability to identify red flags can differentiate nonspecific and pathologic etiologies, allowing the AGACNP to choose the appropriate treatment.
- Nonpharmacologic measures should be used whenever possible.
- There is often a psychosocial component to low back pain.

- NSAIDs are first line analgesics for management of low back pain.
- Care transitions are best facilitated with thorough documentation of the patient visit and a verbal handoff.

EVIDENCE-BASED RESOURCES

National Institute for Health and Care Excellence (NICE) Guideline on Low Back Pain with or without Sciatica (https://www.nice.org.uk/guidance/ng59)

North American Spine Society Evidence-Based Clinical Guidelines for Multidisciplinary Spine Care: Diagnosis and Treatment of Low Back Pain: (https://www.spine.org/Portals/0/assets/downloads/ResearchClinicalCare/Guidelines/LowBackPaiL.pdf)

U.S. Department of Veterans Affairs and the U.S. Department of Defense Evidence-Based Practice Work Group Clinical Practice Guideline: Diagnosis and Treatment of Low Back Pain: (https://www.healthquality.va.gov/guidelines/Pain/lbp/)

15.3: ANKLE STRAINS AND SPRAINS

PRESENTING SIGNS AND SYMPTOMS

Ankle strains and sprains are common injuries seen in patients who participate in sports that involve running, jumping, or dancing, but can occur accidentally with normal daily activities, falls, or motor vehicle collisions (MVC; Delahunt et al., 2018). Injury can include damage to the tendons, which connect muscle to bone; ligaments, which hold bones together; or the cartilage that covers the articular surface (Norris & Lalchandani, 2018c).

Ankle strain and sprain may present similarly; although there is some overlapping of clinical management, there should be differentiation between the etiologies. A strain involves injurious stretching or tearing of a muscle and/or a tendon and is often related to overuse or repeated mechanical overloading (Norris & Lalchandani, 2018b). A sprain is more often related to an acute injury and there is a stretching and/or tearing of ligaments usually caused by excessive involuntary twisting or unusual movement of the joint (Norris & Lalchandani, 2018b; Ortega-Avila et al., 2020). Both types of injury will exhibit signs of inflammation such as localized soft tissue swelling, edema, redness, and tenderness (U.S. Department of Health and Human Resources, National Institutes of Health, National Institute of Arthritis and Musculoskeletal and Skin Diseases, 2015). However, the onset of swelling from a sprain will present more rapidly. In the case of the sprain, there additionally may be signs of acute soft tissue and microvascular injury such as ecchymosis. Patients will describe symptomatology of pain with weight-bearing activities and movements of the ankle. The AGACNP will further see signs of altered gait such as limping or avoidance of using the affected extremity.

HISTORY AND PHYSICAL FINDINGS

The history and physical examination should identify and evaluate for (a) intensity and onset of pain; (b) presence of known injury mechanism versus overuse (c) function, joint stability, and range of motion {ROM}, (d) associated fractures; and (e) neurovascular status (Delahunt et al., 2018; Ortega-Avila et al., 2020; Strudwick et al., 2018). Per the International Ankle Consortium, one should also inquire about history of previous ankle sprain, as chronic joint instability can occur (Delahunt et al., 2018).

History

History preceding a strain may be described as onset of ankle pain that persists or "flares" up with particular activities or movements and may not be associated with a known injury. For example, one may report "ankle pain occurs each time I take a long walk" yet there is no ankle pain with other activities. Strain is typically related to overuse which is excessive or repeated use of the affected body part. For example, in the case of the ankle, overuse could occur with walking, jogging, dancing on a regular basis, or work-related overuse involving walking or standing on a hard surface for long periods.

On the other hand, an ankle sprain is typically acute onset with an identifiable accidental injury, such as "stepped off a curb," "slipped on the ice," "stepped in a hole." A sprain often has a mechanism of injury easily recalled by the patient such as a "sudden twisting" or "rolled the ankle," and some patients report hearing a snapping or popping sound. Twisting injury can occur as pronation with external rotation or supination with internal rotation beyond the structural limits of the joint. Identifying (if known by the patient) the direction of the twisting will help guide the examination and consideration of differentials (Ortega-Avila et al., 2020).

Physical Exam

Considerations with ankle injury will include initial assessment of neurovascular status, palpation of posterior tibial and dorsalis pedis pulses, assessment of capillary refill in toes, as well as skin temperature and movements of the ankle, foot, and toes for signs of neurovascular or functional compromise (Delahunt et al., 2018).

When examining any joint, it is good clinical practice to examine the joints above and below the injury, and all associated structures (Gribble, 2019). Starting with the ankle, one can then progress to the knee and foot. Presence or absence of bony tenderness should be assessed, and this will help determine a need for imaging to rule out associated fractures (Ortega-Avila et al., 2020; Stiell et al., 1993). Starting with the ankle, the Ottawa Ankle Rules (OAR) is an easy, reliable, evidence-based examination technique to employ (Gribble, 2019; Stiell et al., 1993; Strudwick et al., 2018). The AGACNP will palpate

the bones of the lateral malleolus posterior edge and tip, and base of the fifth metatarsal laterally, followed by the medial malleolus posterior edge and tip plus the navicular bone medially (Figure 15.5). Per the OAR: If bony tenderness is identified in one of the four areas, plain film or digital ankle x-rays are indicated; if there is no bony tenderness yet the patient is unable to bear weight or walk at least four steps on the affected ankle, ankle x-rays are indicated (Stiell, 2021a). Otherwise, imaging is done on a case-by-case basis (considering suspected grade of sprain; Box 15.1) and typically is of little use when diagnosing a soft tissue injury such as an ankle

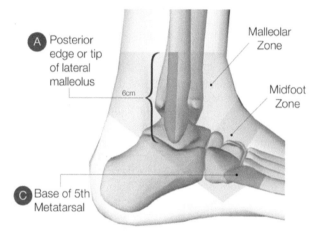

Lateral View

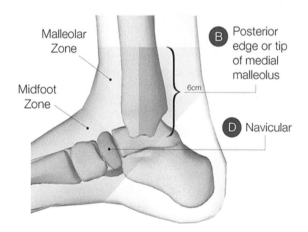

Medial View

FIGURE 15.5: Lateral and medial views of the ankle with Ottawa Ankle Rules. Per the Ottawa Ankle Rules, imaging studies to evaluate for fractures are indicated if there is bony tenderness at any of these sites: (A) posterior edge or tip of the lateral malleolus, (B) posterior edge or tip of the medial malleolus, (C) base of the fifth metatarsal, (D) navicular. In the absence of bony tenderness, x-rays are indicated if the patient is unable to bear weight or ambulate at least four steps on the affected ankle.

Source: Reproduced with permission from Stiell, I. G. (2021a). *The Ottawa ankle rules.* http://www.theottawarules.ca/ankle_rules

BOX 15.1 GRADES OF SPRAIN

Grade 1: Mild sprain of the ligament; slight stretching and microscopic tearing of the ligament fibers; mild tenderness and swelling around the ankle

Grade 2: Moderate sprain with hematoma formation; partial tearing of the ligament; moderate tenderness and swelling around the ankle; abnormal looseness of the ankle joint

Grade 3: Severe sprain with total disruption of the ligament; complete tear of the ligament; significant tenderness and swelling around the ankle; substantial instability of the ankle joint

Grade 4: Severe sprain with avulsion at the bony insertion of the ligament

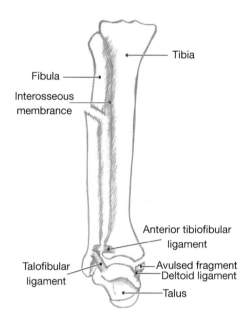

FIGURE 15.6: Maisonneuve fracture. Maisonneuve fracture is unstable, involves a proximal fibula fracture (1), and widening of the medial clear space (2) suggesting ruptured anterior tibiofibular, talofibular, and deltoid ligaments.
Source: Reproduced from Brown, D. P., Freeman, E. D., Cuccurullo, S. J., Maitin, I. B., Parikh, S., & Delavaux, L. (2019). Musculoskeletal medicine. In S. J. Cuccurullo (Ed.), *Physical medicine and rehabilitation board review* (4th ed.). Springer Publishing Company, p. 263, Fig. 4.129.

strain or sprain (Delahunt et al., 2018; Ortega-Avila et al., 2020; Strudwick et al., 2018). This can be used as a teachable moment as patients may question the reasons for not receiving an x-ray for the ankle injury.

In addition to palpating the bones of the midfoot (navicular and fifth metatarsal base), the remainder of the foot and toes should be checked for bony tenderness. Bony tenderness of the metatarsals or toes supports imaging of the foot or toes as indicated by the exam. The focus of the knee exam should include palpation of the fibular head and progress down the length of the fibula to assess for Maisonneuve fracture (Strudwick et al., 2018) which is a fracture of the proximal fibula with an unstable ankle injury (widening of the ankle mortise on x-ray), often comprising ligamentous injury (distal tibiofibular syndesmosis, deltoid ligament [DL]) and/or fracture of the medial malleolus. In the case of a suspected Maisonneuve fracture, a plain film or digital tibia-fibula x-ray series is indicated (the entire fibula should be visualized). Another indication for a tibia-fibula series is a widened medial clear space (the space between the groove of the distal tibial prominence and the medial margin of the distal fibula) of the ankle joint on the ankle x-ray; this widening suggests ruptured anterior tibiofibular, talofibular, and DLs associated with the Maisonneuve fracture (Figure 15.6).

Occasionally a chip of bone may be pulled loose by a ligamentous stretch, commonly known as an avulsion fracture; this type of fracture will be visible on ankle x-rays. If an avulsion is associated with a complete ligament disruption, then it is also consistent with a Grade 4 sprain. Box 15.1 describes Grades 1 to 4 sprains, with Grade 1 considered a mild sprain and Grades 2 to 4 progressing in severity (Haddad, 2016).

Function and ROM are important examinations to determine the extent of the injury and often the extent of the patient's pain. Determining the location of the pain during motion helps in diagnosis and treatment (Gribble, 2019; Haddad, 2016). The patient can be asked to actively perform ROM, or the AGACNP can passively facilitate the movements of the ankle (flexion/extension,

eversion/inversion) noting which movements cause pain. This is key to determining the suspected underlying ligamentous injury and making the appropriate diagnosis (Gribble, 2019; Haddad, 2016). Table 15.5 describes the ligaments anatomically associated with ankle ROM which can be used as a diagnostic guide and Figure 15.7 identifies the ankle joint ligaments medially and laterally.

Anterior Talofibular Ligament Sprain

An anterior drawer test can determine stability of the anterior talofibular ligament (ATFL). The patient can be placed in supine lying or sitting position with the knee in 90 degrees flexed position to relax the calf (gastrocnemius) muscles and prevent the patient from resisting the examiner. One hand stabilizes the distal tibia and fibula while the other hand holds the calcaneus maintaining the ankle in a neutral position or 10 degrees of plantar flexion. The calcaneus is pulled anteriorly while the tibia and fibula are pushed posteriorly; both ankles should be compared. Excessive anterior translation of the talus on the injured side in comparison to the uninjured side indicates a positive test and possible tear of the ATFL (Delahunt et al., 2018; Gribble, 2019).

Calcaneo-Fibular Ligament Sprain

An inversion stress test (also called talar-tilt inversion) examines the stability of the calcaneo-fibular ligament (CFL) on the lateral side of the ankle. The patient can

TABLE 15.5: Determining Ligaments and Tendons Involved in a Strain or Sprain

LIGAMENT OR TENDON	PAIN-ELICITING MOVEMENT OR FUNCTIONAL DEFICIT	STABILITY EXAMINATION(S)
Achilles tendon	Painful, weak, or absent ankle and foot dorsiflexion or extension	Thompson test
Anterior-inferior tibiofibular ligament (AITFL)	Painful dorsiflexion	External rotation test (Kleiger's)
Anterior talofibular ligament (ATFL)	Painful inversion	Anterior drawer test
Calcaneo-fibular ligament (CFL)	Painful inversion	Inversion stress test (talar-tilt inverted)
Deltoid ligament (DL)	Painful eversion or dorsiflexion	Eversion stress test (talar-tilt everted); External rotation test (Kleiger's)
Posterior-inferior tibiofibular ligament (PITFL)	Painful dorsiflexion	External rotation test (Kleiger's)

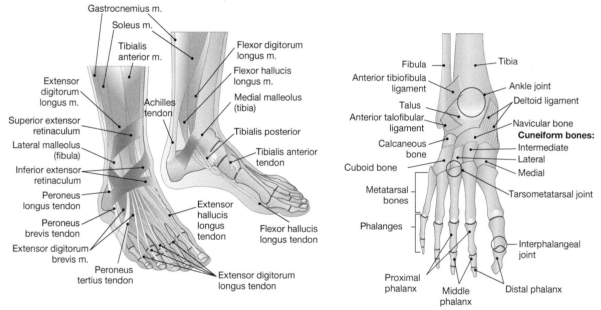

FIGURE 15.7: Ligaments of the medial and lateral ankle joint. Lateral ankle ligaments: anterior and posterior talofibular, calcaneofibular; medial ankle ligaments: deltoid (anterior and posterior tibiotalar, tibiocalcaneal, tibionavicular).
Source: Reproduced from Stutzman, Z., & Gawlik, K. (2021). Evidence-based assessment of the musculoskeletal system. In K. S. Gawlik, B. M. Melnyk, & A. M. Teall (Eds.), *Evidence-based physical examination: Best practices for health and well-being assessment*. Springer Publishing Company, p. 411, Fig. 15.12.

be positioned in supine sitting or lying with the knee in full extension. The distal leg is stabilized with one hand while the other hand holds the heel with the ankle in neutral position. The heel is inverted with respect to the tibia. It is important to hold the talus and calcaneus as one unit to prevent excessive subtalar movement. Pain in the area of the ligament, a clunking sensation, or a spongy feeling indicates a positive test and a possible tear of the CFL (Delahunt et al., 2018).

Deltoid Ligament Sprain

An eversion stress test (also called talar-tilt eversion) is performed to evaluate the DL on the medial side of the ankle. The patient can be positioned similar to the inversion stress

test. The heel is everted and abducted while stabilizing the distal tibia, performed on both sides for comparison. Increased laxity, a spongy feeling, and/or pain on the injured side in comparison to the uninjured side would indicate a positive test and a possible tear of the DL.

Syndesmotic Injury/High Ankle Sprain

External rotation (Kleiger's test) can be used to assess for syndesmotic injury, also noted as a "high ankle sprain." The syndesmosis is the distal tibiofibular joint comprised of the anterior inferior tibiofibular ligament (AITFL), the posterior inferior tibiofibular ligament, interosseous ligament, and the inferior transverse ligament. Ankle dorsiflexion is maintained, and the foot is externally rotated on a stabilized leg. A positive test occurs when pain is recreated in the area over the syndesmosis region (Delahunt et al., 2018).

Achilles Tendon Injury

Weakness or absence of ankle and foot dorsiflexion should prompt examination of the Achilles tendon for possible rupture. This can be done using a Thompson test, which involves squeezing the calf above the level of the injury to see reflexive passive dorsiflexion of the foot. This exam is best done with a prone patient and affected leg bent at 90- degrees; however, a limited exam can be with the dependent extremity. The Achilles tendon integrity should be considered and examined with ankle and foot injuries (Strudwick et al., 2018).

DIFFERENTIAL DIAGNOSIS AND DIAGNOSTIC CONSIDERATIONS

Analysis of the presenting history, pertinent positive and negative examination findings, and differential diagnoses will help the AGACNP develop an appropriate evaluation and treatment plan. Making the appropriate diagnosis will involve performing physical examination techniques and/or imaging studies to exclude differentials. It is imperative that the AGACNP is knowledgeable about the anatomy and physiology of the ankle and adjacent joints to aid in the diagnostic effort.

Differential diagnoses for ankle strain include but are not limited to:

- Sprain
- Stress and occult fractures
- Endonitis

Differential diagnoses for ankle sprain include but are not limited to:

- Stable fractures (avulsions, fibular, unilateral malleolus)
- Stress and occult fractures
- Tendon rupture (Achilles)
- Unstable fractures (bimalleolar, trimalleolar, Maisonneuve)

Special Populations

Consideration of the structural bony and joint changes with aging must also be included. Age-related changes in the ankle joint may include osteoarthritis and degenerative joint disease (Bixby & Puig, 2018). Injuries involving the articular cartilage of any joint may predispose to chronic joint instability and disease (Delahunt et al., 2018). Patients and those with fall risk should be identified for advice on home care and follow-up (Strudwick et al., 2018). Diabetic patients should always receive follow-up with the primary care provider (PCP) and/or appropriate specialist to monitor healing and possibly prevent a Charcot arthropathy (Strudwick et al., 2018) which is a neuropathy of the foot and ankle. Patients that are prone to or have a history of deep venous thrombosis (DVT)

should be counseled regarding the possibility of DVT development following the injury (Strudwick et al., 2018).

Advanced Imaging

Computed tomography (CT) scans may be indicated in the event an unstable ankle injury is suspected, especially for highly traumatic injuries with Grades 3 to 4 sprains (Ortega-Avila et al., 2020; Strudwick et al., 2018). If the AGACNP is properly trained in technique, an ultrasound can detect soft tissue injuries of the ankle differentiating the ankle ligamentous integrity (Allen et al., 2020; Gribble, 2019; Haddad, 2016; Strudwick et al., 2018). However, CT has been shown to be more sensitive in detecting fractures (Allen et al., 2020). MRI is another advanced imaging procedure which can be done for suspected severe injury to the ligaments, damage to the cartilage or bone of the joint surface, or a small bone chip (Gribble, 2019; Haddad, 2016; Strudwick et al., 2018). These types of imaging should be done in the appropriate setting; ultrasound, CT, or MRI can be done in the emergency department, urgent care clinic, or later by the orthopedic specialist. If diagnostic imaging must be delayed, it is best to stabilize the foot and ankle with appropriate splinting to properly limit joint movement (Table 15.6).

TREATMENT

Classic treatment for lower extremity injuries, including the ankle, involves the acronym RICE: rest, ice, compression, elevation (Strudwick et al., 2018). This is the opportunity to determine the extent of the patient's self-care knowledge in this area and advise. The patient should rest the ankle by avoiding weight bearing and generally circumventing activities that cause pain (Strudwick et al., 2018). Healing of the dense connective tissue involved in joint injuries requires time to restore the structures so that they are strong enough to withstand the forces imposed on the joint (Delahunt et al., 2018). Depending on the capability of the patient and presence/absence of concomitant injury, the patient should be removed from weight bearing with crutches, wheelchair, or a knee scooter/walker (Strudwick et al., 2018). Ice should never be applied directly to the skin, it should be applied over clothing, ACE wrap, or splint to avoid skin injury from frostbite. There are many cryotherapy methods such as apply ice "20 minutes on 20 minutes off" or "10 minutes every 1 to 2 hours." Compression can be applied with ACE wrapping or a neoprene ankle sleeve depending on the extent of the patient's initial soft tissue swelling and edema. The patient should be encouraged to elevate the ankle as often as possible during the first week of the injury to mitigate swelling/edema and pain.

Treatment for strains and Grades 1 to 3 sprains can be conservative; while Grade 4 sprains require referral to an orthopedic surgeon (Ortega-Avila et al., 2020; Strudwick et al., 2018). Immobilization for a strain is indicated until the pain and swelling have subsided (may be

TABLE 15.6: Grade of Sprain, Recommended Stabilization, Imaging, Referral

SPRAIN GRADE	RECOMMENDED STABILIZATION	RECOMMENDED IMAGING AND TYPE	RECOMMENDED REFERRAL
1	ACE wrap or neoprene ankle sleeve; may require removable aircast or stirrup splint	Plain film or digital x-ray only if positive OAR	PCP in 1–2 weeks
2	Removable aircast or stirrup splint; may require short leg orthoglass posterior foot/ankle mold splint	Plain film or digital x-ray only if positive OAR	PCP within 1 week
3	Short leg orthoglass splint posterior foot/ankle mold; may also require orthoglass sugar tong mold around ankle	Plain film or digital x-ray or CT scan initially with follow-up MRI; depending on the setting could go straight to MRI	Orthopedic specialist within 1 week
4	Short leg orthoglass splint with sugar tong mold around posterior mold	Plain film or digital x-ray, or CT scan initially with follow-up MRI; depending on the setting could go straight to MRI	Orthopedic specialist within 1 week

CT, computed topography scan; MRI, magnetic resonance imaging; OAR, Ottawa Ankle Rules; PCP, primary care provider.

several weeks to months). In a sprain, the affected joint is usually immobilized for several weeks. Immobilization may be followed by graded active exercises; stabilizing treatment and rehabilitation are essential in preventing chronic ligamentous instability (Ortega-Avila et al., 2020; Strudwick et al., 2018).

For patients with sprain, the appropriate splinting technique should be utilized to stabilize and rest the ankle (Table 15.6). The decision to splint should be based on sprain severity (grade), individual functional requirements, and the patient's preference (Strudwick et al., 2018). Whenever possible, the AGACNP should be involved in applying the splint; however, it is always the NP's responsibility to assess and document neurovascular status post splint application.

Pain management is an essential portion of the treatment plan. This may simply involve recommending RICE; however, it may include OTC analgesics (acetaminophen, ibuprofen, naproxen) and/or prescription analgesics (opioids). Acetaminophen and ibuprofen are highly recommended for mild-moderate pain, and opioids should be reserved for cases with moderate-severe pain (Strudwick et al., 2018). Dosing and frequency recommendations should be provided for the patient. Pain control is essential for patient comfort and recovery. Collaborative decision-making with the patient regarding appropriate and preferred analgesic choices based on subjective levels of pain should be provided.

TRANSITION OF CARE

Naturally, the patient with an ankle strain or sprain would be referred to the PCP for follow-up and additional evaluation and treatment as needed. Recommended follow up time frames can be found in Table 15.6; however, these should be individualized per patient. Minor sprains require thorough patient education only (Strudwick et al., 2018). However, physical therapy (PT) referral can be provided to the patient by the AGACNP if deemed

appropriate for more severe sprains, or defer to the PCP (Strudwick et al., 2018). Referral to an orthopedic healthcare provider, preferably one that specializes in care of the foot and ankle, should be provided for unstable ankle injuries such as Grades 3 to 4 sprains (Ortega-Avila et al., 2020), known or suspected Achilles tendon rupture, or associated fractures (Strudwick et al., 2018).

CLINICAL PEARL

- Consider utilizing a systematic and evidence-based examination technique such as the OAR.

KEY TAKEAWAYS

- Avoid not differentiating between the diagnosis of strain versus sprain; embrace the opportunity to educate your patient about the etiology of their injury.
- Imaging such as x-rays may be indicated to rule out associated fractures. However, if not clearly supported by exam, x-rays are not useful in identifying ligamentous and soft tissue injury which can be ascertained by a thorough physical examination of the ankle which should include ROM assessment.
- Whenever possible, the nurse practitioner should be involved in applying the chosen stabilization method; however, it is always the nurse practitioner's responsibility to choose the method and assess and document neurovascular status post splint application.

EVIDENCE-BASED RESOURCES

Ottawa Ankle Rules (OAR) (http://www.theottawarules.ca/ankle_rules)
Ottawa Rules App for iPad and iPhone (https://apps.apple.com/ca/app/the-ottawa-rules/id1104004722)
Ottawa Rules App for Android (https://play.google.com/store/apps/details?id=ca.ohri.ottawarules&hl=en)

15.4: COMPARTMENT SYNDROME

PRESENTING SIGNS AND SYMPTOMS

Acute compartment syndrome (ACS) is a true surgical emergency needing prompt recognition by the AGACNP to prevent serious patient complications. ACS is most often observed after long-bone fractures, musculoskeletal crush injuries, penetrating wounds, and burns located in the upper and lower extremities. Long-bone fractures account for approximately 75% of the ACS cases with tibial fractures being the most common followed by radial fractures in the forearm (Stracciolini & Hammerberg, 2021). ACS has also been reported in patients with tight circumferential dressings and constrictive orthopedic casts which were applied for fracture management (Sander & Weil, 2016). Onset of ACS symptoms can occur within 4 to 10 hours of an injury but have been observed as late as 1 week (Sander & Weil, 2016). Any swollen or tense extremity should be observed carefully for the development of ACS.

Muscle compartments located in the upper and lower extremities are encapsulated with a strong fascial covering. Within these compartments, the normal intercompartmental pressure (ICP) ranges from 8 to 10 mmHg (Geersen, 2016; Papachristos & Giannoudis, 2018). When an injury occurs to the muscle, the muscle begins to swell within this compartment and, due to the nature of the fascial covering, has limited ability to stretch which impairs the normal venous and lymphatic flow within the compartment. At an ICP pressure of 20 mmHg, arterial flow decreases resulting in diminished perfusion pressure within the compartment. At an ICP pressure of 30 mmHg, a surgical fasciotomy may be warranted due to the great potential for nerve injuries, ischemia, and necrosis in the surrounding tissues (Geersen, 2016; Purcell, Terry, & Sharp, 2019)

HISTORY AND PHYSICAL FINDINGS

To make a rapid clinical diagnosis of ACS, the AGACNP should start with a detailed and thorough history of the injury including time of injury, mechanism, prior history of surgery (including hardware) or injury to affected extremity, use of any anticoagulant therapy, and, in cases of injuries to the arm/forearm/hand, to inquire about dominant handedness. During the physical exam it is important to expose the extremity by removing any clothing, dressings, or casting material to observe for open wounds, ecchymosis, crepitus, pain, point tenderness, deformity, range of motion (ROM) and neurovascular status.

Pain out of proportion (POP) to the injury is one of the early signs of ACS. Patients describe the pain as extreme, constant, deep, and burning (Geersen, 2016) and is also intensified on pain with passive stretch (PPS). Both POP and PPS have definitive indicators of ischemia in the extremities (Oron et al., 2018). Classic clinical findings of ACS include the 6 P's, summarized in Box 15.2 (Collinge et al., 2018; Purcell, Terry, & Sharp, 2019; Stracciolini & Hammerberg, 2021).

Patients who are conscious and able to give trustworthy information regarding their symptoms may be the most reliable monitor for symptoms of ACS. Patients who are unconscious or when the physical exam is not consistent, the AGACNP should prepare for compartment measurements and frequent monitoring.

Intercompartmental Pressure Monitoring

There are several ICP devices currently utilized in the United States. It is important for the AGACNP to familiarize themselves with the ICP device being used at their institution prior to caring for ACS patients. Ideally, to reinforce the correct procedure and use of the equipment a simulated-based learning experience (SBLE) should be completed prior to performing the actual procedure. Performing ICP measurement is easy and safe with a low risk of complications. Contraindications for ICP measurement include areas suspicious for infection or cellulitis in the affected extremity.

In the lower leg, there are four compartments: the anterior compartment, lateral compartment, deep and superficial posterior compartments (Figure 15.8), with the anterior compartment being most common for ACS.

In the forearm, there are four compartments: the deep and superficial volar compartments, dorsal compartment, and the lateral compartment with the volar compartments being most common for ACS due to the high incidence of radial fractures in adults.

Included in most ICP kits:
1. Intracompartmental pressure monitor system
2. Syringe, prefilled with saline
3. Sideport noncoring needle
4. Diaphragm chamber
5. Intracompartmental needle
6. Sterile drapes, gauze
7. Arterial line transducer cable and system (for extended monitoring)
8. Three-way stopcocks

BOX 15.2 6 P'S CLINICAL FINDINGS OF ACUTE COMPARTMENT SYNDROME

1. <u>P</u>ain out of proportion to the injury— described as severe and does not respond to analgesia (early and most common sign).
2. <u>P</u>PS—PPS can be performed easily by flexing the toes in the lower extremity to elicit a pain response.
3. <u>P</u>aresthesias—described as burning, numbness, tingling or the extremity has "pins and needles."
4. <u>P</u>aralysis—decreased movement in the extremity.
5. <u>P</u>allor—pallor or cyanotic color change (late sign).
6. <u>P</u>ulselessness—(late sign).

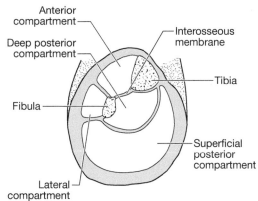

FIGURE 15.8: Four compartments of the lower leg.
Source: Reproduced from Brown, D. P., Freeman, E. D., Cuccurullo, S. J., et al. (2019). Musculoskeletal medicine. In S. J. Cuccurullo (Ed.), *Physical medicine and rehabilitation board review* (4th ed.). Springer Publishing Company, p. 247, Fig. 4.114.

Procedure

1. Gather all equipment and verify that the ICP monitor is functional
2. Set up all equipment per manufacturer's directions
3. Place extremity at the level of the heart
4. Site should be cleaned with betadine and chlorhexidine and sterilely prepped
5. Administer local anesthetic to site (1% lidocaine)
6. Level ICP monitor to zero
7. With dominant hand, insert the intercompartmental needle perpendicularly to the compartment being tested. You should feel the needle go through the fascial layer at about 1 to 3 cm
8. Inject 0.2 to 0.3 mL saline from device
9. Take pressure
10. Multiple sites will need to have ICP; in the event of continuous monitoring site, apply loose fitting dressing

In the event the ICP kit cannot be located, an 18-gauge needle can be attached to an arterial pressure monitor to measure ICP in compartments (Stracciolini & Hammerberg, 2021).

If one or all the compartments evaluated have a positive result (30 mmHg) an emergent surgical consult is warranted for an emergent fasciotomy. An emergent fasciotomy should be performed in less than 2 hours (Papachristos & Giannoudis, 2018).

DIFFERENTIAL DIAGNOSIS AND DIAGNOSTIC CONSIDERATIONS

Differential diagnoses for compartment syndrome include but are not limited to:

- Rhabdomyolysis
- Deep vein thrombosis
- Cellulitis
- Hematoma deep in muscle tissues
- Infiltration of IV fluids or medications
- Necrotizing fasciitis
- Fracture

TREATMENT

Any time ACS is suspected in a patient with a swollen and tense extremity, during the physical exam the AGACNP should maintain the affected extremity at the level of the patient's heart. This assists with normal arterial, venous, and lymphatic drainage as well as avoiding increased ICP from dependent swelling (Stracciolini & Hammerberg, 2021). It is crucial to remove any circumferential bandages or casting material to perform a detailed physical exam of the suspicious extremity. Hypotension should be avoided as it decreases perfusion pressure in the affected extremity. The patient should also be assessed for metabolic acidosis and myoglobinuria to prevent any acute kidney injury (AKI) (Geersen, 2016).

Surgical Intervention

A positive result in one or two compartments is sufficient evidence for an emergent surgical fasciotomy (Sander & Weil, 2016). An emergent fasciotomy may be done at the bedside or completed in the operating room. The AGACNP will be vital in helping to facilitate that the presurgical checklist is ordered and completed prior to the procedure.

CLINICAL PEARLS

- Long-bone fractures account for approximately 75% of the ACS cases with tibial fractures being the most common followed by radial fractures in the forearm.
- Classic clinical findings of ACS include the 6 P's.
- ICP measurement is easy, safe with a low risk of complications.
- Normal ICP ranges from 8 to 10 mmHg.
- With ICP pressure of 30 mmHg, a surgical fasciotomy may be warranted due the great potential for nerves injuries, ischemia, and necrosis in the surrounding tissues.

EVIDENCE-BASED RESOURCES

American Academy of Orthopaedic Surgeons/Major Extremity Trauma and Rehabilitation Consortium Management of Acute Compartment Syndrome Clinical Practice Guideline. https://www.aaos.org/globalassets/quality-and-practice-resources/dod/acs-cpg-final_approval-version-10-11-19.pdf Published December 7, 2018.

15.5: RHABDOMYOLYSIS

Rhabdomyolysis is characterized by the breakdown and necrosis of muscle tissue and the release of intracellular content into the bloodstream. There are multiple different causes of rhabdomyolysis, but the pathophysiology remains consistent involving the destruction of the sarcolemmal membrane (the sheath which wraps and protects skeletal muscle fibers) and release of intracellular components into the systemic circulation. Due to a lack of prospective studies and underreporting of most mild cases, its exact incidence is difficult to determine. Rhabdomyolysis can occur in children and older adults, and in either gender (Cabral et al., 2020).

Rhabdomyolysis is more common in African American males between the ages of 10 and 60 and more frequently in individuals with a body mass index (BMI) of greater than 40 kg/m^2. Depending on the individual's age, the etiology of rhabdomyolysis may also vary (Nance & Mammen, 2015). There are diverse causes of rhabdomyolysis which can be classified as genetic and acquired. The genetic causes include myopathies and enzyme deficiencies while acquired causes among adults include trauma, hypoxic injury, drugs, infections, and hyperthermia. Approximately 10% to 40% of cases of rhabdomyolysis lead to acute kidney injury (AKI), 5% to 15% of AKI cases are attributed to rhabdomyolysis. For patients who develop AKI, their mortality rate is as high as 80%, making AKI one of the most concerning complications of rhabdomyolysis (Yang et al., 2020).

PRESENTING SIGNS AND SYMPTOMS

Depending on the myriad of inciting causes and the extent and severity of muscle damage, the clinical presentation of rhabdomyolysis varies widely. Variation may range from asymptomatic patients with mild muscle breakdown with a slight increase in measured serum levels of enzymes released from muscle cells, to significant muscle destruction associated with metabolic acidosis, electrolyte abnormalities, severe intravascular volume depletion, and AKI. In conscious patients, the most common clinical complaints include pain, cramping, muscle tenderness, stiffness, motor weakness and potential loss of function in the affected muscle groups (Shapiro et al., 2012).

Though rhabdomyolysis presents with many nonspecific symptoms, in approximately 40% to 50% of adult patients, it presents in a triad of symptoms which includes weakness, muscle pain, and dark tea-colored urine (Yang et al., 2020). The proximal muscle groups, such as forearms, biceps, thighs, calves, and the lower back are the most frequently involved muscles. Some patients do not experience pain or swelling until volume resuscitation and reperfusion. In approximately 10% of patients, skin discoloration or blisters appear which are indicative of pressure necrosis (Yang et al., 2020).

HISTORY AND PHYSICAL FINDINGS

In rhabdomyolysis, as with other diseases, a thorough history and physical examination will provide important clues. The history and physical examination should identify and evaluate for (a) intensity and onset of pain, (b) presence of known injury mechanism, (c) presence of muscle weakness, and (d) neurovascular status. However, laboratory tests are still required to confirm the diagnosis. Typically, the history may include a recent traumatic experience, ingestion of alcohol or illicit drugs resulting in unresponsiveness, crush injuries, or electrical injuries (Cabral et al., 2020). The characteristic clinical features of rhabdomyolysis include myalgia, muscle weakness, and soft tissue swelling which develop over hours to days. Some nonspecific presenting symptoms of rhabdomyolysis include nausea and vomiting, fatigue, and fevers (Bosch et al., 2009).

DIFFERENTIAL DIAGNOSIS AND DIAGNOSTIC CONSIDERATIONS

In rhabdomyolysis, a high index of suspicion is needed, and laboratory tests are required to confirm the diagnosis. Differential diagnoses for rhabdomyolysis include but are not limited to:

- Traumatic injuries
- Bacterial infections
- Extreme cold or heat exposures
- Myalgias
- Guillain-Barré syndrome
- Electrolyte imbalance
- Inflammatory or immune-mediated myositis

Several substances are released into the plasma including myoglobin, creatine kinase (CK), electrolytes, and protein due to the muscle cell necrosis. Detection of these substances contribute to the early diagnosis of the syndrome. In rhabdomyolysis, the most sensitive marker of muscle injury is an elevated level of serum creatine kinase from skeletal muscle (CK-MM) isoenzyme subtype. Though the activity peaks within 24 to 72 hours, elevations are noted within 2 to 12 hours of muscle damage. According to De Meijer et al. (2003), after the diagnosis of rhabdomyolysis in patients who had higher admission and peak serum CK levels, AKI was likely to develop.

Other pertinent laboratory findings include an elevated white blood cell count in the presence of active infection, electrolyte imbalances including hyperkalemia, hyperphosphatemia, hypo/hypercalcemia, hyperuricemia, and metabolic acidosis (Yang et al., 2020).

Making the diagnosis of rhabdomyolysis takes into account the presentation of muscle pain and weakness and the presence of darkly colored urine or a heme-positive urine dipstick, in combination with elevated serum and urine myoglobin and increased CK and CK-MM (Yang et al., 2020).

TREATMENT

The main recommendation in treating rhabdomyolysis with the goal of preventing end organ complication is the early and aggressive repletion of fluids with and correction of electrolyte imbalances. In more severe cases of rhabdomyolysis, compartment pressures should be measured when significant muscle injury has occurred. In these situations, emergent fasciotomies are required to manage compartmental compression syndromes characterized by significant neurovascular compromise.

In patients with severe AKI as a complication of rhabdomyolysis, dialysis may be indicated in the presence of oliguria, persistent hyperkalemia, metabolic acidosis, and other electrolyte imbalances (Shapiro et al., 2012).

CLINICAL PEARLS

- The classic triad of rhabdomyolysis includes muscle weakness, myalgias, and dark (tea-colored) urine.
- Elevations in CK and CK-MM are diagnostic of rhabdomyolysis but are not prognostic.
- In the absence of the absence of red blood cells, a heme-positive urine dipstick occurs in rhabdomyolysis.

KEY TAKEAWAYS

- Rhabdomyolysis is potentially life-threatening and should be approached as a severe medical emergency that requires prompt diagnosis so that its life-threatening complications can be avoided.
- Aggressive fluid resuscitation, prevention of complications including AKI, and repletion of serum electrolytes may decrease morbidity and mortality in patients diagnosed with rhabdomyolysis.

A robust set of instructor resources designed to supplement this text is located at **http://connect.springerpub.com/content/reference-book/978-0-8261-6079-9.** Qualifying instructors may request access by emailing **textbook@springerpub.com.**

REFERENCES

Full list of references can be accessed at http://connect.springerpub.com/content/reference-book/978-0-8261-6079-9

CHAPTER 16

NEUROLOGIC DISORDERS

Chris Winkelman, Diane McLaughlin, and Kimberly Ichrist

LEARNING OBJECTIVES

- Describe components of assessment in a comatose patient.
- Differentiate ischemic stroke from other similar conditions.
- Formulate an acute treatment plan that is timely and evidence-based.
- Describe data to collect to recognize intracerebral and intraventricular hemorrhage (ICH; IVH).
- Differentiate ICH from other similar conditions.
- Design an acute treatment plan for ICH with or without IVH that is timely and evidence-based.
- Describe workup of a first-time seizure.
- Discuss medication administration algorithms in a patient with ongoing seizure activity.
- Perform common tests for meningitis.
- Demonstrate treatment strategies when meningitis or encephalitis are suspected.
- Explain Parkinson's disease (PD) assessment and management.
- Determine a drug regimen for ongoing PD management in acute and critical care.

INTRODUCTION

Neurology is a subject that cannot be sufficiently detailed in a single chapter for the AGACNP. Selected topics in this section are common or require time-sensitive assessment and intervention. Acute brain dysfunction is a common presentation to the hospital and a frequent medical or perioperative care complication. Like brain dysfunction, acute weakness can similarly lead to critical care hospitalization. A rapid and focused workup will guide therapies. Distinguishing between focal and generalized processes can narrow differential diagnoses and identify etiology. In acute and critical care, central nervous system (CNS) disorders often require specialized knowledge and skills. Timely diagnosis and intervention are based typically on a focused assessment. Avoiding secondary harm is essential to care.

16.1: ALTERED CONSCIOUSNESS

Diane McLaughlin

PRESENTING SIGNS AND SYMPTOMS

A thorough neurologic examination is needed to help establish a degree of altered consciousness and differentiate between other states of altered consciousness.

To first assess altered consciousness, the patient's arousal level is determined, typically described as alert, lethargic, obtunded, or comatose. Some patients require a high degree of noxious stimuli to elicit a response. Nailbed pressure or supraorbital pressure are two methods that can be utilized to stimulate the patient.

The Glasgow Coma Scale (GCS) is frequently used to help classify patients. This scale was developed in the 1970s to describe the level of consciousness in patients with acute brain injury (Teasdale & Jennett, 1974). It has been found to have high reliability and reproducibility (Reith et al., 2016). It is not necessarily an adequate predictor of mortality. However, the AGACNP should not assume that patients with low GCS scores have nonsurvivable injuries. The GCS comprises three segments: eye, verbal, and motor, with a minimum value of 3 and a high value of 15 (Table 16.1; (Healey et al., 2003). Patients with GCS less than 8 are considered comatose.

Motor response is also useful to assess in patients. Posturing can be present in both structural and metabolic causes of coma. A critical component of motor testing is determining if asymmetry is present, which points toward a unilateral structural lesion. However, symmetry and unilateral damage are not always linked, as Todd's paralysis can also cause this phenomenon.

The pupillary response is assessed using a penlight. Fixed, dilated pupils typically indicate downward herniation. However, there are pharmacologic causes of mydriasis. In these cases, pilocarpine can be administered and there will be no effect on pharmacologic iridoplegia. However, if the cause is hypoxia, pilocarpine will cause miosis.

The loss of corneal reflex is a late sign of coma progression. The absence of gag reflex is not a useful marker of coma severity, as it may be absent in normal people. However, a new loss of gag reflex indicates a worsening picture.

TABLE 16.1: Glasgow Coma Scale

4 YEARS TO ADULTS	
Eye opening	
4	Spontaneous
3	To speech
2	To pain
1	No response
Verbal response	
5	Alert and oriented
4	Disoriented conversation
3	Speaking but nonsensical
2	Moans or unintelligible sounds
1	No response
Motor response	
6	Follows commands
5	Localizes pain
4	Moves or withdraws to pain
3	Decorticate flexion
2	Decerebrate extension
1	No response
3–15	

Note: In intubated patients, the Glasgow Coma Scale verbal component is scored as a 1, and the total score is marked with a "T" (or tube), denoting intubation (e.g., "8T").

Source: Reproduced with permission from Rita, K. C., Cline, D. M., John Ma, O., Fitch, M. T., Joing, S., & Wang, V. J. (2017). *Tintinalli's emergency medicine manual* (8th ed., pp. 721–725) McGraw-Hill Education

HISTORY AND PHYSICAL FINDINGS

History is significant in determining the cause of altered consciousness. The chronicity of change can help differentiate between a worsening metabolic process versus acute structural change (Venkatasubramanian et al., 2020). In patients whose condition has deteriorated over time, metabolic processes or slow structural changes should be considered as a cause for acute changes in consciousness (Venkatasubramanian et al., 2020).

The patient's health history details conditions that contribute to diagnostic reasoning. Significant history of disorders that may lead to altered consciousness includes diabetes, seizures, psychological disorders or previous suicide attempts, substance abuse disorders, recent infections, or malignancy (Venkatasubramanian et al., 2020). The presence of these comorbidities may help guide the examiner in selecting diagnostics.

Medication use is also essential information to obtain, as many medications may alter consciousness when they are at toxic levels.

Locked-in syndromes can occur in Guillain-Barré syndrome, myasthenia gravis, high spinal cord injuries, or damage to the base of the pons (Gress, 2009). Although patients with locked-in syndrome have no motor movement, vertical eye movements are intact. Therefore, it is necessary for all patients without motor function to be assessed to control extraocular eye movements.

DIFFERENTIAL DIAGNOSIS AND DIAGNOSTIC CONSIDERATIONS

Table 16.2 presents the differential diagnoses to be considered by the AGACNP in a patient who presents with an altered or deteriorating level of consciousness.

Diagnostic Testing

Initial laboratory testing to consider includes point-of-care glucose to evaluate for hypoglycemia; complete blood cell count to identify infectious/inflammatory states; basic metabolic profile to identify renal or metabolic dysfunction; toxicology screening (ETOH, urine drug screen); liver function tests and ammonia level to evaluate for encephalopathy; and blood gas for acid/base disturbances such as hypercarbia or hypoxia which many contribute to alteration in mental status.

Noncontrast computed tomography (CT) of the head (CTH) can quickly rule in or rule out acute intracranial hemorrhage, hydrocephalus, and some types of tumors. A CT with contrast can be useful if there is a concern for abscess or extra-axial fluid collection. CT angiogram (CTA) may be indicated if there is a concern for acute ischemic stroke or large vessel occlusion. Magnetic resonance imaging (MRI) can be used in place of CTA when there is a concern for acute ischemic stroke. It also can help identify changes when no other apparent cause of coma is identified. Electroencephalogram (EEG) is ordered when the AGACNP observes a seizure, unexplained motor activity, or determines unresponsiveness with a history of seizures or unclear etiology of unresponsiveness to evaluate for nonconvulsive status epilepticus. A lumbar puncture can be obtained if there is suspicion for central nervous system (CNS) infection, CNS malignancy, autoimmune disorders, neuroinflammatory disorders, or concern for subarachnoid hemorrhage in the presence of a negative CTH.

TREATMENT

Treatment aims to reverse the underlying cause of coma and prevent secondary injury. Supportive care is provided while the differential is investigated. The priorities are ensuring the airway is protected and cardiopulmonary support provided. The AGACNP should consider the use of naloxone, thiamine, and/or glucose—and delay diagnostic tests—in patients whose cause of coma is unclear as these may help quickly improve the patients'

TABLE 16.2: Altered Level of Consciousness and Common Diagnoses

METABOLIC	STRUCTURAL	TOXIDROMES	INFECTIOUS	OTHER

Hypoxia
Hypoglycemia
Hypoperfusion, shock
Hypothermia
Hepatic encephalopathy
  with coma
ICH, IVH, or SAH related
	Mass lesion
	Acute ischemic stroke
	ICH
	Herniation syndromes
	Blood in brain tissue, ventricles,
	  or subarachnoid space
		Drug overdose
		Profound intoxications
			Encephalitis
			Meningitis
			Sepsis
				Nonconvulsive status
				  epilepticus
				Catatonic state
				Locked-in
				Cerebellar and brainstem
				  hemorrhage can
				  present with coma

ICH, intracerebral hemorrhage; IVH, intraventricular hemorrhage; SAH, subarachnoid hemorrhage.

condition, have very few adverse side effects, and are important therapies in the prevention of Wernicke's encephalopathy

TRANSITION OF CARE

There is a wide range of potential outcomes in patients that present with coma. In patients that have metabolic causes, they may recover to their baseline over time with supportive care. A return to baseline function is less likely in patients with structural damage, and discussion of patient wishes and goals of care becomes essential early in the course of a degenerative disease. Many of these patients require tracheostomy, gastric tube, and a high level of care. It is more difficult to predict the prognosis in patients without structural damage. In both scenarios, it is vital to establish an open, honest relationship with the family who will make decisions on the patient's behalf. Early rehabilitative and palliative care consults are crucial in the care of these patients and can help the primary team clarify the goals of care.

CLINICAL PEARLS

- Locked-in patients have low GCS scores and can be missed if only relying upon GCS.
- Lateralizing symptoms are concerning for structural lesions or potentially seizures.

KEY TAKEAWAY

- Low GCS on presentation is not necessarily an indicator of mortality. However, a persistently low GCS is associated with poor prognosis and outcomes.

16.2: ENCEPHALITIS AND MENINGITIS

Diane McLaughlin

Neuroinfectious disorders carry high morbidity and mortality and need to be recognized and treated promptly to improve outcomes. Though meningitis and encephalitis are different disorders, they present similarly and must be considered equally. Meningitis is inflammation of the leptomeninges. Inflammation does not always mean that infection is present. Encephalitis is inflammation of the brain, is defined by major/minor criteria, and can occur concurrently with encephalomyelitis and/or meningoencephalitis (Venkatesan et al., 2013). Encephalopathy is a symptom that can result from various insults such as meningitis, encephalitis, metabolic disorders, postictal states, intoxication, and more.

PRESENTING SIGNS AND SYMPTOMS

Though there can be significant heterogeneity of presentation in meningitis or encephalitis, classic symptoms alert the provider to a possible neuroinfectious disorder. Altered mental status, nuchal rigidity, and fever are considered the "classic" triad of presenting symptoms. However, less than 50% of patients will present with all three of these symptoms. Additional presenting symptoms can include signs and symptoms of increased intracranial pressure (ICP; papilledema, vomiting, mydriasis [dilated pupil]), cranial nerve palsies, or seizures.

There are physical exam findings that can help in the diagnosis of meningitis. Kernig's sign is the patient's inability to straighten their leg greater than 135 degrees without pain (Kernig, 1882). Initially described in patients in the sitting position, this is not easy to replicate in critically ill patients but can be performed by flexing the thigh to the abdomen when supine. Pain is not a necessary feature of this test. Brudzinski's sign describes neck flexion causing leg flexion. Likewise, the extension of the flexed legs caused a reciprocal response (Brudzinski, 1909). Both of these tests are specific for meningitis but have very low sensitivity and lack of these findings should not delay further diagnostics. The jolt test has a patient move their head side-to-side rapidly. If there is meningeal irritation, the headache worsens (Uchihara & Tsukagoshi, 1991). Whereas the presence of positive findings of any of these tests does make meningitis more likely, the absence of positive findings does not rule out meningitis because of the heterogeneity of presentation.

The diagnosis of encephalitis or encephalopathy with an infectious or autoimmune inflammatory etiology is based on one major and two minor findings (Venkatesan et al., 2013). The major finding is subacute onset of impairment in consciousness, memory, and mental status or new-onset psychiatric changes without alternative cause. The minor findings (at least two must be present; Venkatesan et al., 2013) are:

1. Fever ≥ 38° Celsius within 72 hours before or after the presentation
2. Seizures (focal or generalized) not attributable to a previous seizure disorder
3. Cerebrospinal fluid (CSF) pleocytosis (white blood cells >5/cubic mm)
4. Evidence of brain parenchymal inflammation on neuroimaging (acute or subacute)

HISTORY AND PHYSICAL FINDINGS

Once there is suspicion of meningitis, the history and physical is essential for two reasons: (a) to determine if neuroimaging is necessary before proceeding to lumbar puncture, and (b) to determine empiric antibiotics. Key components of the history and physical are

1. Age
2. Immunocompromised state
3. History of CNS disease
4. Seizures—particularly within 1 week
5. Neurologic abnormalities, including vision changes
6. Social risk (e.g., college student)
7. Physical findings (e.g., altered mental status, nuchal rigidity, fever, rash, petechiae)

DIFFERENTIAL DIAGNOSIS AND DIAGNOSTIC CONSIDERATIONS

Differential Diagnoses

Table 16.3 categorizes the differentials associated with infections or inflammation of the CNS.

Diagnostic Testing

CT of the head is indicated in patients at risk for herniation. These patients include those mentioned earlier: immunocompromised host, history of CNS disease, papilledema, new-onset seizures, focal neurologic deficits, and altered mental status. CT can help rule out other causes of symptoms but importantly can warn of possible downward herniation if lumbar puncture is pursued in a patient with significant cerebral edema and mass effect.

CSF analysis is necessary for the diagnosis of meningitis. The CSF is typically obtained by lumbar puncture. Opening pressure is measured to determine if the patient has elevated intracranial pressure. Initial CSF analysis includes glucose, protein, cell count with differential, gram stain, and culture. Additional studies consist of encephalitis panel, including herpes simplex virus (HSV). CSF lactate is at times useful, particularly to help distinguish bacterial meningitis from viral meningitis (Slack et al., 2016).

MRI may be indicated if CSF findings are nonspecific (Venkatesan et al., 2013). MRI is ordered with gadolinium, as certain etiologies of encephalitis have specific MRI findings. Herpes viruses typically invade the temporal lobe. Arboviruses, *Listeria*, brucellosis, and tuberculosis often involve the brainstem (Venkatesan et al., 2013). Mass lesions and/or ring-enhancing lesions can indicate toxoplasmosis, tuberculosis, bacterial abscess, and potentially fungal infections (Venkatesan et al., 2013). MRI is useful to determine the breadth and depth of inflammation and anatomical location.

An EEG can be obtained if there is a concern for ongoing seizures contributing to altered mental status. An EEG can also help localize the seizure focus to a specific anatomical region, such as periodic lateralizing epileptiform discharges in the temporal lobe which are common in HSV encephalitis.

TREATMENT

Treatment is mainly supportive. In viral meningitis fluids, antipyretics and analgesics are the cornerstones of therapy. In bacterial meningitis, antimicrobials are administered to treat the causative pathogen. Before initiating empiric antibiotic therapy for bacterial meningitis, dexamethasone 0.15 mg/kg is administered every 6 hours for 2 to 4 days. Give the first dose of dexamethasone immediately before the antibiotic's first dose (McGill

TABLE 16.3: Differential Diagnoses for Central Nervous System Infection and Inflammation

MENINGITIS	ENCEPHALITIS	ENCEPHALOPATHY	VASCULAR CAUSES	TRAUMA	OTHER
Viral Bacterial Other infectious: Fungal, parasitic, tuberculosis, syphilis Malignancy Chemical irritation IVH or SAH related	Viral Autoimmune Malignancy Paraneoplastic	Wernicke's Hepatic Uremia Sepsis Electrolyte abnormalities Intoxications	Ischemic stroke ICH Venous sinus thrombosis	Concussion SDH EDH	Seizure Postictal Leukoencephalopathy NCSE

EDH, epidural hematoma; ICH, intracranial hemorrhage; IVH, intraventricular hemorrhage; NCSE, nonconvulsive status epilepticus; SAH, subarachnoid hemorrhage, SDH, subdural hematoma.

et al., 2016). Dexamethasone is an adjuvant therapy utilized to impact bacterial meningitis's inflammatory consequences, including cerebral edema, increased ICP, and cerebral vasculitis. Typically, empiric therapy consists of ceftriaxone 2 g IV every 12 hours and vancomycin 15 to 20 mg/kg IV every 8 to 12 hours. If the patient is over 60 years old or immunocompromised, ampicillin 2 g every 4 hours is added to this regimen to provide *Listeria* coverage (McGill et al., 2016).

For suspected encephalitis, infectious causes are treated with appropriate antimicrobial therapy. For example, in HSV, acyclovir (10 mg/kg every 8 hours) is administered until CSF is negative or in the presence of continued positive polymerase chain reaction (PCR) testing for 14 to 21 days, dependent upon disease severity. Acyclovir is typically started empirically until HSV PCR returns negative from the CSF sample. Arbovirus does not have a specific antimicrobial and care is supportive.

In autoimmune encephalitis, supportive care is used in combination with immunosuppressive therapies. However, there is a lack of recommendations, and most recommendations are not based upon high levels of evidence.

TRANSITION OF CARE

The transition of care will occur several times, from the emergency department (ED) to the ICU, ICU to floor, and floor to home. The patient can be safely transferred from the ED to the ICU after the patient has a secure airway, is hemodynamically stable for transport, and any ICP elevation has been managed. Lumbar puncture and antibiotics ideally are started in the ED. However, some patients may not demonstrate signs of meningitis/encephalitis until after admission and treatment begins at that time.

The patient is ready for floor transfer once the patient has had a formal diagnosis and a definitive treatment plan developed. The patient must be neurologically and hemodynamically stable before discharge from the ICU.

Upon admission, disposition needs are assessed and should include rehabilitation services; a case manager may be integral to this process. Once a formal plan for ongoing treatment and follow-up is refined, the patient can be discharged from the ICU. Many patients require neurocognitive rehabilitation, along with physical and occupational therapy. Most patients will have a follow-up with hospital providers to ensure that the underlying cause of meningitis/encephalitis was treated completely.

CLINICAL PEARLS

- Kernig's sign and Brudzinski's sign are physical exam findings associated with meningitis.
- *Streptococcus pneumoniae, Haemophilus influenza,* and *Neisseria meningitides* are common pathogens associated with meningitis.

KEY TAKEAWAYS

- Meningitis or encephalitis is a differential in every patient with fever and altered mental status unless an apparent cause.
- Do not delay antibiotic administration to obtain CT head or lumbar puncture.

EVIDENCE-BASED RESOURCE

https://www.cdc.gov/meningitis/clinical-resources
.html

16.3: INCREASED INTRACRANIAL PRESSURE AND HERNIATION

Kimberly Ichrist

The intracranial vault consists of three main components: brain parenchyma, cerebrospinal fluid (CSF), and blood. The intracranial pressure (ICP) reflects the constant volume sum of brain parenchyma, CSF, and blood. The volumes are comprised of brain parenchyma (80%, approximately 1200 mL), CSF (10%, approximately 250 mL, production rate approximately 250–500/24 hours), blood (10%, approximately 150 mL; Darsie & Moheet, 2017). The Monroe-Kellie hypothesis states that if one volume is increased, it will lead to a decrease in one or both of the remaining volumes (Darsie & Moheet, 2017). A change in intracranial volume that exceeds the compensation mechanism may displace the brain parenchyma resulting in herniation, as the skull is a rigid compartment.

PRESENTING SIGNS AND SYMPTOMS

The common signs and symptoms of ICP include headache, altered mental status, nausea and vomiting, papilledema (leading to visual blurring or visual loss), and Cushing's triad (widened pulse pressure, bradycardia, and irregular respirations). The signs and symptoms of brain herniation may vary according to location (Figure 16.1) and are detailed in Table 16.4.

HISTORY AND PHYSICAL

The clinical presentation may vary according to the underlying etiology. A patient presenting with altered consciousness is first evaluated for conditions associated with ICP.

The AGACNP's focus is on managing the primary cause of brain injury to prevent secondary injury. The underlying etiology is addressed; some conditions are irreversible even with medical or surgical interventions.

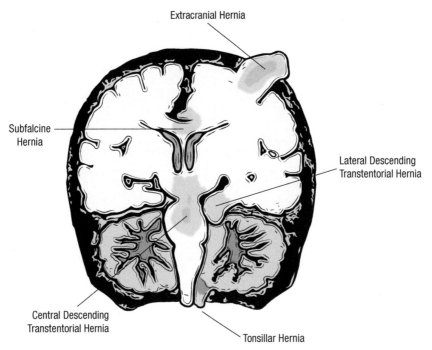

FIGURE 16.1: Visual demonstration of herniation patterns.
Source: Courtesy N. McLaughlin.

TABLE 16.4: Classic Herniation Syndromes

LOCATION	CAUSE	PRESENTATION
Cranial defect	Penetrating head injury or craniotomy site	Dependent on location
Subfalcine	Passage of contents of either the anterior fossa beneath the falx cerebri	Loss of attention and apathy. Inability to recite days of week months of the year
Diencephalic shift or torsion	Compression and distortion of the thalami and midbrain	Alteration of consciousness, small pupils, lack of posturing with flaccid extremities. The presentation can be mistaken for encephalopathy or coma secondary to toxic/metabolic cause
Uncal	The volume of the middle cranial fossa exceeds its capacity; the temporal lobe uncus herniates into the space occupied by the midbrain's adjacent ipsilateral CN III, PCA and cerebral peduncle	Ipsilateral CN III palsy is the localizing feature. As herniation progresses, ipsilateral, contralateral, or bilateral weakness with/without flexor posturing can occur
Transtentorial/central	Direct upward pressure and displacement of the midline structures, including the brainstem, through the tentorial notch. The ascending path of CN VI from the rostral pons to the cavernous sinus will have downward traction	The early clinical feature is asymmetric CN VI palsy. Bilateral upper limb flexion bilateral lower limb extension. As herniation progresses, all limbs will have an extension reflex then the complete absence of motor response
Upward	Posterior fossa lesions cause upward compression of the midbrain, thalami, and superior cerebellar artery. A critical complication is compression of the cerebral aqueduct can lead to obstructive hydrocephalus	Loss of consciousness, superior CN III palsy
Tonsillar	It can result from any herniation but typically results from posterior fossa lesions. The cerebellar tonsil descends through the foramen magnum with direct compression of the medulla	The classic presentation is Cushing's triad: widened pulse pressure, reflex bradycardia, and irregular breathing to apnea

CN, cranial nerve; PCA, posterior cerebral artery.

Source: Adapted from Darsie, M. D., & Moheet, A. M. (2017). *The pocket guide to Neurocritical Care: A concise reference for the evaluation and management of neurologic emergencies.* Neurocritical Care Society.

TABLE 16.5: Differential Diagnoses for Intracranial Hypertension With or Without Herniation

INCREASED INTRACRANIAL PRESSURE DIFFERENTIALS	POSSIBLE ETIOLOGIES	FOCUS WORKUP ON ETIOLOGIES
Intracranial space-occupying mass lesions	Subdural or epidural hematoma, brain tumor, cerebral abscess, intracranial hemorrhage	Injury, anticoagulation therapy, cancer, infection, hypertension, aneurysm, or medical history
Increased brain volume (cytotoxic edema)	Cerebral infarction, global hypoxic-ischemia, Reye syndrome, acute hyponatremia	Stroke, investigate recent events, medical and social history
Increase brain and blood volume (vasogenic edema)	Hepatic encephalopathy, traumatic brain injury, meningitis, encephalitis, eclampsia, subarachnoid hemorrhage	Liver, trauma, infection, encephalopathy, hypertension, aneurysm, coagulopathy, vascular malformations, vasculitis, amyloid angiopathy, or medical history
Increased cerebrospinal fluid volume	Communicating hydrocephalus, noncommunicating hydrocephalus, choroid plexus papilloma	Contributing factors and medical history

Source: Lee, K. (2018). The NeuroICU book. McGraw-Hill Medical.

DIFFERENTIAL DIAGNOSIS AND DIAGNOSTIC CONSIDERATIONS

Differential Diagnoses

The differential diagnoses for intracranial hypertension with or without herniation are summarized in Table 16.5.

Diagnostic Testing

Cranial CT scan is preferred over MRI of the brain due to imaging speed. Obtain initial labs of a basic metabolic panel (BMP), complete blood count (CBC), liver function tests, and a coagulation panel. Further imaging and lab values will be based on the initial workup.

TREATMENT

The treatment strategies are contingent on the underlying etiology of the injury. Prevention of increased ICP is the standard of care. The optimal level of ICP is less than 20 mmHg. Interventions to prevent intracranial hypertension are aimed at altering one of the three main components: brain parenchyma, CSF, and blood volume:

- Avoid internal jugular central venous catheter placement and overly tight C-collars or tracheostomy tie which may restrict venous return.
- Elevate the head of the bed to >30 degrees and keep the head midline to promote venous return.
- Prevent seizures, fever, or shivering; these increase cerebral metabolism and increase ICP.
- Control pain and agitation.
- Maintain $PaCO_2$ 35 to 40 mmHg.

When ICP becomes elevated to greater than 20 mmHg for 5 or more minutes, consider the following interventions to reduce it to the goal:

- If external ventricular drain (EVD) is in place, begin to drain CSF cautiously.

- Short-term hyperventilation to pCO_2 < 35 mmHg to vasoconstrict and decrease vascular volume (duration 1 minute).
- Osmotic therapy to reduce cerebral edema and vascular volume: hypertonic saline and/or mannitol.
  - Hypertonic saline has different concentrations ranging from 2% to 23.4% and doses are administered according to the exam and sodium goals.
    - 23.4% bolus can be given emergently with brain herniation. Hypertonic saline administration requires a central line.
    - Preferred in patients who benefit from volume expansion.
  - Mannitol is a 20% concentrated solution and administration doses 0.5 g/kg to 2 g/kg as scheduled or bolus doses.
    - Not given as a continuous infusion due to rebound cerebral edema.
    - Recommend monitoring serum osmolality and avoid therapy with level >320 mOsm/kg or osmolar gap of more than 20 mOsm/kg.
    - Osmolar gap calculation:

$$Calculated\,Osmolarity \left(\frac{mOsm}{L}\right) = 2Na + \frac{Gluc}{18} + \frac{BUN}{2.8}$$

  - Mannitol is preferred in patients who will also benefit from the drug's diuretic effect.
- For refractory ICP, consider pentobarbital coma, paralytics, and targeted hypothermia to 32°C to 34°C (Darsie & Moheet, 2017; Koenig, 2018).

Surgical Management

The patient may require hemicraniectomy or EVD. A lumbar drain or large volume lumbar puncture may be considered for nonobstructive hydrocephalus.

TRANSITION OF CARE

If the patient presents to the emergency department, initial management includes neurosurgery consult for possible surgical interventions. The patient will be transferred to the ICU (preferably a neurocritical care unit) for close, continuous neurologic management. Code status should be discussed on admission with the team and family. Goals of care are modified when there is irreversible declining status.

CLINICAL PEARL

- Increased intracranial pressure must be corrected quickly to avoid secondary brain injury. Brain herniation is a medical emergency and treatment is emergent and immediate.

BOX 16.1 SIGNS AND SYMPTOMS OF ISCHEMIC STROKE

Balance: Ataxia, decreased/loss of balance or coordination, vertigo
Eyes: Visual loss or visual field deficits, diplopia, nystagmus
Face: Dysarthria, facial droop, facial weakness, decreased consciousness
Arm and/or Leg Weakness: Abrupt onset of paresis (i.e., hemi-, mono-, and, rarely, quadri-paresis), hemisensory deficits
Speech: Difficulty in speaking, slurred speech, dysarthria, aphasia
Time: Sudden onset decreased consciousness, time is brain, activate the stroke system and clock

16.4: ISCHEMIC STROKE

Chris Winkelman

Ischemic strokes are caused by thrombi or emboli in cerebral blood vessels. Risk factors are similar to cardiovascular risk factors, with atherosclerotic plaque rupture leading to thrombosis. Atrial fibrillation is associated with embolic ischemic stroke. Outcomes are dependent on restoring brain perfusion.

Hospital-based, organized stroke care teams save lives for this leading cause of disability in the United States. Stroke care teams are multidisciplinary, clinically trained, and use performance measures regularly to sustain benchmarks (such as onset-to-needle time) and improve care. Efficient prehospital and telehospital care contribute to screening, triaging, and selecting candidates for stroke team assessment and emergent revascularization therapy.

PRESENTING SIGNS AND SYMPTOMS

The classic symptoms of ischemic stroke are acute neurologic deficits or any alteration in level of consciousness. Commonly, symptoms occur in combination. Common ischemic findings are summarized with the BEFAST acronym in Box 16.1 (Herpich & Rincon, 2020).

The National Institutes of Health Stroke Scale (NIHSS) is used in hospital care. There are many prehospital stroke assessment scales to screen, identify, and rate severity in patients with stroke (e.g., the Cincinnati Stroke Triage Assessment Tool, the Los Angeles Prehospital Stroke Screen, and the Rapid Arterial Occlusion Scale; Demaerschalk et al., 2020). However, all stroke centers use the NIHSS in initial and subsequent stroke assessment.

HISTORY AND PHYSICAL FINDINGS

The initial focus for history is to determine the onset of symptoms and record this "last known well" as a 24-hour clock time. If the stroke occurred during sleep, the last known well is recorded as the time to bed.

Once the onset of symptoms has been determined, the provider must conduct a focused neurologic exam. Both vessel size and occlusion duration correlate to the area of ischemia, subsequent brain damage and disability, and mortality risk (Tkacs et al., 2021). Table 16.6 details the large cerebral blood vessels and presenting symptoms when these vessels are occluded. The middle cerebral artery (MCA) is most often occluded in ischemic stroke.

DIFFERENTIAL DIAGNOSIS AND DIAGNOSTIC CONSIDERATIONS

The differential diagnosis for ischemic stroke can be any condition that decreases consciousness or causes focal neurologic changes. Table 16.7 details potential diagnoses and the elements of diagnostic reasoning to narrow the diagnosis. To determine if ischemic stroke can be treated with mechanical thrombectomy (MT), a CT perfusion scan and additional screening, using the rapid arterial occlusion evaluation scale, is done within 6 to 20 hours of presentation (Herpich & Rincon, 2020).

Diagnosis of ischemic stroke is time sensitive. Evidence-supported care indicates best outcomes are achieved with (a) completion of a neurologic assessment using a stroke severity rating scale within 10 minutes of arrival to the hospital and (b) neurologic imaging to exclude intraventricular hemorrhage (IVH), usually a noncontrast CT scan, within 20 minutes of arrival. Serum glucose to rule out hypoglycemia as a stroke mimic is completed on arrival. Blood glucose is treated to achieve values 140 to 180 mg/dL in the 24 hours in patients with suspected or actual acute ischemic stroke.

A serum cardiac-specific troponin and 12-lead EKG are recommended with arrival but should not delay either neurologic assessment or imaging. Continuous EKG monitoring for the first 24 hours following a stroke diagnosis is used to detect cardiac dysrhythmias

TABLE 16.6: Cerebrovascular Anatomy and Associated Clinical Presentation When Circulation Is Disrupted

ARTERY	ASSOCIATED ANATOMICAL SUPPLY	PATIENT PRESENTATION
Internal carotid artery	Cortex and subcortical frontal lobe, anterior temporal lobe	Contralateral hemiparesis or contralateral sensory deficits
Anterior cerebral artery	Cortex of frontal lobe	Contralateral leg and foot paresis/paralysis with sensory deficits Gait impairment Slowed response to tasks Flat affect Impaired new memory formation
Middle cerebral artery	Cortex and subcortical frontal lobe, and lateral temporal and parietal lobes	Left artery: aphasia, right hemiparesis/hemisensory deficit, right homonymous hemianopia, left head and gaze preference Right artery: Left hemispatial neglect, left hemiparesis, hemisensory deficit, left homonymous hemianopia, right head, and gaze preference
Vertebrobasilar arteries	Occipital lobes, cerebellum, thalamus, brainstem, and upper spinal cord	Dizziness, vertigo, diplopia, quadriparesis, ipsilateral face, and contralateral body hemiparesis and sensory deficit, ataxia, visual loss, impaired consciousness
Posterior cerebral artery	Peripheral branch: Superficial temporal and occipital cortex affecting visual function Deep cortical branch: Cerebellum, thalamus, brainstem	Left: Right visual field defect, alexia (AKA acquired dyslexia) without agraphia, right hemisensory disturbance Right: Left visual field deficit, visual neglect, left hemisensory disturbance

Source: Adapted from Demaerschalk, B. M., Scharf, E. L., Cloft, H., Barrett, K. M., Sands, K. A., Miller, D. A., & Meschia, J. F. (2020). Contemporary management of Acute Ischemic stroke across the continuum: From TeleStroke to Intra-Arterial management. *Mayo Clin Proc, 95*(7), 1512–1529. https://doi.org/10.1016/j.mayocp.2020.04.002; Tkacs, N. C., Compton, P. A., & Pavone, K. (2021). Nervous system. In N. C. Tkacs, L. L. Herrmann, & R. L. Johnson (Eds.), *Advanced physiology and pathophysiology*. Springer Publishing Company.

TABLE 16.7: Differential Diagnoses for Ischemic Stroke and Unique Considerations

DIAGNOSIS	CONSIDERATIONS
Intracranial hemorrhage (ICH); hemorrhagic stroke	Hemorrhagic stroke and ICH have a greater association with headache, nausea and vomiting, and coma
Seizure	Focal deficits are reversible, with spontaneous resolution over 1–48 hours Associated with seizure-induced neuronal dysfunction
Hypoglycemia	Blood glucose <45 mg/dL with symptom resolution immediately following IV glucose administration. Often presents with aphasia and drowsiness or obtundation; deficits may be focal or general
Metabolic encephalopathy or drug toxicity	Consider illicit drug use, drug overdose, alcohol poisoning, thiamine deficiency (Wernicke encephalopathy), hyperosmolar hyperglycemia, hyponatremia, and hepatic disease. It is often associated with decreased consciousness, poor attention, or acute confusional states (e.g., delirium)
Conversion disorder; psychiatric disease	Comorbid psychiatric problems are common. Symptoms of paresis, paralysis, and movement disorders are common. Diagnosis of exclusion
Sepsis	Symptoms of exposure to infectious agents, signs of systemic inflammation (e.g., malaise, hypotension, tachycardia), or infection (e.g., fever, leukocytosis) are congruent with sepsis
Other diagnoses that can be considered are complicated migraines, intracranial tumor, intracranial abscess, hypertensive encephalopathy, exacerbation of neurodegenerative disease (e.g., multiple sclerosis, Guillain-Barré, others), and syncope.	

associated with stroke etiology (i.e., atrial fibrillation) or dysrhythmic complications following a stroke. EKG abnormalities, including ST-segment, T wave, and QRS complex abnormalities, can occur in 16% to 20% of patients with ischemic stroke (Khechinashvili & Asplund, 2002). However, only 1% to 2% of patients with ischemic stroke have a concomitant myocardial infarct (Alqahtani et al., 2017). The 12-lead EKG changes can be accompanied by increased serum troponin and both can be unrelated to myocardial ischemia. The EKG and troponin findings in ischemic stroke are thought to be related to stroke-induced autonomic dysfunction from brain injury (Alqahtani et al., 2017). Without associated infarct symptoms of chest pain, shortness of breath, new heart failure, or new-onset dysrhythmias, there is a limited need for urgent consultation with cardiology.

While evidence for benefit is lacking, other standard laboratory tests done with assessment included a CBC (platelet count), a comprehensive metabolic panel (CMP), and coagulation studies (i.e., the international normalized ratio [INR], and activated partial thromboplastin time [aPTT]). A pro-Type B natriuretic peptide (pro-BNP) can be added for patients with a history of heart failure. Serum tests are prioritized when there is a suspicion of coagulopathy or kidney dysfunction.

General supportive care for airway and breathing includes maintaining peripheral oxygen saturation (SpO_2) greater than 94%. Typically, these intimal steps of imaging and obtaining baseline laboratory values occur in the emergency department (ED) with stroke team member involvement. Also, fibrinolytic therapy may be initiated in the field if a portable CT scan can be obtained or in the ED. If they meet eligibility criteria, the patient may be transported to an interventional radiology suite for further endovascular intervention.

TREATMENT

The AGACNP, in the initial phase of care, will likely admit the patient to the ICU for frequent surveillance of neurologic symptoms and blood pressure (BP). Maintain systemic BP to support organ function. Avoid hypotension and hypovolemia. Consider BP goals of <220/110 for all patients. If the patient is to be treated with IV fibrinolytic therapy or MT, keep the BP <185/110, managing both systolic (SBP) and diastolic (DBP) values. Drugs used to achieve BP goals include IV labetalol, nicardipine, or clevidipine. Hydralazine and enalaprilat may be considered.

The emergent treatment for ischemic stroke treatment is revascularization with either IV alteplase or MT. Tenecteplase is emerging as an alternative to alteplase, as it is more fibrin specific and has a longer duration of activity than alteplase. These therapies require time-dependent determination of eligibility, interpretation of the noncontract CT, and clinical judgment. Shared decision-making, to include a discussion of the risks and benefits of these therapies, is recommended in guidelines (Powers et al., 2019).

Alteplase, a fibrinolytic that causes thrombolysis via the tissue-plasminogen activation (tPA), is administered within 4.5 hours of moderate-to-severe stroke symptom onset or "last known well." However, data suggest IV alteplase is most effective at reversing symptoms when administered within 3 hours of symptoms. It can be effective and safe up to 9 hours following moderate-to-severe ischemic stroke symptom onset (Herpich & Rincon, 2020). Alteplase is administered as 0.9 mg/kg, with a maximum dose of 90 mg over 60 minutes. An initial 10% of the dose is given as a bolus over 1 minute. Although there are other tPa drugs (i.e., tenecteplase), only alteplase has Food and Drug Administration (FDA) approval for use in ischemic strokes. Tenecteplase is administered as a single bolus dose of 0.25 to 0.4 mg/kg (Warach et al., 2020).

When the patient wakes with stroke symptoms or has an unclear onset time, a diffusion-weight magnetic resonance imaging sequence (DW-MRI) may be used in comprehensive stroke centers to guide treatment decisions. In patients with DW-MRI lesions smaller than one-third of the MCA territory and no visible signal on fluid-attenuated inversion recovery (FLAIR), alteplase is recommended (Grosch et al., 2020).

AGACNPs involved with acute ischemic stroke care are prepared to manage alteplase therapy complications in the immediate hours following drug administration. These complications are bleeding, including ICH and angioedema. ICH can occur in as many as 2% to 7% of patients up to 10 hours after alteplase administration, particularly in patients with large strokes, diabetes, and older age. An ischemic stroke's conversion to a hemorrhagic stroke is associated with high mortality and more significant disability than ischemic stroke alone. Angioedema caused by tissue plasminogen increasing bradykinin production can occur in 1% to 5% of patients with sufficient severity to require intubation (Sczepanski & Bozyk, 2018).

MT requires expertise and specialized equipment, which are present in many comprehensive stroke centers. It is indicated for patients with a large artery occlusion in the anterior cerebral circulation, a condition that occurs in about 30% of patients who experience an acute ischemic stroke. It must be initiated within 24 hours of the last known well and can be used regardless of alteplase administration.

There are two sets of eligibility criteria for MT. One set of eligibility criteria is for early presentations—within 6 hours of symptom onset. The second set is for a late presentation. Because of late presentation and ineligibility, only about one quarter of patients with large anterior cerebral vessel occlusion are eligible for MT. The most effective MT approaches use stent-retrievers and/or aspiration to achieve fast first-pass complete reperfusion (Ospel et al., 2020). The typical access site is femoral. The AGACNP may provide site access and monitor or treat femoral site complications such as prolonged bleeding, hematoma formation, pseudoaneurysm formation, retroperitoneal bleeding, thrombosis or emboli, and limb ischemia (Shapiro et al., 2020).

Additional considerations for ICU care include not only management of stroke but interventions to avoid secondary brain injury. The AGACNP provides neurologic assessment, guidance for drug titration to achieve BP or hemodynamic goals, determination of intracranial hypertension, the need to drain CSF from hydrocephalus, glycemic control, new-onset seizure management, new-onset dysrhythmia treatment, determination of complex or frequent ineffective airway self-management, identification of respiratory failure and subsequent ventilatory management, and early recognition of infection (McNett & McLaughlin, 2019).

Intracranial hypertension is recognized by worsening mental status, respiratory abnormalities, and pupil size changes and reaction to light. The AGACNP will determine if symptomatic cerebral edema or hydrocephalus requires external CSF drainage. If the patient has a large hemispheric infarct or uncontrollable intracranial hypertension, the neurosurgeon may elect to perform a decompressive hemicraniectomy.

Both hypo- and hyperglycemia can extend brain injury and interfere with repair and recovery. Suspected or witnessed seizure can be evaluated in the ICU with a continuous EEG.

Dysrhythmias can alter brain perfusion. Notably, atrial fibrillation is associated with embolic stroke and requires rate control and long-term anticoagulation.

Ineffective airway management is manifested with copious oral secretions and/or dysphagia. The AGACNP's goal is to prevent aspiration. Respiratory failure can result from ineffective airway clearance and brain injury leading to central hypoxemia or combined hypoxia and hypercarbia. Infection can be related to aspiration, line placement, comorbidities, or surgical interventions.

Fever has a detrimental effect on stroke-related mortality and morbidity and the AGACNP must manage fever aggressively (Herpich & Rincon, 2020).

Nutrition and early rehabilitation occur in the ICU setting within 24 to 48 hours of admission. Comorbid and chronic care management also is addressed throughout critical and acute care hospitalization. For example, prolonged immobility related to hemodynamic instability or intracranial hypertension may require the addition of venothromboembolism event (VTE) prevention, such as intermittent pneumatic compression of lower extremities. The benefit of low molecular weight heparin (LMWH) is not clear in stroke patients.

TRANSITION OF CARE

Once the risk for acute neurologic deterioration decreases and neurologic exams stabilize, transfer from ICU to the acute care unit is planned. The AGACNP coordinates de-escalation of ICU care, including changing IV to oral or enteral drugs, providing a period of spontaneous respiration for at least 24 hours, determining aspiration risk (airway self-management), evaluating whether there is an absence of mental status changes that require frequent neurologic assessments.

If external diversion of CSF is necessary to prevent secondary brain injury, the AGACNP coordinates care to place a ventriculoperitoneal shunt. Generally, this is determined by decreased mental status when the external drainage device is clamped for increasingly extended periods before removal.

The AGACNP coordinates care for a tracheostomy and percutaneous endoscopic gastrostomy (PEG) when aspiration risk occurs. Referral to physical medicine can help determine the appropriate level of care to transition from inpatient to rehabilitation (Olson & Juengst, 2019; Thompson & Ifejika, 2019). Physical medicine includes physical, occupational, and speech therapy, access to rehabilitation specialists (e.g., physiatrist), and other specialists to enhance and restore functional ability and quality of life. A coordinated team approach is essential to meet patient-centered goals.

The stroke care team will transition the patient to rehabilitation after the ICU and acute care stay, often 5 to 7 days following ischemic stroke. If no neurologic deficits are present at acute care discharge, the transition will be outpatient provider follow-up. If there are neurologic deficits, rehabilitation improves functional outcomes. There is no single, best site for rehabilitation. Options include inpatient rehabilitation, skilled nursing facility rehabilitation, and home/outpatient rehabilitation.

Best practices include hand-off communication that is detailed and structured, provided before the transfer so that equipment and supplies, if needed, can be obtained, additional communication on the day of transfer, and a third contact 24 to 48 hours the following transfer to ensure that continuity of care, medication adherence, and sustainable strategies to reduce stroke risk is established (Olson & Juengst, 2019; Thompson & Ifejika, 2019). Screening for depression is advocated for any patient with a chronic condition.

Generally, two drug categories are prescribed for stroke risk reduction in the post-ICU phases of care. The first is an antiplatelet and the second is a statin.

Antiplatelet: Aspirin, dosed at 81 to 325 mg daily, is started 2 to 14 days after symptom onset (Kleindorfer et al., 2021). When atrial fibrillation or in patients with severe stenosis of a major intracranial artery, the addition of clopidogrel 75 mg daily for 90 days is recommended (Kleindorfer et al., 2021). Clopidogrel is a pro-drug. A small but significant population with metabolizing enzyme genetic inheritance cannot convert this drug to its active form. Ticagrelor 90 mg twice daily may be an alternative to clopidogrel for high-risk patients (Kleindorfer et al., 2021). Other direct-acting anticoagulants (DOACs) may be indicated, particularly for the patient with atrial fibrillation and selected inherited or acquired hypercoagulopathy. LMWH may be an alternative to antiplatelet therapy for patients who do not tolerate or cannot afford DOACs. However, the evidence for efficacy and safety in the stroke population is unclear (Neumann et al., 2020).

Statin: Statins reduce the risk of recurrent thromboembolic stroke by almost 20%. In patients with complex drug regimens, rosuvastatin and pravastatin do not undergo metabolism by cytochrome P450 enzymes and may be safer to use. However, no data support one statin's selection over another in stroke risk reduction (Tramacere et al., 2019).

CLINICAL PEARLS

- Use a point-of-service serum glucose test to rule out hypoglycemia, possible stroke mimic.
- Establish the time of symptom onset for stroke; record symptom onset as clock time (i.e., "11 a.m.," *not* "30 minutes ago").
- Use the NIHSS to provide baseline and trend data for neurologic changes.
- Stroke symptoms depend on the ischemic area of the brain and the site of cerebrovascular occlusion.
- IV alteplase (administered within 4.5 hours of symptom onset) and MT (delivered within 24 hours of symptom onset only when a large vessel is occluded) are associated with reversal of stroke symptoms, reduced disability, and lower mortality but are often not delivered due to delays in patient arrival to a stroke center.

KEY TAKEAWAYS

- The diagnosis and ICU management of stroke is time sensitive.
  - Complete a focused neurologic assessment with the NIHSS score within 10 minutes of patient presentation
  - Obtain a non-contrast head CT within 20 minutes of patient presentation.
- Early access to a primary or comprehensive stroke center improves outcomes.
- Early physical medicine during hospitalization can improve functional patient outcomes.
- A coordinated approach for rehabilitation transition, including a standard hand-off tool, recurrent communication before and after a change in care settings, and a resource guide based on patient-centered experiences with rehabilitation facilities, is recommended for all patients with ischemic stroke.

EVIDENCE-BASED RESOURCES

Powers, W. J., Rabinstein, A. A., Ackerson, T., Adeoye, O. M., Bambakidis, N. C., Becker, K., Biller, J., Brown, M., Demaerschalk, B. M., Hoh, B., Jauch, E. C., Kidwell, C. S., Leslie-Mazwi, T. M., Ovbiagele, B., Scott, P. A., Sheth, K. N., Southerland, A. M., Summers, D. V., Tirschwell, D. L., & on behalf of the American Heart Association Stroke Council. (2019). Guidelines for the early management of patients with acute ischemic stroke: 2019 update to the 2018 guidelines for the early management of acute ischemic stroke: A guideline for healthcare professionals from the American Heart Association/American Stroke Association. *Stroke, 50*(12), e344–e418. https://doi .org/10.1161/STR.0000000000000211

Standards for Neurologic Critical Care Units; Prophylaxis of Venous Thrombosis in Neurocritical Care Patients; *and* Evidence-based Guidelines for the Management of Large Hemispheric Infarction: https://www.neurocriticalcare .org/resources/guidelines

16.5: INTRACEREBRAL AND INTRAVENTRICULAR HEMORRHAGE

Chris Winkelman

Intracerebral hemorrhage (ICH) is defined as brain parenchymal bleeding. Most commonly caused by hypertension, ICH causes 10% to 20% of all strokes worldwide (An et al., 2017). Besides hypertension, other causes of ICH are cerebral amyloid angiopathy, tumor, vascular abnormalities (e.g., saccular aneurysm, arteriovenous malformations, and cavernous malformations), anticoagulation/antiplatelet therapy, illicit sympathomimetic drug use, and trauma (McGurgan et al., 2020). Mortality for patients with ICH is 25% to 30% within 21 to 30 days in the United States and over 50% at 1 year (McGurgan et al., 2020).

Intraventricular hemorrhage (IVH), defined as blood in the cranial ventricles, can occur in as many as half of patients with spontaneous ICH (Trifan et al., 2019). The severity of IVH, measured by the volume of ventricular blood (i.e., Graeb score; Graeb et al., 1982), contributes to both mortality and poor functional outcome when associated with ICH (Trifan et al., 2019). It is rare to see adults with primary IVH as a presenting pathology. The most common conditions related to IVH are hypertensive ICH and subarachnoid bleeding. Vascular malformations may account for as many as half of patients who experience ICH. Anticoagulant or antiplatelet therapy is also a cause of ICH and IVH.

PRESENTING SIGNS AND SYMPTOMS

The presentation of ICH is similar to ischemic stroke (see Section 16.4, Ischemic Stroke). The onset of symptoms is abrupt and typically manifests as a focal deficit. Focal symptoms evolve over minutes to hours, similar to ischemic stroke. Headache, reduced consciousness (i.e., a reduced Glasgow Coma Score [GCS] by two or more points during acute evaluation), seizure, vomiting, and very high blood pressure (BP) are somewhat more likely with ICH or IVH than ischemic stroke (Ai et al., 2018). Still, these symptoms are neither specific nor sensitive to ICH or IVH diagnoses. Focal signs are minimal or absent with IVH. The focal dysfunction depends on the bleeding vessel's location, blood volume, and the degree of mass effect (see Section 16.4, Ischemic Stroke).

HISTORY AND PHYSICAL EXAM

Ask for the time of symptom onset and ask a witness if the patient cannot reply. Obtain crucial information about whether trauma is associated with this change in function since traumatic ICH and IVH may require neurosurgical management. Determine if the patient has a coagulopathy or is taking anticoagulation or antiplatelet medications. If the patient is taking one of these agents, obtain the agent's name, the dose, and the most recent administration time.

Evaluate baseline status, typically using the GCS or the National Institutes of Health Stroke Scale (NIHSS). While neither of these tools was normed for patients diagnosed with ICH or IVH, they are simple to use and have prognostic value. The FOUR score is a potential alternative and does not require verbal ability (Almojuela et al., 2019). Obtain a baseline ICH severity score, such as the ICH score (Gregorio et al., 2018; McGurgan et al., 2020).

DIFFERENTIAL DIAGNOSIS AND DIAGNOSTIC CONSIDERATIONS

The AGACNP's acute care focus is on *rapid* diagnosis. The first 24 to 48 hours after admission are challenging. The AGACNP will want to consider incorporating patient and family preferences and values early to avoid nihilism (i.e., undertreatment) and prolonged suffering (i.e., futile or ineffective treatment). Differential diagnoses to be considered with ICH are listed in Table 16.7.

Diagnostic Testing

Rapid neuroimaging is essential to care during admission. Both noncontrast CT and MRI are highly sensitive and specific in diagnosing ICH and IVH and considered reasonable for initial diagnosis (Hemphill et al., 2015). However, the time (i.e., greater time to prepare and more prolonged duration), costs, and patient tolerance for MRI may preclude its use as the first diagnostic image. The image is assessed for ICH location. MRI can also detect brain atrophy or leukoaraiosis (pathological appearance of the brain white matter); lacunes consistent with small vessel disease or cerebral amyloid angiopathy; subtle signs of mass effect such as midline shift; hydrocephalus; IVH extension; and the size of the hematoma, using the ABC/2 formula (Figure 16.2; McGurgan et al., 2020). The CT scan will quickly and accurately narrow differential diagnoses to ICH with or without IVH extension.

Collect blood for coagulation studies, a complete blood count (CBC) with differential, a comprehensive metabolic panel (CMP), hemoglobin A1C (HbA1C), cardiac-specific troponin, and a toxicology screen. A pro-brain natriuretic peptide (BNP) may be useful for prognostication in a patient with either a history of atherosclerotic cardiovascular disease or heart failure.

Patients with a stroke diagnosis are at risk for EKG abnormalities in repolarization and ischemia-like injury patterns. Intracranial hemorrhage, particularly with blood in the subarachnoid space, is associated with ST-segment elevation, hyperacute T waves, and QT prolongation in as many as 70% of adults (Khechinashvili & Asplund, 2002). Tropinin elevation is also common (Lasek-Bal et al., 2014). Generally, these findings are associated with autonomic dysfunction, not myocardial ischemia or infarct. Without concurrent symptoms of myocardial infarction such as angina, diaphoresis, new-onset dysrhythmias, or hemodynamic instability, the clinician can monitor the patient with serial EKGs and troponin and continuous EKG monitoring rather than request urgent cardiology consult. Patients with underlying cardiac disease are more likely to exhibit EKG, troponin and pro-BNP abnormalities (Lasek-Bal et al., 2014; Khechinashvili & Asplund, 2002). Some authors report a poorer prognosis or greater risk for readmission to the hospital and ICU with these findings, regardless of actual damage to the myocardium (Khechinashvili & Asplund, 2002; Myint et al., 2008).

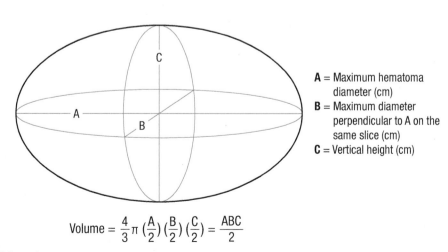

$$\text{Volume} = \frac{4}{3}\pi\left(\frac{A}{2}\right)\left(\frac{B}{2}\right)\left(\frac{C}{2}\right) = \frac{ABC}{2}$$

A = Maximum hematoma diameter (cm)

B = Maximum diameter perpendicular to A on the same slice (cm)

C = Vertical height (cm)

FIGURE 16.2: ABC/2 formula.

Follow-up imaging is recommended for all patients with ICH. Computed tomography angiography (CTA) is usually performed within 2 days of the initial noncontrast CT to determine macrovascular causes of bleeding (aneurysmal sac or arteriovenous malformation) and predictors of hematoma expansion. MRI is useful after the acute phase of ICH, providing information about small vessel disease.

TREATMENT

ICH is a medical emergency. Full provision of high-quality, bundled care includes managing BP, reversing coagulopathy (if present), and consulting or communicating with the neurosurgeon. Management of ICH complications and preventing secondary brain injury are the additional foci for acute and critical care. Despite a lack of effective treatments and high rates of poor outcomes associated with ICH, experts advocate the full provision of bundled care for at least 24 to 48 hours after admission since prognosis is difficult to determine in this timeframe (Gregorio et al., 2018; McGurgan et al., 2020).

The initial priority is to rapidly achieve systolic BP (SBP) value less than 140 mmHg (Hemphill et al., 2015). No single IV agent is superior to accomplish this goal, although labetalol is commonly used (Lattanzi et al., 2017). Patients with ICH often arrive with SPBs greater than 200 mmHg. During the first hour of admission, an SBP 120 to 140 mmHg is associated with reduced death and disability. Several IV agents are used in practice, detailed in Box 16.2. There is no evidence one is superior to another.

BOX 16.2 AGENTS TO MANAGE ARTERIAL HYPERTENSION IN PATIENTS WITH INTRACRANIAL HEMORRHAGE

Labetalol IV bolus 10 to 20 mg IV over 1 to 2 min, may repeat one time. Then 40 to 80 mg IV every 10 minutes; total dose not to exceed 300 mg. Continuous IV dose: 1 to 8 mg/min.

Nicardipine IV continuous, start at 5 mg/hour, titrate up by 2.5 mg/h every 5 to 15 min, maximum 15 mg/h; when desired, BP reached and adjusted to maintain proper BP limits.

Clevidipine IV continuous, start at 1 to 2 mg/h, titrate by doubling the dose every 2 to 5 min until desired BP reached; maximum 21 mg/h.

Hydralazine IV bolus may be considered. 5 to 20 mg/dose every 6 hours. No continuous administration.

Enalaprilat IV bolus may be considered. 1.25 mg/dose over 5 minutes every 6 hours. No continuous administration.

Sodium nitroprusside may be considered as a continuous drip, titrated to BP goal.

BP, systemic blood pressure; IV, intravenous; mg, milligram; min, minute

---

If the patient has a coagulopathy, such as thrombocytopenia, blood products can improve the status, although normalizing values is controversial. It may be acceptable to aim for values that are not dangerous. If uremia is contributing to coagulopathy, consider nephrology consultation and early dialysis. Anticoagulation therapy accounts for at least 20% of all ICH cases (McGurgan et al., 2020). If the coagulopathy is acquired from prescriptive drugs, use reversal agents to minimize rebleeding.

Intensive ICP monitoring is recommended for patients with a GCS <9, evidence of herniation, or hydrocephalus (Hemphill et al., 2015; McGurgan et al., 2020). If there are clinical signs of mass effect or increased ICP, adjusting BP targets is an appropriate intervention. However, the level of evidence for specific measures to reduce ICP (i.e., positioning the head of the bed to 30-degrees elevation, using mannitol and hypertonic saline, prescribing mild sedation and analgesia) is not robust for patients with ICH.

Neurosurgical/neurologic expertise positively contributes to intensive, bundled care. Specialty care in a stroke or neuro unit decreases mortality following ICH (McGurgan et al., 2020). If CTA imaging reveals vascular malformations, early intervention with coiling or repair is indicated. If there are no macrovascular abnormalities, consider MRI/ARI-angiography after the acute phase of care. If the hematoma is lobar, accessible, and creating a significant shift, acute hemicraniectomy may be indicated; deeper hematomas are not amenable to surgical removal (McGurgan et al., 2020). Similarly, neurosurgical intervention is recommended for infratentorial ICH. Neurosurgery timing must balance the risk of rebleeding (high, when done early) with secondary brain injury (high, when done late). Minimally invasive surgery is emerging as an efficient and safe treatment for clot removal in patients with ICH and IVH (Tang et al., 2018).

Other interventions recommended during intensive acute care are more generic to brain health. Provide glycemic control, generally with goals of 140 to 180 mg/d and avoid hypoglycemia. Consider fever prevention interventions and aggressively reduce fever when ICH is associated with severe brain injury (Hemphill et al., 2015). Be prepared for early-onset seizures that occur in about 14% of patients with ICH. Routine prophylactic antiepileptic drugs are not recommended (Hemphill et al., 2015). Start enteral feeding within 48 hours of admission as in the care of any critically ill neurologic patient.

TRANSITIONS OF CARE

As with ischemic stroke, multiple factors influence decisions about transitioning patients. First, the AGACNP must de-escalate care from the ICU to prepare the patient for transfer to acute care. Then hospital length of stay, age, insurance status, comorbidities, and patient or family preferences influence the next steps. While there is some information that early discharge to inpatient rehabilitation is beneficial for patients with ischemic stroke, there are few data to support best practices when the patient has been diagnosed with ICH, IVH, or both. Because patients with ICH are more likely to have prolonged decreased consciousness or the need for ICP management, early transfer from ICU is less likely than with ischemic stroke. The AGACNP must be aware of the high readmission rates for this population, often associated with respiratory deterioration. Involve the case manager or stroke treatment team early to plan for transfers such that equipment and staff or family support are engaged to minimize readmission.

ICH is associated with significant mortality. An early conversation with the family about patient preferences and values is useful for decisions around care transitions. However, the AGACNP is cautioned that early do-not-resuscitate (DNR) orders are associated with fewer supportive care interventions (McGurgan et al., 2020). Avoid using a single assessment, measure or finding to guide decisions acutely and remain focused on patient values, particularly in discussions about transitioning to palliative and end-of-life care.

CLINICAL PEARLS

- As with ischemic stroke, neurologic signs reflect the location of bleeding.
- Bleeding into the brain is associated with uncontrolled hypertension and cerebral vascular disease.
- Noncontrast imaging is fast and used early for ICH and IVH confirmation.
- Extension of ICH into the ventricles (IVH) is a dire complication.
- Patients with ICH need a neurosurgical consult.
- After ICH, BP control is controversial; guidelines recommend SBP <140 mmHg within 1 hour of presentation for best outcomes.

KEY TAKEAWAYS

- Rapid identification and timely management are hallmarks of guideline-recommended care.
- A focused, rapid neurologic exam and non contrast CT scan are essential to differentiate this condition from other, similar presentations.
- Attaining an SBP of 120 to 140 mmHg rapidly and treating acquired or inherited coagulopathy improves survival.
- Avoid secondary brain injury, particularly from increased ICP.
- Provide care in a specialized unit to improve functional outcomes and reduce mortality, although evidence is limited.

EVIDENCE-BASED RESOURCES

Guidelines for the Management of Spontaneous Intracerebral Hemorrhage: https://www.ahajournals.org/doi/10.1161/str.0b013e3181ec611b

Standards for Neurologic critical Care Units and Guidelines for Reversal of Antithrombotics in Intracranial Hemorrhage: https://www.neurocriticalcare.org/resources/guidelines

16.6: PARKINSON DISEASE

Chris Winkelman

Parkinson disease (PD) is the most common movement disorder and is progressively neurodegenerative. PD is caused by the degeneration of dopamine-producing neurons in the substantia nigra, part of the midbrain's basal ganglia (Tkacs et al., 2021). Degeneration of the dopamine pathway is accompanied by relative overactivity of acetylcholine in the subcortical basal ganglia, the striatum (Tkacs et al., 2021). PD is considered idiopathic with known genetic and environmental exposure (e.g., pesticides, solvents, metals) contributions (Armstrong & Okun, 2020). It is more common among men and those over 50 years.

Neuroleptic malignant syndrome (NMS) can present after abrupt discontinuation of dopamine agonists, a class of drugs used to treat PD. This syndrome also occurs in up to 3% of patients who take dopamine antagonists such as antipsychotics and metoclopramide. NMS is thought to result from neurotransmission derangements in central (i.e., thalamic) and peripheral (i.e., skeletal muscles) structures (Velosa et al., 2019).

For patients with PD, reasons for admission include (a) disease-related complications such as autonomic dysfunction, motor fluctuations, psychiatric symptoms, and adverse effects of drug therapy; (b) indirect disease-related complications, particularly pneumonia and injury from fall; and (c) systemic diseases unrelated to PD including cardiovascular disease and infection (Ramirez-Zamora & Tsuboi, 2020).

PRESENTING SIGNS AND SYMPTOMS

PD has variable symptoms with variable intensity. Akinesia and bradykinesia on one side of the body with resting tremor, often in wrists, and rigidity are consistent PD manifestations. These symptoms result in changes in posture, walking, and facial expression. Early nonmotor symptoms are orthostatic hypotension, hyposomia (reduced sense of smell), hypophonia, sleep disorders, and constipation. Motor and nonmotor symptoms progress in late disease. They include postural instability leading to falls, psychiatric disorders (e.g., depression, anxiety, apathy, hallucinations, delusions), and cognitive impairment affecting attention, executive, and visuospatial functions (Armstrong & Okun, 2020). A family history of PD increases the likelihood of this diagnosis. PD is staged 1 to 5 as symptoms interfere with daily activities and independence, with Stage 1 as the least severe. The Unified PD Rating Scale is a comprehensive tool to trend motor and nonmotor symptoms.

HISTORY AND PHYSICAL FINDINGS

PD is diagnosed with a history and physical exam. To meet clinical diagnostic criteria, the patient must demonstrate bradykinesia with rest tremor, rigidity, or both (Balestrino & Schapira, 2020). Combined with symptoms, a clear benefit of dopamine agonists defines PD. There are diverse presentations of PD, suggesting that several subtypes occur in this progressive neurodegenerative condition. However, subtype categorization is not used clinically.

NMS related to PD is distinguished by exposure to a dopamine antagonist or a dopamine agonist's withdrawal within the 72 hours preceding the onset of symptoms (Ware et al., 2018). Exhaustion, dehydration, and malnutrition can increase the risk of NMS. Symptoms include (Ware et al., 2018):

- Hyperthermia of greater than 100.4°F/38°C degrees (oral)
- Rigidity
- Reduced or fluctuating mental status
- Elevated creatine kinase (CK)
- High systolic or diastolic BP more than 25% from baseline or more than 20–25 mmHg
- Heart rate elevated more than 25% over baseline
- The respiratory rate increased by 50% or more from baseline
- Diaphoresis
- Urinary incontinence
- Absence of infection, toxin exposure, metabolic or neurologic cause

DIFFERENTIAL DIAGNOSIS AND DIAGNOSTIC CONSIDERATIONS

Differential Diagnoses

The differential diagnoses for PD include essential tremor, drug-induced PD, vascular parkinsonism, multiple system atrophy, and progressive supranuclear palsy. Liver disease, dementia, Huntington disease, and prion diseases (e.g., Creutzfeldt-Jakob disease, bovine spongiform encephalopathy and others) can also mimic PD. These alternative diagnoses are likely to have been established before the patient is admitted to acute or critical care.

Since NMS is a diagnosis of exclusion, the AGACNP first rules out alternative diagnoses before NMS. Because NMS is an emergent condition, quick actions to rule out alternatives must occur. Alternative diagnoses to be considered are thyrotoxicosis, pheochromocytoma, heatstroke, serotonin syndrome, CNS infections or mass lesions, toxin exposure or drug-drug adverse interactions, exposure to inhalation anesthetic, stimulant or hallucinogen use, and alcohol withdrawal.

Diagnostic Testing

Dopamine transporter single-photon emission computed tomography (DaT SPECT) may be used when PD is uncertain with a physical exam. In this imaging, a radioactive tracer is taken up to dopamine transporters in the basal ganglia; there is reduced uptake in PD. Myocardial scintigraphy (using iodine-123-meta-iobensylguanidine) can be used to establish confirmation of a PD diagnosis. This test assesses cardiac norepinephrine uptake, which is low due to postganglionic sympathetic neuron dysfunction in PD.

There is no single serum or image test for the diagnosis of NMS. Serum CK may indicate rhabdomyolysis associated with NMS. Neuroimaging is usually normal during NMS symptom occurrence.

TREATMENT

Available treatment for PD offers motor symptom control and supportive care but does not alter disease progression. Multidisciplinary teams effectively diagnose and manage PD (Radder et al., 2020). Physical, occupational, and speech therapy can maintain motor ability and speech, improve balance and gait, address dysphagia, and contribute to functional adaptation. Regular, intense exercise results in less worsening of motor function and may mitigate bothersome symptoms (Armstrong & Okun, 2020; Martignon et al., 2020).

Motor symptoms of PD are treated pharmacologically and surgically. Levodopa is the most effective drug for motor symptoms (Balestrino & Schapira, 2020). Other drugs used are dopamine agonists and monoamine oxidase-B (MAO-B) inhibitors. Anticholinergic agents can be used to treat prominent tremors. Deep brain stimulation (DBS) is a surgical intervention to improve on-medication motor symptoms. Leads are placed in the subthalamic nucleus or globus pallidus interna and attached to a battery pack in the chest, similar to a cardiac pacemaker.

Nonmotor symptom treatment has fewer data to support treatment. Selective serotonin reuptake inhibitors and cognitivebehavioral therapy treat depression and anxiety. If psychosis presents, wean contributing drugs such as anticholinergic, amantadine, dopamine agonists, and MAO-B inhibitors. The challenge is that weaning PD treatment drugs may result in the reemergence of debilitating symptoms. It is possible to add antipsychotic drugs (i.e., clozapine, quetiapine) with weekly monitoring for adverse effects. Treatment for orthostatic hypotension and constipation is not unique to PD. Low-quality evidence supports treating insomnia with melatonin or clonazepam. There are no evidence-based treatments for apathy. Several clinical trials are investigating the use of cannabinoids for nonmotor PD symptoms.

For patients with PD hospitalized in acute and critical care, the priority treatment is to maintain home medications (e.g., formulation, dose, frequency) and administration schedule from home settings (Ramirez-Zamora & Tsuboi, 2020). This priority is within the AGACNP's scope of practice. When PD drugs are stopped, omitted, or prescribed differently, there is a great probability of significant adverse events. Medication errors are common in as many as 75% of patients with PD (Ramirez-Zamora & Tsuboi, 2020). Adjusting dopaminergic drugs to manage psychosis or orthostatic hypotension while in the hospital requires expertise; consultation with a movement disorder neurologist or specialist is recommended. When starting new drugs, consultation with a knowledgeable pharmacist is advised; there is evidence that pharmacists in hospital settings reduce inappropriate prescribing and add safety, although these data are not specific to patients with PD in the United States (Lertxundi Etxebarria et al., 2020; Patel & Gurumurthy 2019). Dopamine-blocking agents, such as antipsychotics and metoclopramide, should not be given as they worsen motor symptoms. Serious drug-drug interactions, especially with MAO-B inhibitors, are common and avoidable. Patients with PD are at high risk for delirium from anticholinergic effects of some antibiotics and many drugs used to manage acute hypertension or dysrhythmias. The Parkinson's Foundation offers a Hospitalization Letter to communicate essential information about drug administration and other priorities in care (https://www.parkinson.org/blog/tips/advanced-directives).

Other priorities include heightened surveillance for aspiration related to dysphagia, increased falls, the risk from postural instability and autonomic dysfunction, avoiding drug-drug interactions, especially with MAO-B inhibitors, and implementing a bowel regimen to avoid all-too-common constipation. An interprofessional approach is best and the AGACNP can work with the dietician, speech therapist, pharmacist, and nursing staff to minimize the risk of aspiration, falls, and constipation. Sleep disturbances are commonly associated with PD and are addressed first with nonpharmacologic interventions. Patients with DBS devices may need the device turned off during diagnostic tests such as an EKG. The Joint Commission offers disease-specific care certification to ensure adherence to established standards for specific inpatient populations. There is one hospital's report that using this format improved care for patients with PD in inpatient settings (Azmi et al., 2019).

NMS treatment is supportive. For the patient with PD, either withdraw the antidopaminergic drug or re-start the dopamine antagonist. Consider volume replacement, monitoring and correcting serum electrolytes, physical cooling measures to manage hyperthermia (Velosa et al., 2019; Ware et al., 2018). Intensive monitoring for complications is indicated for at least 24 hours. While not based on high-quality evidence, treatment with a trial of lorazepam at 1 to 2 mg every 4 to 6 hours may reduce rigidity and fever (Ware et al., 2018).

TRANSITION OF CARE

Hospitalization may be an opportunity to introduce palliative care to patients with PD. Palliative care focuses on symptom management to improve the quality of life for both patients and their families. Ensuring that the patient receives interprofessional care during transitions in settings is essential to minimize complications and adverse events. Planning and communicating changes in care settings and supporting independence are crucial to safely discharging patients with PD from critical and acute care settings.

CLINICAL PEARLS

- Many drugs act as neuroleptics and interfere with PD treatment; the pharmacist and movement disorder specialist can advise the AGACNP who is starting a new drug in the inpatient setting for the patient with PD.
- Maintain the home drug, dose, frequency, and schedule for drugs used to manage PD.
- Work closely with team members to minimize risk from aspiration, falls, and constipation as these are common conditions in patients with PD.

KEY TAKEAWAYS

- PD is diagnosed clinically and typically in outpatient settings.
- Sudden withdrawal of dopamine agonists, used to manage PD, can result in NMS and patient harm.
- Management of patients with PD prioritizes the home medication regimen.
- Work closely with experts to deliver safe, high-quality care for the patient with PD admitted to acute or critical care to avoid harm from aspiration, falls, and constipation.

EVIDENCE-BASED RESOURCE

https://www.parkinson.org/understanding-parkinsons

16.7: SEIZURES, EPILEPSY

Diane McLaughlin

PRESENTING SIGNS AND SYMPTOMS

There are many different seizure types, and each presents differently. The most commonly observed seizure is the generalized tonic-clonic seizure, characterized by an acute loss of consciousness with stiffening followed by jerking/twitching motor movement. Other types of generalized seizures include absence, which occurs in childhood. Atonic is an acute loss of motor tone, sometimes called "drop" attacks. Clonic seizures involve rhythmic jerking, usually in the upper hemisphere. Tonic seizures are often accompanied by impaired consciousness and present as an acute muscle stiffening.

Partial seizures make up the other category of seizures. These include focal seizures, which can vary significantly in presentation dependent upon the part of the cortex from which the seizure originates. An aura often precipitates these. Some focal seizures occur with intact awareness and some with impaired awareness. In patients with impaired awareness, the patient appears awake but cannot interact with their environment. Automatisms (chewing, lip-smacking) may be present.

The post-ictal period is the time immediately following seizures, which can last minutes to hours. During this time, the patient gradually arouses. The patient often has slow, deep respirations but is minimally responsive to external stimuli. Confusion and agitation can be present in some patients.

Some patients have Todd's paralysis following a seizure. Todd's paralysis is a temporary focal weakness that occurs on one side of the body following seizures and can last minutes to hours.

HISTORY AND PHYSICAL FINDINGS

History and physical exam in these patients supply essential information about the underlying cause of the seizure. For example, a patient with known seizures is most likely subtherapeutic on medication, typically noncompliant. Structural abnormalities are the most likely cause of new-onset seizures in patients with no known history. In children, the most common cause is febrile seizures.

Important information to gather includes the time that the seizures started and stopped.

DIFFERENTIAL DIAGNOSIS AND DIAGNOSTIC CONSIDERATIONS

Many labs can be useful in diagnosing the underlying cause of seizures. Substrates, such as glucose, SpO2, complete blood count (CBC) to evaluate potential infection, comprehensive metabolic panel (CMP) to include electrolyte abnormalities, lactate, urinalysis (UA), toxicology screen to assess for illicit substances, alcohol level, and drug levels to determine compliance or appropriate dosing of existing antiepileptic regimen are useful. Prolactin can help differentiate between seizure and psychogenic nonepileptic seizures (PNES) as it rises two to three times for 10 to 60 minutes following most complex partial or generalized seizures. Cerebrospinal fluid (CSF) can be sent if there is a concern for encephalitis or meningitis. Seizures are often the presenting symptom in patients with encephalitis. One mnemonic used is SICK DRIFTER, shown in Figure 16.3.

Differential Diagnoses

- Migraines (typically gradual onset over 5–10 minutes)
- Psychogenic nonepileptic seizures (PNES)
- Encephalitis/meningitis
- Tumor

SICK DRIFTER

S — Substrates (Sugar, oxygen)

I — Isoniazid Overdose

C — Cations (Na, Ca, Mg)

K — Kids (Eclampsia)

D — Drugs (CRAP: Cocaine, Rum [Alcohol], Amphetamines, PCP)

R — Rum (Alcohol withdrawal)

I — Illness (Chronic seizure disorder or other chronic disorder)

F — Fever (Meningitis, encephalitis, abscess)

T — Trauma (Epidural, subdural, intraparynchymal hemorrhage)

Extra: Toxicologic (TAIL: Theo, ASA, Isoniazid, Lithium) and 3 Anti's: (Antihistamine overdose, Antidepressant overdose, Anticonvulsants (too high dilanitin, tegretol) or benzo withdrawal

R — Rat Poison (Organophosphates poisoning—not actually rat poison!)

FIGURE 16.3: Differential diagnoses to consider when evaluating seizures.
Source: Courtesy N. McLaughlin.

Diagnostic Testing

Neuroimaging is obtained in every first-time seizure patient to evaluate for the structural cause of the seizure. If there is a concern for acute findings, such as intracranial hemorrhage (ICH), CT imaging is preferred due to the availability to obtain quickly. MRI is best to get the most information, including possible mesial temporal sclerosis, infarcted tissue, tumors, or cortical dysplasia.

If the patient does not return to baseline, EEG is obtained to evaluate status epilepticus and the need for continued intervention. A nonemergent EEG can be scheduled in patients who return to baseline.

TABLE 16.8: Antiepileptic Bolus Guide

	FOSPHENYTOIN	VALPROIC ACID	LEVETIRACETAM
Bolus dose	20 mg PE/kg	40 mg/kg	60 mg/kg
Max. dose	1,500 mg	3,000 mg	4,500 mg

TREATMENT

There are two crucial components of management: patient safety and monitoring. Most single seizures are self-limiting (Krumholz et al., 2015). The priority is ensuring that the patient's airway, breathing, and circulation are supported (Glauser et al., 2016). Protecting the airway does not necessarily mean intubation, but the patient's ability to maintain an airway is evaluated. However, supplemental oxygen is applied to attain a SpO_2 greater than 92% to 94% (Glauser et al., 2016). Patients are not restrained or held immobile during a seizure. Provide a safe environment by clearing the area of hard or sharp objects. Place the patient on their side to help prevent aspiration. Place no items in the patient's mouth during a seizure. Monitor the patient during the seizure and until the postictal state, if it occurs, resolves.

In patients with persistent seizures (>5 min), medical management starts with administering a benzodiazepine. In the hospital, IV lorazepam can be administered at a dose of 0.1 mg/kg/dose with a max of 4 mg/dose, which can be repeated once (Krumholz et al., 2015). If IV access is not available, intramuscular midazolam can be administered as a single dose of 10 mg for patients weighing >40 kg (Krumholz et al., 2015).

If seizures continue to persist and/or there is a concern for status epilepticus, second-line therapy is administering antiepileptic medication such as fosphenytoin, valproic acid, or levetiracetam (Table 16.8; Krumholz et al., 2015).

If seizure control is still not achieved, the patient typically requires intubation for anesthetic dosing of midazolam, propofol, or pentobarbital and continuous EEG monitoring. The overall treatment goal in patients with status epilepticus is avoiding secondary brain injury, preventing decreased cerebral perfusion, and seizure termination.

TRANSITION OF CARE

The transition from EMS or emergency department to managing service includes the time and nature of seizure and stabilizing therapies administered.

In patients with first-time unprovoked seizures, a discussion should be had regarding the need for antiepileptic medications. The highest risk for recurrence is during the first 2 years. Up to one third of patients experience adverse effects from theirantiepileptic drugs (AEDs; Venkatasubramanian et al., 2020).

Most states require patients to be seizure-free to maintain driving privileges. Some states require providers to report a seizure condition to the state motor vehicle department.

CLINICAL PEARLS

- Most seizures end within 2 minutes.
- Lateral tongue bite has high specificity in distinguishing between PNES and generalized seizures.

KEY TAKEAWAYS

- Evaluate patients with unexplained unresponsiveness for status epilepticus.
- Status epilepticus that is unresolved in <20 hours has a mortality >80%, as opposed to cases resolved in <10 hours, which carry a mortality of <10%.
- Provoked seizure due to an acute neurologic cause is unlikely to recur.

EVIDENCE-BASED RESOURCES

Guidelines for the Evaluation and Management of Status Epilepticus: https://www.neurocriticalcare.org/resources/guidelines

Krumholz, A., Wiebe, S., Gronseth, G. S., Gloss, D.S., Sanchez, A. M., Kabir, A. A., Liferidge, A. T., Martello, J. P., Kanner, A. M., Shinnar, S., Hopp, J. L., & French, J. A. (2015). Evidence-based guideline: Management of an unprovoked first seizure in adults: Report of the guideline development subcommittee of the American Academy of Neurology and the American Epilepsy Society. *Neurology, 84*(16), 1705–1713. https://doi.org/10.1212/WNL.0000000000001487

A robust set of instructor resources designed to supplement this text is located at **http://connect.springerpub.com/content/reference-book/978-0-8261-6079-9.** Qualifying instructors may request access by emailing **textbook@springerpub.com.**

REFERENCES

A full list of references can be accessed at http://connect.springerpub.com/content/reference-book/978-0-8261-6079-9

CHAPTER 17

PSYCHOSOCIAL, BEHAVIORAL, AND COGNITIVE HEALTH DISORDERS

LEARNING OBJECTIVES

- Identify signs, symptoms, and risk factors indicative of agitation, delirium, anxiety, and insomnia in hospitalized adults.
- Discuss management strategies to mitigate agitation, anxiety, delirium, and insomnia in hospitalized adults.
- Demonstrate understanding of causes of dementia.
- Implement appropriate diagnostic testing and treatment for dementia.
- Demonstrate understanding of treatment strategies for geriatric depression.
- Apply best practices to reduce the incidence and severity of post-ICU syndrome in patients and families recovering from critical illness.
- Demonstrate understanding of the risk factors for developing posttraumatic stress disorder (PTSD).
- Apply evidence-based treatments for PTSD.
- Differentiate between different withdrawal syndromes and identify corresponding treatment strategies.
- Demonstrate understanding of the risk factors for developing Wernicke's encephalopathy.

INTRODUCTION

This chapter equips the adult-gerontology acute care nurse practitioner (AGACNP) with the information needed to successfully manage psychosocial, behaviorial health, and cognitive disorders encountered in acute care settings. Signs and symptoms of various disorders are discussed, in addition to risk factors and management strategies. An overview of both pharmacologic and nonpharmacologic strategies to mitigate the disorders and syndromes are provided.

17.1: AGITATION

Brayden Kameg

Agitation or combative behavior is a common complication within acute care settings. Rates of agitation within acute care settings consistently exceed 50%; thus, AGACNPs must be familiar with the identification and management of agitation (Gravante et al., 2020; Williamson et al., 2020). Risk factors for the development of agitation within acute care settings include older age over 65 years, obesity, tobacco use, postsurgical status and intraoperative complications, and endotracheal intubation (Kang et al., 2020; Lawson et al., 2020). The nature of critical care environments, including frequent nursing care procedures, such as oral and ophthalmic care, pressure area care, endotracheal tube and catheter care, can also precipitate agitation in adults who are hospitalized (Lesny et al., 2020). In addition to increased healthcare expenditures, hospital-related agitation increases the risk of longer hospital stay, longer duration of mechanical ventilation, and increased risk for self-extubation (Burk et al., 2014). Given the both the frequency of agitation and adverse outcomes related to agitation, AGACNPs must ensure that agitation is swiftly identified and adequately managed.

PRESENTING SIGNS AND SYMPTOMS

Early signs of agitation include restlessness or tremulousness. Individuals might appear visibly anxious. Agitation can progress to pacing in those who are ambulatory, or frequent nonpurposeful physical movement and psychomotor agitation. Individuals may attempt to remove tubes or catheters and may also attempt to self-extubate. In more severe cases, individuals who are experiencing acute agitation might become overtly combative and violent toward themselves, staff, or others (Ely et al.; 2003).

HISTORY AND PHYSICAL FINDINGS

AGACNPs must be astute in their assessment for those hospitalized and at risk for agitation. Careful attention should be paid to the aforementioned risk factors, and AGACNPs should evaluate for psychiatric or substance use disorders or traumatic brain injuries (TBI) that might predispose adults to impulsivity and subsequent agitated or combative behavior (Burk et al., 2014). The Richmond Agitation Sedation Scale (RASS) or the Riker Sedation Agitation Scale (SAS) can also be utilized to evaluate for agitation and augment history and physical exam findings (Ely et al., 2003).

DIFFERENTIAL DIAGNOSIS AND DIAGNOSTIC CONSIDERATIONS

For adults experiencing agitation while hospitalized, substance intoxication, psychosis, or mania should be considered. Furthermore, individuals exhibiting signs and symptoms of agitation should be evaluated for delirium. Consideration of infectious, neurologic, metabolic, and endocrine etiologies is also needed.

TREATMENT

Prevention of agitation is critical and can improve outcomes for hospitalized adults. Prevention measures include nonpharmacologic interventions, such as early mobilization, cognitive stimulation, and facilitation of adequate sleep. These prevention interventions should be done universally in critical care settings.

The Society of Critical Care Medicine (SCCM) has developed clinical practice guidelines for the management of agitation in adults who are hospitalized (Devlin et al., 2018). When using pharmacologic treatment for those mechanically ventilated, such as sedatives, the risks versus benefits of such use must be carefully weighed, as sedative use can increase risk of mortality in those who are hospitalized. When a sedative is indicated, sedation status should be assessed routinely and frequently via reliable and valid instruments, such as the RASS or the Riker SAS. Light degrees of sedation and daily awakening trials are recommended. Regarding the choice of sedative, nonbenzodiazepines are preferred, including propofol or dexmedetomidine (Devlin et al., 2018).

Antipsychotics can be utilized for adult patients who are experiencing agitation in acute care settings (Wang et al., 2020). These medications can be administered intramuscularly or intravenously. Agents include haloperidol, olanzapine, risperidone, and ziprasidone, and cautious monitoring of extrapyramidal symptoms, which can sometimes worsen agitation, should ensue (Aubanel et al., 2020).

Physical restraints can also be used in individuals experiencing agitation, but are generally considered a last-line approach, as such use can contribute to worsening functional decline, increased length of stay, and increased rates of morbidity and mortality (Chou et al., 2020). When restraints are utilized, close monitoring is warranted. In severe, intractable agitation, collaboration with consultation-liaison psychiatric providers may also be prudent (Ortiz, 2020).

KEY TAKEAWAYS

- Agitation is a frequently encountered complication of acute illness and correlated with poor health outcomes in hospitalized patients.
- Vigilant monitoring for agitation is critical, and preventive strategies should be implemented universally.
- Pharmacologic options include sedatives or neuroleptics, although these are considered a last-line approach.
- Physical restraints should be used with caution.

EVIDENCE-BASED RESOURCE

Devlin, J. W., Skrobik, Y., Gélinas, C., Needham, D. M., Slooter, A. J. C., Pandharipande, P. P., Watson, P. L., Weinhouse, G. L., Nunnally, M. E., Rochwerg, B., Balas, M. C., van den Boogaard, M., Bosma, K. J., Brummel, N. E., Chanques, G., Denehy, L., Drouot, X., Fraser, G. L., Harris, J. E., … Alhazzani, W. (2018). Clinical practice guidelines for the prevention and management of pain, agitation/sedation, delirium, immobility, and sleep disruption in adult patients in the ICU. *Critical Care Medicine, 46*(9), e825–e873. https://doi.org/10.1097/CCM.0000000000003299.

17.2: ANXIETY

Brayden Kameg

Given the stress of hospitalization, anxiety symptoms are common among adults within acute care settings. Furthermore, due to community prevalence of anxiety disorders, AGACNPs are likely to encounter those with anxiety disorders across the care continuum. In general, rates of anxiety disorders among adults in the United States are estimated at 7% (Goodwin et al., 2020). Patients with chronic health problems who struggle with comorbid anxiety are more likely to utilize healthcare resources and are at increased risk for hospitalizations (Benderly et al., 2019; Mannes et al., 2019). Risk factors for the development of anxiety disorders include substance use, physical comorbidities and previous hospitalization and associated greater duration of stay (Huang et al., 2020; Zimmermann et al., 2020). Consequences of anxiety include lack of adherence and poor follow-up with aftercare (Mendes et al., 2019), thus highlighting the importance of recognizing and addressing anxiety within the acute care setting.

PRESENTING SIGNS AND SYMPTOMS

Individuals experiencing anxiety may report feeling anxious, and may exhibit restlessness, insomnia, and irritability. These individuals may be more likely to endorse somatic complaints, including gastrointestinal discomfort or related symptoms and headaches or muscle tension. Individuals who are anxious may present with increased rate of speech and may appear scattered and inattentive. Vital signs may be within normal limits or elevated, and individuals might appear diaphoretic. In severe cases, individuals may develop panicky symptoms including nausea or vomiting, tremulousness, and pallor. Individuals may report feeling out of control or fearful (Sanson et al., 2018).

HISTORY AND PHYSICAL FINDINGS

AGACNPs must be astute in their assessment for those hospitalized and at-risk for anxiety. History should be gathered with consideration to anxiety disorders that preceded hospitalization, including panic disorder, generalized anxiety disorder, and social phobia. Furthermore, AGACNPs should inquire about new onset anxiety symptoms, such as those mentioned previously, since hospitalization. Physical exam findings are typically within normal limits, although those experiencing acute anxiety may present with tachycardia, tachypnea, and hypertension.

DIFFERENTIAL DIAGNOSIS AND DIAGNOSTIC CONSIDERATIONS

It is critical that AGACNPs consider medical comorbidities that can mimic signs and symptoms of anxiety, including chronic obstructive pulmonary disease, hyperthyroidism, tachyarrhythmias, hypoxemia, hypoglycemia, and pheochromocytoma. Other differential diagnoses include adjustment disorders or other trauma-related disorders, depression with anxious distress, and personality disorders. AGACNPs can utilize standardized screening tools, such as the Generalized Anxiety Disorder seven-item scale, to further aid in and support the diagnosis (Williams, 2014).

TREATMENT

Nonpharmacologic treatment interventions are the first line for the treatment of anxiety. On an inpatient basis, effective and therapeutic communication strategies can mitigate anxiety among those hospitalized and their family members (Seaman et al., 2017). Other non pharmacologic strategies include music therapy and aromatherapy (de Witte et al., 2022; Rafii et al., 2020; Rambod et al., 2020).

Regarding pharmacologic interventions, AGACNPs can utilize psychotropic medications or anxiolytics on an as-needed basis for acute anxiety and panic. Medications such as benzodiazepines can be utilized with caution and are a time-limited and as-needed intervention. For those with more longstanding anxiety, first-line medications such as selective serotonin reuptake inhibitors or serotonin norepinephrine reuptake inhibitors can be initiated while an individual is hospitalized, with follow-up care for therapy and medication management planned prior to discharge (Garakani et al., 2020). Collaboration with psychiatric consultation-liaison services may also be prudent (Oldham et al., 2021).

TRANSITION OF CARE

Whether an individual had longstanding anxiety symptoms, or developed them secondary to hospitalization, mental health aftercare should be offered. Individuals can be referred to an outpatient mental health provider, such as a psychiatric-mental health nurse practitioner (PMHNP), psychiatrist, psychologist, or counselor.

KEY TAKEAWAYS

- Anxiety is common and hospitalization course may worsen anxiety in adults.
- Pharmacologic interventions, such as benzodiazepines, can be used on an as-needed basis for patients in which it is safe and appropriate.
- Long-term pharmacotherapy, including selective serotonin reuptake inhibitors, can be initiated on an inpatient basis.

17.3: DELIRIUM

Adrienne Markiewicz and Alyssa Profita

Delirium, one of the most common mental disorders seen in hospitalized patients and the critically ill, is associated with many comorbid conditions and is at times difficult to diagnose. Delirium has an astounding prevalence in hospitalized patients, affecting up to 20% of general inpatients and up to 80% of critically ill patients requiring mechanical ventilation (Nikooie et al., 2019). The financial implications of delirium incidence are likewise astronomical, costing older adults in the United States $38 billion annually (Leslie & Inouye, 2011). Given this challenge, the ability to correctly diagnose and treat delirium has been reliant on the application of standardized diagnostic methods and evolving research that includes a multidisciplinary approach to care.

PRESENTING SIGNS AND SYMPTOMS

Based on the *Diagnostic and Statistical Manual of Mental Disorders, Fifth Edition* (*DSM-5*) criteria, delirium is characterized by the rapid onset of altered level of consciousness, with an inability to focus, sustain, or shift attention, and a change in cognition or development of a perceptual disturbance that is not explained by dementia (American Psychiatric Association [APA],

2013a). Additionally, there must be evidence from the patient's history, physical examination, or diagnostic workup that the disturbance is the direct result of a medical condition, substance intoxication/withdrawal, or multifactorial. This definition covers a broad clinical spectrum of symptoms while implying great nuance and complexity. As delirium is characterized by sudden and acute onset and fluctuating course, it is important to establish the patient's level of prior cognitive functioning and carefully elicit the course of cognitive deterioration. Consciousness disturbance is typically the earliest sign, manifesting as a hypo- or hypervigilant state (Boustani et al., 2014). The patient may be easily distractible by irrelevant happenings in the environment, or have difficulty remembering recent events. Basic information must often be repeated due to wandering attention. Disorientation, short-term memory loss, disorganized thinking, and language difficulties are common. Symptoms may be unpredictable, intermittent, and can become worse at night (Martins & Fernandes, 2012). Box 17.1 lists diagnostic criteria for delirium. For full diagnostic criteria, consult the *DSM-5*.

HISTORY AND PHYSICAL EXAMINATION

The history is of paramount importance in differentiating acute delirium in hospitalized patients from dementia and other psychiatric disorders. Particular attention to risk factors in the context of hospitalization is important. Box 17.2 gives risk factors for delirium in hospitalized patients (Tilouche et al., 2018). Delirium is an acute disorder, precipitated by medical conditions, substances, and/or medication effects. The clinician should elicit history of established neurocognitive disorders, any evidence or suspicion of pre-existing dementia, and obtain a thorough medication history.

BOX 17.1 POSSIBLE CHANGES NOTED WITH ACUTE DELIRIUM

Acute Delirium:
- An acute disturbance in attention and awareness with cognitive changes including disorientation, visual, or perceptual alterations.
- Develops over hours to days.
- Represents a change from baseline, fluctuates during the day.
- Not better explained by another pre-existing, evolving, or established neurocognitive disorder.
- Physical examination or laboratory evidence that support that the disturbance is caused by a medical condition, substance use or withdrawal, or medication side effect.

May Include:
- Hypoactivity or hyperactivity
- Sleep disturbances

BOX 17.2 RISK FACTORS FOR DELIRIUM IN CRITICAL ILLNESS

Modifiable
Benzodiazepine and morphine analgesic use
Corticosteroid use
Blood transfusions
Immobility

Nonmodifiable
Age (>65 years)
Underlying dementia
Underlying hypertension
Underlying chronic obstructive pulmonary disease (COPD)
Prior coma
Elevated or increasing high acute physiology and chronic health (APACHE) scores

Postoperative Patients
Undertreated or overtreated pain
Frailty
Sleep disruption
Intraoperative blood loss
High serum cortisol levels

The physical examination may produce a variety of findings. Patients may display acute agitation, attention deficits, and may be resistant to care. Alternatively, patients may appear sedate, noninteractive, or display fear. The clinician should establish the absence of coma, as this state excludes delirium as a differential diagnosis. The neurologic examination is often confounded by inattention and altered consciousness; however, the clinician should focus on cranial nerve assessment to rule out focal findings indicative of structural neurologic disease. Nonconvulsive status epilepticus may be misdiagnosed as delirium. Physical examination findings which would lead the clinician to suspect seizure activity include bilateral facial twitching, unexplained nystagmus, lip smacking, chewing, or swallowing movements and acute aphasia or neglect. As physical examination findings in delirious patients will vary, use of objective, validated assessment tools is key (Kalabalik et al., 2014; Tilouche et al., 2018).

DIFFERENTIAL DIAGNOSIS AND DIAGNOSTIC CONSIDERATIONS

The differential diagnosis of acute altered mental state is broad, necessitating a thorough history and physical examination. As always, ruling out life-threatening pathology should take utmost priority. Exacerbation of psychiatric illness and underlying dementia must be ruled out; however, it is possible for these patients to develop delirium when acutely ill. Thus, when the diagnosis is unclear, the clinician should presume delirium and look for an underlying etiology. Laboratory evaluation in patients with delirium should include serum electrolytes, creatinine, glucose, calcium, complete blood count, and a urinalysis. In patients with suspected infection or sepsis, urine culture, sputum culture, blood cultures (as appropriate) and workup of the suspected source should be done. Toxicology screen, liver function test, and arterial blood gas could be considered if the initial laboratory evaluation is not high yield. Patients with focal neurologic findings should undergo neuroimaging as part of the initial workup, however, further investigations such as lumbar puncture or electroencephalogram (EEG) should only be done if there is a specific indication (i.e., suspicion of central nervous system infection or evidence of seizures) or if the cause of delirium remains unclear despite a thorough initial screening.

Validated tools can be helpful in establishing the diagnosis of delirium. These tools presume absence of coma and the ability of the patient to answer the questions. Although several have been proposed and studied, the Confusion Assessment Method (CAM) and its surrogate for critically ill patients, the Confusion Assessment Method for the Intensive Care Unit (CAM-ICU), have been the most consistently reliable and widely used. CAM-ICU has demonstrated high inter rater reliability, sensitivity and specificity (Ely et al., 2001; Inouye et al., 1990) and can be used in patients receiving sedation and mechanical ventilation. Delirium is considered present when a patient has positive acute change or fluctuating course of mental status and inattention with either altered level of consciousness or disorganized thinking. Figure 17.1 shows the CAM-ICU algorithm. A patient is CAM-ICU positive when the patient has both features 1 and 2 and either feature 3 or 4. Though CAM-ICU can be used in lightly sedated patients, the patient must be able to follow commands and participate in the assessment.

TREATMENT

Nonpharmacologic Interventions

The SCCM Guidelines for Pain, Agitation, Delirium, Immobility and Sleep Disruption (PADIS) provides best practice related to the treatment of delirium in critically ill patients. This consensus statement makes the conditional recommendation that delirium be addressed with a multicomponent, nonpharmacologic approach that includes all disciplines to minimize modifiable risk factors for delirium, improve cognition, and optimize sleep, mobility, hearing, and vision (Devlin et al., 2018). Box 17.3 lists these interventions in further detail.

Treatment of delirium begins with prevention. Patients should be in rooms with windows where possible, with lights and environment mimicking a day-night cycle.

CONFUSION ASSESSMENT METHOD (CAM) ALGORITHM

(1) acute onset and fluctuating course
-and-
(2) inattention
-and either-
(3) disorganized thinking
-or-
(4) altered level of consciousness

[Score based on cognitive testing. See details at: www.hospitalelderlifeprogram.org]

FIGURE 17.1: Confusion Assessment Method for the Intensive Care Unit (CAM-ICU).
Source: Confusion Assessment Method. Copyright 2003, Hospital Elder Life Program, LLC. Permission granted by the American Geriatrics Society, 2019.
Note: No responsibility is assumed by the AGS or the Hospital Elder Life Program, LLC for any injury and/or damage to persons or property arising out of the application of any of the content at help.agscocare.org.

BOX 17.3 INTERVENTIONS FOR ACUTE DELIRIUM IN CRITICALLY ILL PATIENTS

Nonpharmacologic Interventions to Reduce Incidence and Severity of Delirium
Frequent reorientation
Maintain day-night cycles
Use of digital clocks and information boards
Minimize light and noise
Reduce sedating agents
Early mobilization
Use of assistive devices (e.g., hearing aids, eyeglasses)
Family presence

Overly bright lights and loud noises should be avoided. Digital clocks can also assist in maintaining a sense of time and staff should frequently orient the patient. Sedatives, particularly benzodiazepines should be avoided unless absolutely indicated to treat the primary diagnosis or if there is concern of possible withdrawal. Patients should be mobilized early in the hospital course by nursing staff with consultation from skilled physical and occupational therapists as necessary. Any assistive devices used by the patient should be also utilized in the hospital to facilitate sensorium including glasses and hearing aids (Ely, 2017). If acute delirium develops, these interventions compound in importance. Restraints should be avoided. If possible, familiar objects from home can be brought in to assist with orientation. Family presence can also reorient the patient, provide comfort, and give the clinician a more thorough history and knowledge of baseline functioning (Barnes-Daly et al., 2018; Devlin et al., 2018; Pun et al., 2019). In one study, a 1-minute video message from family members significantly decreased agitation in elderly patients with hyperactive delirium (Waszynski et al., 2018).

Pharmacologic Interventions

There is no medication approved by the U.S. Food and Drug Administration (FDA) for the prevention or treatment of ICU delirium. This section briefly discusses two classes of medications used in clinical practice to ameliorate the symptoms of delirium in hospitalized and/or critically ill patients, however no guidelines exist that support the routine use of pharmacologic intervention in acute delirium. Consider the use of pharmacologic agents only if the patient poses a risk of harm to themselves or others.

Antipsychotics

The routine use of antipsychotic medications for treatment of delirium in hospitalized adults is controversial, with mixed data. A more recent systematic review on the subject found no difference in delirium duration, hospital length of stay, or mortality between antipsychotics (Haldol and second-generation antipsychotics) and placebo with potential for increased frequency for harmful cardiac side effects (Nikooie et al., 2019). This same review found no significant mortality benefit or had insufficient data for a direct comparison of the second-generation antipsychotics. SCCM PADIS guidelines make conditional statements that antipsychotics should not be used in low doses to prevent delirium in ICU patients (Devlin et al., 2018).

Dexmedetomidine

Dexmedetomidine is an alpha-2-adrenoceptor agonist with anesthetic and sedative properties used in the ICU setting as continuous sedation for mechanical ventilation, treatment of selected substance withdrawal, and to manage agitation in hyperactive delirium. Several studies show superiority of dexmedetomidine to lorazepam and other benzodiazepines in the ICU for sedation with mechanical ventilation, with clear outcomes data demonstrating reduced ventilator days, delirium incidence, delirium duration, and mortality (Kalabalik et al., 2014). However, outcomes data regarding the use of dexmedetomidine solely for treatment of delirium are much less robust. The SCCM PADIS guidelines make the distinction that no pharmacologic management option has demonstrated an effect on delirium-related outcomes (Davidson et al., 2013; Pun et al., 2019).

KEY TAKEAWAYS

- Delirium has a high prevalence in hospitalized adults and is associated with adverse outcomes.
- A multidisciplinary approach is critical to reducing incidence and severity of delirium, particularly in the elderly and critically ill.

17.4: DEMENTIA

Michelle Wade

The World Health Organization defines dementia as a syndrome, usually of a chronic or progressive nature, where there is deterioration in cognitive function beyond what might be expected from normal aging (Global action plan on the public health response to dementia, 2017). Dementia affects one's memory, visuospatial skills, thinking, comprehension, language, and judgment. The National Collaborating Centre for Mental Health goes on to say that "The impairment in cognitive function is commonly accompanied, and sometimes preceded, by a deterioration in emotional control often evidenced by behaviors, social behavior, and/or motivation but each must be evaluated independently" (Pal et al., 2018).

Dementia results from a variety of diseases and injuries that primarily or secondarily affect the brain, such as Alzheimer's disease, traumatic brain injury,, or stroke. Dementia is often grouped under neurocognitive disorders. Neurocognitive disorders are another classification for dementia and are characterized by deficits in cognitive function, with a significant decline from a previous level of function. Decline may be evident in one or more areas of function including activities of daily living (ADLs) and impairment in instrumental activities of daily living (IADLs). This decline is often displayed as inattention, language issues, memory issues, decreased visuospatial skills, or changes in executive function. Knowing the key features and pathology of each type of dementia can help in the accurate diagnosis of patients; this is essential so the patients and the caregivers will receive the treatment and support services appropriate for their condition in order to maintain the highest possible quality of life.

Diagnoses in this grouping include vascular dementia, Lewy body dementia, frontal temporal dementia, Parkinson's dementia, HIV dementia, neurosyphilis, and Korsakoff's dementia. Down's syndrome is also a known precursor to dementia (Pal et al., 2018). It is important to think about underlying illness when diagnosing dementia. For example, a person with hypertension (HTN) and coronary artery disease (CAD) may be predisposed to vascular dementia; a person found to have high levels of serum beta-amyloid is generally found to develop Alzheimer's dementia. Knowing such things will assist you with your diagnosis and ICD-10 coding.

There is no single test for dementia; instead, providers (often with the help of specialists such as neurologists, neuropsychologists, geriatricians, and geriatric psychiatrists) use a variety of approaches and tools to help make a diagnosis. This includes basic lab tests, basic and sometimes advanced imaging, as well as neurocognitive testing.

There are multiple types of dementia and the differentiation and boundaries of each are not distinct and often cross over into each other, making diagnosis a challenge and showing the importance of a full and thorough history and physical.

PRESENTING SIGNS AND SYMPTOMS

The clinical features are the key to understanding the type of dementia. Some of the different types of dementia are characterized:

Alzheimer's dementia
1. Gradual onset and course of progressive decline
2. Memory, language, visuospatial defects
3. Depressive symptoms, which may precede diagnosis
4. Delusions, hallucinations, agitation, and apathy

Vascular dementia
1. Abrupt onset and stepwise course of progression
2. Aphasia
3. Often with history of CAD and/or HTN

Lewy body dementia
1. Visual hallucinations and delusions
2. Extrapyramidal symptoms
3. Fluctuating mental status
4. Increased sensitivity to antipsychotic medications

Frontotemporal dementia
1. Change in personality
2. Hyperorality
3. Impairment and executive function, with relatively well-retained visuospatial skills

HISTORY AND PHYSICAL FINDINGS

Diagnosing dementia requires a history evaluating for cognitive decline and impairment in daily activities, with corroboration from a close friend or family member. This is often done during a triad office visit or interview where the patient is the focus but the friend or family member is there to supplement or verify information. In addition, a mental status examination by a clinician must be undertaken and will help to delineate impairments in memory, language, attention, visuospatial cognition such as spatial orientation, executive function, and mood. This testing can be accomplished with any of the screening tools that are commercially available; some examples are the Montreal Cognitive Assessment (MOCA), the Mini Mental State Examination (MMSE), or the Mini-Cog© (Borson et al., 2003). Each of these is validated and each has a specific population in which they are best used.

There are modifiable and nonmodifiable risk factors for dementia. The modifiable risk factors include hypertension and diabetes, diet, obesity, tobacco use, and limited cognitive, physical, and social activities. The nonmodifiable risk factors for dementia include female sex, Black race, Hispanic ethnicity, and genetic factors such as the apolipoprotein E (*APOE*) gene (Pal et al., 2018). There is a growing body of evidence suggesting an increased diagnosis of dementia in patients with modifiable risk factors. Because of this there is growing consensus that modifiable risk factors must be addressed early in life. This includes increasing physical activity, preventing and reducing obesity, promotion of balanced and healthy diets, increased social engagement, and promotion of cognitively stimulating activities. The cessation of tobacco use and harmful use of alcohol is imperative for cognitive health. The prevention and management of diabetes, hypertension, especially in midlife, and depression can slow and delay onset of dementia.

DIFFERENTIAL DIAGNOSIS AND DIAGNOSTIC CONSIDERATIONS

Dementia diagnoses must be differentiated from delirium. As discussed in the earlier section, delirium is defined as a disturbance in cognition that develops over a short period of time and is characterized by an alteration in attention that fluctuates in severity during the course of the day. Delirium may be the consequence of an acute medical condition, being hospitalized, or can be medication or substance induced (Kalish et al., 2014).

History taking and the physical examination are especially important in the identification of the etiology of dementia. For example, focal neurologic abnormalities suggest stroke. Brain neuroimaging may demonstrate structural changes including, but not limited to, focal atrophy, infarcts, and tumor that may not be identified on physical examination. Additional evaluation with cerebrospinal fluid assays or genetic testing should be considered in atypical dementia cases, such as age of onset under 65 years, rapid symptom onset, and/or impairment in multiple cognitive domains but not episodic memory. Medication side effects must also be ruled out as a cause of memory impairment that can mimic dementia. This is done during history taking by asking about start dates of all medications, infusions, and over-the-counter herbals or supplements. One then must try to correlate the change in behavior to the time around a medication initiation.

Metabolic derangements or reversable causes must also be considered (Box 17.4). Differential diagnosis is important, and a complete differential list must be considered to identify potential reversible causes.

BOX 17.4 DIAGNOSTIC STUDIES TO RULE OUT METABOLIC DERANGEMENT IN SETTING OF DEMENTIA

Ammonia level
Complete blood count
Comprehensive metabolic panel
Computed tomography (CT) of head and neck for masses and flow
Liver function tests
Magnetic resonance imaging (MRI)
Positron emission tomography (PET) scan to rule out Lewy body dementia
Syphilis serology
Thyroid function testing
Urinalysis and culture
Vitamin B_{12} and folate levels

TREATMENT

Currently there are no curative treatments for dementia (Koller et al., 2016); the medications available are for use in early stages and to promote independence of the patient for as long as possible. Treatment is guided at supportive levels for both the patient and the family/caregivers. Antidepressants are often used as a supportive treatment for depression in dementia; sertraline and citalopram may help to reduce agitation as well as address depression. Mood stabilizers have been used in the past but are under review at this time for dementia patients who develop behavioral issues. Pharmacologic and nonpharmacologic treatments are summarized in Table 17.1.

The principal goals for dementia care include:
- Early diagnosis in order to promote early and optimal management
- Optimizing physical health, cognition, activity, and well-being
- Identifying and treating accompanying physical illness
- Detecting and treating challenging behavioral and psychological symptoms
- Providing information and long-term support to caregivers

TRANSITION OF CARE

The global action plan on the public health response to dementia (2017) states that people with dementia should be empowered to live in the community and to receive care aligned with their wishes and preferences as long as it remains safe for the patients and the caregivers. To ensure that people with dementia can maintain a level of functional ability consistent with their basic rights and human dignity, they will need integrated, person-centered, accessible, affordable health and social care. This includes home health services as well as senior

TABLE 17.1: Nonpharmacologic and Pharmacologic Treatments for Dementia

NONPHARMACOLOGIC MAINSTAY OF SUPPORTIVE TREATMENT	PHARMACOLOGIC
Cognitively engaging activities	Cholinesterase inhibitors (donepezil, galantamine, rivastigmine)
Socialization such as family gatherings	NMDA receptor antagonist (memantine)
Fall precautions	
Reading	Antidepressants are often helpful as over 1/3 of patients will develop depression
Physical exercise, walking	
Consistent environment with supportive care for ADLs	Mood stabilizers have been used in the past but are under review at this time
Reminiscence therapy: family pictures, memory-evoking memorabilia	
Physical therapy, occupational therapy, or speech language services for therapy and cognition supportive services	Antipsychotics should be reserved for dementia patients that fail nonpharmacologic options and are a threat to self or others

ADL, activities of daily living; NMDA, N-methyl-D-aspartate.

living environments and long-term care. Palliative care is a core component of the continuum of care for people living with dementia from the point of diagnosis through to the end of life and into the bereavement stages for families and caregivers. These services provide physical, psychosocial, and spiritual support for people with dementia and their caregivers, including support with advance care planning.

CLINICAL PEARLS

- Dementia is not a normal part of aging.
- Modifiable risk factors need to be addressed early in adulthood.
- A thorough search for a potentially reversible cause is required.
- Caregivers need support in addition to the patient.

KEY TAKEAWAYS

- The history is the key to the diagnosis of dementia.
- Family and caregivers are instrumental in the history.
- Your patient needs to feel involved and validated.

17.5: GERIATRIC DEPRESSION SYNDROMES

Thomas Farley

Geriatric depression, also known as late life depression, affects adults aged 65 years and older. Approximately 5% to 15% of older patients in primary care have symptoms of clinically significant depression (Kok & Reynolds, 2017; Park & Unützer, 2011). A subset of approximately 5% of these patients will have symptoms of major depression (Park & Unützer, 2011). Geriatric depression is known to increase the risk of death including by suicide (Aziz & Steffens, 2013).

PRESENTING SIGNS AND SYMPTOMS

Geriatric depression syndromes typically present with sadness, low energy, fatigue, loneliness, anhedonia, avolition, and unexplained physical symptoms in the patient.

HISTORY AND PHYSICAL FINDINGS

The patient history may include chronic physical pain, myocardial infarction (MI), coronary artery disease (CAD), stroke, obesity, dementia, diabetes, and Parkinson disease.

DIFFERENTIAL DIAGNOSIS AND DIAGNOSTIC CONSIDERATIONS

The following disorders may present with depressive symptoms and should be ruled out:
- Atypical presentation of depression
- Concurrent medical illness
- Minor depression
- Dysthymic disorder
- Depression without sadness
- Subthreshold depression
- Bipolar disorder
- Mixed anxiety depressive disorder
- Bereavement
- Adjustment disorder
- Vascular dementia
- Substance- or medication-induced depression

The diagnosis of geriatric depression should be made by a trained mental health specialist.

TREATMENT

Pharmacologic

- A meta-analysis performed in 2013 found that pharmacotherapy benefited moderately to severely depressed geriatric patients with long-illness duration (Nelson et al., 2013).
- Clinicians need to be vigilant to prevent drug-drug interactions from polypharmacy.
- First-line therapy is SSRIs/SNRIs and include sertraline, paroxetine, and duloxetine (Beyer & Johnson, 2018).

- Illness duration is a factor in response to pharmacotherapy. Increased benefit with pharmacologic antidepressants is more prevalent in patients with depression duration greater than 10 years (Nelson et al., 2013).

Electroconvulsive Therapy

- Electroconvulsive therapy (ECT) not accepted by all patients
- Requires anesthesia
- Reserved for severe depression or depression refractory to other treatments

Psychotherapy, Physical Therapy, and Exercise

- Limitations to physical therapy and psychotherapy due to health insurance status and availability of therapists. Exercise for geriatric patients may be hindered by physical limitations.
- Systemic review and meta-analysis demonstrated efficacy of psychotherapy for geriatric depression (Huang et al., 2015).
- Generally recommended for patients with mild to moderate depression (Kok & Reynolds, 2017).

TRANSITION OF CARE

Transition of care may apply the concept of collaborative care where primary care providers communicate closely with patients and mental health specialists to treat depression. This model has shown to be effective in several clinical trials (Park & Unützer, 2011). Patient outcomes are tracked over time. Treatment plans are adjusted using evidence-based treatments and therapies.

CLINICAL PEARLS

- Dysphoric mood is less evident and not as reliable an indicator for depression in geriatric patients (Park & Unützer, 2011).
- Poorly controlled pain is associated with depression (Park & Unützer, 2011).
- Patients with depressive disorders who do not meet criteria for major depressive disorder can still have major psychosocial impairment.

KEY TAKEAWAYS

- Evaluation of suspected geriatric depression should be performed by a mental health specialist qualified to differentiate between depressive disorders.
- SSRI/SNRIs are first line pharmacotherapy for geriatric depression.
- Geriatric depression is not a normal aging process.
- Collaborative care between primary care providers and mental health specialists is vital.

17.6: INSOMNIA

Brayden Kameg

Hospitalizations often include periods of acute sleep disturbances in adults due to a variety of environmental, medical, and individual risk factors (Stewart & Arora, 2018). The very nature of inpatient medical-surgical units or intensive care units (ICUs) can contribute to disrupted sleep in those hospitalized, due to increased noise, frequent awakenings, lack of windows or natural light, and routine disruptions (Simons et al., 2018). In adults, community prevalence of insomnia is nearing 20%, and those with chronic health problems are at increased risk for insomnia (Ford et al., 2015). The prevalence of obstructive sleep disorders, including sleep apnea, exceeds 15% in adults (Senaratna et al., 2017). Consequences of insomnia or poor sleep include anxiety, pain, reduced quality of life, depressive symptoms, cognitive deficits, hypertension, cardiovascular disease, obesity and metabolic syndrome, and type 2 diabetes mellitus (Medic et al., 2017). Given the number of individuals with sleep problems in the community, compounded by hospital-related risk factors for sleep disturbances and associated comorbidities, AGACNPs should be familiar with managing insomnia in hospitalized adults.

PRESENTING SIGNS AND SYMPTOMS

Individuals who are struggling with insomnia and sleep disturbances might present with fatigue, excessive daytime sleepiness, increased blood pressure, hyperglycemia, and delirium (Stewart & Arora, 2018). Other presenting signs and symptoms include drowsiness, decreased attention, and physical weakness. Those experiencing significant sleep disturbances may also develop anxiety and mood lability (Bjorøy et al., 2020).

HISTORY AND PHYSICAL FINDINGS

AGACNPs should consider the aforementioned signs and symptoms of insomnia and sleep disturbances when caring for adults who are hospitalized. A history of sleep disorders and associated treatment prior to hospitalization should be considered. Additionally, details related to new onset sleep disturbances since hospitalization should be obtained. Physical exam findings are typically within normal limits, although those experiencing insomnia or sleep disturbances might present with hypertension and hyperglycemia (Stewart & Arora, 2018).

DIFFERENTIAL DIAGNOSIS AND DIAGNOSTIC CONSIDERATIONS

Differential diagnoses should include alternative sleep disorders, including obstructive sleep apnea, parasomnias, narcolepsy, and restless legs syndrome. Furthermore, AGACNPs should evaluate for other psychiatric disorders that can precipitate sleep disturbances, including mood disorders, anxiety disorders, and trauma-related disorders. Some individuals with longstanding sleep disturbances may benefit from referral to sleep medicine and associated sleep studies, including polysomnography.

TREATMENT

Nonpharmacologic treatment interventions are the first line for the treatment of insomnia for hospitalized individuals. Such interventions can include ensuring a quiet environment, music therapy, aromatherapy, and light therapy to ensure adequate regulation of circadian rhythms (Cho et al., 2017; Elías et al., 2019; Feng et al., 2018).

Regarding pharmacologic interventions, AGACNPs can utilize pharmacologic interventions on an as-needed basis to promote sleep. Such agents include melatonin and melatonin receptor agonists (ramelteon), orexin receptor antagonists (suvorexant), and antidepressants (doxepin and trazodone; Buysse et al., 2017). Benzodiazepines and sedative hypnotics should generally be avoided and used as a last-line intervention due to risks related to oversedation, falls, tolerance, and dependence.

TRANSITION OF CARE

For those with longstanding insomnia, cognitive behavioral therapy for insomnia is recommended as a first-line treatment, and referral for this modality on an outpatient basis should be considered (Soong et al., 2021).

> **KEY TAKEAWAYS**
> - Hospitalizations place adults at risk for insomnia and sleep disturbances.
> - Pharmacologic interventions can be utilized, but benzodiazepines and sedative hypnotics should generally be avoided.
> - Cognitive behavioral therapy for chronic insomnia is recommended as a first-line treatment.

17.7: POSTINTENSIVE CARE UNIT SYNDROME

Adrienne Markiewicz

Approximately 5 million American adults are admitted to the ICU annually (Khan et al., 2015) and 50% will survive 1 year after ICU admission (Davidson et al., 2013). As more patients survive, the consequences of lifesaving measures become more apparent. Post ICU care syndrome (PICS) is a cluster of persistent deleterious physical, emotional, social, cognitive, and functional symptoms following critical illness which decrease the ICU survivor's quality of life in a plethora of ways (Needham et al., 2012). PICS has been recognized formally as a sequelae of critical illness and was given its current name following a consensus meeting of stakeholders in

2012. Further consensus among key multidisciplinary stakeholders, including ICU survivors, has established ongoing need to risk stratify and intervene early in this patient population (Elliott et al., 2014). Despite this agreement, it remains unclear exactly what intervention will provide reproducible benefit (Devlin et al., 2018). As critical care research directs attention to patient-centered outcomes beyond ICU mortality, translation of the current best evidence to practice is needed.

PRESENTING SIGNS AND SYMPTOMS

Table 17.2 describes symptoms clinicians may observe in patients with PICS. It is important to note that PICS also affects the families of ICU survivors beginning with the onset of critical illness and continuing for months or years following ICU survivorship (Elliott et al., 2014). As families struggle to process rapidly changing information and navigate complex emotions surrounding the near death of a loved one, a struggle for sensemaking occurs (Davidson & Zisook, 2017). If traumatic experiences are not properly processed, PICS may occur in a family member and present as depression, anxiety, or PTSD (Rosenberg et al., 2019).

HISTORY AND PHYSICAL FINDINGS

On physical exam, patients may have muscular atrophy due to prolonged immobility, poor nutritional status, or neuromuscular weakness. Patients may have signs of cognitive impairment such as impaired attention span, mental processing, and executive function. Additionally, patients may be withdrawn or show signs of depression and anxiety. The history of each patient will vary according to experience, and physical examination for this population should be based on patient-centered priorities. A qualitative study of critical illness survivors found 12 core patient priorities for critical illness recovery through secondary analysis of patient interviews. Box 17.5 lists these priorities, which span from basic survival during the acute phase of critical illness to more aspirational wishes as the patient moves toward discharge and begins reassimilation at home (Scheunemann et al., 2020). Clinicians should bear these priorities in mind, with the understanding that the recovery process may not be entirely linear. Focused questions and examination to determine patient priorities will lead to optimal comprehensive care during recovery.

DIFFERENTIAL DIAGNOSIS AND DIAGNOSTIC CONSIDERATION

Though any patient with a recent ICU stay should be evaluated for PICS, it is important that the clinician rules out other pathology playing a role in presenting symptoms. Symptoms can be palliated while alternative diagnoses are explored. Particular attention should be given to the patient's acceptable quality of life, any pre-existing functional deficits prior to critical illness, and concomitant psychiatric morbidity. ICU survivors do not exist in a vacuum and may have psychological or cognitive barriers to physical rehabilitation causing long-term attrition. In these cases, it may be helpful to involve a rehabilitation psychologist to identify specific needs and barriers (Merbitz et al., 2016).

TREATMENT

Inpatient Interventions

The first step to addressing the complex issues faced by patients and families who experience PICS is through mitigation. The ABCDEF bundle was designed by the Society of Critical Care Medicine (SCCM) to reduce delirium, weakness, and prolonged mechanical ventilation, all of which are known inputs to PICS. This group of interventions targets daily actions by the care team including pain management, sedation holidays, spontaneous breathing trials, environmental interventions to normalize sleep/wake cycle, delirium prevention, and family presence (Barnes-Daly et al., 2018). Unlike other ICU intervention bundles, ABCDEF does not target a specific disease process but rather symptoms common to the vast majority of the critically ill and is therefore applicable to any patient in the ICU regardless of level of required support (Pun et al., 2019). Other strengths include its multicomponent and multiprofessional construction, incorporating in a single bundle the most important aspects of many of the other inpatient interventions targeting PICS reduction. Despite high level evidence of effectiveness, the challenges of implementation and continued adherence cannot be understated. ABCDEF requires trained, dedicated staff to implement and a unit culture that adopts the elements as best practice. A worldwide survey for bundle compliance found significant variation in practice, reducing bundle efficacy (Morandi et al., 2017).

Inpatient consult teams have been proposed as a PICS reduction and mitigation strategy with the idea that provision of information to the patient related to ICU stay and early risk assessment may impact the onset of PICS. In most studies, this took the form of a formal consultation within an inpatient service line provided to the patient at some point following ICU stay. Though this idea has high face value, it has failed to translate into reproducible outcomes affecting quality of life, depression, or incidence reduction. Variation in consult team strategy, purpose, and target outcomes and single center trials all contribute to an overall low quality of evidence. To date, the only single-center, randomized pilot trial of an inpatient consult service found that patients randomized to the consult service received more intervention and had increase in median tie to hospital readmission as compared to usual care (Bloom et al., 2019). Consult teams require additional infrastructure and trained personnel. Further multicenter studies of similar design should be undertaken to ascertain whether consult teams could provide any benefit to ICU survivors.

TABLE 17.2: Selected Potential Long-Term Patient and Family Outcomes After Intensive Care

COMPLICATION	DESCRIPTION	SELECTED RISK FACTORS	NATURAL HISTORY
PATIENT OUTCOMES			
Pulmonary	Impairment in spirometry, lung volumes, and diffusion capacity	Diffusion capacity; duration of mechanical ventilation	Generally mild impairment with improvement during first year, but can persist 5 years or more
Neuromuscular/ICU-acquired weakness	Includes critical illness polyneuropathy and myopathy	Hyperglycemia; Systemic inflammatory response syndrome; Sepsis; Multiorgan dysfunction	Polyneuropathy may recover more slowly than myopathy; can extend to 5 years
Physical function	Disease atrophy; Impairment in activities of daily living (ADL/IADL) and 6-min walk distance	Immobility/bed rest; Systemic corticosteroids; ICU-acquired illness; Slow resolution of lung injury; Age; Preexisting IADL impairment	Some improvement in ADL within months, but impairments may be seen in ADL at 1 year and IADL at 2 years; Long-lasting impairment in 6-minute walk distance vs. population norms
Psychiatric	Depression	Traumatic/delusional memories of the ICU, sedation, psychiatric symptoms at discharge, impairment of physical function	May decrease over first year
	Posttraumatic stress disorder	Sedation, agitation, physical restraints, traumatic/delusional memories	Little improvement in first year
	Anxiety	Unemployment, duration of mechanical ventilation; Overall risk factors: Female gender, younger age, less education, and pre-ICU psychiatric symptoms, and personality	May persist past first year
Cognitive	Impairments in memory, attention, executive function, mental processing speed, visuo-spatial ability	Lower pre-ICU intelligence; ICU delirium; Sedation; Hypoxia; Glucose dysregulation	Significant improvement during first year, with residual deficits up to 6 years later
FAMILY OUTCOMES			
Psychiatric	Depression	Overall risk factors: Female gender, younger age, less education, pre-ICU psychiatric symptoms, and personality, distance to hospital, restricted visiting	Depression and anxiety decrease over time, but are higher than population norms at 6 months
	Posttraumatic stress disorder	Dissatisfaction with communication, ICU physician perceived as "un-caring," passive preference for decision-making and preferences	Posttraumatic stress disorder and complicated grief can persist 4 years or more after death or discharge and may not decrease over time
	Anxiety	Severity of illness not associated with development of symptoms	

Source: Reproduced with permission from Davidson, J. E., Harvey, M. A., Bemis-Dougherty, A., Smith, J.M., & Hopkins, R. O. (2013). Implementation of the pain, agitation, and delirium clinical practice guidelines and promoting patient mobility to prevent post-intensive care syndrome. *Critical Care Medicine, 41*(9 Suppl. 1), S136–S145. https://doi.org/10.1097/CCM.0b013e3182a24105

BOX 17.5 PATIENT PRIORITIES DURING ICU RECOVERY

1. Feeling of safety
2. Being comfortable
3. Ability to mobilize
4. Participation in self-care
5. Maintaining personhood
6. Connection with others
7. Ensuring family well-being
8. Going home
9. Restoration of psychological health
10. Restoration of physical health
11. Resumption of previous roles and routines
12. New life experiences

ICU mobility programs have been well studied and shown to decrease ICU length of stay, reduce days of mechanical ventilation, and reduce incidence of delirium as well as increase functional status (Hopkins et al., 2016). Mobility in critically ill adults therefore targets several inputs to PICS and it can be extrapolated that those survivors with higher functional status following critical illness are more likely to recover without significant morbidity. Within the last 10 years, consistent integration of physical and occupational therapy into the multidisciplinary ICU team with forward follow-up on the general ward and continuing to outpatient settings has become the clear best practice (Bemis-Dougherty & Smith, 2013). Less evidence is available regarding the continuity of early mobility in the ICU to continued mobility programs and rehabilitation in the outpatient setting.

ICU diaries are an emerging tool in the fight to decrease incidence and severity of PICS. Like mobility programs and the ABCDEF bundle, diaries have higher level evidence support in the form of prospective trials as compared to other PICS interventions. These diaries try to "fill in the gaps" of patient memory and assist in psychological recovery from critical illness (Aitken et al., 2013). Even when ICU survivors remember details surrounding their course, diaries can serve as an affirming and trust-building tool (Glimelius Petersson et al., 2018). Real-time recording of ICU events to preserve patient memories is not without some controversy as well as ethical and legal concerns. Most paramount is the question of ultimate benefit. Patient selection, variations in diary content, patient privacy laws, information sharing, and choice of metrics all present challenges to successful implementation and do inhibit factual conclusion that ICU dairies uniformly provide benefit to all adult ICU survivors.

Outpatient Interventions

PICS clinics are outpatient centers dedicated to ICU recovery and are staffed with multidisciplinary ICU providers, including in some examples rehabilitation psychologists. These clinics do not attempt to replace the patient's primary care provider but rather expand on critical illness recovery in the outpatient setting to ensure access to community resources, physical and cognitive rehabilitation, and medication management (Sevin et al., 2018). Some clinics offer a venue for peer support groups and could be an ideal place to review ICU diaries. In addition, critical care pharmacists also complete medication reviews and screen for adverse drug reactions. Two articles describe the role of the critical care pharmacist in mitigating medication-induced deleterious side effects when performing duties in this setting (Stollings et al., 2018). Development of a PICS clinic requires either creation of a new dedicated service line or reconstruction of an existing ICU care delivery model, which can be cost prohibitive. Without solid outcomes data that also benefit operational goals, organizations may find it difficult to make the financial case for PICS clinics.

CLINICAL PEARLS

- PICS is a cluster of physical, emotional, and cognitive symptoms persisting in survivors of critical illness.
- Incidence of PICS is increasing as more patients survive critical illness.
- Several inpatient and outpatient interventions have been explored to mitigate the effects of PICS; however, high-level evidence is lacking and further research is required.

17.8: POSTTRAUMATIC STRESS DISORDER

Thomas Farley

Posttraumatic stress disorder (PTSD) is a disorder that may develop after exposure to even a single major traumatic event (Bisson et al., 2015). Symptoms of re-experience, avoidance, changes in cognition, and hyperarousal may be found in any combination (Miao et al., 2018). High quality evidence for effective therapies is lacking. The most promising therapies are non pharmacologic and focus on the specific trauma event.

PRESENTING SIGNS AND SYMPTOMS

Signs and symptoms include hypervigilance, persistent intrusive memories, avoidance of triggering stimuli, alterations in mood, and emotion regulation dysfunction. PTSD can present in a delayed fashion even years after the trigger event (Bisson et al., 2015).

HISTORY AND PHYSICAL FINDINGS

History includes exposure to, or witnessing of, a major traumatic event. Examples include natural disasters, war, interpersonal violence, rape, or sexual abuse. Exposure to the critical care environment as a patient is an emerging risk factor (Righy et al., 2019).

DIFFERENTIAL DIAGNOSIS AND DIAGNOSTIC CONSIDERATIONS

Must fulfill either 20 *Diagnostic and Statistical Manual of Mental Disorders, Fifth Edition* (*DSM-5*; American Psychiatric Association, 2013) criteria or six proposed ICD-11 criteria (Bisson et al., 2015). A common feature is exposure to, or the witnessing of, a severely traumatic event.

TREATMENT

There are currently no recommended pharmacologic or cannabinoid-based treatments based on lack of evidence in clinical trials (Astill Wright et al., 2019; Black et al., 2019). Meditation, yoga, and cognitive behavioral therapy have demonstrated some treatment effect in meta-analyses (Carpenter et al., 2018; Gallegos et al., 2017). A Cochrane review demonstrated very low quality evidence that eye movement desensitization and reprocessing (EMDR) therapy may be effective (Bisson et al., 2013).

CLINICAL PEARLS

- Low evidence that pharmacologic therapies have beneficial effect.
- Symptoms may present before clinician has knowledge that patient witnessed or experienced stressful event.

KEY TAKEAWAYS

- PTSD can develop in any person exposed to a traumatic event including patients who survived critical illness.
- Presentation may be delayed, even years after event.
- Consultation with trained mental health provider is recommended for accurate diagnosis.

17.9: SUBSTANCE WITHDRAWAL

Jacqueline Ferdowsali

PRESENTING SIGNS AND SYMPTOMS

Substance withdrawal is a problematic behavioral change, with physiological and cognitive concomitants that occur with cessation, reduction, or use/abuse of a substance. The condition causes clinically significant distress or impairment in social, occupational, or other areas of functioning. The signs and symptoms cannot be better explained by another medical or mental health condition (American Psychiatric Association [APA], 2013a).

The presenting signs and symptoms for each specific substance can vary based on the underlying mechanism of action of the substance (Table 17.3). While there are many different potential substances that patients can experience withdrawal from, the most common and/or life-threatening substances are covered in greater detail in this text.

TABLE 17.3: Physical Signs and Symptoms Associated With Substance Withdrawal

SUBSTANCE	WITHDRAWAL SYMPTOMS	ONSET
Opioids*	• Dysphoric mood • Nausea or vomiting • Muscle aches • Lacrimation or rhinorrhea • Pupillary dilation • Piloerection or sweating • Diarrhea • Yawning • Fever • Insomnia • High blood pressure	Short-acting opioids: 6–12 hours Long-acting opioids: 2–4 days
Alcohol**	• Autonomic hyperactivity: Sweating or pulse rate greater than 100 bpm • Increased hand tremor • Insomnia • Nausea or vomiting • Transient visual, tactile, or auditory hallucinations or illusions • Psychomotor agitation • Anxiety • Generalized tonic-clonic seizures	Typically, within 4–24 hours
Benzodiazepines	• Autonomic hyperactivity: Sweating or pulse rate greater than 100 bpm • Hand tremor • Insomnia • Nausea or vomiting • Transient visual, tactile, or auditory hallucinations or illusions • Psychomotor agitation • Anxiety • Grand mal seizures	Fast-acting benzodiazepines: Within 6–8 hours Long-acting benzodiazepines: 1–2 days or 7 or more days
Stimulant***	• Dysphoric mood • Fatigue • Vivid, unpleasant dreams • Insomnia or hypersomnia • Increased appetite • Psychomotor retardation or agitation	A few hours to several days

*According to the *DSM-5*, three or more of the listed findings need to be present in order to constitute opioid withdrawal (excludes high blood pressure).

** According to the *DSM-5*, two or more of the listed findings need to be present in order to constitute alcohol withdrawal.

***According to the *DSM-5*, two or more of the listed findings need to be present plus dysphoric mood in order to constitute stimulant withdrawal.

Source: Data from the American Psychiatric Association. (2013b). Substance-related and addictive disorders. In *Diagnostic and statistical manual of mental disorders* (5th ed.). American Psychiatric Association. https://doi-org.unr.idm.oclc.org/10.1176/appi.books.9780890425596.dsm16; Arroyo-Novoa, C. M., Figueroa-Ramos, M. I., & Puntillo, K. A. (2019). Opioid and benzodiazepine iatrogenic withdrawal syndrome in patients in the intensive care unit. *AACN Advanced Critical Care, 30*(4), 353–364. https://doi.org/10.4037/aacnacc2019267

Opioids

The onset of withdrawal symptoms for opioids may be observed as soon as 6 to 12 hours for short-acting opioids or as long as 2 to 4 days for long-acting opioids after the last use of the substance. If an opioid antagonist has been administered, the withdrawal symptoms may occur much more quickly. For short-acting opioids, the symptoms peak in about 1 to 3 days and can last up to 7 days. It is possible to develop subacute symptoms which last for weeks or months and include anxiety, dysphoria, anhedonia, and insomnia (APA, 2013b). The initial symptoms are anxiety, restlessness, irritability, increased sensitivity to pain, and subjective reports of muscle aches. There are several available scales to measure opioid withdrawal symptoms including the Clinical Opiate Withdrawal Scale (COWS), Subjective Opiate Withdrawal Scale (SOWS), and the Short Opioid Withdrawal Scale-Gossop (SOWS-Gossop).

Alcohol

The onset of alcohol withdrawal symptoms may occur as early as 4hours after the last alcohol consumption. Symptoms typically peak within 24 hours and start improving by the fourth or fifth day (APA, 2013b). The initial signs and symptoms are often tremulousness and anxiety. If left untreated these symptoms can quickly result in the development of delirium tremens and seizures (Caputo et al., 2020). Using the Alcohol Use Disorders Identification Test (AUDIT) or the Alcohol Use Disorders Identification Test-Piccinelli Consumption (AUDIT-PC), every patient in the acute care setting should be screened for potential alcohol withdrawal. There are several tools available that may be helpful in assessing the patient's risk for severe alcohol withdrawal. These include Prediction of Alcohol Withdrawal Severity Scale or the Luebeck Alcohol-Withdrawal Risk Scale (Alvanzo et al., 2020; Wood et al., 2018). Assessment of alcohol withdrawal symptoms can be done using the Clinical Institute Withdrawal Assessment of Alcohol Scale, Revised (CIWA-Ar; Pribék et al., 2021). However, it should be noted that the CIWA-Ar does not perform equally in all types of patient populations experiencing alcohol withdrawal symptoms, especially in the acutely ill, and therefore should be interpreted with caution (Higgins et al., 2019). For those patients with alcohol withdrawal delirium the CAM-ICU, Delirium Detection Score (DDS), RASS, or Minnesota Detoxification Scale (MINDS) should be used over the CIWA-Ar scale (Alvanzo et al., 2020).

Benzodiazepines

The initial signs and symptoms of benzodiazepine withdrawal presentation are dependent on the type of benzodiazepine used. If short acting, signs and symptoms may present within hours (6–8 hours) or if long acting, withdrawal may not begin for 1 to 2 days. Initial signs and symptoms include insomnia, anxiety, irritability, nightmares, altered mood, tremor, autonomic hyperactivity, nausea or vomiting, hallucinations, psychomotor agitation, seizures (APA, 2013b; Arroyo-Novoa et al., 2019; Jobert et al., 2021).

Stimulants

This category includes amphetamine-type substances and cocaine. The most common symptom is a dysphoric mood and is accompanied by physiologic changes (Table 17.3). The onset of signs and symptoms can be within hours up to days after last use.

HISTORY AND PHYSICAL FINDINGS

When conducting a history with a patient it is imperative to fully understand the complete picture of their substance use. A nonjudgmental approach is imperative as patients are often reluctant to disclose this sensitive information. One strategy to facilitate complete documentation of their substance use is to ask about substance use in the medication history section (Turner et al., 2017). As part of the history gathering it is important to document the substance taken, how much is usually consumed, and the time of the last use.

The physical exam findings associated with withdrawal for each substance is summarized in Table 17.3.

DIFFERENTIAL DIAGNOSIS AND DIAGNOSTIC CONSIDERATIONS

The potential differential diagnosis for a patient presenting with signs and symptoms associated with a withdrawal syndrome can be long and varied. They range from potential infection to another psychiatric condition such as depression. If the substance causing withdrawal symptoms is not known, a urine drug screen and alcohol level may be helpful. Additionally, consideration of other potential differential diagnoses may be needed to ensure a different physiological explanation for the withdrawal symptoms is not present, such as a complete blood count (CBC) or imaging if infection is suspected.

TREATMENT

Treatment approaches for substance withdrawal depend on what substance the patient is withdrawing from. Additionally, understanding the patient's intentions related to withdrawal and discontinuation of the substance is important as administration of the substance may be the ethical treatment option to avoid and/or stop the withdrawal syndrome. A detailed approach to withdrawal symptom management is provided for several common substances in the following sections.

Opioids

Treatment of opioid withdrawal may be complicated by the fact that a clear understanding of the patient's prior use of opioids may not be known. There are several approaches a clinician may need to implement. For the patient with known opioid use who does not wish to withdraw, continuation of an opioid in the acute setting is appropriate to prevent withdrawal (Prunty & Prunty, 2016). In patients for whom opioid use is suspected and signs of withdrawal begin, it may also be appropriate to start or continue the patient on a maintenance opioid dose. For those patients who decide to begin opioid withdrawal in the hospital, consultation with a mental health specialist is advised as the two medications used to treat opioid withdrawal, buprenorphine and methadone, may require special prescribing privileges (Prunty & Prunty, 2016). Best practice is to wait for signs of opioid withdrawal prior to prescribing either buprenorphine or methadone (Srivastava et al., 2020). Clonidine is an alternative treatment option for those facilities where prescribing buprenorphine or methadone is not an option (Prunty & Prunty, 2016; Turner et al., 2017). Dexmedetomidine and ketamine may be helpful in avoiding severe withdrawal symptoms in the intensive care setting but

have not been as robustly investigated (Arroyo-Novoa et al., 2019). The physical symptoms associated with opioid withdrawal can be managed with other pharmacologic treatments as well (Table 17.4).

Alcohol Withdrawal Syndrome

There are two general approaches to managing alcohol withdrawal. The first, and considered best practice, is the symptom-triggered approach. The second is the fixed dosing approach which may be appropriate if assessment is limited. The symptom-triggered approach incorporates assessment from the CIWA-Ar scale and administration of benzodiazepines (Alvanzo et al., 2020). Benzodiazepines are considered the first-line treatment of alcohol withdrawal management. Any benzodiazepine may be used, but longer acting agents are preferred in most cases. Alternative and/or adjunctive treatment regimens may include clonidine, carbamazepine, gabapentin, phenobarbital, or valproic acid. New research is investigating if a phenobarbital treatment strategy may

TABLE 17.4: Symptomatic Relief of Withdrawal Symptoms

SYMPTOM	DRUG	DOSAGE	ROUTE OF ADMINISTRATION	NOTES
Insomnia	Trazodone	50–100 mg	Oral	At bedtime for 4 days and then as needed
	Promethazine	25–75 mg	Oral	At bedtime as needed
	Temazepam	10–30 mg	Oral	At bedtime as needed
Nausea/vomiting	Metoclopramide	10 mg	Oral or IM	Every 4 to 6 hours as needed for a total of 30 mg daily
	Dimenhydrinate	50–100 mg	Oral or IM	Every 4 hours as needed not to exceed 400 mg daily
	Prochlorperazine	5–10 mg	Oral or IM	Every 8 hours as needed not to exceed 40 mg
Abdominal cramps	Propantheline	15 mg	Oral	Every 8 hours as needed
	Hyoscine butylbromide	20 mg	Oral	Every 8 hours as needed
Diarrhea	Loperamide	4 mg initially	Oral	2 mg after each unformed stool
Muscle cramps	Acetaminophen	325–650 mg	Oral	Every 4 hours as needed, a maximum daily dose of 4,000 mg
	Naproxen	500 mg	Oral	Every 12 hours with meals for 4 days, then reduced to as needed
	Quinine sulfate	300 mg	Oral	Every 12 hours as needed
Headaches and pain	Ibuprofen	400 mg	Oral	Every 8 hours as needed
	Acetaminophen	325–650 mg	Oral	Every 4 hours as needed, a maximum daily dose of 4,000 mg
Agitation and anxiety	Hydroxyzine	25–50 mg	Oral	Every 8 hours as needed
	Diazepam	5 mg	Oral	Every 8 hours as needed, taper over 3 to 5 days

IM, intramuscularly.

Source: Reprinted from Turner, C., Fogger, S., & Frazier, S. (2017). Opioid use disorder: Challenges during acute hospitalization. *The Journal for Nurse Practitioners, 14(2)*, 61–67. https://doi.org/10.1016/j.nurpra.2017.12.009

provide enhanced outcomes (Tidwell et al., 2018). Data are limited at this point to suggest a complete practice change, but future research may direct an alternative treatment approach. A suggested symptom-based approach is summarized in Table 17.5. Additionally, thiamine and folate/folic acid should be administered to all patients. Magnesium may need to be replaced in those with hypomagnesemia or history of alcohol withdrawal seizures (Alvanzo et al., 2020). Patients in the ICU may require prophylactic treatment for alcohol withdrawal if there is known or suspected dependence on alcohol.

TABLE 17.5: Suggested Symptom-Based Prescribing Approach for Alcohol Withdrawal

Thiamine 100 mg IV/IM for 3–5 days Consider magnesium and phosphorus replacement in select populations*	
CIWA-Ar <10 (and low risk of developing severe or complicated alcohol withdrawal)	Supportive care or pharmacotherapy Benzodiazepines, carbamazepine, phenobarbital, or gabapentin Adjunctive: Carbamazepine, gabapentin, or valproic acid
CIWA-Ar 10-18	Pharmacotherapy Benzodiazepines (first¹ line therapy) Alternatives: Carbamazepine, phenobarbital, or gabapentin Adjunctive: Carbamazepine, gabapentin, or valproic acid
CIWA-Ar ≥19	Pharmacotherapy Benzodiazepines (1ˢᵗ line therapy) Alternatives: phenobarbital Adjunctive: Phenobarbital, carbamazepine, gabapentin, or valproic acid
Alcohol seizure	Fast-acting benzodiazepines
Alcohol withdrawal delirium	Delirium onpharmacologic interventions Pharmacotherapy recommended to achieve a light somnolence Benzodiazepines either short- or long-acting IV (1ˢᵗ line therapy) Alternative: Phenobarbital Adjunct: Antipsychotics (not used as monotherapy)
Adjunctive therapy (should not be used alone to control symptoms) Autonomic hyperactivity and anxiety Persistent hypertension or tachycardia	Clonidine or dexmedetomidine Beta-blockers

*For patients with hypomagnesemia or previous history of alcohol withdrawal seizures, magnesium should be administered. For patients with hypophosphatemia (<1 mg/dL), replacement should be provided.

Source: Data from Alvanzo, A., Kleinschmidt, K., Kmiec, J., Kolodner, G., Marti, G., Murphey, W., Tirado, C., Waller, C., & Nelson, L. (2020). The ASAM Clinical Practice Guideline on alcohol withdrawal management. *Journal of Addiction Medicine, 14*(3S Suppl. 1), 1–72. https://doi.org/10.1097/ADM.0000000000000668

Benzodiazepines

If the patient is not actively seeking withdrawal from benzodiazepines continuation of the benzodiazepine is the most appropriate strategy to avoid severe withdrawal. Benzodiazepines should never be abruptly stopped and if discontinuation is desired a slow taper and consideration of transition to long-acting benzodiazepine, such as diazepam, is recommended (Brett & Murnion, 2015; World Health Organization, 2009). Robust evidence to support alternative treatment strategies is lacking (Fluyau et al., 2018).

Stimulants

There are no specific treatment recommendations for individuals going through withdrawal secondary to stimulant use (Siefried et al., 2020). General symptom withdrawal management can be used (Table 17.4). Nonpharmacologic strategies should also be implemented if the individual becomes angry or aggressive.

TRANSITION OF CARE

An acute interface with the healthcare system may be an opportunity to transition patients into substance treatment programs. Discussing available options with patients can help facilitate this transition in care (Turner et al., 2017; Weimer et al., 2019).

KEY TAKEAWAYS

■ Substance withdrawal is highly variable and dependent on the substance used.
■ Every patient should be approached individually and a nonjudgmental ethical approach to substance withdrawal should be employed.

EVIDENCE-BASED RESOURCE

American Psychiatric Association. (2013b). Substance-related and addictive disorders. In *Diagnostic and statistical manual of mental disorders* (5th ed.). American Psychiatric Association. https://doi-org.unr.idm.oclc.org/10.1176/appi.books.9780890425596.dsm16

17.10: SUICIDAL BEHAVIOR AND SCREENING

Helena Turner

PRESENTING SIGNS AND SYMPTOMS

Patients at risk for suicide are identified by multiple factors. These may include the patient presenting for care following a suicide attempt or displaying characteristic signs and symptoms, especially in combination with known risk factors. They may also include patient self-report or through the reports of family, friends, or other concerned individuals or via screening (Suicide Prevention Resource Center, 2015). Behavioral changes that may precede a suicide attempt are correlated with many of the symptoms of depression, including insomnia, loss of appetite or reduced dietary intake, withdrawal from others and/or from hobbies and activities, decreased attention to personal hygiene, or neglect of medical care (McGirr et al., 2006; Rudd et al., 2006). Other behavioral changes can include agitation, aggressive behaviors, and impulsive, dangerous, or self-harmful behaviors such as driving recklessly or increased substance use (Popovic et al., 2015; Rudd et al., 2006; Schuck et al., 2019). Patients may begin making preparations for death such as giving away belongings, cleaning and tidying their home or room, writing goodbye notes, writing a will, making visits to friends and family, or obtaining a gun or stockpiling medications (National Institute of Mental Health, n.d.-b).

Affective symptoms that may indicate increased risk for suicide include feelings of hopelessness, anhedonia, despair, guilt or shame, anxiety or panic, anger or rage, a persistent sad affect and depressed mood, feeling trapped or without reason to live, and extreme mood swings (McLean et al., 2008; Rudd et al., 2006; Schuck et al., 2019). Patients may verbalize some or all of these feelings, including a desire to die, or a sense of being a burden on others (Hill & Pettit, 2014). Suicidal behavior is often precipitated by experiencing a recent trauma or a life crisis. These may include events leading to shame or despair such as the death of a loved one (including pets), the demise of a relationship, the loss of a job, experiencing a financial or legal crisis, or loss of health status (McLean et al., 2008; Pitman et al., 2020; Schiff et al., 2015).

Signs and symptoms of increased risk for suicide are especially relevant within the context of risk factors for suicide. A history of a previous suicide attempt is a strong predictor of future attempts and death by suicide (Office of the Surgeon General & National Action Alliance for Suicide Prevention, 2012b). Most deaths by suicide occur in those with a mental illness, primarily unipolar or bipolar depression, psychosis (especially with command hallucinations), and substance use disorders (especially alcohol use disorder; Bachmann, 2018; Baldessarini, 2020; Poorolajal et al., 2016). Other mental illnesses associated with suicide include eating disorders, personality disorders, and anxiety disorders (Bachmann, 2018; Baldessarini, 2020). Additional risk factors include having a family history of suicide, a history of child abuse or neglect, having a serious medical illness or pain, social isolation, and being single, widowed, or divorced (Angelakis et al., 2019; Baldessarini, 2020; Pitman et al., 2020; Tidemalm et al., 2011).

Women attempt suicide more frequently than men, but men use more lethal means and thus have a higher rate of suicide (Han et al., 2016). Suicide rates increase with age and are highest among men aged 45 to 64 years old and 75 years and older in the United States (Hedegaard et al., 2018). Other populations at high risk for suicide are American Indians, Alaska Natives, veterans, and members of a sexual or gender minority (Bachmann, 2018; Office of the Surgeon General & National Action Alliance for Suicide Prevention, 2012a).

HISTORY AND PHYSICAL FINDINGS

Patients presenting to the hospital who are being evaluated or treated for a behavioral health disorder as their primary concern are required by The Joint Commission to undergo a comprehensive suicide risk assessment (The Joint Commission on Accreditation of Healthcare Organizations, 2015). Patients who are being treated primarily for a medical condition may be at risk for suicide due to their illness or other risk factors and should also be screened for suicidal thoughts (Boudreaux et al., 2020). Validated, rapid screening tools include the Patient Safety Screener 3 (PSS-3), the Patient Health Questionnaire-9 (PHQ-9), and the Ask Suicide-Screening Questions (ASQ) tool (Boudreaux et al., 2015; National Institute of Mental Health, n.d.-a; Rossom et al., 2017). These tools may be used in the emergency department, on medical units, or in the outpatient setting.

If a patient screens positive for suicidal ideation, further assessment should be made of the patient's suicidal thoughts, plans, intent, and past attempts, as well as their mental health history and current symptoms, history of substance use disorder(s) and recent substance use, and anxiety, agitation, or irritability (Suicide Prevention Resource Center, 2015). Assessment also includes an evaluation of the patient's protective factors, such as responsibility to children or pets, strong relationships with friends or family, existing supportive relationships with care providers, good coping and problem-solving skills, and cultural or religious beliefs that discourage suicide (McLean et al., 2008). Additional collateral information may be obtained from the patient's outpatient provider, from the medical record, and, with the patient's permission, from friends and family (Suicide Prevention Resource Center, 2015). The ED Safe Secondary Screener developed by the Suicide Prevention Resource Center, or the SAFE-T (Suicide Assessment Five-Step Evaluation and Treatment) guide developed by the Substance Abuse and Mental Health Services Administration (SAMHSA) are tools that may be used for this assessment (SAMHSA, n.d.; Suicide Prevention Resource Center, 2015). According to these guides, a patient is considered to be high risk for suicide if they have made a nearly lethal suicide attempt, have persistent ideation with strong intent and a specific plan, have access to lethal means, have a severe mental illness with presenting symptoms, have experienced a precipitating event as described previously, display or have a history of impulsive or agitated behavior, and are lacking protective factors.

DIFFERENTIAL DIAGNOSIS AND DIAGNOSTIC CONSIDERATIONS

Differentiating a suicide attempt from nonsuicidal self-injury is accomplished through assessment of the lethality of the behavior and through patient interview to ascertain the presence or absence of suicidal intent. Nonsuicidal self-injury involves cutting, burning, scratching, prevention of wound healing, and banging or hitting (Bentley et al., 2014; Cipriano et al., 2017). Injuries are typically superficial, and patients most often act upon their arms, legs, wrists, and thighs (Cipriano et al., 2017). Upon interview, the patient denies suicidal intent and instead frequently expresses a desire to relieve negative emotions or tension, or to feel sensation (Klonsky, 2011).

TREATMENT

Treatment of suicidal thoughts and behaviors is focused on establishing safety for the patient and staff and instilling hope (Wheat et al., 2016). Place patients identified as high-risk for suicide in a private space that is clear of items that could be used to harm themselves, initiate suicide precautions according to facility regulations, and request a psychiatric consultation for comprehensive suicide risk assessment (Betz & Boudreaux, 2015; Suicide Prevention Resource Center, 2015). Suicidal patients under the influence of alcohol or other drugs should be closely monitored until the effects of the substance have resolved and a further risk assessment can be made (Betz & Boudreaux, 2015). Patients treated on a medical unit for injuries resulting from a suicide attempt should be reevaluated for suicide risk once stabilized.

Lithium and clozapine are the only medications with evidence of reducing suicidal behaviors, but neither is immediately effective (Riesselman et al., 2015; Wheat et al., 2016). If verbal deescalation techniques are unsuccessful, psychotropic medications such as sedatives, anxiolytics, antipsychotics, and ketamine are used to calm and stabilize the agitated patient until the patient can be evaluated by a behavioral health specialist (Deal et al., 2015; Guerrero & Mycyk, 2020; Wheat et al., 2016). Physical restraints may also be used as a last resort, according to facility policies, if clinically indicated, but patients must always be treated in the least restrictive manner possible (Deal et al., 2015; Guerrero & Mycyk, 2020; Wheat et al., 2016).

Patients at risk for suicide who do not require inpatient psychiatric hospitalization should receive brief suicide prevention interventions to modify risk factors (National Action Alliance for Suicide Prevention, 2018; Suicide Prevention Resource Center, 2015). These interventions include providing verbal and written information about local and national crisis centers and hotlines, education about treatment options, lethal means counseling, and safety planning (National Action Alliance for Suicide Prevention, 2018; Suicide Prevention Resource Center, 2015). While being respectful of the patient's autonomy and privacy, ask permission to include family members or close friends in the discussion so that they can provide support to the patient in future (National Action Alliance for Suicide Prevention, 2018).

Lethal means counseling is based upon the understanding that reducing access to the means of suicide can provide time for the immediate crisis to subside and give the patient the opportunity to access supportive resources (Harvard School of Public Health, n.d.). Many suicide attempts occur during a crisis with very little planning, and the majority of those who attempt suicide do not make subsequent attempts (Harvard School of Public Health, n.d.). Firearms, suffocation, and poisoning, respectively, are the most frequently used means of suicide in the United States for both men and women (Harvard School of Public Health, n.d.). Assess whether the patient has access to firearms or medications and work with the patient and their friends and family to reduce the patient's access to these means until they have recovered (National Action Alliance for Suicide Prevention, 2018). Firearms can be stored away from the home. Unused, expired, and unnecessary medications should be disposed of safely, and current medications can be kept in a medication lock box to be dispensed as necessary (Suicide Prevention Resource Center, 2015).

Safety planning involves working with the patient to develop a list of resources the patient can use to cope during a suicidal crisis (National Action Alliance for Suicide Prevention, 2018; Suicide Prevention Resource Center, 2015). There are various templates and apps available to help with this process. All templates generally include a list of the patient's warning signs of a developing crisis, coping skills, friends' and family members' phone numbers, phone numbers of providers and agencies, reminders of things important to the patient, and ways to make the environment safe (Suicide Prevention Resource Center, 2015). Emphasize to the patient that making a safety plan is a positive step in recovery, but that it is necessary to participate in outpatient mental health care to address underlying issues that lead to suicidal feelings (Suicide Prevention Resource Center, 2015).

TRANSITION OF CARE

Effective transition of care is especially important for survivors of a suicide attempt, as the risk for a subsequent attempt is particularly high following discharge from an acute care setting (Hogan & Grumet, 2016). Prior to discharge, communicate with other providers involved in the patient's care, and make an appointment for follow-up care with a provider skilled in the treatment of suicidal ideation and behaviors (National Action Alliance for Suicide Prevention, 2018; Suicide Prevention Resource Center, 2015). Collaborate with the patient to address barriers to outpatient care such as lack of insurance or transportation (Suicide Prevention Resource Center, 2015). Educate the patient and their friends and family about the importance of attending follow-up appointments (Suicide Prevention Resource Center, 2015). Finally, after discharge, at least one supportive contact should be made by the provider or staff who have provided care (Hogan & Grumet, 2016; Miller et al., 2017; National Action Alliance for Suicide Prevention, 2018; Suicide Prevention Resource Center, 2015). These caring contacts may be in the form of a call, text, postcard, email, or letter, and can help prevent self-harm and increase engagement in follow-up care (Doupnik et al., 2020; Miller et al., 2017; Suicide Prevention Resource Center, 2015).

17.11: WERNECKE'S ENCEPHALOPATHY

Thomas Farley

Wernecke's encephalopathy (WE) is the well understood complication of thiamine deficiency that is often associated with alcohol use disorder. However, WE can occur in any patient at risk for nutritional deficiency including disorders of the gastrointestinal tract. A variety of bariatric procedures can precipitate WE, including sleeve gastrectomy and intragastric ballooning (Oudman et al., 2018). Since symptoms can be vague, many cases are diagnosed after death (Sinha et al., 2019). WE should be considered a neurologic emergency when diagnosed and treated immediately.

Glucose metabolism depends on thiamine. In the absence of thiamine, glucose is metabolized through anaerobic pathways, generating lactate and creating acidosis. The acidosis affects periventricular structures accounting for the observed neurologic symptoms.

It is crucial to make the clinical diagnosis early. Up to 80% of patients with untreated WE will develop Korsakoff syndrome characterized by memory impairment with confabulation. Korsakoff syndrome presents with short-term memory loss, long-term memory preservation, and confabulation. It is generally chronic and irreversible. Up to 20% of patients with untreated WE may die from the disorder (Latt, 2014).

PRESENTING SIGNS AND SYMPTOMS

WE is described as having the classic triad of mental status changes, ocular abnormalities, and gait disturbance. However, the classic triad is not found in all patients. Symptoms are often more diffuse and nonspecific including headache, fatigue, speech disturbances, inattentiveness, anorexia, and weakness (Okafor et al., 2018).

HISTORY AND PHYSICAL FINDINGS

Patient history may include:
- Excessive alcohol use
- Intestinal obstruction
- Malignancy
- Vomiting
- Bariatric surgery
- Malnutrition

Physical findings may include:
- Hypothermia
- Hypotension
- Spectrum of altered mental status
- Oculomotor abnormalities
- Ataxia
- Decreased fine motor function
- Decreased deep tendon reflexes

DIFFERENTIAL DIAGNOSIS AND DIAGNOSTIC CONSIDERATIONS

WE is a clinical diagnosis. Estimation of thiamine levels is not routinely performed (Latt & Dore, 2014).

Patients with any portion of the classic triad of mental status changes, ocular abnormalities, and gait disturbance in combination with history of nutritional deficiency should prompt the clinician to initiate treatment.

Caine criteria for diagnosis of WE is useful since it demonstrates sensitivity of nearly 100% in patients with alcohol abuse disorder without hepatic encephalopathy (Caine et al., 1997). Diagnosis is made in any patient with two of the following:
- Nutritional deficiency
- Altered mental status or impaired memory
- Oculomotor abnormalities
- Cerebellar dysfunction

Normal computed tomography (CT) of the brain does not rule out WE. Magnetic resonance imaging (MRI) of the brain commonly includes findings of cytotoxic and vasogenic edema (Okafor et al., 2018) with hyperintense signals in the dorsal medial thalamic nuclei, periaqueductal grey area, and the third or fourth ventricles (Figure 17.2; Fujikawa & Wernicke, 2020).

TREATMENT

Primary treatment of WE is thiamine (vitamin B1) and should be administered via parental route within 48 to 72 hours after onset of symptoms (Latt & Dore, 2014). A comprehensive literature review recommends avoiding initial administration of thiamine orally due to poor bioavailability. Recommended IV dosing is thiamine 200 to 500 mg IV every 8 hours for 3 days (Flannery et al., 2016). Additional resources recommend tapering dosing after 3 days in patients with definitive diagnosis of WE to thiamine 100 mg PO every 8 hours for 7 to 14 days (Latt & Dore, 2014).

Magnesium is an important cofactor of thiamine and should be repleted along with thiamine if treating for WE. Suggested dosing of 1 mEq/kg in divided doses in first 24 hours of treatment then 0.5 mEq/kg/day in divided doses for 3 days (Flannery et al., 2016).

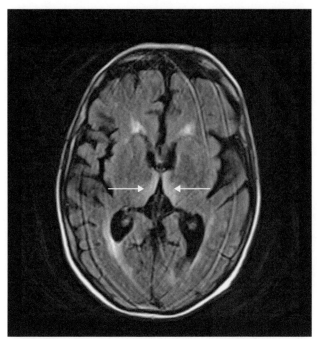

FIGURE 17.2: Fluid-attenuated inversion recovery magnetic resonance images of the brain of a 28-year-old woman with Wernicke encephalopathy showing hyperintense signals in the bilateral medial thalami (arrows).
Source: Jto410.

CLINICAL PEARLS

- WE can present in any patient with nutritional deficiency.
- The diagnosis is made clinically. Imaging is not necessary.
- A delay in treatment can result in prolonged or persistent neurologic dysfunction.
- A low threshold to treat is recommended given the relative safety of thiamine administration.

KEY TAKEAWAYS

- Clinical diagnosis of WE is missed in upward of 80% of patients (Okafor et al., 2018)
- Always treat WE if suspected in clinical presentation given grim prognosis of untreated disease.
- Use parental thiamine over oral form for initial treatment.
- Ideal dosage of thiamine is not clear but 500 mg IV every 8 hours for 3 days appears sufficient.

SPRINGER PUBLISHING **CONNECT**™

A robust set of instructor resources designed to supplement this text is located at **http://connect.springerpub.com/content/ reference-book/978-0-8261-6079-9.** Qualifying instructors may request access by emailing **textbook@springerpub.com.**

REFERENCES

Full list of references can be accessed at http://connect .springerpub.com/content/reference-book/978-0-8261-6079-9

PART III

GENERAL CLINICAL TOPICS FOR THE ACUTE CARE NURSE PRACTITIONER

CHAPTER 18

INFECTIOUS DISEASES

R. Brandon Frady, Gail Lis, and Susanna (Sue) Sirianni

LEARNING OBJECTIVES

- Explain specific infectious diseases affecting patients in the acute care setting.
- Relate risk factors associated with select infectious diseases with particular attention to immunocompromised individuals.
- Develop differential diagnoses based on history and physical findings.
- Identify key diagnostic studies to develop working diagnosis for patients with infectious diseases.
- Determine treatment, based on evidence-based guidelines, for patients with infectious diseases.
- Integrate principles of microbiology and antibiotic stewardship in prescribing treatment for select infectious diseases.
- Differentiate the unique presentation for older adult populations.

INTRODUCTION

This chapter focuses on select infectious diseases that are likely to be encountered by the adult-gerontology acute care nurse practitioner (AGACNP). The illnesses discussed in this chapter are not comprehensive but provides common etiologies that are primary reasons for hospital admission, have a significant morbidity and mortality if not recognized appropriately or treated efficiently and effectively (sepsis), have a potential to cause a public health concern or result from public health compromise (tuberculosis, infectious diarrhea), or cause life-altering complications (diabetic foot infections [DFI]). Many of the illness presented in this chapter have subtle presentations or multiple etiologies that require a comprehensive patient history in order to assist in differentiation. In addition, several conditions discussed are complications secondary to hospitalization and antibiotic use (*Candidiasis, Clostridioides difficile*), and others a result of infections that have seeded to other places (spinal abscess, endocarditis).

Differential diagnoses and diagnostic workups can be extensive in the case of infectious diseases, especially when there are multiple possibilities to consider, or because the etiology is unclear secondary to subtle or atypical presentation. An example is an infection in the older adult population. The presentation among older adults is similar for all underlying infections without specific symptoms directed at the body system affected. Fever of unknown origin (FUO) is also presented as a separate section because of the diagnostic challenge to healthcare providers in both adult and older adult populations.

Evidence-based interventions are discussed that integrate the principles of microbiology and antimicrobial stewardship and have been extrapolated from the appropriate clinical practice guidelines. These principles will assist the provider in understanding the likely microbial pathogen and, therefore, use appropriate antimicrobial therapy that supports antibiotic stewardship.

18.1: FEVER OF UNKNOWN ORIGIN

Fever of unknown origin (FUO) is defined as a body temperature ≥38.3°C (101°F) for 3 weeks or longer without a clear etiology after appropriate evaluation (Cunha et al., 2015). Fever is one of the most common presenting symptoms in both the outpatient and inpatient settings. Most febrile conditions are readily diagnosed or resolve after a short period of time. FUO, however, presents a diagnostic challenge to healthcare providers and the differential can be extensive and the workup expensive. The workup should be based upon a thorough history (symptom driven) and physical examination. FUO is typically classified into four categories based on their etiology (Table 18.1). Within each of the classifications there are examples of specific etiologies. Note that the specific etiologies are not comprehensive and provide the most common causes. If the practitioner understands these classifications, the history can be tailored to the symptoms within these classifications, the physical examination focused to findings that support what is indicated within the history, and the appropriate diagnostic workup used to rule the working diagnosis in or out (Bush, 2020) The workup should entail the context of the fever (e.g., recent travel, immune status). Since this section has the potential to elicit many differential diagnoses, common classifications of etiologies are discussed. Common diagnostics are also identified for all patients presenting with FUO in addition to expanded diagnostics should this be necessary.

TABLE 18.1: Classification of Fever of Unknown Origin, Possible Etiologies, and Pertinent Positives

CLASSIFICATION	POSSIBLE ETIOLOGIES	HISTORY OF PERTINENT POSITIVES
Infections (25%–50%)	Consider opportunistic infections in immunocompromised persons (cytomegalovirus), HIV, endocarditis, Epstein-Barr virus, abscess (abdominal/dental), Lyme disease, TB, osteomyelitis (vertebral), toxoplasmosis	Prior or recent invasive procedures or surgeries (include dental, endoscopies), presence of hardware from orthopedic surgery, prosthetic joints, valve replacement, pacemaker, cosmetic implants Animal exposure (new pets, trip to petting farm/zoo) Chills Immunosuppressant medications Mosquito or tick exposure Blood transfusions Painful lymph nodes
Connective tissue disorders (10%–20%)	SLE, giant cell arteritis, rheumatoid arthritis, polyarteritis nodosa, Still's disease, polymyalgia rheumatica	Fever Headache Oral ulcers Malar rash Acalculous cholecystitis Joint pain Generalized lymphadenopathy
Neoplasms (5%–35%)	Lymphoma, leukemia, colon cancer, renal cell carcinoma, hepatoma, metastatic cancer, myeloproliferative disorder	Significant weight loss–especially if associated with anorexia Painless enlarged lymph nodes
Miscellaneous (15%–25%)	Deep vein thrombosis, drug fever, cirrhosis, inflammatory bowel disease, subacute thyroiditis	Neck/jaw pain (thyroiditis) Bowel pattern changes Medication history Generalized extremity pain Alcoholism

SLE, systemic lupus erythematous; TB, tuberculosis.

Source: Adapted from Bush, L. (2020, July). *Fever of unknown origin*. https://www.merckmanuals.com/professional/infectious-diseases/biology-of-infectious-disease/fever-of-unknown-origin-fuo

HISTORY OF PRESENT ILLNESS

The history of present illness (HPI) will vary depending on the underlying etiology. The HPI should focus on duration, pattern (occurs daily at specific time, every other day, insidious or acute onset) and associated symptoms (chills, headache, fatigue, nausea, vomiting, diarrhea, anorexia, night sweats, myalgias, arthalgias, rashes). The pattern of fever is essential to determining the etiology. It is recommended that the history is repeated more than once and often by another practitioner, especially if the etiology remains unclear after the initial workup. It may also be useful to obtain additional history from family members or friends to elicit details that the patient may not recall.

Subjective

A thorough history is required for patients presenting with FUO. The practitioner should conduct a general history that includes medical, surgical, medication, social, and family history. This should then be followed by a more specific, detailed review of systems. Pertinent positives are highlighted for each of the classifications and corresponding etiologies in Table 18.1.

Medication History

Drug fever is well documented in the literature and often overlooked as an etiology of fever. Fever related to drug therapy can occur at any time during the course of treatment and may last up to 1 week for the fever to resolve especially if the medication is metabolized slowly and has a long half-life. Medications may also mask the actual degree of the fever and include drugs such as steroids, nonsteroidal anti-inflammatory drugs (NSAIDs), acetaminophen, and antimicrobial use. It is important to obtain prescribed medications, new medications, over-the-counter, and herbal remedies.

Social History

- Patients' country of origin, previous countries of residence
- Living conditions
- Employment history
- Vaccination status
- Recent travel (e.g., exploring caves, food and water consumption, destinations, prophylactic medications, vaccinations)
- Recreational drugs (e.g., IV drug use)

- Recreational activity (e.g., gardening, swimming in lakes)
- Sexual history
- Animal and insect exposure (e.g., new pets, exotic pets, visit to petting farm/zoo)
- Unusual dietary habits (e.g., unpasteurized mild or cheese, improperly/undercooked food [poultry, eggs])

Family History
- May reveal a genetic link (e.g., connective tissue disorders, autoimmune disease)
- Exposure to same infectious agent

Objective

The physical exam should also be thorough with focus on clues obtained from the history. Pertinent positives are identified to assist the provider in associating exam findings with historical clues to determine the underlying etiology (see Table 18.1).

DIFFERENTIAL DIAGNOSIS AND DIAGNOSTIC CONSIDERATIONS

Routine diagnostic tests are ordered to assist in differentiating the etiology of FUO. Once results from these studies are obtained, further testing may be necessary (see "Expanded Diagnostic Testing").

Laboratory
- Blood cultures
- Urinalysis (presence of red blood cells clue to endocarditis, renal cell carcinoma); urine culture (presence of fungal organisms)
- Complete blood cell count with differential—leukocytosis, leukopenia (hematologic malignancies), thrombocytopenia (hematologic malignancies, malaria, rickettsial, viral infections); atypical lymphocytosis, blasts (leukemia, lymphoma), eosinophils (parasites), lymphopenia (HIV)
- Blood chemistry including alkaline phosphatase (isolated elevation—lymphoma), lactate dehydrogenase, bilirubin, and liver enzymes (hepatobiliary abnormalities), increased lactate dehydrogenase (lymphoma, leukemia, histoplasmosis, pneumocystis)
- Antinuclear antibodies and rheumatoid factor—connective tissue, auto immune
- HIV fourth generation tests
- Serum protein electrophoresis—multiple myeloma, lymphoma, systemic lupus erythematous (SLE)
- Creatinine kinase—myositis
- Erythrocyte sedimentation rate (ESR) and C-reactive protein (CRP)—inflammatory markers, not specific for infectious etiology
- Fecal occult—colon cancer, inflammatory bowel disease (IBD)
- Ferritin—thyroid function
- Angiotensin-converting enzyme (ACE)—malignancy, multiple myeloma, miliary tuberculosis, lymphoma, cirrhosis

Imaging
- Chest x-ray (CXR)

Expanded Diagnostic Tests

If history and physical findings provide evidence to further differentiate etiology of FUO, the following laboratory and imaging tests can be ordered. This is not an all-inclusive list.

Laboratory
- Tuberculin skin test
- Sputum acid fast bacillus
- Q fever, *Brucella, Salmonella* IgM/IgG titers
- Carcinoembryonic antigen (CEA); elevated in cancerous and noncancerous (cirrhosis) conditions
- Stool cultures, ova, and parasites
- Fungal panel
- Epstein-Barr virus (EBV)/cytomegalovirus (CMV) IgM/IgG titers

Imaging
- Transthoracic echocardiogram (TTE)/transesophageal echocardiogram (TEE)
- Chest computed tomography (CT)—may detect small nodules suggestive of malignancy, fungal mycobacterial or nocadial infection, hilar and/or mediastinal lymphadenopathy (lymphoma, histoplasmosis, sarcoidosis)
- Abdominal CT—intraabdominal infections, lymphoproliferative disorders
- Nuclear imaging (gallium-67 scintigraphy and technetium-99m, indium-111 tagged white blood cell scan) able to screen entire body for possible abscess/inflammatory focus
- Panorex of jaw
- Magnetic resonance imaging (MRI)—spinal epidural abscess (SEA), malignancy
- F-fluorodeoxyglucose positron emission tomography (FDG-PET) CT scans—anatomic sites of inflammation and malignancy
- Lymph node biopsy
- Bone marrow biopsy (neoplastic disorders, intracellular infections, miliary tuberculosis)

TREATMENT

Treatment is typically limited until the etiology of the fever, if any, is determined. Supportive care is recommended; however, antipyretics should be used cautiously as continued use may mask occurrence of fevers. Empiric antibiotics or steroids are not recommended unless there are specific clinical indications. Early, initial treatment with antimicrobials is not recommended and may interfere with culture results. If the patient presents with a life-threatening illness (such as a septic picture), then empiric antibiotics could be initiated. Consultations with subspecialties are typically necessary (especially infectious disease when the etiology remains unclear) to assist in the diagnosis and treatment. Additional subspecialties may include hematology and rheumatology.

18.2: *CLOSTRIDIOIDES DIFFICILE (CLOSTRIDIUM DIFFICILE)*

Clostridium difficile infection (CDI) is considered one of the most common healthcare-associated infections in the United States (McDonald et al., 2018). CDI has been recently reclassified and now renamed as *Clostridioides difficile* (CD) (Centers for Disease Control and Prevention [CDC], 2019) CD is typically acquired in the hospital or an extended care facility. Patients hospitalized for more than 2 weeks are at greater risk for contracting CD secondary to fecal colonization. Pertinent history includes prior history of CD colitis, risk factors, and symptoms supportive of current infection. Patients with prior history of CD colitis are more likely to experience a recurrence in 15% to 30% of cases (Gerding & Johnson, 2018). Recurrence may be related to relapse of the same strain or reinfection with new strain. There are several risk factors associated with CD (Box 18.1) but recent exposure to antimicrobial therapy is significant. The following factors related to antimicrobial therapy should be considered to assist in the prevention of CD: Minimize the frequency and duration of high-risk antibiotic therapy and the number of antibiotic agents prescribed, implement antibiotic stewardship programs to minimize overuse and support evidence-based antibiotic prescribing practices. Antibiotics targeted should be based on epidemiologic data.

It is unclear if proton pump inhibitors increase a patients' risk for CD, some studies have shown an epidemiologic association but others have not; additional studies to examine causality are needed (Sucher et al., 2021).

COMPLICATIONS

Patients with CDI can develop severe or fulminant infection. Severe infection is defined as a WBC ≥15,000 or a serum creatinine >1.5 mg/dL; fulminant infection is defined as patients meeting criteria for severe CDI plus the presence of hypotension, shock, ileus or hypotension. Patients with fulminant CDI may not have diarrhea and their illness may imitate that of a surgical abdomen and/or sepsis (Kelly et al., 2021). Toxic megacolon is a sequelae of fulminant CDI and associated with a higher mortality rate.

PRESENTING SIGNS AND SYMPTOMS

Frequent malodorous nonbloody diarrhea with urgency.

HISTORY AND PHYSICAL FINDINGS

Subjective

Pertinent Positive

- Prior history of CD colitis
- Risk factors associated with CD colitis (Box 18.1).
- Diarrhea
  - Soft and unformed to watery or mucoid, malodorous
  - Nonbloody
- Fever

BOX 18.1 RISK FACTORS ASSOCIATED WITH *CLOSTRIDIOIDES DIFFICILE*

1. Recent hospitalization or nursing home placement
2. History of prior CD infection
3. Antibiotic exposure (most antimicrobials carry risk); most common:
   - Clindamycin
   - Ampicillin
   - Cephalosporin (3rd/4th generations)
   - Fluoroquinolones
   - Carbapenems
4. Inflammatory bowel disease (especially ulcerative colitis)
5. Older age (>65)
6. Significant immunocompromised state (solid organ transplant recipients, hematopoietic stem cell transplant patients, chemotherapy, advanced HIV patients)
7. Chronic kidney disease, end stage renal disease
8. Gastrointestinal surgery
9. Enteral tube feedings
10. Acid-suppressing medications

Source: Adapted from Shane, A. L., Mody, R. K., Crump, J. A., Tarr, P. I., Steiner, T. S., Kotloff, K., Langley, J. M., Wanke, C., Warren, C. A., Cheng, A. C., Cantey, J., & Pickering, L. K. (2017). 2017 Infectious Diseases Society of America Clinical Practice Guidelines for the diagnosis and management of infectious diarrhea. *Clinical Infectious Diseases*, 65(12), e45–e80. https://doi.org/10.1093/cid/cix669.

- Abdominal pain
- Constipation

Pertinent Negative

- Recent exposure to food/toxin that may cause diarrhea
- Recent exposure to viral gastroenteritis outbreak
- Risk factors suggestive of inflammatory bowel disease (IBD) or history of IBD

Objective

Pertinent Positive

- Fever
- WBC ≥15,000 or serum creatinine >1.5 mg/dL (indicates severe infection)
- Abdominal pain
- Frequent episodes of malodorous diarrhea
- Hypotension, shock, ileus or megacolon (indicates fulminant infection)

Pertinent Negative

- Bloody diarrhea

DIFFERENTIAL DIAGNOSIS AND DIAGNOSTIC CONSIDERATIONS

- Inflammatory bowel disease (IBD)
- Viral gastroenteritis

- Food-borne associated diarrhea
- Enteral tube feedings
- Overuse of laxatives

Diagnostic Tests

Stool for *C. difficile* toxin—Patients should be screened for clinical symptoms (at least three loose or unformed stools in less than 24 hours with history of antibiotic exposure and not on laxatives). Testing is completed using either a one-step or multistep process.

- One-step
  - **Nucleic Acid Amplification Test (NAAT):** PCR method tests for toxic genes. Test is rapid and sensitive.
- Multistep
  - **Glutamate Dehydrogenase (GDH):** Initial screen that tests for antigen (GDH). Sensitive, but not specific (indicates if *C. difficile* is present but not if bacteria is producing toxins).
    - If positive, a confirmatory test is completed to detect presence of toxins.
      - Toxins by enzyme immunoassay assay (EIA), or
      - Nucleic acid amplification (NAAT; if positive GDH and negative EIA).
  - Alternative multistep
    - NAAT with EIA.
- Fecal lactoferrin should not be ordered to diagnose CDI.

Repeat testing is not recommended within 7 days during the same episode of diarrhea and should not be done on asymptomatic patients. Repeat testing may be recommended in an epidemic setting where CD acquisition is more frequent. Repeat testing to establish clinical cure has no value and is not recommended (McDonald et al., 2018).

Imaging

- Plain abdominal imaging is typically unnecessary and will unlikely demonstrate any pathology until the disease progresses. Bowel dilatation, mural thickening, and thumbprinting may be viewed in advanced or recurrent disease. If toxic megacolon is present, free intraperitoneal air may be seen if perforation has occurred.

TREATMENT

Oral vancomycin or fidaxomicin (Dificid) is recommended for the treatment of CD across the spectrum of illness (Table 18.2). Metronidazole (Flagyl) should be used only as an alternative for non-severe CDI when oral vancomycin or fidaxomicin are unavailable or as adjunctive therapy with oral vancomycin in patients who have fulminant CD. Intravenous vancomycin is ineffective in the treatment of CD; however, rectal instillation of vancomycin is recommended in patients with fulminant CD who have an ileus (Shane et al., 2017). The use of fecal transplantation does have a role in patients with recurrent CD and patients have demonstrated improved outcomes. Surgical management may be necessary in patients who are severely ill. Subtotal colectomy is recommended in this case with preservation of rectum. Additional treatment recommendations include discontinuance of inciting antibiotic agent(s) as soon as possible, and fluid and electrolyte replacement as needed.

Recurrent Clostridioides difficile

Fifteen percent to 30% of patients will experience recurrence of CD and patients who have a first recurrence are at an increased risk of a second recurrence. CD recurrence is significantly lower in patients treated with fidaxomicin than those treated with vancomycin. Risk for recurrence includes those ≥65 years of age, those who continue antibiotics while being treated for CD, and those who remain in the hospital after being diagnosed with CD. See treatment for recurrent CD in Table 18.2. Taper and pulse therapy are recommended for recurrent episodes and include decreasing dosing over time and administering oral vancomycin or fidaxomicin as every other day dosing (McDonald et al., 2018).

Infection prevention and control measures should be implemented. Patients with CD should be placed in a private room with a dedicated toilet to decrease transmission. Healthcare personnel should institute contact plus precautions that include gown and gloves upon entry to a room. Patients with suspected CD (have symptoms and stool sample ordered) should also be placed in contact plus isolation with the same precautions as identified previously. Disposable patient equipment should also be utilized (e.g., stethoscope, thermometer, blood pressure cuff). Hand hygiene is crucial with soap and water for both patients and staff. Patients and family members should be educated regarding hand hygiene prior to discharge.

TRANSITION OF CARE

If a patient with CD is to be transferred to another unit of care or facility, ensure that the diagnosis is made clear with the necessary precautions in place. Patients with active symptoms should not be discharged until their diarrhea is controlled and are metabolically and physiologically stable (electrolytes and vital signs are normalizing).

CLINICAL PEARLS

- Minimize frequency and duration of high-risk antibiotic therapy and number of antibiotics prescribed (fluoroquinolones, clindamycin, cephalosporins [unless used as surgical prophylaxis]).
- Adhere to an antibiotic stewardship program.
- Consider CD as differential in patients with new-onset leukocytosis and/or fever.
- Patients may not always have diarrhea.
- Oral vancomycin or fidaxomicin is considered standard treatment across the illness spectrum.
- Discontinue antimicrobial therapy as soon as feasibly possible.
- Severe CDI may present as surgical abdomen without presence of diarrhea.

TABLE 18.2: Recommendations for the Treatment of *CDI* in Adults

CLINICAL PRE- SENTATION	RECOMMENDED AND ALTERNATIVE TREATMENTS	COMMENTS
Initial CDI episode	Preferred: Fidaxomicin 200 mg given twice daily for 10 days Alternative: Vancomycin 125 mg given 4 times daily by mouth for 10 days Alternative for nonsevere CDI, if above agents are unavailable: Metronidazole, 500 mg 3 times daily by mouth for 10–14 days	Implementation depends upon available resources Vancomycin remains an acceptable alternative Definition of nonsevere CDI is supported by the following laboratory parameters: White blood cell count of 15,000 cells/μL or lower and a serum creatinine level <1.5 mg/dL
First CDI recurrence	Preferred: Fidaxomicin 200 mg given twice daily for 10 days, OR twice daily for 5 days followed by once every other day for 20 days Alternative: Vancomycin by mouth in a tapered and pulsed regimen Alternative: Vancomycin 125 mg given 4 times daily by mouth for 10 days Adjunctive treatment: Bezlotoxumab 10 mg/kg given intravenously once during administration of SOC antibiotics[a]	… Tapered/pulsed vancomycin regimen example: 125 mg 4 times daily for 10–14 days, 2 times daily for 7 days, once daily for 7 days, and then every 2 to 3 days for 2 to 8 weeks Consider a standard course of vancomycin if metronidazole was used for treatment of the first episode Data when combined with fidaxomicin are limited. Caution for use in patients with congestive heart failure[b]
Second or subsequent CDI recurrence	Fidaxomicin 200 mg given twice daily for 10 days, OR twice daily for 5 days followed by once every other day for 20 days Vancomycin by mouth in a tapered and pulsed regimen Vancomycin 125 mg 4 times daily by mouth for 10 days followed by rifaximin 400 mg 3 times daily for 20 days Fecal microbiota transplantation Adjunctive treatment: Bezlotoxumab 10 mg/kg given intravenously once during administration of SOC antibiotics[a]	… … … The opinion of the panel is that appropriate antibiotic treatments for at least 2 recurrences (i.e., 3 CDI episodes) should be tried prior to offering fecal microbiota transplantation Data when combined with fidaxomicin are limited. Caution for use in patients with congestive heart failure[a]
Fulminant CDI	Vancomycin 500 mg 4 times daily by mouth or by nasogastric tube. If ileus, consider adding rectal instillation of vancomycin. Intravenously administered metronidazole (500 mg every 8 hours) should be administered together with oral or rectal vancomycin, particularly if ileus is present	Definition of fulminant CDI is supported by: Hypotension or shock, ileus, megacolon

The recommendations are based on the 2017 guidelines and these current focused guidelines. Abbreviations: CDI, *Clostridioides difficile* infection; SOC, standard of care.
[a]Bezlotoxumab may also be considered for patients with other risks for CDI recurrence but implementation depends upon available resources and logistics for intravenous administration, particularly for those with an initial CDI episode. Additional risk factors for CDI recurrence include age >65 years, immunocompromised host (per history or use of immunosuppressive therapy), and severe CDI on presentation.
[b]The Food and Drug Administration warns that "in patients with a history of congestive heart failure (CHF), bezlotoxumab should be reserved for use when the benefit outweighs the risk."

Source: Johnson, S., Lavergne, V., Skinner, A. M., et al. (2021). Clinical practice guideline by the Infectious Diseases Society of America (IDSA) and Society for Healthcare Epidemiology of America (SHEA): 2021 focused update guidelines on management of *Clostridioides difficile* infection in adults. *Clin Infect Dis, 73*(5), e1029-e1044.

18.3: INFECTIOUS DIARRHEA

PRESENTING SIGNS AND SYMPTOMS

Acute diarrhea is the passage of three or more loose or liquid stools per 24 hours (or more frequently) than what is considered normal for an individual person.

HISTORY AND PHYSICAL FINDINGS

Diarrhea can be caused by a variety of factors including infectious and noninfectious etiologies. The most common causative factors are viruses, bacteria, and protozoa, with viruses being of highest incidence. These pathogens can cause a variety of symptoms and can be further differentiated into inflammatory versus noninflammatory diarrhea syndromes (Chin-Hong & Guglielmo, 2021). Inflammatory diarrhea is typically bloody, small volume caused by invasive bacteria or parasites or by toxin production, and predominantly affects the large intestine. Patients may also report significant abdominal discomfort, fecal urgency, and fever. Noninflammatory diarrhea is typically caused by viruses or toxins that affect the small intestine and interfere with salt and water balance. This causes large-volume watery diarrhea that is associated with nausea, vomiting, and abdominal cramping (Chin-Hong & Guglielmo, 2021).

Although acute diarrhea has many etiologies, including noninfectious causes, there are epidemiologic clues to determining its etiology. A detailed clinical and exposure history is imperative for persons presenting with diarrhea. A common risk factor for infectious diarrhea is related to the introduction and transmission of pathogens through mass production and distribution of food, contact with infected persons, water systems, recreational water facilities, day care centers, global travel, animal exposure (feces), hospitalization, and some sexual practices (Shane et al., 2017). Travelers diarrhea is most common in developing countries; 40% to 60% of travelers will develop diarrhea associated with contact of contaminated food or water. Diarrhea will develop within 10 days of contact. Although travelers diarrhea can be caused by viruses, bacteria, and protozoan, bacteria is the most common etiology and includes enterotoxic *Escherichia coli Salmonella, Campylobacter,* and *Shigella.* Coinfection with an additional pathogen is likely to occur in 20% of those infected (Graves, 2013).

Patients with diarrhea are likely to present with a variety of symptoms depending on the severity. The bacterial pathogens are often associated with bloody diarrhea. Several pathogens express a toxin that can cause severe symptoms and/or significant sequelae. These pathogens include *Shigella dysenteriae* and several *E. coli* strains. *Escherichia Coli* O157:H7 is the most common and is referred to as Shiga toxin-producing *E. Coli* (STEC). The *E. Coli* O157:H7 is also referred to as *enterohemorrhagic E. Coli (EHEC)* because of the bloody diarrhea that this particular strain produces. The *E. Coli* O157:H7 can also cause hemolytic uremia and/or thrombotic thrombocytopenia purpura (Cohen, 2016). The American College of Gastroenterology suggests that additional medical evaluation should take place for individuals presenting with profuse watery diarrhea that results in hypovolemia, bloody stools, fever >38.5°C, more than six stools in a 24-hour period for more than 48 hours, severe abdominal pain, diarrhea in the elderly and those significantly immunocompromised (Riddle et al., 2016). The sequelae of infectious diarrhea is often benign, but it can also lead to severe dehydration as well as systemic manifestations and complications especially if related to toxin-producing pathogen and/or if the patient is immunocompromised.

Subjective

Pertinent Positive

- >3 loose, liquid stools within a 24-hour period and change from usual bowel pattern
- Fever
- Abdominal pain/cramping
- Bloody versus nonbloody diarrhea
- Incubation period (time of exposure to time of symptoms)
- Immune status
- Recent travel/vacation/cruising
- Exposure to pet feces
- Day care center
- Recreational water/untreated water
- Dietary habits (foods recently consumed), catered events, restaurant dining
- Close contact to persons with similar symptoms

Pertinent Negative

- Food allergies
- Recent change in medications, diet
- Recent antimicrobial therapy
- Enteral feedings
- Chemotherapy or radiation

Objective

Pertinent Positive

- Liquid stools, may be bloody
- Abdominal pain
- Fever
- Leukocytosis/lymphocytosis (bacterial versus viral)
- Dehydration
  - Elevated blood urea nitrogen (BUN)/creatinine
  - Elevated hematocrit
  - Mental status changes
  - Tachycardia/hypotension
  - Dry mucosa/skin tenting
  - Weak pulses
  - Decreased urinary output
- Sepsis
- Nongap metabolic acidosis/electrolyte imbalances (hypernatremia/hypokalemia)

Pertinent Negative

- Fecal impaction
- Ischemic colitis
- Thyrotoxicosis
- Chronic illness/malignancy
- IBD

DIFFERENTIAL DIAGNOSIS AND DIAGNOSTIC CONSIDERATIONS

Infectious Etiologies

- Viruses
  - **Rotavirus:** Common in infant/children and transmitted to adults, self-limiting vomiting, nonbloody diarrhea, fever.
  - **Norovirus:** Most common cause of gastroenteritis in adults. Common outbreaks seen in restaurants, catered events, long-term care facilities, schools, day care centers, vacation destinations. Vomiting, nonbloody diarrhea and is self-limiting.
- **Protozoan:** Less likely of an occurrence, should be considered when diarrhea progresses from persistent to chronic. Protozoan pathogens include *Cryptosporidium, Giardia, Cyclospora,* and *Entamoeba histolytica. Cryptosporidium* is most common parasitic cause of foodborne etiology. Transmission occurs from an infected person or animal or a fecally contaminated food or water source. *Giardia* is associated with day care outbreaks. *Cyclospora* is a small bowel pathogen

TABLE 18.3: Etiology of Infectious Diarrhea by Bacterial Pathogens

PATHOGEN	SOURCE	SYMPTOM	TESTING	TREATMENT	COMPLICATIONS
Campylobacter	Raw or undercooked poultry, seafood, meat, produce, unpasteurized dairy, contact with animals, and by drinking untreated water	Bloody diarrhea, fever, severe abdominal pain	Routine stool culture	Supportive care Azithromycin (first choice), fluoroquinolone alternative	Erythema nodosum, glomerulonephritis, hemolytic anemia, Guillain-Barre syndrome, immunoglobulin A nephropathy, reactive arthritis, postinfectious irritable bowel syndrome, intestinal perforation
Listeria	Bacteria, fruits, unpasteurized fruit juices, vegetables, leafy greens, sprouts	Fever, diarrhea		Mild, no transmission Systemic	Meningitis
Salmonella—Depending on species causes typhoid fever (enteric) or gastroenteritis	Gastroenteritis from unpasteurized milk, dairy products, fruit juices; undercooked eggs; vegetables, leafy greens, sprouts; undercooked poultry Typhoid from swimming/drinking untreated fresh water, or ingestion of food contaminated by chronic carriers	Sudden-onset diarrhea (may be bloody); fever, abdominal cramps within 6 hours of intake, may last 4–7 days Typhoid: 5–21-day incubation period; prolonged fever, headache, chills, symptoms as noted previously	Routine stool culture, blood, bone marrow	Supportive care; Antimicrobial for typhoid only: ceftriaxone or ciprofloxacin (first choice); ampicillin or TMP-SMX or azithromycin (alternate)	Erythema nodosum, reactive arthritis, postinfectious irritable bowel syndrome, intestinal perforation, hepatosplenomegaly, aortitis, osteomyelitis, extravascular deep tissue focus (typically seen with typhoid)
Shiga toxin-producing *E. Coli* (STEC)	Bacteria: Unpasteurized milk, dairy products, fruit juices, vegetables, leafy greens, and sprouts, undercooked beef; visiting petting farm/zoo	Bloody diarrhea, severe abdominal pain	*E. Coli* O157:H7 and Shiga toxin; NAAT for Shiga gene	Supportive care: Antibiotics can cause hemolytic uremic syndrome	Hemolytic uremic syndrome, postinfectious irritable bowel syndrome
Shigella	Uncooked eggs, swimming or drinking untreated water; anal-genital, oral-anal, or digital-anal contact	Bloody diarrhea, severe abdominal pain	Routine stool culture	Supportive care Azithromycin, ciprofloxacin, (first choices); TMP-SMX or ampicillin (alternate if susceptible)	Erythema nodosum, glomerulonephritis, reactive arthritis, postinfectious irritable bowel syndrome, intestinal perforation, lethal toxic encephalopathy and/or seizure
Yersinia	Bacteria; unpasteurized milk or dairy products, undercooked pork	Fever, bloody diarrhea, abdominal pain (similar to appendicitis)	Specialized stool culture or molecular assay or NAAT; also isolated from blood, bile, throat swab, CSF	TMP-SMX (first choice); cefotaxime or ciprofloxacin (alternate)	Erythema nodosum, hemolytic anemia, reactive arthritis, intestinal perforation, aortitis, osteomyelitis extravascular deep tissue focus
Staphylococcus aureus	Bacteria; unpasteurized milk or dairy products, undercooked poultry	Nausea, vomiting, diarrhea, abdominal cramps that begin within 30 minutes; typically symptoms last 24 hours	Specialized stool culture	Supportive	

CSF, cerebrospinal fluid; NAAT, nucleic acid amplification test; TMP/SMX, trimethoprim/ sulfamethoxazole.

Source: Data from Centers for Disease Control and Prevention. (n.d.-b). *Foodborne diseases active surveillance network.* Retrieved October 24, 2020, from https://www.cdc.gov/foodnet/surveys/index.html; Shane, A. L, Mody, R. K., Crump, J. A., Tarr, P. I., Steiner, T. S., Kotloff, K., Langley, J. M., Wanke, C., Warren, C. A., Cheng, A. C., Cantey, J., & Pickering, L. K. (2017). 2017 Infectious Diseases Society of America Clinical Practice Guidelines for the diagnosis and management of infectious diarrhea. *Clinical Infectious Diseases, 65*(12), e45–e80. https://doi.org/10.1093/cid/cix669;

with a duration of greater than 3 weeks and causes excessive fatigue. *Entamoeba histolytica* typically occurs in migrants from and travelers to endemic countries.

■ Bacterial pathogens are differentiated in Table 18.3.

Noninfectious Etiologies

■ Fecal impaction
■ Ischemic colitis
■ Thyrotoxicosis
■ Malignancy
■ IBD
■ Malignancy/chemotherapy/radiation
■ Pharmacology
■ Diet/enteral feeding
■ Runner's diarrhea

Diagnostic Tests

■ Stool cultures should be obtained on persons presenting with fever, bloody or mucoid stools, severe abdominal cramping or tenderness, or signs of sepsis. Specific diagnostic tests are identified in Table 18.3. A stool culture will identify the presence of pathogens; however, specific toxin tests are necessary if a particular pathogen is suspected
■ Ova and parasites—if a parasite is suspected based on history, eosinophils on differential, travelers with diarrhea lasting more than 14 days
■ Viral stool culture—enteric adenovirus
■ Enzyme induced assay—rotavirus
■ Blood cultures—systemic manifestations (sepsis), enteric fever suspected, immunocompromised, high-risk conditions (hemolytic anemia), travel to enteric fever-endemic areas
■ Complete blood cell count—leukocytosis bacterial pathogens, sepsis, leukopenia (virus, severe sepsis), eosinophilia (parasites)

■ Comprehensive metabolic panel—dehydration, renal function (especially if hemolytic uremic syndrome is a concern)
■ Peripheral blood smear—hemolytic uremia syndrome (red blood cell fragments)
■ Imaging—may not assist with diagnosis but is useful to assess for complications
   ● Abdominal series, abdominal CT—intraabdominal free air, toxic megacolon
   ● MRI/ultrasound—aortitis, mycotic aneurysms

TREATMENT

The recommended treatment for infectious diarrhea is outlined in Table 18.3. It is important to note that antimicrobial therapy is not recommended as empiric treatment in many cases. Following are general guidelines to the use of antibiotics in the treatment of infectious diarrhea:

Immunocompetent Patients

■ Fever documented in medical setting
■ Abdominal pain
■ Bloody diarrhea
■ Bacillary dysentery (frequent scant bloody stools, fever, abdominal cramps, tenesmus)
■ Persons who have recent international travel with body temp ≥38.5°C and have signs and symptoms of sepsis
■ Empiric treatment should be based upon antibiograms and travel history using either fluoroquinolones (ciprofloxacin), macrolides (azithromycin), or cephalosporins. Alternative choices are also listed in Table 18.4 should the patient have intolerance to first-line drugs
■ Antimicrobial therapy for persons with infections related to Shiga toxin-producing *E. Coli* (STEC) strains should be avoided

TABLE 18.4: Comparison of Sepsis Definitions

CONDITION	CRITERIA IN 1991/2003 (SEPSIS-1/ SEPSIS-2)	CRITERIA IN 2016 (SEPSIS-3)
Systemic inflammatory response syndrome (SIRS)	Temperature <36°C (96.8°F or >38°C [100.4°F]) Heart rate >90 Respiratory rate >20/min or $PaCO_2$ <32 mmHg WBC <4 × 10⁹/L (<4000/mm³), >12 × 10⁹/L (>12,000/mm³), or ≥10% bands	
Sepsis	2 SIRS + actual or suspected infection	Suspected or documented infection and acute increase in ≥2 sepsis-related organ failure assessment (SOFA) points
Severe sepsis	Sepsis + sepsis-induced organ dysfunction or hypotension (SBP <90 mmHg) or lactate >4 mmol	
Septic shock	Severe sepsis + persistent hypotension (SBP <90 mmHg or 40 MmHg below baseline) despite fluid administration of 20 cc/kg or lactate >4 mmol	Suspected or documented infection + vasopressor therapy required to maintain MAP ≥65 mmHg and lactate >2 despite adequate fluid resuscitation of 30 cc/kg

MAP, mean arterial pressure; SBP, systolic blood pressure; WBC, white blood cells.

- Persons who have signs and symptoms of sepsis and suspected of having enteric fever should be treated with broad spectrum antibiotics after blood, stool, and urine cultures have been obtained. De-escalation of therapy should occur as soon as culture results are available (Shane et al., 2017)

Immunocompromised

- Empiric antimicrobial treatment is recommended for patients with severe illness and bloody diarrhea
- The same recommendation for specific antimicrobial use applies to the immunocompromised patient as the immunocompetent patient

Supportive Care for Immunocompetent and Immunocompromised Patients

- Supportive treatment is the cornerstone of therapy in patients with infectious diarrhea
- The ISDA recommends reduced osmolarity oral rehydration solution (ORS) as first-line therapy for mild to moderate dehydration in adults with acute diarrhea from any cause (Shane et al., 2017)
- A nasogastric tube may be placed to administer ORS unless the patient has an ileus or some type of obstruction
- Most individuals admitted to the hospital may require IV lactated Ringer's or normal saline if there is severe dehydration, signs/symptoms of shock, mental status changes, and patient is not able to consume the ORS
- Antiemetics for nausea
- Antimotility drugs (e.g., loperamide) can be prescribed for acute watery diarrhea in immunocompetent persons
  - Contraindicated in toxic megacolon

CLINICAL PEARLS

- A detailed exposure history is essential (e.g., food, pets, travel, recreational water venues, patient care, day care).
- Viral pathogens are the primary etiology of infectious diarrhea and are typically self-limiting.
- Persons with bloody diarrhea should be assessed for enteropathogens.
- Enteric fever should be considered when a febrile person has a travel history to an endemic area, consumed foods by persons of endemic exposure.
- Routine antimicrobial therapy is not recommended unless exhibiting signs of sepsis, severe abdominal pain, bloody diarrhea, febrile, or immunocompromised.
- Antimicrobial therapy is contraindicated in patients with Shiga toxin-producing pathogens.
- Treatment is centered around supportive care.

18.4: SEPSIS

Sepsis is one of the most prevalent diseases worldwide affecting over 30 million people (Fleischmann et al., 2016) with an estimated mortality of 11 million deaths annually (Rudd et al., 2020). In the United States it affects approximately 1,031/100,000 persons (Kempker & Martin, 2016). It is the leading cause of morbidity and mortality in hospitalized patients with an estimated mortality rate of 5.6% for patients with sepsis; 14.9% for those with severe sepsis; and up to 34.2% for those with septic shock (Paoli et al., 2018). The older adult (≥65 years of age) accounts for >60% of sepsis cases (Centers for Disease Control and Prevention [CDC], n.d.-a). The economic burden of sepsis varies greatly depending on the severity of illness and whether sepsis was present on admission or developed in the hospital. Costs of care range from >$16,000 for sepsis to as high as >$68,000 for those who develop septic shock in hospital (Paoli et al., 2018).

CHANGING DEFINITIONS

Sepsis is the body's overwhelming response to infection that leads to deadly organ dysfunction (Singer et al., 2016). While sepsis has been around for many years the definition has evolved over time. Sepsis was originally defined as a systemic inflammatory response (SIRS) to an actual or suspected infection (Bone et al., 1992). A continuum of sepsis was proposed that started with two SIRS criteria plus an actual or suspected infection (sepsis) progressing through various stages including severe sepsis, septic shock, and eventually multiorgan dysfunction syndrome (MODS) and eventually death. The definitions were updated in 2001 to include lab and clinical variables (Levy et al., 2003). In 2016, the Sepsis Definition Task Force proposed the Third International Consensus Definition (Sepsis-3) to describe the current understanding of pathobiology of sepsis as a dysregulated host response to an infection that results in organ dysfunction (Table 18.4). The Sepsis-3 consensus was intended to replace SIRS criteria with the sepsis-related Organ Failure Assessment (SOFA) score and the qSOFA, an abbreviated version that does not require any laboratory data (Singer et al., 2016). While using SIRS criteria is sensitive but not specific to sepsis, it is superior to qSOFA for diagnosing sepsis whereas the qSOFA is better at predicting mortality from sepsis (Serafim et al., 2018). The 2021 sepsis guidelines recommend against using qSOFA as a screening tool for sepsis and using SIRS, National Early Warning Scores (NEWS) or Modified Early Warning Scores (MEWS) as a screening tool for sepsis (Evans et al., 2021).

PRESENTING SIGNS AND SYMPTOMS

While the disease is commonly encountered, it remains a somewhat elusive disease for healthcare providers to identify, largely because it can easily be mimicked by other diseases.

Presenting signs and symptoms for sepsis can vary greatly depending on the cause of sepsis, host, and host response to the infection. Patients presenting with symptoms of infection such as fever, malaise, cough, or abdominal pain are easy to identify, as are those that present with signs of organ dysfunction such as hypotension, altered mental status, or acute kidney injury. However, those who are immunocompromised, elderly, or young can present atypically with vague symptoms (Vincent, 2016). Vague symptomatology coupled with the everchanging definition of sepsis make identification difficult.

HISTORY AND PHYSICAL FINDINGS

History and physical exam findings are variable depending on the health of the host, type of infection, infecting organism, and when the patient presents in the disease process. Table 18.5 describes the various organ functions and symptoms.

DIFFERENTIAL DIAGNOSIS AND DIAGNOSTIC CONSIDERATIONS

Since sepsis can be precipitated by many different organisms and can affect multiporgan systems, it stands to reason that many disease processes can mimic it. Conditions other than sepsis can produce a SIRS and many differentials need to be considered. Differentials include, but are not limited to, intracranial hemorrhage; myocardial infarction; pulmonary embolism; pancreatitis; shock; and trauma. When considering a differential diagnosis based on the presence of SIRS criteria, the presence or absence of infection needs to be established to identify whether the diagnosis is sepsis.

TABLE 18.5: Sepsis Presentations by Organ System

SYSTEM	ORGAN FAILURE MANIFESTATIONS
Central nervous system	Altered mental status
Pulmonary system	PaO_2/FiO_2 ratio <200 or ARDS Acute respiratory failure
Cardiovascular system	Hypotension (SBP <90 mmHg, MAP <65 mmHg or decrease of 40 mmHg from baseline) Chest pain Unexpected metabolic acidosis (pH <7.30)
Hematologic system	Thrombocytopenia (platelet count <100,000 cells/mm^2) Coagulation abnormalities (INR >1.5 or aPTT >60 sec)
Gastrointestinal system	Hyperbilirubinemia:Total bilirubin >2.0 mg/dL or 35 mmol/L Shock liver (elevated ALT/AST)
Renal system	Acute oliguria Creatinine >2 mg/dL or >2 times upper limit of normal

ALT, alanine transaminase; aPTT, activated partial thromboplastin time; ARDS, acute respiratory distress syndrome; AST, aspartate aminotransferase; INR, international normalized ratio; SBP, systolic blood pressure.

Patient Evaluation

The initial patient evaluation needs to include the following:

- Blood cultures × two from two different sites
- Lactic acid (LA) (which can be obtained from either an arterial or venous sample) or by using point of care technology
- Complete blood count (CBC) with differential
- Coagulation profile
- Comprehensive metabolic panel (CMP)
- Urinalysis (UA)
- Cultures of any potentially infected sites
- Chest radiograph if pneumonia is suspected
- Other diagnostic imaging will be based on presenting signs and symptoms

TREATMENT

Once a diagnosis of sepsis or septic shock has been made, timely interventions must be completed including identification of the possible source. Providing optimal sepsis care has been summarized into groups of interventions that should be completed within 3 and 6 hours of sepsis identification. The components of the bundle are as follows.

3-Hour Bundle

- Blood cultures x2, prior to antibiotic administration
- Serum lactate
- Source control
- Fluid resuscitation with 30 mL/kg if systolic blood pressure (SBP) is <90 mmHg or mean arterial pressure (MAP) <65 mmHg or decrease in baseline SBP by >40 mmHg or LA >4.0
- Broad spectrum antibiotics (ideally within 1 hour of identification)

6-Hour Bundle

- Re-evaluation of volume status
- Vasopressor therapy if SBP is <90 mmHg or MAP<65 mmHg
- Repeat LA if original LA >2.0

Source control and site of infection is an integral component of treatment of the septic patient. The two most common sources of sepsis are the lungs or urine; however, other less obvious sources need to be considered. Other sites to consider are intraabdominal sources, skin and soft tissue infections, endocarditis, and septic joints. In a patient with an invasive line or hardware, those must also be considered as potential sources. While identification and treatment of the possible source is imperative, so is removal of any offending agent. Patients with necrotizing fasciitis will require emergent debridement and patients with bowel perforation will require an emergent exploratory laparotomy.

Antimicrobial Therapy

Prompt appropriate antimicrobial therapy is administered immediately, ideally within 1 hour when sepsis is definite or probable and/or sepsis is possible with the presence of shock (Evans et al., 2021). Initial therapy must take into consideration and include factors such as recent exposure to antibiotics, suspected site, as well as patient- and pathogen-related factors. Important patient-related factors to consider include severity of illness, comorbid conditions, recent exposure to antibiotics, likelihood of multidrug resistant organisms, age, weight ,and patient allergies. Furthermore, a history of organ dysfunction must also be considered as many antibiotics are cleared renally or hepatically (Green & Gorman, 2014).

The initial antimicrobial of choice should target the most likely infectious organism. Initial coverage should include coverage for both gram-positive and gram-negative organisms, as well as anaerobic coverage if intraabdominal pathology is suspected. Immunocompromised or patients receiving prolonged antimicrobial therapy may also require antifungal coverage. Timeliness of antimicrobial therapy, ideally within 1 hour ("door-to-needle") of presentation and before blood cultures are drawn, has demonstrated improved patient outcomes (Laupland & Ferrer, 2017). If blood cultures are unable to be drawn, antimicrobials should not be delayed.

Initial antibiotic coverage should include broad-spectrum, multidrug regimens in septic shock (Table 18.6) dependent upon the most likely source. In the event that other pathogens are suspected such as *Clostridioides difficile*, vancomycin (oral or rectal) should be added.

De-Escalation of Antimicrobials

It is important to evaluate antimicrobial therapy daily and de-escalate broad-spectrum antimicrobials as soon as possible. In patients with no evidence of infection, empiric antibiotics should be stopped. If culture data are available, antimicrobial therapy should be narrowed based on the identified organism and sensitivities. Lastly, consideration of patient response to antimicrobial therapy must also be considered when considering de-escalation. Most infections will not require more than 7 to 10 days of therapy unless there are indications for longer use such as undrained sources of infection, *Staphylococcus aureus* bacteremia, and neutropenia (Rhodes et al., 2017).

Fluid Resuscitation

Patients with sepsis or septic shock should receive a 30 mL/kg bolus of crystalloids within the first 3 hours of sepsis identification in order to restore intravascular volume and increase oxygen delivery to the tissues (Singer et al., 2016). Reassessment of volume status using dynamic measures is required as part of ongoing patient resuscitation and is part of the 6-hour bundle. Dynamic measures such as administering a fluid bolus or a straight leg raise have been deemed superior to static measures such as central venous pressure monitoring. Direct measurement of cardiac output (CO) or surrogate measurements such as pulse pressure variation will

TABLE 18.6: Treatment Regimens for Community-Acquired and Healthcare-Associated Sepsis by Likely Source

POSSIBLE SOURCE	COMMUNITY ACQUIRED	HEALTHCARE-ASSOCIATED
Lungs	• Third generation cephalosporin with a macrolide or respiratory fluoroquinolone *If risk for Pseudomonas or MDR:* • Cefepime or piperacillin/tazobactam *If critically ill or high risk for MRSA or necrotizing pneumonia* • Vancomycin	• Third or fourth generation cephalosporin or extended spectrum penicillin *Plus/Minus* • Aminoglycoside or fluroquinolone • PCN allergy carbapenem • Beta-lactam–beta-lactamase inhibitor • Vancomycin or linezolid
Urinary tract infection	• Third or fourth generation cephalosporin (if critically ill)	• Extended spectrum beta-lactam *Plus/Minus* • Aminoglycoside or fluroquinolone *Add for history of or suspected MDR:* • Cefepime or carbapenem
Intraabdominal	• Carbapenem or piperacillin/tazobactam *Or* • Third or fourth generation cephalosporin + metronidazole	• Carbapenem or piperacillin/tazobactam *Or* Third or fourth generation cephalosporin + metronidazole
Necrotizing skin and soft tissue infections	• Vancomycin and piperacillin/tazobactam *Plus* • Clindamycin if necrotizing infection suspected	• Vancomycin and piperacillin/tazobactam *Plus* • Clindamycin if necrotizing infection is suspected

MDR, multidrug resistant organism; MRSA, methicillin-resistant *Staphylococcus aureus*.

identify if a patient is fluid responsive. Dynamic measures include passive leg raising combined with CO measurement, fluid challenges against stroke volume (SV), systolic pressure or pulse pressure, and increases of SV in response to changes in intrathoracic pressure.

Vasopressor Therapy

Patients with persistent hypotension that is unresponsive to fluid resuscitation should be started on vasopressor therapy to target a MAP >65 mmHg (Singer et al., 2016). Vasopressors are necessary to restore the sympathetic tone of the vascular system and to improve myocardial depression and mitochondrial dysfunction. The initial vasopressor of choice is norepinephrine titrated to MAP >65 mmHg. If a second vasopressor is required either vasopressin or epinephrine can be added.

TRANSITION OF CARE

Approximately 85% of patients with sepsis come through the emergency department (ED), so it is imperative that patients with sepsis are identified, and that treatment is begun promptly in the ED (Filbin et al., 2018). While many patients will complete the 3-hour bundle while in the ED, it is important that a handover occur between the ED RN and the receiving unit RN.

CLINICAL PEARLS

- Early identification and treatment of sepsis is paramount for patient survival.
- Administer broad-spectrum antibiotics as soon as possible, ideally within 1 hour of the diagnosis of septic shock.
- De-escalate antibiotics based on culture results and patient response.
- Source control is achieved by removing infected foreign objects (such as hardware or tissues), draining abscesses, and removing any invasive lines or tubes.
- Fluid resuscitation and re-evaluation of fluid volume status are key to ensuring adequate tissue perfusion.
- Vasopressor therapies should be initiated in patients with a MAP <65 mmHg after adequate fluid resuscitation.

EVIDENCE-BASED RESOURCES

Survivingsepsis.org

18.5: HUMAN IMMUNODEFICIENCY VIRUS/ACQUIRED IMMUNODEFICIENCY SYNDROME

HIV is estimated to affect more than 1.1 million people aged 13 and older at the end of 2019 (Centers for Disease Control and Prevention [CDC], 2021). HIV and acquired immunodeficiency syndrome (AIDS) presentation may range from asymptomatic healthy individuals to end-stage AIDS symptoms. HIV infections have an acute phase where the patient is symptomatic, followed by an asymptomatic period. It is during this asymptomatic phase that people are more likely to transmit HIV to other people. Patients are less likely to be diagnosed during the acute phase of the infection.

Patients in the acute phase of infection often have a fever, rash, swollen lymph nodes, and malaise. This acute phase can last from 72 hours to a few weeks. Patients may associate these symptoms with a viral-type illness and not seek medical attention. Once the acute phase is over, the patient will again become asymptomatic and remain asymptomatic for years. During the asymptomatic stage, the patient's immune system is undergoing damage (Hess et al., 2017). Patients who are diagnosed during the initial acute phase—or at the time of laboratory testing—should have prompt initiation of antiretroviral therapy (ART) upon confirmation of disease. Patients who initially test negative for HIV with symptoms of acute illness should be tested again in 2 weeks. During these 2 weeks, patients may seroconvert and have a positive HIV antibody test.

Differentiation between HIV1 and HIV2 is necessary for ART selection. A full outline of ART therapy is discussed later in this chapter. HIV1 infections have a faster disease progression and are the most commonly seen form of HIV infection worldwide (Wu et al., 2017). HIV2 infections are seen more commonly in people from West Africa, Spain, Portugal, and Goa, India. HIV2 infections have lower HIV viral loads, a slower decline in CD4 counts, and a long asymptomatic period (Wu et al., 2017).

AIDS is the final stage of HIV infection. The CDC outlines the criteria for AIDS-defining illnesses which include opportunistic infections and malignancies that rarely occur in immunocompetent patients (CDC, 2016b). AIDS definitions include definitive diagnosis with or without laboratory evidence of HIV infection, AIDS diagnosis with laboratory evidence of HIV infection, and presumptive AIDS diagnosis with laboratory evidence of HIV infection (CDC, 2016b). Box 18.2 provides a detailed review of the CDC definition. Patients with CD4 counts less than 200 cells/mcL or a CD4 lymphocyte less than 14% are at increased risk for development of AIDS within 3 years in the absence of effective ART (CDC, 2016b).

EPIDEMIOLOGY

HIV was estimated to have affected more than 1.1 million people aged 13 and older at the end of 2019 (CDC, 2021). A closer look at age, race, ethnicity, and transmission category reveals that people 25 to 29 years old make up 20% of patients with new HIV diagnoses, and 79% of new cases are age 20 to 49 ("HIV surveillance report," 2008). Black or African American people make up nearly

BOX 18.2 CENTERS FOR DISEASE CONTROL AND PREVENTION AIDS CASE DEFINITIONS: PATIENTS OVER THE AGE OF 6 YEARS

Confirmatory AIDS Diagnosis (With or Without Laboratory HIV Confirmation)

- Candidiasis of esophagus, trachea, bronchi, or lungs
- Cryptococcosis, extrapulmonary
- Cryptosporidiosis with diarrhea for longer than 1 month
- Cytomegalovirus of organs other than spleen, liver, and or lymph nodes
- Herpes simplex virus with mucocutaneous eruption lasting for more than 1 month, or bronchitis, pneumonitis, esophagitis of any duration
- Kaposi sarcoma under the age of 60 years
- Primary lymphoma of the brain under the age of 60 years
- *Mycobacterium avium complex* or *Mycobacterium kansasii*, disseminated
- *Pneumocystis jirovecii* pneumonia
- Progressive multifocal leukoencephalopathy
- Toxoplasmosis of the brain

Confirmatory AIDS Diagnosis (With Laboratory Confirmation of HIV)

- Disseminated coccidioidomycosis
- HIV encephalopathy
- Histoplasmosis, disseminated
- Isosporiasis (also known as cystoisosporiasis) with diarrhea persisting longer than 1 month
- Lymphoma of the brain (primary) at any age
- Other non-Hodgkin lymphoma of B cell or unknown immunologic phenotype
- Any mycobacterial disease caused by mycobacteria other than *Mycobacterium tuberculosis*, disseminated
- Disease caused by extrapulmonary *M. tuberculosis*
- Salmonella septicemia
- HIV wasting syndrome
- CD4 lymphocyte count below 200 cells/mcL or a CD4 lymphocyte percentage below 14%
- Pulmonary tuberculosis
- Recurrent pneumonia
- Invasive cervical cancer
- Dementia
- Wasting

Possible AIDS Diagnosis (With laboratory HIV Confirmation)

- Candidiasis of esophagus
- Oral candidiasis
- Cytomegalovirus retinitis
- Mycobacteriosis
- Kaposi's sarcoma

- *Pneumocystis jirovecii* pneumonia
  a) History of dyspnea on exertion or nonproductive cough of recent onset (within the past 3 months); and
  b) Chest film evidence of diffuse bilateral interstitial infiltrates or gallium scan evidence of diffuse bilateral pulmonary disease; and
  c) Arterial blood gas analysis showing an arterial oxygen partial pressure of <70 mmHg or a low respiratory diffusing capacity of <80% of predicted values or an increase in the alveolar-arterial oxygen tension gradient; and
  d) No evidence of bacterial pneumonia.

- Toxoplasmosis of the brain:
  a) Recent onset of a focal neurologic abnormality consistent with an intracranial disease or a reduced level of consciousness; and
  b) Brain imaging evidence of a lesion having a mass effect or the radiographic appearance of which is enhanced by injection of contrast medium; and
  c) Serum antibody to toxoplasmosis or successful response to therapy for toxoplasmosis.

- Recurrent pneumonia
  a) More than one episode in 1 year
  b) Acute pneumonia

- Pulmonary tuberculosis
  a) Apical or miliary infiltrates
  b) Radiographic and clinical improvement with antituberculosis treatment

Source: Adapted from Papadakis, M. A., McPhee, S. J., & Rabow, M. W. (2021). *Current medical diagnosis & treatment 2021*. McGraw-Hill Education LLC

half of new diagnoses at 42%, followed by Hispanic/Latin American and Caucasian. Of note, between 2014 and 2018, Native American/Alaskan American had a 15% increase in HIV rates, along with a 78% increase in HIV rates for Native Hawaiian/Pacific Islander (HIV surveillance report, 2008). Transmission rates for 2018 men who have sex with men has the highest percentage of new infections at 66%, followed by heterosexual partner transmission at 24%, then IV drug use at 6.6%. In 2018, 42% of patients with HIV died from all-cause reasons ("HIV surveillance report," 2008). Globally 1.7 million new HIV cases were reported in 2018. It is estimated that 37.9 million people worldwide have HIV, with 770,000 deaths of HIV patients globally in 2018.

In the United States, 65 per 100 patients received HIV care, 50 per 100 maintained some form of ongoing HIV care, and 56 per 100 are virally suppressed ("HIV surveillance report," 2018). The lifetime risk for males is

1 in 61 and 1 in 253 in females (Hess et al., 2017). There are also racial and ethnic disparities associated with lifetime risk. Black/African American men have the highest lifetime risk at 1 in 22. Data analyzed based on risk group were highest among men having sex with men at 1 in 6, and the lowest risk is men having sex with women at 1 in 524 (Hess et al., 2017). States in the South have an overall higher lifetime risk (Hess et al., 2017).

PRESENTING SIGNS AND SYMPTOMS

Patients with HIV may be asymptomatic for years, even without any treatment. Up to 60% of patients with HIV will be initially asymptomatic (Henry et al., 2014). Patients' initial presentation may be vague and are often associated with the acute retroviral syndrome. Initial symptoms include fever, lymphadenopathy, chills, rash, night sweats, muscle aches, sore throat, myalgia, arthralgia, diarrhea, and headache. A closer look at each symptom reveals the following distinguishing features.

Head, Eyes, Ears, Nose, and Throat

Lymphadenopathy typically occurs in the second week of infection and includes axilla, cervical, and occipital areas. Sore throat includes pharyngeal edema and hyperemia without tonsillar swelling or exudate (Freedberg et al., 1994). Mucocutaneous ulcerations are a distinct feature of HIV infection. These ulcerations can occur orally, anally, esophageal, and/or on genitals. Sexually transmitted infections must be considered. Prolonged illness and mucocutaneous ulcerations are also suggestive of symptoms associated with HIV infection.

Skin

A rash is a common presenting symptom. The rash is generalized occurring 48 to 72 hours after a fever and lasts 5 to 8 days. The rash is located on the upper thorax, collar region, face, and occasionally extends to the feet, palms, and soles. The rash is well-circumscribed, round to oval in shape, pink to deep red, and without pruritus (Papadakis et al., 2021).

Gastrointestinal

Gastrointestinal (GI) symptoms include nausea, diarrhea, anorexia, and weight loss.

Neurologic

Headache is common and described as retro-orbital pain worsening with eye movements.

Acquired Immunodeficiency Syndrome Symptoms

Patients with AIDS have symptoms of opportunistic infections and unusual malignancy, as outlined in Box 18.2.

HISTORY AND PHYSICAL FINDINGS

A complete history and physical for suspected HIV infection and follow-up for HIV-confirmed patients are necessary to establish infection and monitor for development of AIDS. Also, the history and physical is used to determine comorbid conditions affecting prognosis and ART therapy choices.

Chief Complaint and History of Present Illness

Initially, chief complaints are vague and may have a broad differential. The presenting symptoms as described previously make chief complaints ambiguous. Patients with high-risk behaviors and/or accidental exposure need to have a thorough history of present illness, including risk-taking behaviors. For unintentional exposures, the timing and type of exposure are essential to the history of present illness (HPI). Additionally, for opportunistic infections and knowledge of the most recent CD4 and HIV viral load counts are included in the HPI (CDC, 2016b).

Past Medical and Surgical History

Past medical and surgical history are focused on evaluation of comorbid condition such as viral hepatitis, cardiovascular risk, disease, tuberculosis, sexually transmitted infections, gynecological history and pregnancy, malignancy, psychiatric history, chronic renal failure, peripheral neuropathy, and metabolic bone disease, essential for all patients (Bernard et al., 2006). The thorough medical and surgical history are to aid the ART pharmacologic considerations.

Social History

Social history features should include risk factors for HIV transmission and additional exposures that increase the risk of developing opportunistic infections. Travel and employment are essential to assess opportunistic infection exposure and to assess the patient's insurance status. Social history should include history of substance use, including current substance use behavior. Substance use can lead to HIV transmission by sharing needles and increase the risk of exposure to bloodborne pathogens. Sexual history is focused on past and present sexual habits and practices, including condom and contraceptive use. Family history should review cardiovascular health, cancer history, diabetes, and hyperlipidemia.

Review of Symptoms

A comprehensive review of symptoms should elicit pertinent positives such as fever, night sweats, weight loss, and localized pain. In severely immunocompromised patients, assess for floaters or changes in vision, thrush, dysphagia cough, shortness of breath, diarrhea, skin rash, headache, inability to concentrate, muscle weakness, and paresthesia (CDC, 2016b).

Physical Exam

While a comprehensive physical exam is essential for the initial evaluation, the following specific body systems are necessary to assess for the common findings for HIV patients. They are critical to the setting of advanced immunosuppression. Skin examination includes evaluation for seborrheic dermatitis, eosinophilic folliculitis, psoriasis, superficial fungal disease, molluscum contagiosum, herpes simplex, herpes zoster, and Kaposi's sarcoma. Also, evaluation of body morphology for malar fat atrophy and thinning of extremities or buttocks. Conversely, inspection for prominent cervicodorsal fat deposition is an important exam finding.

Head, Eyes, Ears, Nose, and Throat

Patients with advanced immunosuppression are at risk for cytomegalovirus retinitis and should be referred to ophthalmology as needed. The oral mucosal should be examined for evidence of candidiasis, oral hairy leukoplakia, aphthous ulcerations, herpesimplex virus pustules, oral Kaposi's, and periodontal disease. The anogenital examination focuses on evaluation for STI and *Candida* infections. Finally, conduct a focused neurologic examination for peripheral neuropathy, muscle weakness, cognitive function, and neurologic infections.

DIFFERENTIAL DIAGNOSIS AND DIAGNOSTIC CONSIDERATIONS

Patients presenting with HIV/AIDS have similar signs and symptoms to other diseases. The differential diagnoses for patients presenting with constitutional symptoms of fatigue, weight loss, and fever are noted in Box 18.3 (Ghosn et al., 2018).

BOX 18.3 DIFFERENTIAL DIAGNOSES FOR HUMAN IMMUNODEFICIENCY VIRUS/ ACQUIRED IMMUNODEFICIENCY SYNDROME

- Cancer
- Chronic infections
- Cytomegalovirus
- Disseminated gonococcal infection
- Endocarditis
- Endocrine disorders
- Epstein-Barr virus
- Mononucleosis
- Rubella
- Syphilis
- Toxoplasmosis
- Tuberculosis
- Viral illness other than HIV
- Viral hepatitis
- Other viral infections

Patients presenting with pulmonary symptoms need to have chronic lung infections, interstitial lung diseases, and other pulmonary inflammatory diseases evaluated as a part of the workup. Also, differentials within the neurologic system associated with altered mental status or neuropathy must include alcoholism, liver dysfunction, kidney dysfunction, thyroid disease, and vitamin deficiencies in the workup. If there is headache associated with neurologic symptoms, meningitis must be included. If the patient presents with diarrhea as the primary complaint, GI etiologies are included like colitis, inflammatory bowel disease, and malabsorptive syndrome must be considered.

Laboratory and Diagnostic Testing

For patients suspected to have HIV/AIDS HIV antibody testing; CD4 T lymphocyte cell count; plasma HIV RNA viral load; complete blood count; comprehensive metabolic panel; hepatitis serology for A, B, and C;, fasting glucose; and fasting lipids. Patients may need further genotypic resistance testing for low viral loads and screening for sexually transmitted infections.

Standard labs for HIV testing are HIV-1/2 antigen/antibody immunoassay which detects antibodies for HIV-1 and HIV-2 along with HIV-1 p24 antigen. HIV-1/HIV-2 antibody differentiation confirms the diagnosis between HIV-1 and HIV-2. HIV viral loads measure the amount of actively replicating HIV. Patients with negative HIV-1/HIV-2 antigen/antibody testing but who have a positive viral load are most likely to have an active infection in progress. HIV viral loads are useful for detecting acute infection and the response to ART. Absolute CD4 lymphocyte counts are the best for determining the stage of HIV infection. CD4 lymphocyte percentage (normal 25% to 65%) is more reliable than CD4 count (normal 500 to 1500 cells/mm^3) and is useful in assessing the risk of developing opportunistic infection and or malignancy (Battistini Garcia & Guzman, 2021).

TREATMENT

Treatment of HIV infections is categorized into three types: (a) prevention, (b) opportunistic infection management, and (c) treatment of HIV infection.

Prevention of Transmission

Preventive strategies include correct and consistent use of condoms, oral pre-exposure prophylaxis, and post exposure prophylaxis (Baggaley et al., 2015). Studies have shown that using effective ART to consistently suppress the HIV RNA plasma levels to less than 200 viral copies/mL prevents the transmission of HIV to sexual partners (CDC, 2016b). Patients using treatment as prevention are educated on the need to maintain adherence with ART therapy. Interruptions or lack of adherence to the ART regimen can pose a risk to the patient's sexual partner(s).

Harm Reduction

In addition to prevention, the World Health Organization (WHO) recommends access to sterile injection equipment for IV drug user via needle and syringe programs. Opioid-addicted people should be offered access to opioid substitution therapy, and people that are likely to encounter opioid overdose situations should have access to naloxone. Patients with alcohol or other substance abuse problems should have access to evidence-based interventions.

Prevention of Complications

The decision to initiate prophylaxis is based on the CD4 T count, HIV RNA viral load, and history of opportunistic infections. Data suggest that patients with increased CD4 T counts and low viral loads can have prophylactic regimes discontinued. There are three primary opportunistic infections discussed here: (a) *Pneumocystis jirovecii* pneumonia (PJP), (b) *Mycobacterium avium complex*, and (c) *Toxoplasma gondii* (toxoplasmosis). Pneumocystis pneumonia prophylaxis is offered to patients with CD4 T counts less than 200 copies/mL, a CD4 T lymphocyte percentage less than 14%, weight loss, or oral candidiasis (Papadakis et al., 2021). Table 18.7 outlines the treatment options for prophylaxis for PJP, *M. avium*, and toxoplasmosis. Patients with a history of PJP should receive secondary prophylaxis until viral loads are undetectable and a CD4 T count is maintained at greater than 200 cells/mcL. Prophylaxis against *M. avium* should be initiated when the patient's CD4 T count is less than 75 to 100 cells/mcL. Treatment options are clarithromycin and azithromycin. Studies have demonstrated a 75% reduction in *M. avium* cases with treatment (Papadakis

TABLE 18.7: Prophylaxis Medication Regimes

ORDER RANK	MEDICATION	DOSE	SIDE EFFECTS	LIMITATIONS
— *PNEUMOCYSTIS JIROVECII*				
1	Trimethoprim-sulfamethoxazole	One double-strength tablet three times a week to one tablet daily	Rash, neutropenia, hepatitis, Stevens-Johnson syndrome, hyperkalemia	Hypersensitivity is common
2	Dapsone	50–100 mg orally daily *Or* 100 mg 2 or 3 times per week	Anemia, nausea, methemoglobinemia, hemolytic anemia	Less effective than trimethoprim-sulfamethoxazole, check G6PD level before initiation, check methemoglobinemia level 1 month after treatment
3	Atovaquone	1500 mg orally daily with a meal	Rash, diarrhea, nausea	Less effective than trimethoprim-sulfamethoxazole, equipotent to dapsone, more expensive
4	Aerosolized pentamidine	300 mg monthly	Bronchospasm (Pretreat with bronchodilator)	Apical *P. jirovecii*, pneumothorax, extrapulmonary *P. jirovecii* infections
— *MYCOBACTERIUM AVIUM COMPLEX*				
1	Azithromycin	1,200 mg orally weekly		Preferred due to increased compliance and low cost
2	Clarithromycin	500 mg orally twice daily		
— *TOXOPLASMOSIS*				
	Trimethoprim-sulfamethoxazole	One double-strength tablet daily	Rash, neutropenia, hepatitis, Stevens-Johnson syndrome, hyperkalemia	Hypersensitivity is common
	Pyrimethamine, dapson and leucovorin combination therapy	Pyrimethamine 25 mg orally once a week PLUS dapsone 50 mg orally daily PLUS leucovorin 25 mg orally once a week	Anemia, nausea, methemoglobinemia, hemolytic anemia	A glucose-6-phosphate dehydrogenase (G6PD) level should be checked prior to dapsone therapy, and a methemoglobin level should be checked at 1 month. Prophylaxis can be discontinued when the CD4 cells have increased to greater than 200 cells/mcL for more than 3 months

DS, double strength; mg, milligrams

Source: Adapted from Papadakis, M. A., McPhee, S. J., & Rabow, M. W. (2021). *Current medical diagnosis & treatment 2021*. McGraw-Hill Education LLC.

et al., 2021). Prophylaxis should be continued until CD4 counts rise above 100 cells/mcL in response to ART therapy for a minimum of 3 months. Finally, toxoplasmosis prophylaxis is considered when there is a positive IgG toxoplasma serology and CD4 counts fall below 100 cells/mcL. The therapy outlined in Table 18.7 should be continued until the CD4 counts are greater than 200 cells/mcL for 3 months or more.

Antiretroviral Therapy

ART has improved the morbidity and mortality associated with HIV infection. The current options for ART include six categories and 25 medications. Most current regimens consist of dual or triple therapies. Initiation of therapy should follow the following principles. First, when starting ART, a primary goal is to have complete suppression of viral replication as measured by the HIV viral load due to antiretroviral medication resistance. Second, ART that achieves undetectable viral load is considered durable therapy. Finally, partial suppression should be avoided, and if toxicity develops, change the offending medication instead of dose reduction.

The rapid detection and initiation of ART have a profound impact on the risk reduction for patients. Initiation of therapy should be started as soon as possible for all patients. ART can be started immediately upon a positive diagnosis. While waiting on additional testing to assess drug resistance, initiation of one of the following regimens is acceptable: dolutegravir/tenofovir alafenamide or tenofovir disoproxil fumarate/emtricitabine (Mounzer et al., 2019). Additionally, a patient who is started on abacavir should have a negative HLA-B*5701 allele testing before initiation due to increased risk for severe allergic reaction. HIV treatment protocols have been focused on triple therapy from at least two different classes. There are new expectations to triple therapy. The combination of dolutegravir plus lamivudine was found to be noninferior to dolutegravir plus tenofovir disoproxil fumarate and emtricitabine as initial therapy in patients with HIV viral load of fewer than 500,000 copies/mL. Another exception is dolutegravir and rilpivirine. This drug combination is an alternative treatment for patients with successful viral suppression for at least 6 months, no history of treatment failure, and are not resistant to either medication. ART medications are broken into five major categories: nucleoside and nucleotide reverse transcriptase inhibitors (NRTIs), nonnucleoside reverse transcriptase inhibitors (NNRTIs), protease inhibitors (PIs), early inhibitors including fusion inhibitors and chemokine coreceptors 5 (CCR5), and integrase inhibitors. Table 18.8 outlines the class with the selected agents.

TABLE 18.8: Classification of Antiretroviral With Select Agents for Each Class

CLASS: NUCLEOSIDE REVERSE TRANSCRIPTASE INHIBITORS (NRTIs)			
MEDICATION (ABBREVIATION)	**DOSE**	**COMMON SIDE EFFECTS**	**SPECIAL MONITORING/ CONSIDERATIONS**
Abacavir (ABC)	300 mg orally twice daily	Rash fever	None
Emtricitabine (FTC)	400 mg orally daily (>60 kg) 250 mg orally daily for (30-59 kg)	Mild discoloration of the palms and soles of feet	None
Lamivudine (3TC)	150 mg orally twice daily or 300 mg daily	Rash, peripheral neuropathy	None
Zidovudine (AZT)	600 mg orally daily in two divided doses	Anemia, neutropenia, nausea, malaise, headache, insomnia, and myopathy	Complete blood count including differential 4–8 weeks after starting therapy
CLASS: NUCLEOTIDE REVERSE TRANSCRIPTASE INHIBITORS (NRTIs)			
Tenofovir alafenamide (TAF)/emtricitabine	25 mg of TAF with 200 mg of emtricitabine once daily	Nephrotoxicity, hepatoxicity, bone resorption, if hepatitis B (HBV) positive ;HBV exacerbation after discontinuing	Urine studies at baseline, including serum creatinine, urinalysis, liver enzymes, HBV antigen, bone density. Repeat studies between 2 and 8 weeks and then every 3–6 or as needed.
Tenofovir (TDF)	300 mg orally daily	Kidney dysfunction, bone resorption, gastrointestinal distress	Urine studies at baseline, including serum creatinine, urinalysis, liver enzymes, HBV antigen, bone density. Repeat studies between 2 and 8 weeks and then every 3–6 or as needed

(continued)

TABLE 18.8: Classification of Antiretroviral With Selected Agents for Each Class *(continued)*

CLASS: NUCLEOSIDE REVERSE TRANSCRIPTASE INHIBITORS (NRTIs)			
MEDICATION (ABBREVIATION)	**DOSE**	**COMMON SIDE EFFECTS**	**SPECIAL MONITORING/ CONSIDERATIONS**
CLASS: NON-NUCLEOSIDE REVERSE TRANSCRIPTASE INHIBITORS (NNRTIs)			
Delavirdine	400 mg orally three times per day	Rash	None
Doravirine	100 mg orally daily	Headache, fatigue, abdominal pain	None
Efavirenz	600 mg orally daily	Neurologic disturbances, rash, hepatitis	None
Etravirine	200 mg orally daily	Rash, peripheral neuropathy	None
Rilpivirine	35 mg orally daily	Depression, rash	None
CLASS: PROTEASE INHIBITORS (PIs)			
Atazanavir	400 mg orally daily *Or* 300 mg atazanavir with 100 mg ritonavir orally daily	Hyperbilirubinemia	Bilirubin level monitoring every 3–4 months
Atazanavir/cobicistat	300 mg atazanavir with 150 mg cobicistat orally daily	Hyperbilirubinemia	Bilirubin level monitoring every 3–4 months
Darunavir/cobicistat	800 mg darunavir and 150 mg cobicistat orally daily	Rash	None
Darunavir/ritonavir	**Experienced treatment patients:** 600 mg darunavir and 100 mg ritonavir orally twice daily	Rash	None
	Naïve Patients: 800 mg darunavir and 100 mg ritonavir orally daily		
Ritonavir	600 mg orally twice daily or in lower dosing if used for boosting other PIs	Gastrointestinal distress, peripheral paresthesia	None
CLASS: FUSION INHIBITOR			
Enfuvirtide	90 mg subcutaneously twice daily	Injection site pain, allergic reaction	None
CLASS: CCR5 INHIBITOR			
Maraviroc	150 mg orally twice daily or 300 mg orally twice daily	Cough, rash, fever	None
CLASS: INTEGRASE STRAND TRANSFER INHIBITORS (INSTIs)			
Bictegravir	50 mg orally daily. Used on combination medications only	Diarrhea, nausea, and headache	None
Dolutegravir	**Treatment- naïve patients:** 50 mg orally daily **Integrase-experienced patients:** suspected to have resistance 50 mg orally twice daily	Hypersensitivity, insomnia, fatigue, headache, rash	No special monitoring If given in combination with efavirenz, fosamprenavir/ritonavir, tipranaavir/ ritonavir, or rifampin give 50 mg orally twice daily
Raltegravir	400 mg orally twice daily	Diarrhea, nausea, headache	None

Source: Adapted from: Papadakis, M. A., McPhee, S. J., & Rabow, M. W. (2021). *Current medical diagnosis & treatment 2021.* McGraw-Hill Education LLC.

SPECIAL CONSIDERATIONS

Most PIs and integrase inhibitors are administered with other agents to increase plasma levels. This boosting allows for improved potency, lower dosing, and less frequent dosing of ART therapy. For hemodialysis patients dosing on dialysis days there should be at least one daily ART given after dialysis. Additionally, there are many forms of fixed dosing formulation of ART medications. Table 18.9 outlines a selected list of fixed-dose combinations.

CLINICAL PEARLS

- Modes of transmissionare sexual contact, parenteral exposure, perinatal exposure.
- Presenting complaints are fever, night sweats, weight loss, and sore throat.

- Initial and ongoing evaluation of CD4 count and HIV viral loads to assess and manage ART.
- Patient education on initiation and maintenance therapy, including notification of partners with exposure risk.

KEY TAKEAWAYS

- Early detection and treatment are critical to viral suppression and limiting transmission.
- Medication adherence is an essential part of HIV/AIDS treatment.
- Patient education on medication side effects and the need to report these symptoms to a clinician are essential to care.

TABLE 18.9: Fixed Antiretroviral Therapy Dose Medications

MEDICATION	DOSING AND SPECIAL CONSIDERATIONS
TDF 300 mg, emtricitabine 200 mg, efavirnez 600 mg	One pill daily is a complete ART regimen
Emtricitabine 200 mg, TAF 25 mg, bictegravir 50 mg	One pill daily is a complete ART regimen. Recommended initial treatment regimen
TDF 300 mg, emtricitabine 200 mg, rilpivirine 25 mg	One pill daily is a complete ART regimen. Only for patients with HIV viral load <100,000 copies/mL
TDF 300 mg, lamivudine 300 mg, doravirine 100 mg	One pill daily is a complete ART regimen
TAF 25 mg, emtricitabine 200 mg	One pill daily with NNRTI, PI, integrase inhibitor, or CCR5. ess effect on the kidney and bone. They are approved for single-agent in males for pre-exposure prophylaxis, not studied in females.
Dolutegravir 50 mg, lamivudine 300 mg	One pill daily is a complete ART regimen in treatment naïve patients or resistance
Abacavir 600 mg, lamivudine 300 mg	One pill along with NNRTI, PI, Integrase inhibitor, or CCR5
TAF 10 mg, emtricitabine 200 mg, elvitegravir 150 mg, cobicistat 150 mg	One pill daily is a complete ART regimen
Dolutegravir 50 mg, rilpivirine 25 mg	One pill daily with food for patients virally suppressed with viral load <50 copies/mL
TAF 25 mg, emtricitabine 200 mg, rilpivirine 25 mg	One pill daily. Only for patients with a history of viral loads ≤ 100,00 copies/mL. Or for replacement for patients stable on treatment for 6 months with no resistance
TDF 300 mg, emtricitabine 200 mg, elvitegravir 150 mg, cobicistat 150 mg	One pill daily is a complete ART regimen
TAF 10 mg, emtricitabine 200 mg, darunavir 800 mg, cobicistat 150 mg	One pill daily is a complete ART regimen. Recommended initial treatment regimes
Abacavir 600 mg, lamivudine 300 mg, dolutegravir 50 mg	One pill daily is a complete ART regimen. Recommended initial treatment regimens
Abacavir 300 mg, lamivudine 150 mg, zidovudine 300 mg	One pill twice daily with NNRTI, PI, integrase inhibitor, CCR5. While there are three medications, this formulation does not constitute a full treatment
TDF 300 mg, emtricitabine 200 mg	One pill daily with NNRTI, PI, integrase inhibitor, or CCR5. Approved as single pre-exposure prophylaxis.

ART, antiretroviral therapy; NNRTI, nonnucleoside reverse transcriptase inhibitor; PI, protease inhibitor.

Source: Adapted from Papadakis, M. A., McPhee, S. J., & Rabow, M. W. (2021). *Current medical diagnosis & treatment 2021*. McGraw-Hill Education LLC.

EVIDENCE-BASED RESOURCES

Division of HIV/AIDS Prevention: https://www.cdc.gov/hiv/default.html

National Center for HIV/AIDS, Viral Hepatitis, STD, and TB Prevention: https://www.cdc.gov/nchhstp/default.htm?CDC_AA_refVal=https%3A%2F%2Fwww.cdc.gov%2Fnchhstp%2Findex.html

Centers for Disease Control and Prevention: https://www.cdc.gov/

Clinical Info HIV: https://clinicalinfo.hiv.gov/en/guidelines

18.6: MYCOBACTERIUM TUBERCULOSIS

Tuberculosis (TB) is one of the world's most widespread illnesses and infects approximately one third of the world's population (Chesnutt et al., 2021). The majority of TB cases (95%) are estimated to occur in developing countries, and include regions of Southeast Asia, Africa, and the Western Pacific. Smaller numbers of cases have been reported in the Eastern Mediterranean, Americas, and Europe (World Health Organization [WHO], 2021). The United States has one of the lowest TB case reports in the world, and has primarily experienced a decline in cases since 1993 (Raviglione, 2018). The majority of TB cases in the United States are reported among individuals born outside of this country, adults infected with HIV, and disadvantaged populations (Raviglione, 2018; WHO, 2021). Mexico (22%) and the Philippines (12%) are two countries of origin that account for the incidence of TB among individuals currently residing in the United States (Doucette & Cooper, 2015). While the occurrence of TB is widespread across all states, over half of the confirmed cases come from California, Texas, New York, and Florida (Chesnutt et al., 2021). The TB burden among individuals born in the United States reflect both incarcerated and indigenous populations (Doucette & Cooper, 2015).

TB is caused by inhalation of *Mycobacterium tuberculosis* bacterium (MTB). *M. tuberculosis* is an obligate aerobic, nonmotile, nonspore-forming intracellular bacteria that is transmitted via airborne contained within droplet nuclei (Doucette & Cooper, 2015; Levinson et al., 2022). *M. tuberculosis* is also classified as *acid fast bacilli.* This organism has a high content of mycolic acid and this prevents the decolorization of the bacillus once it is stained (Bayot et al. 2021; Raviglione, 2018). *M. tuberculosis* is resistant to many classes of common antimicrobials and has the ability to survive in many extreme conditions (Levinson et al., 2022).

Inhalation of *M. tuberculosis* can cause a spectrum of responses depending on the immune state of the person that is infected. Refer to Table 18.10 to differentiate among the stages of TB and the pathophysiologic response. In the majority of cases, in immunocompetent persons the inhalation of *M. tuberculosis* causes an inflammatory response that recruits macrophages and T cells to "wall off" the infection by forming a granuloma. Presenting signs and symptoms will depend on stage of tuberculosis (Table 18.10). Typical signs and symptoms include fatigue, weight loss, fever, night sweats, and productive cough (Raviglione, 2018).

HISTORY AND PHYSICAL FINDINGS

Note these symptoms are likely to occur with primary progress or active tuberculosis.

Subjective

Pertinent Positives

- History of latent TB
- History of recent global travel to areas of significant epidemiologic risk
- History of recent domestic travel to states with high significance of TB (see overview)
- Exposure to person recently diagnosed with TB
- Slow progressive constitutional symptoms: malaise, anorexia, weight loss, fever, and night sweats
- Chronic cough—typically dry but may become productive if disease progresses
- Blood-streaked sputum; frank hemoptysis is unlikely
- Dyspnea is unusual unless there is extensive disease
- Immunocompromised either from illness or pharmacology:
  - HIV
  - Cancer
  - Corticosteroids
  - Tumor necrosis inhibitors
  - Monoclonal antibodies
  - Diabetes
  - Gastrectomy
  - Chronic kidney disease requiring dialysis

Pertinent Negatives

- Acute onset of symptoms
- High fever
- Productive cough copious expectorant, frank hemoptysis
- Absence of weight changes
- Absence of night sweats
- Dyspnea on exertion
- Paroxysmal nocturnal dyspnea
- No recent travel or exposures
- Exposure to animals

Objective

Pertinent Positives

- Chronically ill
- Cough
- Malnourished
- Adventitious breath sounds (crackles and rhonchi); depending upon severity of illness

TABLE 18.10: Differentiating Tuberculosis Stages of Infections, Symptoms, and Treatment

STAGE	PATHOPHYSIOLOGY	SYMPTOMS/TREATMENT
Primary	• *M. tuberculosis* is inhaled via droplet nuclei, bypasses respiratory defense mechanism and deposits within the alveoli • Inflammatory response occurs, bacilli are ingested by the alveolar macrophages; T cells are also recruited • In an immunocompetent person the bacilli are engulfed by macrophages and T cells that form a granuloma; this limits multiplication and spread • It is possible that infected macrophages may migrate to regional lymph nodes and access the bloodstream causing spread to other areas of the body (apical-posterior aspect of the lung, epiphyses of the long bones, vertebrae, kidneys, and meninges) • The infection at this point is contained but not eradicated; the tubercle bacillus may remain dormant for years OR • Patient may go on to develop progressive primary TB	Asymptomatic/infectious Treatment will be determined by course of disease (either latent or progressive primary)
Progressive Primary	• Immune system unable to contain primary infection • Symptomatic/infectious • Fatigue, fever, weight loss, night sweats, productive cough	6- to 9-month treatment (6 month preferred) 2 months INH, rifampin, PZA, ETHM (see Table 18.11); if isolate is sensitive to INH and rifampin, discontinue PZA and ETHM after 2 months and continue with INH and rifampin for 4 months
Latent	• Occurs postprimary infection in 95% of cases • Immune system is able to suppress bacillary replication • Foci of the bacilli resolve into epithelial cell granulomas which may have caseous and necrotic centers • Reactivation of disease may occur if immune system is suppressed • Asymptomatic/noninfectious	**Treatment reduces risk that infection will progress to active disease:** INH, rifampin, rifapentin can be used as either monotherapy or dual therapy; 3-month therapy for dual, 4- to 9-month therapy for monotherapy
Active	• Develops in approximately 6% of persons with latent tuberculosis infection who are not given treatment • Preventive treatment with 50% occurrence within a 2-year time period • Risk factors to develop active tuberculosis include gastrectomy, diabetes mellitus and those with diminished immune response (e.g., HIV, treatment with immunosuppressive medications – corticosteroids, tumor necrosis factor inhibitors) • Symptomatic/infectious–fatigue, fever, weight loss, night sweats, productive cough	Same as progressive primary

ETHM, ethambutol; INH, isoniazid; PZA, pyrazinamide.

Source: Data from Chesnutt, A. N., Chesnutt, M. S., Prendergast, N. T., & Prendergast, T. J. (2021). Pulmonary tuberculosis. In M. A. Papadakis, S. J. McPhee, & M. W. Rabow (Eds.), *Current medical diagnosis & treatment 2021.* McGraw-Hill. https://accessmedicine-mhmedical-com.sladenlibrary.hfhs.org/content.aspx?bookid=2957&sectionid=249369915; Nahid, P., Dorman, S. E., Alipanah, N., Barry, P. M., Brozek, J. L., Cattamanchi, A., Chaisson, L. H., Chaisson, R. E., Daley, C. L., Grzemska, M., Higashi, J. M., Ho, C. S., Hopewell, P. C., Keshavjee, S. A., Lienhardt, C., Menzies, R., Merrifield, C., Narita, M., O'Brien, R., … Vernon, A. (2016). Official American Thoracic Society/Centers for Disease Control and Prevention/Infectious Diseases Society of America Clinical Practice Guidelines: Treatment of drug-susceptible tuberculosis. *Clinical Infectious Diseases, 63*(7), e147–e195. https://doi.org/10.1093/cid/ciw376

Pertinent Negatives

- Hypoxia
- Tachypneic
- Lungs clear to auscultation
- Oral thrush

DIFFERENTIAL DIAGNOSIS AND DIAGNOSTIC CONSIDERATIONS

- Lung cancer
- Hodgkin's lymphoma
- Sarcoidoisis
- Mycoplasma pneumonia
- Community-acquired bacterial pneumonia
- Fungal pathogens
- Brucellosis

Definitive diagnosis depends on isolation of *M. tuberculosis* from cultures or identification of the organism by DNA or RNA amplification technique (Nahid et al., 2016).

- **Sputum (Acid-Fast Smear):** Three consecutive morning sputum specimens; if patient is unable to produce adequate sputum expectorant, sputum induction with 3% saline should be ordered. Early morning sampling increases sensitivity by 12%. Bronchoscopy could also be ordered to obtain bronchial washing for sputum sample if the above two methods are not sufficient (Lewinsohn et al., 2017).
- **Sputum (Genetic and Nucleic Acid Amplification Test [NAAT]):** Especially valuable for those who are immunocompromised as there is a higher incidence of false negative. This method enables identification

of bacteria or bacterial particles by making use of DNA-based molecular techniques. A positive NAAT is considered adequate for diagnosis of *M. tuberculosis* irrespective of AFB results. These tests can also identify resistance markers (Doucette & Cooper, 2015; Lewinsohn et al., 2017; Nahid et al., 2016).

- **Tuberculin Skin Test (Mantoux):** Asymptomatic latent and active TB. Positive reaction is based upon millimeters of induration and the criteria for test positivity varies among different groups:
  - **≥5 mm:** HIV positive, recent contacts of a person with infectious TB disease, persons with radiographic changes suggestive of TB, immunocompromised patients (organ transplants)
  - **≥10 mm:** Recent immigrants with high prevalence of TB, HIV negative injection drug users, residents and employees in high-risk congregate settings (correctional facilities, hospitals, homeless shelters, long-term care facilities)
  - **≥15 mm:** Persons with no known risk factors for TB (Doucette & Cooper, 2015; Nahid et al., 2016).
- **Interferon Gamma Release Assay (IGRA; QuantiFERON/T-SPOT):** Useful in persons who have been vaccinated for TB (fewer false positives) and to achieve better discrimination of positive responses secondary to non-TB *mycobacterium*. Sensitivity is decreased in HIV patients with low CD4 counts. The CDC recommends that these tests can be used interchangeably with tuberculin skin tests (CDC, 2016a; Doucette & Cooper, 2015; Lewinsohn et al., 2017; Raviglione, 2018).
- **CXR:** Routine CXR imaging is typically done to evaluate etiology of presenting symptoms or to assess for inflammatory response secondary to known exposure. CXR findings in primary disease do not differentiate TB as the imaging pattern but may identify small unilateral infiltrates, hilar and paratracheal lymph node enlargement, atelectasis, and pleural effusions. In reactivated disease, apical cavitary lesions are typically seen in addition to discrete nodules and pneumonic infiltrates. Healed TB lesions appear as a fibrotic scar with shrinkage of lung parenchyma and calcification. Persons with HIV will often present with normal radiographic findings (Doucette & Cooper, 2015; Raviglione, 2018).

TREATMENT

The focus of treatment is on curing the individual patient and decreasing the spread of *M. tuberculosis* to the community at large. This is achieved through a multidrug regimen that rapidly kills multiplying bacteria, attains a relapse-free cure, and protects against the development of drug resistance. See Table 18.11 for pharmacology used in the treatment of *M. tuberculosis* and regimen options. Treatment is based on the type of TB a person has (primary, latent, progressive). Drug susceptibility testing

should be completed on isolates and managed through consultation with infectious disease and/or pulmonary experts. Additional factors that may impact the overall treatment regimen include patient factors (age, comorbidities, immune and nutrition status, history of alcohol abuse), diagnostic findings (microbiologic, genetic, and radiographic features), pharmacokinetic factors (drug–drug interactions with other medications), and regimen factors (numbers of medications prescribed, length of treatment, adherence). Patient education and interprofessional collaboration are essential in supporting positive outcomes. It is imperative that patients understand the importance of the intensity of the drug regimen and the personal accountability to manage drug treatment (Nahid et al., 2016).

As with other diseases that are treated with antimicrobials, resistance can occur even with the recommended four medication regimens. Drug-resistant TB is classified as *M. tuberculosis* that is resistant to at least one first-line TB medication (rifampin or isoniazid; CDC, 2021). Individuals who have resistance to one of the first-line medications (rifampin or isoniazid) are typically prescribed a fluoroquinolone with favorable outcomes. Fluoroquinolones are also used in persons who are unable to tolerate first-line TB medications (CDC, 2021; Doucette & Cooper, 2015). Multidrug-resistant TB (MDR-TB) is defined as resistance to more than one anti-TB medication that includes isoniazid and/or rifampin. "Extensively drug-resistant TB" is also defined by the CDC as resistance to isoniazid and rifampin, in addition to a fluoroquinolone and three of the injectable second-line medications (CDC, 2021). There are several medication regimens that can be used in the treatment of MDR-TB or extensively drug-resistant TB. It is recommended that an expert in tuberculosis management be consulted for persons with drug-resistant bacilli. There are a few treatment options that are now part of clinical practice guidelines specifically targeting drug-resistant organisms. These treatment recommendations include fluoroquinolones (if sensitive) (levofloxacin or moxifloxacin), bedaquiline and linezolid (Doucette & Cooper, 2015; Mase & Chorba, 2019; Nahid et al., 2019).

TRANSITIONS OF CARE

Patients who are diagnosed and started on treatment in the acute care setting will be discharged once a plan is put in place. As with all discharge plans, the focus for patients with TB should be on patient-centered care. This means that the patient should be involved in making decisions related to pharmacologic management and overall plan of care. Case management is key to this transition and should include the following: understanding patient literacy and improving treatment literacy, discuss outcomes of treatments, assess, and evaluate the extent of supervision required for good outcomes, discuss infectiousness and infection control measures, and determine support systems in place. Because pharmacology is key

TABLE 18.11: Pharmacology Used in the Treatment of Tuberculosis

DRUG	STAGE USED/LENGTH OF TREATMENT	SIDE EFFECTS	CONSIDERATIONS
Isoniazid (INH) Bactericidal	Latent Active post latent (6–9 months) Progressive primary (6–9 months)	Peripheral neuropathy Hepatitis Rash Mild CNS	AST/ALT **Pyridoxine 25–50 mg PO daily prophylaxis for neuropathy** Potent inhibitor of CYP isoenzymes; can cause increase in concentrations of medications
Rifampin Bactericidal	Latent Active post latent (6–9 months) Progressive primary (6–9 months)	Hepatitis Rash Flulike symptoms Discoloration of body fluids (urine, tears) Renal failure GI upset Bleeding	AST/ALT BUN/creatinine/GFR CBC with platelets Inhibits effect of several medications (oral contraceptives, warfarin, corticosteroids, digoxin, methadone, oral hypoglycemics) Significant interactions with drugs used to treat HIV: protease inhibitors and nonnucleoside reverse transcriptase inhibitors (NNRTI)
Rifapentine Bactericidal	Latent	Bone marrow suppression Hepatitis GI upset Flulike symptoms Hematuria/pyuria Discoloration of body fluids	CBC, AST/ALT Strong cytochrome P450 inducer with multiple drug interactions
Ethambutol Bacteriostatic; mainly used to inhibit development of resistant mutants	Active post latent (first 2 months) Progressive primary (first 2 months) **If resistance to INH, then given for 9 months**	Optic neuritis; reversible with discontinuation of drug	Rare drug interactions
Pyrazinamide Bactericidal	Active post latent (first 2 months) Progressive primary (first 2 months)	Hyperuricemia, Hepatoxocity Rash GI upset Joint aches	Uric acid AST/ALT Rare drug interactions
Streptomycin Bactericidal		Eighth nerve damage Nephrotoxicity	BUN/Creatinine

ALT, alanine transaminase; AST, aspartate aminotransferase; BUN, blood-urea-nitrogen; CBC, complete blood count; CYP, cytochrome P450; GFR, glomerular filtration rate; NNRTI, nonnucleoside reverse transcriptase inhibitors.

Source: Data from Burchum, J. R. (Ed.). (2018). Antimycobacterial agents. In L. D. Rosenthal & J. R. Burcham (Eds.), *Lehne's pharmacotherapeutics for advanced practice providers* (pp. 833–847). Elsevier; Nahid, P., Dorman, S. E., Alipanah, N., Barry, P. M., Brozek, J. L., Cattamanchi, A., Chaisson, L. H., Chaisson, R. E., Daley, C. L., Grzemska, M., Higashi, J. M., Ho, C. S., Hopewell, P. C., Keshavjee, S. A., Lienhardt, C., Menzies, R., Merrifield, C., Narita, M., O'Brien, R., ... Vernon, A. (2016). Official American Thoracic Society/Centers for Disease Control and Prevention/Infectious Diseases Society of America Clinical Practice Guidelines: Treatment of drug-susceptible tuberculosis. *Clinical Infectious Diseases, 63*(7), e147–e195. https://doi.org/10.1093/cid/ciw376; .

to cure, prevention of spread, and decreased resistance, adherence to treatment regimens must be included in all transition-of-care decisions. If there is concern regarding adherence to treatment, one management approach includes the use of direct observed therapy (DOT). The use of DOT has been widely used and is supported in the literature as fostering good outcomes. This practice can be easily adopted in today's electronic environment with the use of web-based modalities. It is also imperative that patients maintain follow up appointments to review drug therapy and monitor for adverse effects (see Table 18.11 for adverse effects and diagnostic studies; Nahid et al., 2016).

CLINICAL PEARLS

- The majority of TB cases in the United States are reported among individuals born outside the United States.
- Symptoms are associated with the classification of primary, progressive, or recurrent/reactivation TB.
- Diagnosis of TB is confirmed based on identification of *Mycobacterium tuberculosis* via acid fast staining and/or molecular testing.
- Treatment should be patient centered using multi-drug regimen for an extended period.

18.7: INVASIVE CANDIDIASIS

PRESENTING SIGNS AND SYMPTOMS

Fever, myalgia, visual changes, symptoms related to localized candida infection(s)

HISTORY AND PHYSICAL FINDINGS

Candidiasis is a fungal infection caused by yeast species *Candida*. *Candida*, like some bacteria, are normal flora that live on the skin and inside the body (e.g., gut, vagina, mouth). Similar to bacterial pathogens, yeast can also cause illness if there are too many pathogens. Many patients have localized fungal infections secondary to proliferation of yeast that do not cause significant illness; however, these localized infections can contribute to fungal systemic infections. Some localized fungal infections include oral thrush, skin yeast infections, vaginosis, esophagitis, and funguria. In isolation, these infections are easily treated by oral or topical medications, but multiple sites of infection often lead to fungal overgrowth that can cause systemic fungemia or invasive candidiasis (IC; bloodstream infection). It is suggested that there is a link between *Candida* colonization and IC. Additional risk factors for IC include parenteral nutrition, use of broad-spectrum antimicrobials over a prolonged period of time, central venous catheters, immunocompromised host, prolonged stay in hospital (especially ICU), and abdominal surgery. Patients who have gastroduodenal perforation, anastomotic leak, or necrotizing pancreatitis are a known population to be at high risk for IC. Rarely, patients may develop *Candida* meningitis, vertebral osteomyelitis, endocarditis, and hepatosplenic candidiasis (immunocompromised cancer patients post chemotherapy). The focus of this section is on IC as this often occurs in intensive care settings, especially in patients with longer stays, and is associated with increased mortality (35%–75%; Al-Dorzi et al., 2018; León et al., 2014). The primary *Candida* species is *albicans,* but non *albicans species* are also increasing in occurrence. These include *C. glabrata, C. parapsilosis, C. tropicalis,* and *C. krusei. C. auris* is an emerging multidrug resistant *Candida* species that presents a serious global health threat because it can cause outbreaks, is difficult to isolate, and is problematic to treat because it can be resistant to all three classes of antifungals. In addition to *Candida* species, there are additional fungal pathogens that can cause illness. These fungal pathogens include *Histoplasmosis and Coccidioidomycosis* and are typically isolated in immunocompromised individuals (Pappas et al., 2016).

Subjective

May relate to localized fungal colonization and/or infection.

Pertinent Positives

- Fever
- Myalgia
- Visual changes
- White oral patches
- Sore throat/difficulty swallowing
- Heartburn
- Vaginal discharge/itching
- Rash
- Recent long-term exposure to antimicrobial therapy
- Recent prolonged hospital stay
- Immunocompromised/immunosuppressive medications
- Total parenteral nutrition
- History of recent GI surgery for gastroduodenal perforation, anastomotic leak
- History of necrotizing pancreatitis
- Headache

Pertinent Negatives

- Works with soil (histoplasmosis)
- Exposure to bird droppings (histoplasmosis)
- Cough, shortness of breath (histoplasmosis, coccidioidomycoses)
- Hemoptysis (aspergillosis)
- Recent travel, night sweats (tuberculosis [India, China, Pakistan, Philippines], coccidioidomycoses [southwest United States, northern Mexico, Central and South America])
- History of mold exposure (aspergillosis)
- Rash on upper body and legs (coccidioidomycoses)

Objective

May relate to local fungal infection or sequelae from invasive candidemia.

Pertinent Positives

- Fever
- Oral thrush
- Vaginal discharge
- Rash – intertriginous areas; central erythema and maceration; papular/pustular satellite lesions
- Total parenteral nutrition
- Central venous catheters
- Funguria
- Yeast isolated from sputum
- New onset murmur (endocarditis)
- Back pain
- Retinal changes
- Nuchal rigidity

Pertinent Negatives

- Diffuse macular erythematous rash (aspergillosis)
- Hemoptysis (aspergillosis, tuberculosis [blood streaked])
- Tachypnea (aspergillosis, coccidioidomycoses)
- Ronchi, crackles (aspergillosis)
- Lymphadenopathy (esophageal cytomegalovirus)

DIFFERENTIAL DIAGNOSIS AND DIAGNOSTIC CONSIDERATIONS

Differential Diagnoses

- Candidemia
  - Histoplasmosis
  - Coccidiodomycosis
  - Bacterial tuberculosis
  - Aspergillosis
- Esophageal candidiasis
  - Herpes simplex virus
  - Cytomegalovirus
  - Varicella zoster
  - Gastroesophageal reflux disease (GERD)

The diagnosis of IC is difficult as diagnostic tests lack sensitivity (blood cultures <50%). Suspicion for IC centers around the risk factors identified previously and observed physical assessment findings and other diagnostics that support the presence of yeast (oral thrush, skin yeast rash, funguria). A skin biopsy can be used to ascertain the presence of fungal elements, urine culture to assess for *Candida* or other fungal pathogens, and vaginal culture, KOH (potassium hydroxide) smear or wet prep to diagnose vaginal infection. In addition to blood cultures, the (1,3) β-D-glucan assay is utilized as an indirect measure of *Candida* species but has limited sensitivity similar to that of blood cultures. The D-glucan is an antigen assay that is a constituent of the cell wall of many fungi. The T2Candida Panel© (T2 Biosystems), is a magnetic resonance assay that directly detects *Candida* species in whole blood samples in 3 to 5 hours. This test is highly sensitive and has an excellent negative predictive value (Pappas et al., 2016).

Additional testing may be warranted to rule out other pathogens that may cause similar symptoms (see "Differential Diagnoses"). This includes fungal serology (specific IgM and IgG antibody testing) for coccidioidomycoses and aspergillosis, antigen testing for histoplasmosis, skin PPD or QuantiFERON-TB Gold Plus© (Qiagen) for tuberculosis, and/or sputum analysis for all fungal pathogens, and acid-fast staining for tuberculosis. Oral endoscopy may be warranted to evaluate the esophagus for fungal pathogens and obtain a biopsy (Pappas et al., 2016).

TREATMENT

Primary treatment for candidemia or suspected IC is identified in Table 18.12. Indications for specific illnesses are also provided. Duration of treatment for candidemia without complications is 2 weeks after documented clearance of *Candida* species. Blood cultures should be obtained to ascertain clearance of candidemia and establish point of reference for duration of therapy. See Table 18.12 for drug classes and indications for invasive candidemia. It is also recommended that all patients who have had candidemia follow up with an ophthalmologist post treatment as ocular dissemination and endophthalmitis may occur.

Candida species localized from a respiratory secretion is typically a result of colonization and does not require antifungal therapy. In addition, patients with funguria should also not be treated unless the person is neutropenic or will be undergoing urologic manipulation. The treatment for vulvovaginal candidiasis is a topical agent or a single 150 mg dose of fluconazole. For severe cases of vulvovaginitis fluconazole, 150 mg every 72 hours for 3 to 4 doses is prescribed and treatment for 10 to 14 days for recurring infections. Oral pharyngeal candidiasis can be treated with clotrimazole troches (5 times daily), nystatin suspension, or oral fluconazole 100 to 200 mg daily for 7 to 14 days for moderate to severe disease (Nahid et al., 2016).

TABLE 18.12: Primary Treatment for Candidemia or Suspected Invasive Candidiasis

DRUG CLASS	INDICATION	SIDE EFFECTS
AZOLE		
Fluconazole • Fluconazole IV or oral: 12 mg/kg loading dose then 400 mg (6 mg/kg) daily • Broad-spectrum fungicide • For neutropenic patients, fluconazole 400 mg daily can be used for step down therapy during persistent neutropenia in clinically stable patients who have susceptible isolates and documented bloodstream clearance **Voriconazole** • Offers little advantage over fluconazole. Recommended as step down therapy for *C. krusei* fungemia	• Neutropenic/non-neutropenic candidemia; invasive candidiasis in intensive care unit; intraabdominal suspected candidiasis, septic arthritis, and osteomyelitis (duration of treatment will be longer), esophageal candidiasis • Acceptable alternative to echinocandins as initial therapy in selected patients, those not critically ill and unlikely to have fluconazole resistance • Testing for susceptibility is recommended for all bloodstream and clinically relevant infections; unable to use in neutropenic patients with *C. krusei*	• Inhibitor CYP3A4 and CYP2C9 – multiple drug interactions • GI (nausea, vomiting, diarrhea, abdominal pain), headache, skin rash • Hepatotoxicity especially with underlying liver dysfunction

(continued)

TABLE 18.12: Primary Treatment for Candidemia or Suspected Invasive Candidiasis *(continued)*

DRUG CLASS	INDICATION	SIDE EFFECTS
ECHNIOCANDINS		
Caspofungin • Loading dose 70 mg, then 50 mg daily **Micafungin** • 100 mg daily **Anidulafungin** • Loading dose 200 mg then 100 mg daily	• Neutropenic/non-neutropenic candidemia; invasive candidiasis in intensive care unit; intraabdominal suspected candidiasis, septic arthritis, and osteomyelitis (duration will be longer), esophageal candidiasis • Testing for echinocandin susceptibility should be considered in patients who have had prior treatment with echinocandin and those who have infection with *C. glabrata* or *C. parapsilosis* • Transition from echinocandin to fluconazole (within 5–7 days) for patients clinically stable, isolates susceptible to fluconazole and have negative repeat cultures	• Well tolerated • Infusion-related effects include headache, GI distress, fever, rash, and flushing (histamine release)
Amphotericin • 3–5 mg/kg daily • Wide-spectrum fungicide; 2 week half-life, not dialyzable	• Use If there is intolerance to azole or echinocandins, limited availability, or resistance. Native valve endocarditis; pacemaker and implantable defibrillators, central nervous system infections (step down to fluconazole if isolate is susceptible, patient is clinically stable and blood cultures are negative)	• Infusion-related effects include fever, chills, hypotension (slow down rate of infusion or premedicate with antihistamines or glucocorticoids) • Nephrotoxicity with prolonged use, potassium wasting

Source: Data from Pappas, P. G., Kauffman, C. A., Andes, D. R., Clancy, C. J., Marr, K. A., Ostrosky-Zeichner, L., Reboli, A. C., Schuster, M. G., Vazquez, J. A., Walsh, T. J., Zaoutis, T. E., & Sobel, J. D. (2016). Clinical Practice Guideline for the management of candidiasis: 2016 update by the Infectious Diseases Society of America. *Clinical Infectious Diseases, 62*(4), e1–e50. https://doi.org/10.1093/cid/civ933; Rosenthal, L. D. (Ed.). (2018). Antifungal agents. In L. D. Rosenthal & J. R. Burcham (Eds.), *Lehne's pharmacotherapeutics for advanced practice providers* (pp. 855–866). Elsevier

CLINICAL PEARLS

■ Invasive *candidiasis* is a complication that occurs in patients with prolonged hospital stays, have invasive catheters, are receiving parenteral nutrition, are exposed to broad spectrum antimicrobial therapy for an extended period, have a localized *Candida* infection, and/or undergone significant GI surgery.

■ The best serologic test for the diagnosis of candidemia is T2Candida Panel©.

■ Treatment for IC include the use of drugs from one of the following classes; polyenes (amphotericin B, nystatin), echinocandins (e.g., caspofungin, micafungin), azoles (e.g., fluconazole, clotrimazole, miconazole, ketaconazole).

■ A significant complication in patients with candidemia is endophthalmitis; patients should have an ophthalmology consult upon discharge.

18.8: DIABETIC FOOT INFECTIONS

PRESENTING SYMPTOMS

Nonhealing ulcer, erythema, warmth, purulence, swelling, pain.

HISTORY AND PHYSICAL FINDINGS

Foot infections are a common problem in diabetic patients and if not assessed appropriately and treated effectively can lead to several complications including osteomyelitis and/or amputation (Embil & Trepman, 2017). Patients with diabetic foot infections (DFIs) are also at increased risk for necrotizing fasciitis. Many factors predispose the diabetic patient to foot ulceration, and infections are typically the result of decreased sensation secondary to neuropathy and foot deformity. Diabetic ulcers typically occur in areas of increased pressure (soles of feet), friction (due to footwear), or trauma (lack of footwear). Patients often do not recognize the presence of an ulcer because they do not perform daily foot assessments and it is not until systemic signs and symptoms of infection develop that medical care is pursued (Lipsky et al., 2012).

DFIs should be classified using a validated classification system according to severity of symptoms and systemic involvement (Table 18.13). Most DFIs are polymicrobial with *Staphylococcus* being the primary organism. In patients with a mild or moderate infection the staphylococcal pathogen may be methicillin-sensitive (MSSA) and therefore treated accordingly with antibiotics that target this pathogen. Patients who have been

TABLE 18.13: Diabetic Foot Infections Classification of Severity of Infection International Working Group of Diabetic Foot (Perfusion, Extent, Depth, Infection, Sensation [PEDIS]) and Infectious Diseases Society of America (IDSA) and Treatment Recommendations

CLINICAL MANIFESTATION	PEDIS	IDSA	ANTIBIOTIC TREATMENT RECOMMENDATIONS
No signs/symptoms of infection	1	Uninfected	No treatment
• Two or more manifestations of inflammation (purulence, pain, warmth, erythema, tenderness, induration) • Cellulitis/erythema that extends <2 cm around ulcer • Infection is limited to skin or superficial subcutaneous tissue • No other local or systemic illness	2	Mild	Not recently received antibiotic treatment; target gram-positive cocci **Most common:** Cephalexin, amoxicillin-clavulanate **Alternatives:** Clindamycin,* doxycycline,* levofloxacin
Infection as above; person has no systemic illness and is metabolically stable; has one or more of the following: • Cellulitis extending >2 cm • Lymphatic streaking • Spread beneath the superficial fascia • Deep tissue abscess • Gangrene • Involvement of muscle, tendon, joint, or bone	3	Moderate	**Most common:** Amoxicillin-clavulanate, ertapenem, imipenem-cilastatin **Alternatives:** Cefoxitin, ceftriaxone, levofloxacin, moxifloxacin, tigecycline Levofloxacin or ciprofloxacin plus clinidamycin **If concern for MRSA add:** Vancomycin, linezolid, or daptomycin to one of above **If concern for pseudomonas or ESBL:** Imipenem-cilastatin
Infection in person with systemic toxicity or metabolic instability (fever, chills, tachycardia, hypotension, confusion, vomiting, leukocytosis, acidosis, severe hyperglycemia, azotemia)	4	Severe	Same as moderate, will likely require MRSA coverage May also require extended spectrum gram-negative and anerobic coverage (this will provide *pseudomonal* coverage) Piperacillin-tazobactam Imipenem-cilasatitin (useful for pseudomonas and/or ESBL)

*Has MRSA coverage.

ESBL, extended spectrum beta lactamase; MRSA, methicillin-resistant *Staphylococcus aureus*; PEDIS, perfusion, extent, depth, infection, sensation, developed by International Working Group of Diabetic Foot (IWGDF).

Source: Adapted from Lipsky, B. A., Berendt, A. R., Cornia, P. B., Pile, J. C., Peters, E. J. G., Armstrong, D. G., Deery, H. G., Embil, J. M., Joseph, W. S., Karchmer, A. W., Pinzur, M. S., & Senneville, E. (2012). 2012 Infectious Diseases Society of America Clinical Practice Guideline for the diagnosis and treatment of diabetic foot infections. *Clinical Infectious Diseases, 54*(12), e132–e173. https://doi.org/10.1093/cid/cis346.

exposed to antibiotics over time because of chronic recurrent infections will be at risk for staphylococcal pathogens that are resistant to methicillin (MRSA) and therefore may require MRSA coverage. Gram-negative bacilli are often present as copathogens in patients with chronic wound infection who have received antimicrobial therapy in the past. Extended spectrum gram-negative bacilli (*pseudomonas, extended spectrum beta lactamase [ESBL]*) should be a consideration in individuals who have had extensive antimicrobial exposure, have a deep invasive wound infection with malodorous drainage and systemic manifestations, or prior cultures that identify these pathogens. Anaerobes should also be a consideration for deep wound infections (Lipsky et al., 2012).

Subjective

Pertinent Positives

■ Presence of ulcer
■ Erythema, warmth, swelling affected limb
■ Drainage—may or may not be purulent, may be malodorous
■ Pain
■ Confusion
■ Fever, chills
■ Peripheral neuropathy
■ Prior history of wound infection
■ High blood sugars
■ Foot deformity

Pertinent Negatives

■ Normoglycemia
■ Normothermia
■ Clear drainage
■ Pain
■ Purple discoloration without warmth
■ Intermittent claudication
■ History of peripheral arterial disease or venous insufficiency
■ History of recent trauma

Objective

Pertinent Positives

- Mental status changes, confusion
- Hypotension, tachycardia, hyperpyrexia
- Erythema, swelling, crepitus along affected limb
- Purulent secretions
- Decreased sensation to touch
- Wound with friable or discolored granulation tissue, undermining of wound edges
- Positive probe to bone (PTB) test
- Charcot foot deformity

Pertinent Negatives

- Superficial ulceration with irregular edges
- Superficial ulceration with regular edges
- Blackened discoloration
- Pulselessness of affected limb
- Bilateral erythema and swelling without warmth
- Hyperpigmentation
- Ecchymosis

DIFFERENTIAL DIAGNOSIS AND DIAGNOSTIC CONSIDERATIONS

Differential Diagnoses

- Venous insufficiency ulceration
- Peripheral arterial ulceration
- Gangrene
- Hematoma

Diagnostic Tests

- Complete blood count with differential
- Comprehensive metabolic panel
- Blood cultures
- Inflammatory markers—see osteomyelitis
- Wound culture—should be obtained post cleansing and/or debridement, deep tissue; swab specimens are discouraged especially in inadequately debrided wounds or wounds that have been open for more than 24 to 48 hours
- Plain foot films—to assess for bony abnormalities, soft tissue gas, and radio-opaque foreign bodies
- MRI if abscess or osteomyelitis is suspected (see osteomyelitis)

TREATMENT

The primary determinant of whether a patient requires hospitalization is dependent upon the severity of the infection. All patients assessed to have a severe infection should be hospitalized in addition to select patients classified as having a moderate infection with complicating features (severe peripheral arterial disease). Patients who have failed outpatient treatment, and little or no improvement is assessed, may also require hospitalization for further diagnostic evaluation and IV therapy. It is also reasonable to hospitalize any patient who is unable to comply with an outpatient treatment regime until an appropriate plan of care can be established. Treatment is multifactorial and includes wound care, pharmacology, and surgical intervention.

Initial antimicrobial treatment instituted in the hospitalized patient is typically empiric and is based upon the severity of the infection, what pathogens are likely present, patient's recent history of antimicrobial exposure, local prevalence of pathogens, and available microbiologic data from recent cultures. See Box 18.4 for considerations prior to prescribing antibiotics and to assist in understanding the importance of antibiotic stewardship principles. It is essential for providers to understand the microbiology of common organisms present in DFIs, and risk factors for *Pseudomonas* and other multidrug resistant pathogens prior to prescribing antimicrobial therapy (Lipsky et al., 2012). Prescribing broad-spectrum antibiotics may not be necessary, even initially, and may

---

BOX 18.4 ANTIBIOTIC SELECTION CONSIDERATIONS FOR DIABETIC FOOT INFECTION

- Is there clinical evidence of an infection?
  - Fever
  - Erythema/warmth
  - Swelling
  - Leukocytosis
  - Purulence
- Is there a high risk for MRSA?
  - Recent/recurrent antibiotic use for chronic diabetic foot ulcer
  - Recent hospitalization
  - Colonization with MRSA pathogens/prior history of MRSA infection
  - Long-term care facility
  - Immunosuppression/multiple comorbidities
- Has the patient received antimicrobial therapy in the past month?
  - If so, include agents against gram-negative bacilli
- Is there a high risk for *pseudomonas*?
  - Recent hospitalization
  - Recent/recurrent antibiotic use for chronic diabetic foot ulcer
  - Colonization with *Pseudomonas*
  - Immunosuppression
  - Exposure to healthcare procedures

Source: Adapted from Lipsky, B. A., Berendt, A. R., Cornia, P. B., Pile, J. C., Peters, E. J. G., Armstrong, D. G., Deery, H. G., Embil, J. M., Joseph, W. S., Karchmer, A. W., Pinzur, M. S., & Senneville, E. (2012). 2012 Infectious Diseases Society of America Clinical Practice Guideline for the diagnosis and treatment of diabetic foot infections. *Clinical Infectious Diseases*, *54*(12), e132–e173. https://doi.org/10.1093/cid/cis346

support the proliferation of multidrug resistant organisms in the future. Table 18.13 identifies antibiotic treatment recommendations. The recommended course of antimicrobial therapy in a patient without osteomyelitis is 1 to 2 weeks for a mild infection and 2 to 3 weeks for moderate to severe infections.

All patients with DFI should have a foot specialist/surgeon/podiatrist consultation to evaluate the wound for debridement and additional surgical intervention that may be necessary. Urgent surgical intervention is required for foot infections accompanied by gas, an abscess, or necrotizing fasciitis. A vascular surgery consult may be necessary if there is significant vascular insufficiency or if higher limb amputation is required.

Wound care is also essential to treatment of diabetic foot ulcerations. Wound "off-loading" is recommended to redistribute pressure off of the wound and is an essential aspect of care (Lipsky et al., 2012).

DIABETIC FOOT OSTEOMYELITIS

Diabetic foot osteomyelitis (DFO) is a common complication of DFI. DFO occurs from a soft tissue infection that spreads to the bone; first it involves the cortex and then the marrow. All aspects of the foot can be affected but it most frequently affects the forefoot. Healthcare providers should consider osteomyelitis for any infected deep or large foot ulcer that is chronic in nature, recurs after initial healing, or overlies a bony prominence. The pathogens involved in osteomyelitis are essentially the same as those identified in the soft tissue and reflect the microorganisms identified under DFIs (Giurato et al., 2017). At this point in the infection trajectory, the pathogens are typically polymicrobial and may include methicillin-resistant *Staphylococcus aureus* (MRSA), *Pseudomonas,* and/or extended spectrum beta-lactamases (ESBL)-producing organisms. These organisms typically occur secondary to prolonged and/or recurrent antibiotic therapy and empiric treatment without culture-based knowledge. Osteomyelitis is a significant risk factor for minor and major amputations, especially if the patient has concurrent peripheral arterial disease (PAD; Giurato et al., 2017).

DIFFERENTIAL DIAGNOSIS AND DIAGNOSTIC CONSIDERATIONS

Osteomyelitis is the result of chronic infection and may not consistently show signs and symptoms of inflammation. Healthcare providers should consider osteomyelitis as a diagnosis based on criteria listed in the preceding. Additional criteria include probe-to-bone (PTB) test, radiographic images, bone culture and histology. The PTB test involves probing the ulcer to assess whether it reaches the bone; if so, this is considered positive and is highly suggestive of osteomyelitis. MRI has the highest sensitivity and specificity in the diagnosis of DFO. If MRI is contraindicated, a leukocyte

(white blood cell) tagged scan can be used to assist in making the diagnosis. The leukocyte tagged scan has better specificity than the triple phase bone scan. Plain radiographs have low sensitivity and specificity for confirming or excluding osteomyelitis. Serum inflammatory markers will usually be elevated in osteomyelitis, although, white blood cells may be normal if the patient has received recent antimicrobial therapy. A C-reactive protein (CRP), erythrocyte sedimentation rate (ESR), and procalcitonin (PCT) may also be elevated; however, CRP and PCT will return to their normal ranges about 3 weeks post infection. The ESR will continue to remain elevated. The criterion standard for diagnosing DFO is isolation of bacteria from a bone sample and histologic findings of inflammation. The bone culture may provide a false negative secondary to sampling error or recent antibiotic therapy. There could also be a false positive secondary to wound colonization or skin flora. Based on these issues, clinical history, wound evaluation, radiology, and inflammatory markers provide the best evidence to support the diagnosis of DFO (Lipsky et al., 2012).

TREATMENT

- **Surgical:** Bone resection is considered the extensiveness of surgery.
- **Medical:** Antibiotics are used in the treatment of osteomyelitis with or without surgical intervention. In select cases, surgery may not be necessary or there may be circumstances when surgical intervention is not in the best interest of the patient. Selection of antibiotics is based on the availability of culture (bone or soft tissue) or empiric treatment of suspected organism if culture is not available. The treatment of osteomyelitis correlates with the most likely pathogens (same as for DFIs), the patients' antimicrobial exposure history (see Table 18.13), and community pathogens. Duration of treatment depends on whether surgery was performed and the extensiveness of the resection (Lipsky et al., 2012).
- Antibiotics 2 to 3 days post op for complete removal of infected bone
- Antibiotics 4 to 6 weeks post op for incomplete removal of infected bone
- 3 months if no surgery

TRANSITION OF CARE

A comprehensive discharge plan is necessary for patients with diabetic wound infections. Patients may need to be transitioned to a rehabilitation center if they have undergone reconstructive surgery or any type of amputation to learn how to adjust to changes in mobility. Patients may need to be transitioned to an extended care facility if they are unable to manage the complex care needs at home, especially if complex wound care and IV antimicrobial therapy is required. The achievement of glycemic control should occur prior to discharge and the maintenance of glycemic control is absolutely necessary to support wound healing and prevent further complications. Outpatient follow-up will be necessary related to the various disciplines of care (e.g., infectious disease, surgery, wound care). Many of the surgical procedures (including amputations) and complexity of care can be detrimental to a patient's overall mental well-being. It is important that AGACNPs ensure the psychological aspect of care is assessed prior to discharge with the appropriate resources in place to assist the patient in adjusting to body image changes.

CLINICAL PEARLS

- Classification of severity of DFI is essential to guide treatment.
- Treatment of DFIs should target common pathogens (*Staphylococcal aureus* and gram-negative bacilli).
- Risk factors for MRSA and *Pseudomonas* should be assessed prior to prescribing antibiotic coverage for these pathogens.
- Osteomyelitis and amputation are common complications.
- Patient care should be multifaceted with an effective care transition in place.

18.9: SPINAL EPIDURAL ABSCESS

PRESENTING SIGNS AND SYMPTOMS

Back pain, fever, fatigue.

HISTORY AND PHYSICAL FINDINGS

Spinal epidural abscess (SEA) is an accumulation of purulent material in the space between the dura matter and the osseo-ligamentous boundaries of the vertebral canal. Epidural abscesses that are located in the anterior epidural space are typically associated with discitis and/or vertebral osteomyelitis (Hauser, 2018). Discitis is inflammation that occurs between the intervertebral discs and is a result of the inflammatory response from the infection. Discitis may or may not cause osteomyelitis (Tunkel & Scheld, 2014).

There are three primary mechanisms that cause SEA.

1. Hematogenous spread via the bloodstream from another source of infection. Skin and soft tissues are typically the primary source, with IV drug use being a significant risk factor. Other causes of hematogenous spread include respiratory tract infection (pneumonia), genitourinary (urinary tract infections), abdominal viscera, oral cavity (dental infections), and heart valves (endocarditis). Oftentimes patients are not aware of recent infections and the source of inoculation remains unknown.
2. Direct extension occurs through spread of an infection near the spinal canal that colonizes the epidural space. This may occur if the patient has a prior history of vertebral osteomyelitis.

3. Iatrogenic inoculation occurs through invasive procedures, both therapeutic and diagnostic. This would include spinal surgery and percutaneous spinal procedures (epidural catheterization; Lyons et al., 2020).

The most common causative organism of SEA is *Staphylococcus aureus* (70%), followed by *Streptococcal* species (7%). Both *S. aureus* and *Streptococcal* species correlate with skin, soft tissue, and respiratory infection etiologies. Gram-negative bacilli could also cause SEA especially if related to IV drug use, abdominal etiologies, and urinary tract infections. *Mycobacterium tuberculosis* and fungal pathogens also contribute as causative organisms; however, both are rare in occurrence. Additional factors that predispose a person to SEA include diabetes mellitus (DM), end stage renal disease, sepsis, malignancy, morbid obesity, alcoholism, hepatic cirrhosis, indwelling catheters, and recent distant site of infection as indicated earlier. Patients who are immunocompromised because of the conditions listed in the preceding or take medications that suppress the immune system are also at risk (Lyons et al., 2020).

Subjective

Pertinent Positives

- Back pain, insidious onset, worsens at night, constant aching
- Radiculopathy
- Back spasms
- Persistent low-grade fever
- Chills
- Fatigue, malaise
- Abdominal pain
- Bladder dysfunction, incontinence
- Bowel dysfunction, incontinence
- Weakness, paralysis
- Pertinent medical history/risk factors—DM, alcohol use (ETOH), malignancy, cirrhosis, chronic kidney disease, immunosuppression, transplant
- Pertinent surgical history—recent spinal surgery or procedure, dental procedure, invasive procedure (arteriogram, catheterization)
- Medication history—drugs that suppress the immune system

Pertinent Negatives

- Pain subsides over time
- Pain relief when leaning forward
- Wide-based gait
- Loss of height
- Primary pain in the buttocks, thighs, legs
- Neurogenic claudication

Objective

Pertinent Positives

- Fever
- Tachycardia

- Hypotension
- Spinal tenderness; local point percussion
- Muscle weakness, sensory abnormalities (e.g., hypesthesia, paresthesia, dysethesia)
- Hyporeflexia lower extremities
- Gait disturbance

Pertinent Negatives

- Loss of lordosis
- Stooped posture
- Total paralysis lower extremities

Interval between onset of pain and onset of neurologicadeficit varies. A combination of fever and back pain in an immunocompromised patient or someone with a history of IV drug use should increase suspicion of SEA.

DIFFERENTIAL DIAGNOSIS AND DIAGNOSTIC CONSIDERATIONS

Differential Diagnoses

- Muscle strain
- Herniated disc
- Lumbar spinal stenosis
- Compression fracture
- Degenerative joint disease
- Vertebral metastases
- Ankylosing spondylitis
- Ruptured or symptomatic abdominal aortic aneurysm
- Renal colic

Diagnostic Tests

- Complete blood cell count—leukocytosis
- Erythrocyte sedimentaion rate (ESR)—inflammatory marker, most sensitive screen; slow to return to normal
- C-reactive protein (CRP)—inflammatory marker; will rise faster at initial onset and return to normal faster
- Blood cultures
- Urinalysis and urine culture—possible source of seeding
- Echocardiogram—if endocarditis is suspected especially in cases of IV drug use
- Tuberculin skin test or QuantiFERON if risk factors for TB
- MRI with IV contrast—first choice; include complete spinal imaging
- MRI without contrast—if unable to administer contrast
- CT myelogram—if unable to obtain MRI
- CT with IV contrast if CT myelogram unable to be performed

TREATMENT

- Surgical decompression and drainage of abscess is treatment of choice.

- The administration of antibiotics should be delayed until cultures can be obtained and then tailored based upon culture results.
- Antibiotics can be started prior to the operative treatment/abscess drainage under the following circumstances:
  - Substantial delay of surgery
  - Significant neurologic dysfunction
  - Sepsis/bacteremia
- Empiric antimicrobial coverage should provide broad spectrum coverage for the most common causative organism (*Staphylococcus* and *Streptococcus* species); *Mycobacterium tuberculosis* should also be considered in the appropriate context. If antibiotics are started empirically prior to cultures being obtained, and cultures are obtained at a later date, organisms may not be present on culture. In this case, continue with empiric therapy: vancomycin and ceftriaxone.
- Additional gram-negative antimicrobial coverage should be prescribed in the following circumstances:
  - Immunocompromised—vancomycin and cefepime
  - History of IV drug use—vancomycin and cefepime
  - History of recent infection or manipulation of the genitourinary tract—vancomycin and ceftriaxone or cefepime
- If cultures identify an *S. aureus* that is MSSA, the following antibiotics are recommended:
  - High dose nafcillin
  - Cefazolin as alternative
- Pain management

Vertebral osteomyelitis is likely in most patients with SEA. Treatment is typically 6 weeks in patients with lesser degree of bone infection and up to 8 weeks in those patients with osteomyelitis. Relapses may occur in up to 15% of those treated within a 6-month period (Chenowith et al., 2018).

TRANSITIONS IN CARE

Patients who experienced significant neurologic dysfunction as a result of the SEA may require extended physical therapy as either an inpatient or outpatient. In addition, the administration of long-term IV antibiotics also complicates treatment plans. Case managers will need to collaborate with the AGACNP to arrange for home care follow-up or adequate placement in an extended care facility depending upon patient circumstances. Education regarding IV antibiotic administration upon discharge is imperative to ensure positive outcomes; both patients and families should be included. Noncompliance with antibiotic administration in the home setting may set the patient up for treatment failure and recurrence as antimicrobial resistance may emerge.

18.10: INFECTION IN THE ELDERLY

PRESENTATION OF INFECTION IN OLDER ADULTS

Infections in older adults may vary in appearance from what is considered typical to that of an atypical presentation. Many of the symptoms that an older adult would present with are vague and may not relate to the underlying disease process. AGACNPs must be keenly aware of possible infectious etiologies without specific signs and symptoms that would normally assist in determining the diagnosis (Goldrich & Shah, 2021).

HISTORY OF PRESENT ILLNESS

Frequently, the history of present illness is obtained from a family member, friend, or caregiver. The older adult patient may not be aware of changes in behavior that have others concerned. The following symptoms are often observed by family members and that is what brings the patient to the emergency department for further evaluation: change in functional status, fatigue, altered mental status, inability to carry out activities of daily living, increased lethargy, agitation in a patient with underlying dementia, and decreased appetite. Older adults may not have fevers but may report chills and rigors.

Exacerbations of comorbidities may also reflect an underlying infectious etiology (High, 2017). As with other assessments, the onset, duration, associated symptoms, and location of pain (if applicable) should be explored. AGACNPs should also be aware that older adults may have more than one underlying infection.

Subjective

There are common findings among older adults that are pertinent to infections. As previously mentioned, pertinent history may be reported by the patients but are more likely to be provided by a family member or caregiver from another facility. While most patients present with mental status changes, weakness, and fall, it is what the patient does not present with that needs to be investigated. Table 18.14 identifies typical symptoms associated with common infectious etiologies that differ from a "normal" disease presentation. Please note that some older adults may have normal presentation of illness (refer to specific illness presentation for this discussion).

Objective

From a physical examination standpoint, older adults may have minimal overt symptoms suggestive of underlying infection. Abdominal exams are typically benign thus causing practitioners to eliminate the GI tract as a

TABLE 18.14: Differential Diagnosis of Common Infectious Disease Syndromes in Older Adults

SYNDROME	ETIOLOGY/SYMPTOMS/DIAGNOSTIC CONSIDERATIONS	PERTINENT POSITIVES/DIAGNOSTIC
Bacteremia/sepsis	Likely source genitourinary or gastrointestinal – urinary tract infections (gram-negative rods), diverticulitis (gram-negative rods/Enterococci) *Mortality much higher in those >65 years of age*	UTI symptoms–weakness, fall, mental status changes, pelvic pressure Diverticulitis symptoms–weakness, fall, mental status changes, constipation, poor appetite, abdominal exam may be normal Cholangitis–weakness, fall, mental status changes, poor appetite, sclerae icteric if obstruction Fever, leukocytosis may or may not be present; may have leukopenia, hypotension, tachycardia (may not be present if on beta-blockers) Blood cultures may be positive Lactic acidosis, elevated liver panel UA/urine cultures positive Abdominal CT–if diverticulitis/cholangitis suspected (positive gram-negative blood cultures with negative urinalysis)
Infective endocarditis	Degenerative valve disorders–*Streptococcus/Staphylococcus/HACEK (Haemophilus species, Aggregatibacter actinomycetemcomitans, Cardiobacterium hominis, Eikenella corrodens, and Kingella kingae)* Prosthetic valves–coagulase negative *Staphylococcus* Pacemakers–*Staphylococcus* Genitourinary/gastrointestinal–bacteremia from UTI, perforated diverticulum (gram-negative bacillus/*Enterococcus*)	Weakness, fatigue, dizziness, fall, mental status changes. Fever/leukocytosis unlikely; could have low grade fever New murmur Blood cultures–likely positive ESR/CRP elevated Presence of RBC in urine Transthoracic echocardiogram not useful for diagnosis secondary to degenerative, calcified valves; transesophageal echocardiogram recommended

(continued)

TABLE 18.14: Differential Diagnosis of Common Infectious Disease Syndromes in Older Adults *(continued)*

SYNDROME	ETIOLOGY/SYMPTOMS/DIAGNOSTIC CONSIDERATIONS	PERTINENT POSITIVES/DIAGNOSTIC
Prosthetic device infection	Prosthetic joints, cardiac pacemakers, artificial heart valves, intra-ocular lens implants, vascular grafts, penile prostheses Early infections are typically caused by contamination at time of surgery or as a result of nosocomial pathogen (IV access, urinary catheters); likely pathogens skin-related (*Staphylococcus/Streptococcus*) or nosocomial (MRSA, gram-negative rods) Late infections are typically a result of seeding from another bacterial infection (e.g., gram- negative rod from bacteremia caused by urinary tract infection)	History of prosthetic device, history of recent UTI or hospitalization Weakness, fall, mental status changes, may have tenderness/erythema at site of prosthetic joint Fever/leukocytosis unlikely but could have low grade fever and mild leukocytosis Blood cultures may or may not be positive UA–may be positive if recent or current infection ESR/CRP elevated
Pneumonia	*Streptococcus* most common pathogen; atypical pathogens less common in older adults; increased susceptibility for post viral secondary bacterial pneumonia; gram-negative and MRSA should be a consideration if recently hospitalized, from a facility, or immunocompromised	Altered mental status, acute functional impairment, falls, dizziness, weakness, anorexia, dehydration, incontinence, exacerbation of chronic diseases Cough, shortness of breath Vital signs may be normal except for respiratory rate (tachypneic); may or may not be hypoxic CBC within normal limits or mild leukocytosis CXR may be normal initially especially if patient is dehydrated or neutropenic
Tuberculosis (TB)	Advanced age major risk factor; risk of reactivation secondary to compromised immune system	Prior history of TB–especially with recent history of cancer with treatment Nonspecific dizziness, mental dullness (less likely to present with cough, night sweats) Fever/Leukocytosis unlikely CXR–wide spread pulmonary parenchymal infiltrates Tuberculin skin test has decreased sensitivity in older adults and should be repeated if initial result is negative and there is high suspicion for TB; QuantiFERON® has slightly improved sensitivity than skin test and should be repeated in older adults if first result is negative
Fever of unknown origin (FUO)	Typically has different causes than those <65 Most FUO relate to an infectious etiology as noted previously Additional etiologies–connective tissue disorder (temporal arteritis) malignancy, drug fever	Symptoms as noted previously

CBC, complete blood count; CRP, c-reactive protein test; CXR, chest x-ray; ESR, erythrocyte sedimentation rate; FUO, fever of unknown origin; RBC, red blood cells; TB, tuberculosis; UA, urinalysis; UTI, urinary tract infection.

Source: Adapted from High, K. P. (2017). Infection: General principles. In J. B. Halter, J. G. Ouslander, S. Studenski, K. P. High, S. Asthana, M. A. Supiano, & C. Ritchie (Eds.), *Hazzard's geriatric medicine and gerontology* (7th ed.). McGraw-Hill. https://accessmedicine-mhmedical-com.sladenlibrary.hfhs.org/content.aspx?bookid=1923&sectionid=144563653.

possible etiology. Refer to Table 18.14 for typical findings in older adults related to common infectious diseases.

DIFFERENTIAL DIAGNOSIS AND DIAGNOSITC CONSIDERATIONS

Older adults will present with similar symptoms for all infectious etiologies. The common infectious syndromes are identified in Table 18.14 along with key pertinent positives that may occur. Practitioners should consider that there may be more than one infectious etiology occurring and therefore it is prudent to be comprehensive in the workup. The following diagnostics should be part

of any initial workup for an elderly presentation of mental status and/or functional status changes. Once differential diagnoses have been established, further specific testing can be undertaken to investigate the etiology. Some of these specifics are provided in Table 18.14.

- Complete blood cell count
- Comprehensive metabolic panel
- Procalcitonin
- Lactic acid
- Urinalysis, urine culture
- Blood cultures
- CXR
- Head CT

TREATMENT AND ANTIBIOTIC STEWARDSHIP

Treatment for infections in older adults are subsumed under the appropriate clinical practice guidelines for disease-specific interventions. Broad-spectrum antibiotics should be prescribed in patients who are septic and the source of infection is not clear. Additional elements should be considered prior to selecting antibiotics:

- Patient exposure history to antibiotics
- Hospital- and community-based antibiograms for resistance patterns
- Review patient medication profile to ascertain possible interactions with other medications

Antibiotic dosing should be reviewed with pharmacy. Dosing reduction may be necessary secondary to a decrease in renal function; however, the assumption should not be made that all antibiotic doses should be decreased. There are several antibiotics that are concentration dependent in order to work effectively (fluoroquinolones) and by decreasing the dose unnecessarily may set the patient up for future resistance. There are also other factors associated with aging that may impact efficacy if not dosed appropriately (altered gastric motility, decreased absorption, increased adipose tissue). As with all other antibiotics prescribed, de-escalation of therapy should occur as soon as possible (Debias & Wright, 2018).

TRANSITIONS OF CARE

Depending on the source of infection and course of treatment, older adults may require long-term antibiotic therapy. This often includes IV therapy for diseases such as osteomyelitis or endocarditis. The case manager will need to work with the patient and family to determine the best option for this therapy once discharged. It is important to stress that antibiotic administration continues as scheduled in order to prevent recurrence of the infection or resistance. This plan may require placement in an extended care facility or family support to administer the antibiotic at home or transport the patient to an infusion center.

CLINICAL PEARLS

- Older adults with infectious diseases will often have an atypical presentation that is manifested by mental status changes and functional impairment.
- Older adults are less likely to experience fever or have leukocytosis.
- Infections that typically occur in older adults emerge from the genitourinary and gastrointestinal systems.
- Prior antibiotic exposure history and hospital/community antibiogram should be evaluated to determine best antimicrobial agent.
- The AGACNP should consult with pharmacy to ensure proper dosing of antibiotic(s) selected.

 SPRINGER PUBLISHING CONNECT™

A robust set of instructor resources designed to supplement this text is located at http://connect.springerpub.com/content/reference-book/978-0-8261-6079-9. Qualifying instructors may request access by emailing textbook@springerpub.com.

REFERENCES

Full list of references can be accessed at http://connect.springerpub.com/content/reference-book/978-0-8261-6079-9.

CHAPTER 19

MANAGEMENT OF TRAUMATIC INJURY IN ADULTS AND OLDER ADULTS

Melinda Hodne, Jessica S. Peters, and Abbye Solis

LEARNING OBJECTIVES

- Appraise scientific knowledge, methodology, and evidence-based practice to assess the impact of traumatic injury in adults across the lifespan.
- Utilize evidence-based management strategies to diagnose and manage various disease states for adults and older adults following traumatic injury.
- Prioritize accurate differential diagnoses of acutely and critically ill adults following traumatic injury across the lifespan based on the synthesis of subjective and objective clinical data.

INTRODUCTION

All-cause unintentional injury was the leading cause of death for patients between the ages of 15 and 44 in 2018. For those 45 years of age and older, all-cause unintentional injury was the third leading cause of death in the United States. The prevalence of traumatic injuries, both intentional and unintentional, in the United States supports that the acute care provider be proficient in the initial evaluation of trauma patients seeking care in the emergency department. Central to advanced practice trauma care is the identification of life-threatening injury coupled with knowledge of resuscitation and definitive management. Trauma is broadly classified into three groups: penetrating, blunt, and deceleration (Dumovich & Singh, 2019).

TRAUMA SYSTEMS

In 1990 Congress passed the Trauma Care Systems Planning and Development Act with the aim of improving emergency medical services and trauma care in the United States. Guidelines of care were developed by the American College of Surgeons (ACS) Committee on Trauma and the American College of Emergency Physicians. A designation process was outlined and developed which included a verification process. Trauma centers were verified and designated as Levels 1 to 5, with Level 1 providing a comprehensive regional center with total care from prevention through rehabilitation. Level 2 provides definitive care for all injured patients, Level 3 provides immediate 24-hour emergency coverage with availability of general surgeons but may have limited specialty care requiring transfer to a tertiary center, Level 4 provides Advanced Trauma Life Support (ATLS) with transfer to a higher level of care once stabilized, and Level 5 provides stabilization and diagnostics with transfer to a higher level of care. No facility may market itself as a trauma center without designation and verification through the ACS (Cameron et al., 2020).

19.1: TRAUMA EVALUATION AND SURVEY

While the presenting signs and symptoms of the patient requiring trauma care differ by etiology of traumatic event, patients often experience mortal or morbid symptoms, including hypotension, hypoxia, hypothermia, acute blood loss, penetrating trauma, or injuries to limbs. ATLS is a widely accepted program developed by the ACS that trains providers to immediately treat trauma patients to improve patient outcomes (as opposed to prioritization of trauma care). ATLS provides a structured approach for management of the trauma patient with standard algorithms of care and emphasis on the first hour after a traumatic injury, considered to be the most critical, commonly referred to as the "golden hour" (ACS, 2018; Cothren & Moore, 2019).

PRIMARY SURVEY

Traumatic injury patients require immediate attention in the acute care setting; the emergency department setting is often high-paced and anxiety provoking for even the most experienced providers. To assist the provider in managing this high-intensity environment, ATLS supports the use of the "ABCDE" methodology for the initial assessment, or primary survey, of trauma patients. The World Health Organization also supports the "ABCDE" approach as a systematic way to assess trauma patients (Ali, 2014). This sequential algorithm is:

- Airway maintenance with restriction of cervical spine motion
- Breathing and ventilation

- Circulation and hemorrhage control
- Disability (assessment of neurologic status)
- Exposure/environmental control

Airway Maintenance With Restriction of Cervical Spine Motion

The adult-gerontology acute care nurse practitioner (AGACNP) must rapidly assess for airway patency. This can be quickly evaluated by asking the patient their name and asking what happened prior to the traumatic event. Lack of response, stridor, vocal abnormalities, pain during vocalization, or bloody secretions give clues to immediate airway compromise. Frequent airway patency assessment is vital, as initial patency of the airway could change as the patient's status changes.

If the patient has a decreased level of consciousness (Glasgow Coma Scale [GCS] score of 8 or lower) or is unconscious, endotracheal intubation is necessary. Restricting cervical spine motion while securing the airway prevents development and/or progression of spinal injury sequelae, typically with a cervical collar. If endotracheal intubation is necessary, maintaining alignment of the spine is prudent during the intubation process.

Breathing and Ventilation

Airway patency alone does not ensure proper oxygenation and ventilation. AGACNPs must monitor their patient's oxygen saturation levels and intervene appropriately. Proper ventilation must be confirmed to alleviate hyperventilation and hypoventilation. Common causes of hypoventilation after a traumatic event include a blunted level of consciousness or unconsciousness, pain, or flail chest. Auscultation of the chest and assessment of thoracic expansion can aid in the diagnosis of a thorax abnormality. Additionally, lung ultrasound can accelerate the diagnosis of an intrathoracic abnormality, for example, a pneumothorax or hemothorax, that may require immediate intervention for normalizing oxygenation and ventilation.

Circulation and Hemorrhage Control

Compromise of the circulatory system, or shock, is exhibited by hypotension, delayed capillary refill, and cool extremities. This can be seen with or without tachycardia. Hemorrhage is the most common culprit of hypotension in traumatic patients and identification of the location/cause of hemorrhage is essential. Rapid, external hemorrhage can be obvious and direct pressure can help slow bleeding. However, identification of internal bleeding is not always apparent upon initial presentation. Computed tomography (CT) scan should be considered for hypotensive patients when external or internal trauma is suspected. A focused assessment with sonography in trauma (FAST) exam, or systematic ultrasound assessment, can identify fluid in the abdomen, potentially leading to surgical intervention. Regardless of the origin of bleeding, controlling and/or stopping the bleeding is crucial to the treatment of hemorrhagic shock.

Adequate IV access is necessary when trauma patients present with circulatory compromise of any origin. Two large bore catheters are preferred for judicious fluid replacement; initial access could include peripheral IVs, intraosseous catheters, or central lines. Rapid replacement of blood loss with blood products and IV fluids should be performed until hemodynamic stability is reached.

Disability (Assessment of Neurologic Status)

Rapid assessment of the trauma patient's neurologic status is also a part of the primary survey. The GCS (Table 19.1) is a simple and objective method to determine level of consciousness. Alterations in a normal GCS scale

TABLE 19.1: Glasgow Coma Scale for Adults

	4 YEARS TO ADULTS
EYE OPENING	
4	Spontaneous
3	To speech
2	To pain
1	No response
VERBAL RESPONSE	
5	Alert and oriented
4	Disoriented conversation
3	Speaking but nonsensical
2	Moans or unintelligible sounds
1	No response
MOTOR RESPONSE	
6	Follows commands
5	Localizes pain
4	Moves or withdraws to pain
3	Decorticate flexion
2	Decerebrate extension
1	No response
3-15	

Note: In intubated patients, the Glasgow Coma Scale verbal component is scored as a 1, and total score is marked with a "T" (or tube) denoting intubation (e.g., "8T").

Source: With permission from Cydulka, R. K., Cline, D. M., John Ma, O., Fitch, M. T., Joing, S., & Wang, V. J. (2017). *Tintinalli's emergency medicine manual* (8th ed., pp. 721–725). McGraw-Hill Education

should immediately clue the provider of a potential head injury, hypoxia, hypercarbia, among other things like hypoglycemia, alcohol, narcotics, and other toxins that might alter level of consciousness. However, neurologic alterations should always be assumed to be an intracranial injury until proven otherwise, unless a bystander can give a detailed report of the traumatic event thus eliminating an intracranial and/or spine injury.

Exposure/Environmental Control

Proper assessment of the patient during the primary survey requires visualization of the entire body. Removing and/or cutting of the clothes might be necessary to fully appreciate an exposure injury, including thermal or chemical burn. Loose clothing can hide many injuries, such as a compound bone fracture. Additionally, bleeding sources could be identified if ecchymosis or discoloration is seen.

Normothermia is a goal of resuscitation. Warming blankets, warmed blood products or IV fluids may be necessary to prevent negative effects from hypothermia, which includes coagulopathy and acidemia.

HISTORY AND PHYSICAL FINDINGS

Secondary Survey

The secondary survey is a complete subjective history and objective head to toe assessment. It begins when patient stabilization is achieved with the primary survey. However, a thorough medical history is often delayed or not achievable during a life-threatening event. The mnemonic "SAMPLE" is an efficient means of obtaining a history from a conscious and oriented patient, even if the patient is acutely decompensating. Prehospital personnel and/or bystanders can assist in gathering this information for the providers, particularly when the patient has a decreased level of consciousness.

SAMPLE includes:

- <u>S</u>igns and symptoms
- <u>A</u>llergies
- <u>M</u>edications (current)
- <u>P</u>ast illnesses/pregnancy
- <u>L</u>ast meal and PO intake
- <u>E</u>vents and environment related to the injury

Understanding the mechanism of injury (or events/environment) is key for the provider anticipating potential injuries and enhancing understanding of physiological responses. Blunt trauma events, as in motor vehicle accidents, falls, or interpersonal violence, should include information about seat-belt use, speed of accident, ejection from the vehicle, height of fall, and type of weapon used. Penetrating trauma, such as gunshot or knife wounds, should be detailed with number of wounds, entrance and exit locations, and caliber and size of bullet or knife. Burn injury treatment is heavily dependent on location and propellant (e.g., gasoline, grease, chemicals). Electrical burns, inhalation injuries, and hazardous material injury details can greatly alter a provider's immediate response.

SPECIAL CONSIDERATIONS

Care of the patient after a traumatic event is influenced by the type of injury sustained and level of physiologic instability. The AGACNP must assume that all patients are to receive resuscitative efforts, including cardiopulmonary resuscitation (CPR) and intubation. Informed consent is often not achievable. For interpersonal violence events, clothing and personal items could be considered forensic evidence. Bullets, guns, and other weapons should be safeguarded until given to law enforcement. Hospitals have policies regarding obtaining blood alcohol levels and drug screening for all trauma patients. Signs or verbalizations of abuse should be taken seriously from all patients; elder abuse or neglect, intimate partner violence, and rape should lead to more detailed assessments by properly trained providers and/or hospital personnel, such as a forensic nurse.

TRANSITION OF CARE

Prehospital and Interhospital Transfer

Prehospital emergency personnel have protocols from which to make decisions about the destination of trauma patients. Sometimes this is to the nearest emergency department for immediate treatment. All emergency departments must accept trauma patients, regardless of ability to pay, as outlined in Medicare requirements tied to reimbursement. However, a hospital might not have the capacity to properly care for the patient after obtaining stability. That hospital must then transfer the patient to an accepting facility capable of providing adequate longer-term care, according to the Emergency Medical Treatment and Active Labor Act (EMTALA).

Intrahospital Transfer

Transfer of the trauma patient within a hospital is highly dependent upon the patient's injuries, acuity, and interventions required for patient stability. Outcomes from traumatic injuries are improved when patients are assigned to inpatient units specializing in the type of trauma sustained; for example, a neurologic intensive care unit (ICU) for a traumatic brain injury (TBI) (Bukur et al., 2015).

CLINICAL PEARLS

- Use the "ABCDE" methodology for the initial assessment, or primary survey, of trauma patients.
- The secondary survey is a complete subjective history and objective head-to-toe assessment and begins when the primary survey is completed.

19.2: HEAD INJURY/TRAUMATIC BRAIN INJURY

HISTORY AND PHYSICAL FINDINGS

Traumatic brain injury (TBI) is estimated to cause approximately 150 deaths per day in the United States. The Centers for Disease Control and Prevention (CDC) defines a TBI as a bump, blow, or jolt to the head that disrupts normal functions of the brain. Since 2014, four out of five TBI-related emergency department encounters for those 65 years of age or older were caused by falls. For those adults less than 65 years of age, motor vehicle collisions (MVC) accounted for the majority of hospitalizations from TBI (CDC, 2019). Of note, intentional injury is a contributing reason for mortality from a head trauma in adults (Capizzi et al., 2020).

Presenting signs and symptoms differ on the cause of head injury, or primary injury, but should always include the initial assessment for circulation, airway, and breathing (CAB). Prehospital assessment within these CAB categories should aim interventions to avoid hypoxemia, hypotension, and abnormalities in temperature at all costs (Capizzi et al., 2020). Figure 19.1 diagrams a flowchart of cellular injury after TBI.

The varying presenting symptoms of TBIs complicate attempts to classify injuries (Teasdale & Jennett, 1974). TBIs have historically been categorized by the Glasgow Coma Scale (GCS) into three diagnoses: mild (GCS 13–15), moderate (GCS 9–12), and severe (GCS <9). However, the initial GCS can change due to secondary injury effects or insults. Patients with an initial mild category of injury can rapidly decline with a GCS defined as a severe TBI; frequent neurologic assessments are necessary to detect early signs of neurologic compromise leading to life-threatening complications. Prehospital details of the mechanism of injury, GCS, and pupil examination should be clearly communicated to providers upon hospital presentation (Eapen & Cifu, 2018; Whitfield et al., 2020). But solely using the GCS is widely criticized. The provider must also ascertain length and loss of alteration of consciousness, length of posttraumatic amnesia, and presence or absence of imaging finding are essential components of determining treatment for head injury patients (Eapen & Cifu, 2018). See Table 19.2 for the classification of TBI severity.

Mild TBIs are most often described as a concussion but the effects of these types of injuries can be substantial. Concussions, or mild TBI, account for 10% to 15% of all sports-related injuries. The majority of TBIs are mild and can be monitored in the emergency department, often released the same day under established concussion protocols (CDC, 2019). Approximately 70% of TBIs occur with polytrauma and incidences in the United States are increasing each year (CDC, 2019). Moderate to severe TBIs are often subcategorized into focal injuries/

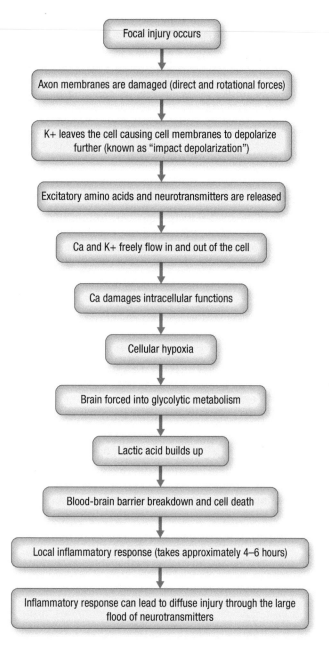

FIGURE 19.1: Pathophysiology of cellular injury after traumatic brain injury (TBI).
Source: Reproduced with permission from Capizzi, A., Woo, J., & Verduzco-Gutierrez, M. (2020). Traumatic brain injury: An overview of epidemiology, pathophysiology, and medical management. *Medical Clinics of America, 104*(1), 213–238. https://doi.org/10.1016/j.mcna.2019.11.001

contusions and diffuse axonal injury (DAI; Eapen & Cifu, 2018; Whitfield et al., 2020).

Cerebral Perfusion Pressure

Cerebral perfusion pressure (CPP) is the product of mean arterial pressure (MAP) and intracranial pressure (ICP).

TABLE 19.2: Classification of Traumatic Brain Injury Severity

	BEST GCS IN FIRST 24 HOURS	LOSS OF CONSCIOUSNESS	ALTERATION OF CONSCIOUSNESS/ MENTAL STATE	IMAGING	POSTTRAUMATIC AMNESIA
Mild	13-15	0-30 min	Up to 24 hours	Normal	<1 day
Moderate	9-12	>30 min to <24 hours	>24 hours	Normal or abnormal	>1 day and <7 days
Severe	3-8	>24 hours	>24 hours	Normal or abnormal	>7 days

Source: Eapen, B., & Cifu, D. (2018). *Rehabilitation after traumatic brain injury.* Elsevier, p. 14.

ICP is determined by the volume of the three intracranial compartments: (a) brain parenchyma (<1,300 mL in the adult); (b) cerebrospinal fluid (100–150 mL); and (c) intravascular blood (100–150 mL). When one compartment expands, there is a compensatory reduction in the volume of another, and/or the baseline ICP will increase. Elevations in ICP are life-threatening and may lead to a phenomenon known as Cushing reflex (hypertension, bradycardia, and respiratory irregularity).

With brain injury autoregulation may be impaired, so even modest drops in blood pressure can decrease brain perfusion and result in cellular hypoxia. A goal CPP of <60 mmHg is considered the lower limit of autoregulation in humans. Traumatic hypotension leads to ischemia within low-flow regions of the injured brain, so aggressive fluid resuscitation may be required to prevent hypotension and secondary brain injury. It is important to maintain a MAP of ≥80 mmHg because low blood pressure in the setting of elevated ICP will result in a low CPP and brain injury (Wright & Merck, 2020). With a TBI, autoregulation is lost and the goals of treatment are to regulate ICP by addressing one of these three components (Ramayya et al., 2019; Wright & Merck, 2020).

Focal Injuries

Scalp Injury

Close examination should be performed when patients present with injuries to the scalp region. Abrasions and lacerations are clues to the site of impact, object causing the injury, and potential for secondary brain parenchymal injury. Openings in the epidermis and dermis of the scalp bleed heavily, possibly leading to hemorrhagic shock requiring colloid resuscitation. Polymicrobial infections are common and prophylactic antibiotics should be considered. Impact locations should not be determined by bruising pattern alone, as contrecoup injuries can cause tracking of blood (Whitfield et al., 2020).

Skull Fractures

Significant blows to the skull can result in skull fractures and are classified as linear, comminuted, compound, and skull base fractures. Linear fractures are the most common type of skull fracture. Comminuted fractures can produce multiple bone fragments with a "depressed" appearance at the site of injury. Lacerations to overlying skin make infections a concerning complication to compound fractures. Bones of the base of the skull are relatively thin and several additional classifications exist: hinge, ring, and basilar (Whitfield et al., 2020).

Brain Contusions

Contusion injuries to the brain are often described as a coup and contrecoup. Coup injuries occur near or at the site of injury due to direct force on the brain tissue. Contrecoup injuries result as the brain is moved to abnormal parts of the skull by the force of injury, specifically as rapid deceleration of movement happens when the skull hits a solid surface. For example, blunt trauma to the occipital region may cause a contrecoup injury to the frontal region of the brain (Whitfield et al., 2020).

Intracranial Hemorrhage

Epidural Hemorrhage

Blood between the outer layer of the dura and the skull is an epidural hematoma. This type of hemorrhage does not cross suture lines and is most often in the lateral, especially the coronal, sutures. MVCs, physical assaults, and accidental falls are the most common causes of epidural hemorrhage and often coincide with a skull fracture. Bleeding from the anterior meningeal artery or dural venous sinus causes collection of blood within the temporal region, found in up to 75% of epidural hemorrhages (Capizzi et al., 2020; Figure 19.2).

Subdural Hemorrhage

Although subdural hemorrhage, or hematomas inside of the dural space, can occur as a result of rapid acceleration or deceleration of the head, they can also occur in the elderly as the brain atrophies. This bleeding usually is due to tearing of the cortical bridging veins, or those adjacent to the superior sagittal sinus, and can cross suture lines. This bleeding can occur acutely at the time

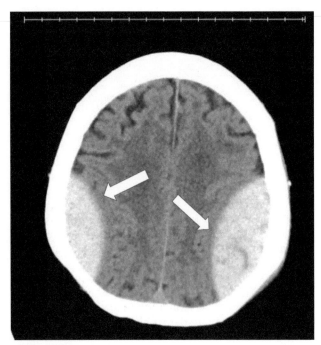

FIGURE 19.2: Epidural hemorrhage.
Source: Reproduced with permission from Capizzi, A., Woo, J., & Verduzco-Gutierrez, M. (2020). Traumatic brain injury: An overview of epidemiology, pathophysiology, and medical management. *Medical Clinics of America, 104*(1), 213–238. https://doi.org/10.1016/j.mcna.2019.11.001

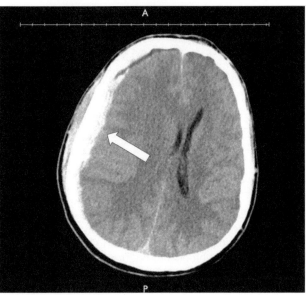

FIGURE 19.3: Subdural hemorrhage.
Source: Reproduced with permission from Capizzi, A., Woo, J., & Verduzco-Gutierrez, M. (2020). Traumatic brain injury: An overview of epidemiology, pathophysiology, and medical management. *Medical Clinics of America, 104*(1), 213–238. https://doi.org/10.1016/j.mcna.2019.11.001

of injury, subacutely (1–2 weeks postinjury), or chronic (>2 weeks postinjury). Chronic subdural hematomas are most common in low intracranial physiological states, such as the elderly, alcoholics, or postdrainage of hydrocephalus. For all subdural hematomas, presentation varies at time of event. However, it is known that volume of the hemorrhage itself is important; clinical deterioration occurs at 40 mL with death occurring around 90 mL of blood (Capizzi et al., 2020; Figure 19.3).

Subarachnoid Hemorrhage

Bleeding in the subarachnoid space varies in severity from small collections, common after head injuries, to large hemorrhages resulting after impact to the head or neck in an assault. If such an assault causes massive subarachnoid hemorrhage due to laceration of the vertebral artery, basilar artery, or one of the smaller arteries, and causes immediate collapse, the injury is often fatal (Capizzi et al., 2020; Figure 19.4).

Intraventricular Hemorrhage

Intraventricular hemorrhage from trauma is most often secondary to contusions or moderate to severe subarachnoid hemorrhage. It is often considered life-threatening due to the degree of obstructive hydrocephalus that occurs because of the hematoma (Capizzi et al., 2020).

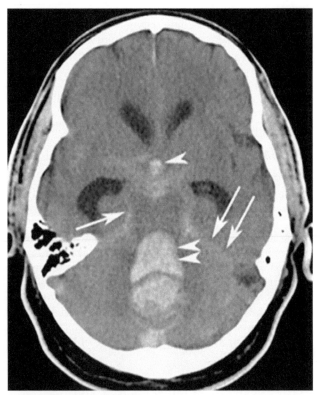

FIGURE 19.4: Subarachnoid hemorrhage.
Source: Reproduced with permission from Shazia Mirza and Sankalp Gokhale (2016-07-25). Neuroimaging in Acute Stroke, http://www.smgebooks.com/neuroimaging/chapters/NI-16-06.pdf

Diffuse Axonal Injury

DAI is a term used when widespread axonal damage occurs. Although this term is also used to describe irreversible brain damage from hypoxia, ischemia, and hypoglycemia, traumatic causes of DAI are from rapid acceleration/deceleration injuries, particularly when rotational or coronal movement of the head occurs at the time of injury. Injury to the axons results when fibers are transected or tortuous throughout the white matter of the brain, particularly in the corpus callosum and brainstem. The cause of these traumatic injuries are typically MVCs, assaults, or falls from a substantial height. Patients with DAIs are unconscious from the time of injury, with persistent vegetative state or immediate death as the most common outcomes. If someone survives such an injury, substantial morbidity and disability results (Whitfield et al., 2020).

DIFFERENTIAL DIAGNOSIS AND DIAGNOSTIC CONSIDERATIONS

For trauma patients without obvious head trauma, acute or dull headaches, photosensitivity, nausea/vomiting, changes in GCS, pupillary abnormalities, or loss of consciousness should all clue the provider that a head injury could have occurred at the time of the trauma. Clinical presentation with a lucid interval between the time of injury and neurologic deterioration should cause concern for epidural hematoma (CDC, 2019; Whitfield et al., 2020).

CT of the head is the gold standard for diagnosing the intracranial pathologic conditions previously mentioned. Emergent CTs are noncontrast to evaluate for active bleeding. In multisystem trauma and when a head injury is suspected, noncontrast head CTs are performed and examined first before contrast studies of other body parts are obtained. Magnetic resonance imaging (MRIs) will give more detailed information about the extent of brain injury but its use is limited due to the length of time MRI requires (Capizzi et al., 2020).

Battle's sign is a physical assessment finding of ecchymosis over the mastoid process, often with tenderness, and is indicative of basilar skull fracture (75% positive predictive value). Rhinorrhea and bruising over the eyes (raccoon eyes) can also be associated with the postauricular discoloration. Physical examination should also include assessment for hemotympanum. Battle's sign warrants further brain imaging with non contrast CT. Up to 15% of patients with Battle's sign also have a cervical spine injury. However, it should be noted that this sign is often a delayed finding and can take 1 to 2 days postinjury to appear (Whitfield et al., 2020).

TREATMENT

The primary trauma survey allows the provider to gain a GCS score, determine if mechanical intubation is necessary for airway protection, and to stabilize other life-threatening conditions. Monitoring and treatment for posttraumatic seizures, often seen with moderate to severe head trauma, is necessary and could occur up to 2 years after the injury (Whitfield et al., 2020). Neurosurgical consultation should not be delayed in patients with obvious head trauma in the event that ICP monitoring or emergent intracranial decompression is necessary.

Further damage caused by the impact results in a series of cellular events known as the secondary neurotoxic cascade. This cascade causes ongoing damage to the brain resulting in outcomes more severe than what may have occurred from the primary injury. Preventing secondary injury needs to be included in the treatment of traumatic head injuries (Oropello et al., 2014). Delayed complications from head trauma include posttraumatic amnesia, seizures, syndrome of inappropriate antidiuretic hormone secretion (SIADH), diabetes insipidus (DI), adrenocorticotropic hormone (ACTH) deficiency, and hydrocephalus. AGACNPs should monitor for signs and symptoms of these conditions in both acute and subacute settings. Post traumatic agitation, mood or personality changes, and delirium occur in up to 96% of TBI patients—most commonly agitation—and can persist long term, complicating rehabilitation efforts. Pharmacologic intervention and psychological therapy can assist in managing verbal or physically aggressive behaviors (Capizzi et al., 2020; Whitfield et al., 2020). Frequent assessments for self-harm should be a part of TBI recovery plans. Rehabilitation begins upon admission and involves an interprofessional team.

19.3: THORACIC TRAUMA

PRESENTING SIGNS AND SYMPTOMS

Thoracic trauma represents the second most common traumatic injury and is associated with significant morbidity and mortality. Early identification and management are associated with improved out-of-hospital survival rates. For example, rib fractures alone occur in up to 10% of all traumatic injuries and are associated with a mortality rate upward of 13% (Burguete et al., 2015). Thoracic traumatic injuries are associated with increased hospitalization rates and lengths of stay because of the secondary effects of thoracic trauma including pneumonia and severe pain.

Thoracic traumatic injury represents a cascade of injuries that occur secondary to both blunt and penetrating traumatic injuries. Blunt trauma can occur secondary to acceleration and deceleration, compression, and blast injuries. Penetrating chest traumatic injury is dependent on the penetrating pathway (bullet and/or stab wounds) and more commonly involve lung tissue versus thoracic vessel injury; however, this is directly dependent on the proximity and mechanism of injury. Blunt trauma injury that occurs secondary to acceleration and deceleration injuries is associated with significant in-field mortality; however, early identification of significant injury and potential thoracic vessel injury prompting airway stabilization and resuscitation are dependent on understanding of the mechanism of injury and associated with improved patient outcomes.

HISTORY AND PHYSICAL FINDINGS

When evaluating a patient for suspected chest trauma it is important to first consider the degree of hemodynamic instability and potential airway compromise associated with the suspected injury. Immediate life-threatening thoracic trauma represents a significant source of morbidity and mortality if not immediately detected and stabilized. The second category of thoracic traumatic such as pulmonary contusion includes injuries that occur in a relatively hemodynamically stable patient that is not immediately presenting with hypoxia. While less severe on immediate trauma injury survey, if these injuries are not supported in posttraumatic injury care, they represent a significant source of delayed traumatic injury morbidity and mortality (Eckhardt et al., 2020).

DIAGNOSTIC TESTING IN SUSPECTED CHEST TRAUMA

Chest radiographic studies are typically easily obtained and can determine presence of pneumothorax or hemothorax, fractures of the ribs, clavicles, and sternum following traumatic injury. The quality of the film is directly dependent on patient positioning and penetration. The availability of ultrasound and CT technology has decreased dependence on chest radiographic studies as immediate diagnostic tools. CT studies are considered superior to chest radiographic studies for diagnosis of chest traumatic injury. Utilization of contrast with imaging allows for the evaluation and identification of contrast extravasation, vessel injury, and hemorrhage source. This is particularly significant if interventional radiology and vessel ligation is considered to obtain hemostasis. Thoracic ultrasound is a readily available, noninvasive method that has increased utilization as part of the abdominal FAST (focused assessment with sonography in trauma) exam for retroperitoneal trauma. Advances in technology have allowed for increased accessibility, portability, and real-time evaluation and diagnosis. Limitations of thoracic ultrasound include training and competence in the tactile skill of probe placement and interpretation of images. It is important to note that diagnostic testing is not a replacement for obtaining a comprehensive history, physical examination, and laboratory analysis. Furthermore, diagnostic testing needs to consider the time-sensitive nature of traumatic injury and should not delay interventions such as definitive surgical repair or embolization necessary for hemostasis and recovery (Nicks et al., 2020).

SPECIFIC THORACIC TRAUMATIC INJURIES

Thoracic traumatic injuries that require immediate intervention include flail chest, tension, and open pneumothorax, massive hemothorax from large vessel injury, and cardiac tamponade. Regardless of the underlying etiology, all these life-threatening forms of thoracic trauma will present with hypoxia and hemodynamic instability, and often result in prehospital cardiac arrest following traumatic injury. The goal of care is determination of underlying etiology and stabilization until definitive and potential surgical management can occur.

Flail Chest

Flail chest occurs secondary to rib fractures of three or more ribs adjacent to each other. Flail chest should be suspected in patients following blunt trauma, particularly if localized to a certain thoracic region. The adjacent rib fractures destabilize the chest wall and thus the patient develops paradoxical movement that interferes with ventilation. It is important to evaluate a patient for pulmonary contusion, hemothorax, pneumothorax, and great vessel injuries since these frequently are seen in a patient with flail chest. Flail chest is considered a life-threatening thoracic injury since patients often present with significant respiratory distress and associated pulmonary contusions and thus, hypoxia. Inspection of the chest wall is notable for paradoxical chest wall movement and often auscultation of adventitious breath sounds depending on whether flail chest is in associated with contusion, hemothorax or pneumothorax. Management of flail chest is dependent on the amount of respiratory failure and hypoxia present if patients are in severe respiratory distress; immediate intubation and mechanical ventilation is often warranted. If hypoxia and respiratory failure are not present, the mainstay of therapy is pain management and pulmonary hygiene. Patients with flail chest are at a higher risk of developing secondary traumatic injury including pneumonia and thrombosis secondary to immobility and poor pain control inhibiting adequate pulmonary hygiene. The impact of flail chest injury is significant. More than 80% of patients with flail chest require admission to the ICU and nearly 60% will require mechanical ventilation (Bradley et al., 2017). The injury has a significant effect on inhospital complications because 20% of patients will develop pneumonia and up to 7% will develop sepsis (Bradley et al., 2017).

Patients with flail chest may benefit from nerve blocks or placement of an epidural catheter to aid in pain control and promote effective mobilization. Appropriate utilization of these therapies is dependent on a multitude of patient specific factors including hemodynamic stability or instability, hemorrhage, or neurologic and/or spinal cord injuries and should be evaluated on an individual basis. Furthermore, early utilization of continuous positive airway pressure (CPAP) therapy or high flow nasal cannula can support patients with mild respiratory distress and potentially avoid mechanical ventilation. Patients with flail chest regardless of systemic injuries should be admitted to the critical care unit initially for airway and oxygenation monitoring, secondary to the concern of developing respiratory decompensation, and aggressive pulmonary toilet and pain control nursing care needs.

Tension Pneumothorax

Tension pneumothorax occurs secondary to expiratory air trapping (air is able to enter the pleural space but is unable to fully exit) in the pleural space under positive pressure. Elevated pleural pressures can interfere with venous return and result in hypotension, tachycardia, cyanosis, severe dyspnea, and hemodynamic instability. As pressure rises, it causes a mediastinal shift toward the contralateral (opposite) side resulting in pressure on the lungs, heart, trachea, and mediastinal vessels. Physical exam findings (in addition to those noted) may include decreased chest excursion, tracheal deviation, agitation, diaphoresis, jugular venous distention, diminished breath sounds, absent tactile fremitus, and hyperresonance to percussion.

Treatment is time sensitive and requires immediate chest tube placement or needle decompression in the second intercostal space in the midclavicular until a chest tube can be placed for delimitative treatment and management (Burguete et al., 2015).

Open Pneumothorax

Open pneumothoraxes are often referred to as sucking chest wounds. Large open pneumothoraxes become sucking chest wounds secondary to air entering the chest cavity through the wound versus the trachea, therefore the patient loses the ability to generate negative pressure within their chest cavity for inspiration and expiration. Diagnosis is based on physical exam findings and include hypoxia, hemodynamic instability, and auscultation of sucking within the chest cavity with attempted inspiration and expiration. Primary treatment includes supplementation oxygen therapy, placement of an occlusive dressing over the chest wound, and immediate placement of a thoracostomy tube. Placement of an occlusive dressing without chest tube placement can cause the open pneumothorax to rapidly transition to a tension pneumothorax resulting in further hemodynamic instability (Burguete et al., 2015).

Massive Hemothorax

Massive hemothorax occurs following blunt or penetrating trauma that results in damage to the large pulmonary vascular system. Often injury of the great vessels including the pulmonary arteries and aorta results in significant prehospital hemorrhage and mortality. In an average sized adult, a hemothorax can hold up to 40% of a patient's circulating blood volume. Massive hemothorax is considered life-threatening if the volume is greater than 1,500 cc. Massive hemothorax is life-threatening for several reasons. Large volume hemothorax can cause hypovolemia. This decrease in circulating volume can lead to hypovolemic shock with a decrease in preload, resulting in left ventricular dysfunction and inadequate cardiac output. Furthermore, accumulation of blood within the lung parenchyma leads to hypoxia secondary to alveolar hypoventilation, ventilation–perfusion mismatch, and anatomic shunting. Patients will present with paradoxical inspiratory pattern upon inspection. In addition to hypoxia and hemodynamic instability, auscultation and physical exam findings are associated with decreased or absent breath sounds and asynchronous to minimal chest movement noted with respiratory effort. Immediate treatment for massive hemothorax is placement of a chest tube; if drained volume is greater than 1000 cc immediate surgical consultation is warranted for definitive management of bleeding.

Cardiac Tamponade

The three principal features of tamponade (Beck's triad) are hypotension, distant or muffled heart sounds, and jugular venous distention. The limitations to ventricular filling are responsible for reductions of cardiac output and arterial pressure. The quantity of fluid necessary to produce cardiac tamponade may be as small as 200 mL when the fluid develops rapidly as seen in tamponade secondary to traumatic injury. The accumulation of fluid causes restriction during diastole and thus a decrease in venous filling pressures which ultimately lead to a decrease in cardiac output. Traumatic injury tamponade is most commonly associated with penetrating chest trauma. However, any patient that presents with suspect or known high speed blunt sternal chest trauma (e.g., unrestrained driver) that results in sternal fractures needs to be ruled out for cardiac tamponade. The incidence of tamponade with sternal fractures is as high as 20% (Nicks & Manthey, 2020). Bedside echocardiography demonstrating a large cardiac silhouette, pericardial fluid collection with associated hypotension, and elevated jugular venous pressure should be suspicious of tamponade. Treatment is dependent on the degree of patient decompensation present. Patients with hemodynamic variability and imminent cardiac arrest warrant performing bedside pericardiocentesis to immediately remove compressive hematoma until management including surgical pericardial window can be performed to definitively manage bleeding (Zulfiqar & Veerasamy, 2017).

Pulmonary Contusions

Pulmonary contusions are damage or injury to lung parenchyma that result in hemorrhage and edema without direct laceration injury. Pulmonary contusions occur secondary to direct injury and as a secondary effect to the resuscitation with crystalloid that occurs following traumatic injury and suspected hypovolemia secondary to blood and volume loss following traumatic injury. Increased capillary hydrostatic pressures result in leakage of blood and fluid into the interstitium and alveoli. This then leads to intrapulmonary shunting and further increase in hydrostatic pressure which decreases lung elasticity and recoil. Ultimately this can progress to hypoxic and hypercarbic respiratory failure that requires mechanical ventilation. Physical exam findings in patients with pulmonary contusions may include a pleural friction rub however this can quickly progress to decreased or absent breath sounds. Patients may complain of chest pain and tachypnea with hypoxia. CT scan findings often demonstrate patchy, ground glass opacities similar to findings with aspiration pneumonitis that can progress to consolidation as edema and infiltration progress. Large lung parenchyma contusions can progress to acute respiratory distress syndrome. Treatment is mainly supportive including implementing pain control measures and mechanical ventilation that uses lung protective strategies (Zulfiqar & Veerasamy, 2017).

TREATMENT OF THORACIC TRAUMA

Thoracostomy Tube Insertion and Management

Management and monitoring of chest tubes will vary significantly depending on indication, presence or appearance, and volume of drainage. Management of pneumothorax and tension pneumothorax without hemothorax includes placement of tube thoracostomy, with low continuous wall suction to facilitate re-expansion and to monitor for pulmonary adema. Once the majority of the pneumothorax is evacuated, suction is applied for the next 24 hours. If an air leak exists, as evidenced by continual or intermittent bubbling through the water seal chamber, suction is maintained. This should be evaluated and differentiated by fluid level fluctuations noted throughout the respiratory cycle. Once there is no evidence of an ongoing air leak, the tube may be placed to water seal while performing intermittent chest radiographic studies to evaluate for any reaccumulation of the pneumothorax. If the patient experiences tachypnea, tachycardia, hypoxia, or hypotension following placement of the chest tube to water seal, the chest tube should be returned to continuous suction, the patient should be given supplemental oxygen, and an immediate radiographic study should be performed. If the patient does not experience reaccumulation of the pneumothorax following patient observation for 12 to 24 hours, the chest tube may be considered for removal. Persistence of an air leak for more than 72 to 96 hours warrants further investigation for definitive management including surgical repair or potential chemical or mechanical pleurodesis, a procedure to promote adhesion of the visceral and parietal pleura together to obliterate the pleural space and prevent future air leaks and pneumothorax re-expansion (Bradley et al., 2017).

Surgical and Interventional Radiology Consultation

Patients with blunt or penetrating trauma who present with hemodynamic instability warrant immediate surgical trauma evaluation and management. All resuscitative techniques and stabilization interventions such as placement of advanced airway, chest tubes, and pericardiocentesis are supportive measures until hemostasis can be established through surgical repair or interventional radiology embolization. Procedures are highly variable based on trauma presentation or penetrating trauma trajectory (Bradley et al., 2017).

CLINICAL PEARLS

- Regardless of underlying etiology all life-threatening forms of thoracic trauma will present with hypoxia and hemodynamic instability, and often result in prehospital cardiac arrest following traumatic injury.
- Early identification and management of thoracic trauma is associated with improved out of hospital survival rates.

19.4: ABDOMINAL AND PELVIC TRAUMA

Abdominal and pelvic trauma represent a broad classification system that occurs secondary to blunt or kinetic injury and penetrating trauma. Injuries can occur singularly or as part of multisystem traumatic injury. Injuries are typically classified based on the structure injured including abdominal wall, solid organ (spleen, liver, pancreas, and kidney), hollow viscus (stomach, intestines, bladder, and uterus) and vasculature injury. Both blunt and penetrating trauma can lead to organ laceration or rupture. Laceration injuries can lead to significant hemorrhage while organ rupture or laceration can lead to translocation of intraabdominal contents into the peritoneal space. Abdominal trauma can be challenging since it can be occult and often occurs with other injuries easily identifiable (thoracic trauma or head injuries). Young, healthy patients may be able to compensate for intraabdominal hemorrhage before clinical signs become overt; significant intraabdominal hemorrhage can occur prior to the presence of physical exam findings and hemodynamic alterations. Delayed identification of intraabdominal traumatic injury can lead to the development of intraabdominal hematoma, biliary leakage and biloma, bowel obstruction or ileus, abscess, or hematoma (Jones, 2015).

PRESENTING SIGNS AND SYMPTOMS

Inspection of a patient with abdominal injury may reveal abrasions or a seat belt mark. Cullen's sign of periumbilical bruising may be indicative of peripancreatic hemorrhage and Grey-Turner's sign of flank ecchymosis may be indicative of retroperitoneal hematoma. Light and deep palpation may or may not elicit peritonitic pain and general or regional tenderness or signs of acute abdomen (e.g., rigidity, rebound, guarding) may relate to other co existing injuries. Serious intraabdominal injury should not be ruled out based on inspection and physical exam findings alone, particularity if the mechanism of injury is highly suspicious. Studies suggest that 45% of blunt trauma patients thought to have a benign abdomen on initial physical exam are later found to have a significant intraabdominal injury (Ferroggiaro & Ma, 2020). However, any blunt abdominal trauma patient with diffuse peritonitis or who is hemodynamically unstable should be taken urgently to the operating room for laparotomy and exploration (Zulfiqar & Veerasamy, 2017).

DIAGNOSTIC TESTING ABDOMINAL TRAUMA

FAST Exam and CT Scans

The FAST (focused assessment with sonography in trauma) exam utilizes bedside ultrasound techniques to quickly identify pathological fluid in the peritoneum or pericardium in patients with blunt or penetrating traumatic injury. The exam focuses on the following four areas: (a) the right upper quadrant (RUQ) which visualizes Morison's pouch, the right pericolic gutter, the hepato diaphragmatic area and the left lobe of the liver; (b) the subxiphoid view which evaluates the pericardial space; (c) the left upper quadrant (LUQ) which visualizes the splenorenal recess, subphrenic space, left paracolic gutter, and the left lower hemithorax; and (d) the suprapubic view to evaluate the rectovesical pouch in males and rectouterine pouch in females (Bloom & Gibbons, 2022). The FAST examination is accurate, rapid, noninvasive, repeatable, and portable, and involves no nephrotoxic contrast material or ionizing radiation. Massive hemoperitoneum can be quickly detected with a single view of Morison's pouch. FAST also evaluates for free pericardial or pleural fluid and for pneumothorax. As with any ultrasonography, the strength of the exam is based on the operator skill and technique. Abdominal and pelvic CT scan with contrast are superior in the ability to identify the exact source of the intraabdominal free fluid including specific vessel injuries with contrast extravagation or solid organ injury or perforation. CT scans can provide superior assessment and evaluation of the retroperitoneal space. Limitations to CT imaging are patient stability and need for time-sensitive surgical intervention.

SPECIFIC ABDOMINAL TRAUMATIC INJURIES

SPLENIC INJURIES

Splenic injuries account for over 50% of all intraabdominal injuries (Nicks & Manthey, 2020). Splenic injuries can be classified as contusions (bruising), lacerations, hematomas, and fractures. Splenic injuries are graded from 1 to 5 based on severity of injury, the size and location of the laceration or hematoma, and the presence of active bleeding. Higher grade splenic injuries are associated with significant morbidity and mortality. Treatment of splenic injury is dependent on the degree of injury, presence of intraabdominal hemorrhage, and hemodynamic instability and are typically evaluated on a case-by-case basis. While damage control surgery and splenectomy may be warranted in some patients, observation and nonoperative treatment (such as splenic embolization) may be appropriate in patients with lower-grade injury.

LIVER INJURIES

The liver is the most commonly injured solid organ in penetrating trauma and the second most common abdominal organ injured in blunt trauma mainly due to its size and location. Similar to splenic injuries, liver injuries can include contusions, lacerations, and hematomas and are also graded for severity and management. The majority of Grade 1 or 2 liver lacerations are managed nonsurgically, however all patients who present with evidence of a liver laceration should be evaluated and managed by a trauma surgeon. All decisions to non surgically manage liver lacerations should be made at the discretion of trauma surgery since delays in intervention are associated with significant morbidity and mortality. The most significant consequence of liver injuries is hemorrhage. Patients who present with significant blunt or penetrating liver injury and hemodynamic instability typically require laparotomy or selective arterial embolization to attempt hemorrhage control (Rozycki & Root, 2018).

BOWEL INJURIES

Duodenal injuries may initially present asymptomatically or be immediately overlooked during primary assessment or damage control when they occur concurrently with multisystem traumatic injury. As the duodenal hematoma expands, signs and symptoms of obstruction may develop (abdominal pain, distention, and vomiting). Patients may also develop delayed abscess development from spillage of enteric contents into the abdominal cavity. Delayed development of fever and leukocytes and potential sepsis can be an associated development of an abscess and bacterial translocation. Bowel perforation should be suspected with the presence of penetrating trauma with the small bowel being injured most often. Radiographic findings of free fluid or free air are highly suspicious for bowel perforation and injury (Rozycki & Root, 2018).

KIDNEY AND URETERAL INJURIES

Kidney injuries are the third most common abdominal organ injured in blunt abdominal trauma. Similar to the liver and spleen, kidneys can sustain lacerations, contusions, and fractures. Injuries that involve capsular rupture or vascular supply can result in significant intraabdominal hemorrhage. The most suspicious finding for ureteral injury is presence of gross hematuria upon initial evaluation. Both macroscopic and microscopic presence of hematuria should be monitored and evaluated (Rozycki & Root, 2018).

BLADDER INJURIES

Bladder injuries can occur in both blunt and penetrating traumatic injury. Bladder rupture has a mortality rate up to 20%, mainly due to the high correlation of rupture associated with presence of pelvic fractures. The presence of bladder rupture warrants immediate surgical consultation and repair (Rozycki & Root, 2018).

CLINICAL PEARLS

- Significant intraabdominal injury can present initially with benign abdominal exam findings.
- Positive FAST and radiographic exam findings with evidence of free fluid or free air is highly suspicious of bowel perforation and injury.

19.5: TRAUMATIC FRACTURES

Traumatic fractures cause disability, death, and significant cost to society (American College of Surgeons [ACS], 2018). Assessment of traumatic fractures follows the same evaluation pathway of all trauma-related evaluations: airway, breathing, circulation, disability, and exposure. While many traumatic fractures may appear dramatic, it is important to rule out life-threatening and limb-threatening injuries quickly and systematically. A fracture is described based on location: proximal, midshaft, or distal. A fracture is characterized as open or closed. An open fracture is a fracture in which there is direct communication with the external environment (Li et al., 2020). This section concentrates on extremity, pelvis, hip, and spine fractures. There are many types of traumatic fractures and they are further described in Table 19.3.

Extremity Fracture

Patients with extremity fractures may have an isolated injury or the extremity fracture may be part of a multisystem injury. All trauma evaluations begin with the systematic approach of a primary and secondary survey. Extremity fractures can be associated with significant blood loss. Closed fractures to the long bones of the femur and humerus may result in a 500 mL to 1500 mL blood loss (Lee & Porter, 2005).

TABLE 19.3: Types of Fractures

TYPE OF FRACTURE	DESCRIPTION OF FRACTURE
Comminuted	Two or more fracture pieces
Transverse	A transverse fracture through the bone
Oblique	An angled fracture
Segmental	Two distinct areas of fracture leaving a segment of bone in discontinuity of the rest of the bone
Compression	One vertebral body is compressed into the adjacent vertebral body
Impacted	Bony fragments are compressed

Source: Adapted from Morgan, S. (2018). Disorders of musculoskeletal function: Trauma, infection, neoplasm. In T. Norris (Eds.), *Porth's pathophysiology: Concepts of altered health status* (pp. 1349–1374). Wolters Kluwer

PRESENTING SIGNS AND SYMPTOMS

The chief complaint for extremity fractures is pain. Signs of an extremity fracture include hematoma, edema, lacerations, deformity, decreased or loss of motor and/or sensation, and tenderness over the injury site (Feichtinger et al., 2020).

HISTORY AND PHYSICAL FINDINGS

History

A detailed history is obtained when extremity fractures are suspected. Information of mechanism of injury, location, timing, and prehospital signs and symptoms are gathered. The mechanism of injury includes the manner in which the injury occurred. Common mechanisms of injury for extremity fractures include motor vehicle crashes, falls, crush injury, blast injury, motor vehicle striking of pedestrians, and penetrating injuries. Based on the mechanism of injury, specific patterns of injury may occur. For example, a pedestrian struck by a car may be associated with lower extremity injuries including tibia and fibula fractures. Distinguishing the location of where the injury occurred assists with the possibility of contamination of an open fracture (Li et al., 2020). Knowledge regarding the timing of the injury assists with ongoing bleeding or time a tourniquet was applied. Information on timing of tourniquet application assists in determining distal ischemia of the extremity. History obtained regarding the prehospital situation assists in plan of care including immobilization of the extremity and evidence of a decrease in motor function and sensation of the extremity (ACS, 2018).

Physical Examination

The identification of any life-threatening injuries is the first step in the physical exam. A systematic approach to the secondary survey assists in identifying extremity injuries. The extremities should be fully exposed for adequate assessment. The extremity assessment begins with inspection of the extremity skin for bleeding, ecchymosis, lacerations, abrasions, pallor, edema, and asymmetry while noting spontaneous motor function of the extremities. It is important to note any distal motor function of an extremity with a deformity. Palpation is the next assessment tool. Palpation includes the identification of areas of tenderness, crepitus, variations in temperature, and tense compartments of the extremity. If the patient is able to communicate, asking the patient to identify areas of tenderness should be incorporated into the assessment. Sensory evaluation of the extremity is performed to identify any potential nerve injury. Sensory deficits can also be present with expanding hematomas, spine injuries, and inadequate perfusion to the extremity. Distal pulse assessment ensures proper distal perfusion. If the patient is hypotensive, alternative pulse assessment such as Doppler is used to confirm adequate distal blood flow (ACS, 2018).

DIFFERENTIAL DIAGNOSIS AND DIAGNOSTIC CONSIDERATIONS

Any pertinent positive finding on history and/or physical examination should warrant further investigation. Differential diagnosis of an extremity injury include fracture, dislocation, ligamentous injury, tendon injury, nerve, or vascular injury. An x-ray should be obtained of the extremity. Other diagnostic imaging utilized may include CT and MRI to assess soft tissue, ligamentous, tendon, and vascular injuries (ACS, 2018).

TREATMENT

If an extremity fracture is diagnosed, referral to a surgical specialist is indicated. If there is a delay in the treatment, the extremity should be immobilized until the surgical consultation can occur. The surgical consultation will determine if the fracture is best treated with external immobilization or an internal fixation and/or reduction. If the fracture is an open fracture, a surgical consult should be done immediately. IV antibiotics, such as a first-generation cephalosporin, should be considered for all open fractures. Open fracture management includes operative exploration and debridement (Rodriguez et al., 2014). Tetanus immunization status should be ascertained in the presence of an open fracture (ACS, 2018).

PELVIC FRACTURES

Pelvic fractures are associated with a high energy impact to the body. Patients with a pelvic fracture and hypotension have a high rate of mortality. The mortality rate of pelvic fractures is estimated at 25% (Abdelrahman et al., 2020). An open book fracture is a fracture pattern where there is an anterior posterior compression injury. The compression causes disruption of pubic symphysis and thus opens the pelvic ring. This disruption causes injury to the arterial and venous systems. Figure 19.5 demonstrates the vascular anatomy within the pelvic ring.

Three other common classifications of pelvic fractures include lateral compression, vertical shear, and complex type. The lateral compression occurs with a lateral impact closing the pelvic ring. The closing of the ring is associated with less vascular injury hence a decrease in mortality (Skitch & Engels, 2018). The lateral compression fracture is the most common type of pelvic fracture. A vertical shear injury occurs when there is vertical disruption causing pelvic instability. The last type of pelvic fracture is a complex injury type where there is a combination of at least two types of pelvic fractures (Morgan, 2018).

PRESENTING SIGNS AND SYMPTOMS

The chief complaint related to a pelvic fracture is pain. Signs of a pelvic fracture include hematoma; hypotension; edema; lower extremity deformity; decreased or loss of distal motor function and/or sensation; blood at the rectum, vagina, or urethral meatus; hematuria; instability of the pelvis or tenderness of the pelvis (ACS, 2018).

HISTORY AND PHYSICAL FINDINGS

History

A detailed history is important when a pelvic fracture is suspected. Information should include mechanism of injury, location, timing, and prehospital signs and symptoms. Common mechanisms of injury for pelvic fractures include motor vehicle crashes, falls, crush injury, blast

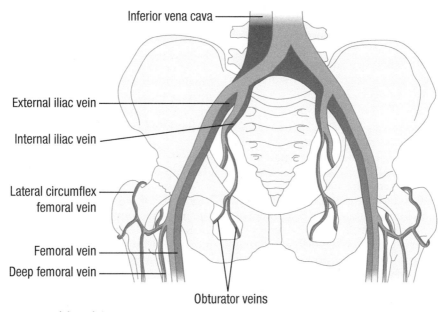

FIGURE 19.5: Vascular anatomy of the pelvis.

injury, or struck pedestrian (Abdelrahman et al., 2020). Important information regarding the prehospital care include vital signs, especially if there is hypotension, the use of a pelvic stability device, and resuscitation such as IV fluid or blood products prior to arrival (ACS, 2018).

Physical Examination

The first step in assessing a pelvis is to determine hemodynamic stability. Tachycardia, hypotension, and change in mental status can all be signs of hypovolemic shock (ACS, 2018). The assessment of the pelvis begins with the inspection of the pelvic region. Evidence of blood at the rectum, the vagina or the urethral meatus, scrotal hematoma, and hematuria are signs of urethral disruption which is a sign of a pelvic fracture. Lower extremity shortening or rotation without deformity are consistent findings with a pelvic fracture. Palpation is used to elicit tenderness of the bony prominence as well as manual manipulation of the pelvis. Manual manipulation of the pelvis consists of gentle equal pressure over the iliac wings in a downward fashion. If there is laxity of the pelvis, it is considered an unstable pelvis. Once a pelvis is classified as unstable, no other manual manipulation exams should be performed for concern of further disruption of vasculature. If a fracture of the pelvis is suspected, a rectal and internal vaginal exam are indicated to ensure there are no obvious bony protrusions from the pelvic fracture (ACS, 2018).

DIFFERENTIAL DIAGNOSIS AND DIAGNOSTIC CONSIDERATIONS

A pelvic fracture is suspected based on the mechanism of injury when there is unexplained hemodynamic instability and with the complaint of pain in the pelvic area. Other potential diagnoses include intrabdominal injury, hip fracture, and femur fracture. If a patient is hemodynamically unstable, an AP pelvic x-ray is performed. However, due to the risk of having coinciding abdominal injuries, patients that are hemodynamically stable may undergo a CT of the abdomen and pelvis generally to rule out fracture as well as vascular injuries and abdominal injuries (Skitch & Engels, 2018).

TREATMENT

Initial treatment of a pelvic fracture is focused on the hemodynamic stability of the patient. If the patient is classified as hemodynamically unstable, fluid resuscitation and control of the hemorrhage are the priorities. If a pelvis is classified as unstable, mechanical stabilization of the pelvis is indicated to decrease the potential hemorrhage. A pelvic binder or a sheet may be wrapped around the pelvis to try to control hemorrhage within the pelvis. Surgical consultation is warranted for any pelvic fracture and hemodynamic instability. The pelvis is a difficult area to obtain operative control of bleeding. Angiography can be used to assist with ongoing bleeding in the pelvis. Other treatment options include

traction, operative internal fixation and/or reduction, and nonoperative treatment (Skitch & Engels, 2018).

HIP FRACTURES

Hip fractures are an increasing health concern with the aging population. The continuous increase in hip fracture incidence is related to the increase in the older adult population. Hip fractures are associated with significant morbidity and mortality. There is a 5% to 10% increase in mortality within 3 months of a hip fracture (Mukherjee et al., 2020). Females are at higher risk than males for having a hip fracture. Ninety-five percent of hip fractures are caused by falls (Centers for Disease Control and Prevention [CDC], 2016).

Hip fractures are classified based on the location of the fracture. The most common types of hip fractures are femoral neck and intertrochanteric fractures. Femoral neck fractures have the potential to disrupt blood supply to the area. The disruption of blood supply is linked to complications including nonunion and avascular necrosis (Morgan, 2018).

PRESENTING SIGNS AND SYMPTOMS

Most hip fractures in the older adult occur from a minimal impact trauma such as a fall from standing. Some hip fractures occur as a result of a fall due to weakened bone (American Academy of Orthopaedic Surgeons, 2015). The associated chief complaint with hip fractures is generally pain in the affected hip. Other signs of a hip fracture include a hematoma, edema, and rotated or shortened lower extremity (ACS, 2018).

HISTORY AND PHYSICAL FINDINGS

History

As with other traumatic fractures, understanding the mechanism of injury and timing is important in hip fractures. Identifying patients risk factors such as osteoporosis or known neoplasm is important aspect of their past medical history. If the mechanism of injury was a fall, further inquiry regarding frequency of falls, possibility of abuse, and use of assistive devices are important (American College of Surgeons [ACS], 2018).

Physical Examination

The hip assessment begins with inspection of the extremity skin for bleeding, ecchymosis, lacerations, abrasions, pallor, edema, and asymmetry. Observation of spontaneous movement of the extremity is part of the inspection. Motor assessment of the extremity should be performed unless there is an obvious deformity. Palpation is the second aspect of the examination. Palpation of the hip includes the identification of areas of tenderness, crepitus, variations in temperature and firmness of the extremity. Distal pulse assessment ensures proper distal perfusion (ACS, 2018).

DIFFERENTIAL DIAGNOSIS AND DIAGNOSTIC CONSIDERATIONS

The differential diagnosis of a hip fracture includes contusion or sprain of the hip joint. Other potential diagnoses include pelvic fractures and a distal femur fracture. A radiographic x-ray is the first-line diagnostic imaging for a hip fracture. CT or MRI may be obtained if soft tissue, vascular, or missed injury on radiographic x-ray are suspected (Rehman et al., 2016).

TREATMENT

Initial treatment of a hip fracture includes pain control, fracture reduction if indicated with traction or splinting, and consultation with an orthopedic surgeon. Surgical treatment within 48 hours of the hip fracture remains the preferred approach to hip fractures. The type of surgical treatment is based on the type of hip fracture. Surgical treatment options include total hip arthroplasty, hemi-arthroplasty, nail and screw fixation. Besides the type of hip fracture, preexisting conditions and fraility of the patient are also considered. Osteoporosis and arthritis are important factors for type of treatment (American Academy of Orthopaedic Surgeons, 2015). Non operative treatment is considered when the older adult is frail with comorbidities. However, nonoperative treatment has been linked to a higher complication and mortality rate (Kim et al., 2020). Other treatment regimens include osteoporosis treatment, fall prevention, and exercise programs (Mukherjee et al., 2020).

SPINE FRACTURES

Spine fractures occur in 5% of the population over the lifetime. Cervical spine fractures comprise 55% of all spinal fractures. The other spine fractures are distributed equally between the thoracic and lumbar regions (Cosman et al., 2017).

PRESENTING SIGNS AND SYMPTOMS

Similar to other traumatic fractures, spine fractures have a chief complaint of pain. However, the chief complaint may vary depending on the severity of injury. Other symptoms of a spine fracture include loss of motor or sensation. Signs of spinal fractures are hematoma over the posterior spine, hypotension, edema, decreased or loss of distal motor and/or sensation, shortness of breath, or bradycardia, bowel, and bladder dysfunction (ACS, 2018).

HISTORY AND PHYSICAL FINDINGS

History

Understanding the mechanism of injury and timing is important in spine fractures. Common mechanisms of injury for spine fractures include motor vehicle crashes, falls, crush injury, blast injury, and penetrating trauma. Timing of the injury is important especially when the patient is hypotensive. Information regarding the pre-hospital care includes vital signs, the use of a cervical collar, and the maintenance of inline stabilization of the entire spine. Vertebral fractures are also associated with osteoporosis. Hence, a detailed review of the patient's past medical and past functional history is indicated (Cosman et al., 2017).

Physical Examination

All suspected trauma patients should receive a full trauma evaluation to identify life-threatening injuries. Regarding a suspected spine fracture, spinal stabilization must continue until the potential of a spine fracture or other spinal injury has been eliminated. During the secondary survey, assessment of the entire spine is indicated for deformity, ecchymosis, lacerations, abrasions, or lack of spontaneous motor function. Palpation requires a team to provide inline stabilization while the examiner palpates the entire spine. Proper palpation includes the removal of the cervical collar while maintaining cervical immobilization. Any tenderness with palpation, crepitus, or laxity of the bony prominence are suggestive of a spinal fracture. A neuromuscular exam and rectal exam should also be performed and documented when there is a suspected spinal fracture (ACS, 2018).

DIFFERENTIAL DIAGNOSIS AND DIAGNOSTIC CONSIDERATIONS

Differential diagnoses for spinal fractures include dislocation, ligamentous injuries, hematoma, sprain, and disc injury. While emergency radiographic x-rays may be used to assess for fractures, the preferred imaging for traumatic spine injuries is CT scan. If the CT scan is negative, however, and the patient continues to have pain with range of motion of the neck, an MRI is indicated. A spinal MRI assesses for injuries to the ligaments, discs, spinal cord, and other injuries to the soft tissue (Tins, 2017).

TREATMENT

The treatment of a spine fracture varies based on the injury type. Treatment of an isolated transverse process fracture of the thoracic spine may consist of pain control. A cervical spine fracture with neurologic deficits may require immediate operative decompression of the spinal cord. If there is an unstable fracture that cannot be immediately operated on, spinal traction can be used to temporarily realign the spine and decompress the spinal cord.

A halo device maintains cervical alignment. Halo devices have relatively effective clinical outcomes for spinal fusion. However, the halo device is linked to complications of aspiration, dysphagia, and increased falls (Sharpe et al., 2016). Surgical decompression and fusion are operative options to repair malalignment and allow fusion of the fractures. Cervical collars and thoracic braces may be used as treatment to reduce the range of motion of the injured spine segment for clinically stable fractures.

19.6: FACIAL FRACTURES

Facial fractures occur globally at a rate of 98 per 100,000 people. Facial fractures cause disability as well as the potential for airway obstruction, breathing difficulties, and bleeding. Falls are the most common mechanism of injury associated with facial fractures (Lalloo et al., 2020).

ORBITAL FRACTURE

Orbital fractures commonly occur due to a blunt injury to the eye region. The orbit is a bone that surrounds the eye. It encases the eyeball as well as the eye's vascular and nerve matrix.

PRESENTING SIGNS AND SYMPTOMS

Similar to other traumatic fractures, orbital fractures may have a chief complaint of pain. Symptoms may include a sensation of a foreign object or discomfort with eye movement. Signs of orbital fractures include ecchymosis, edema, crepitus, tenderness with palpation, and decreased visual acuity (American College of Surgeons [ACS], 2018).

HISTORY AND PHYSICAL FINDINGS

History

The mechanism of injury and timing are significant pieces of the history for orbital fractures. Common mechanisms of injury for orbital fractures include falls, motor vehicle crashes, assault, and penetrating trauma (Lalloo, 2020). Specific history for a suspected orbital fracture includes baseline visual acuity, use of corrective lenses, current use of contact lenses, and history of increased intraocular pressure (ACS, 2018).

Physical Examination

The eye exam begins with inspection of pupil for size, shape, reactivity, ecchymosis, lacerations, abrasions, hemorrhage of the conjunctiva, and visual acuity testing. An examination of the extraocular movements of the eye is performed to assess for muscle or nerve entrapment within the fracture. Palpation of the bony ridges is performed to elicit tenderness, crepitus, or to detect instability (ACS, 2018).

DIFFERENTIAL DIAGNOSIS AND DIAGNOSTIC CONSIDERATIONS

Differential diagnoses of orbital fractures include other facial fractures as well as frontal bone fractures, traumatic brain injury, and cervical spine injuries. Globe rupture, extraocular muscle entrapment, nerve injury, and

hemorrhage may also be part of the differential diagnosis. While radiographic x-ray is able to show the bony structure of the face, the preferred diagnostic tool is a CT scan. CT allows for visualization into the orbital socket. Other diagnostic considerations with orbital fractures include intraocular pressure measurement (Lalloo et al., 2020).

TREATMENT

The treatment of orbital fractures should be focused on the physical exam findings. A consultation to an ophthalmologist is recommended for any orbital fractures. If the fractures are stable they may be treated with nonoperative management. If the fractures include displacement, entrapment of muscle, or increased intraoperative pressure, surgical treatment is indicated (Lalloo et al., 2020).

LE FORT FRACTURES

Le Fort fractures were first described by Rene Le Fort. Le Fort fractures describe injury patterns to the face. A Le Fort fracture is not correlated with a high mortality rate in isolation; however, it is associated with concurrent traumatic brain injuries and cervical spine injuries. The most common mechanisms of injury associated with Le Fort fractures include motor vehicle crashes, assaults, and falls (Phillips & Turco, 2017). There are three types of Le Fort fractures: Le Fort I, Le Fort II, and Le Fort III. Figure 19.6 illustrates these fracture patterns.

Le Fort I is described as a horizontal fracture of the maxilla above the root of the teeth. The fracture extends to nasal septum and the pterygoid plate. It can be unilateral or bilateral. Le Fort II is described as a fracture superiorly in the midface which includes the nasal bridge, maxilla, orbital floor, and orbital rim. The pattern is one of a triangle where the teeth are the base and nasal bridge is the tip. Le Fort II is usually considered

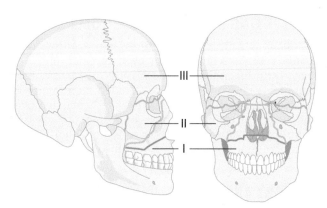

FIGURE 19.6: Le Fort fractures. Type I, horizontal, alveolar ridge; Type II, pyramidal, nasofrontoal suture; Type III, horizontal, craniofacial dislocation.

Source: Cahoon, T. M., & Redden, K. (2022). Le Fort Osteotomy. In J. S. Furstein (Ed.), *Pediatric anesthesia: A comprehensive approach to safe and effective care*. Springer Publishing Company, Fig. 80.2.

bilateral. Le Fort III is described as a fracture through the nasal bridge through the medial floor and lateral orbital walls extending to the zygomatic arch. Le Fort II and III are associated with other associated injuries such as epistaxis, cerebral spinal fluid drainage, and extraocular muscle or nerve entrapment (Phillips & Turco, 2017).

PRESENTING SIGNS AND SYMPTOMS

Symptoms of Le Fort fractures include pain, difficulty breathing, and decreased vision. Signs of the fractures are dependent on the location of the fractures. Common signs include edema, malocclusion of the jaw, ecchymosis, deformity, and distortion of facial structures, leakage of cerebrospinal fluid (CSF), dentition fractures, and epistaxis (Phillips & Turco, 2017).

HISTORY AND PHYSICAL FINDINGS

History

As with other fractures, understanding the mechanism of injury and timing are significant pieces of the history for Le Fort fractures. Information about mechanism of injury, location, timing, and prehospital signs and symptoms guide the clinical diagnosis. Common mechanisms of injury include motor vehicle crashes, assaults, and falls. Prehospital information should include potential airway obstruction, difficulty breathing, epistaxis, and any discharge from the nose or ears (ACS, 2018).

Physical Examination

Le Fort fractures are associated with other injuries including traumatic brain injuries and cervical spine fractures. A systematic trauma evaluation identifies life-threatening injuries. Examination of the Le Fort fractures begins with inspection of pupil size and reactivity, ecchymosis, lacerations, abrasions, epistaxis, drainage from nose or ears. Examination of the oral pharynx assists in identification of dental fractures, discoloration of the upper palate or posterior CSF/blood drainage. An examination of the extraocular movements of the eye is performed to assess for muscle or nerve entrapment plus palpation of the bony areas of the face to assess for tenderness or obvious instability (Phillips & Turco, 2017).

DIFFERENTIAL DIAGNOSIS AND DIAGNOSTIC CONSIDERATIONS

Le Fort fractures differential diagnoses include isolated fractures of the face. Other diagnosis to consider include traumatic brain injury (TBI) and cervical spine injuries. Similar to orbital fractures, globe rupture, extraocular muscle entrapment, nerve injury, and hemorrhage may also be present. As with the orbital fractures, radiographic x-ray allows visualization of the bony structures; however, CT scan is the preferred diagnostic tool. It is suggested that a CT of the brain and cervical spine is also done due to the correlation of Le Fort fractures and other significant head and neck trauma (Phillips & Turco, 2017).

TREATMENT

Initial treatment is focused on identification of injuries, bleeding, and airway protection. If airway protection is a concern, the patient should receive a definitive airway through either endotracheal tube or tracheostomy. Twenty-two percent of patients with a Le Fort fracture receive a tracheostomy. Le Fort fractures require consultation of a facial surgeon. Surgical treatment for Le Fort fractures occur in 60% of all Le Fort fractures. Le Fort I fractures require less surgical intervention when compared to Le Fort II and Le Fort III (Phillips & Turco, 2017).

TRANSITION OF CARE AFTER TRAUMATIC FRACTURES

Traumatic fractures cause significant disability and morbidity. Many traumatic fractures are treated, and the patient is not admitted to the hospital. Of those admitted trauma patients, 36% do not go home at time of discharge. Factors identified with an increased risk of a nonhome discharge included older age, female gender, higher injury severity score (ISS), concurrent comorbidities, and Medicare insurance (Graham et al., 2020). As with all admitted patients, discharge should begin at time of admission.

19.7: MULTISYSTEM TRAUMA

PRESENTING SIGNS AND SYMPTOMS

Seldom does the traumatic patient present with just one isolated injury. Trauma involving two or more anatomical systems such as a chest stab wound with a pneumothorax and subclavian vein injury is an example of multisystem trauma. The most frequent cause of multisystem trauma is blunt injury from a motor vehicle collision (MVC). Vehicle type, seat-belt use, and speed of collision impact outcomes from MVCs; patients can present with head, spine, thoracic, abdominal, and extremity injuries. The physical exam allows the provider to make differential diagnoses based on region of the body in multisystem trauma; for example, a "lap belt and bucket handle" (ACS, 2018, p. 85) injury from a seat belt leads the provider to suspect colon, spleen, aorta, and thoracic injuries.

The injury severity score was first introduced in 1974 by Susan Baker and colleagues; it assesses the combined effects of multisystem trauma and is based on an abbreviated injury scale classification (AIS). Each injury is assigned an AIS score in the range of 1 to 6 (see Table 19.4) in one of six body regions. Only the highest AIS score in each body region is used. The three most severely injured body regions with the highest scores have their AIS score squared and added together for the total ISS (Table 19.5). The total ISS is between 0 and 75, with the higher the score the poorer the outcome. This internationally recognized scoring system directly correlates with trauma mortality and morbidity. Although

TABLE 19.4: Abbreviated Injury Scale

SCORE	ABBREVIATED INJURY SCALE (AIS)	EXAMPLE
1	Minor	Facial abrasion
2	Moderate	Subcapsular liver hematoma
3	Serious	Subarachnoid hematoma
4	Severe	Bilateral femur fracture
5	Critical	Flail chest
6	Unsurvivable	Decapitation

TABLE 19.5: Injury Severity Score

BODY REGION	INJURY DESCRIPTION	ABBREVIATED INJURY SCALE (AIS)	SQUARE THE TOP THREE
Head and neck	Cerebral contusion	3	9
Face	No injury	0	
Chest	Flail chest	5	25
Abdomen	Severe splenic rupture	5	25
Extremity	Unilateral femur fracture	3	
External	Minor abrasions	1	
TOTAL Injury Severity Score: 59 ISS = Sum of (3 highest AIS values)^2 ISS = $a^2 + b^2 + c^2$			

updated iterations of the ISS have been developed, the ISS continues to be the most commonly used in U.S. emergency departments (Shi et al., 2019).

Prioritization of the "ABCDE" methodology for the primary survey is key for multisystem trauma patients in shock as they could be experiencing several types of shock requiring differing interventions. However, fundamental concepts to resuscitation of a multisystem trauma patient are constant; identification of injuries is paramount (Ali, 2014).

Computed Tomography

CT can provide diagnostic information to specific organs injured and extent of injury. Modern CT scanners are fast, provide immediate imaging for the emergency department provider, and are the examination of choice for patients that are hemodynamically stable but whose suspected multisystem injuries require further evaluation. For example, retroperitoneal, pelvic, and major vessel

injuries are difficult to assess with a traditional physical exam. CT exams require availability of a CT machine, patient transport, considerations for IV contrast, and patient cooperation—all of which could delay this diagnostic tool (Menaker & Boswell, 2020).

Ultrasound

In a skilled provider, the use of ultrasound in multisystem trauma patients is part of the primary survey and can be a lifesaving diagnostic tool in patients both hemodynamically stable and unstable. The FAST exam is a protocolized ultrasound of the abdomen and thorax regions, designed to detect free fluid in the peritoneum and pericardium. The protocol requires four total views: three views of the abdomen and one of the heart (Figure 19.7). Blood in the pericardial sac can be detected by the subcostal view of the heart. Abdominal views can detect free fluid in the RUQ, LUQ, and the pelvis. However, it should be noted that ultrasound cannot distinguish between what type of fluid exists in these areas, for example blood versus urine versus bowel contents.

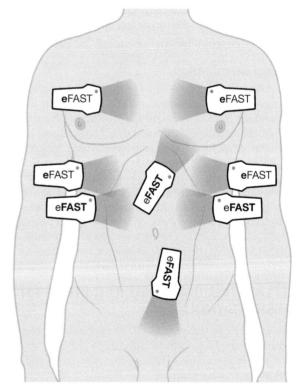

FIGURE 19.7: Ultrasound probe location for FAST and eFAST exams.
Source: Campo, T. M., & Lafferty, K. A. (2021). *Essential procedures for emergency, urgent, and primary care settings: A clinical companion* (3rd ed.). Springer Publishing Company, Fig. 5.1.

The eFAST exam (extended focused assessment with sonography in trauma) is an extension of the FAST exam. In addition to the four basic FAST views, the eFAST adds one view of the anterior and dorsolateral on each side of the thorax, for four views total of the lungs. These views allow for detection of a hemothorax and/or pneumothorax.

Additional ultrasound applications exist for the diagnosis of injuries in the multisystem trauma patient, such as examining for hydronephrosis, examining the aorta for dissection, bone fracture identification, and ocular injuries (Weile et al., 2017; Whitson & Mayo, 2016).

X-Ray

Emergency departments often have x-ray machines in their trauma bays. Simple x-rays with immediate electronic visualization of images can allow for the rapid diagnosis of life-threatening injuries throughout the body; pneumothorax, pelvic fracture, retained bullets, and bony fractures are just a few examples. Although ultrasound evaluation from a skilled provider can diagnose some of these injuries, x-ray remains a vital aspect of the care of the traumatic injury patient, especially when the patient is so hemodynamically unstable that transporting to a CT scanner is too dangerous (Menaker & Boswell, 2020).

CLINICAL PEARLS

- Identifying injuries in multisystem trauma can be achieved using the "ABCDE" algorithm during the primary survey.
- Diagnostic tools can assist the provider in identifying life-threatening traumatic injuries but should not delay treatment for hemodynamically unstable injuries.

19.8: TRAUMA IN THE ELDERLY

In 2016, 22.8% of the U.S. population were 65 years of age or older. It is predicted that by 2060, 25% of our population will be older than 65 years of age. Furthermore, the number of individuals expected to be 85 years or older is expected to triple by 2060. While our older adults are living longer, they are also living with more comorbidities. Seventy-five percent of individuals aged 65 and older have at least one comorbidity (Hamidi & Joseph, 2019).

CHANGES IN PHYSIOLOGY

The physiology of the older adult changes over time. Many of these physiologic changes place an older adult trauma patient at risk for higher morbidity and mortality. The changes in physiology coupled with comorbidities increase the mortality rate in the older adult trauma

patient. Decreased muscle mass and decreased respiratory vital capacity increase the risk of aspiration, atelectasis, and pneumonia. The decrease in cardiac stroke volume and heart rate associated with aging does not allow the physiologic response to hemorrhagic shock. In some cases, older adults are on medications such as beta-blockers that do not allow for a compensatory increase in heart rate seen with hemorrhagic shock. The older adult may have altered renal function that increases the risk of developing acute kidney injury. Decreased elasticity of skin and thinning epidermis leads to tears in the skin and difficulty in wound healing. The thermal regulatory response of the older adult also impairs the ability to regulate body temperature leading to an increased risk of hypothermia (American College of Surgeons [ACS], 2018). Due to co morbidities, older adults are more likely to be on antiplatelet or anticoagulants which increases risk for traumatic brain, thoracic, abdominal, and pelvic hemorrhage. Frail older adults have a 25% mortality rate within 1 year of a trauma (Benoit et al., 2019).

MECHANISM OF INJURY

Falls are the most common mechanism of injury in geriatric trauma. One in four older adults fall each year (Bollinger et al., 2015). A fall raises the risk of a future fall in the older adult. Other fall risks for the older adult include medication effects, changes of the nervous and musculoskeletal systems, sensory impairments, and environmental hazards. Motor vehicle crashes are the second most common mechanism of trauma injury in the older adult. Other mechanisms of injury include pedestrian strikes, suicide, and abuse (Benoit et al., 2019).

INJURY

Many injuries have specific considerations for the older adult. Chest injuries such as rib fractures have a higher morbidity and mortality rate than in younger patients. The physiologic changes of the chest plus the pain of the rib fractures lead to a higher rate of atelectasis and pneumonia leading to a higher mortality rate. The risk factors of osteoporosis, osteoarthritis, degenerative disc disease, and spinal stenosis make spinal fractures and thus spinal cord injuries more prevalent in the older adult. Osteoporosis contributes to the spontaneous fractures of the vertebral body and hip. Adults over the age of 85 years have a 1% occurrence of spontaneous fracture of the vertebral body or hip every year (ACS, 2018).

CONCLUSIONS

While the older adult has an increased risk of disability and death, care should be taken to create individual plans of care to overcome the physiologic changes including multimodal pain control to decrease the risk of delirium, early operative management to allow for increased morbidity, and eliciting specialists to assist with early mobilization. Specialists such physiatry (rehabilitation specialist), palliative care, and geriatrics should be considered as part of the multispecialty team. Social work should be involved for transition of care and to ensure that the elderly are safe in their community settings. Whenever possible, older adults should be part of the goals of care. The older adult faces incredible challenges. However, dedicated and focused care can overcome many of the challenges the older trauma patient faces.

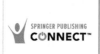

A robust set of instructor resources designed to supplement this text is located at **http://connect.springerpub.com/content/ reference-book/978-0-8261-6079-9.** Qualifying instructors may request access by emailing **textbook@springerpub.com.**

REFERENCES

Full list of references can be accessed at http://connect .springerpub.com/content/reference-book/978-0-8261-6079-9.

CHAPTER 20

FLUID, ELECTROLYTES, AND ACID-BASE DISORDERS

Maggie Thompson

LEARNING OBJECTIVES

- Describe the homeostatic mechanisms controlled by electrolytes.
- Recognize common presentation, diagnosis, and management of various electrolyte imbalances.
- Discuss the importance of homeostasis in acid-base balance.
- Evaluate different types of IV fluids and the indications for each.

INTRODUCTION

Fluid, electrolyte, and acid-base derangements are frequently encountered pathologies in the acute care setting. A pathologic process leaves the patient's body unable to compensate for the disease state, and in turn, the body is unable to regulate fluids and electrolytes as it normally would. It is essential for the adult gerontology acute care nurse practitioner (AGACNP) to understand the normal physiologic processes sustained by these balances and subsequently the alterations driven by acute and critical illnesses. In order to understand the implications of volume and acid-base management, it is important to first understand the normal functioning of electrolytes and the implications of their derangements. Electrolytes such as sodium, potassium, and calcium are essential for normal cellular functioning.

ELECTROLYTE–SODIUM

Sodium abnormalities, hypo- and hypernatremia, are the most frequently encountered electrolyte derangements in clinical practice. Additionally, the development of either hypo- or hypernatremia has been correlated with an increase in morbidity and mortality. In order to understand why sodium disorders have such serious implications for patient outcomes, it is important to understand sodium regulation and its function within the body.

Sodium is the most abundant cation within the body and determines the plasma osmolality. Osmolality is the concentration of dissolved particles within a kilogram of water. Normal serum osmolality is between 280 and 295 mmol mOsm/kg H_2O. Tonicity is determined by the concentration of osmoles that do not freely cross the cell membrane, or effective osmolality (Seay et al., 2020). The tonicity of the plasma determines the concentration of water within the cell and can expose cells to stress when not in homeostasis. For cell volume to remain stable, extracellular, or plasma, sodium levels should remain between 135 and 145 mmol/L. If tonicity of extracellular plasma is greater than that of intracellular tonicity (i.e., there is a higher concentration of osmoles outside of the cell), the cell is disposed to *hypertonic stress*. Water will shift from intracellular to the plasma to dilute the surrounding plasma, causing cell shrinkage. Conversely, if the extracellular tonicity is low, the cell is exposed to *hypotonic stress*, water will shift to intracellular in an attempt to reach an equal concentration of water and solutes. This will cause cell edema. Because serum and intracellular sodium and water concentration are closely intertwined, sodium disorders are frequently called water metabolism disorders. Additionally, derangements in sodium are often driven by changes in total body water rather than by changes in the concentration of the cation itself (Braun et al., 2015).

Tonicity within the body is regulated by the pituitary gland and kidneys. The primary hormone responsible for tonicity regulation is antidiuretic hormone (ADH), also known as arginine vasopressin (AVP). The pre-prohormone of ADH is created within the hypothalamus, cleaved into ADH, then stored within the pituitary gland. When plasma tonicity increases, osmoreceptors within the hypothalamus cause the release of ADH. ADH then acts on the collecting ducts of the kidneys to promote water reabsorption and retention to counteract the increase in serum tonicity. As tonicity increases, ADH secretion increases (Balanescu et al., 2011). ADH secretion is also triggered by decreased blood volume or blood pressure via activation of baroreceptors within the cardiovascular system. Conversely, when serum tonicity decreases or sodium plasma falls below 135 mmol/L, vasopressin secretion is inhibited.

Without vasopressin present the collecting ducts within the kidneys are impermeable to water and the kidneys produce dilute urine. Solute-free urine production is known as aquaresis. When present, vasopressin binds to the V2 receptor within the collecting duct to increase the permeability of the collecting duct. This allows the reabsorption of water rather than the excretion of water. In turn, with vasopressin present, the kidneys produce concentrated urine with high osmolality. Urine osmolality can be used as an indirect marker of vasopressin activity (Seay et al., 2020). The ability to concentrate urine as a result of plasma tonicity is often impaired in patients with chronic kidney disease.

The brain exists within a fixed space in the skull and is particularly sensitive to volume shifting due to changes in sodium and water concentration. Subsequently, the most feared complications of hypo- and hypernatremia are of neurologic consequence. The brain can adapt to chronic changes in osmolality (i.e., >48 hours), but is unable to adapt when changes in sodium occur abruptly (i.e., <48 hours). This concept has critical implications for sodium derangements and their treatments including osmotic demyelination syndrome (ODS) which will be discussed in detail in this chapter.

HYPONATREMIA

Hyponatremia is the most frequently encountered electrolyte disorder in clinical practice with 15% to 30% of hospitalized patients demonstrating a decrease in serum sodium (Upadhyay et al., 2006). The direct cost of hyponatremia on an annual basis in the United States alone is estimated to be between $1.6 and $3.6 million (Boscoe et al., 2006). Hyponatremia is also associated with increased morbidity and mortality outcomes for patients. When compared to normonatremic hospitalized patients over 65 years of age or older, hyponatremic hospitalized patients of this age group were found to be twice as likely to die during their hospitalization (Terzian et al., 1994). Patients with heart failure who develop hyponatremia have an increased risk of mortality (Verbalis et al., 2013). Hyponatremia concurrent with liver disease leads to an increased risk of hepatorenal syndrome, hepatic encephalopathy, and overall mortality (Ginès & Schrier, 2009; Ginès et al., 1993; Guevara et al., 2010). Furthermore, any patient with severe hyponatremia is at risk for osmotically induced cerebral edema.

Hyponatremia is defined as a serum sodium of <136 mmol/L and severe hyponatremia defined as serum sodium <125 mmol/L (Hoorn & Zietse, 2017). The clinical manifestations and implications for hyponatremia vary based upon rate of derangement development and the degree of impairment. Acute hyponatremia develops in a timespan of <48 hours, while chronic hyponatremia occurs in a timeframe >48 hours. Plasma tonicity typically correlates with hyponatremia. Most hyponatremias are hypotonic hyponatremias which will primarily be discussed within this chapter. This indicates a plasma osmolality of <280 mOsm/kg H_2O (Table 20.1). The patient's history, physical exam, and laboratory diagnostics will further define the type of hyponatremia.

Hypovolemic Hypotonic Hyponatremia

Hyponatremia can occur in the setting of volume depletion with associated solute loss. Thiazide diuretics are often associated with hyponatremia as they impair the ability of the kidney to concentrate urine. Extensive gastrointestinal losses in the setting of a low-sodium diet may also cause hyponatremia. Cerebral salt wasting following head trauma or neurosurgical procedures may cause hypovolemic hyponatremia. Primary adrenal insufficiency with mineralocorticoid deficiency will cause hyponatremia due to renal sodium wasting (Seay et al., 2020).

Euvolemic Hypotonic Hyponatremia

Syndrome of inappropriate antidiuretic hormone (SIADH) is the leading cause of euvolemic hyponatremia (Verbalis et al., 2013). This includes both cerebral and nephrogenic SIADH. SIADH causes renal salt wasting with associated water reabsorption. Bartter & Schwartz (1967) proposed criteria to diagnose SIADH that are still used today (Box 20.1; Bartter & Schwartz, 1967). Tumors with ectopic hormone production, such as small-cell lung cancers, central nervous system disorders, and pulmonary diseases are at high risk for development of SIADH.

Another common cause of this form of hyponatremia is drug administration. The mnemonic CAR DISH is used to identify the common medications associated with hyponatremia: chemotherapy, antidepressants/antipsychotics, anticonvulsants, antiinflammatory drugs, recreational drugs, diuretics, inhibitors, sulfonylureas, hormones and hypnotics (Box 20.2; Tee & Dang, 2017).

TABLE 20.1: Hyponatremia and Serum Tonicity

EVALUATION OF HYPONATREMIA AND TONICITY		
	SERUM SODIUM CONCENTRATION (mmol/L)	PLASMA OSMOLALITY (mOsm/kg H_2O)
Hypotonic	<135	Low (<280)
Isotonic	<135	Normal (280–295)
Hypertonic	<135	High (>295)

BOX 20.1 SIADH DIAGNOSTIC CRITERIA

- Decreased serum osmolality (<275 mOsm/kg)
- Inappropriate urine concentration—increased urine osmolality (>100 mOsm/kg)
- Clinical euvolemia
- Increased urine sodium excretion (>20–30 mmol/L)
- No other cause for euvolemic hyponatremia (severe hypothyroidism, hypocortisolism, normal renal function)

SIADH, syndrome of inappropriate diuretic hormone.

BOX 20.2 MEDICATIONS ASSOCIATED WITH HYPONATREMIA

- **C**hemotherapy
- **A**ntidepressants, **A**ntipsychotics, **A**nticonvulsants, **A**nti-inflammatory
- **R**ecreational drugs
- **D**iuretics
- **I**nhibitors (angiotensin-converting enzyme inhibitors, selective serotonin reuptake inhibitors)
- **S**ufonylureas
- **H**ormones, **H**ypnotics

Exercised-induced hyponatremia (EAH) results following endurance athletics such as marathons and ultramarathons. It is thought that nonosmotically stimulated AVP secretion due to excessive ingestion of water during these activities leads to euvolemic, rather than hypovolemic, hyponatremia.

Low-solute intake hyponatremia results from large volume intake with low solute content. Patients who drink large quantities of beer with little food intake over a prolonged period (beer potomania) limits solute-free water excretion given the low solute load in beer, causing water retention and hyponatremia. Primary polydipsia, or excessive water intake, can be seen in psychiatric patients, especially those with psychosis due to schizophrenia. Polydipsia has been reported in up to 20% of inpatient psychiatric patients (de Leon et al., 1994).

Pituitary disorders that impair normal ACTH secretion lead to secondary adrenal insufficiency that may also cause euvolemic hyponatremia. Hypothyroidism is also a rare cause of hyponatremia.

Hypervolemic Hypotonic Hyponatremia

Hypervolemic hyponatremia is caused by conditions that promote renal salt and water reabsorption. Edema is caused by the water and sodium retention. Heart failure, cirrhosis, acute kidney injury (AKI), chronic kidney injury, and nephrotic syndrome impair the kidneys' ability to maximally excrete water, and in turn, cause hyponatremia.

Pseudohyponatremia

Significant elevations in plasma lipids and proteins can cause an artificial decrease in the measured serum sodium. It is important to note if either of these conditions is present prior to diagnosing hyponatremia to prevent unnecessary testing and/or treatment.

Isotonic/Hypertonic Hyponatremia

Iso- to hypertonic hyponatremia occurs when there are excessive solutes within the serum. This solute gradient causes water to shift from the intracellular space to the extracellular space and subsequently causes a dilutional hyponatremia. Hyperglycemia is the most common etiology of this form of hyponatremia. The sodium can be corrected based on the serum glucose. For every 100 mg/dL increase in serum glucose, the concentration of sodium decreases by around 1.6 mEq/L. In instances where the serum glucose is >400 mg/dL, the concentration of sodium may decrease by 2.4 mEq/L per 100 mg/dL of glucose (Seay et al., 2020). As the glucose improves, the hyponatremia will resolve.

The administration of mannitol, radiographic contrast agents, or glycine from surgical irrigation can also cause hyponatremia. Each of these substances introduces additional solutes into the plasma and does not allow for accurate measurement of serum sodium (Verbalis et al., 2013).

PRESENTING SIGNS AND SYMPTOMS

The presentation of a patient with hyponatremia varies based on the acuity of the presentation and the degree of hyponatremia. Neurologic manifestations of hyponatremia are the most readily recognizable due to an increase in cerebral edema. With chronic hyponatremia, patients may present with mild cognitive impairments, such as gait instability, attention impairments, and falls (Renneboog et al., 2006). Patients who develop acute hyponatremia may present with lethargy, headaches, confusion, and muscle cramps. These symptoms can very rapidly progress to seizures, coma, brainstem herniation, and neurogenic pulmonary edema with subsequent respiratory arrest.

HISTORY AND PHYSICAL EXAM FINDINGS

Hyponatremia is not a disease state on its own but rather a manifestation of an underlying condition. The AGACNP should perform a thorough history and physical to help guide the assessment and diagnosis of hyponatremia in addition to the underlying pathology. Particular focus should be shown to the patient's volume status. If the patient has symptoms such as peripheral or sacral edema, jugular venous distention, or pulmonary crackles, hypervolemia should be suspected. It is often difficult to differentiate between euvolemia and subtle hypovolemia at which time diagnostics may be helpful.

DIFFERENTIAL DIAGNOSIS AND DIAGNOSTIC CONSIDERATIONS

The initial diagnosis of hyponatremia is made through evaluation of serum sodium. Sodium concentration is <135 mmol/L. After determining that the patient is hyponatremic, the AGACNP should ascertain the cause and type of hyponatremia. Serum osmolality should be drawn, especially if the patient appears hypo- or euvolemic, to determine the serum tonicity. The AGACNP should also determine if this change is acute (e.g., following endurance exercise) or chronic (e.g., outpatient utilization of diuretics).

Once it is determined that the AGACNP is evaluating a hypotonic hyponatremia, urine osmolality should be measured. This will assist in evaluating the concentrating ability of the kidneys. If the urine osmolality is low (<100 mOsm/kg), the AGACNP can suspect increased water intake. If the urine osmolality is ≥100 mOsm/kg, a urine sodium should be measured. If the urine sodium is <30 mmol/L and the patient is hypervolemic, the patient may have a hypervolemic hyponatremia with ongoing sodium retention. If the urine sodium is <30 mmol/L and the patient is hypovolemic, the hyponatremia may be due to diarrhea or vomiting. If the urine sodium is ≥30 mmol/L, the clinician should assess for the use of diuretics. If the patient is not on diuretics, they are inappropriately excreting sodium, either via urinary or GI losses. Low urine sodium could also be due to SIADH or adrenal insufficiency (Verbalis et al., 2013).

TREATMENT

Prior to treating hyponatremia, it is essential for the AGACNP to determine whether the hyponatremia is acute (onset <48 hours) or chronic (onset >48 hours). It should also be determined if the patient is symptomatic with manifestations of cerebral edema (e.g., confusion, seizures, coma). The AGACNP should also take steps to treat the underlying cause of hyponatremia (e.g., withholding diuretics, treatment of GI illness, or initiation of mineralocorticoid replacement).

Acute Hyponatremia

Patients who acutely develop hyponatremia are at the highest risk of developing devastating neurologic manifestations such as brain herniation. The goal of treating acute hyponatremia is to prevent or reverse these consequences. In order to reverse the consequences of acute hyponatremia, such as in the setting of ecstasy (3–4 methylenedioxymethamphetamine [MDMA]) use, acute psychosis, or endurance exercise, a 4 to 6 mmol/L increase in serum sodium is adequate to reverse neurologic manifestations (Verbalis et al., 2013). The treatment for acute hyponatremia is a 100 mL bolus of 3% saline infused over 10 minutes for severe symptoms. This can be repeated twice if needed. The sodium can then be allowed to autoregulate.

The secretion of AVP will stop and a large volume of dilute urine should be produced by the kidneys to promote homeostasis.

Chronic Hyponatremia

While the acute decrease in sodium can lead to neurologic injury, the opposite is true in patients with chronic hyponatremia. Neurologic sequelae are associated with rapid increases in sodium in the chronically hyponatremic patient. The most feared consequence of rapidly corrected sodium is the development of ODS. ODS is a biphasic illness caused by the rapid correction of hyponatremia. The symptoms of hyponatremia initially resolve with the rapid correction of hyponatremia; however, days later, new progressive neurologic findings, such as seizures, behavioral disturbances, swallowing dysfunction, paralysis, or movement disorders, occur. Demyelinating lesions in the central pons and symmetrical lesions outside the pons drive this neurologic illness and can be seen on properly timed MRI 1 to 3 weeks following the incident. Alcoholism, hypokalemia, malnutrition, and liver disease are present in a high percentage of patients who develop ODS. It is important to note that normalization of acute hyponatremia does not carry a risk of ODS when the duration is known to be <48 hours (Seay et al., 2020).

The goal of sodium correction for patients with chronic hyponatremia should be 4 to 8 mmol/L/day for patients with a low risk of ODS. Those at high risk of developing ODS should be corrected at an even slower rate of 4 to 6 mmol/L/day. The longer the duration of hyponatremia and the lower the serum sodium, the greater the concern for iatrogenic neurologic injury due to rapid or overcorrection. Serum sodium measurements should be obtained at a 4- or 6-hour interval to closely monitor correction.

If the sodium rises too rapidly and the starting serum sodium was ≥120 mmol/L, the sodium likely does not need to be lowered to prevent ODS. However, if overcorrection occurs (>8 mmol/L in 24 hours) and the starting serum sodium was <120 mmol/L, the serum sodium will need to be lowered due to the risk of ODS. Interventions to raise sodium should be held for 24 hours. Additionally, to relower the sodium, the AGACNP should consider the administration of vasopressin. Water losses should be replaced with electrolyte-free water, and the serum sodium should be checked frequently until the target serum sodium is reached (Hoorn & Zietse, 2017).

Volume Expansion

In the case of hypovolemic hyponatremia, volume expansion will correct hyponatremia. When the volume deficit is corrected, the body will initiate aquaresis to normalize the serum concentration of sodium. However, it is often difficult to elucidate a patient's volume status by clinical exam alone. In this instance, an isotonic fluid challenge can be both diagnostic and therapeutic

(Verbalis et al., 2013). For patients who are hypovolemic this will cause both an increase in urine and serum sodium. When continuing with volume resuscitation, the serum sodium should be closely monitored to prevent overcorrection. However, in patients with SIADH, following a volume bolus the urine sodium will increase, the serum sodium may fall because the water will be retained by the kidneys. If the serum sodium is ≥120 mmol/L or there are neurologic symptoms and SIADH is suspected, hypertonic saline, such as 3% saline, should be utilized for the volume challenge to prevent an acute drop in serum sodium.

Vaptans

There are currently two FDA-approved vasopressin receptor antagonists (vaptans) available for use in the United States: conivaptan and tolvaptan. These medications act by blocking endogenous AVP from binding to V2R receptors within the kidneys. In turn, the kidneys produce solute-sparing water. Conivaptan is an IV infusion indicated for euvolemic and hypervolemic hyponatremic patients in the hospital settings. Tolvaptan is an oral V2R antagonist indicated for euvolemic and hypervolemic hyponatremia. Tolvaptan should not be given to patients with liver disease. These medications should be administered in conjunction with a specialist (e.g., hepatologist).

Hypervolemic Hyponatremia

In contrast with patients with hypo- or euvolemic hyponatremia, the patient with hypervolemic hyponatremia should be treated with sodium restriction and diuretic therapy. Vaptans may also play a role in the treatment plan. The patient should also be referred for specialty management of their underlying condition, such as heart failure or end-stage liver disease.

HYPERNATREMIA

Hypernatremia is associated with increased morbidity and mortality in both the inpatient and outpatient settings. Hypernatremia is caused by either renal or non-renal water loss that outpaces the salt loss or sodium intake. The body experiences water deficiency compared to the total body sodium and potassium. The most common cause of hypernatremia is water loss (Seay et al., 2020).

The thirst mechanism prevents hypernatremia in healthy individuals. Slight elevations in plasma tonicity stimulate thirst and vasopressin release. By triggering the thirst mechanism to increase free water intake, the body is able to prevent hypernatremia. In the outpatient setting, patients at highest at risk for development of hypernatremia are the elderly and those residing in nursing homes who are unable to regulate their own free water intake (Palevsky et al., 1996). Hospitalized patients who develop hypernatremia are similar to the ages of the

overall hospitalized patients but lack access to free water. The free water prescription for these patients does not meet their losses and is often an iatrogenic hypernatremia. Renal concentrating ability may be present due to the administration of diuretics or osmotic diuresis. The subsequent diagnosis of hypernatremia falls into three categories: hypovolemic, euvolemic, or hypervolemic (Braun et al., 2015).

Hypovolemic Hypernatremia

Hypovolemic hypernatremia typically occurs when free water loss exceeds salt loss or sodium intake. Risk factors and causes include body fluid loss (e.g., burns, diaphoresis), diuretic use, gastrointestinal losses, heat injuries, and osmotic diuresis (e.g., mannitol use or enteral feeding). Hypovolemic hypernatremia can also be caused by a lack of access to water, as with elderly patients, those with cognitive deficits, or individuals in assisted living.

Euvolemic Hypernatremia

Diagnoses associated with euvolemic hypernatremia include central and nephrogenic diabetes insipidus, fever, hypodipsia, and sickle cell disease. Many medications are associated with sodium retention, including (but not limited to) amphotericin, aminoglycosides, lithium, and phenytoin.

Hypervolemic Hypernatremia

Diagnoses associated with hypervolemic hypernatremia include Cushing syndrome, hyperaldosteronism, and iatrogenic administration of sodium.

PRESENTING SIGNS AND SYMPTOMS

As with hyponatremia, the most distressing symptoms from hypernatremia are neurologic in nature. Patients with acute hypernatremia, such as from acute salt intoxication, may present with seizures, coma, or high fever. Cell shrinking can occur within the brain with hypernatremia which can lead to vascular rupture or intracranial bleeding. These patients may present obtunded or with intracranial bleeding. These symptoms are most likely to occur with a serum sodium of >160 mEq/L (Braun et al., 2015).

Chronic hypernatremia causes a reversible encephalopathy (Sterns, 2015). Patients may also complain of anorexia, generalized muscle weakness, restlessness, nausea, and vomiting (Braun et al., 2015). They may present with irritability or altered mental status.

HISTORY AND PHYSICAL FINDINGS

When examining a patient with suspected hypernatremia, the AGACNP should evaluate for signs and symptoms of the patient's volume status. With hypervolemia the patient may demonstrate pulmonary or peripheral edema. If hypovolemic the AGACNP may appreciate orthostatic hypotension, tachycardia, hypotension, dry mucous membranes, or decreased skin turgor. The duration of the hypernatremia should also be determined. An onset of <48 hours indicates acute hypernatremia, while an onset of >48 hours indicates chronic hypernatremia. In acute hypernatremia, physical exam and diagnostics may demonstrate hypertonia, intracranial hemorrhage, or thrombosis of dural sinuses.

DIFFERENTIAL DIAGNOSIS AND DIAGNOSTIC CONSIDERATIONS

Hypernatremia is a manifestation of an underlying pathologic process or iatrogenic cause. Diagnostics to determine the cause of hypernatremia should be guided by the patients' history and physical. Diagnosis of hypernatremia is made through serum sodium concentration of >145 mM; severe is considered >152 mM.

TREATMENT

For both acute and chronic hypernatremia, the patient's physiologic free water deficit should be calculated (Box 20.3). The AGACNP should consider this total deficit when creating a care plan to correct hypernatremia. Rapid correction is indicated for acute hypernatremia to prevent neurologic sequelae of hypernatremia. This should be done with correction of the free water deficit through use of either enteral free water or a hypotonic solution, and discontinuation of salt-containing agents (Seay et al., 2020).

The goal for treatment of chronic hypernatremia is to restore normal serum sodium concentration while preventing iatrogenic injury. With rapid rehydration of the brain due to aggressive sodium correction, the patient is at risk of cerebral edema. Treatment involves repletion of free water, preferably orally or enterally, in the setting of water loss. Historically, the recommendation has been to lower the serum sodium at no greater than 0.5 mEq/L/h. A recent retrospective study found no difference in mortality or complications with more rapid correction at >0.5 mEq/L/h (Chauhan et al., 2019; Sterns, 2019). No randomized control trials currently exist to compare the two interventions, and current recommendations include correcting chronic hypernatremia over a 48-hour period to prevent complications (Seay et al., 2020).

BOX 20.3 FREE WATER DEFICIT

Free-water deficit: TBW (L) × ([Na$^+$/140 mEq/L] − 1)

TBW = 0.6 × body weight (kg)

CLINICAL PEARLS

- Sodium imbalances are the most frequently observed electrolyte imbalances and are associated with increased morbidity and mortality for patients.
- The most profound consequences of sodium disorders are a direct result of water shifting in the brain that results in neurologic sequelae.
- The AGACNP should elicit the underlying pathophysiology causing the sodium imbalance in order to treat both the electrolyte imbalance and the disease.
- Evaluating both the serum osmolality and urine electrolytes can assist in determining the type of sodium imbalance and the involvement of the kidneys in the disorder.
- Too rapid correction of severe hyponatremia presents high risk of neurologic injury and too rapid correction of severe hypernatremia may carry a risk for neurologic injury.

EVIDENCE-BASED RESOURCE

Seay, N. W., Lehrich, R. W., & Greenberg, A. (2020). Diagnosis and management of disorders of body tonicity-hyponatremia and hypernatremia: Core curriculum 2020. *American Journal of Kidney Diseases*, 75(2), 272–286. https://doi.org/10.1053/j.ajkd.2019.07.014

ELECTROLYTE–POTASSIUM

Potassium (K$^+$) is the most abundant cation within the body and regulation is essential to normal cellular functioning. Normal plasma levels of potassium are maintained within a narrow therapeutic range of 3.5 to 5.0 mmol/L. Within the body approximately 98% of potassium is found within intracellular compartments while only 2% is found extracellularly (Palmer & Clegg, 2019). Normal potassium levels are necessary to regulate not only action potentials of cardiac, neuronal, and muscular tissue, but also hormone secretion, vascular tone, systemic blood pressure control, gastrointestinal motility, acid-base homeostasis, glucose and insulin metabolism, mineralocorticoid action, and renal concentrating ability (Gumz et al., 2015).

Homeostasis of potassium is primarily regulated by the kidneys with some excretion via the gastrointestinal tract. Potassium is filtered by the glomerulus and reabsorbed within the proximal tubule and loop of Henle (Palmer, 2015). Secretion begins in the early distal nephron and into the collecting duct. This process takes hours to occur following ingestion of potassium (Kovesdy et al., 2017). However, given such a narrow therapeutic window needed to sustain life, the body has developed multiple mechanisms to temporize potassium levels to prevent hyper- or hypokalemia as the kidneys excrete the electrolyte. Insulin release following a meal shifts dietary potassium intracellularly until the kidneys are able to excrete it. Catecholamines and beta-adrenergic stimulation increase the activity of Na+/K+ ATP-ase. Dyskalemias, either hypokalemia (serum K$^+$ <3.5 mmol/L) or hyperkalemia (serum K$^+$ >5 mmol/L), are associated with worsened outcomes for patients (Kovesdy et al., 2017).

HYPERKALEMIA

Hyperkalemia is defined as a serum potassium >5.0 mEq/L. Risk factors for development of hyperkalemia include the presence of chronic kidney disease, diabetes, heart failure, and in those receiving renin-angiotensin-aldosterone system inhibitors (Palmer et al., 2021). An increase in serum potassium increases the risk of morbidity and mortality for patients.

The causes of hyperkalemia can be divided into three different categories: cellular shifting, excessive intake of dietary potassium, or decreased renal excretion (Palmer & Clegg, 2017). Notably, it is important to first rule out pseudohyperkalemia that can be caused by cell lysing due to either phlebotomy or to specimen processing.

Changes in cellular concentration of potassium can lead to acute hyperkalemia. Patients who present with a tissue injury such as rhabdomyolysis, trauma, hemolysis, or tumor lysis syndrome are at high risk for the development of hyperkalemia due to a release of potassium from cells (Palmer & Clegg, 2017). As previously discussed, excretion of insulin by the body drives potassium into cells. Therefore, patients with an insulin deficiency are at risk of hyperkalemia. Heavy exercise may cause hyperkalemia due to potassium sequestration outside the cell to promote a vasodilatory effect. Hyperchloremic acidosis can drive hyperkalemia. Lastly, hypertonic states, such as hyperglycemia and administration of hypertonic solutions may lead to hyperkalemia.

In the setting of chronic kidney disease or adrenal disorders, an increase in the dietary intake of potassium can lead to hyperkalemia. This can be due to foods rich in potassium, such as bananas, potatoes, melons, citrus, and avocadoes. Additionally, salt substitutes and clay ingestion can also lead to hyperkalemia (Palmer & Clegg, 2017).

Lastly, renal impairment can lead to hyperkalemia. Decreased distal delivery of sodium negatively impacts the sodium/potassium pumps and leads to a decrease in the secretion of potassium. This can occur with AKI and chronic kidney disease. Additionally, deficiencies in mineralocorticoids can lead to hyperkalemia. This is often due to medication administration or disease states. Renin-angiotensin-aldosterone system blockers, nonsteroidal antiinflammatory drugs (NSAIDs), calcineurin-inhibitors, and beta-blockers all have the potential to lead to hyperkalemia. Additionally, potassium-sparing diuretics, trimethoprim, pentamidine, spironolactone, eplerenone, and drosperinone all have the potential to cause hyperkalemia due to an impact on the renal distal tubules (Palmer & Clegg, 2017).

PRESENTING SIGNS AND SYMPTOMS

Presenting signs and symptoms for hyperkalemia can be nonspecific and include neuromuscular symptoms and metabolic acidosis. Patients with severe hyperkalemia may prevent with flaccid paralysis, paresthesias, depressed deep tendon reflexes, or shortness of breath (Panchal et al., 2020).

HISTORY AND PHYSICAL FINDINGS

EKG findings change as hyperkalemia worsens. First, the EKG of a patient with hyperkalemia will demonstrate peaked T waves. As the hyperkalemia worsens, the P wave will broaden and eventually disappear, and the QRS will widen. Severe hyperkalemia may precipitate heart block, idioventricular rhythms, sine-wave patterns, asystole, ventricular tachycardia, or ventricular fibrillation (Panchal et al., 2020; Weiss et al., 2017).

TREATMENT
Acute Hyperkalemia

Pharmacologic agents for the treatment of hyperkalemia are indicated with EKG changes or with muscle weakness. These signs and symptoms may vary based on potassium levels, but a serum concentration of potassium greater than 5.5 mEq/L is often a threshold utilized for treatment (Palmer et al., 2021). Urgent hemodialysis is considered with associated kidney injury or dysfunction.

Myocardial Cell Membrane Stabilization

The utilization of IV calcium stabilizes the myocardial cell membrane. Parenteral calcium, either gluconate or chloride, should be administered as an IV bolus or via interosseous access (Panchal, et al., 2020). The duration of this drug is around 30 to 60 minutes, and the AGACNP should proceed with therapy to shift insulin intracellularly and eliminate potassium. Though lacking evidence, repeat administration may be necessary if the EKG does not normalize following the first administration.

Potassium Shifting

Regular insulin with dextrose, either alone or with a beta-2 agonist, is utilized to shift potassium intracellularly to prevent dysrhythmias. Regular insulin with glucose can be utilized as a single dose to shift potassium. Nebulized salbutamol should also be administered to shift potassium. The AGACNP should closely monitor for hypoglycemia with this treatment.

Potassium Excretion

For potassium secretion, use of a loop diuretic, such as furosemide, will precipitate secretion of potassium. Intermittent hemodialysis should be utilized for those with a renal impairment disorder.

Potassium binders utilized in the management of hyperkalemia are not absorbed by the gut and facilitate the elimination of bound potassium in feces (Palmer et al., 2021). The use of sodium gluconate polysterene is no longer recommended due to poor efficacy and risk of bowel ischemia and colonic necrosis (Panchal et al., 2020). Two potassium binders are currently FDA approved for this indication: patiromer sorbitex calcium (Veltassa) and sodium zirconium cyclosilicate (Lokelma). These agents should be considered in the setting of life-threatening hyperkalemia (Palmer et al., 2021).

Chronic Hyperkalemia

Hyperkalemia may present as a chronic problem for patients with chronic kidney disease, heart failure, or those who receive RAAS inhibitor medications. These patients should be counseled in a low-potassium diet. Titration of RAAS medications may be indicated. Prescription of loop diuretics, sodium bicarbonate tablets, or a potassium binder may be indicated (Palmer et al., 2021).

HYPOKALEMIA

Hypokalemia is defined as a serum potassium <3.5 mmol/L (Clase et al., 2020). This imbalance impacts 1% to 3% of the general population. However, the incidence is much higher in hospitalized patients, with some studies noting up to 21% of hospitalized patients experiencing hypokalemia (Viera & Wouk, 2015). This derangement is associated with worsening hypertension and increased mortality in patients with heart disease, chronic kidney disease, and cerebrovascular disease (Asmar et al., 2012).

PRESENTING SIGNS AND SYMPTOMS

Hypokalemia is driven by either a deficit in total body potassium or a shift from extra- to intracellular potassium. Clinical manifestations of hypokalemia are nonspecific in nature. Hypokalemia may drive polyuria due to an inability for the kidney to concentrate urine and an increased risk of nephrolithiasis (Asmar et al., 2012). Patients may complain of cramps, myalgias, weakness, or in severe cases, paralysis or paresthesias. Hypokalemia may cause altered gastrointestinal mobility with subsequent nausea, vomiting, constipation, or paralytic ileus.

HISTORY AND PHYSICAL FINDINGS

One of the most common causes of hypokalemia is use of diuretic medications. Patients who utilize thiazide diuretics are at a five times increased risk of developing moderate to severe hypokalemia (Rodenburg et al., 2014). Additionally, mineralocorticoid-driven hypertension and gastrointestinal losses place patients at high risk for hypokalemia (Clase et al., 2020). If a patient presents with hypokalemia, the AGACNP should take a thorough history to determine potential causes.

The presentation of hypokalemia is typically nonspecific. It is estimated that EKG abnormalities such as U waves and ventricular dysrhythmias are present in 25% to 66% of severe cases (Clase et al., 2020). Patients may demonstrate worsening hypertension, respiratory acidosis due to respiratory muscle weakness, and hyperglycemia due to insulin resistance and an impairment in insulin release (Asmar et al., 2012). Arterial blood gas may demonstrate a chloride-depletion metabolic alkalosis.

TREATMENT

The goal of treatment of hypokalemia is to achieve a normal serum potassium level without causing hyperkalemia. With potassium depletion, every 0.3 mEq/L deficit in serum potassium concentration corresponds to a >100 mEq in total body potassium depletion (Asmar et al., 2012). It is important to note that this does not account for ongoing potassium losses. Potassium chloride is the preferred potassium formulation for repletion given the concurrent repletion of chloride. It is available in liquid, slow-release tablet, or capsule. In the event the AGACNP is unable to administer PO medications, or the patient demonstrates symptomatic severe hypokalemia with symptoms, such as skeletal weakness, paralysis, or diaphragmatic muscle paralysis, IV administration of potassium may be warranted. This intervention should only be performed with continuous cardiac monitoring.

Serum magnesium should be assessed concomitantly with potassium levels. Hypomagnesemia may worsen potassium wasting and should be corrected for adequate therapy. Patients at risk for chronic hypokalemia due to medication may require prophylactic administration of oral potassium.

CLINICAL PEARLS

- Dyskalemias increase the risk of morbidity and mortality for patients, especially those with chronic kidney disease and heart failure.
- Presentation of dyskalemias may be chronic and insidious or acute and fulminant.
- Development of severe dyskalemias predispose patients to cardiac sequelae.
- Treatment of hypo- or hyperkalemia should be both diagnostic and symptom based.
- Response to treatment of hypo- or hyperkalemia should be frequently monitored for efficacy and side effects.

EVIDENCE-BASED RESOURCES

Palmer, B. F., Carrero, J. J., Clegg, D. J., Colbert, G. B., Emmett, M., Fishbane, S., Hain, D. J., Lerma, E., Onuigbo, M., Rastogi, A., Roger, S. D., Spinowitz, B. S., & Weir, M. R. (2020). Clinical management of hyperkalemia. *Mayo Clinic Proceedings, 96*(3), 744–762. https://doi.org/10.1016/j.mayocp.2020.06.014

Palmer, B. F., & Clegg, D. J. (2019). Physiology and pathophysiology of potassium homeostasis: Core curriculum 2019. *American Journal of Kidney Diseases, 74*(5), 682–695. https://doi.org/10.1053/j.ajkd.2019.03.427

ELECTROLYTE–CALCIUM

Calcium is an essential cation within the body that serves an important role in nerve impulse transmission, muscle contraction, blood coagulation, and hormone secretion (Blaine et al., 2015). At any given time, the total amount of calcium in the human body is between 1,000 and 1,200 g, and the average human adult should average 800 to 1,000 mg intake daily (Blaine et al., 2015). Approximately 99% of calcium within the body is found in the skeleton with approximately 1% circulating within the intra- and extracellular spaces. Furthermore, only 1% of the calcium within the bones is exchangeable with plasma calcium. In order to maintain homeostasis, calcium must exist within a very narrow therapeutic range (Hassan-Smith & Gittoes, 2017).

Ingested calcium is primarily absorbed by the intestine, primarily within the duodenum, jejunum, and ileum. Reabsorption occurs within the kidneys. The net absorption of ingested calcium is around 20% when 1 g of calcium is ingested. The remaining calcium is excreted via feces (approximately 80%) with the remainder being excreted by the kidneys (approximately 20%; Blaine et al., 2015).

There are three forms of calcium within the body: ionized (48%), protein bound (46%), and complex molecules (7%). Within the extracellular calcium the complex-fractioned calcium is bound to negatively charged molecules such as albumin and proteins. Ionized calcium is the biologically active form of calcium and responsible for physiologic changes (Aberegg, 2016). Normal serum calcium is around 8.9 to 10.1 mg/dL, and normal ionized calcium concentration is 4.7-5.6 mg/dL. Because serum calcium is often bound to albumin, hypoalbuminemia can lead to a decrease in calcium concentration. For every 1.0 g/dL decrease in serum albumin, there is a total serum calcium decrease of 0.12 mg/dL. Alkalosis decreases the concentration of ionized calcium with over a 0.1 change in pH leading to a 0.12 mg/dL change in ionized calcium (Blaine et al., 2015).

While many physiologic processes have an impact on calcium homeostasis, parathyroid hormone (PTH) is the most important regulator. The parathyroid gland releases PTH in response to changes in calcium and PTH stimulates calcium absorption within the kidneys and calcium release from the bone. Many factors influence the controlled release of PTH into the bloodstream. Hypocalcemia, glucocorticoids, estrogen, dopamine, and adrenergic agonists influence the transcription or secretion of PTH. Hypercalcemia, conversely, can promote degradation of PTH within the cells (Blaine et al., 2015).

Vitamin D also plays an important role in calcium absorption (Blaine et al., 2015). Vitamin D is primarily synthesized by the skin with exposure to sunlight. Vitamin D3, created by the skin, is transported to the liver and converted to 25-hydroxyvitamin D. Parathyroid hormone (PTH) then stimulates the production of active 1,25-dihydroxyvitamin D (1,25(OH)2D) from 25-hydroxyvitamin D. This complex then acts on the gastrointestinal tract to promote calcium absorption. With a lack of vitamin D, there is a decrease in the amount of calcium absorbed by the intestine (Blaine et al., 2015).

HYPOCALCEMIA

Hypocalcemia is defined as total serum calcium concentration <8.8 mg/dL (<2.20 mmol/L) in the presence of normal plasma protein concentrations or as a serum ionized calcium concentration <4.7 mg/dL (<1.17 mmol/L).

PRESENTING SIGNS AND SYMPTOMS

Because calcium is essential for consistent nerve impulse transmission and muscle contraction, a reduction in serum calcium will lead to neuromuscular excitability. Patients may complain of muscle twitching, spasms in the extremities or face, or perioral or digital paresthesias. Patients may complain of irritability, depression, or anxiety (Velasco et al., 1999). Severe hypocalcemia may present with bronchospasm or laryngospasm with subsequent respiratory arrest. Severe hypocalcemia may also cause either generalized tonic-clonic seizures or focal-typical seizures (Cusano & Bilezikian, 2018).

HISTORY AND PHYSICAL FINDINGS

Patients with hypocalcemia are likely to manifest Trosseau's sign. This is the induction of a carpopedal spasm through the inflation of a blood pressure cuff on the upper arm for 3 minutes. A carpopedal spasm will manifest as flexion of the metocarpophalangeal joints and wrist, adduction of the fingers, and extension of the distal and proximal interphalangeal joints (Cusano & Bilezikian, 2018). This finding is between 94% and 99% sensitive for hypocalcemia and is present in only 1% of normocalcemic patients. Chvostek's sign, a fascial muscle spasm induced by tapping over the facial nerve and parotid gland, is neither sensitive nor specific for hypocalcemia. Patients may also demonstrate papilledema (Cusano & Bilezikian, 2018).

Patients with hypocalcemia are at high risk for cardiovascular compromise. Hypocalcemia may induce hypotension, bradycardia, or arrhythmias. An EKG may demonstrate an increase in the ST segment or the QT interval. EKG findings due to hypocalcemia can mimic a myocardial infarction with changes in the ST segments, QS segments, and T-waves (Cusano & Bilezikian, 2018).

DIFFERENTIAL DIAGNOSIS AND DIAGNOSTIC CONSIDERATIONS

There are many causes of hypocalcemia, but generally this disorder results from inadequate PTH secretion or receptor activation, insufficient vitamin D levels or receptor activity, abnormal magnesium metabolism, or clinical scenarios with multifactorial causes (Shoback, 2008). In order to assist in determining the cause of hypocalcemia, a serum PTH should be measured. If the serum PTH is low and the patient is hypocalcemic, the diagnosis is likely hypoparathyroidism. The most common cause of hypocalcemia in the hospital is disruption of the parathyroid gland due to total thyroidectomy (Turner et al., 2016). A lack of sufficient PTH can drive hypocalcemia. This can be caused by hypoparathyroidism, surgical destruction of the parathyroid gland for hyperparathyroidism, autoimmune conditions such as sarcoidosis, and radiation. A reduction in vitamin D activity can result from reduced intestinal absorption, reduced exposure to ultraviolet (UV) light, and chronic renal disease. Large volume blood transfusion may also cause hypocalcemia as the citrate used as a preservative in blood products binds with free calcium in the plasma.

TREATMENT

The goal of treatment of hypocalcemia is to restore normal calcium levels and prevent complications manifesting from hypocalcemia. For mild hypocalcemia oral supplementation should be initiated. If vitamin D deficiency is the cause, vitamin D should also be supplemented. In severe hypocalcemia or mild hypocalcemia with associated symptoms, the goal is to normalize the serum calcium quickly. Calcium gluconate 10% 10 to 20 mL in 50 to 100 mL 5% dextrose should be given over 10 minutes with EKG monitoring (Hassan-Smith & Gittoes, 2017).

HYPERCALCEMIA

PRESENTING SIGNS AND SYMPTOMS

The presenting signs and symptoms of hypercalcemia are often vague and nonspecific. Patients may complain of anorexia, nausea, or constipation. They may admit polyuria and increased thirst. Neurologic manifestations range from mood disturbances, confusion, easy fatiguability and muscle weakness to myalgias, decreased memory, cognitive dysfunction, and coma.

HISTORY AND PHYSICAL FINDINGS

On exam, the AGACNP may appreciate a heart block, shortened QT waves, or ST elevation on telemetry or EKG. Patients will likely be hypertensive. Labs and diagnostics may demonstrate renal abnormalities, such as insufficiency or inability to concentrate urine, nephrolithiasis, pancreatitis, or peptic ulcer disease.

DIFFERENTIAL DIAGNOSIS AND DIAGNOSTIC CONSIDERATIONS

Diagnostics to evaluate hypercalcemia should include a serum calcium, albumin, and PTH level. A basic metabolic panel should also be drawn. If the patient has high calcium and a detectable to high PTH, the most likely diagnosis is hyperparathyroidism. If the patient is hypercalcemic but has a low PTH, the hypercalcemia is likely due to a malignancy or less common cause.

Around 90% of cases of hypercalcemia are due to either primary hyperparathyroidism or a malignancy. When hypercalcemia is a manifestation of malignancy, it is a poor prognostic indicator. It indicates that there is likely either a large primary tumor or diffuse skeletal involvement of the cancer. The AGACNP should perform a thorough history and physical to rule this out as a cause when diagnosed unexpectedly. Granulomatous disorders, particularly sarcoidosis, and thyrotoxicosis may cause hypercalcemia. Multiple medications, including thiazide diuretics, calcitriol, and lithium, may cause hypercalcemia. Ingestion of a large amount of calcium carbonate, such as with milk-alkali syndrome, may cause hypercalcemia. There has also been an increase in hypercalcemia associated with over-the-counter use of calcium carbonate for osteoporosis prevention.

TREATMENT

A calcium level of ≥11.5 typically causes no symptoms. A serum calcium level >12.5 mg/dL will cause patients to begin to become symptomatic, and a calcium level >14 mg/dL is considered a medical emergency.

Intravenous Fluids

The first treatment consideration is to initiate IV fluid repletion. Hypercalcemia causes the kidneys to decrease renal tubular reabsorption and results in polyuria. Associated nausea and vomiting may prevent enteral water intake (Maier & Levine, 2015). Subsequently, hypercalcemic patients will often be volume depleted and need IV fluids for volume resuscitation and repletion. The recommendation is often to infuse 3 to 6 L of IV fluid in the initial 24-hour period following diagnosis, and this should lower the serum calcium by 1 to 2 mg/dL (Hosking et al., 1981). However, particular caution should be paid to the rate of the infusion, especially in the setting of malignancy. The clinician should balance the rate of volume infusion with the potential for fluid volume overload.

Calcitonin

In addition to IV fluids, subcutaneous calcitonin is often administered to reduce serum calcium. Calcitonin works to lower serum calcium by inhibiting bone resorption (Maier & Levine, 2015). The medication begins to lower plasma calcium levels by 1 to 2 mg/dL within several hours. There is an associated tachyphylaxis over several days with calcitonin due to the downregulation of calcium receptors (Maier & Levine, 2015).

Bisphosphonates

Bisphosphonate medications are pyrophosphate analogues that are deposited within the bone. The medications work to lower calcium levels by inhibiting bone resorption. Bisphosphonates are the mainstay of treatment for malignancy-induced hypercalcemia. The mean time to normocalcemia with bisphosphonate administration is 2 to 6 days. While they have not been extensively studied for hypercalcemia not associated with malignancy, these agents should be considered for hypercalcemia of other etiologies.

When administering bisphosphonates the AGACNP should be aware that rapid infusions may lead to renal injury due to precipitant of a solid phase in the blood. This risk increases with concurrent chemotherapy, dehydration, and use of other nephrotoxic medications. The patient may be at risk of transient asymptomatic hypocalcemia. When used repeatedly, bisphosphonates have been associated with osteonecrosis of the jaw.

Additional Therapies

Dialysis is employed when patients demonstrate refractory hypercalcemia. There are no randomized control trials to compare the efficacy of dialysis with other modalities of treatment. However, while this effectively reduces the serum calcium level, it does not correct the underlying cause of hypercalcemia. Denosumab, a monoclonal antibody used for the treatment of osteoporosis, has also shown promise for the treatment of refractory hypercalcemia (Karuppiah et al., 2014).

Hyperparathyroidism

Hyperparathyroidism is one of the primary causes of hypercalcemia. While many patients may be asymptomatic for years, some may need a parathyroidectomy due to symptomatic hypercalcemia. Box 20.4 lists the criteria for parathyroidectomy (Bilezikian et al., 2014).

CLINICAL PEARLS

- Calcium derangements place patients at high risk of both cardiac and neurologic sequelae.
- Mild hypo- and hypercalcemia can be monitored while severe hypo- and hypercalcemia are medical emergencies.
- Calcium derangements are the result of a pathologic process such as parathyroid dysfunction.

BOX 20.4 INDICATIONS FOR PARATHYROIDECTOMY

- Increase in serum calcium >1 mg/dL above upper limit of normal
- Decrease in bone mineral density that is significantly decreased versus the baseline measurement
- Vertebral fracture present
- Nephrolithiasis present
- Decrease in creatinine clearance <60 mL/min

EVIDENCE-BASED RESOURCES

Hassan-Smith, Z., & Gittoes, N. (2017). Hypocalcaemia. *Medicine, 45*(9), 555–559. https://doi.org/10.1016/j.mpmed.2017.06.006

Turner, J. J. O. (2017). Hypercalcaemia—Presentation and management. *Clinical Medicine, 17*(3), 270–273. https://doi.org/10.7861/clinmedicine.17-3-270

ACID-BASE IMBALANCE

Normal cellular functioning is dependent on a strictly defined pH balance. A normal pH for the human body is 7.35 to 7.45. At a cellular level, a normal pH is essential for fertilization, cell growth and volume regulation, and protein synthesis (Seifter & Chang, 2017). The central nervous, digestive, cardiac, respiratory, and urinary systems are all particularly vulnerable to changes in pH (Romero & Rossano, 2019). A drift in pH of even 0.1 alters the activity and activation of metabolic enzymes. Acidemia is defined as a decrease in the blood pH below 7.35, whereas acidosis is a physiologic process characterized by a primary decrease in HCO_3 level (metabolic acidosis) or a primary increase in $PaCO_2$ (respiratory acidosis). Conversely, alkalemia is defined as an increase in the blood pH above 7.45, whereas alkalosis is a physiologic process characterized by a primary increase in HCO_3^- level (metabolic alkalosis) or a primary decrease in the $PaCO_2$ (respiratory alkalosis; Woodrow, 2010).

PATHOPHYSIOLOGY

Movement of hydrogen (H^+) ions across the cell membrane gradient determines both intra- and extracellular pH. Hydrogen ion donors are known as acids, while hydrogen ion acceptors are known as bases. The flux of hydrogen ions between acids and bases maintains homeostasis within the body. The physiologic approach to acid-base management, often used in clinical practice, focuses on the carbonic acid/bicarbonate buffer system. The chemical equation is as follows: $CO_2 + H_2O \leftrightarrow H_2CO_3 \leftrightarrow H_2CO_3^- + H^+$. This equation ties carbon dioxide, the volatile acid form of carbonic acid, to bicarbonate within the body. A change in the partial pressure of carbon dioxide (P_{CO2}) causes a shift in serum bicarbonate and vice versa to maintain a pH of 7.35 to 7.45. The kidneys act as the primary regulator of bicarbonate while the lungs serve as the regulator for carbon dioxide. Derangements can occur due to physiologic processes. Accumulation of acids causes acidosis, or an abnormally low pH. Accumulation of bases causes alkalosis, or an abnormally high pH. There are four main categories of acid-base imbalances in the human body: metabolic acidosis, respiratory acidosis, metabolic alkalosis, and respiratory alkalosis. The treatment for each type of derangement should be to treat the underlying disorder.

DIFFERENTIAL DIAGNOSIS AND DIAGNOSTIC CONSIDERATIONS

When an acid-base balance is suspected, an arterial blood gas should be drawn along with serum electrolytes. A systematic approach to interpretation of the blood gas and chemistries should be taken for diagnosis (Kaufman, n.d.).

1. Is the pH high, low, or normal? (acidosis, alkalosis, compensated, or no derangement)
   a. pH <7.35 = acidosis
   b. pH >7.45 = alkalosis
2. Is the derangement primarily respiratory or metabolic?
   a. In primary respiratory disorders, the pH and $PaCO_2$ change in opposite direction, while in primarily metabolic disorders, the pH and $PaCO_2$ change in the same direction (Table 20.2).
3. Is the derangement appropriately compensated?
   a. If not, more than one acid-base derangement may be present.
   b. Compensation can be determined through formulas listed in Table 20.3.
4. For metabolic acidosis: Calculate the anion gap.
   a. Then, calculate the ratio in change for the anion gap to the decrease in bicarbonate:
      i. ΔAG: $\Delta[HCO_3^-]$
         1–2: Uncomplicated metabolic acidosis
      ii. <1: Concurrent nonanion gap metabolic acidosis likely present
      iii. >2: Concurrent metabolic alkalosis likely present

TABLE 20.2: pH/$PaCO_2$ Disturbance in Simple Acid-base Disturbance

ACID-BASE PRIMARY DISTURBANCE		
CONDITION	pH	$PaCO_2$
Respiratory acidosis	↓	↑
Metabolic acidosis	↓	↓
Respiratory alkalosis	↑	↓
Metabolic alkalosis	↑	↑

TABLE 20.3: Expected Compensation in Acid-base Derangement

Metabolic acidosis	$PaCO_2 = (1.5 \times [HCO_3^-]) + 8$
Acute respiratory acidosis	Increase in $[HCO_3^-] = \Delta PaCO_2/10$
Chronic respiratory acidosis	Increase in $[HCO_3^-] = 3.5(\Delta PaCO_2/10)$
Metabolic alkalosis	Increase in $PaCO_2 = 40 + 0.6(\Delta HCO_3^-)$
Acute respiratory alkalosis	Decrease in $[HCO_3^-] = 2(\Delta PaCO_2/10)$
Chronic respiratory alkalosis	Decrease in $[HCO_3^-] = 5(\Delta PaCO_2/10)$ to $7(\Delta PaCO_2/10)$

METABOLIC ACIDOSIS

Metabolic acidosis is one of the most frequently encountered acid-base derangements found in acutely ill patients. Incidence of metabolic acidosis in critically ill patients has been reported to be as high as 64% of patients with a 45% mortality rate (Gunnerson et al., 2006). Metabolic acidosis is defined as a primary decrease in serum concentration of bicarbonate with a resulting decrease in the partial pressure of arterial carbon dioxide ($PaCO_2$). This occurs as a result of an increase in nonvolatile acids within the body or a loss of bicarbonate and an inability of the body to compensate for these changes.

Once a metabolic acidosis has been diagnosed with a low bicarbonate and low pH, the respiratory response must be determined. Hyperventilation is initially triggered by metabolic acidosis in an attempt to compensate by decreasing the serum $PaCO_2$. This attempt will likely be blunted or incomplete in patients with lung disease (Seifter & Chang, 2017). Once a steady state is reached, the clinician is able to calculate a predictable change in (Δ) between HCO_3^- and $PaCO_2$. When metabolic acidosis lasts for 24 hours or longer, Winter's formula can be utilized to determine the expected $PaCO_2$ for any value of HCO_3^- (Box 20.5). If the $PaCO_2$ is greater than anticipated based on this formula, then a concurrent respiratory alkalosis is present. Next, the serum anion gap should be calculated.

Anion Gap Metabolic Acidosis

The serum anion gap is the difference between the anions and cations within the serum. For clinical purposes, the formula used is as follows: $[Na^+] - ([Cl^-] + [HCO_3^-])$. A normal anion gap is 12 ± 4 mEq/L. It is important that this value varies slightly depending on the laboratory as some formulas include the concentration of serum potassium in the equation. When the anion gap is high, an additional compound is driving the acidosis in addition to the imbalance of sodium bicarbonate and carbon dioxide. An elevated anion gap is definitive for presence of a metabolic acidosis.

Causes of anion gap metabolic acidosis can be remembered utilizing the mnemonic CAT MUDPILES (Figure 20.1). Two of the most common causes of death in either industrial or home fires are carbon monoxide and cyanide poisoning (Kaita et al., 2018). Toulene is a hydrocarbon found in solvent, paints, paint thinners, glues, and disinfectants that is broken down into an acid when ingested. Patients can become intoxicated after "glue sniffing." Methanol is a wood alcohol found in windshield washer fluid and some unregulated hand sanitizers (Yip et al., 2020). Uremia in the setting of chronic kidney disease causes gap acidosis with the retention of phosphate

BOX 20.5 WINTER'S FORMULA

$PaCO_2 = 1.5[HCO_3^-] + 8 \pm 2$

Causes of high anion-gap metabolic acidosis

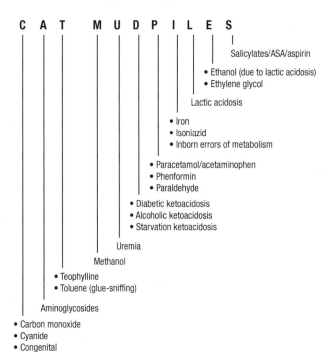

FIGURE 20.1: Causes of high anion-gap metabolic acidosis.
Source: Courtesy of Savvas Radevic.

and sulfate (Kraut & Madias, 2016). Diabetic ketoacidosis is associated with ketogenesis and lipolysis, causing an increase in acid production. Propylene glycol is a preservative found in medications administered in the hospital setting, such as IV lorazepam (Zar et al., 2007). Iron toxicity causes mitochondrial dysfunction and cellular death resulting in metabolic acidosis. Isoniazid inhibits the conversion of lactate to pyruvate in the liver and depletes vitamin B6 resulting in metabolic acidosis. Lactic acidosis is the most frequent cause of metabolic acidosis. There are two types of lactic acidosis. Type A lactic acidosis is associated with tissue hypoxia, such as in severe trauma or cardiogenic shock. Type B lactic acidosis occurs with no evidence of tissue hypoxia (Kraut & Madias, 2014). Ethylene glycol is used in the manufacturing of antifreeze and toxic when ingested (Narita et al., 2017). When ingested, it produces the toxic metabolites of alcohol dehydrogenase and aldehyde dehydrogenase causing acidosis. Salicylate toxicity is typically associated with a high anion gap acidosis (Jacob & Lavonas, 2011).

Nonanion Gap Acidosis

Metabolic acidosis can also develop in the absence of an anion gap. Loss of bicarbonate through the gastrointestinal tract, such as with diarrhea or ureteral diversion, causes a metabolic acidosis. Laxative abuse has also been associated with its development. Renal loss of bicarbonate through mechanisms such as tubular renal acidosis and

the utilization of carbonic anhydrase inhibitors may cause acidosis. Each of these conditions leads to hyperchloremia with subsequent acidosis.

Respiratory Acidosis

Respiratory acidosis is most often driven by a process impairing a patient's ability to effectively ventilate. A slow respiratory rate with ineffective ventilation causes an increase in the $PaCO_2$ leading to an acidosis. A decrease in serum pH with an increase in $PaCO_2$ indicates a respiratory acidosis. This may be caused by a disease process such as chronic obstructive pulmonary disease or obstructive sleep apnea. It can also be due to ingestion of centrally acting medications, such as opioids, sedatives, or benzodiazepines.

The goal of treatment should be to normalize the serum $PaCO_2$ to correct the acidosis. The AGACNP should focus on airway management, effective ventilation, and reversal of the cause of central depression.

METABOLIC ALKALOSIS

Metabolic alkalosis is characterized by an increase in serum bicarbonate causing an increase in serum pH to >7.45 (Emmett, 2020). There are two separate forms of metabolic alkalosis: chloride-depletion metabolic acidosis and nonchloride depletion metabolic acidosis.

Chloride Depletion Metabolic Alkalosis

Chloride depletion is the most common cause of alkalosis (Soifer & Kim, 2014). Risk factors for development of metabolic acidosis include nasogastric suctioning or vomiting. Chloride-wasting diarrhea, as seen with laxatives, is also a common cause. Prior diuresis may also cause an alkalosis. Total parenteral nutrition (TPN) with increased acetate places patients at risk for alkalosis. Lastly, renal hypoperfusion with alkali ingestion may cause alkalosis, as seen with massive transfusion or bicarbonate administration. Clinical presentation often manifests with signs and symptoms of hypovolemia, such as orthostatic hypotension, tachycardia, or dry mucous membranes.

Nonchloride Depletion Metabolic Alkalosis

Active diuresis is a common cause of this form of alkalosis. Renal excretion of free water outpaces the loss of bicarbonate. Hypokalemia and potassium depletion lead to a shift of H^+ ions intracellularly and place patients at risk of alkalosis. Mineralocorticoid excess of any etiology, such as with Cushing's syndrome, places patients at risk for this derangement.

TREATMENT

As with the other acid-base disturbances, the primary treatment for alkalosis is to treat the underlying cause. Carbonic anhydrase inhibitors (acetazolamide) can promote renal excretion of bicarbonate to lower serum levels (Soifer & Kim, 2014). In the instance of chloride losses, chloride should be replaced through IV fluids. In the event that nasogastric suctioning incited the event and cannot be stopped, an H_2 blocker or proton pump inhibitor may help to prevent further chloride losses.

In very rare cases, rapid reversal is indicated in severe metabolic alkalosis with pH >7.55 or in patients with altered mental status or cardiac arrhythmia. In this instance, a hydrochloric acid infusion can be considered (Gooch, 2015). Dialysis can also be considered for treatment of patients with renal failure.

Respiratory Alkalosis

In respiratory alkalosis, the arterial $PaCO_2$ falls to a lower level than expected. This is always due to hyperventilation and an increase in alveolar ventilation. Hyperventilation can be due to a neurologic cause, as with stroke, anxiety, pain, fear, or physiologic processes such as sepsis. It can also be secondary to pulmonary etiology, such as with pulmonary embolism, pneumonia, pulmonary edema, or asthma. The AGACNP should focus on airway management, decreasing alveolar ventilation, and management of the underlying cause to correct respiratory alkalosis.

CLINICAL PEARLS

- Acid-base derangements are associated with increased mortality and frequently encountered in clinical practice.
- Acid-base derangements are due to an underlying pathology rather than existing as a primary disorder. The underlying cause should be recognized and treated to correct the derangement.
- Arterial blood gas interpretation should be approached systematically to determine primary and concurrent acid-base disorders.

EVIDENCE-BASED RESOURCE

Gooch, M. D. (2015). Identifying acid-base and electrolyte imbalances. *Nurse Practitioner, 40*(8), 37–42. https://doi.org/10.1097/01.NPR.0000469255.98119.82

INTRAVENOUS FLUID MANAGEMENT

Fluid management is essential in the hospital setting. IV fluid administration is the most common intervention administered in the acute care setting (Semler & Kellum, 2019). Both too little intravascular volume (hypovolemia) and too much intravascular volume (hypervolemia) are associated with increased mortality (Balakumar et al., 2017). Hypovolemia occurs with a decrease in intravascular volume and can be precipitated by a variety of causes: gastrointestinal losses, renal free water loss, hemorrhage, and so forth. A decrease

in intravascular volume leads to decreased cardiac output that can result in organ hypoperfusion, renal failure, confusion, splanchnic ischemia, and multiorgan failure (Vincent, 2019). Hypervolemia occurs with an excess of intravascular volume, which can lead to edema, intraabdominal hypertension, respiratory failure, impaired healing, and multiorgan failure. Volume management can be categorized into four phases: salvage and resuscitation, optimization, stabilization, and de-escalation (Vincent, 2019).

SALVAGE AND RESUSCITATION

When patients lose a high volume of intravascular volume due to conditions such as with trauma or sepsis, the initial goal of fluid administration is to restore tissue perfusion. Loss of circulating volume places organs at high risk for malperfusion and damage. Patients profoundly hypovolemic may present with hypotension, tachycardia, or oliguria. This clinical picture should prompt the clinician to initiate fluid administration. Intravascular volume repletion increases cardiac output and subsequently improves organ perfusion. The initial resuscitation can be guided by frequent assessment of heart rate, blood pressure, and urine output. While labs may demonstrate evidence of hypovolemia, fluid salvage and resuscitation should be initiated by the patient's clinical picture.

OPTIMIZATION

Following initial resuscitation and restoration of end organ perfusion, the next goal is to optimize ongoing fluid resuscitation. At this time, the AGACNP should carefully examine the patient and assess for ongoing volume deficits and volume responsiveness. Serum lactate levels should be monitored to evaluate tissue oxygenation and can be used as a marker for response to therapy. Central venous pressure monitoring may also be utilized to evaluate volume responsiveness. Bedside echocardiography is also a useful tool in assessing volume status.

STABILIZATION

It is essential that volume status is frequently reassessed and that administration of fluids cease once euvolemia is reached. Positive fluid balance in sepsis patients has been linked with an increased risk of death (Sakr et al., 2017). Routine maintenance fluids are only indicated for the patient that is euvolemic, hemodynamically stable, and unable to maintain their own daily fluid intake requirement enterally (Barlow et al., 2020).

DE-ESCALATION

After a patient's condition has stabilized, the de-escalation phase of fluid maintenance can commence. This involves removing excess fluid administration, and often with the administration of loop diuretics to promote a negative volume balance.

TYPES OF FLUIDS

It is essential that the clinician consider IV fluids as medications and that a thoughtful approach is taken with the prescription of fluid. Table 20.4 demonstrates the electrolyte composition of frequently utilized fluids in the acute care setting (Moritz & Ayus, 2015).

CRYSTALLOID SOLUTIONS

Saline

Saline, also known as normal saline or 0.9% saline, is the most commonly prescribed IV fluid (Finfer et al., 2010). Saline contains equal parts sodium and chloride at 154 mEq/L. The solution lacks a buffer, and for this reason it is known as an "unbalanced" solution. Because of the supraphysiologic concentration of sodium and chloride, it is a slightly hypertonic solution. The high chloride concentration also predisposes patients to the development of hyperchloremic acidosis. Large volume resuscitations with normal saline have been associated with an increased risk of acute kidney injury and ICU-related mortality (Semler et al., 2018). However, in certain clinical scenarios such as head trauma, saline may be indicated given its slightly hypertonic properties.

Balanced Solutions

Balanced solutions, such as lactated Ringer's, Hartmann solution, or PlasmaLyte A (Baxter), were created to mimic the concentrations of electrolytes in human plasma. The excess chloride of normal saline was replaced with a buffering agent, such as lactate, acetate, or gluconate. This helps to reduce the tonicity of the solution and neutralize the pH (Barlow et al., 2020).

HYPOTONIC SOLUTIONS

Hypotonic solutions, such as 5% dextrose in water, are often indicated for repletion of free water. Hypotonic fluids are often utilized for the correction of hypernatremia or in diabetic ketoacidosis. This type of fluid should be avoided in patients with central nervous diseases.

HYPERTONIC SOLUTIONS

Hypertonic fluids, such as 3% sodium chloride or 23.4% sodium chloride, have a significant supraphysiologic concentration of both sodium and chloride. These fluids are often utilized as volume expanders to promote movement of water into the intravascular space from the extravascular space and for patients with elevated intracranial pressures or with symptomatic hyponatremia.

COLLOID SOLUTIONS

Colloid solutions contain large, insoluble molecules that do not readily cross the cell membrane. This establishes a high oncotic pressure that promotes the movement of fluid from the extravascular to intravascular space (Barlow et al., 2020). Albumin is frequently utilized as a colloid. This fluid is available in both a 5% and 25% concentration. The 5% concentration effectively increases intravascular fluid volume by 100%, while the 25% solution increases intravascular volume by 400% (Barlow et al., 2020). While this volume expansion is appealing when attempting to avoid fluid volume overload in acutely ill patients, randomized control trials have yet to consistently demonstrate reduced mortality risk with the use of albumin versus an isotonic solution.

TABLE 20.4: Electrolyte Concentration in Frequently Utilized Fluids

	GLUCOSE	SODIUM	CHLORIDE	POTASSIUM	BUFFER	CALCIUM	MAGNESIUM	pH	OSMOLARITY	OSMOLALITY
	G/dL	Mmol/dL							mOsm/L	mOsm/kg
Plasma	0.07-0.11	135-145	95-105	3.5-5.0	23-30	2.2-2.6	0.8-1.2	7.35-7.45	308	288
5% Dextrose in water	5	0	0	0	0	0	0	3.5-6.5	252	
Ringer's lactate	0	130	109	4	28	1.35	0	6-7.5	273	254
Hartmann solution	0	131	111	5	29	2	0	5.0-7.0	278	
0.9% Saline	0	154	154	0	0	0	0	4.5-7	308	286
Multiple electrolytes injection, type 1, USP	0	140	98	5	50	0	1.5	4.0-6.5	294	

CLINICAL PEARLS

- Administration of IV fluids is the most common intervention in the hospital and should be approached with caution.
- IV fluids should be chosen with consideration of their indication and necessity.
- The AGACNP should frequently reassess volume status during ongoing resuscitation to determine hypo-, hyper-, or euvolemia.

EVIDENCE-BASED RESOURCES

Moritz, M. L., & Ayus, J. C. (2015). Maintenance intravenous fluids in acutely ill patients. *New England Journal of Medicine, 373*(14), 1350–1360. https://doi.org/10.1056/NEJMra1412877

Vincent, J. L. (2019). Fluid management in the critically ill. *Kidney International, 96*(1), 52–57. https://doi.org/10.1016/j.kint.2018.11.047

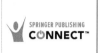

A robust set of instructor resources designed to supplement this text is located at **http://connect.springerpub.com/content/reference-book/978-0-8261-6079-9.** Qualifying instructors may request access by emailing **textbook@springerpub.com.**

REFERENCES

Full list of references can be accessed at http://connect.springerpub.com/content/reference-book/978-0-8261-6079-9.

CHAPTER 21

SHOCK

LEARNING OBJECTIVES

- Define historical referents for shock and current definitions of the following forms of shock: hypovolemic, cardiogenic, distributive: anaphylactic/neurogenic and obstructive.
- Describe commonalities in all forms of shock.
- Relate pathophysiologic variants that occur in different forms of shock.
- Analyze current evidence-based treatment based on pathogenesis of shock.
- Evaluate effective shock treatment based on current recommendations.
- Hypothesize current shock treatment and future management implications of the various forms of shock.

INTRODUCTION

Steven Branham and Patrick A. Laird

As a clinical syndrome, shock has plagued clinicians for years. Part of the confusion is that shock is not an isolated disease, but a syndrome that is a manifestation of the effects of hypoperfusion resulting in a cellular oxygenation debt. Historically, shock was viewed purely as a dysfunction in a body system, such as the cardiovascular, hepatic, and renal systems (Best & Taylor, 1945). This view was fatally flawed, as cellular impact was not considered the primary problem in shock. A great deal of research has been conducted to understand shock better. Rice (1991) outlined the current thoughts of that time, describing the stages of shock as initial, compensatory, progressive, and refractory. These stages remain clinically useful but do little to address changes germane to shock at the cellular level. The current lexicon classifies shock using four distinct systems: hypovolemic, distributive, cardiogenic, and obstructive. Some authors, however, combine cardiogenic and obstructive shock as a single entity (Day & Whitmore, 2020; Standl et al., 2018). For this chapter, the four-stage classification system is used, as it provides a global grouping of the physiologic alterations resulting from shock.

Hypovolemic shock is related to circulating volume status and includes hemorrhagic conditions. Distributive

shock includes impediments to vascular tone such as sepsis, anaphylaxis, or nervous system derangements affecting tone. An entire chapter of this book is dedicated to septic shock, which is not covered in detail in this chapter. Cardiogenic shock (CS) encompasses factors impacting cardiac output (CO) such as pump failure, rate disturbance, or heart valve disorders. Obstructive shock includes defects in preload, afterload, and right heart ability causing a direct effect on CO, tissue perfusion, and oxygenation. Each type is covered in detail in this chapter.

Shock state classification systems are useful for creating global groupings based on physiologic alteration resulting in a state of hypoperfusion. One commonality among all forms of shock is the result: cellular hypoperfusion and oxygenation. Preferred methods of cellular metabolism that employ the aerobic oxidative reductive pathway are reduced or lost. The result is anaerobic cellular metabolism that results in metabolic acidosis. Typical biomarkers and physiologic markers have limited utility when diagnosing shock, as the respective attenuation can occur in nonshock states. Exact epidemiologic rates of shock are difficult to find, as the underling disease process is often cited as the cause of mortality and morbidity, or the underlying shock state is reported rather than the global classification of shock.

Hemodynamic parameters associated with the various shock states are found in Table 21.1.

TABLE 21.1: Hemodynamic Parameters of Various Shock States

TYPE OF SHOCK	MAP	CO/SV	CVP	MPAP	PCWP	SVR
Cardiogenic	↓→	↓	↑	↑	↑	↑
Distributive	↓	↑	↓	↓	↓	↓
Hypovolemic	↓→	↓	↓	↓	↓	↑
Obstructive	↓	↓	↑	↑	↑	↑

↑ Increased; ↓ Decreased; → No change.

CO/SV, cardiac output/stroke volume; CVP, central venous pressure; MAP, mean arterial pressure; MPAP, mean pulmonary arterial pressure; PCWP, pulmonary capillary wedge pressure; SVR, systemic vascular resistance.

21.1: HYPOVOLEMIC/HEMORRHAGIC SHOCK

Daniel O'Neill and Tara C. Hilliard

Hypovolemic/hemorrhage shock is a dynamic process and AGACNPs must be able to recognize the subtle changes in physiology in order to commence early aggressive treatment to promote optimal recovery. No single vital sign or laboratory test can diagnose hemorrhagic/hypovolemic shock. Therefore, emphasis is based on clinical recognition and the presence of inadequate tissue perfusion, which is the definition of shock. This section reviews the pathophysiology of hemorrhagic/hypovolemic shock and current treatment options available.

PRESENTING SIGNS AND SYMPTOMS

A 28-year-old male electrician and army reservist with no past medical history presents via ambulance to the local emergency department (ED). The patient was involved in a head-on motor vehicle crash. In the ED his vital signs are: P 115, BP 80/70, RR 20, SaO_2 on 100% NRB 100%, T 36.9°C. Initial evaluation by emergency medical services (EMS) reveals bruising over the chest and abdomen and a deformed right forearm. EMS applied oxygen, started one IV of normal saline at 100 mL/h, and splinted the arm.

On arrival at the ED, the AGACNP considers the differential diagnosis while evaluating the patient. As the AGACNP proceeds through the primary survey reviewing airway, breathing, and circulation, the initial impression is hypovolemic/hemorrhagic shock.

HISTORY AND PHYSICAL FINDINGS

CO is defined as the volume of blood pumped by the heart per minute and is determined by multiplying heart rate (HR) by stroke volume (SV) so that CO = HR × SV. It is important to remember that the volume of blood returned to the heart determines myocardial muscle fiber length after ventricular filling at the end of diastole. In addition, muscle fiber length is related to the contractile properties of myocardial muscle which is known as Starling's law (Colwell, 2022).

The AGACNP suspects the patient is bleeding, and the key focus now is correcting blood loss which caused the hemorrhage/hypovolemic shock. As blood volume is depleted early on, altered mental status is common. Thready pulses, tachycardia, and tachypnea are frequently present. Patients in shock often exhibit cool, pale, or ashen skin with decreased capillary refill and dry mucous membranes; compensatory mechanisms commence which include vasoconstriction and an increased HR in an attempt to preserve CO. This is noted within the measurable vital signs of tachycardia and tachypnea. Then, a release of catecholamines occurs causing peripheral vascular resistance, which in turn, increases diastolic blood pressure and reduces pulse pressure. Early in hemorrhagic shock, venous return is preserved by compensatory mechanisms; however, these mechanisms are limited. Effective methods to treat hypovolemic/hemorrhagic shock are to restore CO, promote end organ perfusion and venous return by arresting the bleeding, and initiating appropriate volume replacement. Without adequate volume replacement cells are inadequately perfused and deprived of essential substrates for aerobic metabolism leading to a shift to anaerobic metabolism. Anaerobic metabolism results in lactic acid formation and subsequent development of metabolic acidosis.

If hemorrhagic/hypovolemic shock is not treated adequately, adenosine triphosphate (ATP) production becomes inadequate, cells lose membrane integrity, and the electrical gradient is lost. This leads to a deleterious process of cellular destruction with inducible nitric oxide synthase (iNOS), cytokines, and tumor necrosis factor (TNF) production leading to end organ dysfunction. Thus, the key is early correction with isotonic electrolyte solutions to avoid progressive cellular damage leading to cell death (International ATLS Working Group, 2013).

DIFFERENTIAL DIAGNOSIS AND DIAGNOSTIC CONSIDERATIONS

When diagnosing hypovolemic/hemorrhagic shock, hemodynamic collapse will be evident. After securing the airway and breathing, circulatory assessment is paramount to identify shock. History, mechanism of injury, and assessment of vital signs all must be quickly evaluated to identify shock. Overreliance on systolic blood pressure as an indicator of the shock state can cause a delay in diagnosis as most healthy individuals can compensate for a fall in systolic pressure until 30% of the blood volume is lost. Attention should be directed to pulse rate, respiratory rate, and skin circulation. Any injured patient who is cool and has tachycardia is considered to be in shock until proven otherwise.

When assessing the patient with hemorrhagic/hypovolemic shock, a common pitfall is to wait for a patient to fit specific physiologic classifications before initiating volume replacement. Hemorrhagic/hypovolemic shock can be categorized into four classes of shock (Table 21.2).

Trauma Triad of Death

After reviewing the patient's vital signs and noting the HR and blood pressure, this patient would fit within the parameters of Class II hypovolemic/hemorrhagic shock. With this stage of shock, the trauma triad of death should be considered. Within this triad, if the patient continues to bleed and transitions through the classes of shock then a lethal triad will occur. Once the patient is in the lethal triad it is very difficult to reverse and promote an optimal outcome. This is particularly important when thinking about the golden hour, which is a concept

TABLE 21.2: Four Classes of Shock

CLASS OF SHOCK	DESCRIPTION
Class I	Volume loss of up to 15%. A patient in this class will demonstrate minimal signs of complications. There are no measurable changes in blood pressure, pulse, or respiratory rate. Healthy patients with this amount of blood loss usually tolerate the loss and do not require significant volume replacement.
Class II	Volume loss of 15% to 30%. A patient in this class will start demonstrating measurable vital sign changes such as increased heart rate above 100, increased respirations, and some changes in level of consciousness when 750 to 1500 mL of blood loss occurs. With a blood loss of 15% to 30%, cardiovascular changes and urine output are only mildly affected. During Class II shock is the optimal time to initiate stabilization therapy with crystalloid solutions according to evidence-based guidelines.
Class III	Volume loss of 30% to 40%. The blood loss is approximately 1500 to 2000 mL in an adult. This amount of blood loss is devastating and patients in this class of shock will show classic signs of shock such as altered mental status, hypotension, and tachycardia. At this stage, fluid and blood products are essential in the management of the patient in order to prevent further deterioration in condition.
Class IV	Volume loss of more than 40%. The degree of blood loss is immediately life-threatening and symptoms include no negligible urine output, hypotension, loss of consciousness, and marked tachycardia. This condition requires immediate blood products and surgical intervention.

Source: International ATLS Working Group. (2013). Advanced trauma life support (ATLS®): The ninth edition. *The Journal of Trauma and Acute Care Surgery, 74*(5), 1363–1366. https://doi.org/10.1097/TA.0b013e31828b82f5

generally accepted in trauma care where the optimum outcome for injured patients is definitive care within 60 minutes.

The trauma triad of death consists of three key components: hypothermia, acidosis, and coagulopathy. Hypothermia in hemorrhagic shock can result in devastating physiologic consequences and predicts a poor outcome. Hypothermia notably affects coagulation and impairs platelet function and initiation of clotting factors which lead to increased bleeding. Acidosis occurs due to inadequate tissue perfusion and cells start to utilize an anaerobic pathway. As perfusion worsens, lactic acid accumulates in tissues and leads to disruption of coagulation and further increased anaerobic metabolism. Finally, a combination of acidosis and hyperthermia leads to depletion of platelets and clotting factors resulting in early coagulopathy and severe hemorrhage (Keane, 2016).

Coagulopathy is noted in up to 30% of severely injured patients on admission. Fluid resuscitation with resultant dilution of platelets and clotting factors with adverse effects of hypothermia on platelet aggregation and clotting cascade can occur. Prothrombin time, partial thromboplastin time, and platelet count are valuable baseline studies to obtain in the first hour of care. Therefore, it is important to be guided by the coagulation parameters to assist decision-making for transfusion.

TREATMENT
Crystalloids and Colloids

Treatment decisions are based on patient assessment and condition and classification of shock. Treatment for hemorrhagic/hypovolemic shock typically includes administering 30 mL/kg body weight of a fluid challenge and assessing response.

Ideally warm isotonic crystalloids such as Ringer's lactate or normal saline (0.9%), 1 to 2 L for adults and 20 mL/kg for children is indicated. A ratio of 3:1 for adults should be used which means 3 L of crystalloids for each unit of blood lost. After each fluid challenge, the patient's response should be assessed by monitoring vital signs. Crystalloids are readily available and inexpensive; however, they generally leave the intravascular space within 30 minutes necessitating the need for larger volume administration. Colloids on the other hand provide a lengthier time period of volume expansion and are replaced on a 1:1 ratio. However, colloids are more expensive and not as readily available as crystalloid fluids.

Much debate has occurred over the last 20 years on which fluid such be initiated for initial fluid resuscitation, crystalloid or colloid. Research from the last two decades has shown colloids are no more effective (on a volume-for-volume basis) in restoring blood volume. A systematic review of 37 randomized controlled trials of fluid resuscitation using either colloid or crystalloid preparations in critically ill patients found that colloids could cause pulmonary edema, anaphylactic shock, and lead to a small increase in risk of death (Schierhout & Roberts, 1998). Authors of this systematic review concluded that continued use of colloids was not supported for volume replacement. A similar review conducted by Bisonni in 1991 (Bisonni et al., 1991), looked at 26 randomized controlled trials of colloids versus crystalloids in fluid resuscitation of hypovolemic patients. The study identified similar results, and the author concluded colloids were not favored in initial fluid resuscitation. A recent multicenter randomized trial CRISTAL (Colloids versus crystalloids for the resuscitation of the critically ill) compared mortality in critical patients with colloid versus crystalloid use and found no difference in 28-day mortality (Annane et al., 2013). In clinical practice crystalloids generally tend to be more favored and more readily used than colloids which are used more cautiously.

The goal of resuscitation is to restore end organ perfusion; however, if blood pressure is raised rapidly before bleeding is controlled, then this can be detrimental. This has led to alternative treatment pathways with one example being permissive/controlled hypotension.

Permissive hypotension was described by Bickell et al. (1994) in his landmark study in which patients with penetrating trauma were randomized into groups receiving fluids versus no fluids in the prehospital group. Bickell et al. (1994), noted that the group that did not receive fluids had improved outcomes versus the group that received fluids.

The group that received fluids demonstrated issues with dilution, clot formation, and increased coagulopathy versus the nonfluid group. This led to the birth of permissive hypotension, which was translated into practice and used in the Iraq and Afghanistan wars. Medics were instructed to palpate for a radial pulse, and if a pulse were present, no fluid was given in the prehospital setting and the patient was transferred to surgical care. If pulseless upon presentation the patient was given a fluid bolus in 250 mL bolus increments until return of a pulse, at which time further fluid administration was discontinued (Kudo et al., 2017). Some debate still exists that questions the practice, suggesting that permissive hypotension is still inconclusive and requires further research.

Blood

Blood replacement should be considered for those patients in Class III, Class IV, transient, and nonresponsive patients. Replacement should ideally occur with packed red blood cells (RBCs), plasma, and platelets in a 1:1:1 ratio. Initial blood therapy is initiated with O negative blood type until type-specific blood is available. Type-specific is preferred and can be achieved in most healthcare systems within 30 minutes (Holcomb et al., 2007).

Tourniquets

Tourniquets should be used to assist in stopping blood loss in an extremity injury causing hypovolemic shock. Tourniquets have been used robustly by the military in the Iraq and Afghanistan wars with significant success in controlling blood loss. Studies by Kragh et al. (2008) demonstrated that when a tourniquet is placed early in a combat casualty before the onset of shock there is a 10% mortality. When tourniquets are applied after the signs of shock are present the mortality rate increases dramatically to 90%.

Tourniquets have been shown to be very effective in controlling hemorrhage from extremity injuries and have been subsequently implemented into civilian EMS systems.

Tourniquets should be placed high, tight, and at a site proximal to the injury/wound to control blood loss. McNickle et al. (2019), determined that survivability was higher when prehospital tourniquets were applied. It is imperative that the provider assess and reassess the effectiveness of tourniquet after every application and patient movement including every head-to-toe examination. It must be emphasized that limb tourniquets should be converted to hemostatic or pressure dressing within 2 hours only if bleeding can be controlled (TECC, 2019).

Tranexamic Acid

Tranexamic acid (TXA) has become widely popular since the CRASH-2 study (Roberts et al., 2013) which demonstrated that TXA reduces blood loss by inhibiting the enzymatic breakdown of fibrin. Initiation of TXA treatment within 3 hours of injury reduces the risk of hemorrhage death by about one third, regardless of baseline risk. Because TXA does not have any serious adverse effects, it can be administered to a wide spectrum of bleeding trauma patients and should be considered in the treatment of hypovolemic/hemorrhagic shock (Roberts, 2015).

Resuscitation

Underresuscitation and overresuscitation can be fatal and careful transition to postresuscitation phase is important to improve outcomes (Ramesh et al., 2019). The postresuscitation phase is defined as the period where microcirculatory flow is improved postcorrection of coagulopathy with the systolic blood pressure (SBP) >100 mmHg and mean arterial pressure (MAP) >65 mmHg. Response to fluid resuscitation should be monitored closely, and if a patient is fluid responsive then no further administration should be considered as the risk of fluid overload outweighs hemodynamic benefits (Ramesh et al., 2019).

Special Considerations

When managing patients in hypovolemic/hemorrhagic shock, AGACNPs must consider advanced age, level of physical fitness status, pregnancy, and medications. Advanced age results in depletion of physiologic reserve, most notably cardiac compliance decreases with age. Due to the lack of adequate physiologic reserve, elderly patients are unable to effectively increase their heart rate to compensate for blood loss and certain medications such as beta-blockers should be considered which will affect ability to increase heart rate.

Athletes and healthy young people must be treated with caution as this group generally tolerates blood loss well and can compensate for longer periods without showing classical signs of hypovolemic/hemorrhagic shock. Similarly, pregnant patients have an increase in blood volume and will compensate for blood loss for extend periods before showing clinical signs. Patients on medications such as beta-blockers will not demonstrate increased heart rate with increasing blood loss.

TRANSITION OF CARE

Bleeding control, maintenance of tissue oxygenation, and coagulation support is key to improving outcomes of hemorrhagic shock patients. Hemorrhagic shock can be fatal if not recognized early, appropriate volume resuscitation is not initiated, and bleeding not controlled. Early transition from prehospital care to definitive care is imperative for optimal outcome. Failure to recognize early signs of hypovolemic shock and class of shock reduce survivability. Therefore, rapid assessment, control of hemorrhage, and early volume-controlled resuscitation and transfer to surgical care as quickly as possible increase optimal outcomes. Future therapies for the treatment of hemorrhagic/hypovolemic shock will hopefully be developed in the coming years, such as the development of artificial blood products, hypertonic colloids, and recombinant products (Angele et al., 2008).

CLINICAL PEARLS

- Control hemorrhage.
- Use minimal volume of IV fluids to maintain adequate hemodynamic response.
- Use blood products as soon as clinically indicated.
- Blood ratio of 1:1:1 with packed red blood cells, fresh frozen plasma, and platelets.
- TXA should be given within 3 hours of injury.

KEY TAKEAWAYS

- Be suspicious of the trauma triad.
- Avoid overreliance on pulse and blood pressure in the young and fit, as they tolerate blood loss well.
- If you suspect hemorrhagic/hypovolemic shock start treatment immediately.

21.2: CARDIOGENIC SHOCK

Amanda Bergeron

Cardiogenic shock (CS) occurs when the heart is not able to adequately deliver blood to the body resulting in inadequate tissue oxygenation, organ hypoperfusion leading to multisystem organ failure and death. The definition of CS varies, but generally is expressed as hypotension with systolic blood pressure (SBP) <90 mmHg, cardiac index <2.2 L/min/m², pulmonary capillary wedge pressure (PCWP) >18 mmHg, and signs of organ hypoperfusion in the form of altered mental status, oliguria, cold extremities. In CS, a vicious cascade occurs that it initiated by myocardial ischemia leading to decreased cardiac output (CO). The decrease in CO further decreases myocardial perfusion, leading to further damage. In addition, the body's compensatory mechanism of increasing heart rate (HR) and afterload in attempts to increase CO and blood pressure may cause further impairment to the already damaged myocardium. Decreased CO leads to end organ damage, initiating a systemic inflammatory response thereby increasing the demand of the heart causing further ischemia. If not interrupted, this cycle leads to progressive organ dysfunction and ultimately may lead to death (Hollenberg, 2019). There are many causes, with the most common cause being left ventricular (LV)

failure secondary to acute myocardial infarction (AMI). Other causes of LV or right ventricular (RV) dysfunction may lead to cardiogenic shock (CS), which may include myocarditis, cardiac tamponade, end-stage cardiomyopathy, mechanical complication of myocardial infarction (MI), such as ventricular septal defect (VSD) or mitral regurgitation (MR), prolonged cardiopulmonary bypass, acute valvular regurgitation secondary to endocarditis, pulmonary embolism causing RV failure, or stressed-induced (Takotsubo) cardiomyopathy (Hollenberg, 2019). Although mortality in CS remains high, guidelines for defining, identifying, and managing CS have improved inhospital management (van Diepen, 2017).

PRESENTING SIGNS AND SYMPTOMS

Signs and symptoms of CS are due to decreased myocardial contractility following an insult, thus decreasing CO, and causing hypotension, systemic vasoconstriction, and further cardiac ischemia. Ineffective stroke volume (SV) and inability of the body to effectively compensate lead to hypoperfusion. The body attempts to improve coronary circulation by increasing peripheral vasoconstriction. Consequently, increased peripheral vasoconstriction results in diminished blood flow to peripheral tissues and other organs, as well as increasing cardiac afterload, increasing the workload on an already damaged heart (Vahdatpour, 2019). Signs of hypoperfusion include altered mental status, cold clammy skin, and mottled extremities, although symptoms may vary among patients. Patients in CS may complain of chest pain, palpitations, weakness, dizziness, deceased exercise tolerance, and nausea or vomiting. Commonly patients will present with signs of volume overload such as dyspnea, peripheral edema, cough, and orthopnea.

HISTORY AND PHYSICAL FINDINGS

A detailed history and physical exam are essential in diagnosing CS. LV failure due to AMI or pump failure due to loss of cardiac function from previous MI is the most common cause of CS (Hollenberg, 2019). There is an increased risk of developing CS in those patients with ST-elevation myocardial infarction (STEMI) as compared to non-ST-elevation myocardial infarction (NSTEMI), although the mortality is higher in NSTEMI patients who develop CS (Vahdatpour, 2019). Obtaining a detailed history to include any presence of recent MI or chest pain, recent viral illness, or history of heart failure or other cardiac condition is essential in diagnosing CS. Cardiac risk factors should also be assessed for, such as diabetes mellitus, tobacco use, hypertension, family history of cardiac disease, age >45 in men and 55 in women, as well as decreased physical activity.

Patients in CS will typically present with hypotension (SBP <90 mmHg) and signs of organ hypoperfusion. Findings suggestive of low perfusion may include narrow pulse pressure, altered mental status, cool extremities, and renal/hepatic dysfunction. Compensatory mechanisms include an increased sympathetic response, resulting in tachycardia, which can increase myocardial oxygen demand further increasing cardiac ischemia.

Symptoms of congestion such as orthopnea, paroxysmal nocturnal dyspnea, edema, and abdominal tenderness (usually right upper quadrant) may also be present (Hollenberg, 2019).

On physical exam, patients may have jugular vein distention (JVD), cool and/or mottled extremities, rales, gallop rhythm or new heart murmur, faint, or rapid peripheral pulses, abdominojugular reflex, or hepatomegaly. Although hypotension is common in CS, the SHOCK trial registry did find that about 5.2% of patients did not have hypotension (SBP <90 mmHg), although signs of hypoperfusion did still exist (Hochman et al., 1999).

Manifestations of CS may be different in patients where shock is due to RV dysfunction in the setting of inferior wall infarct or pulmonary embolism. In this patient population, signs of pulmonary vascular congestion may be absent. Hypotension, signs of hypoperfusion, and JVD will likely be present.

In cases where a right heart catheterization is performed, or a pulmonary artery catheter is placed, more information may be obtained to help diagnose CS. Hemodynamic profiles can vary in patients diagnosed with CS (Table 21.3) Low cardiac index (<2.2) is common to all profiles, but systemic vascular resistance (SVR), PCWP, and central venous pressure (CVP) can vary. CS involving LV failure typically presents as "cold-wet," which according to the SHOCK trial, occurs in two thirds of patients (Hochman et al., 1999). These patients have high SVR and are volume overloaded and congested.

DIFFERENTIAL DIAGNOSIS AND DIAGNOSTIC CONSIDERATIONS

Early diagnosis to allow for early initiation of treatment, in order to prevent irreversible damage to vital organs is essential (Hollenberg, 2019). All types of shock present with similar features such as hypotension, tachycardia, altered mental status, and organ dysfunction, making diagnosing CS challenging. Differential diagnoses include hypovolemic shock, distributive, and obstructive shock (Vahdatpour, 2019).

TABLE 21.3: Hemodynamic Presentations of Cardiogenic Shock

	WET	DRY
WARM	↓ SVR ↑ PCWP ↑ CVP	↓ SVR ↓ PCWP ↓ CVP
COLD	↑ SVR ↑ PCWP ↑ CVP	↑ SVR ↓ PCWP ↓ CVP

CVP, central venous pressure; PCWP, pulmonary capillary wedge pressure; SVR, systemic vascular resistance.

Electrocardiogram

ECGs should be immediately performed when a patient arrives in presumed shock. With the most common cause of CS being acute MI, it is important to identify ECG changes such as ST elevation or ST depression. In cases of suspected RV infarct, a right-sided ECG may be performed to identify ST elevations in right-sided leads (Hollenberg, 2019). Identification of pathologic Q waves may indicate extensive damage, or MI with delayed presentation. In the setting of STEMI, emergent cardiac catherization should be performed to attempt revascularization, potentially reducing further myocardial damage. ACS may also present as sustained arrhythmias, such as ventricular tachycardia, ventricular fibrillation, atrial fibrillation, new bundle branch block, or high-grade atrioventricular block (Vahdatpour, 2019).

Laboratory Testing

Routine laboratory tests should include complete blood count (CBC), basic metabolic panel (BMP), liver function tests, cardiac biomarkers, arterial blood gases, and lactic acid levels. Signs of end organ damage such as elevated creatinine, elevated transaminases, and lactic acidosis may indicate organ hypoperfusion secondary to CS. N-terminal pro-B-type natriuretic peptide levels should also be checked, as elevated levels can arise from an acute decompensation of chronic heart failure (Vahdatpour, 2019). Arterial blood gases may reveal reduced peripheral oxygenation, resulting in lower PaO_2 levels and higher CO_2 levels (Vahdatpour, 2019). A serum lactate level >2 mmol/L also reflects inadequate tissue oxygenation/metabolism due to shock. Although serum lactate levels may be elevated in other types of shock, this finding along with other signs and symptoms may aid in the diagnosis of CS (Chioncel, 2020). Ruling out other causes of lactic acidosis such as diabetic ketoacidosis (DKA), liver insufficiency, and medication use such as propofol or epinephrine is also important (Chioncel, 2020).

Chest Radiograph

Chest radiographs should be done on all patients who present with signs of shock. A finding of congestion or pulmonary edema on chest radiographs may help in differentiating CS from other types of shock (Hollenberg, 2019). Although not all pulmonary edema is cardiac related, this finding in combination with the physical exam and other diagnostic findings may lead to a diagnosis of CS. In cardiogenic pulmonary edema, chest radiographs will show fluffy air-space opacities in central as well as peripheral lungs, whereas noncardiogenic pulmonary edema will have batwing opacities with air bronchograms. Cardiomegaly may also be present in CS (Sureka et al., 2015).

Echocardiography

Echocardiography is a critical tool to aid in diagnosing CS and should be done as soon as possible. Echocardiograms can help determine causes of CS such as cardiac tamponade, mechanical complications of AMI, or acute valvular abnormalities. Other important information obtained from echocardiograms include assessment of both RV and LV function, wall motion abnormalities, and an estimation of left and right filling pressures (Chioncel, 2020).

Right Heart Catheterization

In some cases, right heart catheterization may be deemed appropriate when other findings do not clearly suggest CS as in cases of mixed shock, or if the patient does not respond to initial therapy (Chioncel, 2020). The use of right heart catheterization or Swan-Ganz catheter placement remain controversial, but the hemodynamic information provided can help guide treatment, especially in cases of RV failure. Its use can also provide accurate information on filling pressures, as well as close monitoring of CO (Hollenberg, 2019).

TREATMENT

Initial Management

Initial management to improve outcomes should focus on treating the underlying cause. When acute coronary syndrome (ACS) is determined as the cause of CS, early revascularization in the cardiac catheterization lab should be initially performed. According to the SHOCK trial, early coronary interventions (<12 hours) significantly lowered mortality at 6, 12, and 60 months, leading to a class I/B recommendation (SHOCK, 1999). Next, the status of congestion should be determined (wet vs. dry) by use of echocardiography, or invasive monitoring in the form of central line or pulmonary artery (PA) catheter. Central line use is recommended for central venous pressure (CVP) monitoring, central venous saturation measurements, and for administration of vasoactive drugs (Chioncel, 2020). If it is determined that the patient is hypovolemic, small boluses of crystalloids can be used. For patients who are considered hypervolemic or "wet," loop diuretics such as furosemide should be given early. Initial doses of furosemide should be 0.5 mg/kg or double the patient's home oral dose. Close monitoring of response to diuretics should be performed and repeat or higher doses given as needed (Mebazaa, 2016).

If a PA catheter is present, mixed venous oxygen saturations (SVO_2) should be monitored closely, as low SVO_2 may indicate reduced CO, hypoxemia, anemia, or increased oxygen consumption. Although SVO_2 will likely be low in CS, monitoring this parameter can allow one to evaluate the response to therapies to determine its effectiveness (Vahdatpour, 2019). The use of PA catheters for close hemodynamic monitoring may help the provider determine the need for mechanical circulatory support (MCS) if medical therapy is failing. Although studies suggest that the use of PA catheters have no mortality benefit and are associated with complications such as pulmonary infarcts, arrhythmias, infection and balloon rupture, they may be useful in select patients (Vahdatpour, 2019).

Oxygenation and ventilation should also be closely monitored, and a continuous pulse oximeter should be used. A goal oxygen saturation of >90% is used, although may vary depending on patients underlying conditions (e.g., COPD). The use of invasive ventilation may be needed if other methods are inadequate. Low tidal volume ventilation is recommended, as it is considered lung protective and reduces stress on the RV (Vahdatpour, 2019).

Vasopressors and Inotropes

Vasodilators, inotropes, and vasopressors are used in CS to maintain coronary and systemic profusion, until mechanical circulatory support is placed or until shock resolves. These medications are required in 80% to 90% of patients who present in CS (Chioncel, 2020). Use of vasopressors should be titrated at the lowest dose possible to maintain a mean arterial pressure (MAP) of >65 mmHg, reducing associated negative side effects (Vahdatpour, 2019). Norepinephrine (0.02–1.0 mcg/kg/min) is considered the preferred first-line agent for CS, as it provides vasoconstriction with a mild inotropic effect. Vasopressin may be indicated in patients with acute RV failure, as it has less pulmonary vasoconstriction than norepinephrine. Dopamine is typically considered a second-line drug, as it has inotropic effects at lower doses (3–10 mcg/kg/min) and causes vasoconstriction only at higher doses (10–20 mcg/kg/min). Norepinephrine is preferred, as dopamine has been shown to produce more arrhythmias, as well as the need to use higher doses to produce vasoconstriction (van Diepen, 2017).

Inodilators have both inotropic effects as well as vasodilatory effects, making it an effective treatment in CS. These drugs, such as milrinone, dobutamine, and isoprotererol, have strong inotropic effects, while reducing SVR and peripheral vascular resistance (PVR). They can be used in normotensive and hypertensive patients, as well as in combination with a vasopressor (Table 21.4).

Mechanical Circulatory Support Devices

MCS devices have become more common in the treatment of CS and should be considered early in patients with refractory CS. MCS is associated with significant complications, therefore expertise in both insertion and management is necessary to reduce the risk of complications (Chioncel, 2020). Patients in refractory CS should be transferred to centers with MCS capabilities early on to give the highest chance of survival.

Intraaortic Balloon Pump

The intraaortic balloon pump (IABP) increases CO by about 0.5 to 1 L/min and works via counterpulsation. IABP is inserted in the femoral or axillary artery via a sheath and is able to be inserted either in a cardiac catheterization laboratory or at the bedside. IABPs reduce myocardial oxygen consumption, decrease afterload, increase coronary artery perfusion, and improve

TABLE 21.4: Mechanism of Action and Effects of Common Vasoactive Drugs Used in Cardiogenic Shock

MEDICATION	EFFECTS ON RECEPTOR	HEMODYNAMIC EFFECTS	INDICATION	CAUTIONS
VASOPRESSORS				
Norepinephrine	Alpha-1 > beta-1 agonist	↑↑SVR, ↑CO, ↑HR, ↑↑BP	Initial choice in CS and other forms of shock	May cause tachyarrhythmias Infuse in large vein, preferably via a central line
Dopamine	Dopa, beta-1, beta-2, alpha-1 (dose dependent agonist)	↑CO (all doses) ↑↑SVR (10–20 mcg/kg/min), ↑↑CO, ↑↑HR, ↑BP	CS	May cause Tachyarrhythmia (more frequently than other agents)
Vasopressin	V1 agonist	↑↑SVR, ↑↑BP	CS, RV failure	May cause hyponatremia
Epinephrine	Alpha-1 = beta-1 > beta-2 agonist	↑↑SVR, ↑↑CO, ↑BP, ↑↑HR	CS	May cause tachyarrhythmias
Phenylephrine	Alpha-1 agonist	↑↑SVR, ↑↑BP	CS secondary to aortic or mitral stenosis`	Increases afterload concern if LV dysfunction
INODILATORS				
Milrinone	PD-3 inhibitor	↑CO, ↓SVR, ↓PVR, ↓BP	Normotensive or hypertensive cardiogenic shock, RV failure	May cause atrial arrhythmias and hypotension
Dobutamine	Beta-1 > beta-2 agonist	↑↑CO, ↓SVR, ↓PVR, ↓BP	Normotensive or hypertensive cardiogenic shock, RV failure	Caution in recent MI as it may increase myocardial oxygen demand and causes tachycardia; may cause hypotension
Isoproterenol	Beta-1 > beta-2 agonist	↑↑CO, ↓SVR, ↓PVR, ↑↑HR, ↓BP	Off-label use for CS	Can worsen tachyarrhythmias

AV, atrioventricular; BP, blood pressure; CO, cardiac output; CS, cardiogenic shock; HR, heart rate; LV, left ventricle; MI, myocardial infarction; PD-3, phosphodiesterase 3; PVR, pulmonary vascular resistance; RV, right ventricle; SVR, systemic vascular resistance; v1, vasopressin.

Source: Vahdatpour, C. (2019). Cardiogenic shock. *Journal of the American Heart Association, 8*(8), e011991–e011991. https://doi.org/10.1161/JAHA.119.011991; van Diepen, K. (2017). Contemporary management of cardiogenic shock: A scientific statement from the American Heart Association. *Circulation, 136*(16), e232–e268. https://doi.org/10.1161/CIR.0000000000000525

CO (Vahdatpour, 2019). IABPs also moderately unload the left ventricle and improve systemic blood pressure. While IABPs provide some support, there must be some degree of native cardiac function as well as stable electrical function for the IABP to be effective.

Both positioning of the IABP and timing of inflation and deflation are key in optimizing its use. IABP has been widely used in management of CS, although recent data do not support this practice. In the setting of AMI-CS, the IABP-SHOCK-II randomized control trial did not show mortality benefit of IABP support as compared to medical treatment alone. IABP may be considered in select patients with mechanical complications of AMI (such as acute mitral regurgitation [MR] or ventricular septal defect [VSD]), or as a means to stabilize them in order to transfer to a center that can provide higher levels of mechanical circulatory support (MCS) (Chioncel, 2020; van Diepen, 2017).

Percutaneous Ventricular Assist Devices

Percutaneous MCS, or ventricular assist devices, can provide more support to patients in CS as either a bridge to recovery or a bridge to a more durable device or cardiac transplantation. These devices halt hypoperfusion and ischemia associated with CS by improving CO, decompressing the LV, reducing afterload and providing coronary perfusion (Chioncel, 2020; Hollenberg, 2019). Several percutaneous devices exist including the Impella (RP, 2.5, CP, 5.0, 5.5) and TandemHeart (RA-PA and LA-FA). Device selection should be based on acuity of illness, degree of support required, anatomy, and operator expertise (Tehrani, 2020; Table 21.5).

Venoarterial Extracorporeal Membrane Oxygenation

Venoarterial extracorporeal membrane oxygenation (VA ECMO) may be used in the setting of refractory CS, cardiac and pulmonary failure, and cardiac arrest. VA ECMO provides support for both the heart and lungs by using a membrane oxygenator in the circuit, which pulls deoxygenated blood from a vein and returns oxygenated blood in the aorta. Cannulation is done via femoral artery and femoral vein, or central cannulation can occur in the operating room usually following cardiac surgery. Complications with VA ECMO include bleeding, limb ischemia,

TABLE 21.5: Mechanical Circulatory Support Devices

	IABP	IMPELLA RP	TANDEMHEART (RA-PA)	IMPELLA (2.5, CP, 5.0, 5.5)	TANDEMHEART (LA-FA)	VA ECMO
Flow	0.5–1 L/min	4.0 L/min (max)	4.0 L/min (max)	2.5–5.5 L/min	4.0 L/min (max)	Up to 7.0 L/min
Use	CS, AMI	Acute RV failure following AMI, LVAD insertion, cardiac surgery or cardiac transplantation	Acute RV failure following AMI, LVAD insertion, cardiac surgery or cardiac transplantation	CS, AMI, LV failure, high risk PCI	CS, AMI	Bi-V failure, cardiac arrest, refractory CS, myocarditis, or allograft rejection
Mechanism	Counterpulsation	Axial flow continuous pump (RA to PA)	Continuous centrifugal pump	Axial flow continuous pump (LV to aorta)	Continuous centrifugal pump (LA to femoral artery)	Continuous centrifugal pump
Placement/ position	Placed in femoral artery, sits in aorta with tip of balloon 2–3 cm below origin of left subclavian artery	Placed in femoral artery, pump in right ventricle, crossing pulmonic valve pushing blood into the pulmonary artery	Dual lumen cannula (Protek Duo) inserted in the internal jugular vein	Placed in femoral artery (2.5, CP) or axillary artery (5.0, 5.5), pump in left ventricular crossing aortic valve pushing blood into aorta	Cannula placed in femoral vein, across transseptal puncture and into LA, blood flow returns to femoral artery	Cannula placed in femoral vein returning blood to aorta via femoral artery, or central cannulation
Effects	Reduce afterload, increase coronary perfusion	Right ventricular support, reduction in RV filling pressures	Reduces RA and RV preload by moving blood from RA to PA, increases PA pressures, increases LV preload	Reduces LVEDP, decreases myocardial oxygen consumption, increases CO, MAP, coronary perfusion and end-organ perfusion	LV unloading, improvement in cardiac output, increase afterload	Provides full cardiac and pulmonary support, RV unloading, increases CO, increases LV afterload
Contraindications	Unstable cardiac rhythm, aortic regurgitation (moderate>severe), aortic dissection or aneurysm, severe PVD	Mechanical valves, stenosis or regurgitation of TV or PV, anatomical abnormalities limiting ability for proper placement, RA or IVC thrombus, IVC filter, contraindication to anticoagulation	Mechanical valves, stenosis or regurgitation of TV or PV, RA thrombus, contraindication to anticoagulation	RV failure, LV rupture, ASD or VSD, mechanical aortic valve or severe aortic stenosis or severe aortic regurgitation, LV thrombus, severe PVD, contraindication to anticoagulation	RV failure, contraindication to anticoagulation, anatomic abnormalities limiting ability for proper placement, LA thrombus, aortic regurgitation	Moderate to severe aortic regurgitation, severe PVD, advanced age (>75 years), life expectancy <1 year, contraindications to systemic anticoagulation, neurologic injury

Less support → More support

ASD, atrial septal defect; AMI, acute myocardial infarction; CO, cardiac output; IABP, intraaortic balloon pump; IVC, inferior vena cava; LV, left ventricle; LVAD, left ventricular assist device; LVEDP, left ventricular end-diastolic volume; MAP, mean arterial pressure; PA, pulmonary artery; PV, pulmonic valve; PVD, peripheral vascular disease; RA, right atrium; RV, right ventricle; TV, tricuspid valve; VSD, ventricular septal defect; VA ECMO, venoarterial extracorporeal membrane oxygenation.

Source: Tehrani, T. (2020). A standardized and comprehensive approach to the management of cardiogenic shock. *JACC. Heart Failure, 8*(11), 879–891. https://doi.org/10.1016/j.jchf.2020.09.005

stroke, thromboembolism, hemolysis, infection, and aortic valve insufficiency (van Diepen, 2017). Although VA ECMO can provide a higher level of support, increased LV afterload caused by VA ECMO can lead to LV distention and pulmonary edema. Often, LV unloading devices such as Impella or IABP are used in conjunction with VA ECMO to reduce these effects (van Diepen, 2017).

TRANSITION OF CARE

When treating CS, cardiac recovery is the ultimate goal. In patients who recover and are discharged home, a high rate of early rehospitalizations exists. When discharging patients who were hospitalized with CS, a multidisciplinary approach is necessary in order to provide adequate education, follow-up, and appropriate management of comorbidities. Based on heart failure guidelines, and if appropriate, the following therapies should be initiated or continued: beta-blockers, angiotensin converting enzyme (ACE) inhibitors (or angiotensin receptor blockers [ARBs]), and mineralocorticoid receptor antagonists (MRAs). Education on salt and fluid restrictions are necessary, as well as education on comorbidities that may not have been managed well in the past. Close follow-up in clinic should be scheduled for a week following discharge. It is important to provide education on all medications as well as signs or symptoms of worsening heart failure and indications to return to the hospital (Mebazaa, 2016). Rehabilitation or long-term acute care may be necessary in select patients (Chioncel, 2020).

For patients who are unlikely to recover, consideration of long-term support in the form of a durable MCS device is recommended (van Diepen, 2017). Several devices are approved as a bridge to cardiac transplantation, or as destination therapy for those who are not candidates for transplant. Studies have shown the use of durable MCS can improve survival over 2 years when compared to medical therapy (van Diepen, 2017).

Palliative care should be openly discussed with patients and their families in situations where there is a poor chance of recovery, or in patients with end-stage heart failure who are not candidates for advanced therapies such as cardiac transplantation or durable VAD. Although palliative care is not studied well in CS, its use of palliative care can reduce physical and emotional distress (van Diepen, 2017). It is important to provide education to patients and families on the goal of palliative care, as well as both the barriers and benefits.

CLINICAL PEARLS

- The definition of CS varies, but generally is defined as hypotension with SBP <90, cardiac index <2.2, and PCWP >18 and signs of organ hypoperfusion.
- AMI is the most common cause of CS.
- Obtaining a detailed history and physical is essential for early diagnosis and differentiation from other types of shock.

- "Cold and wet" profile is most common, which consists of high SVR, high PCWP, and high CVP.
- Norepinephrine is often considered the first-line agent for CS but should be used for the shortest time and lowest dose needed.
- MCS should be considered early in the treatment of CS before organ damage occurs.

KEY TAKEAWAYS

- CS is characterized by low CO that often leads to multiorgan failure and death.
- Mortality remains high, exceeding 40%.
- Rapid diagnosis, early intervention, and ongoing hemodynamic evaluations of response to treatment are important in improving outcomes and decreasing mortality.
- If patients are not candidates for long-term MCS or cardiac transplantation, palliative care should be consulted to assist patients and families.
- Multidisciplinary approach at discharge should include education and close follow-up as the rate of readmissions are high in this patient population.
- Transferring patients in CS to centers with MCS capabilities early is key in improving survival in this patient population.

EVIDENCE-BASED RESOURCES

Contemporary Management of CS: A Scientific Statement from the American Heart Association
Epidemiology, pathophysiology, and contemporary Management of CS - a position statement from the Heart Failure Association of the European Society of Cardiology
SHOCK Trial (1999)
IABP SHOCK II Trial (2012)
IMPRESS Trial (2017)
CULPRIT-SHOCK Trial (2017)

21.3: DISTRIBUTIVE SHOCK

Distributive shock is associated with the decreased ability to deliver oxygen to the tissues related to the dramatic decrease in systemic vascular resistance (SVR) (Massey et al., 2018) The most common forms are anaphylactic shock, neurogenic shock, and septic shock.

ANAPHYLACTIC SHOCK

Rita A. DelloStritto

Anaphylaxis is a severe, life-threatening, systemic reaction to an allergen such as medication, food, and insect stings. Anaphylactic shock is classified as a distributive shock (Fudge & Viswesvaraiah, 2021). Before an ana-phylactic reaction can occur, there must have been a previous exposure to the allergen that resulted in the production of IgE antibodies which were produced by the B-cells. After repeated exposure to the allergen, the IgE antibodies, along with the IgE antigens will attach to the IgE receptors on the mast cells and basophils. This results in the release of a mediator called histamine from the granules located in the cytoplasm of the mast cells. Other mediators that may be released are prostaglandins, tryptase, and platelet-activating factors (Fudge & Viswesvaraiah, 2021; Levinson et al., 2020). Histamine release is the primary cause of flushing, pruritis, urticaria, hypotension, and tachycardia. The release of prostaglandin D_2 leads to bronchoconstriction and microvascular permeability (Hong & Boyce, 2018). An increase in vascular leakage and systemic vasodilatation results in a distributive shock.

PRESENTING SIGNS AND SYMPTOMS

The initial presentation of anaphylaxis starts with urticaria, skin flushing, and pruritis. Within minutes to hours, patients can progress to respiratory distress which includes throat fullness, hoarseness, chest tightness, shortness of breath, and anxiety. Symptoms can quickly escalate to worsening respiratory distress and circulatory collapse/shock. If untreated, anaphylaxis may progress to cardiac arrest (Cardona et al., 2020; Fudge & Viswesvaraiah, 2021; Hong & Boyce 2018; Rowe & Granau, 2020).

HISTORY AND PHYSICAL FINDINGS

When assessing patients with anaphylaxis, obtaining a detailed past medical history, including a history of previous allergic reactions is important. If time allows, determine what the patient may have been exposed to or ingested prior to the onset of symptoms. Many times, patients are unable to tell the provider what triggered the allergic reaction (idopathic). When patients are in anaphylactic shock, the provider may not be able to obtain the information. Patients in anaphylactic shock will have a decreased level of consciousness, respiratory distress, tachycardia, tachypnea, and severe hypotension. Significant swelling of the airway and the presence of generalized urticaria may also be present (Cardona et al., 2020; Hong & Boyce, 2018; Rowe & Granau, 2020).

DIFFERENTIAL DIAGNOSIS AND DIAGNOSTIC CONSIDERATIONS

- Carcinoid syndrome results in acute flushing
- Asthma exacerbation
- Aspiration of a foreign body
- Anxiety or panic attack
- ACE inhibitor induced angioedema
- Hereditary angioedema
- Idiopathic erythema multiforme
- Cardiogenic or hypovolemic shock

TREATMENT OF ANAPHYLACTIC SHOCK

All allergic reactions must be treated quickly in order to avoid progression to anaphylactic shock and potential death. Anaphylactic shock should be treated with first-line therapies focused on maintaining a patient airway, effective breathing, and respiration, and to stabilize circulation. IV access should be initiated quickly; supplemental oxygen, IV crystalloids, and epinephrine are essential first steps (Cardona et al., 2020; McLure et al., 2020; Pattanaik et al., 2014; Rowe & Granau, 2020).

- Epinephrine 1:1000 dilution 0.3 to 0.5 milligrams IM
  - Administration into the thigh muscle results in better peak blood levels when compared to injections into the deltoid muscle.
- IV crystalloids, such as 0.9% normal saline or lactated Ringer's
- 1- to 2-liter bolus of second-line therapy includes histamine (H_1 and H_2) blockers, corticosteroids, and short-acting beta-adrenergic agents (Cardona et al., 2020; McLure et al., 2020; Pattanaik et al., 2014; Rowe & Granau, 2020).
- H_1 blocker
  - Diphenhydramine 25 to 50 mg IV or IM
- H_2 blocker
  - Cimetidine 300 mg IV
- Corticosteroids
  - Hydrocortisone 250 to 500 mg IV, or
  - Methylprednisolone 80 to 125 mg IV
  - Prednisone 40 to 60 mg tablets by mouth daily
    - Upon discharge 3 to 5 day tapering dose
  - Short-acting beta agonist
  - Albuterol via nebulizer, 0.5 to 1.0 mL of 0.5% solution
- Vasopressor of choice may be used to reverse severe hypotension that is resistant to the initial treatment with epinephrine and fluids.
- Glucagon should be considered in patients who routinely use beta-blockers and have continued hypotension after the initial treatment with epinephrine and fluids.
  - 1 mg IV every 5 minutes until the hypotension resolves.
  - Continue with 5 to 15 mcg/min continuous IV infusion
  - Monitor for hypokalemia and hyperglycemia

CLINICAL PEARLS

- Patients who present with anaphylaxis may present with hypotension only.
- Epinephrine should be administered via IM route.
- Patients who use beta-blockers may have hypotension refractory to epinephrine and may require glucagon to correct the hypotension.

KEY TAKEAWAYS

- Anaphylaxis is an acute, life-threatening, systemic reaction to a specific antigen.
- Any allergic reaction can rapidly progress to anaphylactic shock.
- Airway support is essential.
- Rapid administration of epinephrine and fluid resuscitation are paramount in reducing the chance of death.

NEUROGENIC SHOCK

Karen Salazar and Sarah M. Muller

Neurogenic shock is a complex, life-threatening, and particularly difficult condition to identify. Neurogenic shock triggers circulatory failure, poor oxygen delivery, increased oxygen consumption, insufficient use of oxygen, and reduces the ability to meet metabolic demands at a cellular level, all of which eventually lead to cellular and tissue hypoxia (Jia et al., 2013). Neurogenic shock results from damage to the central nervous system and disrupts the regular circulation of blood throughout the body. The nerves that control the blood vessels become injured causing smooth muscle in blood vessels to relax, leading to a decrease in vascular tone and vasodilation. Vasodilation with pooling causes a decrease in preload, a decrease in stroke volume (SV), and a decrease in cardiac output (CO).

Circulatory failure is manifested by hypotension, but a clinician must be able to recognize that a patient in neurogenic shock can present with hypertension or normotension also. Neurogenic shock can be very difficult to recognize because pain and anxiety due to injury and trauma can cause a false elevation in blood pressure and heart rate. Therefore, it can be difficult to appreciate the classic signs of bradycardia and hypotension that occur in neurogenic shock making it difficult to diagnose.

Sympathetic discharges are initiated in the lateral horn of the spinal cord segments T1 to L2. Sympathetic innervation of the heart occurs in T1–T5 so it is thought that neurogenic shock can only occur above the level of T5 (Taylor et al., 2017).

PRESENTING SIGNS AND SYMPTOMS

Much like septic shock and anaphylactic shock, neurogenic shock is distributive in nature and the effects are initially reversible but can quickly become irreversible and can lead to multiorgan failure and death. It occurs exclusively in patients with spinal cord injuries and results from loss of sympathetic tone in the heart and vasculature. The necessary energy supplied by the nervous system is then challenged leading to a deadly triad of hypotension, bradycardia, and peripheral vasodilation. Unlike other forms of distributive shock that create a permeable environment in the vascular system, neurogenic shock is a condition in which low SVR leads to a decrease in blood pressure in the presence of normal or elevated CO.

HISTORY AND PHYSICAL FINDINGS

Initial clinical evaluation in all trauma patients is the primary survey; it focuses on life-threatening conditions. Assessing airway, breathing and circulation are the first steps in the primary survey; spinal cord injuries must also be considered at the same time.

Asking questions about the patient's history is essential and the clinician must focus on symptoms related to the vertebral column and noting any motor or sensory deficits. Determining the mechanism of injury is also very important and can help identify a spinal cord injury (SCI) also.

The patient should be physically assessed to identify unstable spinal fractures so that treatment can be initiated immediately. Patients should be carefully log rolled to examine each spinous process from the occiput to the sacrum to help pinpoint the injury. The cervical spine and paraspinal muscles should be assessed for swelling, tenderness, ecchymosis, and alterations in alignment. Bilateral loss of sensation or bilateral loss of motor function confirms a complete SCI.

The assessment of pulmonary function in acute SCI begins immediately. Clinicians should take a history on respiratory symptoms or underlying cardiopulmonary comorbidities. Physical injuries to the chest wall, respiratory rate, chest expansion, breath sounds, abdominal movement, and cough should all be assessed. Pulse oximetry and arterial blood gas are useful and can identify hypoxia or hypercapnia.

The level of respiratory dysfunction depends on the level of the SCI, preexisting pulmonary conditions, chest injury or lung injury; if any of these situations apply, the patient is at greater risk for respiratory dysfunction. Ventilatory muscle function can be affected from denervation associated with chest wall injury. A pneumothorax, hemothorax, or pulmonary contusion can also worsen pulmonary function in the setting of SCI. In the presence of a head injury, or when alcohol and drugs are involved, the central ventilatory drive can become depressed.

Hemorrhagic shock in SCI patients may be difficult to diagnose because the clinical findings may be affected by autonomic dysfunction. Disruption of autonomic pathways from injury to the spinal cord prevents peripheral vasoconstriction and tachycardia which is typical in hemorrhagic shock. This can cause a clinician to miss an associated hemorrhage in the setting of SCI (Jia et al., 2013).

In a study showing a high incidence of autonomic dysfunction, including orthostatic hypotension and impaired cardiovascular control following SCI, it was recommended that an assessment of autonomic function be routinely used, along with the American Spinal Injury Association

(ASIA) assessment, in the neurologic evaluation of patients with SCI (Claydon et al., 2005).

One must conduct a thorough neurologic exam and assess motor function, sensory evaluation, deep tendon reflexes, and perineal evaluation. The most important assessment is being able to establish the presence or absence of an SCI and lesion.

Sacral sparing is a key prognostic indicator; the presence of sacral fibers defines the completeness of the potential for motor recovery. The clinician must be able to determine the level of injury in order to differentiate nerve root injury from SCI. Multilevel involvement suggests SCI as opposed to nerve root injury. Motor weakness with intact reflexes indicates SCI in patients without spinal shock while motor weakness without reflexes suggests a nerve root lesion.

The ASIA established that the most caudal level of injury with normal sensory and motor function is the lowest level of injury. So, if a patient with quadriplegia has a C5 injury one would expect that the patient has abnormal motor and sensory function from C6 down.

The provider should perform sensory function testing in order to establish the different pathways for light touch, proprioception, vibration, and pain. The sensory level is the most caudal dermatome with a normal score of 2/2 for pain and light touch. When assessing muscle strength, the clinician must always score on the maximum strength attained, regardless of how brief that strength was maintained. The patient's motor level is examined when the most caudal muscles have a muscle strength score of 3 or above. Neurologic level of injury is the most caudal level at where motor and sensory levels are intact. The clinician should perform a rectal examination to check motor and sensation. The extent of injury is defined by the ASIA.

DIFFERENTIAL DIAGNOSIS AND DIAGNOSTIC CONSIDERATIONS

Spinal shock is acute loss of motor, sensory, and reflex functions below the level of injury and can occur with neurogenic shock. Diagnosing neurogenic shock requires a detailed examination. Being able to identify SCI is essential to diagnosing neurogenic shock. The AGACNP must be able to determine the mechanism of injury and be able to identify tenderness of the midline spine, the level of consciousness and mental status, as well as any neurologic deficits or intoxication which can change the neurologic exam. Hemorrhagic shock must be ruled out before neurogenic shock can be diagnosed in all trauma patients and neurogenic shock must be considered in all fractures or dislocations of the vertebrae.

Bradycardia, arrhythmias, hypotension, and flushed warm skin should always raise awareness as they are typical signs of neurogenic shock. The joint committee of the ASIA and the International Spinal Cord Society proposed the definition of a neurogenic shock to be general autonomic nervous system dysfunction that also includes symptoms such as orthostatic hypotension, autonomic dysreflexia, temperature dysregulation and focal neurologic deficits are not necessary for the diagnosis of neurogenic shock (Dave, 2020). Hypovolemic shock, obstructive shock, cardiogenic shock, and septic shock are all associated with tachycardia; however, neurogenic shock is associated with bradycardia (Dave, 2020). Table 21.6 includes common symptoms associated with level of cord injury.

Although neurogenic shock is a rare condition it is imperative to consider it in the differential diagnosis for patients with a mechanism of injury or when shock is recognized but the cause is unclear; this is known as undifferentiated shock (Taylor et al., 2017). Neurogenic shock is unpredictable, and its onset can vary greatly. Patients with injuries involving the entire spinal cord are more likely to experience neurogenic shock compared to patients whose injuries are incomplete (Taylor et al., 2017). It is difficult to identify signs upon presentation that predict the severity of neurogenic shock in patients with SCI (Taylor et al., 2017).

Regardless of the anatomical level of injury one must be aware of the possibility of neurogenic shock in order to improve patient outcomes since studies suggest that the entire length of the sympathetic cord supplies innervation to the vasculature so disturbance at any level can lead to shock regardless of the involvement of the heart (Taylor et al., 2017).

Major advancements in radiographic imaging have led to more accurate diagnosis of SCI. However, the diagnosis of neurogenic shock remains a combination of clinical exam, monitoring hemodynamics, and radiographic imaging.

TREATMENT

The goal of treatment in neurogenic shock in SCI is to prevent secondary injury. Secondary injury is complex and not fully understood. Mechanisms contributing to secondary injury are thought to include hypoxia and ischemia, apoptosis, excitotoxicity, inflammation, and edema. Clinical manifestations of these mechanisms are typically seen within the first 8 to 12 hours following initial insult, and peak between the third and sixth day,

TABLE 21.6: Symptoms Associated With Level of Cord Injury

LEVEL OF CORD INJURY	VITAL CAPACITY	COUGH
C1–C2	5%–10% of normal	Absent
C3–C6	20% of normal	Weak and ineffective
T2–T4	30%–50% of normal	Weak
Lower cord	Improves	Improves
T11	Normal	Strong

with recession of symptoms likely occurring around day nine (Jia et al., 2013). Secondary injury, if not intervened upon early, can cause irreversible damage.

Patients with suspected cervical injury should have their neck manually immobilized with a rigid cervical collar (c-collar). Surgery may be required to correct deformities of the spinal canal and decompress the spinal cord and prevent further damage. Disruption of autonomic pathways in neurogenic shock cause vasodilation and unopposed vagal tone, resulting in decreased vascular resistance, hypotension, and bradycardia. Early and adequate management of hypotension is the cornerstone of treatment. An adequate blood pressure is needed for spinal cord perfusion and prevention of secondary injury. Current guidelines indicate a mean arterial pressure (MAP) of 85 to 90 mmHg is sufficient in providing an adequate spinal cord perfusion.

TRANSITION OF CARE

Patients with SCI are at high risk for development of pressure ulcers and deep vein thrombosis (DVT) secondary to reduced mobility. Autonomic dysreflexia is also common in patients with SCI above the T6 level and can be seen in the acute setting but is often a chronic complication of traumatic SCI. The phenomenon is characterized by hypotension, bradycardia, headache, flushing, and sweating. Episodes of dysreflexia are triggered by a noxious stimulus below the level of injury, most often due to a urological source such as a clogged urinary catheter, distended bladder, or urinary tract infection (Allen & Leslie, 2020). A skilled nursing facility, long-term acute care facility, or inpatient rehabilitation center will be required to care for these patients after discharge from the acute care setting.

KEY TAKEAWAYS

- Neurogenic shock is an overwhelming consequence of SCI; it is also known as vasogenic shock.
- SCI can result in a sudden loss of sympathetic tone which causes autonomic instability manifested by hypotension, bradycardia, arrhythmia, and difficulty regulating body temperature.
- Autonomic nervous system dysfunction that includes orthostatic hypotension, autonomic dysreflexia, inability to regulate temperature, and focal neurologic deficits are not necessary for the diagnosis of neurogenic shock.
- Motor weakness with intact reflexes indicates SCI in patients without spinal shock while motor weakness without reflexes suggests a nerve root lesion.
- Complete injury is absence of sensory and motor functions in the lowest sacral segments.
- Incomplete injury is preservation of sensory or motor function below the level of injury, including the lowest sacral segments.

21.4: OBSTRUCTIVE SHOCK

Daniel L. Arellano

Obstructive shock is a clinical syndrome often grouped with cardiogenic shock (CS) (Day & Whitmore, 2020; Standl et al., 2018). Obstructive shock is defined by a physical obstruction to the outflow tract of the cardiovascular system resulting in hemodynamic changes and hypoperfusion, and can be further separated into conditions affecting the pulmonary vascular system, mechanical forces causing alterations in cardiac preload, and other obstructive conditions such as a large mediastinal mass, abdominal compartment syndrome, or aortocaval compression. Etiologies and treatment vary based on the pathophysiology and early recognition.

PRESENTING SIGNS AND SYMPTOMS

Patient presentation in obstructive pathology is similar to other forms of shock. Characteristic hemodynamic patterns in obstructive shock include low cardiac output (CO), abnormally high vascular resistance, and an altered preload state. Pale, cool, and clammy skin, hypotension, tachycardia, shortness of breath, nausea/vomiting, weakness, and syncope are also prevalent. Depending on etiology, there may be other signs and symptoms.

Cardiac causes of obstructive shock include cardiac tamponade, constrictive pericarditis, restrictive cardiomyopathy, and severe valvular stenosis. In each of these clinical scenarios, an obstruction interferes with the ventricular outflow tract and impedes CO. Clinical presentation often reflects the increased preload proximal to the obstruction. Plethoric vasculature such as jugular venous distention (JVD) and telangiectasia may be present in addition to hemodynamic instability and hypotension.

Pulmonary causes of obstructive shock include tension pneumothorax/hemothorax and massive pulmonary embolism. The mechanism for hemodynamic instability in the setting of tension pneumothorax is the rise in intrathoracic pressure causing a shift of the heart and vascular structures impeding ventricular outflow and venous return. In the setting of a massive pulmonary embolism, the right ventricle fails due to high pulmonary vascular resistance. RV failure decreases preload to the left side of the heart and is a large contributor to the common presentation of shock. One unique presentation in pulmonary cases of obstructive shock is hypoxia. Reduction in lung capacity and poor perfusion contributes to poor oxygenation. Pulmonary embolism contributes to hypoxia by decreasing blood flow to the lungs and altering gas exchange. Each of these conditions also manifests with common shock symptoms such as shortness of breath and tachypnea.

Other contributors to obstructive shock include a large mediastinal mass, abdominal compartment syndrome, or aortocaval compression. In these patients, physical obstruction of the great vessels or a rise in abdominal compartment pressure leads to increased vascular resistance and contributes to shock symptoms. In the setting of aortocaval compression, the aorta and inferior vena cava are obstructed in the supine position from the gravid uterus or a large tumor. The conditions in this category commonly lead to hypotension, tachycardia, and syncope.

HISTORY AND PHYSICAL FINDINGS

Key elements of the history and physical exam may assist in rapid diagnosis and appropriate management of obstructive shock. For cardiac causes of obstructive shock, assessment findings such as a loud murmur may indicate the presence of severe valvular stenosis. History findings such as recent infection and IV drug use may be present in these cases as well. Diminished heart sounds, low blood pressure, JVD (known as Beck's triad), and pulsus paradoxus are key physical assessment findings in cardiac tamponade. A history of cancer or recent trauma may be helpful in guiding this diagnosis. Cardiac friction rub and S3 or S4 heart sounds can be present in both cardiac tamponade and constrictive pericarditis. JVD and plethoric vasculature may be present in each of the cardiac causes of obstructive shock. A history of amyloidosis, recent thoracic radiation and scleroderma are all important history findings to gather when considering constrictive pericarditis as a cause of obstructive shock.

Pulmonary causes of obstructive shock will both typically present with hypoxia and tachypnea, though other physical exam findings and history may differ. A tension pneumothorax may have findings of JVD, deviated trachea, absent or reduced breath sounds, and hyperresonance of the affected lung with percussion. Important history elements include recent trauma, recent thoracic procedures, or chronic lung disease. A pulmonary embolism can often present with hypoxia disproportional to exam and diagnostic findings. Eliciting a detailed history including recent travel, hospitalizations, cancer, and surgery will be paramount. Rapid onset of shortness of breath is present in both elements of the pulmonary causes of obstructive shock.

Physical exam findings present in the other contributors to obstructive shock can include abnormal heart and lung sounds, distended abdomen, or gravida. A history of cancer, smoking, liver disease, abdominal surgery, or abdominal trauma are elements to consider. Due to the rapid onset of obstructive shock, it may be difficult to gather these complex history and physical findings. However, the provider must quickly consider some of these elements to formulate a expeditious diagnosis and treatment.

DIFFERENTIAL DIAGNOSIS AND DIAGNOSTIC CONSIDERATIONS

Rapid identification of the type of shock is paramount to ensure appropriate treatment. Formulation of differential diagnoses will assist in considering all possible etiologies of the presenting symptoms. For cardiac causes of obstructive shock, the clinician should consider conditions such as myocardial infarction (MI), heart failure, ruptured chordae tendineae, vascular aneurysm, and vascular dissection. In general, these can be assessed rapidly with bedside echocardiography or even a single view chest x-ray for cardiac tamponade. However, these diagnostics are not a substitute for rapid physical assessment.

Differential diagnosis of the pulmonary causes of obstructive shock can be quite broad. However, given that the patient is in shock, the clinician needs to first consider conditions that are capable of causing rapid hemodynamic instability. Differential diagnoses for these conditions include asthma, pneumonia, mediastinal mass, heart failure, myocardial infarction, pulmonary edema, hemothorax, chronic obstructive pulmonary disease, asthma, and sepsis among others. Diagnostics for a pneumothorax or hemothorax should include a chest x-ray or bedside ultrasonography assessing for lack of lung sliding or absence of comet tail (Nagarsheth & Kurek, 2011). In the setting of rapid patient deterioration, physical assessment and history are often enough to make the diagnosis. Diagnostics for a massive pulmonary embolism are bountiful. There are formal guidelines for the diagnosis of pulmonary embolism (Konstantinides et al., 2020). These diagnostics include clinical presentation, pretest probability, D-dimer, computed tomography of the chest with angiography, ventilation/perfusion scan, pulmonary angiography, magnetic resonance angiogram, echocardiography, and compression ultrasound. However, if the patient is unstable, these tests may be limited to bedside ultrasonography, clinical presentation, pretest probability and/or D-dimer.

Differential diagnoses of a mediastinal mass, abdominal compartment syndrome, and aortocaval compression are broad. Intraabdominal pathology should always be considered in patients with abnormal abdominal assessment findings. Diagnostics should include suspected site of injury (chest and/or abdomen) and utilize ultrasonography, computed tomography, or magnetic resonance imaging. As mentioned, if the patient is unstable, diagnostics may be limited to bedside ultrasonography, x-rays, laboratory testing, and clinical presentation. In most cases, a quick history and physical exam are enough to make the diagnosis of obstructive shock.

TREATMENT

The treatment of obstructive shock should focus on restoring CO, decreasing vascular resistance, and removal/reduction in the obstructive pathology. Tamponade should be treated with removal of fluid in the pericardial sac or other procedures to relieve the pressure around the heart. Judicious administration of IV fluids and vasopressors can be helpful as a bridge to definitive treatment. Constrictive pericarditis and restrictive cardiomyopathy will likely require consultations by cardiology or cardiothoracic surgery for medical management or surgical intervention. Severe valvular disease resulting in obstructive shock will likely need repair with either cardiac surgery or other transcatheter approach.

In the setting of a large pneumothorax contributing to obstructive shock, treatment should include immediate needle or tube thoracostomy. A large-bore thoracostomy may be required in the setting of a hemothorax to prevent clotting of the drainage system. Administration of fluids and vasopressors can also be considered while awaiting tube placement.

There are formal guidelines for the treatment of a massive pulmonary embolism (Konstantinides et al., 2020). However, in the setting of hemodynamic instability and shock, treatment should include thrombolysis, embolectomy, or mechanical circulatory support. The guidelines also emphasize oxygenation, cautious volume replacement, vasopressors, and inotropes as needed (Konstantinides et al., 2020).

Treatment of a mediastinal mass can be complicated. Goals should surround rapid reduction or removal of the contributing mass with surgery, steroids, or radiation. Proper patient positioning may also be helpful to improve hemodynamics and oxygenation. Abdominal compartment syndrome should be treated by interventions to lower the pressure in the abdominal cavity. This can be obtained surgically or by placement of tubes in the causative area to remove fluid or air. Aortocaval compression is best treated with proper patient positioning and avoiding the supine position. However, the afflicting obstruction within the abdomen will need removal or evacuation if hemodynamic instability persists.

Reversing obstructive shock relies heavily on early recognition and rapid treatment. A quick history and physical assessment may be enough to help guide the clinician in the removal of the obstructive pathology and restoration of hemodynamics.

CONCLUSION

Steven Branham and Patrick A. Laird

Shock is a state of cellular hypoperfusion and decreased oxygenation that results in anaerobic metabolism and metabolic acidosis. Shock state classification systems are useful, as they provide insight into the physiologic causes of cellular disruption. These states provide guidance and management for the underlying cause of shock. Physiologic changes such as hypotension, markers of preload or afterload, and lactate production are all impacted as a result of underlying shock states and have limits, as changes often appear to other conditions that are unrelated to shock. A prime example of this is lactate elevation, which occurs not only in shock, but also in shivering, seizure, or episodes of physiologic stress such as a distance marathon. In all forms of shock, typical shock-related physiologicaresponses occur. These protective mechanisms often do not stop once the underlying shock state is corrected and can result in significant mortality and morbidity. Early identification of shock is essential to engage in prompt treatment, thereby preventing a hyperphysiologicaresponse, which is often detrimental even after the underlying shock state is corrected. Shock remains an area of intense study with the application of new diagnoses and treatment modalities.

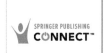

A robust set of instructor resources designed to supplement this text is located at http://connect.springerpub.com/content/reference-book/978-0-8261-6079-9. Qualifying instructors may request access by emailing textbook@springerpub.com.

REFERENCES

Full list of references can be accessed at http://connect .springerpub.com/content/reference-book/978-0-8261-6079-9.

CHAPTER 22

POISONING AND DRUG TOXICITY

Dawn Carpenter and Alexander Menard

LEARNING OBJECTIVES

- Differentiate between the common toxidromes.
- Compare/contrast clinical presentations and clinical findings of different toxicities.
- Differentiate between acute and chronic types of overdose.
- Construct treatment plans for a variety of toxicities and types of overdose.
- Identify and manage complications of toxic ingestions.

INTRODUCTION

This chapter provides an overview of toxicological issues frequently encountered by adult-gerontology acute care nurse practitioners (AGACNPs). An overview of toxidromes sets the stage for AGACNPs to organize and categorize presenting symptoms, clinical signs, toxicological agents, and their treatments. Subsequent sections provide additional details of a variety of toxic ingestions and overdoses, which can be acute or chronic, intentional, or accidental in nature. Additionally, therapeutic medication misuse and overprescribing may be encountered. Regardless of manner of ingestion, the clinical management remains consistent.

22.1: TOXIDROMES

A toxidrome represents patterns of clinical signs and symptoms that are associated with toxicity from a specific classification of chemical agents. Prescription medications, illicit drugs, household chemicals, poisons, and chemical warfare agents can be encountered in clinical settings. Table 22.1 outlines specific toxidromes, provides examples of agents, vital signs, and physical exam findings seen with the toxidrome.

HISTORY AND PHYSICAL FINDINGS

A thorough history from patients may not always be possible, due to impaired mental status or unwillingness to share information. Thus, interviewing family and friends is important to attempt to identify ingested substance(s), quantity, and timing of ingestion.

A detailed history is critical; seek information from those living with the patient or closest to the patient. Consider that legal next of kin may not have this information, thus encourage them to engage friends and/or roommates.

Identify the agent and inquire if an ingestion was accidental or intentional as this information will affect the plan of care for the patient. Ask them to search the environment where the patient was found. Specifically look for pill bottles and perform pill counts along with searching for drug paraphernalia or other empty bottles of chemicals or cleaning agents which can be useful to identify toxic agents. Obtain a thorough social history in an attempt to identify life stressors, including recent changes in relationships such as divorce or death of close friend/family member, changes in employment, arrest or interaction with the legal system, and substance use disorder/relapse. These events or situations can all lead to depression, suicidality, or an increase in substance use. Provide reassurance that this information is essential to care for the patient and will not be shared with law enforcement which will build trust to obtain necessary information (McKean et al., 2017).

Physical examination can provide clues to the substance ingested. A comprehensive exam of any critically ill patient is expected. Specifically review vital signs, skin and temperature, mental status, pupils, bowel and bladder function, reflexes, muscule tone, and odors as these can all be clues to a specific toxidrome or chemical agent. Initial diagnostic workup is included in Table 22.2.

DIFFERENTIAL DIAGNOSIS AND DIAGNOSTIC CONSIDERATIONS

The AGACNP must always consider medical emergencies as a cause of change in mental status or behavior. Do not presume that an altered mental status results from an overdose or toxic ingestion. Sepsis or septic shock, traumatic injury, stroke, seizures, cerebral tumors or aneurysms, meningitis, encephalitis, anemia, and/or diabetic ketoacidosis can easily be missed.

TREATMENT

Treatment of overdose is specific to the agent ingested. The category of agents is specifically addressed in the following sections. Consultation with a toxicologist or

TABLE 22.1: Common Toxidromes

TOXIDROME	EXAMPLES	VITAL SIGNS	MENTAL STATUS	PUPILS	OTHER
Anticholinergic	Atropine, antihistamines, TCAs, scopolamine, antispasmodics, jimson weed, psychedelic mushrooms	Hyperthermia, tachycardia, hypertensive, tachypnea	Hypervigilant, agitated, hallucinating	Mydriasis	Dry flushed skin, urinary retention
Cholinergic	Organophosphates, carbamate pesticides, cholinesterase inhibitors, nerve agents, physostigmine	Bradycardia, tachycardia, hypertension	Confused, coma	Miosis	SLUDGE (salivation, lacrimation, urination, diarrhea, GI upset, emesis)
Opioid	Opioids (morphine, oxycodone, hydrocodone, hydromorphone, fentanyl, codeine, methadone, heroin)	Hypothermia, bradycardia, hypotension, bradypnea	CNS depression, coma	Miosis	Hyporeflexia, pulmonary edema
Sedative/hypnotic	Benzodiazepines, nonbenzodiazepine GABA agonists, barbiturates, chloral hydrate, alcohols	Hypothermia, bradycardia, hypotension, bradypnea	CNS depression, confusion, coma	Miosis	Hyporeflexia
Sympathomimetic	Cocaine, amphetamines, pseudoephedrine, phenylephrine, ephedrine	Hyperthermia, tachycardia, tachypnea	Agitated, hyperalert, paranoia	Mydriasis	Diaphoresis, tremors, hyperreflexia, seizures
Serotonergic	MAOIs, SSRIs, buspirone, tramadol dextrometh-orphan	Hyperthermia, tachycardia, hypertension, tachypnea,	Confused, agitated, coma	Mydriasis	Tremor, myoclonus, diaphoresis, hyperreflexia, trismus, rigidity, muscular hypertonicity
Neuroleptic	Haloperidol, olanzapine, quetiapine, chlorpromazine, promethazine, prochlorperazine, fluphenazine, perphenazine	Hypotension, arrhythmias			Trismus, dystonia, ataxia, parkinsonism, neuroleptic malignant syndrome

MAOi, monoamine oxidase inhibitor; TCA, tricyclic antidepressant; CNS, central nervous system; SSRIs, selective serotonin reuptake inhibitors.

TABLE 22.2: Initial Diagnostic Testing for Patients Suspected of Overdose or Toxicological Exposure

DIAGNOSTIC TEST	RATIONALE
Finger stick blood glucose	Assess for hypoglycemia
ECG	Assess for QTc prolongation/widening
Arterial blood gas	Assess for acidosis, alkalosis, hypoxia, hypercarbia
Chem 7, BUN/creatinine	Assess anion gap, renal impairment, electrolyte imbalances
Serum CPK, urine myoglobin	Assess for rhabdomyolysis
Acetaminophen level	Assess for acetaminophen overdose
Liver function panel, INR	Assess liver function, clearance of agents
Aspirin level	Assess for aspirin ingestion
Alcohol level	Assess for ethanol intoxication
Serum osmolality	Evaluate for toxic alcohol ingestion
Urine drug of abuse screen	Identify commonly abused illicit substances

BUN, blood-urea-nitrogen; CPK, creatine phosphokinase; INR, international normalized ratio.

Source: McKean, S. C., Ross, J. J., Dressler, D. D., & Scheurer, D. B. (2017). *Principles and practice of hospital medicine* (2nd ed.). McGraw Hill Education.

poison control center can be helpful in diagnosing and treating overdoses and ingestions (McKean et al., 2017). Identifying if this was an accidental ingestion will aid in preventing recurrence by developing educational or other interventions to manage the patient's environment. For purposeful overdoses, consultation with psychiatry is essential to diagnose psychiatric, substance abuse, or dual diagnoses and aid in treatment and development of discharge plans with appropriate psychological treatment and follow-up post discharge.

22.2: ACETAMINOPHEN TOXICITY/ POISONING

Acetaminophen is the most common analgesic/antipyretic prescribed. Introduced in 1955, it has become the most ingested poisoning substance and the most common cause of acute hepatic failure in the United States. Many opioid agents are combined with acetaminophen; thus, unknowingly patients take additional over-the-counter acetaminophen concomitantly causing unintentional overdoses. Additionally, given acetaminophen is over the counter, patients commonly believe it poses minimal risk. Acetaminophen is typically safe at 4000 mg/day for adults, 3000 mg/day in elderly (Ye et al., 2018).

PRESENTING SIGNS AND SYMPTOMS

Acetaminophen overdose has four defined stages of illness and management.

- **First Stage:** Early, occurs less than 24 hours after ingestion. Patients with an acetaminophen overdose experience nonspecific symptoms such as lethargy, malaise, or gastrointestinal symptoms such as nausea, vomiting. During this time, laboratory studies are normal. Without immediate treatment patients will develop acute hepatic injury.
- **Second Stage:** From 24 to 72 hours postingestion, signs of hepatotoxicity become evident, including right upper quadrant abdominal pain, elevations in transaminases (AST/ALT), bilirubin, and coagulation studies (PT/PTT).
- **Third Stage:** From 72 to 96 hours, patients demonstrate fulminant hepatic failure, including hepatic encephalopathy, jaundice, and coagulopathy. Liver function tests (LFTs) peak with transaminases reaching or exceeding 5,000 to 10,000; lactic acidosis develops and worsens, and patients progress into hepatorenal failure.
- **Fourth Stage:** Occurs from day 4 through 3 weeks and results in either death or recovery, which may require emergent liver transplantation (Agrawal, & Khazaeni, 2020).

HISTORY AND PHYSICAL FINDINGS

A thorough history is needed, including history of present illness for recent illness or injuries and recent emergency department or urgent care visits. Past medical history should seek information on pain syndromes, depression, suicidality to determine accidental versus intentional ingestion. Review medications, including over-the-counter agents along with duration of treatment, dosing, concomitant agents, including alcohol or illicit substances is essential. Coingestion is common, thus serum blood alcohol level, urine drug screen, ECG, arterial blood gas (ABG) and chem 7 are recommended (Agrawal, & Khazaeni, 2020).

DIFFERENTIAL DIAGNOSIS AND DIAGNOSTIC CONSIDERATIONS

Differential diagnoses for acetaminophen overdose include diseases/processes that cause nausea, vomiting, and right upper quadrant pain such as biliary obstruction, viral hepatitis, peptic or duodenal ulcer disease, or pancreatitis. Other differential diagnoses include gastroenteritis, cytomegalovirus infection, Wilson's disease, hepatorenal syndrome, acute tubular necrosis, and amatoxin toxicity (Agrawal & Khazaeni, 2020).

TREATMENT

Acute Ingestion

Acetaminophen is rapidly absorbed; thus, gastric lavage is not indicated unless it is done within the first hour after ingestion. For asymptomatic patients, obtain an initial acetaminophen level and identify ingestion time. If the patient is at or after 4 hours of ingestion and asymptomatic, then monitor and recheck level every 4 hours. Treatment should be initiated within the first 8 hours after ingestion for treatment to fully protect the liver. All patients with elevated acetaminophen levels require hospitalization and treatment with N-acetyl-cystine (NAC). NAC should be initiated for: (a) any acetaminophen level that is in the toxic range according to the Rumack-Matthew nomogram, (b) acetaminophen level greater than 10 mcg/mL with an unknown ingestion time, (c) acetaminophen level greater than 140 mg/mL when ingestion was greater than 8 hours ago, (d) abnormal liver function tests with an ingestion time greater than 24 hours ago, and (e) anyone with an ingestion and any signs of acute hepatic failure (Muñoz Romo et al., 2018).

Patients who present with ingestions of 32 g or more or acetaminophen levels greater than 300 mcg/mL 4 hours postingestion are considered to have a massive intoxication. As such, higher doses of NAC and longer duration of treatment are indicated (Levine, et al., 2017). Consultation with a toxicologist or poison control center is warranted.

NAC can be administered via IV infusion for 20 hours or PO in divided doses Q4h for 18 doses over 72 hours. Oral route may not be well tolerated by awake patients due to NAC's rotten egg odor. IV dosing of IV NAC includes an initial dose of 150 mg/kg over 60 minutes, followed by 50 mg/kg over 4 hours and completed with 100 mg/kg over 16 hours. Continuation of NAC infusion at the latter rate (100 mg/kg over 16 hours) is indicated until transaminases are <800 U/L or acetaminophen levels remain greater than 10 mcg/mL. Stopping NAC therapy in 3 to 5 days is controversial unless the transaminases are normal, international normalized ratio (INR) is less than 2, and acetaminophen level is undetectable. Treatment failure can occur if NAC infusion is stopped before reaching these endpoints (Levine et al., 2017).

Chronic Ingestion

Patients regularly taking acetaminophen may experience chronic ingestion, which typically causes less liver toxicity. In cases of chronic ingestion, the Rumack-Mathew nomogram (Rumack et al., 1981) is not useful, as levels do not correlate with severity of the overdose. Thus, the AGACNP should suspect and treat as an overdose when the acetaminophen level is greater than 20 mcg/mL and/or when transaminases are elevated.

Additionally, the Rumack-Matthew nomogram (Rumack et al., 1981) can fail for the following reasons: inaccurate timing of ingestion, extended or delayed release acetaminophen preparations, chronic ingestion or multiple ingestions, chronic alcoholism, malnutrition, drugs that increase toxicity (INH, rifampin, phenobarbital, phenytoin, carbamazepine, bactrim), delayed gastric emptying, and wrong unit of measure compared with the nomogram.

22.3: TOXIC ALCOHOL INGESTION/POISONING

Toxic alcohol ingestion/poisoning carries a significant increase in morbidity and mortality if not recognized in a timely manner (Ng et al., 2018). Toxic alcohols include methanol, ethylene glycol, and isopropyl alcohol. These alcohols can be found in commercial solvents, parenteral medications, and some are readily available in common everyday products (Table 22.3). The parent forms of methanol, ethylene glycol, and diethylene glycol are relatively innocuous; the metabolites cause the toxicity (McMartin et al., 2016).

Timely recognition of an ingestion with these agents is critical to facilitate treatment and prevent deleterious effects of blindness, renal failure, coma, and death. The patient may be unaware, unwilling, or unable to divulge that an ingestion has occurred. This increases the difficulty in making the diagnosis of toxic alcohol poisoning, identification of the offending agent, as well as determining whether the ingestion was intentional or accidental.

TABLE 22.3: Sources of Toxic Alcohol by Type

Toxic Alcohol	Methanol	Ethylene glycol	Isopropyl alcohol
Source	Windshield washing fluid, antifreeze, paint or varnishes	Antifreeze	Rubbing alcohol, hand sanitizer

PRESENTING SIGNS AND SYMPTOMS

Toxic alcohol ingestion/poisoning can present with a wide range of symptoms. Patients can present with no symptoms and can range from mild symptoms of abdominal pain and altered mental status including drowsiness, euphoria, disinhibition, confusion, slurred speech, up to and including coma. The time from ingestion to presentation, potential for coingestion of other substances, can have impact on the presenting symptoms. It is the metabolites (Table 22.4) of the toxic alcohol that cause the deleterious signs and symptoms of depressed sensorium and then organ dysfunction (Kraut & Mullins, 2018).

Methanol

Early signs and symptoms of methanol poisoning include nausea, vomiting, abdominal pain, confusion, and central nervous system (CNS) suppression. Later signs of methanol poisoning are associated with metabolic acidosis, blurred vision, photophobia, changes in visual field, diplopia, nystagmus, and blindness. Coingestion of ethanol with methanol has the propensity to delay onset of these symptoms up to 72 hours (Hassanian-Moghaddam & Zamani, 2016).

Ethylene Glycol

Ethylene glycol ingestions can present with varying signs and symptoms depending on when the ingestion occurred. These symptoms can range from transient inebriation, flank pain, nausea, and vomiting, to coma and seizures (Table 22.5; McMahon et al., 2009). Coingestion of ethanol can result in delay in recognizing symptoms of methanol, ethylene glycol, and diethylene glycol ingestion.

Isopropyl Alcohol

Isopropyl alcohol ingestions present with headache, dizziness, miosis, stupor, and coma. Gastrointestinal irritation is also common in the form of abdominal pain, nausea, vomiting, diarrhea, and hematemesis (Gallagher & Edwards 2019).

HISTORY AND PHYSICAL FINDINGS

Toxic alcohol ingestion can be challenging to uncover during history taking as the patient may have intentionally ingested the substance or the patient may be unable to take part in an interview. Physical exam findings are similar with all these agents and include inebriation, nausea and vomiting, and CNS depression.

TABLE 22.4: Metabolites of Toxic Alcohol by Type

Toxic alcohol	Methanol	Ethylene glycol	Isopropyl alcohol
Metabolite	Formic acid	Glyoxylic acid, oxalic acid	Acetone

TABLE 22.5: Onset of Clinical Manifestations of Toxic Alcohol by Type

TOXIC ALCOHOL	ONSET OF CLINICAL MANIFESTATIONS
Methanol	0.5–4 h: N/V, abdominal pain, confusion, CNS depression 6–24 h: Blurred vision, photophobia, blindness
Ethylene glycol	1–2 h: Inebriation 12–24 h: Metabolic acidosis, coma, seizure, 24–72 h: Flank pain, ATN, hypocalcemia, kidney failure
Isopropyl alcohol	Within 1 h: Ataxia, LOC, N/V, gastritis, hypotension High osmolar gap ketonemia or ketonuria without acidosis Ketosis/fruity/sweet odor on breath

ATN, acute tubular necrosis; CNS, central nervous system; N/V, nausea and vomiting; LOC, loss of consciousness.

TABLE 22.6: Physical Examination Findings of Toxic Alcohol Ingestion

METHANOL	ETHYLENE GLYCOL	ISOPROPYL ALCOHOL
Inebriation Tachycardia, tachypnea, N/V, abdominal pain, Blurry vision, photophobia, papilledema	Inebriation, CNS depression, Tachypnea, Tetany	Inebriation AMS, respiratory depression Gastritis, acute pancreatitis

AMS, altered mental status; N/V, nausea and vomiting; CNS, central nervous system.

Patients who present within the first 12 to 24 hours after ingestion of methanol may have a completely normal physical exam. Exam findings can progress over time and include tachypnea, CNS depression as well as papilledema, optic disc hyperemia when completing a fundoscopic exam (Table 22.6; Ashurst & Nappe, 2020).

DIFFERENTIAL DIAGNOSIS AND DIAGNOSTIC CONSIDERATIONS

Toxic alcohol ingestion/poisoning should be included as a differential diagnosis on any patient who presents with an altered mental status and acidemia. Differential diagnoses are diverse due to the wide range of symptoms associated with toxic alcohol ingestion/poisoning. Differential diagnosis includes primary neurologic disorders, infection, diabetic ketoacidosis, starvation ketosis, sepsis, uremia, stroke, seizure, other ingestions such as salicylate, acetaminophen, or sedative or hypnotic ingestions. To narrow the differential diagnoses, further diagnostic testing is required along with continued observation and evaluation.

Obtain laboratory data including arterial blood gas (ABG), serum chemistries, creatine kinase, hepatic func-

tion panel, serum and urine osmolality. Specifically look for hyperosmolality and metabolic acidosis which are key findings in toxic alcohol ingestion/poisoning. The creatine phosphokinase (CPK) can be useful in determining if rhabdomyolysis is present and the hepatic function panel can indicate alcohol hepatitis. A urinalysis may be performed for evaluation of oxalate crystals. A patient may not initially have laboratory alterations depending on the time elapsed from ingestion to presentation. Thus, monitoring of serial laboratory tests and follow-up assessments are needed.

TREATMENT

Mainstays of treatment are IV hydration, sodium bicarbonate administration for a pH <7.3, supportive care including securing an airway and ensuring adequate hydration and perfusion, administration of medications, such as fomepizole, targeted to stop the metabolism of toxic metabolites and renal replacement therapy (RRT). A high suspicion of or confirmation of ingestion should prompt immediate consultation with a medical toxicologist. Depending on the symptoms and medical sequelae other consultations may include nephrology, neurology, and ophthalmology.

Fomepizole

Fomepizole prevents the metabolism of ethylene glycol and methanol into their respective toxic metabolites. Fomepizole can be given for methanol and ethylene glycol toxicity if the following criteria are met:

- Methanol or ethylene glycol plasma concentration >20 mg/dL
- Recent methanol or ethylene glycol ingestion with serum osmol gap >10 mOsm/L
- History or strong clinical suspicion of methanol or ethylene glycol poisoning
- And two or more of the following:
  - Arterial pH <7.3
  - Serum bicarbonate concentration <20 mEq/L
  - Osmol gap >10 mOsm/L
  - Presence of oxalate crystals in the urine (ethylene glycol poisoning only)

Renal Replacement Therapy

Renal replacement therapy (RRT) is indicated for the treatment of methanol, ethylene glycol, and isopropyl alcohol toxicity. It is reasonable to consider RRT with isopropyl alcohol toxicity when serum levels >200 mg/dL and coma and/or hypotension are present. The role of hemodialysis for treatment of methanol and ethylene glycol toxicity is controversial particularly with less severe cases. Hemodialysis is recommended for treatment of ethylene glycol toxicity when metabolic acidosis (pH<7.25) persists despite therapy, in the setting of renal failure or ethylene glycol level >50 mg/dL. In the case of methanol toxicity, RRT is recommended when coma, seizures, or new visual disturbance are present, metabolic acidosis <7.15, persistent metabolic acidosis despite treatment, serum anion gap >24, or serum methanol concentrations >70 mg/dL with fomepizole therapy, or renal failure (Gallagher & Edwards, 2019).

22.4: ANTIARRHYTHMIC TOXICITY/ POISONING

Antiarrhythmic drugs are frequently prescribed medications to control irregular heart rhythms. There are numerous options and indications when selecting an antiarrhythmic medication and these options fall within four main classes of antiarrhythmics (Table 22.7). These medications are frequently prescribed and the AGACNP needs to be prepared to identify the signs and symptoms of overdose/toxicity and the treatment options for them. The action of these medications is on the cardiovascular system, thus making these medication overdoses life-threatening.

Overdose related to calcium channel blockers and beta blockers accounts for a small percentage of all poisoning presentations, but carries significant mortality (Graudins et al., 2016). Digoxin is a cardiac glycoside that functions as an antiarrhythmic but also as an inotrope. Given its use it is prudent to include this medication among this group.

PRESENTING SIGNS AND SYMPTOMS

Patients commonly present with a consistent pattern of symptoms when an antiarrhythmic overdose/toxicity is suspected. These medications primarily impact the rate and rhythm of the heart. The majority of the time patients will present with cardiac depression, i.e., bradycardia and hypotension. Other specific signs and symptoms are outlined in Table 22.8.

HISTORY AND PHYSICAL FINDINGS

History taking commonly reveals consumption of a prescribed antiarrhythmic medication. Seek to identify whether the drug was accidentally overconsumed or intentionally overconsumed. While the treatment for a specific overdose does not change based on intentionality, it must be determined as it will impact discharge planning.

TABLE 22.7: Antiarrhythmic Classes

CLASS (DESCRIPTION)	EXAMPLES
Class I (Sodium channel blockers)	Procainamide, lidocaine, flecainide
Class II (Beta-blockers)	Propranolol, metoprolol, esmolol
Class III (Potassium channel blockers)	Dofetilide, amiodarone
Class IV (Calcium channel blockers)	Verapamil, diltiazem, nifedipine
Other (Cardiac glycoside)	Digoxin

TABLE 22.8: Signs and Symptoms of Antiarrhythmic Overdose/Toxicity

CLASS	SIGNS AND SYMPTOMS OF ANTIARRHYTHMIC OVERDOSE/ TOXICITY
Class I	Procainamide: Torsades de pointes, hypotension, lupuslike syndrome (lupus erythematous) Lidocaine: CNS depression or excitation Flecainide: Increased arrhythmia, seizures
Class II	Propranolol, metoprolol, esmolol: Bronchospasm, lethargy, bradycardia, hypotension
Class III	Dofetilide: Torsades de pointes Amiodarone: Hypotension, arrhythmia, thyrotoxicosis, pulmonary fibrosis, optic neuritis
Class IV	Verapamil, diltiazem, nifedipine: Bradycardia, hypotension, constipation
Other	Digoxin: Palpitations, dyspnea, syncope, gastrointestinal upset, visual disturbance described as yellow/green discoloration

All antiarrhythmics have the potential to cause bradycardia and hypotension which can cause a patient to have a wide range of physical exam findings consistent with hypoperfusion and possibly cardiogenic shock. In addition, antiarrhythmic medications can also induce arrhythmias. Patients can present with syncope or a history of syncope. Syncope in the setting of antiarrhythmic medication consumption should be considered for medication toxicity. Patients with toxicity to procainamide can present with lupus erythematosus.

DIFFERENTIAL DIAGNOSIS AND DIAGNOSTIC CONSIDERATIONS

Differentials diagnoses are wide ranging. These medications can present with bradycardia and hypotension which are consistent with many other pathologies. Antiarrhythmics also impact QRS and QT duration which can be implicated in other drug overdoses. Differential diagnoses include cardiogenic shock, hyperkalemia/hypokalemia, hypomagnesemia, myocardial infarction, antidepressant overdose, antipsychotic overdose, and thyrotoxicosis.

When working up the patient with confirmed or suspected antiarrhythmic toxicity an ECG is required along with continuous telemetry monitoring. In addition, laboratory values need to be obtained including a comprehensive metabolic panel, thyroid panel (for suspected amiodarone overdose/toxicity), digoxin plasma level (for suspected digoxin overdose/toxicity). Clinical features of digoxin toxicity are enough to warrant intervention as toxicity can occur when serum levels are within a normal range (Pincus, 2016).

TREATMENT

Treatment of toxicity from antiarrhythmic medications includes cessation of the medication. Activated charcoal can also be administered if the patient is alert and has recently ingested the medication. Address the resulting issues that arise in the form of supportive care with volume expansion and vasopressors as needed; cardiac monitoring is necessary (telemetry, ECG, vital signs). For a widened QRS (>100 ms) complex in the setting of sodium channel blockade the administration of sodium bicarbonate is indicated (Benowitz, 2012). For torsades de points treatment with IV magnesium or overdrive pacing can be warranted (Smollin & Olson, 2021b). Often antiarrhythmic medications can prolong the QT interval necessitating careful monitoring with magnesium and potassium replacement to reduce the risk of arrhythmias.

For calcium channel overdose administration of IV calcium gluconate or chloride can improve cardiac output and vascular tone. For beta-blocker overdose bradycardia can be improved with the administration of glucagon. Treatment for digoxin overdose has life-threatening toxicity; the antidote digoxin-specific antibody antigen-binding fragments (DSFab also called Digibind) can be administered (Pincus, 2016).

22.5: ANTIDEPRESSANT TOXICITY/ POISONING

Antidepressants are among the top 10 most prescribed medications in the United States (Mossop & DiBlasio, 2017). These medications are widely prescribed to treat depression and are also used to treat other conditions including insomnia, migraine prophylaxis, neuralgic pain, and obsessive-compulsive disorder. In this section, we address noncyclic antidepressants, tricyclic antidepressants (TCAs), and monoamine oxidase inhibitors (MAO-Is). The prescribing trend to treat depression shifted to the use of noncyclic antidepressants due to a more favorable side effect profile when compared to TCAs and MAOIs (Table 22.9). Noncyclic antidepressants in general have a larger therapeutic range and are better tolerated than TCAs and MAOIs.

PRESENTING SIGNS AND SYMPTOMS

Noncyclic

Noncyclic antidepressants have a variety of signs and symptoms that can be associated with specific medications within this class (Table 22.10). Notably this class of medications does not have serious anticholinergic effects like TCAs.

Tricyclic Antidepressants

TCAs are rapidly absorbed within the GI tract and have a long half-life ranging from 7 to 58 hours. Symptom onset usually starts 30 minutes after ingestion and overdose

TABLE 22.9: Classification and Examples of Antidepressants

ANTIDEPRESSANT TYPES	EXAMPLES
Noncyclic antidepressant • Selective serotonin reuptake inhibitors (SSRIs) • Serotonin-norepinephrine reuptake inhibitors (SNRIs) • Dopamine-norepinephrine reuptake inhibitors (DNRIs)	• SSRIs (e.g., fluoxetine, sertraline, citalopram, escitalopram, paroxetine, fluvoxamine) • SNRIs (e.g., venlafaxine, duloxetine) • DNRIs (e.g., bupropion, trazadone, mirtazapine)
Tricyclic antidepressant	• Amitriptyline • Doxepin • Imipramine
Monoamine oxidase inhibitors	• Zelapar • Nardil • Parnate • Marpan

TABLE 22.10: Noncyclic Antidepressant Signs and Symptoms of Toxicity

SUBSET OF NONCYCLIC ANTIDEPRESSANTS	SIGNS AND SYMPTOMS
Selective serotonin reuptake inhibitors (SSRIs)	Nausea Vomiting Diarrhea Seizure Clonus or ocular clonus* Diaphoresis* Agitation* Hyperreflexia* Fever*
Serotonin-norepinephrine reuptake inhibitors (SNRIs)	Tachycardia Altered mental status Seizure Vomiting Mydriasis
Dopamine-norepinephrine reuptake inhibitors (DNRIs)	Bupropion: Seizure Trazadone and mirtazapine: Hypotension

*Symptoms consistent with serotonin syndrome.

signs and symptoms are often apparent within 2 hours. Signs and symptoms typically manifest as cardiovascular, anticholinergic, and/or neurologic abnormalities (Table 22.11).

Monoamine Oxidase Inhibitors

The use of MAOIs has decreased as newer antidepressants that are better tolerated have come to the market. This class of antidepressant is well-known for its interactions with tyramine-containing foods (found in aged cheese and red wines), and the increased risk of serotonin syndrome due to medication incompatibilities (linezolid, tramadol, SSRIs to name a few; LoVecchio, 2020).

TABLE 22.11: Signs and Symptoms of Tricyclic Antidepressant Toxicity

Cardiovascular	Hypotension Tachycardia Bradycardia +/− heart block
Anticholinergic	Fever Mydriasis Xerostomia Hypoactive bowel sounds
Neurologic	Agitation Seizure Decreased mental status Coma

MAOI signs and symptoms of toxicity can include agitation, diaphoresis, tachycardia, hyperthermia, altered mental status, tachypnea, vomiting, arrhythmia, hypertension, seizure, coma, muscle rigidity, and myoclonus.

HISTORY AND PHYSICAL FINDINGS

History taking for any suspected ingestion or overdose must include evaluation of the substance, time, amount, and formulation that was consumed. Reports of the physical environment can also be useful and reveal the medication, formulation, and potential amount that was ingested. Pill counts can aid in the identification of quantity of pills ingested. Antidepressant overdose can be spurred by food or drug interaction. MAOI overdose can be spurred by tyramine-containing foods like aged cheese, red wine, aged meats, avocado. Overdose can also be induced by coingestion of SSRIs, such as tramadol and linezolid to name a few (Garcia & Santos, 2020).

Physical findings for antidepressant overdose are wide ranging and vary depending on the substance ingested. These physical findings include diaphoresis, hyperreflexia, mydriasis, clonus, and ocular clonus.

DIFFERENTIAL DIAGNOSIS AND DIAGNOSTIC CONSIDERATIONS

Diagnosis of an antidepressant toxicity/overdose is made with consistent clinical signs and symptoms of toxicity and known consumption of the antidepressant medication and/or identification of a catalyst interaction (food or drug). Diagnostic considerations for antidepressant overdose must include an ECG to evaluate for arrhythmia and prolongation of the QTc and QRS. Other considerations include screening for coingestion by obtaining salicylate, acetaminophen, and ethanol levels. For all women of childbearing age a pregnancy test must be obtained. Radiologic tests are not diagnostic with antidepressant overdose but can be helpful to rule out other causes for altered mental status and seizures.

Serotonin Syndrome

The Hunter Criteria for Serotonin Syndrome can be helpful to diagnose serotonin syndrome. If a patient has taken a serotonergic agent and meets one of the Hunter Criteria, the diagnosis of serotonin syndrome can be made (Figure 22.1). Serotonin syndrome can occur in hospitalized patients who are concomitantly prescribed antibiotics like linezolid and ciprofloxacin; antidepressants like SSRIs, SNRIs, and MAOIs; antifungals like fluconazole; and opiates.

The list of differential diagnoses for antidepressant overdose/toxicity is fairly long given that the presenting signs and symptoms are often seen with other primary diagnoses. Alteration in mental status can be linked to many diagnoses including but not limited to sepsis, stroke, and other forms of overdose/toxicity like alcohol withdrawal, anticholinergic toxicity, sympathomimetic withdraw. The presentation of hyperthermia can potentially be linked to neuroleptic syndrome.

TREATMENT

Treatment for antidepressant overdose is largely supportive care and discontinuation of the offending agent. Activated charcoal can be administered to the awake and alert patient within 2 hours of ingestion.

Supportive care focuses on airway, breathing, and circulation. Discontinuation of serotonergic therapies is the mainstay of treatment followed by symptom management. Symptoms of agitation, muscle rigidity, seizure, and hyperthermia are often responsive to benzodiazepine and topical cooling methods. If benzodiazepines fail to control symptoms, more intensive therapies can include intubation and initiation of paralytic therapies.

Haloperidol should not be used for treatment of agitation in the patient with serotonin syndrome due to its anticholinergic properties potentially leading to

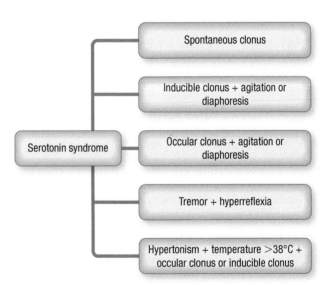

FIGURE 22.1: Hunter criteria for serotonin syndrome.

increased temperature. Acetaminophen and NSAIDs which are commonly used for their antipyreic properties will have little impact on fever from serotonin syndrome as it is not originating from the hypothalamus.

22.6: CANNABIS AND SYNTHETIC CANNABINOIDS TOXICITY/POISONING

With the legalization of marijuana among several states and increasing availability of medical marijuana, cannabinoid intoxication and toxicity has been rising in emergency departments among all age groups. The strength of cannabis-derived products is defined by the concentration of delta-9-tetrahydrocannabinol (THC) has also been increasing in the recent decade (Cooper & Williams, 2019). Illegal forms of THC increased from about 4% to 12%, legal cannabis frequently exceeds 20%, whereas high-concentration products including extracts and resins can be over 65%. Edibles are commonly sold in multidose units averaging 10% per dose; however, multiple doses are commonly consumed at one time. This variability of dosing and edibles that are appealing to children combined with the delayed onset of edibles results in overingestion of THC and thus toxicity (Cooper & Williams, 2019).

Synthetic cannabinoids (SC; e.g., Spice, K2) are commonly confused for cannabis. SC are receptor agonists that bind to the same cannabinoid receptors as THC, Cannabinoid 1, and Cannabinoid 2. SCs are commonly sold as potpourri and incense and ingested by spraying the liquid SC on plant material and smoking rolled in cigarette paper or through a pipe or water pipe. Liquid SC can be vaporized and smoked through electronic cigarettes. SCs are notably more dangerous, with potentially life-threatening consequences (Minns, 2013).

PRESENTING SIGNS AND SYMPTOMS

Ingestion of cannabis and cannabis-derived products can cause relaxation, anxiolysis, euphoria, intensified perception, hyperfocused awareness, and increased appetite. These symptoms are seen within 2 hours of ingestion. Impairment in coordination and motor skills, learning difficulties, and injected conjunctiva are also common. Toxicity signs and symptoms includes anxiety up to and including panic, psychosis and paranoia, illusions, and/or hallucinations (auditory and/or visual) and delirium (Table 22.12). Psychosis may linger for a week or longer (Gonzalez et al., 2018).

Cannabinoid hyperemesis syndrome (CHS), a cyclic vomiting syndrome, presents with intractable nausea and vomiting lasting for days to months. CHS is common in persons with heavy (more than 20 days per month) or high-strength cannabis use occurring in 25% to 40% of these users (Habboushe et al., 2018). CHS poses challenges to control in patients with concomitant migraines, psychosis, and opioid use disorders. CHS has a paucity of data on effective treatments (Gonzalez et al., 2018).

TABLE 22.12: Comparison of Signs and Symptoms of Cannabis and Synthetic Cannabinoids

	CANNABIS AND CANNABINOID PRODUCTS	SYNTHETIC CANNABINOIDS
Psychiatric	Mild: • Inappropriate affect • Depressed mood • Euphoric mood Moderate: • Impaired memory • Disorganized thoughts • Hallucinations • Bizarre or dangerous behavior Severe: • Delusions • Impaired judgment • Dangerous to self/suicidal	Mild: • Dizziness • Altered mental status Moderate: • Memory impairment • Paranoia • Hallucinations Severe: • Delusions/impaired judgment • Agitation • Persistent psychosis • Violence toward self and others • Dangerous to self/others • Suicidal, homicidal
Physiologic	Mild: • Pupil constriction • Nystagmus • Headache • Tachypnea • Tremor • Urinary retention • Ataxia • Sedation • Lethargy Moderate: • Injected conjunctiva • Orthostatic hypotension • Tachycardia • Palpitations • Arrhythmia • Hypotension • Decreased coordination • Increased appetite	Mild: • Increased appetite • Fatigue, sedation, lethargy • Headache Moderate: • Nausea and vomiting • Tachycardia • Hypertension • Orthostatic hypotension • Arrhythmia • Respiratory depression • Pneumonitis • Ataxia Severe: • Acute ischemic stroke • Seizures • Acute myocardial infarction • Rhabdomyolysis/renal failure • Death

Source: Cooper, Z. D., & Williams, A. R. (2019). Cannabis and cannabinoid intoxication and toxicity. In I. Montoya & S. R. B. Weiss (Eds.), *Cannabis use disorders* (pp. 103–111). Springer Publishing Company. https://link.springer.com/chapter/10.1007/978-3-319-90365-1_12

SC intoxication and toxicity is variable. SC toxicity is most noted in young males (Courts et al., 2016). Desired effects include relaxation, disinhibition, euphoria. Nausea and vomiting are common complaints. The most common sign seen in SC intoxication is sinus tachycardia. Toxicity signs include anxiety, agitation, paranoid delusions, hallucinations, violence. Seizures, stroke, coma, and death have been noted with SC toxicity (Courts et al., 2016; Drug Enforcement Administration [DEA], 2020b; Minns, 2013). Death most commonly occurs due to myocardial infarction and organ failure, with acute kidney injury requiring hemodialysis occurring most frequently (DEA, 2020b). Compared to marijuana ingestion, SC ingestions result in more tachycardia, hypertension, hallucinations, severe agitation, and violence (Courts et al., 2016; DEA, 2020b; Minns, 2013).

HISTORY AND PHYSICAL FINDINGS

Common signs and symptoms of adults with cannabis toxicity include paranoia, psychosis, and decreased judgment, perception, and coordination. Common signs and symptoms of SC toxicity signs include anxiety, agitation, paranoid delusions, hallucinations, and potential violence.

DIFFERENTIAL DIAGNOSIS AND DIAGNOSTIC CONSIDERATIONS

Patients presenting with cannabinoid ingestion can be difficult to distinguish from patients with generalized anxiety disorders and panic attacks or psychotic disorders such as schizophrenia. Direct observation of the patient and obtaining direct history as well as collateral information can confirm cannabis use. Urine or blood toxicology testing, if needed, can aid in the diagnosis.

Patients with visual disturbances are more often associated with cannabis, stimulants, and hallucinogens rather than primary psychotic disorders and resolve with cessation of drug use/ingestion resolution. Patients with a history of psychosis or risk factors for schizophrenia are at greater risk of more intense and prolonged psychosis following use of cannabis and SC. SC use is commonly combined with other drugs of abuse by wetting or dipping it in other drugs, such as inhalants or sprinkled with phencyclidine (PCP).

TREATMENT

Treatment of cannabis intoxication typically requires only supportive care, such as supplemental oxygen, cardiac monitoring, IV hydration, electrolyte correction as needed. For intoxication or overdose, sedatives such as risperidone or olanzapine are preferred but benzodiazepines can be used to treat paranoia, delusions, hallucinations, or extreme behaviors. Beta-blockers are effective to manage tachycardia and palpitations. For patients with schizophrenia or at risk of psychosis, cannabinoids can destabilize control of their symptoms; thus, consider increasing their dosage of antipsychotic agents.

Treatment of overdose from SC is commonly more difficult to manage especially in agitated or violent patients. Benzodiazepines are commonly used to manage agitation and antipsychotics are used to manage delirium and/or other psychotic states (Monte et al., 2017). For the most extreme cases of toxicity, admission to critical care units is required for intubation and mechanical ventilation, and if needed vasopressor use to treat hypotension and hemodialysis to treat acute kidney injury (Cooper & Williams, 2019).

22.7: CARBON MONOXIDE TOXICITY/ POISONING

Carbon monoxide (CO) is a colorless, odorless gas that is undetectable to the human senses. CO poisoning accounts for over 50,000 emergency department visits and over 1000 deaths annually (Guzman, 2012; Hampson, 2016). Common causes include smoke inhalation, furnaces, and other heating devices as well as internal combustion engines (vehicles) that create fumes contained within confined spaces without adequate ventilation. CO poisoning results from tissue hypoxia due to CO binding with hemoglobin creating carboxyhemoglobinemia (COhb). CO has over 200 times the affinity for hemoglobin than does oxygen, thus hemoglobin is saturated more readily with inhaled CO than oxygen. COhb is then transported to tissues causing cellular hypoxia. The Haldane effect causes remaining oxygen molecules bound to hemoglobin to have a greater affinity to the hemoglobin, thus remaining attached to the hemoglobin. This affinity results in further impairment of oxygen from cleaving off from hemoglobin to the cells, causing a leftward shift in the oxyhemoglobin dissociation curve and worsening tissue hypoxia (Rose et al., 2017). Additionally, CO binds with other heme-containing proteins including cytochrome C oxidase and myoglobin. The binding to myoglobin, especially cardiac myoglobin, can further reduce oxygen to the myocytes, causing arrhythmias and cardiac dysfunction (Rose et al., 2017). CO also causes inflammation by increasing cytosolic heme levels and heme oxygenase-1 protein, causing increased intracellular oxidative stress. CO binds with platelet heme proteins, causing release of nitric oxide (NO) producing peroxynitrite, which impairs mitochondrial function, worsening cellular hypoxia (Rose et al., 2017). Lastly, CO causes platelet/neutrophil aggregation, releases myeloperoxidase proteases and reactive oxygen species, which leads to oxidative stress, lipid peroxidation, and apoptosis. These effects are primarily observed in the brain, causing neurologic symptoms (Rose et al., 2017).

PRESENTING SIGNS AND SYMPTOMS

Symptoms of CO poisoning are nonspecific and easily missed or misdiagnosed and commonly underreported. Symptoms vary and are associated with the severity of hypoxia caused by the duration of exposure and CO level. The most common presenting symptom of CO poisoning is headache and is frequently associated with dizziness (Guzman, 2012).

HISTORY AND PHYSICAL FINDINGS

CO poisoning is classically diagnosed with a clinical triad including (a) symptoms consistent with CO poisoning, (b) reports of exposure, and (c) elevated COhb level. Many EMS teams can measure ambient air of the patient's environment to aid in diagnosing this condition.

Blood COhb level is the confirmatory test and should be done soon after presentation.

As CO exposure is increased, the more severe neurologica symptoms appear, progressing from headache and dizziness, nausea, and vomiting to confusion, seizures, syncope, strokelike syndromes, and unconsciousness/coma (Table 22.13). Cardiovascular symptoms include tachycardia, elevated cardiac biomarkers due to hypoxia, arrhythmias including supraventricular tachycardia and ventricular tachycardia (VT), and ventricular dysfunction. Patients may present with acute kidney injury due to rhabdomyolysis, as well as noncardiogenic pulmonary edema and cutaneous blisters. The classic description of CO poisoning with "cherry red" skin or mucous membranes is not commonly seen in practice.

The most severe acute CO poisonings have severe cognitive dysfunction with rapidly progressing cerebral edema. The highest mortality is seen in patients who present in an unconscious state requiring intubation, with pH <7.20, have a high COhb level, with fire as a source of CO exposure (Hampson, 2016).

Computed tomography (CT) or magnetic resonance imaging (MRI) of the brain commonly demonstrates white matter hyperintensities in the periventricular area (Hampson, 2016).

DIFFERENTIAL DIAGNOSIS AND DIAGNOSTIC CONSIDERATIONS

The presenting symptoms of CO poisoning are vague and pose challenges as they are nonspecific and can mimic many other disorders such as migraine, influenza, and other viral illnesses. Thus, a thorough and detailed history is critical. NPs need to consider the environment and social history, including the season, as many CO poisonings occur during colder weather when furnaces are running or alternative heat sources are being used, including kerosene heaters and wood stoves. For patients who are found down, explore the location and circumstances of where the patient was found. If the patient was found in a garage, was the car motor running? Did emergency medical services (EMS) report any open egress or ventilation systems? Was there fire in the vicinity of the patient? Are there any other individuals in the home or environment that simultaneously fell ill? Identifying the source is paramount to preventing subsequent poisonings.

Either an arterial or venous COhb level should be obtained immediately upon presentation. A COhb level over 3% confirms CO exposure, whereas in a patient who smokes cigarettes, a COhb level over 10% confirms an exposure. CO levels do not correlate with duration of exposure or clinical signs. A pulse oximetry does not accurately measure the oxygen saturation in patients with CO exposure, as the device cannot distinguish between oxygen and CO molecules in the blood.

TREATMENT

Immediate removal from the source and administration of 100% oxygen via high flow device are the first interventions. Ongoing supplementation of 100% oxygen facilitates the replacement of CO with oxygen on the hemoglobin. Administration of 100% oxygen reduced the 4 to 5 hour halflife of CO by half. Use of hyperbaric oxygen (HBO_2) can decrease the halflife to 30 minutes or less; its use remains controversial but is most often used in patients with CO levels >25% with severe neurologic deficits or cardiovascular symptoms.

Patients with CO poisoning should be placed on telemetry and monitored for cardiac arrhythmias. Serial neurologic exams should be performed. Evaluation for end organ damage should be untaken including serial lactic acid, troponin, ECG, blood-urea-nitrogen (BUN)/ creatinine, liver fuction tests, INR, creatine phosphokinase (CPK).

TABLE 22.13: Signs and Symptoms of Carbon Monoxide Poisoning

SEVERITY	SYMPTOMS	PHYSICAL EXAM
Mild	Headache Fatigue Malaise Dizziness Blurred vision Nausea	Confusion Disorientation Vomiting
Moderate	Syncope Dyspnea Palpitations Chest pain	Ataxia Tachypnea Rhabdomyolysis
Severe	Lethargy	Cardiac arrhythmias Myocardial ischemia Coma Respiratory depression Noncardiac pulmonary edema Seizures

Source: Guzman, J. A. (2012). Carbon monoxide poisoning. *Critical Care Clinics, 28*(4), 537–548. https://doi.org/10.1016/j.ccc.2012.07.007

22.8: CHOLINERGIC TOXICITY/ POISONING

Cholinergic overdose/toxicity is a result of excess acetylcholine which results in cholinergic (nicotinic, muscarinic, and central) receptor overstimulation. The most common form of cholinergic toxicity is from exposure to organophosphates or carbamate insecticides (Lott & Jones, 2021). Organophosphates are chemical substances that are created with alcohols and phosphoric acid and can be found in insecticides but have also been weaponized for use in chemical warfare (sarin gas). Another potential cause of cholinergic toxicity includes commonly prescribed medications used to treat myasthenia gravis, glaucoma, and Alzheimer's disease, such as physostigmine, neostigmine, pyridostigmine, edrophonium, rivastigmine, donepezil, galantamine, although cholinergic toxicity is rare with drugs when taken at therapeutic doses. Cholinergic toxicity/overdose can occur by oral, intravenous, inhaled, ophthalmic eye drops, or dermal exposure.

PRESENTING SIGNS AND SYMPTOMS

Cholinergic toxicity is a result of too much acetylcholine leading to abundant parasympathetic effects. Cholinergic overdose/toxicity presents with signs and symptoms of muscarinic, nicotinic, and central receptor stimulation; see examples in Table 22.14 (Smollin & Olson, 2021a). The cholinergic toxidrome includes hypertension, brady- or tachycardia, confusion to coma, miosis and salivation, lacrimation, urination, diarrhea, GI upset, and emesis.

HISTORY AND PHYSICAL FINDINGS

Presenting physical findings fall in line with cholinergic overdose/toxicity and a history that endorses exposure/ingestion. Physical findings will be consistent with the receptors that are being overstimulated. The patient experiencing toxicity may present with confusion, excessive sweating, lacrimation, salivation, muscle weakness, or even paralysis. There are mnemonics for muscarinic effects of excess acetylcholine; they are SLUDGE and DUMBELS (Table 22.15).

DIFFERENTIAL DIAGNOSIS AND DIAGNOSTIC CONSIDERATIONS

Several different diseases can present similarly to that of cholinergic overdose/toxicity. These differentials include Guillain-Barré syndrome and myasthenia gravis

TABLE 22.14: Cholinergic Receptor Signs and Symptoms

CHOLINERGIC RECEPTOR	SIGNS AND SYMPTOMS
Muscarinic	• Bradycardia • Miosis • Sweating • Hyperperistalsis • Bronchorrhea • Wheezing • Excessive salivation • Urinary incontinence
Nicotinic	• Initial hypertension and tachycardia • Fasciculation • Muscle weakness • Paralysis • Agitation • Anxiety
Central	• Confusion • Headache • Drowsiness

TABLE 22.15: Mnemonics for Muscarinic Effects

MNEMONIC SLUDGE	MNEMONIC DUMBELS
S – Salivation L – Lacrimation U – Urinary frequency/incontinence D – Diaphoresis/diarrhea G – GI cramping E – Emesis	D – Diarrhea U – Urinary Frequency/incontinence M – Miosis B – Bronchospasm/bronchorrhea E – Emesis L – Lacrimation S – Salivation

as the symptomatology of these disease states can present with muscle weakness. Opioid overdose and sepsis may also present with confusion. The patient experiencing an asthma exacerbation will present with wheezing and anxiety.

There are no laboratory tests or radiographic tests to definitely diagnose cholinergic toxicity. The diagnosis is made with the correlation of presenting symptoms consistent with the cholinergic toxidrome and a history of exposure/ingestion.

TREATMENT

The mainstay of treatment is supportive care and removal of the offending agent. Cholinergic toxicity can impact the respiratory system and cardiovascular system resulting in cardiopulmonary collapse (Table 22.16). There is also a risk for significant electrolyte abnormalities which can increase the risk for arrhythmias and death.

Patients who present with cholinergic toxicity from exposure to organophosphates must first be decontaminated and personnel caring for these patients must ensure proper personal protective equipment to avoid self-exposure. If support of the airway is needed by means of an advanced airway, succinylcholine should not be used due to reduced acetylcholinesterase from the overdose, which will result in prolonged paralysis.

Atropine can be given until symptoms improve as atropine improves muscarinic symptoms. Pralidoxime (2 PAM) can also be given and works to restore the activity of acetylcholinesterase, working on the nicotinic effects.

TABLE 22.16: Complication of Cholinergic Toxicity

BODY SYSTEM	IMPACT	COMPLICATION
Respiratory	Bronchospasm, bronchorrhea, respiratory muscle weakness	Respiratory failure
Cardiovascular	Bradycardia, hypotension, hypertension	Arrhythmia, cardiovascular collapse
Renal	Diarrhea, emesis	Arrhythmia, dehydration, electrolyte abnormalities

The result of this medication is improvement in muscle weakness and is particularly indicated with respiratory muscle weakness. The approved dose of pralidoxime for organophosphate toxicity is 1 g to 2 g IV infusion which can be repeated in an hour if muscle weakness persists. Pralidoxime can briefly worsen symptoms, thus atropine needs to be administered first. Atropine can be given in doses of 2 mg to 5 mg IV every 5 minutes in adults until symptoms improve (i.e., bronchorrhea, bronchospasm; Lott & Jones, 2021). Treatment should always include consultation with a medical toxicologist.

22.9: HALLUCINOGEN TOXICITY/ POISONING

Hallucinogenic agents are commonly found in plants and mushrooms or are synthetically produced. Hallucinogens include psilocybin or mushrooms, peyote and mescaline, lysergic acid diethylamide (LSD), ketamine, 3,4 methylene dioxy-methamphetamine (MDMA), or ecstasy and PCP. Each of these is described in more detail. Hallucinogens come in many forms including plants, powders, liquids, and can be ingested through multiple routes as well including orally, smoked, snorted, or injected depending on the product.

Hallucinogenic effects vary with dose, setting, and mood and include distorted thoughts about time and space. Time can seem to stand still, whereas colors change and take on new meanings. Hallucinogenic effects can persist for weeks or months after ingestion with some having "flashbacks" or developing a rare disorder called hallucinogen persisting perception disorder (HPPD). Flashbacks and HPPD include unpredictable recurrence of fragments of the experience in the absence of the drug.

Psilocybin

Psilocybin is a chemical obtained from certain types of mushrooms, also called magic mushrooms, mushrooms and shrooms. The mushrooms that contain psilocybin have long, thin, white-gray stems with dark brown caps on top that have dark gills on the underside. Fresh or dry mushrooms can be eaten or brewed into tea. The effects of psilocybin are hallucinations and the inability to differentiate illusion from reality. Panic and psychoses can also occur.

Peyote and Mescaline

Peyote are small, spineless cacti whose active ingredient is mescaline. Common street names include cactus, mesc, peyote, and buttons. The crown of the cactus is cut off and chewed or ground into powder to be swallowed or smoked or soaked in water to yield an intoxicating liquid. Mescaline causes hallucinations with alterations in space, time, and body image. Feelings of euphoria is common and can be followed by anxiety.

Lysergic Acid Diethylamide

LSD, also known as acid, trips, tabs, microdots, dots, and Lucy, is a synthetic chemical made from a component of ergot, a fungus that infects rye grain. LSD is considered a psychedelic agent and can be made from two types of N-methoxybenzyl derivatives which are quite dangerous due to variations in quality and can result in death (Alcohol and Drug Foundation [ADF], 2020a). LSD is a white odorless crystalline that is very potent and thus diluted. Drops of LSD solution are dried onto gelatin sheets or blotting paper or sugar cubes but can also be sold as liquid, tablets, or capsules. LSD affects everyone differently depending on size, weight, health, quantity ingested, and strength of dose.

Phencyclidine

PCP is also called angel dust, embalming fluid, hog, killer weed, love boat, ozone, peace pill, rocket fuel, super grass, and wack. PCP can be snorted, injected, smoked, and swallowed. PCP can cause euphoria, disconnection from reality, a sense of superhuman strength ,and fearlessness (Medline Plus, 2021).

Methylene Dioxy-Methamphetamine

MDMA, commonly called ecstasy is a synthetic drug that is chemically similar to both a hallucinogen and stimulant, which produces feelings of euphoria, closeness, empathy, sexuality, and increased energy. Effects are seen within 30 to 45 minutes of ingestion, with a duration of 4 to 6 hours. Common names include Adam, beans, clarity, disco biscuit, E, Eve, Go, Hug drug, lover's speed, Peace, STP, X, and XTC. MDMA is primarily distributed in colorful tablets, but can be in capsules, powder, and liquid form. The drug is ingested orally, or crushed and snorted, and occasionally smoked but rarely injected. MDMA causes an increase in the release of serotonin and norepinephrine. MDMA is commonly coingested with other agents such as alcohol or marijuana. Additional risks seen with MDMA includes the illegal manufacturer's inclusion of additives of one or more illicit substances: cocaine, ketamine, methamphetamine, and/or synthetic cathinones called "bath salts" (DEA, 2017).

Ketamine

Ketamine is a dissociative anesthetic with hallucinogenic effects. It distorts the perception of sight and sound, making the user feel disconnected. Ketamine induces sedation, analgesia, and amnesia while under the influence of the drug. For these reasons, ketamine has been used to enable sexual assaults. Common street names include vitamin K, special K, super K, cat tranquilizer, cat valium jet K, kit kat, and purple. Ketamine is distributed as a clear liquid or white/off white powder that can be snorted, smoked, or mixed into drinks. Duration of effects is typically 30 to 60 minutes and is preferred to LSD or PCP because of this short duration. Ketamine is often combined with MDMA, amphetamines, methamphetamine, or cocaine. Overdose of ketamine can induce unconsciousness and life-threatening bradypnea (DEA, 2017).

PRESENTING SIGNS AND SYMPTOMS

Patients with hallucinogen ingestion present with tachycardia, hypertension, mydriasis, nausea, and vomiting. Death related to overdose of LSD, magic mushrooms, and mescaline are uncommon, but when it occurs it is due to suicide, accidents, dangerous behavior ,or erroneously ingesting poisonous plants.

HISTORY AND PHYSICAL FINDINGS

Classic effects of hallucinogens include euphoria, mydriasis, perceptual changes, including visual and auditory illusions (distortion of perception) and confusion, difficulty concentrating, headache, nausea/vomiting, tachycardia, tachypnea, fever, facial flushing, and chills. True hallucinations (no basis in reality) are rare. Overdose signs include panic, paranoia, increased risk taking, psychosis. A "bad trip" commonly manifests as a severe anxiety or panic attack or disturbing hallucinations, which can lead to risky behaviors due to panicked response possibly attempting self-harm. Mind set and environmental setting can strongly affect the psychological and emotional experience and reaction. Coming-down effects following hallucinogen ingestion includes insomnia, fatigue, body and muscle aches, and depressed mood.

DIFFERENTIAL DIAGNOSIS AND DIAGNOSTIC CONSIDERATIONS

Diagnostic and Statistical Manual of Mental Disorders, Fifth Edition (DSM-5) criteria are similar to other intoxications. Additionally, primary psychiatric disorders, including schizophrenia, must be considered as the population who most commonly uses hallucinogens are male adolescents and young adults, who are also in the same age group as those who develop schizophrenia and other psychiatric disorders.

TREATMENT

Hallucinogen use rarely requires medical interventions. Supportive care includes a calm environment, reassurances, treatment of symptoms. Severe reactions including delirium or serotonin syndrome can be managed with benzodiazepines (Khan & Thomas, 2020). First-generation antipsychotics are reasonable second-line agents for persistent concerning behaviors; however, note that haloperidol (Haldol) may decrease seizure threshold. Restraints are not commonly required but may be indicated for patients who are a threat to self or others. Some individuals may experience flashbacks with serotonin reuptake inhibitors, especially sertraline. Risperidone should be avoided as it has been noted to worsen visual hallucinations (Khan & Thomas, 2020).

22.10: INHALANTS TOXICITY/ POISONING

Inhalants are volatile liquids that transform into chemical vapors and are inhaled to create a psychoactive effect (Tables 22.17 and 22.18). Inhalants are typically found in common household or work-related items. Inhalants create a "head rush" followed by euphoria, lightheadedness, dizziness, disinhibition, and impulsivity and a decreased sense of pain that lasts about 15 to 45 minutes. Inhalants are used more commonly by adolescents than adults. However, adults who have ready access to chemicals and anesthetics, including anesthesiologists, nurse anesthetists, dentists, hair stylists, painters, and dry-cleaning workers are at higher risk (Khan & Thomas, 2020). Nitrate use is also commonly seen among men who have sex with men, due to the aphrodisiac effects and relaxation of rectal muscles.

Inhalants rapidly cross the alveolar membranes and blood/brain barrier resulting in near immediate effects as the chemical bypasses hepatic metabolism. For most inhalants, primary elimination is via the lungs and in an unaltered form; however, aromatics, alkyl nitrites, and methylene chloride are cleared hepatically, which can create toxic byproducts such as free nitrites and carbon monoxide (Khan & Thomas, 2020).

TABLE 22.17: Categories of Common Inhalant Agents

INHALANT	EXAMPLES
Aromatic hydrocarbons	Petroleum-based products (gasoline, kerosene), propane, butane
Aliphatic (nonaromatic) hydrocarbons	Toluene (in paint thinners and model glue), xylene
Halogenated hydrocarbons	Hydrofluorocarbons, chlorofluorocarbons (used in many aerosols and propellants), anesthetics, refrigerants, methylene chloride (paint stripper), degreasers, spot removers, dry cleaning agents
Nitrates and nitrites	Amyl nitrate, butyl nitrate, isobutyl nitrite (aka "poppers")
Nitrous oxide	Used in whipped cream canisters as a propellant, power booster in cars and motorcycles, anesthetic agent for medical and dental procedures

Source: Data from Cojanu, A. I. (2018). Inhalant abuse: The wolf in sheep's clothing. *American Journal of Psychiatry, 16*(4), 7–9. https://doi.org/10.1176/appi.ajp-rj.2018.130203; Khan, M., & Thomas, A. (2020). Steroids, dissociatives, club drugs, inhalants, and hallucinogens. In C. Marienfeld (Ed.), *Absolute addiction psychiatry review* (pp. 205–230). Springer Publishing Company. https://link.springer.com/chapter/10.1007/978-3-030-33404-8_13

TABLE 22.18: Methods of Ingesting Inhalants

METHOD/ TERMINOLOGY	DESCRIPTION
Sniffing, snorting	Inhaling from original container through the nose; offers lowest concentration of agent
Huffing	Inhaling from the original container through the mouth or inhaling through a chemically impregnated rag that is held over the mouth
Bagging	Inhalant transferred into a bag (paper or plastic) which is held over mouth or head, seen more commonly in self-harm or suicide attempts; offers highest concentration of chemical
Dusting	Inhaling computer dusting spray via the nose or mouth
Glading	Inhaling air freshener via the nose or mouth

Source: Adapted from Khan, M., & Thomas, A. (2020). Steroids, dissociatives, club drugs, inhalants, and hallucinogens. In C. Marienfeld (Ed.), *Absolute addiction psychiatry review* (pp. 205–230). Springer Publishing Company. https://link.springer.com/chapter/10.1007/978-3-030-33404-8_13

TABLE 22.19: Toxic Effects of Inhalants

SYSTEM	TOXIC EFFECT
Neurologic	Slurred speech, drowsiness, nystagmus, peripheral neuropathy, polyneuropathy, tremor, white matter and cerebellar degeneration
Cardiovascular	Bradycardia, prolonged QT, heart block, myocardial fibrosis, sudden sniffing death syndrome
Pulmonary	Cough, wheezing, dyspnea, emphysema, chemical pneumonitis
Renal	Hypokalemia, acute kidney injury, metabolic acidosis, renal tubular acidosis
Gastrointestinal	Nausea, vomiting, diarrhea, abdominal pain, cramping, hepatotoxicity
Hematologic	Bone marrow suppression, leukemia, aplastic anemia
Integumentary	Perioral rash, eczema, contact dermatitis, burns, angioedema, frostbite injury
Psychiatric	Apathy, depression, insomnia, poor attention, memory loss, psychosis, dementia

Source: Adapted from Khan, M., & Thomas, A. (2020). Steroids, dissociatives, club drugs, inhalants, and hallucinogens. In C. Marienfeld (Ed.), *Absolute addiction psychiatry review* (pp. 205–230). Springer Publishing Company. https://link.springer.com/chapter/10.1007/978-3-030-33404-8_13

PRESENTING SIGNS AND SYMPTOMS

Use of inhalants create a euphoric effect, followed by drowsiness, lethargy, headache, and sleep. Slurred speech, dizziness, diplopia, ataxia, and disorientation can be seen with repeated and increased doses. Prolonged use can cause visual hallucinations, and significant time distortion, commonly cited as reasons for use. Infrequent users report more pleasant experiences, whereas those who use inhalants chronically report both pleasant, unpleasant, and even noxious experiences (Khan & Thomas, 2020).

HISTORY AND PHYSICAL FINDINGS

Inhalant toxicity can affect multiple systems (Table 22.19). Workup includes complete blood count (CBC), basic metabolic panel (BMP), liver function tests (LFT), methemoglobin level, continuous pulse oximetry, ECG. Urine toxicology tests will not identify inhalants but may aid in diagnosing concurrently used agents. Specifically, these tests seek to link findings to inhalant. Elevated methemoglobin level is seen with nitrite use (Khan & Thomas, 2020). Hypoxia, arrhythmias, hypokalemia, hypophosphatemia, and acidosis are seen with toluene use. Liver and renal abnormalities are seen with halogenated hydrocarbon use. Bone marrow suppression is seen with benzene use (Khan & Thomas, 2020).

Death is attributed to asphyxiation or suffocation, aspiration of vomitus, dangerous behavior, or dangerous environment. Sudden sniffing death is rare and exact mechanism is not known but is thought to be related to arrhythmias after inhalation of halogenated hydrocarbons (Cojanu, 2018).

DIFFERENTIAL DIAGNOSIS AND DIAGNOSTIC CONSIDERATIONS

Diagnosis is challenging as these agents are not detected in urine or blood or drug of abuse screening tests. History is paramount in these cases. Seek information from patient, family, and friends.

TREATMENT

Supportive care is the mainstay of therapy for inhalant intoxication. Remove patient from the source and apply supplemental oxygen. For patients who cannot maintain an airway or have respiratory depression, intubation and mechanical ventilation may be required. Give electrolyte replacement as needed and address any arrhythmias based on current ACLS guidelines. For patients with methemoglobinemia, administer high concentrations of oxygen and consider IV methylene blue to accelerate enzymatic reduction of the methemoglobin. Note that methylene blue is contraindicated in patients with G6PD deficiency (Khan & Thomas, 2020).

22.11: OPIOID TOXICITY/POISONING

Opioids, also known as narcotics, is a class of drugs that ise known for their analgesic affects. Opioid overdose has become an all-too-common presenting problem in our healthcare system. In 2017, 68% of the 70,237 U.S.

drug overdose deaths involved an opioid (Wilson et al., 2020). The term *opiate* or *opioid* covers many names of prescription and illicit drugs (heroin, codeine, oxycodone, fentanyl, hydromorphone, methadone, and others). These drugs have a large variation of potencies and durations of action, some of which are regulated in the form of prescription medications and not regulated in the form of illicit opioid drugs.

Opioid medications are prescribed for acute and chronic pain syndromes by a medical provider. This type of drug also has synthetic variations which can be illegally produced, like u-47700, which is a highly potent synthetic opioid. The unregulated production, distribution, and sale of illicit opiates like heroin and fentanyl add to the complexity of treating the patient that presents with an opioid overdose. The concentration of drug and additives is unknown with the illicit forms of opioids.

PRESENTING SIGNS AND SYMPTOMS

Opioids decrease central nervous system (CNS) activity and sympathetic outflow causing patients to present with a range of signs and symptoms. Mild intoxication can present with euphoria, drowsiness ,and miosis; more severe intoxication can cause hypotension, bradycardia, hypothermia, coma, respiratory depression, or even respiratory and cardiac arrest (see Table 22.1). The classic opioid toxidrome is the clinical triad of coma, respiratory depression, and miosis (Williams & Thurman, 2021).

HISTORY AND PHYSICAL FINDINGS

The majority of patients who present for evaluation with opioid toxicity are lethargic or comatose and unable to provide a history; thus family, friends, bystanders, or emergency medical providers supply details. The antidote naloxone (Narcan) for opioid reversal is readily available in the community and it is important to determine if naloxone was given prior to arrival to a healthcare facility and, if so, how much and what the response was. Knowing how the patient responded to the administration of naloxone can inform diagnosis, but do not assume that one dose of naloxone is always sufficient to reverse opioid effects. Obtaining details regarding the surroundings in which the patient was found can inform the provider what preparation of opioid might have been ingested or potential for coingestion. Route of consumption is also important to note as effects might be very quick with IV or nasal insufflation but might take more time if taken by intermuscular injection or oral route. Coingestions like alcohol, benzodiazepines, and other legal or illicit drugs must always be suspected and investigated as this may mask or potentiate presenting signs and symptoms.

Key finding on physical exam will include bradypnea, generalized CNS depression, and miosis. Patients can present differently and the absence of miosis should not exclude opioid overdose. Nausea and vomiting are also physical findings seen with some cases of opioid overdose. Thorough examination of the skin is important and can reveal needle track marks, including punctures, scabs, lesions, and bruising.

DIFFERENTIAL DIAGNOSIS AND DIAGNOSTIC CONSIDERATIONS

Differential diagnoses should include other reasons the patients maypresent with this constellation of symptoms, coma, respiratory depression, and miosis. Differential diagnoses include diabetic ketoacidosis, other poisoning, or toxicity (benzodiazepine, cannabinoid, carbon monoxide, clonidine), ethylene glycol hypercalcemia, meningitis, hypothermia, hypoglycemia, and hypothyroidism/myxedema coma.

The laboratory workup for a patient with opioid toxicity should include complete blood count (CBC), comprehensive metabolic panel (CMP), creatine kinase (CK), arterial blood gas (ABG), and, if concerns over coingestion are present, an acetaminophen, salicylate, alcohol level, and drug screen should also be considered. With concerns for self-harm or coingestion an ECG is recommend to evaluate for arrhythmias. Concerns of injury to the lung or evidence of noncardiogenic pulmonary edema should be investigated with a chest radiograph. An abdominal radiograph needs to be considered if the patient is suspected of swallowing packaged opioids for the purpose of concealment and/or transport. Prolonged periods of respiratory depression and hypoxia can raise the concern for anoxic brain injury and warrant further brain CT scan and MRI and neurology consultation.

TREATMENT

Treatment is focused on administration of the reversal agent, naloxone, and supporting airway, breathing, and circulation. Whole bowel irrigation in the setting of ingestion of extended-release preparations should be considered. Activated charcoal can also be considered for the alert patient up to 3 hours after ingestion (Schiller et al., 2020).

Naloxone is an opioid antagonist and can reverse respiratory and CNS depression within a minute and can be administered via intravenous, intranasal, or intramuscular routes. Due to the short halflife of naloxone, multiple doses can be required. Severe cases of opioid overdose can require a naloxone continuous infusion. The administration of naloxone can cause immediate onset of opioid withdrawal symptoms so careful consideration is required (Table 22.20). One must note that preparations may vary based on availability and institution protocols.

There are two treatment pathways for the provider after the acute overdose has been treated with naloxone and supportive care. These are opioid maintenance and detoxification and need to include referral to treatment and recovery programs. Maintenance can be achieved with an opioid agonist or partial agonist. Detoxification

TABLE 22.20: Naloxone Preparations

Intravenous (bolus)	0.2–2 mg
Intranasal (single dose device)	4 mg
Continuous infusion	Start with 2/3 the dose of naloxone that reversed the patient's symptoms and titrate by 0.1–0.2 mg/h to address symptoms To wean, decrease by 0.1–0.2 mg/h every 2 hours monitoring frequently

is pursued with an alpha-2-adrenergic agonist. Ensuring patients and families have education and access to naloxone is also an element that must be addressed moving on from the acute hospitalization.

22.12: LITHIUM TOXICITY/POISONING

Lithium is a widely utilized treatment option for mood disorders, particularly as an effective therapy for bipolar disorder. Lithium has a narrow therapeutic window and thus can have unintended consequences with small changes in consumption, metabolism, and or excretion of the drug. Like other widely used medications toxicity, can present as acute toxicity, chronic toxicity, and acute on chronic toxicity. Severity of toxicity can be better understood by understanding the duration of lithium exposure and amount ingested (Ford, 2018).

PRESENTING SIGNS AND SYMPTOMS

Clinical presentation of an individual with lithium toxicity or reported lithium ingestion can vary widely from an asymptomatic patient to life-threatening manifestations (Table 22.21).

TABLE 22.21: Signs and Symptoms of Lithium Toxicity

BODY SYSTEM	SIGNS AND SYMPTOMS	
Cardiovascular	• Bradycardia • T wave flattening or inversions and depressed ST segments in the lateral leads • Prolonged QT interval	
Neurologic	• Lethargy • Ataxia • Confusion • Agitation • Hyperreflexia	• Myoclonic jerks • Fasciculations • Hyperthermia • Coma • Seizure/status epilepticus
Gastrointestinal	• Nausea • Vomiting • Diarrhea	
Renal	• Dehydration • Hypernatremia • Acute kidney injury/renal failure	

HISTORY AND PHYSICAL FINDINGS

Careful and complete history taking is crucial when evaluating a patient with suspected or confirmed lithium ingestion/toxicity. As with other ingestions, the two crucial elements to determine are whether the patient is taking lithium as a prescribed medication and if the medication was intentionally or accidentally ingested. These factors will inform the provider on whether the patient has chronic saturation of lithium in the body. Additionally, identify the type of preparation of lithium that was consumed—immediate or delayed release formulation. Identify whether a patient has had a recent illness or changes to oral intake impacts the potential for toxicity. Dehydration is the most common cause of lithium toxicity.

A common and early sign of lithium toxicity is tremor. Tremor is typically noticed in the hands and is symmetric. Tremor is also a known side effect of the medication and often is not a reason for discontinuation of the medication. Additional physical findings of lithium toxicity include confusion, dysarthria, ataxia, hyperreflexia, rigidity, myoclonus, and seizures.

DIFFERENTIAL DIAGNOSIS AND DIAGNOSTIC CONSIDERATIONS

Differential diagnoses to consider with suspected lithium overdose/toxicity include hypoglycemia, delirium and/or dementia, and stroke which all can be linked to the physical finding listed in Table 22.22. Parkinson's may also need to be considered due to the tremor and rigidity that can present with lithium toxicity.

Intentional lithium ingestion can be confirmed by a positive history of consumption. The diagnosis of lithium toxicity is supported by elevated serum lithium levels, noting that in cases of chronic toxicity, lithium serum level may only be slightly elevated. Other useful laboratory studies included a basic metabolic panel (BMP), acetaminophen levels, salicylate levels, and beta-human chorionic gonadotropin level in women of child-bearing age (Baird-Gunning et al., 2017). An ECG should be routinely ordered when the differential includes lithium toxicity given the potential for fatal arrhythmias.

TABLE 22.22: Physical Findings in Suspected Lithium Overdose

	Serum Level	Symptoms
Therapeutic range	0.6–1.2 mEq/L	N/A
Mild toxicity	1.5–2.5 mEq/L	Nausea, vomiting, lethargy, tremor, fatigue
Moderate toxicity	2.5–3.5 mEq/L	Confusion, agitation, delirium, tachycardia, hypertonia
Severe toxicity	3.5 mEq/L and above	Coma, seizures, hyperthermia, hypotension

TREATMENT

No specific antidote for lithium overdose exists; the mainstay of therapy is supportive care. Supportive care includes evaluation and support of a patent and secure airway and circulation support. Fluid resuscitation is common practice with lithium toxicity as lithium is cleared solely through the kidneys. Optimizing renal perfusion will aid in the maximizing lithium excretion. For acute ingestions, gastrointestinal lavage can be helpful particularly when consumption of delayed release formulations is known. The initiation of hemodialysis should be considered based on these clinical manifestations: severe neurologic symptoms, symptoms of toxicity in the setting of renal failure ,and the inability to volume resuscitate. Serum lithium levels should also be evaluated when making the decision to initiate dialysis: a serum level >4.0 mEq/L in acute ingestion and >2.5 mEq/L in acute on chronic or chronic ingestion are significant and should be considered for hemodialysis (Lank et al., 2014).

22.13: SALICYLATE TOXICITY/POISONING

Salicylates are known for their analgesic, anti inflammatory, and antithrombotic properties. Salicylates are found in many prescription and nonprescription medications including bismuth subsalicylate, aspirin, and many topical medication preparations. Salicylate toxicity can result from an acute or chronic ingestion. Chronic ingestions can be confounded by the fact that many medications are combinations of medications which also contain salicylates. Both acute and chronic toxicity are medical emergencies as they are initially associated with respiratory alkalosis which can progress to an anion gap metabolic acidosis. For this topic, the presenting signs and symptoms, pertinent history, physical exam findings and treatments will be broken down into two categories, acute ingestion, and chronic ingestion.

PRESENTING SIGNS AND SYMPTOMS

Acute ingestion/toxicity of salicylates is a medical emergency and requires prompt recognition and treatment. Patients with acute ingestion will have varying signs and symptoms depending on the amount ingested and time since ingestion. Within 1 to 2 hours signs of salicylate ingestion include tinnitus, vertigo, nausea, vomiting, and hyperpnea. These signs can be seen when plasma levels approach or exceed 40 mg/dL. As plasma levels increase to 50–70 mg/dL, symptoms can include fever, diaphoresis, listlessness, and incoordination. Plasma levels that surpass 75 mg/dL increase the risk of hallucinations, seizures, cerebral edema, coma, and noncardiogenic pulmonary edema (Palmer & Clegg, 2020). Importantly, time of ingestion, plasma concentrations, and associated symptoms can vary from patient to patient.

Chronic toxicity presents with small increases in use/consumption of salicylate-containing medications. Thus, chronic toxicity presents in a different manner that often does not correlate well with plasma levels as the patient has a baseline saturation of salicylate-containing medication/s. Chronic toxicity is often seen in older patients due to the higher probability of polypharmacy. Presenting signs and symptoms are similar to acute ingestion but are often attributed other potential sources because there is often no clear indication of an acute ingestion. Symptoms include agitation, confusion, fever, tachypnea, and hallucinations, all of which can be signs and symptoms of other common reasons for presentation including sepsis, dementia or delirium, diabetic ketoacidosis.

HISTORY AND PHYSICAL FINDINGS

When interviewing a patient with suspected acute ingestion of salicylates it is crucial to note when the medication was ingested, how much, what formulation, if other medications or substances were ingested, and if the ingestion was intentional or accidental. The potential for coingestions must be considered, as this can delay gastric absorption. Inquire if the formulation of the salicylate ingested was a delayed- or immediate-release preparation, as this too will affect absorption.

Toxic levels of salicylates directly impact the respiratory center of the medulla and cause increased depth and rate of breathing. Development of a respiratory alkalosis is seen in the early stages following ingestion. The progression of salicylate toxicity has increasing accumulation of ketoacids which are primarily responsible for the increase in the anion gap. Patients with salicylate toxicity are commonly hypovolemic given the excessive losses from hyperpyrexia, diaphoresis, and tachypnea. Physical findings of acute toxicity of salicylates include nausea, vomiting, abdominal pain, tachypnea, dizziness, headache, confusion, hallucinations, seizure, and coma.

DIFFERENTIAL DIAGNOSIS AND DIAGNOSTIC CONSIDERATIONS

The presenting signs and symptoms of salicylate toxicity are similar to many other medical conditions, including sepsis, diabetic ketoacidosis (DKA), asthma, and ethylene glycol toxicity.

Diagnostic considerations pertaining to salicylate toxicity include obtaining a salicylate level, arterial blood gas, comprehensive metabolic panel (CMP), and a lactic acid level. Additionally, an acetaminophen level and ethanol level should be obtained to assess for coingestion. Obtain an ECG, as dysrhythmias are commonly noted with salicylate ingestion. It important to note that serum salicylate levels do not always correlate with the level of toxicity and a multipronged approach is required to evaluate and treat patients with salicylate toxicity. Serial evaluation of salicylate levels and arterial blood gases are required until a consistently improving trend is noted.

TREATMENT

A targeted antidote for salicylate toxicity does not exist. Treatment options for treating salicylate toxicity include supportive care with fluid resuscitation, management of electrolyte abnormalities, ensuring proper respiratory and circulatory support when needed. Further, attention should be paid to prevent further gastrointestinal absorption of salicylates with oral administration of activated charcoal (if the patient is awake, alert, and cooperative). The effectiveness of activated charcoal is beneficial when used within 2 hours of ingestions. Large ingestions of aspirin can slow gastric emptying, with delayed release formulations of aspirin administration of activated charcoal can be done up to 2 hours after ingestion.

The administration of sodium bicarbonate helps in two ways: (a) It promotes salicylate to leave the cell and enter the plasma and (b) urinary alkalization promotes renal excretion of salicylates. Alkalization can be achieved by administration of an infusion of sodium bicarbonate (Palmer & Clegg, 2020). Careful monitoring of potassium levels is required as this intervention can cause hypokalemia.

Hemodialysis is an efficient way to remove salicylate from the serum, correct acidosis, and address electrolyte abnormalities. The threshold for initiating hemodialysis in a patient with salicylate ingestions is multifactorial and requires expert consultation with a medical toxicologist and nephrologist. Consideration for starting dialysis includes an altered mental status, renal insufficiency, acute respiratory distress syndrome requiring supplemental oxygen and failed previous therapy. Patients with a salicylate level of 90 mg/dL should be initiated on hemodialysis regardless of signs and symptoms as the plasma level may precede the onset of symptoms and timely intervention can lessen or prevent the toxic effects to tissues (Palmer & Clegg, 2020). Severe acidosis not responsive to optimal supportive care, evidence of end organ failure such as seizures, rhabdomyolysis, and pulmonary edema should also receive hemodialysis (O'Malley, 2007).

22.14: SEDATIVE-HYPNOTIC TOXICITY/ POISONING

Sedative and hypnotics are prescribed as a sleep aid, to relieve stress and anxiety and muscle spasms, and to prevent seizures (Table 22.23). Primary care providers prescribing antidepressants, anxiolytic sedatives, and benzodiazepines all increased in the last 15 years, with benzodiazepines increasing the most (Maust et al., 2017). These agents are readily found in medicine cabinets and commonly accessed by family and friends. Depressants are combined with other drugs to potentiate or combat the side effects of the other drugs. Specific drugs such as gamma hydroxybutyrate (GHB) and rohypnol are commonly misused to enable sexual assault and rape (DEA, 2020a).

TABLE 22.23: Commonly Prescribed Sedatives and Hypnotics

Over-the-counter sedatives:	• Benadryl (diphenhydramine) • Unisom (doxylamine)
Nonbenzodiazepines	• Ambien (zolpidem) • Belsomra (suvorexant) • Edluar (zolpidem) • Hetlioz (tasimelteon) • Intermezzo (zolpidem) • Lunesta (eszopiclone) • Rozerem (ramelteon) • Silenor (doxepin) • Sonata (zaleplon) • Zolpimist (zolpidem)
Benzodiazepines	• Ativan (lorazepam) • Doral (quazepam) • Estazolam • Dalmane (flurazepam) • Halcion (triazolam) • Klonopin (clonazepam) • Librium (chlordiazepoxide) • Restoril (temazepam) • Rohypnol – illegal in U.S. • Serax (oxazepam) • Tranxene (clorazepate) • Valium (diazepam) • Versed (midazolam) • Xanax (alprazolam)
Barbiturates	• Butalbital (Fiorina) • Butisol (butobarbital) • Phenobarbital • Pentothal • Secobarbital (seconal) • Nembutal
Other central nervous system (CNS) depressants	• Meprobamate • Methaqualone (Quaalude) • Gamma hydroxybutyrate (GHB)

Source: Data from Drug Enforcement Administration. (2020). Drugs of abuse: A DEA resource guide/2020 edition. U.S. Department of Justice Drug Enforcement Administration. https://www.dea.gov/sites/default/files/2020-04/Drugs%20of%20Abuse%20 2020-Web%20Version-508%20compliant-4-24-20_0.pdf; Drug Enforcement Agency. (2020). *Hallucinogens*. https://www.dea.gov/sites/default/files/2020-06/Hallucino gens-2020.pdf

These agents come in the form of pills, syrups, and injectable liquids but are most commonly ingested by swallowing tablets. Hospitalized patients may receive injections during procedures requiring conscious sedation or anxiety-provoking testing such as MRIs.

PRESENTING SIGNS AND SYMPTOMS

Euphoria is common among patients who abuse sedatives. Other effects include lightheadedness, dizziness, nausea, vomiting, depressed mental status, impaired judgment, confusion, slurred speech, weakness, loss of coordination, hypotension, bradypnea, and amnesia, all of which are signs of use of sedatives and hypnotics (DEA, 2020a).

HISTORY AND PHYSICAL FINDINGS

Reports of patients being "found down" are common among sedative overdose victims. Patients often present to the emergency department in an unresponsive state, many with insufficient respirations to support adequate ventilation and oxygenation. Additionally, patients who combine benzodiazepines with narcotics have a higher incidence of overdose as these agents potentiate each other.

DIFFERENTIAL DIAGNOSIS AND DIAGNOSTIC CONSIDERATIONS

Opioid overdose appears similar to sedative overdose and is commonly coingested.

TREATMENT

Supportive care is the mainstay of treatment. Support respiratory function with assisted breathing (ambu bagging), nonivasive ventilation with BiPAP or CPAP; some patients require intubation for inadequate respiratory drive.

Flumazenil (romazicon) is the reversal agent for benzodiazepine overdose. For sedation reversal, Flumazenil 0.2 mg IV Q 5 minutes up to 1 mg total dose or 3 mg per hour. Reassess the patient every 20 minutes for resedation as the halflife of Flumazenil is shorter than that of benzodiazepines. For benzodiazepine overdose start at 0.2 mg IV × 1 and wait 30 seconds; if no improvement, then administer 0.3 mg IV and wait 30 seconds; if no improvement or insufficient improvement administer 0.5 mg IV every minute as needed up to 5 mg total dose. If patient does not respond, consider other sedatives as the causative agent.

22.15: STIMULANT TOXICITY/POISONING

Stimulants are a broad classification of drugs that increase central nervous system activity by increasing catecholamine levels and increase agonistic activity at adrenergic receptors. Stimulants are used for a variety of reasons including medical indications, enhancement of cognitive and physical performance, and recreational use. Caffeine, found in coffee, tea, soft drinks, energy drinks, and chocolate, is the most commonly ingested stimulant in the world, as it promotes cognitive alertness. Nicotine is another commonly used legal stimulant. Amphetamines class of medications can be used for medical therapy and is commonly misused for recreational purposes (ADF, 2020b).

Stimulants can be legal or illegal drugs and are commonly misused and abused by a wide range of sociodemographic populations. College students commonly misuse caffeine for multiple reasons, but mostly to stay awake (Mahoney et al., 2019). Athletes use stimulants to enhance physical performance; many of these agents are banned by the world antidoping agency. Medical indications of stimulants include treatment of attention deficit hyperactivity disorder (ADHD), obesity, nasal and sinus congestion, asthma, hypotension after general anesthesia, and narcolepsy.

Examples of stimulants include amphetamines, methamphetamines, methylphenidate, ephedrine, synephrine, cocaine, methylsynephrine, 1,3-dimethlamylamine (DMAA), mephedrone, khat, synthetic cathinones, and betel nuts. In addition to enhancement of cognitive functions, amphetamines can also cause euphoric and aphrodisiac effects in some users. Methamphetamines are widely distributed illegal drugs solely for recreational purposes. Fentanyl and its analogs are increasingly being found in the illegal stimulant supply, thus causing additional overdose deaths (Park et al., 2020). Dual substance ingestions make diagnosis of the type of overdose more challenging as a patient's symptoms may not resemble just one toxidrome (ADF, 2020b).

PRESENTING SIGNS AND SYMPTOMS

Effects of stimulants when taken in excess include decreased appetite, anxiety, jitteriness, headaches, weight loss, insomnia, psychosis, pruritis, paranoia, diaphoresis, tachycardia, palpitations, chest pain, shortness of breath, hypertension, seizures, arrhythmias, premature atrial contractions (PAC) or premature ventricular contractions (PVC), ventricular tachycardia (VT), stroke, and sudden cardiac death (Table 22.24). If taken intranasally or snorted, rhinorrhea and epistaxis are common.

TABLE 22.24: Severity of Physiologic Stimulant Ingestion/Intoxication

GRADE	PHYSICAL FINDINGS AND SYMPTOMS
1	Enhanced sensory awareness, emotional lability, anxiety, irritability, tremors, diaphoretic, flushing or pallor, mydriasis, insomnia, decreased appetite Vital signs normal Hyperreflexia occasionally
2	Euphoria, agitation, restless, hallucinations, suspiciousness, but can converse and follow commands Vital signs mildly to moderately increased
3	Delirious, unintelligible speech, uncontrollable motor hyperactivity, impaired judgment Moderately to markedly increased vital signs Tachyarrhythmias possible
4	Coma, seizures (more common with cocaine use) Cardiovascular collapse

Source: SAMHSA Treatment for Stimulant Use Disorders. (1999). Chapter 5 medical aspects of stimulant use disorders Treatment Improvement Protocol (TIP) Series, No. 33. Center for Substance Abuse Treatment. Substance Abuse and Mental Health Services Administration (US). https://www.ncbi.nlm.nih.gov/books/NBK64323/

HISTORY AND PHYSICAL FINDINGS

Keen attention to detail is required when taking a history for stimulants. Inquire if patient ever was prescribed or has taken medications for ADHD or weight loss, including borrowed medications from peers or others. Treatment for ADHD includes methylphenidate (Ritalin), lisdexamfetamine, or dextroamphetamine (Adderall) which are stimulants. Diet aids such as didrex, bontril, preludin, fastin, Adipex P, ionomin, and meridian are all stimulants. A thorough social history must explore stimulant use, most specifically caffeine and nicotine, as these come in multiple forms. Caffeine is found in coffee, tea, soda, energy drinks, pills, chocolate, coffee beans, some protein bars, and over-the-counter weight loss pills. Nicotine is also a commonly used stimulant and includes cigarettes, vaping, oral tobacco, gums, and lozenges. Question use of illicit substances, including amphetamines, methamphetamines, cocaine, methcanthinone (khat), and other synthetic cathinones that are referred to as "bath salts." Other common street names for stimulants include: Bennies, black beauties, cat, coke, crank, crystal, flake, ice, pellets, r-ball, skippy, snow, speed, uppers ,and vitamin R (Alcohol and Drug Foundation, n.d.; Department of Justice/ Drug Enforcement Administration Drug Fact Sheet, n.d.).

DIFFERENTIAL DIAGNOSIS AND DIAGNOSTIC CONSIDERATIONS

Stimulants can mimic systemic inflammatory response syndrome (SIRS) that is commonly seen in infectious and noninfectious states. The differential diagnoses are broad and diverse, including sepsis, pancreatitis, generalized anxiety disorder, delirium, stroke, acute coronary syndrome (ACS).

TREATMENT

Treatment of stimulant toxicity depends on the agent ingested and symptoms. Conditions that commonly arise from stimulant ingestion include hypertension, including hypertensive urgency and emergency, acute coronary syndrome, pulmonary edema, agitation, seizures, and intracranial hemorrhage. Treatment options include benzodiazepines, beta-blockers, antiarrhythmic agents, antihypertensive medications, and diuretics. Benzodiazepines are a mainstay of treatment, as they decrease anxiety and agitation, and are required when patients have a seizure. Beta-blockers are useful to aid in controlling tachycardia and can aid in treating hypertension. Antiarrhythmic agents are indicated for treatment of VT.

TRANSITION OF CARE

When transition of care becomes necessary it is crucial to have determined if the ingestion/poisoning was intentional or accidental. If ingestion was accidental, assessment of the home situation is imperative to identify the contributing factors and provide education and resources to the patient and family regarding avoidance and/or removal of the source of the toxin. Information regarding how to contact the poison control center should also be provided.

If ingestion was intentional, a one-on-one sitter while hospitalized should be initiated until further consultation with psychiatry is completed. Evaluation by psychiatry can ensure a safe transition of care to inpatient or outpatient therapy.

The physiologic impact of overdose needs further attention prior to discharge. Patients who required prolonged intubation may need physical therapy or a formal swallow evaluation before eating or discharge. Occupational therapy can assess for any cognitive deficits from potential anoxic events. Patients who developed renal failure from acute tubular necrosis may need ongoing hemodialysis and will need a tunneled hemodialysis line placed prior to discharge and will need follow-up with nephrology after discharge.

Key components of transitional care must be addressed including a complete and accurate discharge summary with diagnoses, testing completed and results, new medication/changes to medication, and follow-up appointments.

CLINICAL PEARLS

- Consult a medical toxicologist or poison control center when overdose/poisoning is suspected.
- On admission, any acetaminophen level above 0 mcg/L should be repeated in 4 hours to assess for ongoing absorption.
- Toxic alcohol ingestion should be suspected with any anion gap acidosis.
- Antiarrhythmic overdose/toxicity requires continuous telemetry monitoring.
- SSRIs should not be prescribed with linezolid to avoid the risk of serotonin syndrome.
- Synthetic cannabinoids (SC) often do not appear on drug of abuse screens.
- Carboxyhemoglobin levels should be obtained on any victim of a structure fire or anyone found down in an enclosed space with a combustion engine running.
- Cholinergic overdose/toxicity is treated with atropine or pralidoxime.
- Hallucinogens rarely require hospital admission.
- Death due to inhalants is most commonly attributed to asphyxiation or suffocation, aspiration of vomitus.
- Perform an SBIRT with every opioid overdose.
- Lithium level are not commonly elevated with chronic toxicity.
- The effectiveness of activated charcoal is beneficial when used within 2 hours of ingestion.
- Patients who are coprescribed benzodiazepines and opioids should have a prescription for naloxone.
- Benzothiazines are the mainstay of treatment for overdose with stimulants.

KEY TAKEAWAYS

- Identification of common toxidromes will aid in diagnosing the overdose/toxicity.
- Coingestion must always be suspected.
- Acute on chronic overdose/toxicity is common among acetaminophen, aspirin and lithium.
- Patients who are coprescribed benzodiazepines and opioids should have a prescription for naloxone.
- Determining whether the overdose/toxicity was intentional or accidental will impact disposition.
- NAC infusion is the preferred treatment for acetaminophen toxicity.
- Respiratory failure and acute kidney injury are the two most common complications of overdose.
- Consultation with a medical toxicologist or poison control center is highly recommended.

EVIDENCE-BASED RESOURCES

Erowid www.erowid.org
American College of Medical Toxicology www.acmt.net
American Academy of Clinical Toxicology www.clintox.org

American Association of Poison Control Centers www.aapcc.org
The Poison Review www.thepoisonreview.com
Poison Control National Capitol Poison Center www.poison.org/
Drug Enforcement Agency DEA.gov

A robust set of instructor resources designed to supplement this text is located at **http://connect.springerpub.com/content/reference-book/978-0-8261-6079-9.** Qualifying instructors may request access by emailing **textbook@springerpub.com.**

REFERENCES

Full list of references can be accessed at http://connect.springerpub.com/content/reference-book/978-0-8261-6079-9.

CHAPTER 23

SOLID ORGAN TRANSPLANTATION

Terri L. Allison and Deborah Ann Hoch

LEARNING OBJECTIVES

- Relate principles of immunology and histocompatibility to transplantation.
- Discuss the role of immunosuppression in preventing rejection.
- Describe the transplant evaluation process and candidate selection.
- Apply transplantation concepts to different types of organ transplants.
- Describe identification and management of transplant-related adverse events and complications.
- Discuss ethical and psychosocial implications of transplantation.
- Integrate solid organ transplant care into adult-gerontology acute care nurse practitioner (AGACNP) practice.
- Describe the importance of a multidisciplinary team approach in transplantation and the contribution of nurse practitioners to patient care.

INTRODUCTION

Solid organ transplantation is a life-saving treatment option for individuals with end-stage organ disease of the heart, lung, liver, pancreas, or kidney; however, care of the transplant patient population is medically complex. The AGACNP must be well-versed in understanding immunology and histocompatibility, immunosuppression, and transplant pharmacology, and must comprehend surveillance strategies to identify myriad posttransplant conditions and complications and apply appropriate management approaches. To optimize transplant outcomes, careful evaluation of potential recipients and donors—whether deceased or living—is essential to ensure the recipient is an acceptable transplant candidate and the donor's organs are suitable for transplantation. To enhance transplantation success, ethical principles and psychosocial implications must also be considered. This chapter presents concepts related to the care of the solid organ transplant recipient.

IMMUNOLOGY AND HISTOCOMPATIBILITY

The immune system is the body's defense against invading pathogens that cause disease. The primary role of the immune system defense mechanisms is to recognize self from nonself, to differentiate between the body's own cells and those that are foreign (Male et al., 2020). Antigens are substances that elicit an immune response and are found on all living cells. Transplanted organs are human but immunologically different from the organ recipient and are therefore perceived by the recipient's immune system as foreigner nonself. A transplanted organ is a nonself-antigen, called an allograft, that can stimulate immune responses in the recipient (Table 23.1). If the immune response is left unchecked, destruction of the allograft and potential death of the recipient can result (Mannon, 2020).

COMPONENTS OF THE IMMUNE SYSTEM

Immune responses involve multiple cell types and complex mechanisms associated with the innate and adaptive immune systems (Male et al., 2020). The innate immune response is nonspecific and is originated by macrophages, neutrophils, and dendritic cells. The adaptive immune response depends on T and B cell lymphocytes (also called T and B cells) and is initiated with recognition of the transplanted organ as nonself by the

TABLE 23.1: Classification of Transplant Grafts: Donor/Recipient Genetic Relationship

TRANSPLANT TYPE	DONOR/RECIPIENT
Autograft	Same individual
Isograft or syngeneic graft	Identical twins
Allograft	Same species, nonidentical individuals
Xenograft	Different species (e.g., pig to human)

Source: Data from Mathias, C. B., & McAleer, J. P. (2020). Transplantation: Immunologic principles and pharmacologic agents. In C. Mathias, J. McAleer, & D. Szollosi (Eds.), *Pharmacology of immunotherapeutic drugs*. Springer Publishing Company. https://doi-org.proxy.library.vanderbilt.edu/10.1007/978-3-030-19922-7_8

cells of the innate immune system (Male et al., 2020). The adaptive immune system is comprised of the cellular and humoral immune systems. The cells of the adaptive immune system respond to a specific antigen, such as an allograft, and confers both specificity and immunity to the antigen.

The process of immunity includes recognition, activation, and response to activation. Initially, the innate immune system cells (macrophages, dendritic cells) recognize an antigen (e.g., a transplanted organ). These cells process the antigen and present the antigen particles to the cells of the adaptive immune system. T and B lymphocytes become activated to propel the cellular and humoral immune responses. The cellular and humoral immune events occur to destroy the antigen, memory cells develop to confer lifelong immunity to the antigen. While these immune responses are essential to protect the body from pathogens and disease, the effects become problematic in the solid organ transplant recipient, and without immune system modulation, the allograft will be destroyed (Lo & Kirk, 2015).

The Innate Immune System

The innate immune cells important to solid organ transplantation are the monocytes, macrophages, and dendritic cells. Neutrophils, a type of granulocyte, are also responsible for innate immune responses (Lees et al., 2016). Monocytes circulate in the blood and migrate into the tissue to become macrophages upon recognition of an antigen, in this case the allograft. Macrophages, dendritic cells, and neutrophils, known as antigen presenting cells (APCs) have phagocytic properties whereby they ingest and process the allograft antigen (alloantigen) for presentation and recognition by the T lymphocytes; thus, APCs are the link between the innate and adaptive immune systems (Lees et al., 2016). Presentation of the alloantigens by the APCs initiates allograft rejection processes.

The Adaptive Immune System

Recognition of the antigen by T lymphocytes is the primary event that initiates the adaptive immune response and is an important step that requires interaction between receptors on the T cells and fragments, or peptides, from the antigen (i.e., allograft; Maltzman et al., 2015). Once activated, the T lymphocytes become cytotoxic to destroy the transplanted organ and stimulate the B lymphocyte response to create antibodies against the antigen. High level specificity and memory are the primary features associated with the T and B lymphocyte responses (Male et al., 2020). Specificity refers to the ability of an immune cell to recognize and respond to a particular antigen. Once stimulated, T and B cells remember the antigen upon subsequent exposure and mount a response to destroy the allograft. In transplantation, the solid organ recipient is chronically exposed to the organ and the immune system perceives the allograft as

nonself and will destroy the organ if the immune responses are not modulated (Lo & Kirk, 2015).

Cellular Immune Response: Types of T Lymphocytes

The cellular immune response is T lymphocyte- mediated. Upon exposure and processing of the alloantigen by the APCs, the activated T cells differentiate into CD8, cytotoxic T lymphocytes and CD4, helper T lymphocytes. Cytotoxic lymphocytes (CD8) induce cytolysis of the allograft cells and destroy the organ (Maltzman et al., 2015). Helper T cells express CD4 and promote CD8 T-cell activities and produce cytokines and chemokines, particularly interleukins, that attract macrophages to destroy the organ and activate B-cells to proliferate and produce antibodies. Memory T cells can mount a rapid secondary response to the allograft and cause more repeated and severe rejection episodes that are less responsive to traditional immunosuppression and thus more difficult to treat (Lo & Kirk, 2015).

Humoral Immune Response: Types of B Lymphocytes

The humoral immune response is mediated by the B lymphocytes which induce humoral allograft rejection, called antibody-mediated rejection (AMR), and is associated with chronic rejection (Lo & Kirk, 2015). AMR is generally resistant to common immunosuppressants and can be predictive of worse posttransplant outcomes. Similar to the cellular immune response, upon activation the B cells expand in numbers and differentiate into plasma cells that generate (a) immunoglobulins (antibodies) to destroy the allograft and (b) memory B cells that circulate in the blood for long periods and have a response time of 3 to 5 days upon subsequent allograft recognition (Lo & Kirk, 2015). The immunoglobulins generated, called donor-specific antibodies (DSAs), are specific to the allograft. Additionally, B lymphocytes have antigen-presenting capabilities and can participate in stimulation of the T-cell response.

Mediators of the Immune Response

APCs release cytokines, particularly interleukin-1 (IL-1), to activate T-lymphocyte differentiation (Su et al., 2015). Interleukin-2 (IL-2) is produced by activated CD4 helper T cells and promotes proliferation of CD4 and CD8 T cells. Cytokines are also involved in production of acute phase proteins, including complement. Complement is a proteolytic enzyme causing cell lysis, destroying the allograft directly (Su et al., 2015).

Summary

Lymphocytes are continuously circulating throughout the tissues and body fluids, as are antigens from the allograft. B lymphocytes are found in the body fluids whereas T lymphocytes are located in the tissues. The alloantigen is recognized and processed by the APCs and presented to the T lymphocytes. In turn, the T lymphocytes are activated, differentiate to CD4 and CD8, and proliferate to destroy the allograft. T lymphocytes also stimulate the release of complement and other effector mechanisms, such as cytokines, that are cytotoxic to the graft. The B lymphocytes differentiate into plasma cells that secrete immunoglobulins, antibodies against the organ. Memory T and B lymphocytes proliferate and remember the allograft upon repeated exposure and are a significant barrier to the recipient's development of tolerance to the allograft (Lo & Kirk, 2015). Differentiation and proliferation of the different types of T and B cells and initiation of their respective functions require approximately 7 to 10 days, creating a delay in the adaptive immune responses (Figure 23.1; Murphy & Weaver, 2017). Graft loss in a solid organ recipient will occur in about 2 weeks if these immune responses are not tempered with immunosuppressant medications.

HISTOCOMPATIBILITY

Major Histocompatibility Complex

All animals express individually unique antigens, or genes, on their cell surfaces. This genetic identity of a species is called the major histocompatibility complex (MHC). In humans, the MHC is labeled human leukocyte antigen (HLA) and determines the inherited genetic identity of an individual (Rajalingham et al., 2015). The deoxyribonucleic acid (DNA) within each cell determines the HLA antigens that are expressed on the outer surface of the body's cells. The HLA is highly polymorphic and is what is used to match organs and tissues in transplantation and controls the acceptance or rejection of a transplanted organ. This polymorphism

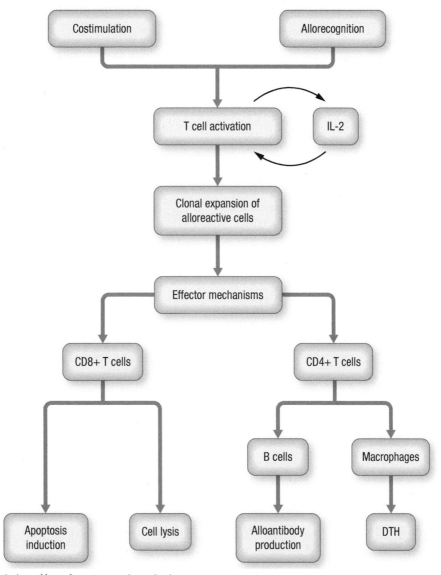

FIGURE 23.1: Differentiation of lymphocytes causing rejection.

is what creates genetic mismatch between donors and recipients (Rajalingham et al., 2015). An organ transplanted between genetically identical persons is recognized as self and accepted by the recipient's immune system. However, an organ from an HLA-mismatched donor is genetically different from the recipient (nonself) and will be destroyed by the recipient immune system without immune modulation. The HLA generates the signaling between the APCs and the lymphocytes. The APC processes and presents the donor HLA (nonself-antigens) to the recipient's T lymphocytes to activate the immune response against the donor organ. The donor's histocompatibility antigens are targets of the recipient's immune responses that cause allograft rejection.

HLA consists of two types of MHC molecules, or proteins. The proteins in the two types are recognized by different functional classes of T lymphocytes; the most important distinction is the source of the peptide fragments processed from the antigen (Table 23.2). Class I MHC molecules are expressed on most nucleated cells and displayed as peptide fragments from cells that are recognized by CD8, cytotoxic, T cells. The recipient's immune response upon recognition of Class I donor MHC mediates cellular rejection. Class II MHC molecules are found on B lymphocytes, dendritic cells and macrophages and are recognized by CD4, helper, T cells. Class II MHC molecules mediate humoral rejection. Expression of MHC Class I and Class II molecules on the body's cell surfaces is regulated by cytokines, interferon in particular. Interferon-2 (IL-2) facilitates T-lymphocyte proliferation to increase the number of sensitized cytotoxic T cells to attack the allograft; whereas IL-6 promotes T and B lymphocyte growth and differentiation into their different functional classes (Su et al., 2015).

TRANSPLANT PHARMACOLOGY

In the mid-20th century, Sir Peter Medawar was awarded the 1960 Nobel Prize in Physiology jointly with Sir Macfarlane Burnet for their "discovery of acquired immunological tolerance" (Ortega, 2012). The researchers presented evidence that rejection of transplanted organs by the recipient was mediated by an immunological response, which could be modified (Ortega, 2012). Since that time, novel immunosuppressive drugs have been developed to block the transplant recipient's reactivity to an allograft, while targeting specific areas of the immune activation pathway. Induction and maintenance therapy are initiated in the pre- and perioperative period and continued for the life of the allograft. Management of immunosuppression requires a balance between sufficient immunosuppression to prevent rejection and sufficient immunity to minimize the opportunity for infection.

The goal of immunotherapy is to block the recipient's immune system from recognizing the allograft as "nonself," leading to rejection. Prior to the early 1980s, immunosuppression was nonspecific and consisted of corticosteroids, the antimetabolite azathioprine, and sometimes total body irradiation. Transplantation became more successful with the advent of cyclosporine, a specific T-cell inhibitor. Three immunosuppressive strategies are utilized in transplantation to modulate the immune system (Table 23.3) and are comprised of induction (high-dose suppression at time of surgery), maintenance therapy (combination of medications for the life of the allograft), and rejection rescue therapy (therapy at time of rejection; Karam & Wali, 2015; Lopez-Larrea & Ortega, 2009).

TABLE 23.2: Relationship of HLA and Allograft Rejection

MHC CLASS	CLASS I	CLASS II
Distribution	Nucleated cells (most body cells) Platelets	Antigen-presenting cells B lymphocytes
Peptide origin	Endogenous, intracellular proteins	Exogenous, extracellular proteins (e.g., blood)
MHC restriction	Seen by cytotoxic T lymphocytes (CD8)	Seen by helper T lymphocytes (CD4)
Rejection type	Cellular	Humoral

Source: Data from Abbes, S., Metjian, A., Gray, A., Martinu, T., Snyder, L., Chen, D. F., Ellis, M., Arepally, G. M., & Onwuemene, O. (2017). Human leukocyte antigen sensitization in solid organ transplantation: A primer on terminology, testing, and clinical significance for the apheresis practitioner. *Therapeutic Apheresis and Dialysis, 21*(5), 441–450. https://doi.org/10.1111/1744-9987.12570; Rajalingham, R., Zhang, Q., Cecka, J. M., & Reed, E. F. (2015). Major histocompatibility complex. In X. C. Li & A. M. Jevnikar (Eds.), *Transplant immunology.* Wiley Blackwell. ProQuest Ebook Central. https://ebookcentral.proquest.com

TABLE 23.3: Definitions of Immunosuppression Strategies

IMMUNOSUPPRESSION STRATEGY	DESCRIPTION
Induction therapy	Pre- and perioperative high dose-immunosuppression at time of transplant surgery
Maintenance therapy	Combination immunosuppression given for life of graft or patient
Rescue therapy	Immunosuppression administered for treatment of rejection

Source: Data from Lake, D. F., & Briggs, A. D. (2017). Immunopharmacology. In B. G. Katzung (Ed.), *Basic and clinical pharmacology* (14th ed.). McGraw-Hill. https://accessmedicine-mhmedical-com.proxy.library.vanderbilt.edu/content.aspx?bookid=2249&sectionid=175224717; Lopez-Larrea, C., & Ortega, F. (2009). Advances in translational transplant immunology. *Transplantation, 88*(3 Suppl), S1–S7. https://doi.org/10.1097/TP.0b013e3181af6473

OVERVIEW OF IMMUNOSUPPRESSIVE AGENTS

The risk of allograft rejection is greatest in the first 6 months following transplantation (Lo & Kirk, 2015); therefore, immunosuppression is maximized during this early period as acute rejection is associated with long-term allograft dysfunction. The further a recipient is from the date of transplant the lower the risk of rejection; however, rejection is always a possibility and immunosuppression is required for the life of the organ and/or recipient. Most transplant centers follow established immunosuppression administration protocols for induction, maintenance, and rescue therapy.

INDUCTION THERAPY

Induction therapy is intense immunosuppression administered at the time of transplant to suppress the immune system and allows a bridge to maintenance immunosuppression (Chouhan & Zhang, 2012; Hricik, 2015). Induction therapy, in combination with maintenance immunosuppression of calcineurin inhibitors (CNIs), mycophenolate acid formulations, and steroids have been shown to reduce the rate of rejection and improve graft and patient survival (Paliege et al., 1994). Use of induction agents can be associated with serious adverse effects such as increased incidence of infections, malignancy, drug toxicity, and cardiovascular burden (Hill et al., 2017; Paliege et al., 1994). The induction agents available are either monoclonal or polyclonal antibodies that deplete expansion of activated T lymphocytes.

Polyclonal Antibodies

Polyclonal antibodies are denoted by their source and include rabbit antithymocyte globulin (R-ATG) and equine antithymocyte globulin (E-ATG; Hardinger, 2006). R-ATG is more effective in preventing acute rejection compared to E-ATG and is the most utilized polyclonal agent in transplantation (Cai & Terasaki, 2011).

R-ATG is a T lymphocyte depleting polyclonal antibody used for induction as well as treatment of acute cellular rejection (ACR). Dosing is 1.5 to 3 mg/kg/day administered IV over 8 hours. Duration of therapy varies for induction and acute rejection (Brennan et al., 2006). Premedication with diphenhydramine, corticosteroids, and acetaminophen is required to reduce cytokine release-associated effects. Adverse reactions include cytokine release syndrome and symptoms, serum sickness, thrombocytopenia, leukopenia, anaphylaxis, infections, and posttransplant lymphoproliferative disease. Reduction in all cell lines may be evident on a complete blood count (CBC). More serious reactions are usually seen with the first dose and with rapid infusion rates. Recipients treated with R-ATG can develop antibodies to the agent, decreasing effectiveness with repeat administration.

Monoclonal Antibodies

Monoclonal antibody agents include alemtuzumab, basiliximab, rituximab, and eculizumab.

Alemtuzumab is a CD52-specific monoclonal antibody that causes profound and sustained lymphocyte depletion. Alemtuzumab induction lowers the risk of biopsy-proven AMR compared with induction with basiliximab (Morgan et al., 2012). Premedication with methylprednisolone, diphenhydramine, and acetaminophen are necessary to reduce the cytokine release effects. Alemtuzumab may be given in two to four divided doses. CBCs are monitored for leukopenia.

Basiliximab immunosuppressive potency is related to the capacity to produce complete binding of the IL-2 receptor sites on T cells. Two IV doses are given, one preoperatively and the second on postoperative day four. Premedication is not necessary. Basiliximab is well tolerated, and side effects are usually minimal; however, anaphylaxis or first dose reactions are occasionally described (Henry & Rajab, 2002).

Rituximab is a monoclonal antibody that targets CD20, resulting in B cell depletion. Rituximab has been used off label for induction and rescue therapy as well as to reduce high levels of preformed anti-HLA antibodies prior to transplantation in a sensitized candidate and to treat posttransplantation lymphoproliferative disease (Herrero & Panizo, 2018; van den Hoogen et al., 2015). Side effects include transient hypotension during infusion, neutropenia, and thrombocytopenia (Wolach et al., 2012). Premedication with acetaminophen and diphenhydramine is recommended.

Eculizumab is a monoclonal antibody used as an induction agent and as a treatment option for postrenal transplant recipients with acute hemolytic uremic syndrome. Common adverse effects include hypertension, diarrhea, headache, anemia, vomiting, nausea, leukopenia, upper respiratory and urinary tract infections, and viral infections (Barnett et al., 2013). *Neisseria meningitides* infection is a life-threatening complication in patients treated with eculizumab; therefore, vaccination against *N. meningitides* before eculizumab administration is strongly recommended (Barnett et al., 2013). Eculizumab is one of the most expensive therapies in the world (approximately $500,000 per patient per year); therefore, insurance authorization prior to treatment with eculizumab is imperative.

MAINTENANCE THERAPY

Maintenance immunosuppression is a multidrug approach with agents that have differing mechanisms so that lower doses of each can be administered to reduce side effects and adverse reactions. Maintenance therapy usually consists of three classes of drugs to include a corticosteroid, a CNI, and an antimetabolite. Therapeutic doses are initially high following transplantation and reduced over time as the likelihood for rejection decreases.

Calcineurin Inhibitors

CNIs are a class of drugs consisting of tacrolimus and cyclosporine that inhibit T lymphocytes (Mueller, 2004). The bioavailability of both drugs is variable and decreased with food. Dosing is twice daily, generally 12 hours apart and the metabolism is through cytochrome P450 3A4 (CYP3A4) and P-glycoprotein. The metabolism is important, as many drugs compete for the CYP 3A4 site, which can affect absorption of these medications (Table 23.4). CNIs have a narrow therapeutic window and 11- to 12-hour trough drug levels are monitored. Suboptimal levels expose patients to rejection and elevated levels can cause neurotoxicity and acute kidney injury. Target drug levels of both cyclosporine and tacrolimus are higher in the early weeks following transplantation and reduced over time as long as the recipient is less likely to have rejection. The CNIs cause renal vasoconstriction and sodium retention and can contribute to hypertension and nephrotoxicity. Gastrointestinal side effects include anorexia, nausea, vomiting, diarrhea, and abdominal discomfort, though these symptoms are more common with tacrolimus. Cyclosporine causes cosmetic side effects including gingival hyperplasia and hirsutism (Thervet et al., 2011). Neurotoxicity may manifest as mild tremor, headache, visual disturbances, and seizures. Common metabolic abnormalities include glucose intolerance, hyperkalemia, hypomagnesemia, and hyperuricemia.

Cyclosporine

There are two formulations of cyclosporine: cyclosporine (Sandimmune) and cyclosporine modified (Neoral, generics). Bioavailability of the two formulations are different, and therefore not interchangeable. Transitioning from one oral formulation to the other requires close monitoring of trough levels. Oral cyclosporine is administered at a consistent time twice daily. If a dose is missed, patients should take cyclosporine as soon as possible and not double the next dose. Dose adjustments are made based on the goal trough levels which are center and organ specific (Gibardi & Tichy, 2012). Optimal dosing and concentrations may be affected by many factors, including pharmacokinetics, underlying infection, drug toxicity and/or rejection. IV cyclosporine is available when patients are not able to take the oral form.

Tacrolimus

Tacrolimus, approved by the Food and Drug Administration (FDA) in 1994, is more potent than cyclosporine and is the preferred agent in most transplant programs. Two extended-release tacrolimus preparations are available with different pharmacokinetics and bioavailability so the formulations are not interchangeable (Tremblay et al., 2017).

Antimetabolite Therapy

Azathioprine (AZA), mycophenolate mofetil (MMF) and mycophenolate sodium (MPA, enteric-coated) are antimetabolites that interrupt the DNA synthesis phase of lymphocyte proliferation (Hui et al., 2014).

Azathioprine

Azathioprine results in the inhibition of DNA, RNA, and protein synthesis in the bone marrow. Leukocytopenia, anemia, and thrombocytopenia are common; therefore, the CBC/differential and platelets should be monitored. Side effects include alopecia, gastrointestinal distress, pancreatitis, and hepatotoxicity, and is more frequently implicated in the increased incidence of skin cancer posttransplant (Holt, 2017).

Mycophenolate

Mycophenolate (either MMF or MPA) has largely replaced AZA as a first-line maintenance antimetabolite in solid organ transplantation (Bardsley-Elliot et al., 1999). Adverse gastrointestinal symptoms (nausea, vomiting, diarrhea) usually elicit a temporary dose reduction in mycophenolate, which can lead to rejection and possibly graft loss (McAdams-DeMarco et al., 2015). The enteric-coated formulation of mycophenolate may be better tolerated. Mycophenolate is given twice daily and dosing targets are dependent on formulation (Langone et al., 2014). Mycophenolate is available for IV administration, and is cytostatic to T and B lymphocytes, and requires frequent CBC monitoring. Mycophenolate carries a boxed warning for embryofetal toxicity and is associated with increased risks of first trimester pregnancy loss and congenital malformations (FDA, 2012). Women of childbearing age must be counseled regarding pregnancy prevention and planning. An FDA-approved patient medication guide,

TABLE 23.4: Dose Conversion Oral to IV Immunosuppression

MEDICATION	ORAL TO IV CONVERSION	NOTES
Cyclosporine	IV 1/3 of oral dose, continuous infusion every 12 hours	Obtain 12-hour trough levels
Tacrolimus	IV 1/3 of oral dose, continuous infusion every 12 hours	IV form can cause anaphylaxis; avoid if possible (e.g., substitute cyclosporine)
Azathioprine	Oral to IV conversion 1:1	
Mycophenolate mofetil	1 g every 12 hours	No IV form for mycophenolate sodium available
Sirolimus		No IV form available

which is available with the product information, must be dispensed with this medication:

- Mycophenolate sodium (Myfortic): https://www .accessdata.fda.gov/drugsatfda_docs/label/2020/ 050791s030lbl.pdf#page=24
- Mycophenolate mofetil (CellCept): https://www .accessdata.fda.gov/drugsatfda_docs/label/2019/05 0722s040,050723s041,050758s037,050759s045lbl .pdf#page=38

Steroid Therapy

Corticosteroids are the cornerstone of maintenance immunosuppressive therapy in solid organ transplantation since they were first used to treat rejection in the 1960s. Steroids block T and B lymphocytes and cytokines (Alloway et al., 2003). Methylprednisolone is administered preoperatively and transitioned to prednisone when oral administration is tolerated. Dosing of corticosteroids varies with type of organ transplant and with transplant center protocols; however, on average, oral prednisone is given at 0.8 to 1 mg/kg/day once daily or in divided doses. Steroids are tapered over weeks or months to a minimal dose or discontinued altogether to mitigate the many side effects of long-term steroid therapy.

REJECTION RESCUE THERAPY

Biopsy-proven acute rejection is treated with high dose oral or IV steroids initially, with the cumulative dosage depending on type and severity of rejection and amount of allograft dysfunction. At times, the addition of a polyclonal antibody (ATG) is added if biopsy pathology is severe. AMR may be treated with rituximab. Basiliximab and alemtuzumab are not used for rescue therapy (Box 23.1).

Rapamycin Inhibitor Therapy

The use of mammalian target of rapamycin (mTOR) inhibitor therapy includes sirolimus or everolimus. These agents are not first-line immunosuppression; rather, they are adjuncts or substitutes in the maintenance immunosuppression regimen. Indications for use are intolerance to CNIs, recurrent rejection, or development of allograft vasculopathy. The mTOR drug class has a long halflife so drug levels should be checked several days

after initiation or a dose adjustment. Potential adverse effects of mToR inhibitors include proteinuria, hyperlipidemia including elevated triglycerides, and impaired wound healing (Asleh et al., 2020; Hays et al., 2015). The mTOR inhibitor must be temporarily discontinued and another agent begun prior to surgery to avoid wound dehiscence and poor healing.

Belatacept

Belatacept is an IV costimulatory inhibitor designed to provide effective immunosuppression while avoiding the toxicity associated with CNIs, such as nephrotoxicity, neurotoxicity, metabolic disorders, and cosmetic effects (Martin et al., 2011). Belatacept is a maintenance agent given initially as loading doses and then every 4 weeks thereafter. Administration of belatacept improves patient adherence by eliminating the need for twice daily CNI dosing. Belatacept cannot be administered to Epstein-Barr virus (EBV) seronegative recipients due to the increased risk of posttransplant lymphoproliferative disease. Belatacept is only indicated in kidney transplant recipients and is used off-label in lung transplantation. The agent is not recommended in liver transplant patients due to increased risk of graft loss and death (Klintmalm et al., 2014).

SUMMARY

The success of organ transplantation is possible due to the availability of effective immunosuppressive agents that modulate the recipient's immune response to the allograft (Box 23.2). The combination of immunosuppressive protocols has significantly reduced the incidence of acute organ rejection. Induction therapy is used in the majority of solid organ transplants. Most maintenance immunosuppressive protocols use a combination of a CNI (e.g., tacrolimus), an antimetabolite (e.g., mycophenolate), and corticosteroid therapy. The mTOR inhibitors were originally introduced to complement cyclosporine therapy, but because of the adverse event profiles, they

BOX 23.1 TREATMENT OF REJECTION

- Pulse steroids may exacerbate hyperglycemia.
- High dose steroids will elevate WBC count in absence of infection.
- Resume infection prophylaxis and gastrointestinal protection while on high-dose steroids.
- The first one to three doses of polyclonal antibody require ICU unit admission due to risk of anaphylaxis and cytokine release syndrome.

BOX 23.2 MANAGEMENT OF IMMUNOSUPPRESSION

- Adjust CNI dosing to achieve goal therapeutic trough level.
- Cyclosporine has two formulations that are NOT interchangeable.
- Administer twice daily immunosuppression every 12 hours.
- Consider potential food and drug interactions with immunosuppressants before prescribing new medications.
- Preferred maintenance immunosuppression combination in most transplants: tacrolimus, mycophenolate, corticosteroids.

are no longer considered a first-line maintenance immunosuppressive agent. Belatacept is currently being used in some settings to replace and minimize the long-term nephrotoxic effects CNIs. Successful posttransplant outcomes are dependent on patient adherence to the medication regimen, in which the AGACNP plays a key role (Karam & Wali, 2015).

EVALUATION OF TRANSPLANT CANDIDATES AND DONORS

Individuals with end-organ disease require timely referral to a transplant center to evaluate for risk stratification and determine candidacy for transplantation. The wait for an organ can be lengthy; therefore, evidence-based management of the patient's disease process and comorbidities while awaiting transplantation is essential. All potential transplant donors undergo evaluation to assess if they meet organ donation criteria. Living donors are evaluated at the transplant candidate's transplant center. Deceased donors are evaluated by an organ procurement organization (OPO) at the donor's location.

TRANSPLANT CANDIDATE EVALUATION

Evaluation of individuals referred for solid organ transplantation is a dynamic process that considers candidate selection criteria against transplant outcomes, including quality of life, life expectancy, and risk (Kazi et al., 2018; Kriss & Biggins, 2021). The purpose of the transplant evaluation is to ensure the candidate meets physiologic criteria for transplantation; that is, the end-organ disease is amenable to transplantation and the comorbid conditions that can compromise successful outcome are absent or manageable. Additionally, psychosocial evaluation is essential to assess the candidate's ability to adhere to the posttransplant regimen, identify availability of psychosocial support to assist the patient throughout the transplantation process, and determine available financial resources (Flattery & Gierlach, 2016). The transplant evaluation process includes extensive education of the patient, family, and support system to ensure the patient makes an informed decision about pursuing transplantation (Flattery & Gierlach, 2016).

Timing of transplant referral should occur early enough in the individual's disease process so that transplantation remains a treatment option before the patient develops comorbid conditions contradictory to transplantation or the person becomes too ill due to end-organ disease to undergo transplantation.

Posttransplant care is medically complex, can be psychosocially demanding, and requires patient adherence to the prescribed regimen for a successful outcome. Patients referred for evaluation undergo a myriad of tests and multidisciplinary consultations (Flattery & Gierlach, 2016). Many laboratory and medical tests are common among all organs and others are specific to the organ being transplanted or the patient's history and comorbidities.

Medical Testing

Conventional labs performed to assess physiologic status include a comprehensive metabolic panel incorporating liver function tests (LFTs) and estimated glomerular filtration rate (excluding kidney candidates), lipid profile, CBC with differential, thyroid panel, urinalysis, rapid plasma reagin (RPR), stool for occult blood, and coagulation studies to include prothrombin time, partial thromboplastin time, and international normalized ratio. Prostate-specific antigen is measured in men >age 50, beta human chorionic gonadotropin in women of childbearing age, and hemoglobin A1C in patients with diabetes mellitus.

Transplant-Specific Laboratory Testing

Transplant-specific laboratory testing is performed to delineate immunologic characteristics of the candidate, assess potential posttransplant infection risk, and identify issues that may impact or preclude listing for transplantation. Prior to wait listing, a transplant candidate's HLA antigens, or genotype, must be identified via DNA analysis (Flattery & Gierlach, 2016). Blood type is confirmed on two occasions from separate blood draws. Successful posttransplant outcome is dependent upon HLA and blood type compatibility between the donor and the recipient.

The panel reactive antibody (PRA) is an immunologic assay that detects the presence of preformed HLA antibodies and determines the degree of a transplant candidate's sensitization. The candidate's serum is mixed with a panel of lymphocytes from potential donors and the result reported as a percentage of the panel with which the candidate's serum reacts (Abbes et al., 2017, Flattery & Gierlach, 2016). Sensitizing events include pregnancy, blood transfusions, prior organ transplantation, and ventricular assist device implantation (Abbes et al., 2017). Preformed HLA antibodies can be a significant barrier to transplantation, causing delays in finding a suitable donor. The higher the PRA percentage, the more likely a transplant recipient is to react to the donor organ. The antigens to which the candidate has developed preformed antibodies are identified and documented when an individual is put on the transplant wait list. When an organ becomes available, a donor with these unacceptable HLA antigens will not be offered to the sensitized recipient. The calculated PRA (cPRA) is an algorithm that uses the kidney, pancreas, or kidney/pancreas candidate's unacceptable antigens to estimate the compatibility of potential donors with the candidate (United Network for Organ Sharing [UNOS], 2020). Highly sensitized individuals may require desensitization while on the transplant waitlist to decrease the burden of circulating anti-HLA antibodies (Box 23.3).

BOX 23.3 TRANSPLANT CANDIDATE SENSITIZATION

- Avoid blood product administration in listed transplant candidates, if possible.
- Use leukocyte-poor filter if blood product administration necessary.
- Repeat PRA 4–6 weeks after any sensitizing event.

Desensitization protocols are center-specific but may include administration of chemotherapy agents such as rituximab or bortezomib, intravenous immunoglobulin (IVIG), and/or plasmapheresis (Abbes et al., 2017; Halloran et al., 2015).

A crossmatch between donor and recipient sera is performed when a potential donor is matched with a candidate. A positive crossmatch indicates HLA incompatibility between the donor and recipient, placing the recipient at higher risk of rejection (Mustian & Locke, 2020). Prospective crossmatches are performed with kidney, pancreas, and kidney/pancreas transplants and when a candidate has a high PRA. A retrospective crossmatch is performed with other organs and candidates with PRA <10%. A virtual crossmatch can be accomplished without actual mixing of donor and recipient sera by matching the candidate's known HLA preformed antibodies against the HLA antigens of the potential donor (Abbes et al., 2017). Recipients transplanted despite a positive crossmatch with a donor organ may undergo a desensitization protocol posttransplant to reduce the incidence of rejection. They are, however, at a higher risk for infection or malignancy (Halloran et al., 2015). Additional transplant-specific labs are found in Table 23.5.

Diagnostic Testing

Evaluation of the candidate's end-organ disease is undertaken to determine if the potential candidate will benefit from transplantation and to consider therapies to support remaining organ function while the candidate is on the waitlist. Various tests are performed to screen for cancer based on the candidate's past medical history, age, gender, and American Cancer Society Guidelines; osteoporosis due to corticosteroid exposure following transplantation; and disease in other organ systems that needs treatment or may preclude transplantation as a treatment option (Tables 23.6 and 23.7).

Contraindications to Transplantation

Evaluation of a transplant candidate considers if the patient meets criteria for transplantation and identifies the presence of absolute or relative contraindications that are weighed against the patient's benefits and risks of undergoing transplantation. Absolute contraindications are problems that preclude transplant. Relative contra-

TABLE 23.5: Food and Drug Interactions With CNIs and mTOR Inhibitors

SUBSTRATES[a]	INDUCERS[b]	INHIBITORS[c]
Amiodarone	Phenytoin, carbamazepine, phenobarbital	Macrolide antibiotics
Statins	Rifampin	Azole antifungals
Dapsone	St. John's wort	Diltiazem, verapamil
Amlodipine, felodipine	Pioglitazone	Antiretroviral protease inhibitors
Clonazepam	Primidone	Conivaptan
Zolpidem	Efavirenz, nevirapine	Cimetidine
Progesterone	Orlistat	Grapefruit juice
Sulfamethoxazole		Nefazodone
Tolvaptan		Nucleoside reverse transcriptase inhibitors
Eplerenone		Hepatitis C virus direct acting antivirals

[a]Substrates compete for metabolism/drug transport; increased concentration of both drugs.

[b]Inducers enhance drug metabolism/drug transport; decreased concentration of immunosuppressant.

[c]Inhibitors decrease drug metabolism/drug transport; increased concentration of immunosuppressant.

CNIs, cyclosporine, tacrolimus; mTOR inhibitors, sirolimus, everolimus.

Source: Data from Correia, M. (2021). Drug biotransformation. In B. G. Katzung & T. W. Vanderah (Eds.), *Basic & clinical pharmacology* (15th ed.). McGraw-Hill. https://accesspharmacy-mhmedical-com.proxy.library.vanderbilt.edu/content.aspx?bookid=2988&sectionid=250594466#250594492; Gibardi, S., & Tichy, E. M. (2012). Overview of immunosuppressive therapies in renal transplantation. In A. Chadrakar, M. H. Sayegh, & A. J. Singh (Eds.), *Core concepts in renal transplantation* (p. 121). Springer Publishing Company; Sparks, T., & Lemonovich, T. (2019). Interactions between anti-infective agents and immunosuppressants-Guidelines from the American Society of Transplant Infectious Diseases Community of Practice. *Clinical Transplantation*, *33*(9), e13510. https://doi-org.proxy.library.vanderbilt.edu/10.1111/ctr.13510

indications are situations whose significance must be considered in the context of the patient's likelihood for successful outcome. Some contraindications are identified as both relative and absolute. Additionally, some contraindications are transplant center or organ-specific (Table 23.8).

DONOR EVALUATION

Solid organ donation occurs when an entire organ or part of an organ is removed from a donor and transplanted into a recipient who meets criteria for transplant. Donors may be deceased or living; organs are matched according to blood group, HLA compatibility (if indicated), body size, severity of candidate medical condition, candidate

TABLE 23.6: Transplant-Specific Laboratory Analysis

TEST	RATIONALE
ABO blood typing	Blood group compatibility required for transplantation Assessment required on two separate occasions Verified by two individuals at listing
Tissue typing/ genotyping (Human leukocyte antigen [HLA])	Identifies genes used to match recipient to donor organ • Required for pretransplant kidney and pancreas recipient:donor matching • Identifies unacceptable donor antigens in sensitized candidate with preformed antibodies
Panel reactive antibody (PRA)	Identifies presence of preformed antibodies against potential donor HLA
Virologies: • Cytomegalovirus • Herpes simplex virus • Varicella-zoster virus • Epstein-Barr virus • Hepatitis B • Hepatitis C • HIV • Toxoplasmosis	• Medical suitability and posttransplant infection risk • Infection can recur in antibody-positive recipient and may require infection prophylaxis following transplant • Antibody-positive donor can transmit viruses to antibody-negative recipients causing de novo disease, contributing to recipient morbidity
C-peptide, glycosylated hemoglobin (HbA1C)	Assess glucose control
Parathyroid hormone	Assess metabolic bone disease risk
Drug/alcohol screen	Assess use/abuse
Urine or serum cotinine	Assess tobacco use

TABLE 23.7: Diagnostic Testing

SCREENING DIAGNOSTIC TESTS	RATIONALE
Abdominal ultrasound	Liver, pancreas, gallbladder, kidney evaluation
Bone densitometry (DEXA)	Osteoporosis screening. Corticosteroids contribute to bone loss
Chest radiograph	Screening for cardiac or pulmonary pathology
Electrocardiogram	Cardiac pathology
Mammogram	Cancer screening, women >age 40
Pap smear	Cancer screening, women >age 21, younger if sexually active
Spirometry or pulmonary function tests	Lung function screening, if indicated; e.g. smoking history

SCREENING DIAGNOSTIC TESTS	RATIONALE
Diagnostic Tests for Indications or Specific Organ Evaluation	Rationale
Cardiac Evaluation • Echocardiogram • Stress testing, exercise or pharmacologic • Left heart catheterization • Right heart catheterization	All patients undergo echocardiogram Other testing as indicated by past medical history and risk factors
Vascular Evaluation • Ankle-brachial Index (ABIs) • Lower extremity Doppler • Peripheral angiography	As indicated by past medical history and risk factors
Colonoscopy or fecal immunochemical test (FIT)	Colon cancer screening age >45
CT of chest, abdomen, pelvis	As indicated by organ, past medical history, and risk factors
Endoscopic retrograde cholangiopancreatography (ERCP)	Liver candidates; suspected biliary duct abnormalities
Liver biopsy	Liver pathology, as indicated
MRI abdomen, heart	Liver: Evaluate blood flow and detection of hepatic iron overload; confirm the presence of vascular lesions (e.g., hemangiomas) Heart: Evaluate cardiac structures and function, coronary artery blood flow, as indicated
Pulmonary function testing	Smoking history
Tuberculosis (TB) testing: PPD, CXR, or QuantiFERON gold	TB screening
Urodynamics study	Evaluate bladder function and capacity in kidney candidates

Source: Data from Flattery, M. P., & Gierlach, J. (2016). Solid organ transplantation: The evaluation process. In S. A. Cupples, S. Kerret, V. McCalmont, & L. Ohler (Eds.), *Core curriculum for transplant nurses* (2nd ed.). Wolters Kluwer; Kazi, S. N., Valsan, D., Schoepe, R., & Superdock, K. (2018). Recipient selection for kidney transplantation. In C. G. B. Ramirez & J. McCauley (Eds.), *Contemporary kidney transplantation* (pp. 25–38). Springer Publishing Company. https://doi.org/10.1007/978-3-319-14779-6_2-1; Kriss, M., & Biggins, S. W. (2021). Evaluation and selection of the liver transplant candidate: Updates on a dynamic and evolving process. *Current Opinions in Organ Transplant, 26*(1), 52–61. https://doi.org/10.1097/MOT.0000000000000829; Smith, R. A., Andrews, K. S., Brooks, D., Fedwa, S. A., Manassaram-Baptiste, D., Saslow, D., & Wender, R. C. (2019). Cancer screening in the United States, 2019: A review of current American Cancer Society guidelines and current issues in cancer screening. *CA: A Cancer Journal for Clinicians, 69*(3), 184–210. https://doi.org/10.3322/caac.21557

wait time, and geographic distance between the donor and candidate (Health Resources and Services Administration [HRSA], 2021, January). Deceased donors are typically matched via the national database of waitlisted candidates based on an organ-specific allocation score.

TABLE 23.8: Absolute and Relative Contraindications to Transplantation

ABSOLUTE	RELATIVE
• Morbid obesity (accepted body mass index [BMI] varies among transplant centers and organ type; generally, BMI 40–45 kg/m^2 or $\geq$ 45 kg/m^2) • Cachexia (BMI <17.5 kg/m^2) • Active systemic infection • Active substance abuse • Active peptic ulcer disease • Psychiatric illness likely to interfere with adherence • Severe uncorrectable cardiac (nonheart candidates) or peripheral vascular disease • Irreversible pulmonary hypertension (heart, heart/lung) • Active malignancy, or within previous 5 years • Poor family/social and/or financial support • Cirrhosis (non-liver candidates) • Nonadherence with current medical regimen • Chronic obstructive pulmonary disease (COPD)/oxygen dependence (nonlung candidates) • Anatomical abnormalities precluding adequate surgical reconstruction or allograft function • Irreversible end-stage organ disease in another organ (other than combined organ transplant) • Uncontrolled HIV or AIDS • Uncorrectable bleeding disorders • Irreversible rehabilitation potential • Current suicidal ideation/multiple suicide attempts/recent suicide attempt, active psychosis or schizophrenia, dementia	• Age >75 (varies by organ and transplant center) • Morbid obesity (accepted body mass index [BMI] varies among transplant center and organ type) • Severe and or symptomatic osteoporosis (compression fracture) • HIV (varies among transplant centers and presence of detectable virus) • Uncontrolled diabetes mellitus • Peripheral vascular disease when presence limits rehabilitation and revascularization not a viable option • Current felony incarceration/history significant criminal behavior • Frailty

Source: Data from Flattery, M. P., & Gierlach, J. (2016). Solid organ transplantation: The evaluation process. In S. A. Cupples, S. Kerret, V. McCalmont, & L. Ohler (Eds.), *Core curriculum for transplant nurses* (2nd ed.). Wolters Kluwer; Wall, A., Lee, G. H., Maldonado, J., & Magnus, D. (2019). Medical contraindications to transplant listing in the USA: A survey of adult and pediatric heart, kidney, liver, and lung programs. *World Journal of Surgery*, 43, 2300–2308. https://doi.org/10.1007/s00268-019-05030-x

Directed donation is allocation of a deceased or living donor organ to a specific candidate named by the person who authorized the donation.

Deceased Donor

The Uniform Determination of Death Act (*Guidelines for the determination of death*, 1981) defines death as "either (1) irreversible cessation of circulatory and respiratory functions, or (2) irreversible cessation of all functions of the entire brain, including the brainstem" established by acceptable medical standards. Organs may be retrieved after declaration of death by neurologic criteria (DDNC) or after circulatory [cardiac] death (DCD).

Definition of Neurologic Death

Imminent neurologic death is defined as the death of a patient who meets both of the following criteria:
1. Meets the eligible death definition with the exception that the patient has not been declared legally dead by neurologic criteria according to current standards of accepted medical practice and state or local law.
2. Has a severe neurologic injury requiring ventilator support who, upon clinical evaluation, has no observed spontaneous breathing and is lacking as least two additional brainstem reflexes.

A patient who is unable to be assessed neurologically due to administration of sedation or hypothermia protocol does not meet the definition of an imminent neurologic death (Aboubakr & Alameda, 2020; Lewis et al., 2020; Organ Procurement and Transplantation Network [OPTN], 2020).

Definition of Donation After Circulatory Death

Donation after circulatory death (DCD) occurs when a decision is made to discontinue mechanical ventilation and other life-sustaining treatments in a critically ill patient who is expected to die quickly after cessation of life support measures. Most OPO have guidelines governing the amount of time between extubation and death; a standard time is 60 minutes. If the patient survives longer than 60 minutes, excessive organ ischemia occurs rendering the patient an unsuitable donor (Lustbader & Goldstein, 2011; UNOS, n.d.).

The practice of DCD considers the quality of end-of-life care for patients and families and includes withdrawal of treatments that are no longer beneficial or that extend suffering. Most patients considered for DCD are in the intensive care unit and ventilator dependent on circulatory support. Quality end-of-life care is a priority and cannot be compromised by the donation process. The decision to forego further life-sustaining therapy is made in accordance with the wishes of the patient and/or identified agent.

Living Donors

The three categories for living organ donation are found in Table 23.9. Living donors are individuals who donate an organ (a kidney, a lung) or part of an organ (lung liver, pancreas, intestine; HRSA, 2021).

Living Donor Paired Donation and Chains

Kidney paired donation (KPD) and living kidney donor chains permit transplantation of candidates who have an identified but incompatible living donor. OPTN policy defines procedures for executing paired donation or donation chains (OPTN, 2021a).

■ **Independent Living Donor Advocate (ILDA):** A person available to assist potential living donors in the living donation process and is a mandated, supportive role in the care of the living organ donor (Hays et al., 2015; OPTN, 2021a).

■ **Kidney Paired Donation (KPD):** Also known as a kidney exchange. This approach is used when candidates with incompatible donors swap donors to receive a blood type or crossmatch compatible kidney. The individuals in each donor/candidate pair enter into a single agreement to donate and receive the kidneys, respectively, according to biological compatibility within the group (Tenenbaum, 2018). KPD may take place within the same transplant center or through a national kidney registry. Patient confidentiality and anonymity are maintained, and many times, the donors will not know each other or the intended recipient.

■ **Living Donor Chains:** A living donor chain is a paired donation where more than two donor/candidate pairs exchange donors to receive a blood type or crossmatch compatible organ. A chain

continues until a living donor donates to an orphan candidate, a wait list candidate, or is a bridge donor (OPTN, 2021a; Tenenbaum, 2018). An orphan candidate is one who does not receive a transplant from a matched donor after the candidate's paired donor has donated. A bridge donor does not have an identified match in the chain and continues to participate in a future chain (OPTN, 2021a).

Donor Evaluation and Organ Eligibility

Each eligible organ must meet certain characteristics prior to donation. If the donor exhibits active infection with a specific diagnosis (e.g., sepsis, COVID-19, tuberculosis), the organ is not acceptable for donation. All donors are screened for infectious disease according to U.S. Public Health Service OPTN Final Rule (Jones et al., 2020).

REGULATION OF CANDIDATE WAIT LISTING AND ORGAN ALLOCATION

To address the nation's shortage of critical lifesaving organs and to improve organ placement and matching, the U.S. Congress passed the National Organ Transplant Act (NOTA:P.L. 98-507) in 1984. This Act established the OPTN to maintain a national registry for organ matching. This Act also required that OPTN be operated by a private, nonprofit organization under federal contract. The UNOS was awarded the initial OPTN contract and continues to administer the OPTN today. UNOS maintains the transplant candidate wait list and is responsible for the fair distribution of organs using a computer rank order algorithm that matches donor and candidate information to allocate organs based on medical urgency, blood group, tissue typing (kidney and pancreas), location of recipient and donor, age, and other organ-specific factors. OPO retrieve organs for transplantation. OPTN, UNOS, and OPOs are subject to federal oversight by the Department of Health and Human Services National Organ Donation Transplantation Program.

Donor Criteria for Donation (Deceased and Living Donors)

1. Blood type must be tested on two separate samples on two separate occasions and submitted separately.
2. The host OPO must accurately document HIV test results for every deceased donor.
3. Blood and urine cultures to rule out infection.
4. Infectious disease testing including HIV (anti-HIV), hepatitis B surface antigen (HBsAg), hepatitis B core antibody (anti HBc), Hepatitis C antibody (anti HCV), hepatitis C RNA or NAT test, cytomegalovirus (CMV) antibody, Epstein-Barr virus, rapid plasma reagin, and toxoplasma immunoglobulin G (IgG) antibody test.
5. Transplant centers may request additional testing based on the organ to be retrieved, the donor's age, and past medical history (OPTN, 2021a).

TABLE 23.9: Categories of Living Donors

Categories	Nondirected Donation (Altruistic)	Paired Donation	Directed Donation
Criteria	The donor is neither related to nor known by the recipient	In kidney transplant only. Can develop into a chain of transplants	Person authorizing donation chooses who will receive the organ
Relationship to transplant candidate	Donor does not specify an intended recipient	Donor may or may not know the intended recipient	Person authorizing donation knows of the intended recipient

Source: Organ Procurement and Transplantation Network. (2021b). *U.S. multi-organ transplant organ procurement and transplant network national data*. U.S. Department of Health and Human Services. https://optn.transplant.hrsa.gov/data/view-data-reports/national-data/

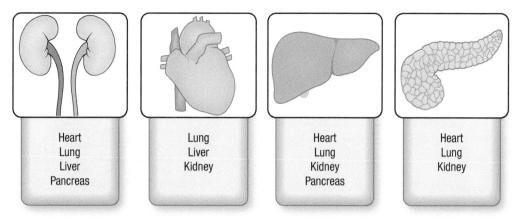

FIGURE 23.2: Multiorgan transplants.

MULTIORGAN TRANSPLANT

Multiorgan transplants are an option for patients with multiorgan failure (Figure 23.2). During multiorgan transplantation, the recipient's diseased organs are replaced with healthy organs, usually from the same donor. More than 1000 multiorgan transplants were performed in 2019 (OPTN, 2021b). The benefits of multi-organ transplant to the recipient are avoidance of multiple surgeries and less exposure to sensitizing events, as the exposure is most often a single donor. The evaluation for a multiorgan transplant requires the candidate meet listing criteria for each specific organ to be transplanted.

POSTTRANSPLANT MANAGEMENT

Immediate posttransplant management is focused on surgical recovery of the recipient, assessment of allograft function, initiation of immunosuppression to achieve therapeutic medication levels, monitoring for adverse events, evaluation of the recipient's functional status, and patient and support person education about medication administration, self-monitoring practices, and manifestations of rejection and infection. Following hospital discharge, patients have frequent outpatient visits, laboratory analysis, and screening tests for allograft rejection (Table 23.10). Additional visits are scheduled as needed to evaluate problems as they present (Flattery & Gierlach, 2016).

COMPLICATIONS AND LONG-TERM CHALLENGES

Successful outcome after solid organ transplantation relies on recipient and provider surveillance for and management of transplant-related complications, sequelae of life-long immunosuppression, and comorbidities. Allograft rejection and infection are two complications that are anticipated and most often occur in the first weeks to months following transplantation. Early recognition

TABLE 23.10: Discharge Planning, Patient Education, and Health Maintenance

TOPIC	POSTTRANSPLANT MANAGEMENT AND EDUCATION*
Rejection	See organ-specific manifestations (Table 23.9)
Vital sign monitoring	• Temperature, heart rate, blood pressure, daily weight, intake/output (kidney), spirometry (lung) • Parameters for reporting abnormal findings to transplant providers
Exercise/physical activity	Weightlifting limits, driving, daily exercise recommendations, rehabilitation
Infection prevention	• Hand hygiene • Avoid people who are ill • Limit contact with crowds • Wear mask in public places 3–6 months posttransplant and when undergoing treatment for acute rejection • Avoid contact with animal feces: avoid cleaning cat litter, bird cages, aquariums • Do not change diapers of children who had recently received live vaccines • Wear gloves and mask while gardening or digging in dirt • Prophylactic medications: antibacterial (toxoplasmosis, *Pneumocystis jiroveci*), antifungal (candida), antiviral (cytomegalovirus, herpes zoster)
Wound care	• Treatment/dressings • Bathing/showering instructions • Parameters to report wound infection, nonclosure, dehiscence
Nutrition/diet	• Avoid unpasteurized foods/dairy/juices, raw seed sprouts • Avoid raw/undercooked meat/seafood. • Avoid raw/undercooked eggs, including cookie dough, batter

(continued)

TABLE 23.10: Discharge Planning, Patient Education, and Health Maintenance *(continued)*

TOPIC	POSTTRANSPLANT MANAGEMENT AND EDUCATION*
Management of new diagnoses	Example: immunosuppression-induced diabetes mellitus
Medications and administration schedule	Provide medication administration record for home use
Food/drug medication interactions	See Table 23.5
Routine health maintenance screening for age, comorbidities	American Cancer Society cancer screening guidelines (Smith et al., 2019) Annual dermatologic exam Age-related/history-appropriate exams US Preventive Services Task Force (USPSTF) Recommended Topics (2021)

* May be organ and transplant center variations.

of these complications is essential to reversing rejection or infection and avoiding long-term sequelae associated with both disease processes.

Transplant-Related Complications

Allograft Rejection

Rejection occurs when the recipient's innate and adaptive immune systems recognize the donor organ as nonself and initiate a cascade of immunologic events intended to destroy the allograft. Rejection can be an acute cellular process mediated by T lymphocytes or an insidious, chronic threat induced by the humoral immune response (Lo & Kirk, 2015). ACR most commonly occurs in the days to months following transplantation but is a possibility for the life of the allograft (kidney, pancreas) or the recipient (heart, lung, liver). Chronic, or humoral, rejection is more insidious, may not be reversible, and is usually associated with the development of donor-specific antibodies (DSAs) to the allograft. Patients are said to be sensitized when DSAs are present.

ACUTE CELLULAR REJECTION

ACR results when T lymphocytes become activated against donor antigens. Activated cytotoxic T cells and complement destroy allograft cells. Symptoms of acute rejection, if present, are manifested as allograft failure (Table 23.11). Transplant recipients are often asymptomatic; therefore, symptom monitoring, laboratory analysis, and surveillance biopsy, depending on organ, are necessary in the first months after transplant. ACR is confirmed with biopsy of the allograft in asymptomatic or asymptomatic recipients and treatment initiated with biopsy-proven rejection. ACR is usually reversible.

TABLE 23.11: Manifestations of Acute Cellular and Antibody-Mediated Rejection

ORGAN	CLINICAL MANIFESTATION	SURVEILLANCE/ CONFIRMATION
Heart	Tachycardia, hypotension, dyspnea, orthopnea, fluid volume overload, edema, ascites, lightheadedness/ dizziness, palpitations, early satiety, activity intolerance Reduced ejection fraction, hemodynamic compromise	Endomyocardial biopsy Echocardiogram
Lung	Reduced spirometry, oxygen desaturation, dyspnea/ tachypnea, cough, radiographic changes (infiltrate, effusion, pulmonary edema), lung pain	Chest radiograph Pulmonary function tests Bronchoscopy Transbronchial biopsy
Liver	Liver pain, abdominal distention, jaundice, abnormal transaminases, pruritus, tea-colored urine	Liver function tests (LFTs) Liver biopsy when LFTs elevated
Kidney	Elevated serum bun-urea-nitrogen and creatinine, abdominal pain over graft site, edema, oligura, hypertension, gross hematuria	Kidney biopsy Renal ultrasound
Pancreas	Severe abdominal pain at graft site, increased serum amylase or lipase, hyperglycemia (not early sign, indicates destruction of islet cells)	CT- or ultrasound-guided percutaneous biopsy C-peptide

Source: Data from Chandraker, A., Sayegh, M. H., & Singh, A. K. (Eds.). (2012). *Core concepts in renal transplantation.* Springer Publishing Company. https://doi .org/10.1007/978-1-4614-0008-0; Cupples, S. A., Lerret, S., McCalmont, V., & Ohler, L. A. (2016). *Core curriculum for transplant nurses* (2nd ed.). Wolters Kluwer. http:// search.ebscohost.com.proxy.library.vanderbilt.edu/login.aspx?direct=true&db =e000xna&AN=20182 44&site=ehost-live&scope=site

Treatment of ACR depends in part on the severity of the rejection and is dictated by the amount of allograft dysfunction and patient signs and symptoms. Biopsy-proven rejection is graded according to the degree of lymphocyte infiltration, edema/inflammation, and tissue and vascular destruction of the allograft. Grading scales are based on guidelines established by the various organ-specific transplant organizations (Demetris et al., 2016). Low-grade or mild ACR is often asymptomatic and may be observed with repeat biopsy in a few weeks without treatment or with increases in doses of one or more of the maintenance immunosuppressive agents. Moderate to severe grade ACR and/or with evidence of organ dysfunction is treated with an oral or parenteral steroid pulse, augmentation of oral immunosuppression with higher doses or change to a different agent, and possibly administration of a mono- or polyclonal antibody (e.g., antithymocyte globulin). Physiologic supportive care of the recipient experiencing organ dysfunction may also be warranted (Cupples et al., 2016).

Manifestations common to all organ rejection include fever, fatigue, malaise, myalgias. Organ-specific signs and symptoms are outlined in Table 23.11.

HUMORAL REJECTION

Humoral, or AMR, is less responsive to antirejection therapy and may not be reversible because of circulating DSAs. Plasma B cells generate DSAs and complement may be fixed, further promoting rejection. Symptoms and diagnosis of rejection with biopsy are similar to ACR; however, treatment is directed toward destruction and removal of circulating DSAs. Evidence related to optimal treatment options is unclear but usual therapies include augmentation of oral immunosuppression, administration of IVIG, and plasmapheresis to remove circulating antibodies (Brennan et al., 2006). With less clear implications but frequently used to treat AMR are administration of rituximab, a monoclonal antibody that depletes B lymphocytes and bortezomib, a proteasome inhibitor that causes apoptosis (Herrero & Panizo, 2018).

Chronic Rejection

Chronic rejection manifests as obliteration or narrowing of tubular structures and/or blood vessels of the graft, ultimately resulting in graft failure. Vascular intimal proliferation causing ischemia and collagen deposition with interstitial fibrosis of the organ ultimately result in graft dysfunction (Lo & Kirk, 2015). Repeated episodes of ACR and/or AMR often lead to chronic rejection. The mechanisms causing chronic rejection are less understood but are considered irreversible with limited treatment options. The outcome of severe graft dysfunction and failure is organ replacement with dialysis (kidney), retransplant, or death of the recipient (Table 23.12).

TABLE 23.12: Manifestations of Chronic Rejection

ORGAN	REJECTION
Heart	Cardiac allograft vasculopathy
Lung	Bronchiolitis obliterans
Liver	Obliterative arteriopathy, bile duct obliteration
Kidney	Chronic allograft nephropathy, chronic renal failure Interstitial fibrosis/tubular atrophy, glomerulosclerosis
Pancreas	Hyperglycemia, decreased C-peptide

Source: Data from Li, X. C., & Jevnikar, A. M. (Eds.). (2015). *Transplant immunology*. Wiley Blackwell. ProQuest Ebook Central. https://ebookcentral.proquest.com

Infection

Infectious complications posttransplant are a major cause of morbidity and mortality, and can lead to allograft dysfunction and graft loss (Martin-Gandul et al., 2015). Infection risk is affected by pre-existing donor infections, reactivation of latent infections, and the recipient's overall health status. Malnutrition, age, frailty, vaccination history, active infection, diabetes mellitus, and cause of the recipient's end organ disease (e.g., cystic fibrosis) can lead to a higher infection risk in the postoperative period (Trachuk et al., 2020). Intraoperatively, long ischemic time and injury to nerves adjacent to the graft implant site have been implicated in increasing infection burden posttransplant. Postoperatively, induction and maintenance immunosuppression to prevent allograft rejection place the recipient at risk for common as well as opportunistic infections.

Central lines, drains, urinary catheters, invasive procedures and implanted devices can also be a source for infection posttransplant secondary to the lymphocyte depression and alteration of the body's ability to mount a response to an infection. Pretransplant infection risk screening is similar for all transplant candidates and is performed to assess infectious risk and guide post transplant need for prophylaxis or treatment. Transplant candidates should be vaccinated prior to transplant for the usual childhood diseases (MMR, varicella, rubeola, pertussis), as live vaccines cannot be given after transplant and vaccination efficacy decreases in the setting of immunosuppression (Stucchi et al., 2018). Annual influenza vaccines are also recommended. Close contacts of transplant recipients should also be fully vaccinated.

Infection Timeline

The timing of an infectious episode after transplantation is critical. Activation of latent infections, opportunistic infections, donor-derived infections, and intraoperative technical issues all are risk factors (Fishman & the AST Infectious Diseases Community of Practice, 2009; Grossi & Fishman, 2009). In the first month, infections are typically related to the technical complications of the surgery (e.g., anastomotic leaks, ischemia) or donor-acquired infections. During months 1 to 6, infections associated with postoperative complications (anastomotic complications) or with augmented immunosuppression can increase risk. Infection prophylactic medications administered the first 3 to 6 months posttransplant are outlined in Table 23.13.

Predominant Viral Infections Posttransplantation

Cytomegalovirus (CMV), a member of the herpesvirus family, is transmitted by direct contact with body fluids, in blood products, or through the transplanted organ. Most transplant centers use a CMV prophylaxis strategy for 3 to 6 months posttransplant for all recipients. At highest risk for developing de novo CMV infection is the CMV seronegative recipient (R-) of a CMV seropositive

TABLE 23.13: Infection Prophylaxis

INFECTION	PROPHYLAXIS AGENT
Herpes viruses: herpes zoster, varicella, cytomegalovirus, Epstein-Barr virus	Valganciclovir, valacyclovir, or acyclovir
Pneumocystis jiroveci, toxoplasmosis	Trimethoprim/sulfamethoxazole (TMP-SMX) Dapsone if sulfa allergy Pentamidine
Candida	Nystatin swish and swallow

Source: Data from Martin, S. I., & Fishman, J. A. (2009). Pneumocystis pneumonia in solid organ transplant recipients. *American Journal of Transplantation, 9*(Suppl. 4), S227–S233. https://doi.org/10.1111/j.1600-6143.2009.02914.x

donor (D+) and can be associated with significant morbidity (Razonable & Humar, 2019). CMV seropositive recipients (R+) are at a lower risk for CMV disease (Raval et al., 2020). Manifestations of CMV infection include fever, malaise, leukopenia, transaminitis, and thrombocytopenia. Invasive CMV disease can cause retinitis, hepatitis, gastrointestinal involvement, or infiltration of the allograft itself (Hartmann et al., 2006).

Varicella zoster virus (VZV) is a member of the herpesvirus family and transmitted via contact with vesicle fluid or respiratory droplets. Primary varicella disease is chicken pox, presenting with fever, vesicles, and pruritus, with rash predominantly on trunk and face. Reactivated disease is herpes zoster or "shingles," presenting with painful vesicles in a dermatomal pattern. The incidence of reactivation of varicella zoster is around 10% in the first 4 years posttransplant (Pergam & Limaye, 2013). Disseminated zoster can affect the skin, retina, and pulmonary system. Diagnosis is based on clinical presentation, positive VZV DNA polymerase chain reaction (PCR) from vesicle fluid, cerebral spinal fluid (CSF), or tissue. Treatment is with oral acyclovir or valacyclovir for VZV and IV acyclovir for primary varicella, disseminated zoster, central nervous system (CNS) or ocular disease (Gourishankar et al., 2004). Herpes simplex is treated similarly with antivirals.

Polyomaviruses associated with solid organ transplant include BK virus and JC virus and can cause acute allograft dysfunction. DNA PCR and/or histology is obtained to monitor for active disease. Treatment includes reducing the net amount of immunosuppression (Thangaraju et al., 2016).

Parvovirus B19 infection can cause severe, refractory anemia, pancytopenia and thrombotic microangiopathy (TMA), hepatitis, encephalitis, and graft dysfunction. Diagnosis is confirmed by detection of B19 virus DNA in the blood. Treatment consists of high dose IVIG, reduction of immunosuppression, and supportive care for symptomatic anemia (Eid et al., 2006).

HEPATITIS C AND DONOR-DERIVED INFECTIONS

Increasing access to the donor pool for transplant candidates shortens wait times and decreases wait list mortality (Schlendorf et al., 2020). Historically, organs from hepatitis C virus (HCV) antibody positive donors generally were not offered to non-HCV infected transplant candidates due to concerns of HCV transmission. HCV-positive donors who are nucleic acid test negative (NAT) have cleared the virus and are less likely to transmit HCV to a transplant recipient; however, HCV-positive, NAT-positive donors have active HCV and viral transmission to the recipient is probable. Development of direct-acting antivirals (DAA) agents that destroy HCV and can cure viremia have allowed expansion of the transplant donor pool. The high cure rate associated with well-tolerated DAAs makes transplant with HCV-positive donors possible (Gonzalez & Trotter, 2018). Transplant candidates must be willing and provide informed consent to accept an HCV-positive donor and institution-specific protocols created to monitor posttransplant HCV viremia and initiate DAA therapy (American Association for the Study of Liver Diseases, & Infectious Diseases Society of America, 2021).

Fungal Infections

Fungal infections can occur with colonization of yeast and molds secondary to the immunocompromised recipient exposure to broad-spectrum antibacterial agents, corticosteroid therapy, and the presence of catheters and endotracheal tubes. Fungal infections in a transplant recipient remain a significant cause of morbidity and mortality with the incidence varying with the type of solid organ transplant and require a reevaluation of the immunosuppressive regimen (De La Cruz & Silveira, 2017). Corticosteroid dosing should be minimized, and target trough levels of cyclosporine and tacrolimus kept at the lower end of the therapeutic range (De La Cruz & Silveira, 2017).

The most common fungal infections are *Candida* species, *Aspergillus*, *Pneumocystis jiroveci* (PJP). *Candida* infections occur most commonly in the first 1 to 3 months following transplantation and are associated with initial high-dose immunosuppression in the early transplant period. Aspergillosis is caused by *Aspergillus fumigatus* found in soil with the respiratory system the predominant site of infection. Presenting symptoms can include wheezing, cough, hemoptysis, chest pain, and weight loss. Providers should have a high index of suspicion for aspergillosis when a transplant recipient presents with these manifestations. A positive galactmannan antigen obtained from serum or bronchial-alveolar lavage (BAL) confirms the infection. Treatment includes an azole antifungal or amphotericin B, and surgical lung resection. Note that antifungal administration requires dose reduction of the CNI to avoid CNI toxicity and renal dysfunction (Table 23.14).

TABLE 23.14: Immunosuppressive Agents and Required Monitoring

	AGENT	MONITORING	RATIONALE	AGENT	MONITORING	RATIONALE
Induction and rescue medications	*Polyclonal antibodies* Antithymocyte globulin (rabbit or equine)	• CBC*/differential/ platelet count • Lymphocyte count (T-cell subset)	• Myelosuppression • Infection • Lymphocyte depletion	*Monoclonal antibodies* Basiliximab Alemtuzumab	• CBC/differential/ platelet count	• Myelosuppression • Infection
	Corticosteroids Methylprednisolone Prednisone	• CBC/differential/ platelet count	• Expect initial ↑ WBC 2° demargination • Infection	Rituximab	• CBC/differential/ platelet count • BMP • IgG	• Myelosuppression • Infection • Renal function • Hypogammaglobinemia
Maintenance medications	*Calcineurin inhibitors* • Cyclosporine • Cyclosporine modified • Tacrolimus Tacrolimus extended release	• BMP* • 12-hour trough level • BMP • 24-hour trough level	• Renal function • Therapeutic blood level • Renal function • Therapeutic blood level	*Antimetabolites* Azathioprine • Mycophenolate mofetil • Mycophenolate sodium	• CBC/differential/ platelet count • CBC/differential/ platelet count • 24-hour trough level (rarely used)	• Myelosuppression • Infection • Myelosuppression • Infection • Therapeutic blood level
	Corticosteroids Prednisone	• CBC/differential/ platelet count	Infection	*mTOR inhibitors* Sirolimus (rapamycin) Everolimus	• CBC/differential/ platelet count • 24-hour trough level • Lipid panel • Urine protein • CBC/differential/ platelet count • 12-hour trough level • Lipid panel • Urine protein	• Myelosuppression • Infection • Therapeutic blood level • Hyperlipidemia • Proteinuria • Myelosuppression • Infection • Therapeutic blood level • Hyperlipidemia • Proteinuria
	Costimulation blocker Belatacept	• CBC/differential/ platelet count	• Myelosuppression • Infection			

BMP, basic metabolic panel; CBC, complete blood count.

Histoplasmosis is caused by the *Histoplasma capsulatum* fungus found in soil contaminated with bat and bird droppings and is endemic to the Ohio and Mississippi river valleys. Transmission is via inhalation of the mold. Onset is an acute illness 3 to 17 days after exposure, presenting with fever, malaise, cough, headache, chest pain, and myalgia. Clinical findings include lymphadenopathy, splenomegaly, hepatomegaly, weight loss, fever, pulmonary nodules, and granulomata. Diagnostic workup includes antigen detection in urine, serum, or BAL aspirate, antibody testing, tissue culture, and microscopy. Treatment for severe disease includes amphotericin B initially, and an azole antifungal.

Pneumocystis pneumonia is caused by the fungus PJP, an infection rarely seen in immunocompetent hosts. Presenting symptoms include fever, hypoxia, dry cough, and fatigue. Clinical workup includes chest imaging, in which "ground glass opacities" can be seen, BAL with a silver stain, and blood for beta D glucan (Martin & Fishman, 2009). First-line treatment is with trimethoprim/sulfamethoxazole (TMP-SMX) for mild disease with the addition of steroids for severe disease. All solid organ recipients typically receive PJP prophylaxis for >4 months and up to 1 year posttransplant. If a patient is sulfa allergic, inhaled pentamidine, atovaquone, or dapsone are alternative agents (Martin & Fishman, 2009).

LONG-TERM COMPLICATIONS

About 3 months posttransplantation, many transplant recipients have had their immunosuppressive target levels reduced. Treatment of underlying comorbidities (hypertension, diabetes mellitus, and hyperlipidemia) and other medical issues are now being addressed secondary to the high level of interaction with their transplant team. Fewer patients lose their grafts in the first year, and many patients will continue to enjoy allograft function for many years to come.

Malignancy

Early cancer screening in transplant recipients follows the same American Cancer Society recommendations for the general population (Smith et al., 2019). Smoking cessation before transplant has led to a reduction in frequency of many malignancies, most notably lung cancer. Resumption of smoking increases lung cancer risk in an immunocompromised patient and contributes to associated disease burden.

Posttransplant Lymphoproliferative Disease

Posttransplant lymphoproliferative disorders (PTLD) are predominantly B-cell mediated and have a high association with Epstein-Barr virus (EBV) infection. EBV is a human herpesvirus that primarily targets B lymphocytes and is associated with disorders such as infectious mononucleosis, Burkitt lymphoma and B cell lymphomas in immunocompromised patients. Clinical presentations of PTLD are variable depending on tumor site. The incidence of PTLD in solid organ transplant is 0.8% to 15% and varies with the type of organ transplanted, the age of the recipient, and the immunosuppression regimen utilized. PTLD is different from lymphomas in the general population in that they are predominantly non–Hodgkin lymphomas. Seronegative recipients of an organ from a seropositive donor are at highest risk for PTLD. Clinical presentation is a mononucleosis-type syndrome with fatigue, fever, and lymphadenopathy (Mendogni et al., 2019). Multiple sites may be involved, including the CNS, liver, lungs, kidneys, and intestines. Tissue biopsy remains the gold standard for PTLD diagnosis and guides staging of disease (Allen & Preiksaitis, 2019). Mortality rate of PTLD is higher than the general population and progression to death can be within months of diagnosis. Treatment of PTLD is a drastic reduction in immunosuppression and chemotherapy consisting of rituximab and cytotoxic therapy (Malyszko, 2019).

Skin Cancer

The need for chronic immunosuppression in the transplant recipient contributes to the risk of cutaneous malignancy. Certain malignancies have a higher association with transplant including Kaposi sarcoma, lip cancer, and nonepithelial skin cancer. Greater than 50% of White organ transplant recipients will develop at least one cutaneous malignancy. Squamous cell carcinoma and basal cell carcinoma account for the majority of skin cancers in organ transplant recipients. Contributing factors include type of transplant, the intensity and type of the immunosuppression, geographic location, and sun exposure. In non-White transplant recipients, tumors are predominantly associated with human papillomavirus infection and occur on sun-exposed areas. The risk of melanoma in the transplant population is threefold higher than the general population (Mittal & Colegio, 2017).

The impact of immunosuppression on development of malignancy is unclear; however, tumor development appears to correlate with intensity and type of immunosuppression (Vajdic & van Leeuwen, 2009). When malignancy occurs, reduction of immunosuppression, particularly the CNIs, and implementation of evidence-based chemotherapy regimens targeting the type of malignancy are warranted (Maggiore & Pascual, 2016).

Chronic Kidney Disease

Chronic kidney disease (CKD) is a common complication after nonrenal transplantation and is associated with increased morbidity and mortality (Ojo et al., 2003). The risk for kidney disease is influenced by many factors in the pretransplant, perioperative, and posttransplantation periods. Serum creatinine is only one marker of kidney function and may be overestimated prior to transplantation, particularly in patients with poor nutritional status, low muscle mass, advanced age, weight loss, and edema. Nonrenal end-organ disease can lead to ineffective circulating fluid volume as with advanced heart failure or hepatorenal syndrome and may not be reversible following organ transplantation (Bloom & Reese, 2007). Pre-existing hypertension and diabetes mellitus increase risk for CKD. HCV infection is recognized as an important risk factor for CKD in liver and heart transplant recipients (U.S. Renal Data System, 2020). In the perioperative period, acute kidney injury may be triggered by hypotension, hypoperfusion, use of radiocontrast, prolonged aortic cross clamp time, poor cardiac output, and aggressive diuresis. Postoperatively, the use of CNIs causes renal vasoconstriction that predisposes patients to acute and chronic kidney injury. Narrow therapeutic CNI drug levels are monitored closely, though type of organ transplanted may necessitate higher drug levels, which lead to longer exposure to the nephrotoxic effects of the CNIs.

Occasionally, CNIs and sirolimus can cause a de novo, drug-induced thrombotic microangiopathy, a pathology that results in thrombocytopenia, anemia (TMA), low haptoglobin, elevated LDH, and acute kidney injury (Miller et al., 1997). The preceding tests would be obtained, including a urinalysis, to rule out other causes of kidney injury. No specific test is available to diagnose drug-induced TMA; therefore, the diagnosis is made clinically with known exposure to a drug previously associated with TMA. TMA may occur rapidly or take several months after introduction of a CNI. Suspect a diagnosis of TMA in any transplant recipient who presents with an elevated serum creatinine, especially if hemolytic anemia and thrombocytopenia are present. Treatment of TMA is discontinuation of the offending medication, switching to another immunosuppressant, and excluding other causes of TMA, including infection with CMV, BK virus, parvovirus, or HIV (Saleem et al., 2018).

Cardiovascular Disease

Cardiovascular events are now the leading cause of morbidity and mortality after liver and kidney transplantation ahead of graft failure and infection (Levy et al., 2021). This trend has gained momentum as the acceptance of older donors with higher comorbidity burden, including those on hemodialysis, has become more common (Gillis et al., 2014). In lung transplant candidates, atherosclerotic disease burden is considered to be a relative contraindication for lung transplantation. Cardiac complications may include myocardial ischemia and infarction, heart failure, arrhythmias leading to sudden death, hypertension, left ventricular hypertrophy, and, in heart transplantation, allograft vasculopathy. The metabolic effects of immunosuppressive agents, infection, and rejection contribute to development of posttransplant cardiovascular disease. A posttransplant metabolic syndrome comprised of hypertension, dyslipidemia, increased fat mass/obesity, and glucose intolerance, combined with other metabolic side effects from corticosteroids and CNIs, requires early recognition and aggressive intervention to minimize the effects of the posttransplant metabolic syndrome (Cohen et al., 2020; Sen et al., 2019). Cardiac evaluation of the transplant candidate is essential for risk stratification, to minimize cardiovascular events and improve long-term survival after transplantation and anticipating the burden of coronary artery disease (Levy et al., 2021; Wild et al., 2015). Risk factor modification, including diet and lifestyle changes, achieving glycemic control, nonpharmacologic and pharmacologic management of hypertension and hyperlipidemia, encouraging weight loss if obese, and tailoring immunosuppressive regimens to prevent complications can improve short- and long-term mortality and graft survival (Tantisattamo et al., 2020; Thomas & Weir, 2015; Warden & Duell, 2019).

Diabetes Mellitus

Posttransplant diabetes mellitus (PTDM) is a serious complication reducing both patient and graft survival after transplantation. Risk factors are multifactorial and include the immunosuppressive regimen (CNIs, corticosteroids), ethnicity, older age, and body mass index (BMI) (Salvadori et al., 2003). Modifiable risk factors should be identified pretransplant, and a multidisciplinary team approach employed to manage hypertension, hyperlipidemia, and metabolic control in the posttransplant phase of care. These patients benefit from a referral to a dietitian and an endocrinology provider. The targets of treatment are the same as for all patients with diabetes mellitus (hemoglobin A1C <7.0), following American Diabetes Association recommendations. Routine surveillance for vascular, ophthalmic, podiatric, and neurologic disease is implemented to reduce risk of diabetic complications, including cardiovascular disease and CKD. Dose reduction of the immunosuppressive regimen, as tolerated by rejection risk, may ameliorate the hyperglycemic effects of immunosuppression.

Metabolic Bone Disease

Osteoporosis and fracture following solid organ transplantation is primarily associated with corticosteroid therapy and can result in a fracture incidence as high as 65% in the posttransplant population (Yu et al., 2014). Long-term corticosteroid exposure reduces bone formation and decreases secretion of androgens and estrogens which increases secretion of parathyroid hormone (PTH). Increased PTH levels result in development of bone mineral disorders. Common pretransplant factors include low bone mineral density secondary to underlying disease (heart failure, CKD, vitamin D deficiency, secondary hyperparathyroidism, chronic use of loop diuretics, and immobility (Maalouf & Shane, 2005; Yu et al., 2014). Excessive alcohol use and chronic cholestasis inhibiting turnover of osteoblast function have been attributed to osteoporosis (Krol et al., 2014). In patients with chronic lung disease, the need for steroid therapy, low body weight, malnutrition, and malabsorption are risk factors for bone mineral disorders (Shane et al., 1996).

Metabolic bone disease is a common complication of CKD and is part of a wide range of disorders of mineral metabolism that result in bone disease. High PTH levels can be observed in approximately one third of patients 5 years after transplantation. Alterations in calcium and phosphorous levels occur in CKD and progress as kidney function deteriorates. Known as "CKD mineral and bone disorders," a clinical syndrome develops as a result of CKD, with abnormalities of calcium, phosphorus, PTH, and vitamin D metabolism. The effects of hyperparathyroidism on bone with mineralization defects can result in a wide range of skeletal abnormalities. Management of patients with CKD-related hyperparathyroidism requires dietary limitation of phosphorus and monitoring of serum phosphorus and calcium levels. Secondary hyperparathyroidism, commonly seen postrenal transplantation, can cause hypophosphatemia due to renal phosphorus wasting.

Steroid-Induced Bone Diseases

Evaluation of transplant candidates for osteoporosis is performed as part of the transplant evaluation. Treatment of secondary causes of osteoporosis (e.g., vitamin D deficiency) is initiated in the pretransplant phase and evaluated at least annually posttransplant. The Fracture Risk Assessment tool (FRAX) is useful to estimate the risk of osteoporotic fracture (Kharroubi et al., 2017; Tsuruda & Kitamura, 2017). Some patients may benefit from bisphosphonates while on the transplant wait list, especially those with a documented fracture history (Ebeling, 2009; Stein et al., 2007). Bisphosphonates should be cautiously used in women of child-bearing age due to potential for fetal harm and are not recommended if creatinine clearance is less than 30 mL/min. If bisphosphonates are contraindicated or not tolerated, calcitriol or hormonal replacement therapy may be options (Fleischer et al., 2008). In the posttransplant period, recommendations to minimize and treat osteoporosis are the same as that of the general population (Table 23.15).

The major bone diseases that affect transplant recipients are osteoporosis and osteonecrosis (avascular necrosis [AVN]), both of which can lead to long-term morbidity. Bone loss occurs rapidly following transplantation primarily in the setting of high dose steroid therapy (Rajapakse et al., 2012). Other factors contributing to increased risk include diabetes mellitus, metabolic acidosis, White race, smoking, impaired nutrition, lack of exercise, and hyperparathyroidism (Bouquegneau et al., 2016: Nikkel et al., 2012). Approximately 90% of AVN occurrences posttransplantation are located at the femoral head. Cyclosporine may contribute to bone loss among patients treated with glucocorticoids; studies on the impact of tacrolimus on bone have not been conclusive. Patient presentation is hip or groin pain exacerbated by weight bearing that may be referred to the knee. Standard radiographs are obtained early in the process with increased clinical suspicion but have low sensitivity unless the AVN is advanced. Magnetic resonance imaging is more conclusive. Nonsurgical management is aimed at preserving the patient's quality of life, considering the patient's age, current mobility, and lifestyle. Maintaining the lowest amount of corticosteroid, bedrest, offloading as tolerated and the use of analgesics as well as newer therapies, such as pulsed electromagnetic field therapy, have been incorporated (Osmani et al., 2017). Approximately 60% of patients with AVN require total hip arthroplasty.

Posttransplantation Reproductive Health

Males

Contemporary solid organ transplantation has improved life expectancy and many recipients want to consider fatherhood as an option. Healthy children have been successfully fathered by lung, liver, pancreas, and heart transplants with the incidence of birth defects ranging from 1.9% to 4.0%, comparable to the general population (Armenti et al., 2001). In renal transplant, uremia is associated with decreased testosterone, sperm counts, sperm quality, hypogonadism, and fertility. After transplantation, testosterone levels and sperm counts improve (Reinhardt et al., 2018). Erectile dysfunction (ED) is common after transplantation and affected by medications and comorbidities. Immunosuppression, particularly tacrolimus and mycophenolate, can affect fertility. Tacrolimus may affect sperm counts. Mycophenolate carries a specific label warning that therapy should be discontinued 90 days prior to having unprotected sex even if the patient has undergone a vasectomy (Semet et al., 2017). Overall health status and physical conditioning of the recipient must be assessed prior to prescribing therapy to treat ED. Phosphodiesterase type 5 inhibitors, intracavernosal injections, and penile implants are safe and effective in transplant recipients (Sun et al., 2018). Fatherhood is possible and safe in transplant recipients with medical evaluation and collaboration with the transplant team.

Females

All women of childbearing age should be counseled concerning the risks of pregnancy posttransplantation. Genetic counseling should be provided to patients with

TABLE 23.15: Management of Osteoporosis

BEHAVIOR MODIFICATION	MANAGEMENT
• Smoking cessation • Weight-bearing and resistance exercise • Fall prevention	• Monitor serum Ca++ and vitamin D levels • Reduce steroid dosing as tolerated • Bone mineral density testing pretransplant, 6–12 months posttransplant and at least biennially • Oral calcium, vitamin D replacement, and bisphosphonates, as indicated

hereditary diseases. Assessment of current allograft function is essential when planning pregnancy. Changes in the immunosuppressive strategy are required and should be planned preemptively. Most transplant centers advise patients to avoid pregnancy the first year posttransplant when the risk of rejection is highest and the immunosuppression therapy most aggressive (Cosia et al., n.d.). Birth defects are not increased with the use of azathioprine, cyclosporine, and tacrolimus during pregnancy. MMF poses a high risk of teratogenicity and carries a U.S. FDA label warning concerning the risk of first trimester fetal loss and congenital malformations (Kim et al., 2013). An FDA-approved medication guide is distributed to patients and includes recommendations to use two forms of birth control while taking mycophenolate (FDA, 2012). Experts disagree on how long patients should delay pregnancy after discontinuing mycophenolate; the FDA recommends a delay of at least 6 weeks. A baseline assessment of renal, cardiac, and liver function should be obtained. The American Society of Transplantation (ATS) recommends criteria for timing of pregnancy, no rejection in past year, adequate and stable graft function, no acute infections that might impact the fetus, and maintenance immunosuppression at stable dosing (McKay et al., 2005). In addition, all other medications should be assessed for teratogenic risk prior to conception. Partnership with a perinatologist and high-risk obstetrician is recommended.

ETHICAL, PSYCHOSOCIAL, AND PROFESSIONAL ISSUES ASSOCIATED WITH SOLID ORGAN TRANSPLANTATION

Solid organ transplantation is unique in that decisions about selection of transplant candidates and donors as well as organ allocation practices are governed not only by federal regulations, evidence-based healthcare practices and provider judgment, but also ethical principles that guide decision-making (OPTN, 2015a). Psychosocial characteristics of the transplant candidate factor into wait listing decisions including life-expectancy, organ failure caused by behavior, compliance/adherence, social support, family dynamics, and repeat transplantation, which can create ethical conundrums for transplant teams (OPTN, 2015b). As a member of the interdisciplinary transplant team, the AGACNP has the opportunity to contribute to transplant candidate discussions and decision-making (Box 23.4).

ETHICAL PRINCIPLES

Utility, justice, and respect for persons are three ethical principles that create the foundational framework for the equitable allocation of scarce human organs for transplantation.

1. Utility holds that an action is good if it is useful in achieving the maximal amount of good or benefit for

> **BOX 23.4 TRANSPLANT TEAM MEMBERS FOR COLLABORATIVE DECISION-MAKING**
> - Transplant surgeon
> - Transplant medical specialist
> - Nurse practitioners
> - Pre- and posttransplant nurses
> - Transplant infectious disease specialist
> - Transplant pharmacist
> - Social worker
> - Psychologist/psychiatrist
> - Physical therapist
> - Financial counselors

a group or community. Organ retrieval and transplantation are undertaken to benefit persons with end-organ disease. The principle of utility as applied to organ allocation should maximize the expected net amount of overall good or benefit; that is, the process of organ allocation should do more good (beneficence) and cause no harm (nonmaleficence) for persons in need of a transplant (OPTN, 2015a).

2. Justice refers to the fairness and equal distribution of scarce resources. Justice as related to organ allocation considers not only the aggregate amount of good (organs) generated but also the way in which the organs are distributed to potential beneficiaries (transplant candidates). Candidates may not be treated the same but giving equal respect and concern to each candidate are required. Race, socioeconomic class, and gender, in general, should not influence organ allocation processes, a practice that is in direct conflict with justice.

3. Respect for persons is a principle upholding that people have a right to autonomy and self-determination. While respect for autonomy is a right, autonomy can be in conflict with organ allocation practices that ensure the fair and equitable distribution of organs and violates the principle of justice. Respect for a person's autonomy is applicable to transplantation in that donors or their surrogates have the right to refuse donation, individuals have the right to refuse an organ, organs can be allocated via directed donation, and allocation processes and rules must be transparent to allow for informed decision-making (OPTN, 2015a).

ETHICAL PRINCIPLES: THE DONOR

The Uniform Anatomical Gift Act, initially passed by Congress in 1968 and revised in 1987 and 2006, established brain death as a legal definition of death. The Act also created a process called "required request" where hospitals were required to offer family members or patient surrogates the option of organ donation; however, this requirement has not substantially increased consent for donation (Siminoff et al., 2013). All 50 states and the District of Columbia have first-person authorization laws which recognize a person's consent to be an organ donor after death via authorization on a driver's license, donor card, or donor registry. Family consent for donation is not required and preserves the principle of respect for autonomy and assures the family of the donor's wishes (Siminoff et al., 2013).

Congress enacted the NOTA in 1984, which established a task force on organ transplantation to examine the ethical, social, and economic aspects of organ procurement. Two principles were established by NOTA: (a) There is no financial compensation for organs or to organ donors, except for medical expenses, and (b) organs must always be donated, explicitly granted by the donor, either living or before death in the spirit of altruism. The two principles established a barrier to exploitation and commercialization of organs and promoted equality in organ distribution. Exploitation and trafficking of organs was addressed internationally with the Declaration of Istanbul (Reed et al., 2009), which clarifies the issues of transplant tourism, trafficking, and commercialism and provides ethical guidelines for practice in organ donation and transplantation. The declaration is endorsed by countries around the world (Jonsen et al., 2006; Reed et al., 2009).

Living donation is the only operation that is performed to specifically help the recipient and provides no medical benefit to the donor. Living donors are subject to harm from the organ retrieval surgery itself and complications and morbidities that can result after the operation. Quality of life and return to work can be impacted. Adverse outcomes may be more likely if the donor is not in perfect health. An uninsured living donor is at risk if postdonation complications occur. Living related donors may be subjected to emotional pressure or coercion to donate a kidney, partial liver, or lung to a family member. Living donors may receive psychological and/or spiritual benefit from helping another person but the associated risks could be viewed as violating the ethical principle to do no harm (Howard & Cornell, 2016).

ETHICAL PRINCIPLES: THE RECIPIENT

Access to the waiting list for an organ transplant is a fundamental prerequisite to organ allocation. Appropriate and timely referral to a transplant center for evaluation must be made by the patient's provider so determination of transplant candidacy is established before the recipient becomes too ill to undergo transplantation and to optimize organ function and functional status or institute a bridge to transplantation interventions (e.g., left ventricular assist device or transjugular intrahepatic portosystemic shunt; Suarez-Pierre et al., 2019; Unger et al., 2017). Listing requirements may differ from center to center and from one organ to another. Allocation

practices based on a waitlist time need to be reviewed to ensure that variable waitlist practices do not discriminate against certain groups of patients. The ethical influence of the race, gender, religion, geography, and the social determinants of health on patient referral patterns, wait listing and delisting decisions, dual transplant center listing, and allocation must be considered by referring providers, transplant centers, and OPTN (Bababekov et al., 2020; Ng et al., 2020; Tsuang et al., 2021).

KEY TAKEAWAYS

- Understanding of immunology and histocompatibility is essential for the AGACNP to provide effective care and management of solid organ transplant recipients.
- Immunosuppressive medications have been developed to target specific areas of the immune system, and therefore each immunosuppressive agent carries a unique medication profile and toxicity risk.
- Successful transplantation requires maintaining balance between effective immunosuppression to prevent rejection and sufficient immunity to prevent infection.
- Posttransplant infections are a complication of a potent immunosuppressive regimen and exceed rejection in incidence.
- Evaluation of candidates for transplant wait listing requires comprehensive assessment of end-stage organ disease, degree of immune sensitization, medical comorbidities, and psychosocial factors.
- Care of the transplant recipient requires management of transplant-related issues (e.g. rejection, infection), as well as long-term sequelae, complications, and comorbidities, including renal insufficiency, hypertension, hyperlipidemia, diabetes mellitus, malignancy, obesity, metabolic syndrome, and cardiovascular disease.
- Solid organ donation and transplantation must consider ethical and psychosocial implications concerning the organ donor and transplant recipient.
- All aspects of transplantation require interdisciplinary collaboration with all members of the team, of which the AGACNP is key; the team has a unique responsibility to provide care that mitigates risk and ensures optimal transplant function and quality of life.

RESOURCES

TRANSPLANT ETHICS WHITE PAPERS

- Go to https://optn.transplant.hrsa.gov/resources/ethics/ for additional white papers on important transplant ethical topics

POSTTRANSPLANT MANAGEMENT GUIDELINES

- ATS: https://www.myast.org/education/guidelines-and-opinionsb
- International Society for Heart and Lung Transplantation (ISHLT): https://ishlt.org/publications-resources/professional-resources/standards-guidelines/professional-guidelines-and-consensus-documents
- Kidney Disease: Improving Global Outcomes (KDIGO): https://kdigo.org/guidelines/

A robust set of instructor resources designed to supplement this text is located at **http://connect.springerpub.com/content/reference-book/978-0-8261-6079-9.** Qualifying instructors may request access by emailing **textbook@springerpub.com.**

REFERENCES

Full list of references can be accessed at http://connect.springerpub.com/content/reference-book/978-0-8261-6079-9.

CHAPTER 24

GERONTOLOGICAL PRINCIPLES OF AGING

LaTricia D. Perry

LEARNING OBJECTIVES

- Differentiate the field of gerontology from geriatric medicine.
- Explore various gerontological theories and articulate implications for practice.
- Describe factors contributing to the complexity of care for aging individuals.
- Explain geriatric syndromes, including frailty and medication-related harm (MRH), and their implications for practice.
- Identify instances of elder abuse, neglect, and mistreatment and articulate implications for practice.
- Define gerontological measures of quality of life.
- Articulate barriers to care for aging individuals.

INTRODUCTION

The care of elders is optimized when adult-gerontology acute care nurse practitioners (AGACNPs) integrate gerontological theory into geriatric practices. Through the incorporation of sociological, biological, and psychological theories of aging into practice, elders are seen as complex individuals with needs that reach beyond the physical being. With full consideration of multifactorial influences on clinical conditions, geriatric syndromes, such as frailty, failure to thrive (FTT), and medication-related harm (MRH), give practitioners insight into the complexity of care for elders. Complex care often results in an increased frequency of interactions with formal and informal caregivers perhaps contributing to a potential for increased incidence of elder abuse/mistreatment, ageism, and FTT. Recognizing these actions and understanding implications for practice is highly valuable to the AGACNP, especially when working to maintain or improve the elder's quality of life. Additionally, AGACNPs should seek opportunities to reduce barriers to care during elderhood by addressing issues leading to avoidance, ensuring access and affordability through policy and program development, improving health literacy, and by embracing the initiative to create age-friendly health systems.

THE INTERSECTION OF GERONTOLOGY AND GERIATRIC MEDICINE

The field of gerontology focuses on the sociological, biological, and psychological aspects of aging as well as policy, research, and practice. Great strides have been made in this growing discipline to better understand the experience of aging from a multidimensional, interdisciplinary approach. Often used interchangeably with the term geriatrics, it is important to recognize that there are distinct differences between gerontology—the study of aging—and geriatrics, a specific branch of medicine or social science that focuses on providing medical care and treatment for elders. Practitioners who embrace the differences and the purpose of each specialty have the distinct opportunity to provide holistic healthcare to aging individuals as a way to potentiate patient outcomes. Ideally, geriatric holistic health assessment includes full consideration of the gerontological aspects of aging across all healthcare disciplines (Figure 24.1).

When assessing a patient in this way, a practitioner demonstrates that the elder's story with all of its complexities and life experience, both past and present, adds a complexity to the health needs as well as the potential compliance with the cocreated healthcare plan.

Nurses have the ability and tools to holistically assess elders in their care. However, when maximizing the approach to care for older adults, consider, whenever possible, an interdisciplinary approach to a healthcare plan. Embracing the knowledge and expertise of other disciplines when considering an appropriate plan of care, creates a multidisciplinary team to maximize patient outcomes especially when addressing the entire individual from a psychological, sociological, and biological perspective. When this type of team approach is used effectively, it has the potential to reduce the burden on the patient and the caregiver, especially if the care is delivered all in one clinic visit (Presley et al., 2020). Additionally, a multidisciplinary team approach offers a comprehensive assessment and management strategy with full consideration of all coexisting conditions to maximize services, improve quality of life, and optimize available resources for the elderly patient (Kar, 2019).

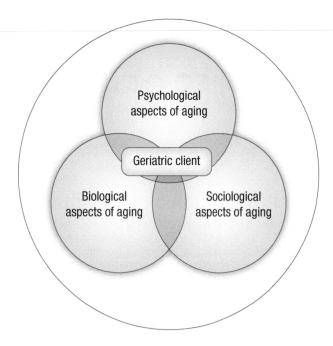

FIGURE 24.1: A geriatric holistic health assessment includes full consideration of the gerontological, biological, sociological, and psychological aspects of aging across all healthcare disciplines.

GERONTOLOGICAL THEORY IN PRACTICE

Although aging has been studied for centuries, gerontology as a formal science is relatively young dating back to the late 1920s with the establishment of the National Institute on Aging and with the first PhD programs in this field existing for just over 25 years. It is important to recognize, however, that various disciplines have studied aging and formed theories for decades and because of increased longevity, the study of aging has been revisited with greater interest in recent years to further advance theory in the field. The field of gerontology has often been considered data rich and theory poor (Bengtson & Settersten, 2016), but theory-based knowledge is being generated at a considerable rate each year to better understand the aging process through a theoretical lens. When exploring gerontological theories of aging, it is important to acknowledge that the various theories have emerged through transdisciplinary science and that all of the science, regardless of whether it is specifically nursing science, can and should be used to provide care for elders holistically. This approach allows for practitioners to consider more comprehensive and complex explanations of how the aging processes and patient outcomes are intertwined (Bengtson & Settersten, 2016). These explanations are best understood through sociological, psychological, and biological theoretical underpinnings.

SOCIOLOGICAL THEORIES OF AGING

At the core of social gerontology is this notion that aging and old age cannot truly be understood or explored without consideration to contributing sociological factors such as life practices and experiences across the life span (Dannefer & Settersten, 2013). Social gerontology considers the impact of a person's aging on their social structure and vice versa. Likewise, social gerontology explores and explains the impact or influence of the social structure on the population of older people as a whole; with significant interest in understanding how aging individuals respond to change within their social structure and the impact of that response to the population as a whole. There are numerous sociological theories of aging, a sampling of sociological theories are explored in this chapter for consideration and application to practice.

Life-Course Perspective

The life-course perspective, one of the most widely used theoretical frameworks in social gerontology, is grounded in the premise that in order to understand why an individual presents the way that they do, we must take into consideration their personal story and specifically understand the psychological and sociological factors as well as the historical and social structural changes through which they have traversed during their life course (Bengtson, 2016). A sociologist, Glen Elder, identified that the life-course perspective was based on the following five premises:
1. Development and aging are lifelong processes.
2. Individuals' lives are interdependently connected over time.
3. The choices that individuals make across their life course affect development.
4. Historical and social structural contexts influence an individual's development.
5. The timing and nature of life transitions affect an individual's development (Bengtson, 2016).
   These principles have been used by a plethora of life-course theorists since inception and serve to drive the quest for defining and ultimately achieving successful aging.

Activity Theory-Disengagement Theory Debate

Social integration in society, and the importance or necessity of such, is at the core of this debate between activity theorists and proponents of the disengagement theory. Activity theorists argued that occupancy in a role (or activity) was imperative for well-being in the later years of life; thus, when activity or role assignment waned in the later years of life as dictated by society (i.e., retirement), so did a sense of well-being for aging individuals (Marshall & Clarke, 2013). This society-imposed decrease in activity was considered to be involuntary; simply expected by societal norms. In contrast, disengagement theorists suggested that aging individuals naturally chose to disengage from activities and that the disengagement was actually an action of self-preservation, an opportunity for self-focus and to turn all energies inward to maintain a personal equilibrium as a mechanism for successful aging (Bengtson, 2016; Marshall & Clark, 2013). The reality is that neither of these theories perfectly explained the differences in individualized aging; however, even to this day, components of each theory are regarded as observable patterns of normal aging and thus, are still referenced and included in gerontological and geriatric practices.

Social Competence/Breakdown Model of Aging

This theoretical model evolved from fundamental principles of ageism and the influence of ageism on an individual's sense of social competence and worth in the social world (Bengtson, 2016). Depending on the level of perceived valuing or labeling across the life course, an individual might consider themselves socially competent or incompetent (Bengtson, 2016). A negative perception of self could lead to a vulnerability to health crises and to negative, dependent situations in later life where individuals begin to act in the way that they understand society expects them to act instead of acting in ways that work to break the cycle of competence breakdown (Bengtson, 2016). Practitioners have the ability to promote actions to counteract or to break this cycle but only when the efforts are set with intention to do just that.

BIOLOGICAL THEORIES OF AGING

It is not uncommon for illness or disease to be considered a normal characteristic of aging. However, it is important for practitioners to recognize that aging is not synonymous with disease or pathology. Indeed, there are certain aspects of the aging process which contribute to an individual's vulnerability to disease or illness, but there is no one pathology that is inevitable with age. Biological aging can be influenced through a variety of both modifiable and nonmodifiable lifestyle variables such as genetics, gender, or chronological age factors. It is the modifiable factors that practitioners can promote when working with elders as ways to influence one's aging experience through personal choices across the life span. It is also important for practitioners to recognize that the nonmodifiable factors must be considered in all plans of care in order for the aging individual to be cared for through a holistic lens.

The potential biological mechanisms of aging are numerous, not completely understood, and are often debated from a theoretical standpoint. Outward physical changes associated with aging and a decline in functionality are often the most common definable characteristics of aging and yet they are just two aspects of the biological mechanisms of change across the life span. At the core of biological changes are two distinct types of theories of aging, stochastic and nonstochastic, where both are based on changes at the cellular level within the human body, but the changes are prompted by different mechanisms. Additionally, as the average life expectancy rate continues to increase, it is important to not only understand the underlying properties of *how* people age by exploring the stochastic and nonstochastic theories, but it is also important to understand the *why* behind aging by exploring evolutionary models as an adaptive role in the aging process (Arbuthnott et al., 2016). Finally, this section weaves implications for advanced nursing practice throughout and as applicable.

Stochastic Theories

Replicative errors due to repetitive adverse changes in cells are the cause of aging in stochastic theories (Saxon et al., 2015). As the name suggests, the cellular changes associated with these theories are not predictable but rather random and due to an accumulation of errors over time. It is because of the accumulation of errors resulting in protein damage that stochastic theories are also known as failure accumulation theories (Barth et al., 2020). There are four common stochastic theories explored in this section: (a) Wear and Tear Theory; (b) DNA Damage Theory; (c) Environmental Theory, and (d) Stress Theory of Aging.

Wear and Tear Theory

Originally introduced in 1882 by Dr. August Weismann, a German biologist, the basic premise of this theory is that vital components of cells and tissue wear out, resulting in aging over time (Saxon et al., 2015). The accumulation of byproducts impedes the normal functioning of cells and tissues and contributes to defects in body parts and/or systems (Saxon et al., 2015). As is characteristic of a stochastic theory, an accumulation of the errors within the cells and tissues from wear and tear is what ultimately contributes to body system failure and death.

DNA Damage Theory

This theory, a generalization of the Free Radical Theory, is based on the notion that cells, once their DNA is damaged beyond repair, enter into a replicative period of senescence (Barth et al., 2020). The cause of such damage is believed to be a variety of internal and external stressors with chemical byproducts known as free radicals being one such stressor (Saxon et al., 2015). The body is typically able to destroy free radicals with protective enzyme systems or naturally occurring antioxidants in the body, but when the enzyme systems fail to protect from free radicals, they may accumulate causing cell membrane damage resulting in replicative senescence (Saxon et al., 2015). The ongoing presence of nonreplicative cells crowds the new and existing fully functioning cells to the point that the functioning cells cease to function and enter senescence (Barth et al., 2020). When cells are no longer able to function as intended, the body is unable to maintain homeostasis and organ failure occurs.

Environmental Theory

This theory is unique as it considers exposure to external stresses as the primary driver of cellular damage and changes that cause aging to occur (Barth et al., 2020). In this theory, these external stresses supersede any contribution that internal sources of cellular stress may have on the aging process and result in epigenetic modifications (Barth et al., 2020). External sources of stress may include but are certainly not limited to environmental factors such as ultraviolet light, toxic chemicals either inhaled or ingested, radiation, or exposure to element extremes but also include psychosocial stresses (Barth et al., 2020).

Stress Theory of Aging

Considered to be one of the most widely accepted theories of aging, this theory recognizes that there is no one specific accelerant of the aging process but rather, a culmination of stressors across the life span which contribute to the rate of aging (Barth et al., 2020). Cellular stress that results from insult to cells from both internal and external sources, accelerate the rate of aging over time in a complex and dynamic way especially when the stressors are chronic in nature (Barth et al., 2020).

Nonstochastic Theories

Unlike the random nature of stochastic theories, non stochastic theories suggest that aging is caused by predetermined or programmed replicated errors in cells within the body (Saxon et al., 2015). While there are many variations of nonstochastic theories of aging, Programmed Aging Theory and Immunological or Immunity Theory are highlighted in this section.

Programmed Aging Theory

Hayflick and Moorehead suggested in 1961 that the aging process was predetermined by the biologic or genetic clock where human fetal fibroblastic cells were only able to divide approximately 50 times in vitro before deteriorating; thus, there was evidence of a programmed aging at the cellular level (Saxon et al., 2015). This theoretical premise implies that life expectancy is intrinsically preprogrammed and independent of outside influence (Saxon et al., 2015).

Immunological or Immunity Theory

This theory posits that as one ages, the immune system becomes less effective in protecting the body from antigens, a process known as immunosenescence (Saxon et al., 2015). Additionally, the body, with age, struggles to differentiate its own tissues from invading antigens resulting in an autoimmune response as well as a decreased immune response in general (Saxon et al., 2015). Autoimmune responses in later life are a significant research interest and have been tied to a number of common disease processes such as Alzheimer's disease, rheumatoid diseases, hypertension, and thromboembolisms (Saxon et al., 2015).

Evolutionary Models of Aging

As the average life expectancy rate continues to increase, it is important to not only understand the underlying properties of *how* people age, but also to understand the *why* behind aging. The *why* is often best explained through evolutionary models of aging (Arbuthnott et al., 2016). Many of the aforementioned biological theories conform to the notion that evolution plays a role in the aging process where the evolution of aging can be best explained through three distinct categories: adaptation, maladaptation, and constraint (Arbuthnott et al., 2016). Each category provides a different perspective on the adaptive role of aging, and each comes with its own set of critics and supporters. At the core of each of these categories is the concept of fitness where *fitness* is when an individual, through the number of offspring they provide, or a gene, is able to prevail to or for future generations (Arbuthnott et al., 2016).

Adaptation

Often considered one of the first defined evolutionary perspectives of aging, the adaptive model posits that the resources consumed by *old* individuals are better used by the *young* leading to the death of the older individuals due to natural selection (Arbuthnott et al., 2016). At the core of this controversial and much debated theory is the notion that natural selection works to improve the fitness of an entire group as opposed to working for the fitness of individuals (Arbuthnott et al., 2016). In this instance, senescence, or deterioration with age, directly increases the fitness of a group where the association between fitness and aging has been determined to be causal in nature (Arbuthnott et al., 2016).

Maladaptation

Peter Medawar, the pioneer of this maladaptive model of aging, suggested that as age increases, there is a decrease in the strength of selection for specific traits at certain ages allowing for the aging process to evolve (Arbuthnott et al., 2016). The notion that genetic mutations could not be adapted for in later life because of the evolutionary principle that survival in late age and fertility have little to no effect on fitness fueled this theory and ultimately became known as the mutation accumulation model, most commonly referred to as simply MA (Arbuthnott et al., 2016). At the core of MA is the hypothesis that selection simply is incapable of removing the mechanisms of aging; thus, accounting for the origins of aging from an evolutionary perspective (Arbuthnott et al., 2016).

Constraint

This evolutionary model, also referred to as the antagonistic pleiotropy (AP), suggests that the relationship between aging and fitness is not causal; instead, aging is a maladaptive byproduct that lends itself to resulting senescence (Arbuthnott et al., 2016). Unlike MA, AP assumes that at a young age, genes exist that increase fitness, and likewise, as one ages, genes exist that decrease fitness (Arbuthnott et al., 2016).

PSYCHOLOGICAL PRINCIPLES OF AGING

With an understanding of select sociological and biological theories of aging, it is important to also consider foundational psychological principles of aging when caring for elders in practice settings. In general, the psychological aspects of aging are connected in large part to sociological influences in the aging process which are undergirded by theories of psychosocial development. These types of theories suggest that the experiences at an early age and across the life span, contribute to one's behavior in later years and that if developmental tasks are mastered at age-specific stages in the life cycle, then an individual is more likely to achieve personal-social adaptation (Saxon et al., 2015). While this premise is debated at times, the foundational premise of development milestones is often advantageous for practitioners when working with older adults to formulate holistic plans of care in practice settings. In this section, two specific psychosocial developmental theories, Maslow's hierarchy of needs and Erikson's stage theory of development, are discussed with a special focus on the application to an aging population.

Maslow's Hierarchy of Needs

Abraham Maslow proposed in the late 1960s that human needs and the ability to have those needs met directly motivated an individual's behavior. Maslow suggested that it wasn't just any random needs, but rather a hierarchy of basic human needs (see Figure 24.2) that had to be met prior to being able to consider the acquisition of higher-level needs where self-actualization/self-fulfillment was known to be the pinnacle of psychosocial

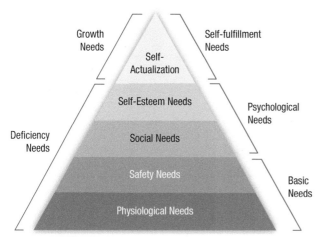

FIGURE 24.2: Maslow's hierarchy of needs.
Source: By Nmilligan.

achievement (Saxon et al., 2015). Maslow suggested that if basic physiologic and safety needs were not met, then it was impossible for an individual to progress to where their psychological needs met. Likewise, if psychological needs such as belongingness, love, and self-esteem were not met, then the individual could not reach their full potential in life to a point of self-actualization. This, in the context of cocreating a plan of care with a patient, bears consideration. Through this psychosocial developmental theory, practitioners are charged to individualize care after gauging the needs of their patient in the context of this defined hierarchy.

Erikson's Stage Theory of Development

In the late 1950s to early 1960s, Erik Erikson suggested that an individual's development could be measured by how they resolved defined developmental crises at distinct stages across the life span (Saxon et al., 2015). The premise behind this theory was that if an individual struggled to resolve a developmental crisis at a particular stage, then their personal development as they approached the next stage could be impacted negatively as well. This was not to imply that development in the future was destined to be negative but rather to suggest that an individual would have to intentionally make personal adjustments in their life to reroute their development in a positive direction. As can be imagined, this would require a great deal of personal reflection and some might argue, if considered in the context of Maslow's hierarchy of needs, would require that self-actualization be achievable.

Erikson posits that there are eight stages of development which are dynamically influenced by biological, psychological, and social factors across the life span (Orenstein & Lewis, 2020). The final two stages, Middle-Age: Generativity Versus Ego Stagnation, and Late Adulthood: Ego Integrity Versus Despair, are the two stages of most significance to the practitioner.

Generativity Versus Ego Stagnation

An acute realization of the finiteness of life, and how that finiteness is perceived, is at the core of this stage of development according to Erikson (Saxon et al., 2015). This stage, occurring primarily in the middle-age years of life (approximately 40–65 years of life), tends to prompt a shift from an ego-centric focus where stagnation can occur to a consideration of others or society as a whole, a sign of generativity (Saxon et al., 2015). With this comes a strong desire to leave a legacy— evidence of one's existence and contribution during one's lifetime as well as a desire to leave the world a better place because of one's existence. If individuals in this stage are unable to move past the ego, they may feel that they lack purpose and value in life rendering them stagnate in their personal development.

Ego Integrity Versus Despair

In Erikson's final stage of development, individuals 65 years of age and older are innately rewinding their life through personal reflection and assigning meaning to their actions over time. It is in this stage that individuals are identifying successes and failures and determining a sense of satisfaction with the accomplishments they have achieved. If their overall feeling is one of self-worth and satisfaction across the life span, then one is likely to achieve ego integrity. Likewise, if there is a sense of failure or inadequacy, then an individual may remain in a state of despair until they set the intention to make amends. At this point, if the individual struggled through any of the defined developmental stages, they may need assistance in the reflection of those unmet developmental stages in order to ultimately achieve a sense of ego integrity. Of particular interest is that Erikson's wife, Joan Erikson, added a ninth stage of development beyond achievement of ego integrity which takes into consideration the expansion of longevity and the unique challenges experienced with continued aging (Orenstein & Lewis, 2020).

IMPLICATIONS FOR NURSING PRACTICE

The application of gerontological theory in nursing practice offers a holistic perspective of aging individuals as they present for care. When there is consideration to the connectedness between the biological, sociological, and psychological aspects of aging, there is a unique opportunity to cocreate interdisciplinary plans of care for and with patients and a robust healthcare team. If practitioners adopt into practice either of the two developmental theories, then there is a strong desire to support patients to an outcome of self-actualization and/or ego integrity recognizing that without a strong sense of health and well-being this may not be achievable. Gerontological theory has the opportunity to guide practice, to guide patient education, to improve communication with patients, to maximize a patient's sense of subjective well-being, and to ultimately elevate patient health outcomes.

COMPLEXITY OF CARE

The U.S. Census Bureau in 2019 projected that by the year 2060, there will be 94.7 million persons aged 65 years or older (Figure 24.3). For perspective, in the year 2018, there were 52.4 million recorded in the same age bracket (U.S. Census Bureau, 2019). In preparation for this continued exponential population growth, practitioners must set the intention to understand the complexities of care that will accompany such growth both for the population as a whole, but also at the individual patient level. With this growing population will come a more diversified set of individuals whom practitioners will need to understand fully with cultural diversity needs, variation

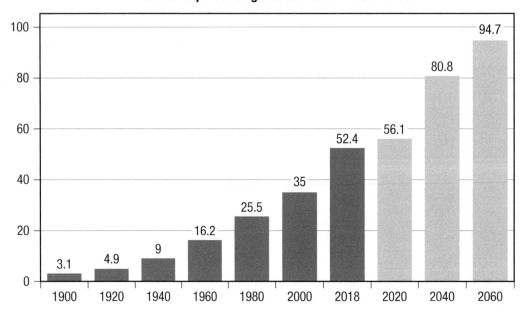

Number of persons age 65 and older: 1900 to 2060

Note: Increments in years are uneven. Lighter bars (2020, 2040, and 2060) indicate projections.

FIGURE 24.3: Number of persons aged 65 and older 1900 to 2060 (numbers in millions).
Source: Reprinted from U.S. Census Bureau. (2019). *2019 profile of older Americans*. https://acl.gov/aging-and-disability-inamerica/data-and-research/profile-older-americans

in needs based on geographic location, complexity of needs based on differing levels of care, just to name a few (Cline, 2015). Because of this, understanding the concept of *complexity of care* will be paramount to providing comprehensive healthcare to aging individuals.

Just as advances in gerontological theory are ongoing, so too are advances in understanding and disseminating information related to the complexities of care associated with aging. The National League of Nursing (NLN) in collaboration with the Community College of Philadelphia began the Advancing Care Excellence for Seniors (ACE.S) project in 2007 for the purpose of improving the dissemination of gerontological education specifically to nursing students (Cline, 2015). The project resulted in the ACE.S framework, defined by Tagliareni et al. in 2012, which emphasized how to provide quality care to and for older adults by defining essential knowledge domains—individualized care, complexity of care, and vulnerability during transitions—and also by defining essential nursing actions in each of the following categories: *A*ssessment of function and expectations, *C*oordination and management of care, *E*vidence-based knowledge (the use of), and *S*ituational decision-making (NLN, 2021). Of significance in the essential nursing actions was this notion of understanding not only geriatric syndromes but also understanding the way in which common diseases uniquely present in older adults. In this section, complexity of care for aging individuals is explored through the lens of geriatric syndromes with a specific emphasis on defining the concept; exploring frailty as a geriatric syndrome; defining FTT as a geriatric syndrome; and emphasizing the potential impact of the geriatric syndrome known as medication-related harm to include a review of the American Geriatrics Society (AGS) Beers Criteria©, and finally, woven throughout the section are implications for advanced nursing practice.

GERIATRIC SYNDROMES DEFINED

Believed to have evolved out of the mid 1960s term *geriatric giant,* a phrase coined by Bernard Isaac, geriatric syndromes are considered the modern giants in the field of geriatrics where value has been placed on early detection and intervention of these syndromes in an attempt to significantly improve patient outcomes by reducing disability, hospitalization, institutionalization, and mortality (Morley, 2017). Geriatric syndromes manifest as clinical conditions most often in frail older adults and are not readily attributed to one specific, underlying disease process. The cause of these syndromes is considered to be multifactorial in nature and the presentation of symptoms is believed to be attributed to an individual's inability to compensate for the culmination of multiple impairments of multiple systems within the body at one time (Magnuson et al., 2019). When an individual's reserves are taxed and they are unable to compensate for these impairments, practitioners are likely to see it

manifest in one of the commonly known geriatric syndromes such as falls, delirium (or other cognitive syndromes), polypharmacy, urinary incontinence, and/or depression. There are three specific geriatric syndromes covered in this section—frailty, FTT, and MRH. While these three syndromes are not more significant or more important than the other syndromes, insight into these syndromes have the opportunity to drive clinical practice in significant ways.

Frailty as a Geriatric Syndrome

Nearly three decades have passed since the concept of frailty was first introduced into the world of geriatric medicine (Church et al., 2020). At that time, the concept of frailty offered a way to define and describe some of the presenting complexities related to the health status of older adults (Church et al., 2020). This definition indicated that an individual was vulnerable to an evolving dependency, deterioration, and even mortality; the inevitability of which increased exponentially when exposed to additional physiologic and psychological stressors (Church et al., 2020). Understanding an individual's level of frailty and factoring that level into the plan of care has become paramount to lessening the vulnerability to poor health outcomes. As such, frailty measurement has become an integral component of geriatric health assessment as it guides practitioners in their determination of interventions which are beneficial versus harmful in providing individualized care to aging individuals (Church et al., 2020).

When evaluating an individual for a level of frailty, a practitioner must consider that assessment includes far more than a review of the prevalence or absence of disease. Frailty is not a result of one disease processes in the body, but rather a culmination of damage or disease processes in the body which contribute to diminished resistance and strength (Ates Bulut, 2018). Frailty, as a geriatric syndrome, manifests as a reduction in physical function compromising strength and endurance which can lead to falls, hospitalizations, long-term disability, dependence, and even mortality (Ates Bulut, 2018). It is important to acknowledge that individuals experiencing frailty will not present with frailty as a chief complaint; instead, practitioners must explore the individual through both gerontological and geriatric lenses to determine a level of frailty and determine how frailty impacts that individual (Ates Bulut, 2018). The key to maximizing the understanding of frailty in patient care with aging individuals is to recognize that frailty, and its implications, must be considered at the individual level, not from a generalized perspective.

A number of screening tools for frailty have been created over the years. One such tool, a clinical judgment frailty tool, aptly named the Clinical Frailty Scale (CFS), was created in the early 1990s for the Canadian Study of Health and Aging (CSHA) as a way to quantify or to summarize the experienced practitioner's perception of an individual's level of frailty or fitness upon completion of a thorough geriatric assessment (Church et al., 2020; Rockwood & Theou, 2020). The original CFS has undergone a number of revisions since it was created with the most recent revision, CFS 2.0, being published in 2020 (Rockwood & Theou, 2020). CFS 2.0 (Figure 24.4) evaluates different domains including cognition, function, and comorbidity where a score of 1 indicates that an individual is categorically *very fit* and a score of 9 indicates that an individual is categorically *terminally ill* (Rockwood & Theou, 2020). The higher the score on the scale, the more predictive of poor health outcomes including mortality, cognitive and/or functional decline, disability, comorbidity, prolonged hospitalization, readmission or admission into other institutions post hospitalization, and falls (Church et al., 2020). While a scoping review conducted by Church et al. (2020)

identified that the CFS has in the past been used most heavily in the hospital setting, the use in both in- and outpatient settings has gained momentum over time as practitioners are recognizing and reporting that the CFS is not only easy to use, but also effective in helping to identify appropriate interventions to form and shape holistic plans of care.

Another common frailty screening tool for use in the clinical setting is the FRAIL scale proposed by the International Association of Nutrition and Aging. This simplistic tool measures five specific components: self-reported *F*atigue, *R*esistance (ability to climb a single flight of stairs), *A*mbulation (ability to walk one block), *I*llness (prevalence of comorbidities—five or more), and *L*oss of weight (more than 5%; Walston et al., 2018). With 1 point possible for each of the 5 areas of assessment in the FRAIL scale, a score of 3 or more indicates

CLINICAL FRAILTY SCALE

	1	**VERY FIT**	People who are robust, active, energetic and motivated. They tend to exercise regularly and are among the fittest for their age.
	2	**FIT**	People who have no active disease symptoms but are less fit than category 1. Often, they exercise or are very active occasionally, e.g., seasonally.
	3	**MANAGING WELL**	People whose medical problems are well controlled, even if occasionally symptomatic, but often are not regularly active beyond routine walking.
	4	**LIVING WITH VERY MILD FRAILTY**	Previously "vulnerable," this category marks early transition from complete independence. While not dependent on others for daily help, often symptoms limit activities. A common complaint is being "slowed up" and/or being tired during the day.
	5	**LIVING WITH MILD FRAILTY**	People who often have more evident slowing, and need help with high order instrumental activities of daily living (finances, transportation, heavy housework). Typically, mild frailty progressively impairs shopping and walking outside alone, meal preparation, medications and begins to restrict light housework.
	6	**LIVING WITH MODERATE FRAILTY**	People who need help with all outside activities and with keeping house. Inside, they often have problems with stairs and need help with bathing and might need minimal assistance (cuing, standby) with dressing.
	7	**LIVING WITH SEVERE FRAILTY**	Completely dependent for personal care, from whatever cause (physical or cognitive). Even so, they seem stable and not at high risk of dying (within ~6 months).
	8	**LIVING WITH VERY SEVERE FRAILTY**	Completely dependent for personal care and approaching end of life. Typically, they could not recover even from a minor illness.
	9	**TERMINALLY ILL**	Approaching the end of life. This category applies to people with a life expectancy <6 months, who are not otherwise living with severe frailty. (Many terminally ill people can still exercise until very close to death.)

SCORING FRAILTY IN PEOPLE WITH DEMENTIA

The degree of frailty generally corresponds to the degree of dementia. Common symptoms in mild dementia include forgetting the details of a recent event, though still remembering the event itself, repeating the same question/story and social withdrawal.

In moderate dementia, recent memory is very impaired, even though they seemingly can remember their past life events well. They can do personal care with prompting.

In severe dementia, they cannot do personal care without help.

In very severe dementia they are often bedfast. Many are virtually mute.

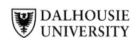

Clinical Frailty Scale ©2005–2020 Rockwood, Version 2.0 (EN). All rights reserved. For permission: www.geriatricmedicineresearch.ca Rockwood K et al. A global clinical measure of fitness and frailty in elderly people. CMAJ 2005;173:489–495.

FIGURE 24.4: Clinical frailty scale.
Source: Reprinted with permission of Rockwood, K., & Theou, O. (2020). Using the Clinical Frailty Scale in allocating scarce health care resources. *Canadian Geriatrics Journal, 23*(3), 254–259. https://doi.org/10.5770/cgj.23.463.

an individual is *frail* whereas, a score of 1 or 2 indicates a status of *prefrail*, and a 0 score finds the individual to be robust or *nonfrail* (Walston et al., 2018). This tool, when used either alone or in conjunction with other frailty screening tools, adds depth to the comprehensive geriatric assessment used to form and shape a holistic plan of care with the goal of optimizing patient care and health outcomes for aging individuals.

When working with aging individuals, it is important to acknowledge that there is often a coexistence of sarcopenia—loss of muscle mass and function—and frailty. The acknowledgment of these two conditions existing simultaneously provides additional insight into plausible interventions or treatment for aging individuals. For example, resistance exercise when performed routinely revealed evidence of increased lean muscle mass, improved grip strength, and improved gait speed (Dodds & Sayer, 2016). As noted in the FRAIL scale, an individual's ability to walk stairs or to walk around a block decreases the score assigned and further demonstrates the correlation between the two conditions. Likewise, if weight loss is indicated on the FRAIL scale, nutritional support and dietary improvements may be indicated. All of these examples give support for an interdisciplinary team approach to meeting geriatric and gerontological needs of aging individuals.

Failure to Thrive as a Geriatric Syndrome

Often defined by the prevalence of characteristics of frailty, FTT is another syndrome for consideration when working with older adults. Individuals with FTT often present with weight loss, decreased appetite and poor nutrition, inactivity, depressive symptoms, impaired immune function, and low cholesterol (Agarwal, 2021). The magnitude of global decline associated with FTT often worsens as the aging individual progresses through the frailty scale which corresponds to, and is compounded by, cognitive impairment and functional disability (Agarwal, 2021). If one were to view FTT in relationship to frailty on a continuum, FTT would be at the endpoint of the continuum with thriving at the opposite endpoint and with frailty somewhere around midpoint (Agarwal, 2021).

FTT, as a diagnosis, must be viewed through a holistic, gerontological lens. When working with older adults who present with conditions associated with FTT, it is important to look for causes of the presentation that are treatable; in essence: Is there a way to address or reverse the biological, psychological, or sociological shortfalls that are leading to this presentation (Agarwal, 2021)? In many instances, even after a comprehensive workup of the individual, evidence of treatable symptoms may not emerge. This further highlights the need to continue the management of underlying chronic conditions and intervene as needed to lessen the severity of symptoms related to FTT (Agarwal, 2021).

To evaluate for FTT, a practitioner may choose to rely on the CFS, previously discussed, to gain a foundational understanding of how the patient presents. Depending on the result of that assessment, a practitioner may choose additional assessment elements to address specific components of this complex syndrome. For instance, a practitioner may choose to run a comprehensive panel of labs, complete an assessment for inappropriate medications, consult with a dietician for the nutrition-related components of the syndrome, and gauge the patient's level of depression using the Geriatric Depression Scale.

Medication-Related Harm as a Geriatric Syndrome

When an individual presents for treatment of a new disease process, and that treatment includes a medication or multiple medications, it is imperative that practitioners review the existing treatment regimens in order to mitigate unintended adverse drug effects from occurring. As life expectancy increases, so, too, does the prevalence of co- and multimorbidity scenarios. In this instance, the likelihood of MRH also increases unless there is an intentional focus to mitigate the potential harm. Before mitigation can occur, there should be an understanding of the factors responsible for MRH such as biopsychosocial factors, polypharmacy, and inappropriate medication use which can then be followed up with a discussion related to harm-reducing efforts including an overview of the AGS 2019 Beers Criteria for Potentially Inappropriate Medication Use in Older Adults.

Biopsychosocial Factors Contributing to Medication-Related Harm

The multifactorial nature of MRH is best understood through a gerontological lens where there is consideration of all potential consequences of a prescribed medication (Figure 24.5). From the moment that a practitioner prescribes a medication, there are a variety of factors that could and will influence the consequence of the prescriber's choice of medication. With this in mind, it is important to assess for the biopsychosocial factors contributing to MRH up front in order for an individualized plan of care to result. From the biological perspective, age-related physiological changes have the ability to influence how drugs are internally processed and to potentially impact a drug's action, where the harm of taking the drug may outweigh the intended benefits (Stevenson et al., 2019).

In addition to biological factors, there are two primary psychosocial factors that have the potential to increase the prevalence of MRH: (a) an individual's ability to adhere to a prescribed medication regimen, and (b) their ability to rebound from insult to their psychosocial being (Stevenson et al., 2019). Other psychosocial factors, such as cognition, functional ability, social support, and/or financial circumstances, may also increase the potential for MRH due to an insult to psychosocial reserves.(Stevenson et al., 2019).

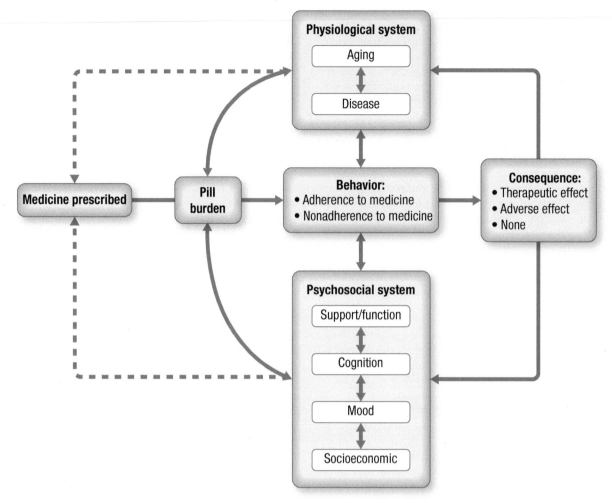

FIGURE 24.5: Simplistic linear visualization of the journey of a medicine from prescription to the effect on a patient.
Source: Republished with permission of Oxford University Press—Journals, from Stevenson, J. M., Davies, J. G., & Martin, C. (2019). Medication-related harm: A geriatric syndrome. *Age and Ageing, 49*(1), 7–11. https://doi.org/10.1093/ageing/afz121; permission conveyed through Copyright Clearance Center, Inc.

Polypharmacy and Inappropriate Medication Use

When considering new medications, it is important to recognize that the effectiveness and safety are typically investigated in controlled groups of research participants where someone with multiple morbidities or frailty is likely excluded (2019 AGS Beers Criteria Update Expert Panel, 2019; Khezrian et al., 2020). *Polypharmacy* is commonly (but not exclusively) defined as taking five or more medications, coupled with frailty or multimorbidities, and where the mechanism of action of each medication and the subsequent interactions between the medications are truly unknown and can lead to significant adverse health outcomes (Khezrian et al., 2020). This fact alone lends support for the prioritization of *individualized care* for aging individuals especially when comorbidities, frailty, and polypharmacy exist

as it ties back to the discourse surrounding complexity of care. There are cases where multiple medications are prescribed based on a holistic geriatric health assessment resulting in polypharmacy or even *excessive polypharmacy,* greater than or equal to 11 medications, and in these instances polypharmacy may be deemed completely appropriate (Khezrian et al., 2020).

Polypharmacy, especially where inappropriate medications are prescribed, has the potential to result in negative consequences for aging individuals (Halli-Tierney et al., 2019; Khezrian et al., 2020). Some of the negative consequences include an increased risk of disability, falls, frailty, adverse drug reactions, medication nonadherence and an increased frequency of accessing the healthcare system (Halli-Tierney et al., 2019). These consequences have the potential to further complicate an individual's well-being by decreasing quality of life, increasing the likelihood of mobility issues, and potentiating increased mortality (Halli-Tierney et al., 2019). The first step in avoiding inappropriate polypharmacy is to understand the risk factors for polypharmacy and to ensure than an assessment tool for polypharmacy and inappropriate medication usage in older adults is included in the practitioner's comprehensive geriatric health assessment methods.

Harm Reduction

In 2017, the World Health Organization (WHO) launched a Global Patient Safety Challenge related to medication safety with the goal of reducing the most severe and avoidable MRH by 50% by 2022 (WHO, 2017). In the call to reduce MRH, WHO shared a vision of improved medication processes including prescribing, dispensing, administering, monitoring, and use (WHO, 2017). It is important to recognize that at the time that WHO charged the healthcare system with this medication safety challenge, attention to potentially inappropriate medication (PIM) use in older adults had existed for a number of years and had now risen to a level of worldwide concern. Originally developed in 1991 by a U.S. geriatrician, Mark Beers, the Beers Criteria for Potentially Inappropriate Medication Use in Older Adults (i.e., at least 65 years of age) continues to be the gold standard for mitigating harm from medications. In 2011, the AGS adopted the charge to continue Beers' work and began to compile and disseminate updated criteria for PIM in what became known as the AGS Beers Criteria, a tool to be used by clinicians, researchers, educators, regulators, and healthcare administrators (2019 AGS Beers Criteria Update Expert Panel, 2019). The intent behind developing this tool was to improve medication selection by clinicians; to act as an education tool for both clinicians and patients; to improve quality of care; and to reduce MRH in the form of adverse drug events (2019 AGS Beers Criteria Update Expert Panel, 2019).

In 2019, the AGS elicited the expertise of an interdisciplinary panel to ensure that the criteria used in 2015 remained relevant. After a review of the evidence, the expert panel determined that the five criteria for inappropriate medication use in older adults should continue to fall into the following categories: (a) PIM use in older adults; (b) PIM use in older adults due to drug-disease or drug-syndrome interactions that may exacerbate the disease or syndrome; (c) drugs to be used with caution in older adults; (d) potentially clinically important drug–drug interactions that should be avoided in older adults; and (e) medications that should be avoided or have the dosage reduced with varying levels of kidney function in older adults. This evidence-based tool is maintained and published for the purposes of being a guide for drugs to avoid in older adults; however, it is not intended to supersede clinical judgment or to deny a patient access to any or all medications (2019 AGS Beers Criteria Update Expert Panel, 2019).

The AGS Beers Criteria is one tool to aid in ensuring that medication is appropriately prescribed, however, there are other explicit and implicit checklists which can be used for medication review such as the *Screening Tool of Older Person's Prescriptions* (STOPP) tool and the *Medication Appropriateness Index* (MAI) tool (2019 AGS Beers Criteria Update Expert Panel, 2019; Halli-Tiernay et al., 2019). When these tools are used by an interdisciplinary team to formulate an individualized holistic plan of care, the effects of their use have the potential to improve patient outcomes in a significant way.

ELDER ABUSE, NEGLECT, AND MISTREATMENT

Assessing for elder abuse is imperative with every comprehensive geriatric encounter. The National Council on Aging (NCOA) reports that approximately 1 in 10 Americans aged 60 and older have experienced some form of elder abuse, with a family member perpetrating 60% of the abuse and neglect incidents (NCOA, n.d.). To better understand the phenomenon of elder abuse, one must be able to first define it, understand potential causes and consequences, be cognizant of screening methods, and understand the nurse's mandatory role in the reporting of such findings.

DEFINING ELDER ABUSE, NEGLECT, AND MISTREATMENT

The National Clearinghouse on Abuse in Later Life (NCALL), a national project of the End Domestic Abuse Wisconsin: The Wisconsin Coalition Against Domestic Violence, was created in 1999 with the intention to provide resources to better understand the connections between domestic violence, sexual assault, and elder abuse, neglect, and exploitation (NCALL, 2021). NCALL defines abuse in later life as "the willful abuse, neglect, abandonment, or financial exploitation of an older adult who is age 50+ by someone in an ongoing, trust-based relationship (i.e., spouse, partner, family member, or caregiver) with the victim" (NCALL, 2021, p. Abuse in Later Life). This definition also includes sexual abuse of an older adult by anyone (including strangers) but excludes self-neglect and other types of abuse committed by strangers (NCALL, 2021). With this definition in mind, NCALL sought to further identify, with input from survivors of abuse, neglect, and/or mistreatment, various tactics which could be included in each of these types of abuse, mistreatment, or neglect and developed a visual of these known as the Abuse in Later Life Wheel (Figure 24.6; NCALL, 2021). For each tactic employed (e.g., threatening, targeting vulnerabilities, denying access to spiritual traditions), perpetrators were reported by survivors to behave in both psychological and emotionally abusive ways (NCALL, 2021). While the Abuse in Later Life Wheel does not encompass all potential

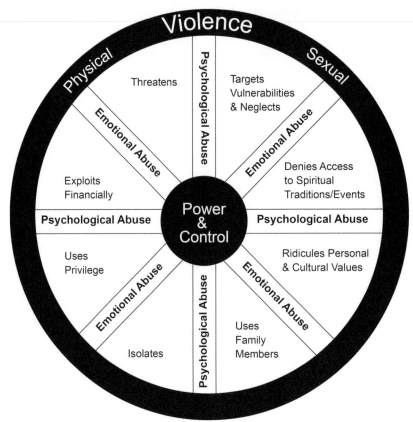

FIGURE 24.6: Abuse in Later Life Wheel.
Source: Published with permission from National Clearinghouse on Abuse in Later Life, an End Domestic Abuse Wisconsin initiative.

forms of abuse, neglect, or mistreatment because it excludes self-neglect and abuse at the hands of strangers, it does provide a conceptual model for practitioners to pause and reflect on when working with aging individuals who may be experiencing (or who have experienced) these acts and are in need of support or intervention (Table 24.1).

Abuse, neglect, and mistreatment can happen in a variety of settings, including an individual's home, a family member's or caregiver's home, in an assisted living facility, or in a nursing home. Given that there are a number of types of elder abuse, neglect, and mistreatment, it is highly possible that an incident could go undetected unless a formal assessment is conducted and even then, some elders may choose not to disclose for fear of retaliation or simply because they have become used to being treated a certain way and have accepted it as a norm. Use of a comprehensive screening tool may be instrumental to identifying and responding to incidences of elder abuse when working with aging individuals.

Risk Factors for Elder Abuse

It is important for all practitioners to be knowledgeable about the risk factors for elder abuse when working with an aging population. Understanding these risk factors

may assist practitioners in identifying opportunities for prevention. In cases of elder abuse the older adult victim and the perpetrator often have some level of risk if the abuse is discovered. The victim is at higher risk when they are dependent upon another for care, when their mental capacity is impaired, and/or if they have a history of being an abuser to the now caregiver (Earlam et al., 2018). Elder abuse can also be a result of self-neglect which may have a variety of risk factors as well. The perpetrator, often a formal or informal caregiver, is at risk for inflicting harm on an older adult when experiencing caregiver stress, fatigue, dissatisfaction with their current arrangement, overwhelmingness, a history of violence or substance-abuse disorders, psychological impairments, lack of coping mechanisms, and/or a lack of support resources (Earlam et al., 2018). At the community level, the risk of perpetration is higher when formal services (e.g., respite care for caregivers) are either limited or unavailable (Centers for Disease Control and Prevention [CDC], 2020). It is also possible that society as a whole plays a role in elevating the risk of perpetration if the cultural norm includes a high tolerance for aggressive behavior, if caregivers are given liberty to make decisions in routine care, if family members are expected to care for elders without outside supports or resources, and finally

TABLE 24.1: Examples of Behaviors per Each Tactic in the Abuse in Later Life Wheel

TACTIC	EXAMPLES OF BEHAVIORS
Physical	Bodily harm caused by hitting, pushing, slapping, choking, burning, pinching, and/or restraining an individual against their will.
Sexual	Sexual harm caused by a caregiver where the individual is either forced into sex acts or is forced to watch sexual acts.
Psychological	Public humiliation, threats of harm
Emotional	Yelling, name calling, degradation
Targets vulnerabilities and neglects	The act of taking away or denying access to items necessary for daily life including food, protection from elements, care and/or medication; refusing to meet or secure transportation needs; deviates from or refuses to follow medical recommendations or plan of care; refuses to dress or dresses inappropriately
Denies access to spiritual and traditional events	Belittles spiritual and/or traditional practices, destroys spiritual or traditional items of importance
Ridicules personal and cultural values	Disrespectful of cultural practices; makes decisions for the individual without consideration for personal or cultural values
Uses family members	Misleads family members regarding condition of older adult; completely excludes or denies access to family
Isolates	Controls all actions of the older adult including who they see and what they do; denies access to modes of communication such as the phone, mail, or other technologies
Uses privilege	Makes all major decisions on behalf of the older adult; speaks for the individual at financial and medical appointments
Exploits financially	Steals money, titles, or possessions; abuses a power of attorney or guardianship
Threatens	Threatens to leave or commit suicide; threatens to institutionalize; abuses or kills pets; displays or threatens with weapons

Source: Adapted from the Abuse in Later Life–Tactic document ©2005 provided by the National Clearinghouse on Abuse in Later Life, an End Domestic Abuse Wisconsin initiative.

if there is a prevalence of ageist beliefs in society (CDC, 2020). Ageist beliefs, when coupled with chronic staffing problems, stressful working conditions, and staff burnout may be significant contributors to increased risk for perpetration of vulnerable elders in institutional settings, thus calling for strong administrative oversight and education in these settings as a protective measure (CDC, 2020). The prevalence of these risk factors does not automatically mean that violence will occur, but they do provide insight into the potential for abuse, if protective factors are not introduced (CDC, 2020).

ELDER ABUSE SCREENING

Screening for elder abuse and mistreatment is essential when conducting a comprehensive geriatric assessment. There are a variety of assessment methods available to practitioners for adoption and integration into routine assessments, such as purposeful interviewing coupled with a thorough skin assessment and the Elder Assessment Instrument (EAI).

Purposeful Interviewing and Thorough Skin Assessment

When a patient presents with physical injuries, it is important to not assume abuse exists, but rather to begin the interview with open-ended questions to determine the cause of the injuries (Earlam et al., 2018). Recalling the various tactics, including behaviors, as defined in the Abuse in Later Life Wheel, may help to direct questions for clarification during the interview. If a caregiver is present during the interview, asking to speak with the individual alone is reasonable but if either the older adult or the caregiver insist on them staying, instead, monitor for inconsistencies in the explanation of how injuries occurred versus the actual presentation of the injury and/or a dismissive attitude related to the injuries (Earlam et al., 2018). An additional cause for concern would be if there is evidence that the dyad had been seeking emergency care from multiple emergency departments with repeated injuries (Earlam et al., 2018). The interview may provide insight or direction into potential protective factors to be implemented or it may drive additional actions for the practitioner. Regardless, a thorough skin assessment is paramount to a comprehensive geriatric assessment. When conducting a full-body skin assessment, the practitioner should assess all skin, including the genitals, documenting all findings, suspicious or otherwise (Earlam et al., 2018). This assessment should also assess for signs of dehydration, malnutrition, and poor dental health (Earlam et al., 2018). Thorough and accurate documentation of findings at present will be helpful in comparing findings to any future assessments as well.

Elder Assessment Instrument

One method for documenting the interview findings of the skin assessment is to employ an assessment tool such as the EAI. This 41-item instrument offers a rapid and sensitive assessment of the signs, symptoms, and subjective complaints associated with elder abuse, neglect, and mistreatment including exploitation and abandonment (Fulmer, 2019). While the tool does not provide a scoring system where a certain score would indicate the need for a referral, it should be noted that a social service referral is considered warranted if the following exist:

1. Evidence of abuse, neglect, or mistreatment,
2. Subjective complaints of elder abuse, neglect, or mistreatment by the older adult, or
3. The practitioner determines through a comprehensive assessment that the older adult is at high risk for mistreatment or abuse (Fulmer, 2019).

This instrument has proven efficacy in ensuring appropriate supports and actions are taken when mistreatment is suspected.

MANDATORY ROLE IN DETECTING AND RESPONDING TO ELDER ABUSE, NEGLECT, AND MISTREATMENT

Patient safety is always a priority responsibility for practitioners. By committing to conducting comprehensive geriatric assessments that include risk factor assessment, practitioners have the opportunity to institute protective factors for elder abuse as a way to reduce the risk for the perpetration of abuse. Identifying and mitigating risk factors may reduce the incidence of abuse in the aging population. Referring individuals, including caregivers of the older adult, to community organizations and agencies may be source of additional support. If an elder presents with evidence of abuse, the practitioner is charged to act on the evidence or suspicion as a mandated reporter (including specifics on how the report is filed). It is important for practitioners to recognize that all states have mandated laws for reporting elder abuse. It is imperative that the AGACNP be familiar with the reporting mandates and statutes in the state(s) in which they work.

QUALITY OF LIFE

When considering the gerontological aspects of aging, it is imperative that consideration be given to how an individual perceives their own sense of well-being or level of life satisfaction as measures of quality of life (van Leeuwen et al., 2019). Quality of life (QoL) is a term that is not easy to define, but through a thematic synthesis of literature, nine QoL domains emerged:

1. Health perception: A positive personal perception of health where there were no limits due to physical condition.

2. Autonomy: Able to manage independently; retaining a sense of dignity; not feeling like a burden to others.
3. Role and activity: Able to allocate personal time to doing activities that result in a personal sense of value, purpose, and involvement with others.
4. Relationships: Engaging in reciprocal relationships where the individual feels supported and also supports others.
5. Attitude and adaption: Having a positive as opposed to a pessimistic outlook.
6. Emotional comfort: Feeling at peace.
7. Spirituality: Believing in something; feeling connected to faith and personal development from beliefs, practicing rituals, and self-reflection.
8. Home and neighborhood: Feeling a sense of security at home with access to neighborhood amenities.
9. Financial security: Feeling comfortable with the financial situation enough that needs are met and a feeling of restriction is avoided (van Leeuwen et al., 2019).

Tying back to the previous discussions related to self-actualization in Maslow's hierarchy of needs as well as Erikson's stage of ego attainment, a strong sense of quality of life may lend itself to improved patient outcomes. Likewise, if an aging individual presents with a sense of a poor quality of life, this will need to be considered when creating a holistic, interdisciplinary-derived plan of care. The intersectionality of each of the domains adds complexity as a change in one domain may have a positive or negative impact on other domains. Understanding where an individual fits into each of the domains may help the practitioner home in on areas of most concern.

BARRIERS TO CARE

When considering barriers to care through a gerontological lens, a plethora of potential challenges for elders emerges. This section covers only a smattering of potential barriers and should not be interpreted as all possible barriers to care. First, it is important to acknowledge that some challenges are personal in nature where an individual prefers to avoid rather than access healthcare for a variety of reasons. Geographic proximity to healthcare resources, lack of transportation, or in the case of telehealth, either a lack of access to technology or an inability to operate the necessary technology to access the care can result in barriers to accessing healthcare especially for individuals living in rural communities or large metropolitan areas but truly could pose challenges for any aging individual. Affordability of healthcare and treatment plans, including medications, continues to be an issue for millions of Americans. Additionally, there are challenges when it comes to health literacy which may loop back around to how we are sharing information with the aging population in the first place. And, finally, there are challenges with access to age-friendly health systems for all individuals. This is not to say that great strides are not being made in improving access, but rather, this is simply to raise awareness to areas where all healthcare providers can continue the efforts for change and equality in access to care.

AVOIDANCE

One might ask why an individual would choose to avoid healthcare, preventive or otherwise, when affordability was not an influencing factor. One theory is that the way in which an individual perceives their aging process, self-perceptions of aging (SPA), or subjective aging (SA), plays a role in whether or not an individual will access care and at what point in a health crisis, they might receive care (Sun & Smith, 2017). Older adults with negative SPA have been found to be less likely to seek preventive care, only seeking care when urgent or emergent care is necessary (Sun & Smith, 2017). This reactive access to healthcare, as opposed to proactive access, lends itself to more serious long-term physical and, potentially, psychosocial sequelae. In these instances, an older adult with a negative SPA may consider their health-related concerns and comorbidities as a normal part of aging; believing that there is nothing a healthcare provider can do for them, so choosing simply to accept the challenges and to avoid accessing healthcare (Sun & Smith, 2017). AGACNPs have the opportunity to counterbalance this mindset during all interactions with older adults by promoting more positive aging self-perceptions and by inviting individuals to share all of their symptoms whether they believe them to be part of the normal aging process or not. By engaging in this way, older adults may recognize that their aging experience is unique to them and that new ailments deserve discussion as opposed to acceptance as part of the aging process (Sun & Smith, 2017).

Communication patterns between healthcare providers and older adults can also contribute to avoidance in seeking healthcare (Galvin & Todres, 2015; Sun & Smith, 2017). Individuals seeking healthcare often enter the clinic settting with a healthy dose of vulnerability and when that vulnerability is met with a communication style that is demeaning, dismissive, or patronizing, even if done unintentionally, a rupture of dignity—the value one places on self—leading or contributing to a negative SPA can result (Galvin & Todres, 2015). This can be especially true for marginalized populations of older adults (i.e., members of the LGBTQ community, members with special needs, ethnically or racially diverse individuals). In addition to having a negative impact on individuals in this way, these communication patterns can lead to health inequities unless the intention is set by practitioners to make an effort to meet individuals where they are and to meet their communication needs in every encounter.

HEALTHCARE ACCESS IN RURAL COMMUNITIES

The proximity to sufficient healthcare services may be compromised based on the geographic location of residence. Access to adequate transportation in rural and urban settings may prove to be a barrier if transportation to and from healthcare appointments is not readily accessible. Individuals in rural areas are more likely to have to travel long distances in order to access the care that may be needed especially when specialty care is needed. In addition, there may be extra financial burdens related to travel expenses, time away from the workplace for self or for caregiver, and lodging if the distance requires an overnight stay (Rural Health Information Hub [RHI Hub], 2019). Practitioners will need to consider these types of barriers when cocreating plans of care with patients as to ensure that the plan is reasonable given the older adult's unique circumstances and geographic location.

DIGITAL INEQUALITY

Technology adoption by older adults has climbed over the past decade or two with roughly two thirds of those 65 years of age and older reporting use of the internet in some fashion (Anderson & Perrin, 2017). Additionally, technology is getting into the hands of older adults through the purchase and use of smart phones or devices at a rate of 42% (Anderson & Perrin, 2017). In spite of these gains, this still leaves one third of older adults who do not use the internet and approximately one half of all elders without broadband services in their home (Anderson & Perrin, 2017). Household income is a predictor of access and use of technology where only 27% of individuals with an annual household income below $30,000 have broadband in their home (Anderson & Perrin, 2017). These scenarios lend themselves to the limitation of access to healthcare services (i.e., telehealth appointments), healthcare literacy materials, and appointment scheduling services which are so readily available and referred to in the healthcare industry today. It is important to consider that even when an individual has access to both a device and to the internet, it does not necessarily indicate that the individual also has the skills, confidence, or desire to use the tools. Practitioners have the opportunity to gauge access and level of comfort with necessary technologies associated with an individualized plan of care.

AFFORDABILITY

Health insurance affordability is a concern shared by aging individuals in the United States especially during a period of time where there are significant legislative, regulatory, and legal challenges to the Affordable Care Act (Tipimeni et al., 2020). The concern lends itself to some aging individuals finding it a necessity to stay in the workforce longer in order to keep existing health insurance in a time of uncertainty (Tipimeni et al., 2020) and leaves other individuals having to rely solely on Medicare, Medicaid, or having to strike a balance between securing supplemental health insurances (known as a "spend down" process) while on a fixed income in order to continue to qualify for Medicaid (Medicare. gov, 2021). Certainly, there are varying levels of coverage including those individuals who are able to secure private insurance to supplement Medicare coverage. Even when health insurance is secured, there are concerns related to meeting out-of-pocket expenses including prescription medication costs (Tipimeni et al., 2020). These barriers can circle back around to avoidance previously discussed; avoidance to accessing healthcare as well as avoidance in filling prescription medications manifesting in an impact to health outcomes (Tipimeni et al., 2020).

HEALTH LITERACY

Another barrier to healthcare for consideration is *health literacy*—an individual's ability to access and subsequently, use information and services to drive personal health-related decisions and actions (CDC, 2021). According to the National Assessment of Adult Literacy (NAAL), print health-related materials posed challenges adults older than 60 years at a rate of 71%; likewise, forms and charts posed difficulties for 80% of the same population (CDC, 2019). Consideration must be given to both the health education content shared with elders, but also the way in which the information is disseminated to the population. The CDC suggests that there is a need for an interdisciplinary approach to improving health literacy with contributors in these efforts coming from business, education, government leaders and agencies, health insurers and providers, the media and many other organizations and individuals who are willing to invest in improved health literacy leading to improved health outcomes (CDC, 2021). The *Healthy People 2030* initiative has expanded the defining characteristics of health literacy to include a public health perspective where both individuals and organizations use their health literacy skills collaboratively to improve the health of the community (CDC, 2021). Practitioners are challenged with understanding how to measure health literacy when working with patients. But there are some basic strategies that can be employed to help meet the health literacy level of most individuals, such as ensuring that all literature is free from jargon and technical language, that the material is presented in an engaging and compelling way, and by defining actual actionable items or steps for older adults to take to promote health and well-being (CDC, 2019).

LACK OF AGE-FRIENDLY HEALTH SYSTEMS

This section offers support to the value of creating and fostering Age-Friendly Health Systems as a mechanism to mitigate or to diminish barriers to healthcare for aging individuals. The Age-Friendly Health Systems, a collaborative initiative of The John A. Hartford Foundation, the Institute for Healthcare Improvement (IHI), American Hospital Association, and the Catholic Health Association of the United States, was created to address the reality that health systems are lagging in their ability to reliably provide evidence-based practice for older adults at every point of care due in large part because of the population boom (IHI, 2021). The aim of this initiative was threefold: (a) to commit to the use of an essential set of evidence-based practices; (b) to cause no harm; and (c) to commit to knowing what is important—what matters—to the older adult and their caregivers (IHI, 2021). This initiative is expressed through a conceptual model known as the 4Ms where each of the Ms stand for an evidence-based element of high-quality care in either a hospital or a practice setting (IHI, 2021). Each of the 4Ms—(What) Matters, Medication, Mentation, and Mobility—is to be adopted and practiced as a full set of actions (IHI, 2021). The What Matters component seeks to ensure that each healthcare entity or practitioner is individualizing care and working collaboratively with the patient to both know and align care with the older adult's care preferences and healthcare goals (IHI, 2021). The Medication component ties back to using an assessment tool such as 2019 AGS Beers Criteria to ensure that appropriate medications are being used and these age-friendly medications are not impeding in any of the other 4M areas; that is, What Matters, Mobility, or Mentation (IHI, 2021). The Mentation component is truly about the prevention, identification, treatment, and management of delirium (IHI, 2021), which can result in a cascade effect of other geriatric syndromes especially when it goes unmanaged. And, finally, maintaining functioning through Mobility in a safe way must be at the forefront of all care in age-friendly settings (IHI, 2021). When the initiative was first launched, the ambition was to spread the 4Ms framework to 20% of U.S. hospitals and medical practices by 2020 (IHI, 2021); ongoing efforts and adoption by more systems and practitioners are paramount to continued success in this arena.

CONCLUSION

This chapter has explored the gerontological aspects of aging as they intersect with geriatric medicine and patient care. When these elements intersect, they provide the AGACNP with the opportunity to conduct a holistic geriatric assessment that includes full consideration of the sociological, biological, and psychological aspects of aging to cocreate an individualized plan of care. As such, this also gives merit to the notion that aging individuals are complex with needs that exceed the physical and/or biological presentation.

EVIDENCE-BASED RESOURCES

Age-Friendly Health Systems: https://hign.org/consultgeri/try-this-series/age-friendly-health-systems-4ms

American Geriatrics Society: https://www.americangeriatrics.org/

American Geriatrics Society Guidelines, Recommendations and Position Statements: https://www.americangeriatrics.org/media-center/news/older-people-medications-are-common-updated-ags-beers-criteriar-aims-make-sure

American Society on Aging: https://www.asaging.org/

Try This©: Series: https://hign.org/consultgeri-resources/try-this-series

Gerontological Society of America: https://www.geron.org/

Hartford Institute of Geriatric Nursing: https://hign.org/

Healthy People 2030 – Older Adults: https://health.gov/healthypeople/objectives-and-data/browse-objectives/older-adults

National Council on Aging: https://www.ncoa.org/

National Institute on Aging: https://www.nia.nih.gov/

National League for Nursing – ACE.S: http://www.nln.org/professional-development-programs/teaching-resources/ace-s

World Health Organization – WHO Global Patient Safety Challenge: Medication Without Harm: https://www.who.int/patientsafety/medication-safety/en/

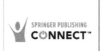

A robust set of instructor resources designed to supplement this text is located at **http://connect.springerpub.com/content/reference-book/978-0-8261-6079-9.** Qualifying instructors may request access by emailing **textbook@springerpub.com.**

REFERENCES

Full list of references can be accessed at http://connect.springerpub.com/content/reference-book/978-0-8261-6079-9.

PART IV

SPECIAL CONSIDERATIONS FOR ADULT-GERONTOLOGY ACUTE CARE NURSING PRACTICE

CHAPTER 25

PALLIATIVE AND END-OF-LIFE CARE

Kristina Kordesch

LEARNING OBJECTIVES

- Identify and understand the difference between hospice care and palliative care.
- Understand the role of palliative and end-of-life care in acute care.
- Define advance care planning, advance directives, living will, and healthcare proxy.
- Understand basic strategies for symptom management for end-of-life care in acute care.

PALLIATIVE CARE AND HOSPICE CARE: DEFINITIONS AND DIFFERENCES

Palliative care is a clinical specialty that focuses on improving quality of life by the prevention and relief of suffering. Palliative care in acute care settings provides patient centric, holistic care that complements the medical care of the acute and critically ill. The World Health Organization (WHO) defines palliative care as "an approach that improves the quality of life of patients (adults and children) and their families who are facing problems associated with life-threatening illness. It prevents and relieves suffering through the early identification, correct assessment and treatment of pain and other problems, whether physical, psychosocial or spiritual" (WHO, 2012). When providing palliative care in conjunction with medical patient care, it is not necessary to stop the curative treatment of illness. Palliative care medicine works alongside and with clinical care and has a focus on a multidisciplinary approach to provide medical, social, emotional, and practical support to patients and families (National Institute on Aging [NIA], 2021).

Palliative care can often transition to hospice care. This transition can occur when the patient and family choose to increase emphasis on comfort care and the medical provider believes the patient is likely to die within 6 months. In hospice care, attempts to cure the person's illness are stopped (NIA, 2021). Support is given to the patient, family/caregivers to provide pain relief, and the emotional and spiritual support needed. Hospice care can be provided in a variety of settings, in the patient's home, in a hospice facility, and often in an inpatient hospital setting.

PALLIATIVE AND HOSPICE CARE: A BRIEF HISTORY

Palliative and hospice care have an intertwined history. The palliative care specialty grew from the practice of hospice care. The history of hospice care as it is now practiced in the United States was first widely documented in the United Kingdom and is largely attributed to nurse/physician Cicely Saunders, who founded many hospice homes. Her model of care was adopted in the United States by Florence Wald, Dean of the Yale School of Nursing after Saunders was an invited speaker and presented her model of hospice care at Yale in 1963. Wald began practicing hospice care and eventually founded a hospice home, which focused on a multidisciplinary approach to alleviate suffering for the dying rather than a focus on curative medicine. Hospice practice developed and gained momentum, which led to the first hospice organization in the United States in 1978: The National Hospice Organization (NHO; Buck, 2011), which, with strong advocacy, demonstrated patient-centered care and increasing popularity in the medical community. The Healthcare Finance Administration (now Centers for Medicaid & Medicare Services [CMS]) conducted a national project to study hospice efficacy, reimbursement, and to establish regulations and standards of hospice care. This study provided the framework and data to create the Medicare Hospice Benefit which was introduced in the United States in 1982 and became permanent in 1986. The Medicare Hospice Benefit is a prospective reimbursement service for hospice care, provides Medicare payment for hospice work, and has facilitated expansion of hospice services nationwide (Connor, 2007–2008).

Palliative care grew from the early hospice work of Saunders and Wald. Dr. Balfour Mount studied Saunders's model and visited Wald's hospice home in the United States. He coined the term "palliative care" and expanded upon the scope of hospice care to patients with chronic illness but not necessarily at the end of life (Clark, 2007). Over the last three decades, palliative care presence in acute care and in the ICU has increased dramatically (Angus et al., 2004). Palliative care has developed into a recognized specialty by WHO, is a recognized subspecialty by the board of American Board of Medical specialties since 2006, and certification is offered for Advanced Practice Registered Nurses by the National Board for Certification of Hospice and Palliative Nurses.

EVIDENCE-BASED RESOURCES

Hospice and Palliative Nurses Association: https://
advancingexpertcare.org//
WHO Palliative Care: https://www.who.int/health-topics/
palliative-care
National Hospice and Palliative Care Organization: https://
www.nhpco.org/palliativecare/

PALLIATIVE CARE

The expansion and wide adoption of palliative care has shown great benefit to the care of chronically ill patients and continues to be a necessary and rapidly growing field of study. There is robust evidence of the contribution palliative care has in patients' lives. Early palliative care has been shown to improve reported quality of life and mood, and these patients have had less aggressive care at the end-of-life in accordance with their wishes (Temel et al., 2010). There is an overall preference to be cared for at home at the end-of-life, and yet the overwhelming majority of U.S. deaths happen in hospitals. However, there has been a shift toward patient preference to die out of the hospital in recent years. Since the widespread adoption of palliative and hospice care, inhospital deaths have decreased and the utilization of hospice facilities and death at home have increased significantly (Cross & Warraich, 2019).

The 2014 World Health Assembly Resolution on Palliative Care designated palliative care as an essential medical service, and their report recommends that every national healthcare system should incorporate palliative care into their continuum of practice. Furthermore, it reiterates that this access to palliative care should be available without discrimination or healthcare coverage status. The broad aim is to recommend revision of local laws and processes to facilitate access to adequate pain control with opioids to patients in need and to include palliative care training and education for all healthcare workers (WHO, 2014).

Multiple national organizations have supported and championed the wide adoption and advancement of the palliative care specialty. The *Lancet* journal has a commission on palliative care and pain relief and has identified lack of pain control and lack of access to palliative care at the end-of-life a global health crisis. This highlights the importance of understanding the global and local need for palliative care, calls for the increased availability of palliative care globally, and advocates to facilitate the availability and appropriate usage of opioids for analgesia (The Lancet Commission Report, 2017).

Many protocols and guidelines to aid the delivery of palliative care exist. Protocol-driven care can improve patient and system outcomes; however, the specifics of each institution and patient population make it challenging to create a universal guideline. The National Coalition for Hospice and Palliative Care has commissioned the National Consensus Project for Quality Palliative Care (NCP) and has worked to establish national guidelines for care. This relays the holistic nature of palliative care by addressing the structure and coordination of care, physical and symptom management, psychological, social, spiritual, and cultural aspects of care (NCP, 2018).

CLINICAL PEARL

- Six elements of quality palliative care: (a) integrated teamwork; (b) management of pain and physical symptoms; (c) holistic care; (d) caring, compassionate, and skilled providers; (e) timely and responsive care; and (f) patient and family preparedness (Seow & Bainbridge, 2018).

PALLIATIVE CARE IN THE INTENSIVE CARE UNIT

While the traditional goal of critical care is to reduce mortality and provide curative care, despite all of our medical capabilities, many patients die in the ICU. In fact, roughly 1 in 5 Americans die after ICU admission (Angus et al., 2004). Despite the focus on curative care, death and end-of-life care is a very present and important event in the ICU. It is imperative that critical care providers are trained and well-versed in the background and scope of palliative care, able to communicate effectively with patients and family about advance care directives, comfort care, and end-of-life. Numerous areas of ongoing research and initiative exist to further incorporate the palliative care specialty into the ICU.

While being well-versed is essential for the critical care provider, palliative care is a specialty unto itself, and consultation and collaboration with a palliative care team for patients in the ICU can be invaluable. Patients who have early palliative care involvement are more likely to have formalization of advance directives and have lower use of nonbeneficial life prolonging treatments at the end-of-life, despite having the same mortality rate (O'Mahony et al., 2010) and are more likely to have comfort care orders placed before the end-of-life (Angus et al., 2004). A close collaboration between the critical care team and the palliative care team provides supportive, patient-centric care.

HOSPICE CARE

The goal of hospice care is "[a death] that is free from avoidable distress and suffering for patients, families, and caregivers, in general accord with patient's families' wishes; and reasonably consistent with clinical, cultural, and ethical standards" (Field et al., 1997).

During their hospital stay, many inpatients shift their goals of care from curative to comfort care. The transition from ICU to hospice ward is a common discharge path; therefore, the transition of care between the critical care provider and the hospice provider should be clearly communicated (NCP, 2018). Despite efforts to accommodate patient preferences—that is, to leave the ICU and transition to home or hospice ward—end-of-life procedures often occur in the ICU (Field et al., 1997). A shared decision-making model (among patients, families, and medical staff) shifts the focus of care to comfort, but ICU patients are often too unstable for transfer to a hospice ward or home. Understanding the basic principles of end-of-life care—and having protocols in place to provide holistic end-of-life care—can facilitate a peaceful end-of-life regardless of the setting.

CHALLENGES IN HOSPICE CARE

Potential or probable nonbeneficial treatment is common at the end of life, frequently in the ICU and oftentimes despite the patient's expressed wishes (Cardona-Morrell et al., 2016; Lee et al., 2020). This is likely due to the traditional curative goal of medicine, or clinician's inclination to provide life-sustaining treatment or "trying everything" despite understanding it may be futile (Visser et al., 2014). In order to provide effective care and recognize the appropriateness of goals of care, training is an essential role in incorporating palliative care in the ICU. Barriers to patient centric end-of-life care are many and include cultural, fiscal, literacy, and access. These barriers may be addressed or avoided with training in a holistic approach to patient care and can provide tools to communicate effectively in end-of-life conversations (Cardona-Morrell et al., 2016; Visser et al., 2014). A lack of preparation and training in providing palliative care can correlate to moral distress at the bedside, affecting both advanced practice providers and nursing staff (Wolf, 2019).

CULTURAL COMPETENCY AND SENSITIVITY

Cultural beliefs, values, and expectations shape a patient's and family's expectation and definition of a "good death" (Martin & Barkley, 2017). Every effort should be made to accommodate and incorporate these values in end-of-life care. Racial disparities exist and have been described in end-of-life care. Challenges and barriers to care of multiethnic patients have been identified and described by both clinicians and patients and families. Families of Black patients versus non-Black patients reported lower satisfaction with communication, concerns of being uninformed, and dissatisfaction with clinician interactions (Welch et al., 2005). Multiethnic patients and clinicians reported significant barriers to end-of-life care despite identifying it as a very important issue (Barwise et al., 2019). Language barriers often impair the ability to have quality end-of-life discussions in the ICU, and non-English-speaking patients have consistently

extended stays before an advance care directive is identified and report less clarity in end-of-life proceedings (Barwise et al., 2019). Clinicians have also reported barriers to effective communication with multiethnic patient populations, including language and interpretation issues, lack of understanding or knowledge of patient's cultural beliefs, limited health literacy, and patients'/families' mistrust of healthcare (Periyakoil et al., 2015).

Hospice usage is also lower for non-White populations, and many socioeconomic and cultural barriers exist (Hughes & Vernon, 2020). Hospice services that had staff-wide cultural sensitivity training and available language services to meet the needs of their diverse patient populations reported better relationships with patients and families of diverse backgrounds. Examples of the reported benefit of cultural training included anticipating and addressing potential mistrust in the healthcare system, understanding differences in perceptions of pain/comfort, and anticipating the differences in amount of family participation in hands-on patient care (Hughes & Vernon, 2020)

ADVANCE CARE PLANNING

Advance care planning is the process of a person communicating their preferences about values and preferences regarding what type of medical care they want, such as emergency treatments and life- sustaining therapies. It involves discussions between the patient, their family or trusted loved ones, and their healthcare providers. There are multiple ways to document and ensure that a person's advance care wishes are known (NIH, 2021). The ICU setting is the exact location advance care planning is meant to account for, and yet only 40% of ICU patients have advance directives documented (Kruser et al., 2019). Effort must be made to obtain advance care planning documents if they exist, or to obtain them if possible. In the case of a critical care provider, the advance care planning conversation is time sensitive. Patients who lack decision-making capacity during their hospitalization and have a surrogate decision maker are more likely to receive aggressive life-sustaining measures prior to death. Many of these patients lose their decision-making capacity during hospitalization, resulting in a missed opportunity to discuss end-of-life with the patient themselves (Zaros et al., 2013). Having an advanceddirective prior to losing the ability to participate would potentially reduce the pain and discomfort of the dying patient and ease the burden of decision-making of surrogates. The clinician's role is to guide the patient in understanding the interventions and treatments they are evaluating, including giving examples and scenarios, and to document their preferences. The clinician can also facilitate identification and notification of an appropriate healthcare proxy who will assist in decision-making if the patient is unable. This conversation is dynamic, ongoing, can be revisited at any time, and can be documented in the form of an advance directive (Silveira, 2021).

Definitions

- *Advance directive*: A legal document documenting a person's preferences and values regarding what medical treatments they agree to (or do not agree to) in the case that they are not able to make their own medical decisions.
- *Living will*: One form of an advance directive. It provides specific instructions for what treatments a person would want if they are dying or permanently unconscious. It often contains treatment or situational-specific questions a person can answer prior to their illness.
- *Healthcare durable power of attorney or healthcare proxy*: This is a legal document that designates a person who can make medical decisions for someone else, should that person become unable to make their own medical decisions. This can provide for unforeseen healthcare decisions that may not have been discussed in a living will (Silveira, 2021).

If a person does not have any advance directives or legal healthcare proxy, there is legislation authorizing who can be designated as a surrogate for a person unable to make their own medical decisions. Local guidelines will inform this designation.

EVIDENCE-BASED RESOURCES

The conversation project: https://theconversationproject .org/nhdd/advance-care-planning/
NIA: National Institute on Aging: Advanced Care Planning https://www.nia.nih.gov/health/advance-care -planning-health-care-directives

END-OF-LIFE CARE

END-OF-LIFE CONVERSATIONS AND COMMUNICATION IN THE INTENSIVE CARE UNIT

Often our critically ill patients do not have advance care directives prior to admission (Kruser et al., 2019) and so discussions with patients or their surrogates must occur in the critical care setting when patients are very sick or at risk of imminent death. Every effort should be made to discuss advance care planning with the patient themselves if they have decision-making capacity. When this is not possible, building a trusting relationship with patients' families can lay the groundwork for successful communication. This is a difficult task in the ICU, with a critically ill patient and a distressed family. Regular structured conversations (sometimes called family meetings) in the ICU, addressing questions and concerns of clinical care, and understanding the patient as an individual have demonstrated a reduction in anxiety, posttraumatic stress disorder (PTSD), and depression scores of family members of ICU patients (Rhoads & Amass, 2013). Word choice and communication style are also important considerations in these conversations. Clinicians must effectively communicate prognosis while appreciating the family's level of understanding of the clinical situation under the toll of a high stress and emotional situation (Berlin, 2017). Delivering honest and consistent messages and acknowledging uncertainty will establish a shared understanding and facilitate conversation (Table 25.1). Consultation and collaboration with a palliative care service will aid in communication and support families and providers in this process (Berlin, 2017).

PAIN, DYSPNEA, AND THIRST

As the focus of care shifts to comfort at the end of life, three main areas of discomfort have been consistently identified and described by patients in the ICU. These are pain, dyspnea, and thirst. Appropriately identifying these discomforts and having strategies to alleviate them are core tenets to end-of-life care. Using an established and validated pain measurement tool can provide better assessment of analgesic and comfort needs (Puntillo et al., 2014).

Pain

Pain at the end of life has been consistently reported and has been identified by patients and families as a fear of end-of-life care (Blinderman, 2015). Opioids are the most common pain medication used in end of life, with morphine and fentanyl being the most common. However, among institutions and providers, significant practice variabilities in pain medication ordering exist (Laserna et al., 2020). Mild pain can first be treated with NSAIDs or acetaminophen, or a low dose opioid. Moderate to severe pain should be treated with opioids, with a combination of long-acting and short-acting formulations. This should provide lasting comfort and the ability to treat episodic or "breakthrough" pain (Blinderman, 2015). Long-acting dosing can then be increased in a stepwise manner.

Dyspnea

Dyspnea is a common and challenging symptom to treat, especially in the critically ill population (Obarzanek & Campbell, 2021). Oxygen therapies such as nasal cannula and noninvasive pressure support ventilation may be employed to treat hypoxemia in various disease states. There is a lack of evidence to support these therapies for the treatment of dyspnea, and therefore they are not regularly used in comfort care (Puntillo et al., 2014). Other drug and nondrug therapies are often employed to help treat dyspnea. Opioids are the most common pharmacologic therapy used, and can have the dual purpose of analgesia and treating dyspnea. Nondrug therapies such as upright positioning, fans, and cold cloths may decrease distress (Table 25.2). In instances where mechanical ventilatory support is removed, the clinician should anticipate and treat dyspnea: A bolus of opioid and a benzodiazepine (as an anxiolytic) is recommended (Blinderman, 2015).

Thirst

Thirst and mouth dryness are significant discomforts of ICU patients. Providing hydration and relief from thirst when possible is an important consideration

TABLE 25.1: Family Meeting/Goals of Care Conversation: Key Objectives and Phrases to Use and to Avoid in the Critical Care Setting

OBJECTIVE	SAMPLE PHRASES TO USE	PITFALLS TO AVOID
Create the right setting and open the family meeting	"Thank you for taking the time to come in to talk about your mom. How are you doing with all of this?" "I want to make sure we all understand what we need to do so that we can give her the best care possible. Before we get started, are there any specific topics you want us to address?"	Setting a dominant tone; delivering an exhaustively detailed clinical summary
Probe for understanding	"Tell me what you know about your mother's condition right now."	Sharing information without assessing prior understanding: "I am not sure if any of the other doctors mentioned this, but your mother [has cancer/had a heart attack/etc.]…"
Deliver prognostic information	"Your mother is very sick. While we are doing everything possible to help her pull through, there is a very serious chance she might not make it…" [pause/allow silence]… …And if she does, she will likely be so weak and debilitated that she will not be able to go home for a very long time, if ever."	Offering false hope or mixed messages: "While things look very grave right now, you never know. Things could always turn around for the better."
Elicit goals/values and fears/worries	"Tell me about your mom. What kind of person is she? What kinds of things are important to her? What do I need to know about her as a person in order to provide the best possible care?" "What do you think she would have to say about this if she could speak for herself right now?" "Was there anything your mom was particularly looking forward to before this all happened?" "What worries you most?" "Can you think of any abilities or activities so crucial to your mom that she would find life without them intolerable?"	Focusing on treatments and procedures: "Do you want us to do the feeding tube or not?" Using language not grounded in reality: "What would your mom have wanted?"
Expect emotion; demonstrate empathy and respect	"Sometimes what is important to you might be different from what would be important to your mom. Is it hard for you to stay focused on her perspective?" "I really respect your ability to put aside your own priorities and be such an amazing advocate for her." "I see your eyes are welling up. This is very hard. Can you tell me more about what you are feeling right now?"	Assuming one understands: "I know how you must feel." Devaluing emotion: "I understand you are angry about what happened, but we need to focus on what to do next."
Make appropriate treatment recommendations grounded in patient goals and values; consider a time-limited trial Affirm commitment to patient and caregiver well-being	"Your mom took the trouble to let us know how she felt about treatments at the end of life. We should honor and respect what she told us." "Based on your mom's priorities, I recommend we start dialysis. Let's see how things go and plan to meet again in the next 48 hours. If by the end of the week things don't turn around, we should discuss a plan B focused on maintaining what you've told me would be most important for her." "We will do everything possible that will help your mom. Her comfort and dignity will be our top priorities." "Let's talk about how we might be able to fulfill your mom's wish to die at home." "Looking back on this 6 months from now, I want you to know in your heart that we all did the best we could–you included." "Can you think of any religious services or spiritual support that would be helpful to you right now?"	Failing to provide a viable alternative; leaving decision up to the surrogate: "Do you still want us to keep doing everything?" Feeding into fears of abandonment and lack of caring: "I think we should stop aggressive therapy." "My recommendation is to withdraw care."
Summarize, strategize, and adjourn	"I know this is a lot of information. It is normal to feel overwhelmed. Would you like some time to process this, before meeting again to discuss some next steps?" "Can you think of anything you wanted to talk about that we haven't addressed?" "I am sure you will think of additional questions. Please write them down so we can discuss them next time we meet." "Thank you so much for sharing what you did with me today. It has helped me understand and appreciate a lot more about your mom and how important she is to you." "Let's get together again on Friday for another update. Would that work for you?"	Prematurely closing the door to further questions or concerns: "If you have no more questions, I think that is about all we have to cover."

Source: Reproduced with permission from Berlin, A. (2017). Goals of care and end of life in the ICU. *Surgical Clinics of North America, 97*(6), 1275–1290. https://doi.org/10.1016/j.suc.2017.07.005

TABLE 25.2: Dyspnea Interventions, Mode of Action, and Rationale

INTERVENTION	DOSE	MODE OF ACTION	RATIONALE
Optimal positioning, usually upright with arms elevated and supported	Whenever patient reports dyspnea or displays respiratory distress	Increases pulmonary volume capacity	Increases air exchange which may improve oxygenation and carbon dioxide clearance and reduce inspiratory effort
Balance rest with activity	Guided by dyspnea/respiratory distress	Decreases excessive oxygen consumption	Prevents hypoxemia
Space nursing care			
Oxygen as indicated by goals of therapy; not useful in normoxemia or when the patient is near death and in no distress	Variable, guided by goals of therapy and patient characteristics	Improves the partial pressure of oxygen; reduces lactic acidemia	Treats hypoxemia
Opioids, such as morphine or fentanyl	Low doses titrated to the patient's report of dyspnea or display of dyspnea behaviors is effective; oral or parenteral; no evidence to support inhaled administration; no evidence on dosing regimens	Uncertain direct effect; reduced brainstem sensitivity to oxygen and carbon dioxide; altered central nervous perception	Strong evidence base supports effectiveness
Benzodiazepines, such as lorazepam or midazolam	Low doses titrated to the patient's report of dyspnea or display of dyspnea behaviors; no evidence for benzodiazepine regimens	Anxiolysis	Fear or anxiety often accompanies dyspnea

Source: Reproduced with permission from Puntillo, K., Nelson, J. E., Weissman, D., Curtis, R., Weiss, S., Frontera, J., Gabriel, M., Hays, R., Lustbader, D., Mosenthal, A., Mulkerin, C., Ray, D., Bassett, R., Boss, R., Brasel, K., & Campbell, M. (2014). Palliative care in the ICU: Relief of pain, dyspnea, and thirst–A report from the IPAL-ICU Advisory Board. *Intensive Care Medicine, 40,* 235–248. https://doi.org/10.1007/s00134-013-3153-z

(NICE, 2015). Often patients are too weak or unable to tolerate eating or drinking, but there are strategies to alleviate the discomfort of dryness. A "bundle" of sprays of water, gauze with cold water, and lip moisturizer has been shown to significantly reduce thirst and dryness in ICU patients (King et al., 2021).

WITHDRAWAL OF SUPPORT

For end-of-life proceedings for the critically ill, there are often multiple life-sustaining treatments to be withdrawn. These can include the ventilator, vasopressors, continuous dialysis, or advanced cardiac devices. The coordination of the withdrawal of these therapies is crucial to providing a peaceful transition for both the patient and the family. Institutions should develop standard protocols for the withdrawal of life-sustaining treatment (Braganza et al., 2017). A meeting at the bedside with the multidisciplinary team and family to create a plan and alleviate any concerns is recommended. A checklist or huddle with nurses, respiratory therapists, clinicians, and families may provide more communication and organization of this process (Lele et al., 2019).

PATIENT-CENTERED CARE

Many initiatives exist to provide emotional and holistic support for patients and families during the dying process. The 3 Wishes Project was designed to celebrate the lives of dying patients by asking about and carrying out three final wishes for dying patients in the ICU. The project aim is to reinforce meaningful human connection at the end of life, even when occurring in the ICU (Vanstone et al., 2020). Another initiative is the program No One Dies Alone, a project started by a critical care nurse which has been adopted at many hospitals nationwide. The goal is to provide compassionate companionship by providing volunteers who come to the bedside for patients in hospice or end-of-life care in the hospital without a family or a support system (Hojat et al., 2020).

EVIDENCE-BASED RESOURCE

The 3 Wishes Project: https://3wishesproject.com/

A robust set of instructor resources designed to supplement this text is located at **http://connect.springerpub.com/content/ reference-book/978-0-8261-6079-9.** Qualifying instructors may request access by emailing **textbook@springerpub.com.**

REFERENCES

Full list of references can be accessed at http://connect .springerpub.com/content/reference-book/978-0-8261-6079-9.

CHAPTER 26

PAIN AND PAIN MANAGEMENT

Jacqueline Ferdowsali

LEARNING OBJECTIVES

- Analyze the pathophysiology of nociception.
- Compare and contrast nociception and pain.
- Differentiate between different components of a pain assessment.
- Construct a multimodal pain management strategy for a patient with acute pain.

INTRODUCTION

Pain is a complex phenomenon that requires an equally nuanced approach to assessment and treatment. Understanding the pathophysiologic process of nociception and the different types of pain experienced informs a multimodal treatment approach. Conducting a comprehensive pain assessment based on a biopsychosocial framework allows for a complete treatment strategy to be developed. Both pharmacologic and nonpharmacologic treatment interventions should be considered when treating acute pain.

PATHOPHYSIOLOGY OF PAIN

Whether a localized event or a more generalized insult there are few other physiologic responses that more profoundly impact the body and person as pain. The concept of pain has been experienced, described, and studied for millennia. Recent advances in neurobiology and clarifying definitions have added to not only the understanding of pain but also the treatment. The structure of this section is to provide a context in which the approach to assessment and treatment of pain can be better understood by drawing on a pathophysiologic framework. To begin, pain and nociception are two different concepts. The International Association for the Study of Pain (IASP, 2017) defines pain as *"an unpleasant sensory and emotional experience associated with, or resembling that associated with, actual or potential tissue damage."* This definition puts forward that pain is not just a biological experience outside of one's control but rather relies on an interaction of the subcortical and cortical systems. The neural process of changing a stimulus into a chemical event in the nervous system is termed "nociception" (Yam et al., 2018). It is imperative to understand that a nociceptive event does not always lead to the perception of pain.

NOCICEPTION

The neural response to a noxious stimulus involves several steps. First, a noxious stimulus, such as tissue damage or temperature extremes, triggers a chemical event that then interacts with a free nerve ending, also termed a nociceptor. This process is known as transduction (Yam et al., 2018). Nociceptors are considered afferent (sensory) neurons and innervate all the areas of the body. The types of nociceptor receptors include mechanoreceptors, thermal, chemical, polymodal, and silent. These receptors are responsible for the transmission in pain signaling. There are two types of afferent neurons: namely A delta fibers and C fibers. A delta fibers contain myelin and are responsible for the initial perception of the noxious stimulus. The C fibers do not have myelin and control the intensity of the stimulation (Kendroud et al., 2020). The chemical event is mediated by neurotransmitters which can be excitatory, inhibitory, or a combination of both. Table 26.1 provides an overview of key neurotransmitters for consideration and their physiologic effect. The afferent neurons then come together at the dorsal root ganglion for the body, the trigeminal ganglion for the face and the pain perception is transmitted through the ascending spinothalamic tracts. Finally, the pain perception travels within the cerebrum to various areas such as the cingulate, somatosensory, insular cortex, and amygdala (Figure 26.1; Yam et al., 2018).

Two important concepts to consider when evaluating responses to noxious stimuli are that of sensitization and modulation. Sensitization implies a change in response of nociceptors than what would be expected. Clinically, this can be demonstrated through hyperalgesia or allodynia. Allodynia is the experience of a painful event by a stimulus that would not normally produce pain and hyperalgesia is an increase in pain beyond what would be expected (IASP, 2017). Modulation is the augmentation of peripheral messages by either the spinal cord or descending outputs. Modulation can either reduce or inhibit the neuronal message. The concept of modulation is integral to the theory of pain described later in this chapter.

TABLE 26.1: Pain-Associated Neurotransmitters

NEUROTRANSMITTER	LOCATIONS OF CHEMICALS	FUNCTION
Prostaglandin E2 and prostacyclin	CNS and PNS	Excitatory/inhibitory
Leukotriene B4	PNS	Excitatory/inhibitory
Nerve growth factor	CNS and PNS	Excitatory
Proton	CNS and PNS	Excitatory
Bradykinin	CNS and PNS	Excitatory
Adenosine triphosphate and adenosine	CNS and PNS	Excitatory/inhibitory
Tachykinins (substance P, neurokinin A, neuokinin B)	CNS andPNS	Excitatory
Hydroxytryptamine	CNS and PNS	Excitatory
Histamine	CNS and PNS	Excitatory
Glutamate	CNS and PNS	Excitatory
Norepinephrine	CNS and PNS	Excitatory/inhibitory
Nitric oxide	CNS and PNS	Excitatory/inhibitory
Calcitonin gene-related peptide	CNS and PNS	Excitatory
Gamm-aminobutyric acid	CNS and PNS	Inhibitory
Opioid peptides	CNS and PNS	Inhibitory
Glycine	CNS	Inhibitory
Cannabinoids	CNS and PNS	Inhibitory

Demonstrates pain-associated neurotransmitters, the location within the central nervous system (CNS) and peripheral nervous system (PNS) and their function.

Source: Data from Yam, M. F., Loh, Y. C., Tan, C. S., Khadijah Adam, S., Abdul Manan, N., & Basir, R. (2018). General pathways of pain sensation and the major neurotransmitters involved in pain regulation. *International Journal of Molecular Sciences, 19*(8), 2164. https://doi.org/10.3390/ijms19082164

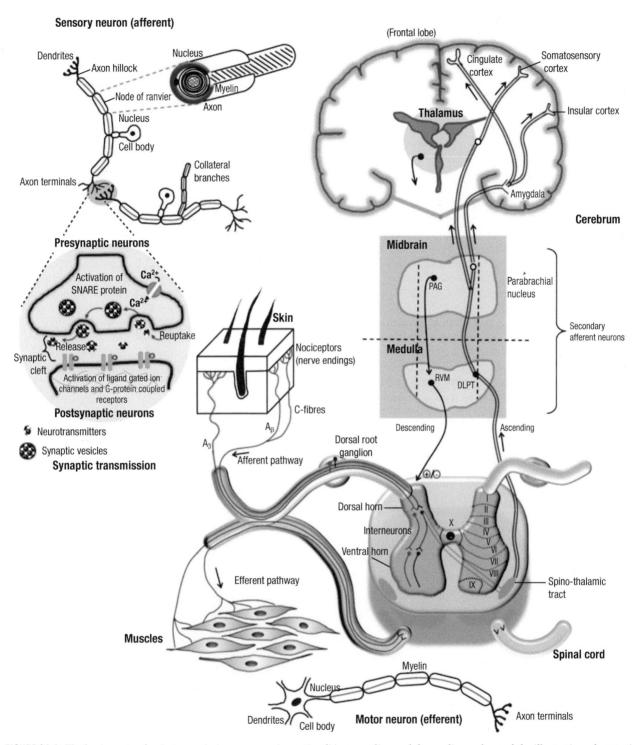

FIGURE 26.1: The basic route of pain transmission upon noxious stimuli in ascending and descending order, and the illustration of synaptic transmission in synaptic cleft.

Source: Reproduced with permission from Yam, M. F., Loh, Y. C., Tan, C. S., Khadijah Adam, S., Abdul Manan, N., & Basir, R. (2018). General pathways of pain sensation and the major neurotransmitters involved in pain regulation. *International Journal of Molecular Sciences*, *19*(8), 2164. https://doi.org/10.3390/ijms19082164, Fig. 1

The pathophysiology of chronic pain is less understood. There are several proposed mechanisms which contribute to peripheral nerve injury and likely chronic pain including altered channel expression, upregulation of markers for neuronal injury, increased expression of receptors, and loss of inhibition (Aronoff, 2016).

MODULATION AND PERCEPTION OF PAIN

As the definition by the IASP indicates, pain is not merely a reflexive, uncontrollable response to a noxious stimulus. Rather, pain is modulated and perceived through biologic, psychologic, and social contexts. Our modern understanding of pain has origins in gate control theory now known as the neuromatrix theory of pain (Frediani & Bussone, 2019). This framework bears witness to the thought that pain is not a simple stimulus/response mechanism but relies on interpretation and consciousness that can result in memories.

The descending pain modulatory system includes the periaqueductal gray area and the rostral ventromedial medulla in the brainstem which have been directly connected to the cerebral cortex areas (Tobaldini et al., 2019). This direct connection further supports the role of conscious control of response to painful stimuli, also referred to as a top-down approach. This provides context to the experience and why some individuals report little pain or have few signs or symptoms of pain while others have significantly different experiences. Also key within the descending pain modulatory system is the endogenous opioid system which inhibits substance P.

Together, transduction, transmission, modulation, and perception form the pillars of the experience of pain. There are several different categories of pain, defined in Box 26.1.

BOX 26.1 DEFINITION OF DIFFERENT TYPES OF PAIN

- **Nociceptive Pain:** Pain that arises from actual or threatened damage to nonneural tissue and is due to the activation of nociceptors
- **Neuropathic Pain:** Pain caused by a lesion or disease of the somatosensory nervous system
- **Nociplastic Pain:** Pain that arises from altered nociception despite no clear evidence of actual or threatened tissue damage causing the activation of peripheral nociceptors or evidence for disease or lesion of the somatosensory system causing the pain.

Source: Reproduced with permission from International Association for the Study of Pain. (2017, December 17). *IASP terminology*. https://www.iasp-pain.org/terminology?navItemNumber=576#Sensitization

COMPREHENSIVE PAIN ASSESSMENT

Every patient reporting pain should undergo an evidence-based comprehensive assessment. A comprehensive pain assessment is based on the biopsychosocial model which informs the biopsychosocial model of pain management (Figure 26.2; U.S. Department of Health and Human Services, 2019). Pain has physical, psychological, social, emotional, and spiritual components which contribute to the individual's perception and tolerance of pain. As the multidisciplinary panel for acute pain management through the American Academy of Pain Medicine highlights, pain assessment is not a singular event related to a numeric scale but rather a comprehensive assessment of the impact of pain on the individual as well as an evaluation of treatment goals (Tighe et al., 2015). Table 26.2 lists patient-reported outcomes (PROs) and suggested reliable and valid scales and instruments from the American Academy of Pain Medicine.

MULTIMODAL THERAPIES

The goal of pain treatment should be to improve the individuals' quality of life and promote functional ability (U.S. Department of Health and Human Services [DHHS], 2019). A multimodal approach to pain treatment is imperative. Placed into broad categories for pain

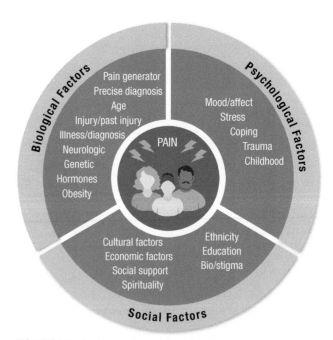

FIGURE 26.2: The biopsychosocial model of pain management.
Source: The Biopsychosocial Model of Pain Management, by U.S. Department of Health and Human Services. (2019, May). *Pain management best practices inter-agency task force report: Updates, gaps, inconsistencies, and recommendations.* https://www.hhs.gov/sites/default/files/pmtf-final-report-2019-05-23.pdf

TABLE 26.2: Pain-Related Patient-Reported Outcomes: Examples of Reliable and Valid Scales, Items, and Instruments

PATIENT-REPORTED OUTCOMES (PROs)	SCALES/ITEMS/ INSTRUMENTS
Pain intensity	NRS, VDS VAS Faces pain scale-Revised, IASP DVPRS PROMIS pain intensity
Pain interference	BPI-SF subscale: Pain interference PROMIS pain interference
Pain relief	BPI item: Pain relief
Pain character and quality	MPQ-SF NPS LANSS NPQ PROMIS pain behavior
Anxiety	HADS APS-POQ-R anxiety item PASS PROMIS anxiety
Depression	HADS APS-POQ-R depression item PROMIS depression
Anger	PROMIS anger
Sleep	ISI PSQI BPI-SF interference subscale item: Sleep PROMIS sleep disturbance PROMIS sleep-related impairment
Pain catastrophizing	Pain Catastrophizing Scale
Pain fear and fear avoidance	FPQ-III PASS TOPS fear avoidance subscale FABQ
Satisfaction with pain care/ outcomes	APS-POQ-R satisfaction item TOPS patient satisfaction with outcomes and health care satisfaction subscales
Social health	BPI interference subscale item: Relations with other people PROMIS social health (ability to participate in social roles and activities) and satisfaction with social roles and activities, social support, social isolation, and companionship
Patient impressions of change	PGIC scale

APS-POQ-R, American Pain Society-Patient Outcomes Questionnaire-Revised; BPI, Brief Pain Inventory; BPI-SF, Brief Pain Inventory–Short Form; DVPRS, Defense and Veterans Pain Rating Scale; FABQ, Fear-Avoidance Beliefs Questionnaire; FPQ-III, Fear of Pain Questionnaire III; HADS, Hospital Anxiety Depression Scale; IASP,

International Association for the Study of Pain; ISI, Insomnia Severity Index; LANSS, Leeds Assessment of Neuropathic Symptoms and Signs; MPQ-SF, McGill Pain Questionnaire-Short Form; NIH PROMIS, National Institutes of Health Patient Reported Outcomes Measurement Information System; NPQ, Neuropathic Pain Questionnaire; NPS, Neuropathic Pain Scale; NRS, Numeric Rating Scale; PASS, Pain Anxiety Symptoms Scale; PGIC, Patient Global Impression of Change; PSQI, Pittsburgh Sleep Quality Index; TOPS, Treatments Outcomes in Pain Survey; VAS, Visual Analog Scale; VDS, Verbal Descriptive Scales.

Source: Reproduced with permission from Tighe, P., Buckenmaier, C. C., Boezaart, A. P., Carr, D. B., Clark, L. L., Herring, A. A., Kent, M., Mackey, S., Mariano, E. R., Polomano, R. C., & Reisfield, G. M. (2015). Acute pain medicine in the United States: A status report. *Pain Medicine, 16*(9), 1806–1826. https://doi.org/10.1111/pme.12760

management these include medication, restorative, interventional procedures, behavioral health approaches and complementary and integrative health. As in any shared decision model the approach to selecting therapies should be guided by risk assessment, stigma, access to care and education (Figure 26.3; DHHS, 2019). The remaining discussion will focus on both nonpharmacologic and pharmacologic considerations for pain management.

Nonpharmacologic Therapies

In 2017, The Joint Commission (TJC) issued new standards related to the management of acute pain in hospitals. It is now a requirement that hospitals provide nonpharmacologic pain treatment options (TJC, 2017). Several nonpharmacologic options, summarized in Box 26.2, have demonstrated benefits similar to or better than pharmacologic treatment (Chou et al., 2020; Tick et al., 2018). Due to the varied and specific recommendations the reader is encouraged to review the recommendations provided for the various nonpharmacologic pain intervention strategies.

Pharmacologic Interventions

Pharmacologic pain treatment can be categorized into nonopioid and opioid. In many cases nonopioid treatment performs similarly if not better than opioid treatment for acute pain management (Chou et al., 2020). In 2018, The Society of Hospital Medicine (Boxes 26.3 and 26.4) released a consensus statement recommending providers reserve using opioids for patients with severe pain or with moderate pain that is not treated by nonopioid therapy or if nonopioid therapy is contraindicated (Herzig et al., 2018). It is therefore imperative that the benefits and risks of nonopioid pharmacologic therapy be well understood.

Nonopioid Pharmacologic Therapy

The general classes of nonopioid pharmacologic therapy include acetaminophen, nonsteroidal antiinflammatory drugs (NSAIDs), antidepressants, muscle relaxants, and anticonvulsants. Depending on the etiology and location of pain—for example low back pain versus post operative pain—different approaches should be considered.

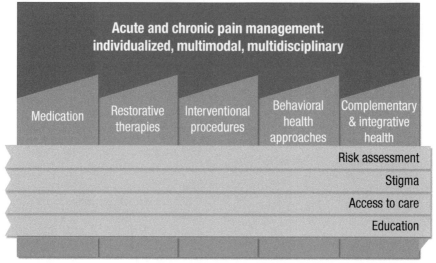

FIGURE 26.3: Comprehensive approach to pain treatment.
Source: From Acute and Chronic Pain Management Consists of Five Treatment Approaches Informed by Four Critical Topics, by U.S. Department of Health and Human Services. (2019, May). *Pain management best practices inter-agency task force report: Updates, gaps, inconsistencies, and recommendations*. https://www.hhs.gov/sites/default/files/pmtf-final-report-2019-05-23.pdf

BOX 26.2 NONPHARMACOLOGIC PAIN THERAPIES

- Restorative therapy
- Therapeutic exercise
- Transcutaneous electric nerve stimulation
- Message therapy
- Traction
- Cold and heat
- Therapeutic ultrasound
- Bracing
- Acupuncture therapy
- Music therapy
- Guided imagery
- Virtual reality-assisted distraction
- Immobilization
- Elevation

Source: Data from Information from Hsu, J. R., Mir, H., Wally, M. K., & Seymour, R. B. (2019). Clinical practice guidelines for pain management in acute musculoskeletal injury. *Journal of Orthopaedic Trauma, 33*(5), e158–e182. https://pubmed.ncbi.nlm.nih.gov/30681429/; Tick, H., Nielsen, A., Pelletier, K. R., Bonakdar, R., Simmons, S., Glick, R., Ratner, E., Lemmon, R. L., Wayne, P., & Zador, V. (2018). Evidence-based nonpharmacologic strategies for comprehensive pain care: The consortium pain task force white paper. *Explore, 14*(3), 177–211. https://doi.org/10.1016/j.explore.2018.02.001; U.S. Department of Health and Human Services. (2019, May). *Pain management best practices inter-agency task force report: Updates, gaps, inconsistencies, and recommendations*. https://www.hhs.gov/sites/default/files/pmtf-final-report-2019-05-23.pdf, The Consortium Pain Task Force White Paper

BOX 26.3 SUMMARY RECOMMENDATIONS FROM THE SOCIETY OF HOSPITAL MEDICINE FOR THE SAFE USE OF OPIOIDS IN THE HOSPITALIZED PATIENT WITH ACUTE PAIN

- Society of Hospital Medicine Consensus Statements
- Limit the use of opioids to patients with 1) severe pain or 2) moderate pain that has not responded to nonopioid therapy, or where nonopioid therapy is contraindicated or anticipated to be ineffective
- Use extra caution when administering opioids to patients with risk factors for opioid-related adverse events
- Review the information contained in the prescription drug monitoring program (PDMP) database to inform decision-making around opioid therapy
- Educate patients and families/caregivers about potential risks and side effects of opioid therapy as well as alternative pharmacologic and nonpharmacologic therapies for managing pain

Source: Herzig, S. J., Mosher, H. J., Calcaterra, S. L., Jena, A. B., & Nuckols, T. K. (2018). Improving the safety of opioid use for acute noncancer pain in hospitalized adults: A consensus statement from the society of hospital medicine. *Journal of Hospital Medicine, 13*(4), 263–271. https://doi.org/10.12788/jhm.2980.

BOX 26.4 SOCIETY OF HOSPITAL MEDICINE CONSENSUS STATEMENTS ONCE DECISION HAS BEEN MADE TO USE OPIOIDS DURING HOSPITALIZATION

- Use the lowest effective opioid dose for the shortest duration possible
- Use immediate-release opioid formulations and avoid initiation of long-acting/extended-release formulations (including transdermal fentanyl) for treatment of acute pain
- Use the oral route of administration whenever possible. Intravenous opioids should be reserved for patients who cannot take food or medications by mouth, patients suspected of gastrointestinal malabsorption, or when immediate pain control and/or rapid dose titration is necessary
- Use an opioid equivalency table or calculator to understand the relative potency of different opioids 1) when initiating opioid therapy, 2) when changing from one route of administration to another, and 3) when changing from one opioid to another. When changing from one opioid to another, clinicians should generally reduce the dose of the new opioid by at least 25% to 50% of the calculated equianalgesic dose to account for inter individual variability in the response to opioids as well as possible incomplete crosstolerance
- Pair opioids with scheduled nonopioid analgesic medications, unless contraindicated, and always consider pairing with nonpharmacologic pain management strategies (i.e., multimodal analgesia)
- Unless contraindicated, clinicians order a bowel regimen to prevent opioid-induced constipation in patients receiving opioids
- Limit coadministration of opioids with other central nervous system (CNS) depressant medications to the extent possible
- Work with patients and families/caregivers to establish realistic goals and expectations of opioid therapy and the expected course of recovery
- Monitor the response to opioid therapy, including assessment for functional improvement and development of adverse effects
- Ask patients about any existing opioid supply at home and account for any such supply when issuing an opioid prescription on discharge
- Prescribe the minimum quantity of opioids anticipated to be necessary based on the expected course and duration of pain severe enough to require opioid therapy after hospital discharge
- Ensure that patients and families/caregivers receive information regarding how to minimize the risks of opioid therapy for themselves, their families, and their communities. This includes but is not limited to: 1) how to take their opioids correctly (the planned medications, doses, schedule); 2) that they should take the minimum quantity necessary to achieve tolerable levels of pain and meaningful functional improvement, reducing the dose and/or frequency as pain and function improve; 3) how to safeguard their supply and dispose of any unused supply; 4) that they should avoid agents that may potentiate the sedative effect of opioids, including sleeping medication and alcohol; 5) that they should avoid driving or operating heavy machinery while taking opioids; and 6) that they should seek help if they begin to experience any potential adverse effects, with inclusion of information on early warning signs

Source: Data from Herzig, S. J., Mosher, H. J., Calcaterra, S. L., Jena, A. B., & Nuckols, T. K. (2018). Improving the safety of opioid use for acute noncancer pain in hospitalized adults: A consensus statement from the society of hospital medicine. *Journal of Hospital Medicine, 13*(4), 263–271. https://doi.org/10.12788/jhm.2980.

A systematic review completed by the Agency for Healthcare Research and Quality (2020) reviewed pain management therapy for acute pain and provided the following results (Chou et al., 2020, p. vii):

- Opioid therapy was probably less effective than NSAIDs for surgical pain and kidney stones
- Opioid therapy might be similarly effective as NSAIDs for low back pain

Additionally, the Opioid Prescribing Engagement Network (2018) recommends nonopioid therapy as the preferred first-line therapy for surgical procedures. For acute musculoskeletal injury a multimodal approach including nonopioid analgesics is preferred (Hsu et al., 2019). General considerations for each nonopioid pharmacologic therapy are summarized in Table 26.3. When deciding about specific treatment options, consideration should be given to other comorbidities such as kidney disease or coagulopathies and medication side effects. Targeted injections may also be an effective intervention for specific pain conditions. The reader is directed to review the DHHS's *Pain Management Best Practices* (2019) section on intervention procedures. Specific recommendations have been summarized from the American Academy of Emergency Medicine for nonopioid pharmacologic treatment in the emergency department (Box 26.5; Motov et al., 2018).

Opioid Prescribing

Recent emphasis on rational opioid prescribing due to the devastating opioid epidemic has changed opioid prescribing practices for acute pain. In most clinical

TABLE 26.3: Nonopioid Pharmacologic Treatment Considerations

PHARMACOLOGIC AGENT	INDICATIONS
Acetaminophen	Acute musculoskeletal injury Kidney stone Postoperative
NSAIDs	Acute musculoskeletal injury and inflammation Postoperative
Antidepressants	Neuropathic pain Chronic pain
Muscle relaxants	Associated spasticity or spasms
Anticonvulsants	Neuropathic pain Acute musculoskeletal injury Postherpetic neuralgia

BOX 26.5 RECOMMENDATIONS FROM THE AMERICAN ACADEMY OF EMERGENCY MEDICINE WHITE PAPER ON ACUTE PAIN MANAGEMENT IN THE EMERGENCY DEPARTMENT

- NSAIDs should be administered at their lowest effective analgesic dose both in the ED and upon discharge. They should be given for the shortest appropriate treatment course. Caution must be exercised when these analgesics are used in patients at risks for renal insufficiency, heart failure, gastrointestinal disorders.
- When a patient's acute painful condition (e.g., sprains, strains, bruises) warrant an NSAID but there are contraindications to their systemic use, strong consideration should be given to topical preparations (e.g., diclofenac gel) or other topical analgesics such as lidocaine patches.
- Oral and rectal forms of acetaminophen either alone or in combination with other analgesics provide similar analgesia to IV acetaminophen but with slower onset of action. For patients who have contraindications to oral and rectal routes, the IV route is preferred.
- Emergency clinicians should consider regional and local nerve blocks for traumatic and nontraumatic painful conditions, alone or in combination with pharmacologic and nonpharmacologicatreatment modalities.
- Subdissociative dose ketamine (SDK), administered alone or as part of a multimodal analgesic approach, may be considered in the ED. Emergency

clinicians should counsel patients that there is a high likelihood of minor but at times bothersome psychoperceptual side effects. Subdissociative ketamine should be administered under the same policies as other analgesics.
- Limited data suggest that administration of IV lidocaine may alleviate specific painful conditions (renal colic, herpetic/postherpetic neuralgia) and should be considered for patients without preexisting structural heart disease and rhythm disturbances.
- Emergency medicine clinicians should consider using trigger point injections with local anesthetics (lidocaine, bupivacaine) for patients with acute myofascial painful conditions such as back pain.
- EM clinicians should consider utilization of nitrous oxide for the treatment of acute painful conditions in the ED either alone or as an adjunct to other analgesics.

Source: Data from Motov, S., Strayer, R., Hayes, B. D., Reiter, M., Rosenbaum, S., Richman, M., Repanshek, Z., Taylor, S., Friedman, B., Vilke, G., & Lasoff, D. (2018). The treatment of acute pain in the emergency department: A white paper position statement prepared for the American Academy of Emergency Medicine. *The Journal of Emergency Medicine, 54*(5), 731–736. https://doi.org/10.1016/j.jemermed.2018.01.020.

scenarios nonopioid nonpharmacologic and nonopioid pharmacologic pain therapies should be tried before opioid pain medications. If opioid pain medications are prescribed, then use of immediate/short-acting (Table 26.4) over long-acting (Box 26.6) is preferred. A key piece of pain management with opioids is the dialogue prior to prescribing. Providing patients with the information about risks and benefits of opioid therapy plus establishing treatment goals for pain and function allow for informed decision-making.

The equivalency of one route of administration or type of opioid is not equal to another route of administration or opioid. Converting the opioid dose into a morphine equivalent dose through an equianalgesic ratio is necessary. This is particularly important when changing from an IV to oral route of administration or to a new opioid. Consideration for incomplete cross tolerance and pharmacokinetics is important to avoid overprescribing. Recommendations are to use a reduction of the equianalgesic dose.

A final key consideration is prescribing strategies postdischarge. Prescribers should use judicious and limited prescription quantities for the outpatient setting. The Opioid Prescribing Engagement Network (2018)

TABLE 26.4: Short-Acting Opioids and Routes of Administration

SHORT-ACTING OPIOIDS	ROUTES
Morphine	PO, epidural, PCA, SC/IV/IM, rectal
Hydromorphone	PO, PCA, SC/IV/IM, rectal
Oxymorphone immediate-release	PO
Oxycodone (can be in combination with acetaminophen, ibuprofen, or aspirin) immediate-release	PO
Hydrocodone (combination with acetaminophen or ibuprofen)	PO
Codeine	PO
Fentanyl	IV/IM, PCA
Meperidine	PO, SC/IV/IM

IM, intramuscular; IV, intravenous; PCA, patient-controlled analgesic; PO, oral; SC, subcutaneous.

Source: Data from Epocrates. (2021). *Epocrates Rx drugs, interaction check, and tables.* www.epocrates.com.

BOX 26.6 COMMONLY PRESCRIBED LONG-ACTING OPIOIDS

- Morphine sulfate controlled-release or extended-release
- Oxycodone controlled-release
- Oxymorphone extended-release
- Hydromorphone extended-release
- Fentanyl transdermal
- Buprenorphine transdermal
- Methadone hydrochloride

Source: From National Institute on Drug Abuse. (June, 2017). *Commonly used long-acting opioids chart.* https://www.drugabuse.gov/sites/default/files/CommonlyUsedLAOpioids.pdf

provides prescribing recommendations for opioid quantities after various surgical procedures in order to reduce the overprescribing of opioids at discharge. This is an important consideration to help stop the diverting of opioids. Another requirement, in most states, prior to prescribing an opioid at discharge is reviewing the prescription drug monitoring program. This is an electronic program that monitors all controlled substance prescriptions provided to an individual. This allows the provider to make an informed decision about prescribing

opioids at discharge. As in the hospital setting, short-acting agents are preferred and only prescribed for a short period of time.

Chronic Opioid Use and Acute Pain

For those patients presenting with acute pain who are chronic opioid users, consideration for opioid tolerance and opioid-induced hyperalgesia is needed. In most situations, continuation of the regularly administered opioid dose plus additional opioid doses is needed (Cooney & Broglio, 2017). Multimodal pain management approaches should also be attempted. The Centers for Disease Control and Prevention recommends using particular caution with dosages greater than or equal to 50 morphine milligram equivalents (MME)/day and avoid increasing to or above 90 MME/day (Dowell et al., 2016) for chronic opioid administration.

KEY TAKEAWAYS

- Nociception is a neural response but pain is modulated and perceived through biologic, psychologic, and social contexts.
- A comprehensive pain assessment is based on the biopsychosocial model.
- The goal of pain treatment should be to improve the individual's quality of life and promote functional ability.
- A multimodal treatment approach to acute pain management should be implemented including nonpharmacologic and pharmacologic interventions.

EVIDENCE-BASED RESOURCES

Chou, R., Wagner, J., Ahmed, A. Y., Blazina, I., Brodt, E., Buckley, D. I., Cheney, T. P., Choo, E., Dana, T., Gordon, D., Khandelwal, S., Kantner, S., McDonagh, M. S., Sedgley, C., & Skelly, A. C. (2020, December). *Treatments for acute pain: A systematic review.* https://doi.org/10.23970/AHRQEPCCER240

Herzig, S. J., Mosher, H. J., Calcaterra, S. L., Jena, A. B., & Nuckols, T. K. (2018). Improving the safety of opioid use for acute noncancer pain in hospitalized adults: A consensus statement from the society of hospital medicine. *Journal of Hospital Medicine, 13*(4), 263–271. https://doi.org/10.12788/jhm.2980

Motov, S., Strayer, R., Hayes, B. D., Reiter, M., Rosenbaum, S., Richman, M., Repanshek, Z., Taylor, S., Friedman, B., Vilke, G., & Lasoff, D. (2018). The treatment of acute pain in the emergency department: A white paper position statement prepared for the American Academy of Emergency Medicine. *The Journal of Emergency Medicine, 54*(5), 731–736. https://doi.org/10.1016/j.jemermed.2018.01.020

Tighe, P., Buckenmaier, C. C., Boczaart, A. P., Carr, D. B., Clark, L. L., Herring, A. A., Kent, M., Mackey, S., Mariano, E. R., Polomano, R. C., & Reisfield, G. M. (2015). Acute pain medicine in the United States: A status report. *Pain Medicine*, *16*(9), 1806–1826. https://doi.org/10.1111/pme.12760

Tick, H., Nielsen, A., Pelletier, K. R., Bonakdar, R., Simmons, S., Glick, R., Ratner, E., Lemmon, R. L., Wayne, P., & Zador, V. (2018). Evidence-based nonpharmacologic strategies for comprehensive pain care: The consortium pain task force white paper. *Explore*, *14*(3), 177–211. https://doi.org/10.1016/j.explore.2018.02.001

A robust set of instructor resources designed to supplement this text is located at **http://connect.springerpub.com/content/reference-book/978-0-8261-6079-9.** Qualifying instructors may request access by emailing **textbook@springerpub.com.**

REFERENCES

Full list of references can be accessed at http://connect.springerpub.com/content/reference-book/978-0-8261-6079-9.

INDEX